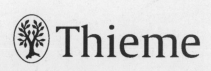

Gallery of Medicinal Plants
(*Dravyaguna Vigyan*)

Monika Sharma, BAMS, MD
Assistant Professor
Department of Dravyaguna
Chaudhary Brahm Prakash Ayurved Charak Sansthan
New Delhi, India

Subash Sahu, BAMS, MD
Associate Professor and Head
Department of Dravyaguna
Chaudhary Brahm Prakash Ayurved Charak Sansthan
New Delhi, India

Thieme
Delhi • Stuttgart • New York • Rio de Janeiro

Publishing Director: Ritu Sharma
Development Editor: Dr Ambika Kapoor
Director-Editorial Services: Rachna Sinha
Project Managers: Prakash Naorem and Apeksha Sharma
Vice President, Sales and Marketing: Arun Kumar Majji
Managing Director & CEO: Ajit Kohli

Thieme Medical and Scientific Publishers Private Limited.
A - 12, Second Floor, Sector - 2, Noida - 201 301,
Uttar Pradesh, India, +911204556600
Email: customerservice@thieme.in
www.thieme.in

Cover design: Thieme Publishing Group
Typesetting by RECTO Graphics, India

Printed in India by EIH Limited – Unit Printing Press

5 4 3 2 1

ISBN: 978-93-88257-57-2
e-ISBN: 978-93-88257-80-0

Important note: Medicine is an ever-changing science undergoing continual development. Research and clinical experience are continually expanding our knowledge, in particular our knowledge of proper treatment and drug therapy. Insofar as this book mentions any dosage or application, readers may rest assured that the authors, editors, and publishers have made every effort to ensure that such references are in accordance with **the state of knowledge at the time of production of the book**.

Nevertheless, this does not involve, imply, or express any guarantee or responsibility on the part of the publishers in respect to any dosage instructions and forms of applications stated in the book. **Every user is requested to examine carefully** the manufacturers' leaflets accompanying each drug and to check, if necessary in consultation with a physician or specialist, whether the dosage schedules mentioned therein or the contraindications stated by the manufacturers differ from the statements made in the present book. Such examination is particularly important with drugs that are either rarely used or have been newly released on the market. Every dosage schedule or every form of application used is entirely at the user's own risk and responsibility. The authors and publishers request every user to report to the publishers any discrepancies or inaccuracies noticed. If errors in this work are found after publication, errata will be posted at www.thieme.com on the product description page.

Some of the product names, patents, and registered designs referred to in this book are in fact registered trademarks or proprietary names even though specific reference to this fact is not always made in the text. Therefore, the appearance of a name without designation as proprietary is not to be construed as a representation by the publisher that it is in the public domain.

Contents

Part II: Nondetailed Plants

Available Online 500+ University Exam Questions

https://medone.thieme.com/images/supmat/9789388257572-sharma-online-content.pdf

Preface

The popularity of Ayurveda is rapidly increasing worldwide because of its holistic approach as well as the insignificant side effects of Ayurvedic or herbal medicines. Most Ayurvedic medicines and other Indian-origin systems of medicine such as Siddha are mainly based on medicinal plants or natural sources. The pharmaceutical industries and educational and research institutes connected to them depend on herbal plants for manufacturing medicines for clinical use as well as for educational and research purposes. However, there is a considerable gap between the demand and supply of medicinal plants due to their insufficient cultivation and swift destruction from their natural habitat. Hence, the chances of adulteration and substitution of genuine drugs are increasing on a daily basis which, in turn, affect the quality and efficacy of Ayurvedic or herbal medicine. In order to nullify or minimize this threat, it is the need of the hour to possess the requisite knowledge concerning the identification of medicinal plants morphologically, microscopically, and by various phytochemical parameters. Against this backdrop, this book entitled *Gallery of Medicinal Plants* has been designed to include all the medicinal plants mentioned in the Central Council of Indian Medicine (CCIM) syllabus, with more than 1,000 colored photographs. The present book contains various details of plants, such as the Latin name, family, vernacular names, synonyms (Sanskrit names), classical classification, distribution, morphology, flowering and fruiting time, key characteristics of identification and propagation, types, *rasapanchaka*, chemical constituents, pharmacological properties, identity, purity and strength, actions, indications, contraindications, therapeutic uses, toxicity, officinal parts used, dose, formulations, substitution, and adulteration.

We have also mentioned the classical and recent data related to these plants which would, in multiple ways, aid Ayurvedic scholars, researchers, as well as the individuals interested in studying medicinal plants. This book makes a very diligent endeavor to present all information in lucid language for it to be easily grasped by the students.

We believe that both the undergraduate and postgraduate students of Ayurveda, pharmacy, Unani, and Siddha, as well as botany will find the book very useful. Suggestions from faculty, researchers, clinicians, and scientists are welcome for improvement in future editions of this book. With this, we humbly submit it to the readers for the betterment of mankind.

Monika Sharma, BAMS, MD
Subash Sahu, BAMS, MD

Abbreviations

A.D.	Anno Domini	C.S.K	Charak Samhita Kalpasthana
A.H	Astanga Hridaya	C.S.Su	Charak Samhita Sutrasthana
A.H.Ci	Astanga Hridaya Chikitshasthana	C.S.Vi	Charak Samhita Vimanasthana
A.H.Su	Astanga Hridaya Sutrasthana	CD	Chakradutta
A.H.U	Astanga Hridaya Uttartantra	GN	Gadanigraha
A.P.I	Ayurvedic Pharmacopeia of India	H.S	Harita Samhita
A.S	Astanga Samgraha	IBS	Inflammatory Bowel Syndrome
A.S.Ci	Astanga Samgraha Chikitsasthana	K. S	Kashyapa Samhita
A.S.Su	Astanga Samgraha Sutrasthana	K.S.K	Kashyapa Samhita Khilasthan
B.C.	Before Christ	R.M.	Raj Martanda
B. P. Ci	Bhava Prakasha Chikitsasthana	S.G.S	Sharangadhara Samhita
B.R	Bhaishajya Ratnavali	S.S.Ci	Sushruta Samhita Chikitsathana
B.S	Bangasena	S.S.Su	Sushruta Samhita Sutrasthana
B.P	Bhavaprakash	S.S.U	Sushruta Samhita Uttaratantra
B.P.N	Bhavaprakash Nighantu	T.L.C.	Thin Layer Chromatography
Bh. S	Bhela Samhita	UTI	Urinary Tract Infection
CNS	Central Nervous System	V.M	Vrinda Madhav
C.S.Ci	Charak Samhita Chikitsasthana	Y.R	Yoga Ratnakara

Introduction

Ayurveda, a system of traditional Indian medicine, is being practiced for over 5,000 years (Garodia et al 2007). Ayurveda elaborates on nature on a whole as a tool for treatment. Acharya Charak proclaimed that there is nothing on the Earth which cannot be used as a medicine. Nature is a rich treasure of valuable remedies in the form of plants, animals, and minerals. Therefore, these are considered as the three resources of Ayurvedic therapeutics. It is not only sufficient to know the power of healing hidden in these resources but it is also equally important to be aware about the form of use, doses, and time of administration, to achieve maximum benefit of these medicaments. Conventional medicines play an important role in health services around the world. About three quarters of the world's population is dependent on different parts of medicinal plants and their extracts for their well-being.

Approximately 80% of the world's population depends wholly or partially on traditional medicine for its primary health care needs (Wambebe 1990). There exist some communities that solely rely on traditional medicines. Despite many allopathic medical facilities being made available by the government and nongovernment sectors, most people still depend on the traditional system of medicine. This might be due to easy accessibility and inexpensive drugs.

India has very rich biodiversity. There are about 47,000 species of plants reported from India. Among 17,500 angiosperms, 5,400 are endemic to India, about 9,500 species are ethnobotanically important, 8,000 are used as medicine, 3,900 are edible, and 880 are in trade (Mittermeier et al 2005). Herbal medicines have been used as a major remedy in the traditional system since antiquity. Their health benefits have made an impact in many parts of the world toward maintaining human health (Patwardhan et al 2005). In the Western world, as many people are becoming aware of the side effects of the synthetic drugs, there is an increasing interest in herbal products (Verma and Singh 2008).

It is also said that 72.19% of the population of India resides in villages (Anonymous 2011). Generally, it is observed that tribes live in deep forests, which are sometimes inaccessible. Such tribes have developed knowledge out of sheer necessity, observation, and experimentation which has been perpetuated from one generation to the next. It is an ongoing process that has continued over the ages (Maheshwari 1983). Considering the limitations of allopathic drugs, the use of herbal medicine has led to a sudden increase in the number of consumers and perhaps herbal drug manufacturers. Certain advantages of the use of herbal medicines are as follows (Singh et al 2015):

a. Easily and sufficiently available, especially in India because of its rich biodiversity.
b. Have a long history of use, good patient tolerance and acceptance, and excellent safety profile.
c. Are cost-effective and constitute a renewable source.
d. Easily cultivated in India owing to its different agro-climatic zones.

Most of the plants are being widely tested and accepted over a period of time and have become part of the codified Indigenous Systems of Medicine viz. Ayurveda, Siddha, Unani, etc. (Jain 2004). A comparison of plant usage across different systems of medicine clearly indicates the difference in the pattern of using them. **Table 1** shows that the number of plants used are the highest in the folk system followed by Ayurveda (Pitroda 2000).

Ayurvedic medicines are completely dependent on the natural sources. People are now realizing the preventive, promotive, and curative effects of Ayurveda that mainly focuse on the use of plant-based medicines for the treatment of various disorders (Parasuraman et al 2014). Herbal medicinal products are complex mixtures that originate from natural sources. Therefore, there is a perception that Ayurvedic formulations are safer than synthetic, chemical-based ones (Patwardhan et al 2005). These plants are used either individually or in formulations. Several applications of a particular plant are used in various formulations for different purposes. For example, a common plant called *Emblica officinalis* Gaertn. has nearly 180 formulations. There are many instances in Ayurveda for the multiple application of a single plant, for instance, Azadirachta *indica* has 42 reported uses, *Centella asiatica* (Linn.) Urban has about 33, *Pergularia daemia* (Forssk.) Blatt. & McCann with

Table 1 Comparison of Plant Use Across Different Systems of Medicine

Medicinal System	Ayurveda	Folk	Homeo	Modern	Siddha	Tibetan	Unani
Ayurveda	**2351**	**900**	189	80	1028	341	880
Folk	900	**5137**	164	86	971	235	573
Homeo	189	**164**	**506**	100	167	77	173
Modern	80	**86**	100	**204**	65	25	75
Siddha	1028	**971**	167	65	**1785**	277	641
Tibetan	341	**235**	77	25	277	**350**	275
Unani	880	**573**	173	75	641	275	**979**

Note: The bold figures indicate the count of plants used in each system and common between folk and other systems.

23, *Aristolochia indica* Linn. has 22, *Alstonia scholaris* R.Br. has 19, and *Holarrhena pubescens* Wall.ex G. Don has 18 reported uses (Ajitkumar 2003).

Shepherds and other forest dwellers know the drugs by name and their habitat as these people are very close to nature. Hence, the knowledge of plants must be obtained from these people. But only knowing the name and habitat of a plant is not sufficient for its medicinal application. A physician ignorant of the plants' habitat or forms can however also be referred to as a Tatwavit (knower of the essence of this science). One who knows the principles of correct application of drugs according to place and time after examining every individual is regarded as the best physician (C.S.Su.1/121-123).

A drug which is not known properly is similar to poison, weapon, fire, or thunderbolt, while the one known is considered as nectar. Proper application of drugs depend upon their proper knowledge. A physician cannot treat a patient without proper knowledge of the drugs. His or her prescription can kill patients. A unknown drug, or known drug administered improperly, leads to bad consequences (C.S.Su.1/124-125).

Even an acute poison can become an excellent medicine if it is properly administered. On the other hand, a drug which is not used in a rational way acts like poison (C.S.Su.1/126). Hence, it is required to plan in a rational way to customize the medicine for clinical use and to obtain success in treatment. Here, a few examples of medicinal plants are provided in accordance with various systems and srotas:

1. **Rasavahasrotas:** Milk, Yava
   a. Shothahara (anti-inflammatory): Dashamool
   b. Shothajanana (causes swelling): Lavana
   c. Gandamalanashak (reduces/cures goitre): Kanchanar, Mundi.
2. **Raktavahasrotas:**
   a. Hridya (cardio tonic): Arjuna, Hritpatri, Karpura, Vanapalandu, Tambula, Karaveera, Taruni
   b. Hridaya uttejaka (cardiac stimulant): Soma
   c. Hridaya avasadak (cardiac depressant): Ahiphena
   d. Raktabharavardhak (increases blood pressure): Kupilu, Hritpatri, Soma
   e. Raktabharashamak (antihyoertensive): Rudraksha, Sarpagandha
   f. Raktasthambhan/Shonitastapana (haemostatics/styptics): Lodhra, Nagakeshar, Priyangu, Parnabeeja, Kukundar, Shaka, Yastimadhu, Mocharasa, Gairik
   g. Raktaprasadana (blood purifier): Sariva, Manjishtha, Chopchini, Shinshapa
3. **Mamsavahasrotas:**
   a. Brimhan (bulk promoting): Kharjura, Madhooka, Aswagandha, Kshiravidari, Kakoli, Kshirakakoli, Vidari
   b. Langhan (mass reducing): Yava, Vacha
4. **Medavaha srotas:**
   a. Medavriddhi (increase fat/obesity): Ghee, vasa (fat)
   b. Medakshapana (reducing fat/antiobesity): Guggulu, Yava, Chanak, Vacha, Pippali, Chitrak

c. Lekhana (scraping): Chirabilwa, Vacha, Musta, Kusta, Haridra, Daruharidra, Ativisha, Chitrak, Katuki

5. **Astivahasrotas:**

   a. Astivardhan (increase bone): Praval, mukta

   b. Astikshapana (reduce bone): no calcium supplement

   c. Astisandhaniya (union of bone): Astishrinkhala

6. **Majjavahasrotas:**

   a. Majjavardhan: Majja (bone marrow)

   b. Majjakshaya: Dry and rough substances

7. **Shukravahasrotas:**

   a. Shukrajanana (spermatogenesis): Jeevak, Aswagandha, Mushali, Shatavari, Talamuli, Makhana, Kokilaksha, Kapikachhu

   b. Kamauttejaka (increase sexual desire in male): Kupilu

   c. Shukrasthambhan (reduces premature ejaculation): Jatiphala, Ahiphena, Akarkarabha

   d. Shukrajanana and rechana (both spermatogenesis and ejaculation of semen): Kshira, Masa

   e. Kamasadaka (anophrodisiac): Kshara, suchi, karpura

   f. Shukrashodhan (purification of semen): Kusta, Katphala, Elavaluka, Kadamba, Ikshu, Kandekshu, Ushir

8. **Pranavaha srotas:**

   a. Chhedan (expectorant): Maricha, Shilajatu, Bibhitaki, Vasa, Talisha, Lavanga, Twak, Yastimadhu, Gojihva, Bola, Vanapsha

   b. Kasahara (bronchial sedatives): Draksha, Haritaki, Pippali, Kantakari, Brihati, Karkatashringi, Kasamarda, Agasthya

   c. Shwasahara (bronchial antiasthmatics): Shati, Puskaramoola, Bharangi, Dugdhika

   d. Kanathya (beneficial for throat): Sariva, Yastimadhu, Sudarsana, Paribhadra, Pippali, Draksha, kantakari, vidari

9. **Annavaha srotas (Pachan santhan/Digestive system):**

   a. Lalaprasekajanana (sialagogues): Tumburu

   b. Lalaprashekashaman (Antisailagogue): Suchi

   c. Trishnanigrahana: Musta, Parpatak

   d. Mukhadaugandhyanashak: Lavanga, Ela

   e. Mukhavaishadyakarak: Tambula, Puga

f. Dantyadhavan/Dantyashodhan: Karanja, Nimba, Karaveera, Tejovati

g. Danyadadhyakar: Babool, Triphala, Bakul

h. Rochan (delish): Vrikshamla, Amlavetash, Dadima, Matulunga, Jambir, Changeri, Tintidika

i. Deepan: Saunf, Marich, Hingu, Ativisha, Chitrak, Jeerak, Krishna Jeerak, Pippali

j. Pachana (digestives): Chitrak, Musta, Eranda Karkati

k. Vidahi: Sarsapa, Lanka.

l. Vistambhi: Kathal, Lonika, Lakucha

m. Vaman (emetics): Madanphala, Ikswaku, Jimutaka, Kutaja

n. Chhardinigrahana (antiemetic): Jambu, Amrapallava, Suchi

o. Shoolaprashamana (antispasmodic): Panchakola, Yavani, Ajamoda, Shandrashura

10. **Drug acts on liver:** Daruharidra, Kakamachi, Bhunimba, Apamarga, Kasni, Bhumyamalaki

    a. Pittasravak (choleratics): Gorachana

    b. Pittasarak (cholagogue): Erand taila, Katuki

    c. Pittasmaribhedan: Ikshuraka mool

    d. Arshoghna: Kutaja, Bhallatak, Daruharidra, Nagakeshar, Chitrak, Mahanimba, Karira, Suran, Sunnisanak

    e. Plihavridhhihara: Rohitaka, Kumari, Indrayan, Sharapunkha, Chirayata, Sharapunkha

11. **Udakavaha srotas:**

    a. Trishnanigrahana: Yavasa, Shanwayasa, Musta, Parpataka, Ushira, Chandan, Dhanyak, Kiratatiktaka, Guduchi, Hribera, Shunthi, Chitrak, Chavya, Vidanga, Murva, Guduchi, Vacha.Musta, Pippali, Patola

12. **Mutravaha srotas: Urinary system:**

    a. Mutravirechaniya (diuretics): Trinapanchamoola, Punarnava, Gokshur, Trapusha, Bhumyalaki, Vasuka

    b. Mutraveerajaniya: Flowers of Kamala, Yastimadhu, Priyangu, Dhataki

    c. Ashmaribhedan (urinary lithontriptics): Kulattha, Pashanabheda, Varuna, Veerataru, Gorakshaganja, Durva, Kasa, Gokshura

    d. Mutrasangrahaniya (urinary astringent): Jambu. Amra, Bhallataka, Vata, Udumbar, Aswattha, Plaksha, Shala, Parisha, Asmantaka, Somavalka

e. Mutravishodhana (urinary antiseptics): Chandan. Kankola

13. **Purishvaha srotas:**

    a. Upashoshan (absorption): Kutaja, Aralu, Shyonak

    b. Purishajanana (formation of faecal matter): Masha, Yava

    c. Rechan (purgative): Trivrut, Aragvadha, Snuhi, Aswagol, Danti, Jayapal, Eranda Taila, Indravaruni, Kutuki, Sanaya, Haritaki

    d. Purishsangrahaniya (faecal astringent): Grahi-Shunti, Jeerak, Gajapippali, Parnayavani

    e. Sthambhan (facecal absorption): Kutaja, Shyonak, Dhataki, Babool, Aavartaki, Shami, Mayaphala, Dhanwan

    f. Purishaveerajaniya (correctives of faecal-pigments): Jambu., Utpala, Tila, Shalakki, Shalmali, Madhooka, Vidari

    g. Anulomana (carminative): Haritaki, Hingu, Yavani

14. **Swedavahasrotas:**

    a. Swedopaga (adjuvant in sudation therapy): Shobhanjana, Erand, Arka, Punarnava, Yava, Til, Kulattha, Masa

    b. Swedapanayana: Ushira

15. **Artavavaha srotas:**

    a. Artavajanana (Emmenagogue): Sarsapa, Ulatkambal, Vansha, Shana

    b. Artavashaman (antiemmenagogue): Nagakeshar, Lodhra, Ashoka, Patranga

    c. Stanyajanana (Galactogogue): Shatavari, Ikshumoola, Rohisha, Nala, Patha

    d. Stanyashaman (antigalactogogue): Mallika

    e. Stanyashodhan (purification breast milk): Devadaru, Sariva, Shunti

16. **Other actions:**

    Kesharanjan: Bhringaraj, mehendi

    Snehopaga: Draksha, Yastimadhu

    Varnya: Sariva, Manjista, Chandan, Nagakeshar, Ushira, Yastimadhu, Durva, Haridra

    Kandughna: Chandan, Ushira, Nimba, Jatamamsi, Latakaranja, Yastimadhu, Daruharidra, Musta

    Kustaghna: Khadir, Bhallatak, Haritaki, Amalaka, Aaragvadha, Vidanga, Karaveera, Jati

    Udardaprashamana: Tinduka

Krimighna (anthelmintic): Palashabeeja, Vidanga, Chauhara, Dadimatwak, Puaga, Ingudi, Tulasi, Barbari, Kampillak, Kitamari

17. **Prajanana santhan** (reproductive system): Female reproductive system:

    a. Prajasthapana: Brahmi, Lakshmana, Durva, Kamal, Kumuda, Kasheruka, Putranjiva

    b. Garbharodhak: Gunja, Patha, Japa

    c. Garbhashaya sankochaka (ecbolics): Kupilu, Arka, Iswari, Kalajaji, Karpasa, Langali, Kebuka,

    d. Garbhashaya shamak (uterine sedative): Suchi

17. **Jwarahara (antipyretics):** Sahadevi, Kiratatikta, Bhunimba, Trayamana, Guduchi, Patola, Sudarsansariva, Haritaki, Bibhitaki, Amalaki, Pilu, Manjista, Draksha

    a. Santapahara (antipyretics): Draksha, Sariva, Vatsanabha

    b. Amapachana: Chirayata, Patola

    c. Vishamajwaraghna (antiperiodic): Karanja, Saptaparna, Quinine, Mamajjaka, Kantaki Karanja, Dronapuspi, tulasi

    d. Dahaprashamana (refrigerants): Kamala, Chandan, Raktachandan, Ela, Gambhari, guduchi, Madhooka, Hrivera

    e. Sheetaprashamana (remove chill)/calefacient: Aguru, Brihat Ela, Tagara, Dhanyak, Shunti, Vacha, Kantakari, Agnimanth, Shyonak, Pippali

    f. Kothaprashamana (antiseptic): Karpur, Chandan, Shrivestak, Sarala, Aswakarna

    g. Rakshoghna (disinfectant): Sarshapa, Nimba, Guggulu

    h. Putihara (deodorants): Loban

    i. Vranashodhan: Gangeruki

19. **Sarvadhatuk karma:**

    a. Jeevaniya (nutrients): Vidari, Munjataka, Kshira, Jeevanti, Jeevak, Rhisabhaka, Meda, Mahameda, Yastimadhu

    b. Sandhaniya(union-promoter): Lajjalu, Yastimadhu, Guduchi, Prishniparni, Patha, Manjista, Dhataki, Lodhra, Priyangu

    c. Balya (tonics): Bala, Atibala, Vidari, Varahi, Shalaparni, Kapikachhu, Shatavari, Arjun (Cardiotonic), Kupilu (tonic for spinal cord), Tagara (nervine tonics)

d. Rasayana (rejuvenatives): Amalaki, Haritaki, Guduchi, Aswagandha, Vridhadaru, Nagabala

e. Vishaghna (antidotes): Shirisha, Nirvisha, Ankola, Patalgarudi

f. Shramahara (antifatigue): Draksha, Kharjura, Priyala, Badara, Dadima, Phalgu, Parushaka, Ikshu

g. Angamardaprashamana (restoratives): Shalaparni, Prishniparni, Brihati, Kantakari, Eranda, Kakoli, Chandan, Ela, Yastimadhu, Ushir

h. Vranaropna (wound healing): Mansarohini

i. Madakari: Ahiphena, Bhanga

j. Sanjasthapana: Vacha, Jatamamshi, Choraka

k. Medhya: Brahmi, Mandookparni, Shankhapuspi, Jyotishmati, Vacha, Kushmanda

l. Chakshusya: Mamira, Kataka

m. Keshya: Narikela, Tila, Bhringaraj, Nilini

n. Varnya: Kumkum, Ketaki

o. Kandughna (antipuritus): Karanja, Koshambra, Nimba, Jayanti, Aranya Jeerak

p. Kusthaghna (antidermatosis): Khadir, Bhallatak, Aaragvadha, Haridra, Tuvarak, Vacha, Jati, Madayantika, Saireyaka, Chakramarda

Suggested Readings

Ajitkumar S. Amruth, the traditional health care. FRLHT 2003;1(1)

Anonymous. Selected Socio-Economic Statistics India. New Delhi: Ministry of Statistics and Programme Implementation, Government of India; 2011

Anonymous. The Ayurvedic Formulary of India. Parts I and II. New Delhi: Department of Indian Systems of Medicine and Homoeopathy, Ministry of Health and Family Welfare, Government of India; 2003

Garodia P, Ichikawa H, Malani N, Sethi G, Aggarwal BB. Feom ancient medicine to modern medicine: Ayurvedic concept of health and their role in inflammation and cancer. J Soc Integr Oncol 2007;5(1):1–16

Jain SK. Credibility of traditional knowledge: The criterion of multilocational and multiethnic use. Indian J Tradit Knowledge 2004;3(2):137–153

Lamoreux J, Fonseca GAB, Seligmann PA, Ford H. Hotspots Revisited: Earth's Biologically Richest and Most Endangered Terrestrial Ecoregions. Monterrey, Mexico: Cemex; 2005

Maheshwari JK. Developments in ethnobotany. J Econ Taxonomic Bot 1983;4(1):I–V

Pandey K, Chaturvedi G. Charak Samhita of Agnivesha. Varanasi: Chaukhambha Bharati Academy; 2019

Patwardhan B, Warude D, Pushpangadan P, Bhatt N. Ayurveda and traditional Chinese medicine: a comparative overview. Evid Based Complement Alternat Med 2005;2(4):465–473

Pitroda S. Annual Report. Bangalore: Foundation for Revitalisation of Local Health Traditions; 2000

Sharma PV Dravyaguna Vigyan. Vol. 1: Basic Concepts. Varanasi: Chaukhamba Bharati Academy; 2001

Singh SP, Singh AP, Singh R, Rai PK, Tripathi AK, Verma NK. A Brief Study on Strebulus asper L.: a Review. Res J Phytomedicine 2015; 1(02):65–71

Verma S, Singh SP. Current and future status of herbal medicines. Veterinary World 2008;1(11):347–350

Wambebe CON. Natural products in developing economy. In AC Igbocchi and IUW Osisign, eds, Proceedings National Workshop on Natural Products; 1990

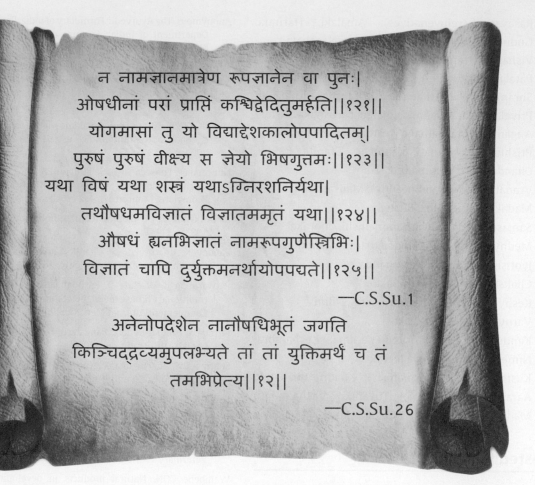

न नामज्ञानमात्रेण रूपज्ञानेन वा पुनः।
ओषधीनां परां प्राप्तिं कश्चिद्वेदितुमर्हति॥१२१॥
योगमासां तु यो विद्याद्देशकालोपपादितम्।
पुरुषं पुरुषं वीक्ष्य स ज्ञेयो भिषगुत्तमः॥१२३॥
यथा विषं यथा शस्त्रं यथाऽग्निरशनिर्यथा।
तथौषधमविज्ञातं विज्ञातममृतं यथा॥१२४॥
औषधं ह्यनभिज्ञातं नामरूपगुणैस्त्रिभिः।
विज्ञातं चापि दुर्युक्तमनर्थायोपपद्यते॥१२५॥

—C.S.Su.1

अनेनोपदेशेन नानौषधिभूतं जगति
किञ्चिद्द्रव्यमुपलभ्यते तां तां युक्तिमर्थं च तं
तमभिप्रेत्य॥१२॥

—C.S.Su.26

Part I

Detailed Plants

1. Agaru [Aquilaria agallocha Roxb.]

Synonym:	*Aquilaria malaccensis Lam.*
Family:	*Thymelaeaceae*
Hindi name:	*Agar*
English name:	*Eagle's wood, Agar wood, Aloe wood*

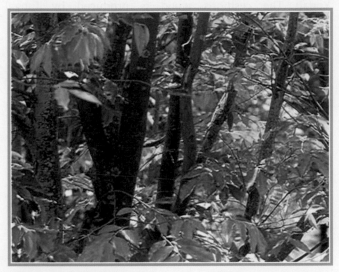

Plant of *Aquilaria agallocha* Roxb.

> *Being highly priced and valuable, Agaru has equaled or exceeded the price of gold; hence, it was often referred to as "black gold" in the past.*

Introduction

The word "Agaru" literally means the one which is the heaviest and no other aromatic wood is heavier (garu) than it.

Since thousands of years, Agaru "The wood of God" has been used for multiple purposes throughout the world. Besides its commercial, historical, spiritual, aromatic, medicinal, and social significance, it is considered as a symbol of high status, wealth, and prosperity. Its use has been reported in many old testaments of Ayurveda, and in Chinese, Tibetan, European, and East-Asian texts. In the ancient Hindu epic, the Mahābhārata, Agaru is referenced as a welcome offering. In the Holy Bible, the spiritual significance of Agaru is demonstrated with it being used along with myrrh in the anointing of Jesus Christ following his crucifixion. The spiritual importance of Agaru in Buddhism was similarly demonstrated when it was used among other fragrant products in the cremation of Buddha.

Agaru is also cited thrice in the Holy Bible as a fragrant product for intimacy and seduction. In Islamic texts, Agaru appears as a conspicuous fragrance used in the ritual burning of incense, for spiritual purification, and as one of the rewards in paradise. Agaru wood mixed with camphor was the preferred scent of the Prophet Muhammad. In Arabian medicines, its oil is used for aromatherapy.

Due to its distinctive fragrance, Agaru is used abundantly for making incense sticks, perfumes, and soaps. Its wood is also used for making sculptures and carvings. In middle-east countries, beads prepared from its wood are used to keep oneself safe from evil spirit and for bringing good luck (Sampson et al 2018).

Medicinal uses of Agaru have been recorded in many pieces of Indian, Greek, Roman, Chinese, Middle Eastern, and European literature since ancient times by people of diverse culture. It is reported to be used as a folklore medicine in inflammatory diseases, skin diseases, headache, arthritis, vomiting, gout, etc. In traditional Chinese medicine, Agaru is used as a chi-regulating drug and carminative medicine

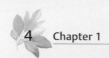

to relieve gastric problems, coughs, rheumatism, and high fever. It can promote chi-circulation to relieve pain, warm the middle energizer to arrest vomiting, and regulate respiration to relieve asthma (National Pharmacopeia Committee 2015).

Acharya Charak has referred to Agaru as an ushna virya dravya in spite of having tikta rasa (C.S.Su. 26/49). Charak also advocated applying paste of Rasna and Agaru to counteract the effect of cold in agraya dravyas (C.S.Su. 25/40). Sushrut used Agaru as dhupan dravya along with Guggulu, Ral, and Shoma in the treatment of karnasweda and vrana.

Because of its consistent high demand and slow natural growth rate, the plant is facing severe scarcity in nature. This is the reason for it being highly priced in trade and for placing it under the category of critically endangered or vulnerable species. Owing to its rapid declining rate, all the species of *Aquilaria* have been placed in the Appendix II list of the Convention on International Trade in Endangered Species of Wild Fauna and Flora since 2004 (CITES 2004).

Vernacular Names

Arabic: Oud, Oodh, Shajarat-al-oudh
Assamese: Sasi, Sashi, Agaru
Bengali: Agar chandan, Agarkastha
Chinese: Chenxiang
Hong Kong: Aloe wood
Indonesia: Gaharu
Japanese: Jinko
Kannada: Krishna Agaru
Malayalam: Akil
Punjabi: Ooda, Pharsi
Tamil: Agalichandanam
Telugu: Agaru
Thailand: Mai kritsana

Synonyms

Anaryaka: It grows abundantly in the forest region of the Northeast of India.
Krimija: The plant is infested by fungus.
Krimijagdh: The gum resin is produced by fungal infestation.
Loha: The infested heartwood is heavy and black like iron.
Pravar: It means a substance which is best among its class.

Rajarha: Due to its valuable nature and great utility, it is used by royal families.
Sheetshaman: It has cold-allaying property.
Shringaj: The plant grows in hilly region.
Vanshika: The plant is gregarious in nature like the bamboo plant and has a nauseating smell.
Varnaprasadana: The heartwood is used to enhance luster of the skin.
Vishvadhupa: The aromatic wood is used for making incense and perfumes.
Yogaj: The resinous wood is produced by fungal association.

Classical Categorization

Charak Samhita: Sheetprasasmana, Shwasahara, Tikta skanda
Sushrut Samhita: Salasaradi, Eladi, Shleshmasansaman
Ashtang Hridaya: Salasaradi, Eladi
Dhanvantari Nighantu: Chandanadi varga
Madanpal Nighantu: Karpuradi varga
Kaiyadev Nighantu: Oushadi varga
Raj Nighantu: Prabhadradi varga
Bhavaprakash Nighantu: Karpuradi varga

Distribution

Agaru is a native plant of China, India, Indonesia, Malaysia, Philippines, Laos, Thailand, Singapore, Sri Lanka, Tibet, Europe, and Africa.

In India, the plant is found growing naturally in evergreen forests of Eastern Himalayas. It grows at an altitude of 700 to 1400 m. It is found in abundance in Assam, Tripura, Meghalaya, Nagaland, Sikkim, Manipur, Bhutan, Khasi hills, etc. Agaru obtained from Sylhet region is considered the best.

Morphology

A large evergreen tree about 70 to 80 ft in height and 4 to 5 ft in girth with a straight and fluted stem. Initially its wood is soft, light, elastic, whitish yellow in color without any characteristic smell. Later as the fungal infection progresses it becomes heavy and black (**Fig. 1.1**).

- **Leaves:** Simple, alternate, ovate-lanceolate to lanceolate-oblong in shape, about 8 to 10 cm long

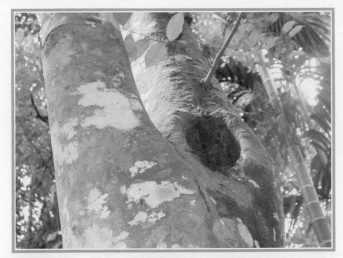

Fig. 1.1 Stem.

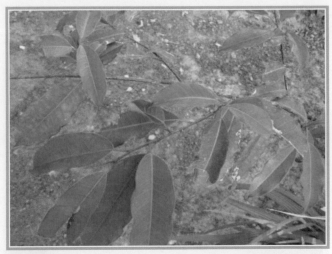

Fig. 1.2 Leaves.

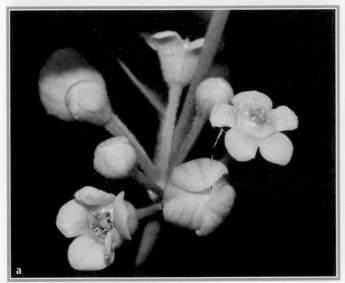

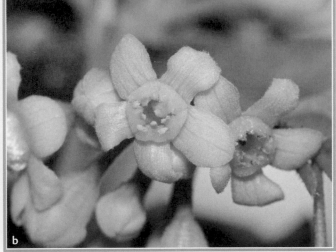

Fig. 1.3 **(a)** Inflorescence and **(b)** flowers.

and 2 to 3 cm broad, short petioled, silky glossy surface, and entire margin (**Fig. 1.2**).

- **Flowers:** Inflorescence of many small, greenish yellow-colored flowers on short peduncle umbels occurring on younger branchlets (**Fig. 1.3a, b**).
- **Fruits:** Capsule, obovoid shape, slightly compressed, yellowish, and tomentose (**Fig. 1.4**).
- **Seeds:** Brownish black colored, ovoid shape with a long tail (**Fig. 1.5**).
- **Heartwood:** Dark resinous wood which is formed when the plant becomes infected with a type of fungus (ascomycetous mold). Species of *Aspergillus*, *Fusarium*, and *Penicillium* are reported to be associated with the development of infection. Prior to infection, the heartwood is odorless, relatively light, and pale colored; however, as the infection progresses, the tree produces a dark aromatic resin in response to the attack, which results in accumulation of a very dense, dark resin in the heartwood. The infected resin–embedded wood is known as Agarwood (**Fig. 1.6**). Infection is more common on the trunk, roots, and area where branches divide. The formation of Agarwood starts when the tree attains the age of 20 years. On an average, approximately 30 mL oil is extracted from 100 kg of infected Agarwood. Oil extracted from the wood is popularly known as Oud oil. The plant is propagated by seeds.

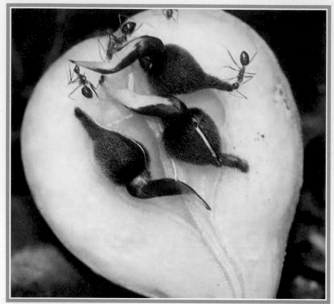

Fig. 1.4 Fruit.

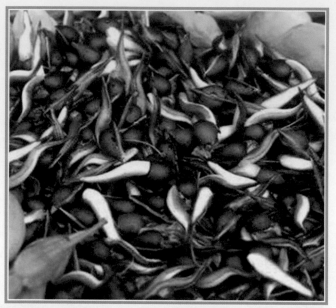

Fig. 1.5 Seeds.

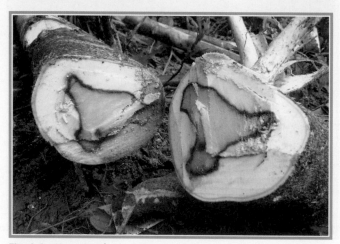

Fig. 1.6 Heartwood.

Phenology

Flowering time: May to June
Fruiting time: July to August

Key Characters for Identification

➤ *An evergreen 70 to 80 ft tree with straight and fluted stem*
➤ *Leaves: simple, alternate, ovate-lanceolate, silky glossy surface*
➤ *Flowers: small, greenish yellow in axillary inflorescence*
➤ *Heartwood: dark, resinous, heavy, aromatic, and is infected with fungus*

Types

- Dhanvantari Nighantu describes Kaleyaka as a type of Agaru
- Sodhala Nighantu describes three types of Agaru: Agaru, Krishna Agaru, and Kakatunda Agaru
- Raj Nighantu describes five types of Agaru: Krishna Agaru, Kasht Agaru, Daha Agaru, Mangalya Agaru, and Agurusaar
- Arthashastra describes three Agaru wood products:
  ➢ Jongaka: Black or variegated black in color and having variegated spots
  ➢ Dongaka: Black in color
  ➢ Parasamudraka: Black in color and smells like navamallika (Shamasastry 1915)

Rasapanchaka

Guna	Laghu, Ruksha, Tikshna
Rasa	Katu, Tikta
Vipaka	Katu
Virya	Ushna

Chemical Constituents

Agaru's heartwood is rich in essential oil, resins, alkaloids (liriodenine), saponins, steroids, terpenoids, tannins, flavonoids (aquisiflavoside, aquilarisinin, aquilarisin, and aquilarixanthone), and phenolic compounds (Satapathy et al 2009). Agaru wood predominantly contains 2-(2-phenylethyl)-4H-chromen-4-one derivatives and sesquiterpenes.

Chromone derivatives include 7,8-dimethoxy-2-[2-(3'-acetoxyphenyl)ethyl]chromones, 6-methoxy-2-(2-phenylethyl)chromones, 6,7-dimethoxy-2-(2-phenylethyl) chromones, aquilarone A-I, aquiseninone A-D, tetrahydrochromone A-M, and quinanone A-D.

Sesquiterpenes include agarol, aquilochin, α & β agarofuran, norketoagarofuran, agarspirol, 10-epi-g-eudesmol, jinkoeremol, jinkohol, kusunol, dihydrokaranone, oxoagarospirol, qinanol A-F, aquilarabietic acid A-K, aquilarin B, aquilacallane A-B, aquimavitalin, abietane ester, gmelofuran apigenin, and 4',7-dimethyl ether (Wang et al 2018; Srivastava et al 2016).

Agaru oil contains selinene, dihydroselinene, agarol, b-agarofuran, vetispira-2(11), valerianol, dihydrokaranone, and tetradecanoic acid (Naf et al 1992, 1995).

Identity, Purity, and Strength

- Foreign matter: Not more than 1%
- Total ash: Not more than 13%
- Acid-insoluble ash: Not more than 0.5%
- Alcohol-soluble extractive: Not less than 1%
- Water-soluble extractive: Not less than 2%

(Source: The Ayurvedic Pharmacopeia of India 2004).

Karma (Actions)

In various samhitas and nighantus, Agaru is described as tikshna, snigdh, sheetprasasmana, varnaprasadan (blood purifier), tvachya (skin tonic), pitta vardhaka (pitta aggravating), shirovirechan (procedure used for head purification), mangalya (auspicious), sugandhik (aromatic), and rochak (relish) in properties. Nighantus recommended its use in the form of lepa (topical application), udvartana (powder massage), and dhum pana (medicated inhalation therapy). Raj Nighantu has described the properties and action of five types of Agaru, which are as follows:

- Krishna Agaru: Katu, tikta rasa, ushna, sheet when applied externally and pittahara when taken orally, slightly tridoshahara.

- Kastha Agaru: Katu, ushna, ruksha, and kaphashamaka
- Mangalya Agaru: Sheet, yogavahi, aromatic
- Daha Agaru: Katu, ushna, keshvardhak, varnya, with persistent aroma
- Agarusaar: Katu, kashaya, ushna, produces aroma on burning, vatashamaka
- Doshakarma: Vata kapha shamaka, pitta vardhaka
- Dhatukarma: Rasayana, tvachya
- Malakarma: Vataanulomaka

Pharmacological Actions

Its heartwood and oil is reported to have antinociceptive, antimicrobial, analgesic, antiinflammatory, antihyperglycaemic, antipyretic, antioxidant, ulcer-protecting, anticancerous, hepatoprotective, antihistaminic, anxiolytic, and thrombolytic properties (Alam et al 2015).

Indications

Traditionally, Agaru's heartwood and oil is used in the treatment of sheet (chill), karna akshi roga (ear and eye diseases), shwasa (asthma), kustha (skin diseases), dustha vrana (chronic ulcers), visha (poison), and shirashool (headache). Charak suggested an external application of Agaru and Rasna to counteract the effect of cold. Sushrut uses Agaru taila for dustha vrana shodhana (cleansing of chronic wound), krimi (microbes), and kustha.

It is also used as a mouth freshener, carminative, and an appetizer in digestive ailments, and it relieves itching, improves blood circulation, and gives relief in cough, bronchitis, and asthma. Agaru oil massage is effective in rigors in fever. Its oil is used to treat toothache, colic pain, and pains during pregnancy (Burfield and Kirkham 2005).

Therapeutic Uses

External Use

1. **Sotha** (edema): Chanda (choraka), Agaru paste is applied externally to decrease edema (A.H.Ci. 17/36, C.S.Ci. 12/70).
2. **Dadru, Kustha** (skin diseases): External application of oil prepared by Agarusaar and Sinshipa is used in chronic nonhealing ulcers and skin diseases like dadru, kitibh, and kustha (S.S.Ci. 31/5).

Internal Use

1. **Shwasa and Hikka** (asthma and hic-cough): Agaru powder mixed with honey twice daily is used as leha to get relief in shwasa and hikka (C.S.Ci. 17/129). Incenses of Agaru wood can also be used to get relief in respiratory congestion and asthma.

2. **Kasa** (cough): Taking 1 to 3 g of Agaru's heartwood powder with honey gives relief in kasa (A.H.Ci. 3/47).

3. **Lavanmeha** (a type of diabetes): Decoction prepared with Patha and Agaru is used to cure lavanmeha (S.S.Ci. 11/8).

4. **Rasayana** (Rejuvinators): Daily intake of Agaru powder with milk gives rasayana effect (A.H.U. 39/104-105).

Officinal Parts Used

Heartwood and oil

Dose

Powder: 1 to 3 g
Oil: 1 to 5 drops

Formulations

Agaruvadi taila, Chandan Agaru kwath, Anu taila, Madhukasava, Chandanadi taila, Shwasahara kasaya churna, Guduchyadi taila, Khadiradi gutika.

Toxicity/Adverse Effects

There are no reported side effects of Agaru when used in recommended dose. Agaru oil being pitta aggravating in nature can cause redness and irritation on local application, while inhalation of excessive fumes or oral intake may result in nausea, dizziness, and burning sensations.

Substitution and Adulteration

Other species of *Aquilaria*, such as *A. crassna, A. malaccensis,* and *A. sinensis*, are used as Agaru's substitutes.

Points to Ponder

Qualities of best Agaru:
- *It should be black in color.*
- *It should be extremely heavy and aromatic.*
- *It should be oily in appearance and taste.*
- *It should sink in water.*
- *It should burn easily with a bright flame giving off a pleasant smell.*

Suggested Readings

Burfield T, Kirkham K. The Agarwood Files. Cropwatch; 2005:6–8

CITES. Amendments to appendices I and II of CITES. In Proceedings of the Thirteenth Meeting of the CITES. Government of India Hosted Asian Regional Workshop on the Management of Wild and Planted Agarwood Taxa; 2004. https://www.Cites.Org/eng/2015_india_agarwood_workshop. Accessed May 5, 2015. Conference of the Parties 2004, Bangkok, Thailand, October 2, 2004

Janey A, Badruddeen MM, Rahman MA, et al. An insight of pharmacognostic study and phytopharmacology of Aquilaria agallocha. J Appl Pharma Sci Vol. 5 (08), pp.- 173-181

Janey A, Mujahid Mohd, Badr B, et al. An insight of pharmacognostic study and phytopharmacology of *Aquilaria agallocha.* J Appl Pharmaceut Sci. 2015;5(8):173–181

Lopez SA, Tony P. History of use and trade of agarwood. Economic Botany. 2018;72(1):107–129

López-Arlene S, Page T. History of use and trade of Agarwood. Econ Bot. 2018;72:107–129

Naf R, Velluz A, Brauchli R, Thommen W. Agarwood oil (*Aquilaria agallocha* Roxb.). Its composition and eight new valencane, eremophilane, vetispirane derivatives. Flav Frag J 1995;10(3): 147–152

Naf R, Velluz A, Busset N, Gaudin JM. New norsesquiterpenoids with 10 epi eudesmane skeleton from agarwood (*Aquilaria agallocha* Roxb.). Flav Frag J 1992;7(6):295–298

National Pharmacopoeia Committee. Pharmacopoeia of the People's Republic of China; 2015 Version; Beijing, Vol. 1. China: Chinese Medical Science and Technology Press; 2015:185–186

Panda H. Aromatic Plants Cultivation, Processing and Uses. Asia Pacific Business Press Inc.; 2009;8:182

Satapathy AK, Gunasekaran G, Sahoo SC, Kumar A, Rodriques PV. Corrosion inhibition by *Justicia gendarussa* plant extract in hydrochloric acid solution. Corros Sci 2009;51(12):2848–2856

Shamasastry R. Kautilya's Arthashastra; 1915. http://libarch.nmu.org.ua/ bitstream/ handle/G e n o f o n d U A /1 9 2 7 3/ f2c8936431b9587a3448e1b3d8eff8e8. Pdf sequence=1

Srivastava B, Sharma VC, Sharma H, Pant P, Jadhav AD. Comparative physicochemical, phytochemical and high performance thin layer chromatography evaluation of heart wood and small branches of *Aquilaria agallocha* Roxb. Int J Ayurveda Pharma Res. 2016;4(1):1–6

The Ayurvedic Pharmacopeia of India. Part I, Vol. 4. New Delhi: Department of AYUSH, Ministry of Health and Family Welfare, Government of India; 2004:4–5

Wang S, Yu Z, Wang C, et al. Chemical constituents and pharmacological activity of Agarwood and Aquilaria plants. Molecules 2018;23(2): 342

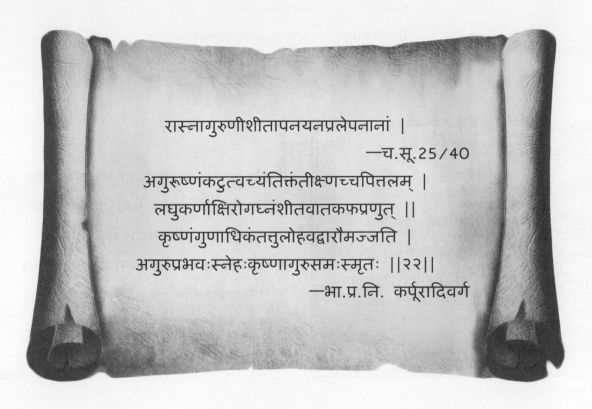

रास्नागुरुणीशीतापनयनप्रलेपनानां |
—च.सू.25/40
अगुरूष्णंकटुत्वच्यंतिक्तंतीक्ष्णच्चपित्तलम् |
लघुकर्णाक्षिरोगघ्नंशीतवातकफप्रणुत् ||
कृष्णंगुणाधिकंततुलोहवद्वारौमज्जति |
अगुरुप्रभवःस्नेहःकृष्णागुरुसमःस्मृतः ||२२||
—भा.प्र.नि. कर्पूरादिवर्ग

2. Agnimantha [*Premna integrifolia* Linn.]

Family:	*Verbenaceae*
Hindi name:	*Arni, Agethu, Tarkari*
English name:	*Indian headache tree*

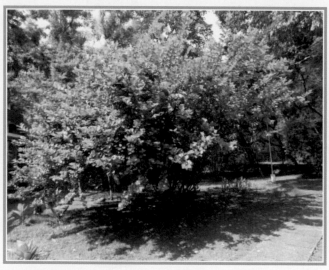

Plant of *Premna integrifolia* Linn.

Laghu and brihat Agnimantha are similar in properties and for lepan (topical application) and upnaah (poultice) in shopha (inflammatory diseases), one should use laghu Agnimantha.

Introduction

The word *Premna* is derived from Greek word *Premnon* which means tree stump, referring to the short and twisted trunk of a tree. Throughout the world the genus *Premna* contains 200 species out of which approximately 30 species are available in India. Common among them are *Premna integrifolia, P. serratifolia, P. mucronata, P. microphylla, P. obtusifolia, P. barbata, P. esculenta*, etc. (De Kok 2013). Since Vedic period its wood is used to ignite the fire (agni) on rubbing together (manthan) in sacrificial ceremonies and yajna. Hence, the tree gets its name as Agnimantha.

In ancient texts there is some controversy about the identity of laghu and brihat Agnimantha. In Charak Samhita, two separate plants Agnimantha and Tarkari are mentioned which are considered as laghu and brihat Agnimantha, respectively, by some writers. Sushrut has included both Agnimantha and Tarkari in varunadi gana which means both are separate plants. In practice *Premna* is used as Agnimantha in southern India whereas *Clerodendron phlomides* is used as laghu Agnimantha in Gujarat and North India.

It is one of the important constituents of a famous formulation called Dashamool that is used to treat a number of ailments. In Charak Samhita, Agnimantha is used for asthapana basti (C.S.Su. 2/11), in the treatment of sthoulya (C.S.Su. 21/24), and as a content of brahma rasayana (C.S.Ci. 1/1/43). Sushrut uses it for the treatment of kustha (S.S.Ci. 10/12), jwara (S.S.U. 39/217), and grahabadha (S.S.U. 36/3). Vagbhatta has included Tarkari in shaka varga and described it as madhur, ishadtikta, and kaphavatashamaka in properties (A.H.Su. 6/96).

Its roots are used in folklore medicine for the treatment of eczema, bone fracture, boils, sores, and gingivitis (Arya and Agarwal 2008).

Vernacular Names

Bengali: Ganibhari, Ganira
Gujarati: Arani, Aranel
Kannada: Takkila, Arani, Taggi
Malayalam: Munja, Munnai
Marathi: Eirani, Eran, Chamari, Takali
Oriya: Ganiyari
Tamil: Pachumullai, Taludalai
Telugu: Nelichett, Nelli, Gabunelli

Synonyms

Arnika: It is used to stimulate the digestive fire.
Ganikarika: It grows along with other trees in groups (gregarious nature).
Jaya, Jayanti: It is used to conquer many diseases.
Nadeyi: It grows on river sides or near a water source.
Shriparni: It has beautiful foliage.
Tarkari: It is praised by people because of its great thera-peutic utility.
Vajyantika, Ketu: The inflorescence of this plant seems to be a flag or banner.

Classical Categorization

Charak Samhita: Shothhara, Sheetprasasman, Anuvasanopaga
Sushrut Samhita: Varunadi, Virtarvadi, Brihat panchmool, Vata sansaman varga
Ashtang Hridaya: Varunadi, Virtarvadi
Dhanvantari Nighantu: Guduchyadi varga
Madanpal Nighantu: Abhyadi varga
Kaiyadev Nighantu: Oushadi varga
Raj Nighantu: Prabhadraadi varga
Bhavaprakash Nighantu: Guduchyadi varga

Distribution

Premna species are distributed throughout tropical and subtropical Asia, Africa, Australia, and the Pacific Islands (Harley et al 2004).

In India the plant is abundantly available near the sea coast of Maharashtra, South India, Andaman and Nicobar Islands, and West Bengal. It is also available in the forest regions of Madhya Pradesh, Gujarat, Karnataka, Assam, and Odisha (Warrier and Nambiar 1997).

Morphology

It is a large shrub or small tree reaching up to a height of 10 m. Trunk is more or less thorny, much branched with multiple spinous branches. Bark is fissured-flaky and brownish-grey in color.

- **Leaves:** Simple, opposite, petiolate, 5 to 8 cm long and 3 to 6 cm wide, glabrous, broadly elliptic, oblong, ovate or subrhomboid, apex shortly acuminate, base rounded or narrowed, entire margin and upper part toothed (**Fig. 2.1**).
- **Flowers:** Inflorescence of terminal pubescent paniculate corymbose cymes, flowers greenish white in color with unpleasant or disagreeable odor, bracts minute and lanceolate. Calyx 2.5 mm long, thick, glabrous, two-lipped, one-lip two-toothed, and the other is subentire. Corolla is glabrous outside, tube 3 × 2 mm, cylindrical, hairy inside the throat, lobes are four in number, oblong, rounded, 1.2 mm long. Stamens have slightly exerted filaments, hairy at the base. Ovary and style is glabrous, stigma has two equal divaricate lobes (**Fig. 2.2a, b**).
- **Fruits:** Drupe, pear shaped, green when unripe and turn black when fully ripe, obovoid-globose shape, 3 to 6 mm long, bony, and four-celled (**Fig. 2.3**). It has pear-shaped seeds.
- **Roots:** Woody, yellowish brown in color, branched, and somewhat tortuous to cylindrical in shape.

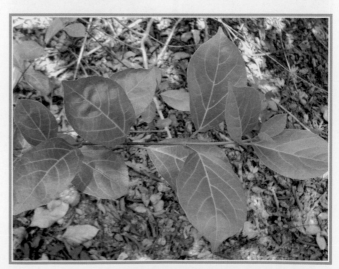

Fig. 2.1 Leaves.

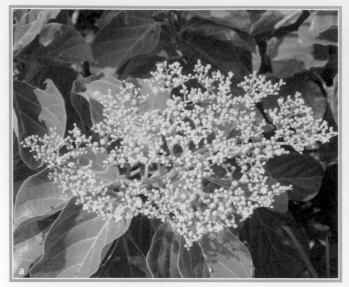

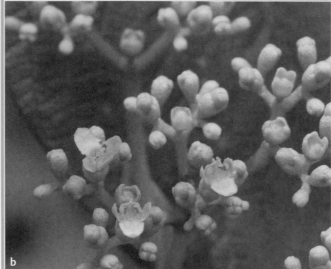

Fig. 2.2 **(a)** Inflorescence. **(b)** Flowers.

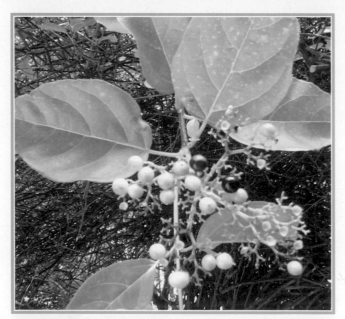

Fig. 2.3 Fruits.

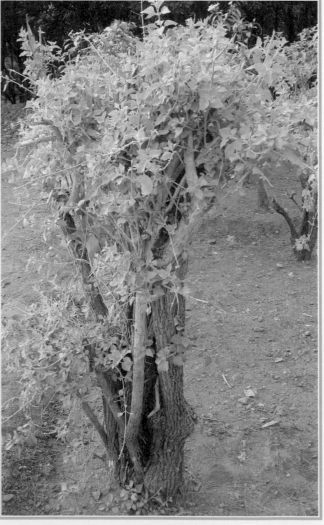

Surface gets exfoliated easily and shows prominent longitudinal striations and wrinkles (Nadkarni and Nadkarni 2005; Kirtikar and Basu 1996). The images of laghu Agnimanth are represented in **Fig. 2.4 to Fig. 2.6**. The plant is propagated by seeds and stem cuttings.

Phenology

Flowering time: April to June
Fruiting time: August to September

Fig. 2.4 Plant of *Clerodendrum phlomidis* L.f.

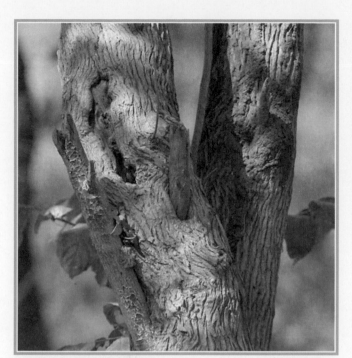

Fig. 2.5 Stem of *Clerodendrum phlomidis L.f.*

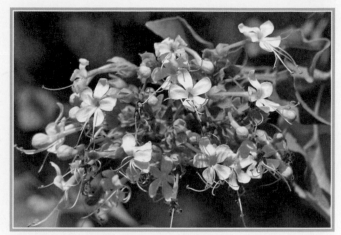

Fig. 2.6 Flower of Arani.

Key Characters for Identification
➤ A large shrub or a small tree with spinous branches
➤ Leaves: simple, opposite, glabrous, elliptic, oblong to ovate shape
➤ Flowers: greenish white in inflorescence of terminal paniculate corymbose cymes
➤ Fruits: small, drupe, obovoid to globose in shape
➤ Roots: yellowish brown, woody with exfoliating wrinkled surface

Types

Nighantu Ratnakar and Raj Nighantu have described two types of Agnimantha:

- Brihat Agnimantha: *Premna integrifolia* Linn.
- Kshudra Agnimantha: *Clerodendrum phlomidis* L.f.

Rasapanchaka

Guna	Laghu, Ruksha
Rasa	Katu, Tikta, Kashaya
Vipaka	Katu
Virya	Ushna

Chemical Constituents

Its roots and bark have premnine, betulin, ganiarine, ganikarine, caryophyllene, premnenol, premnaspirodiene, etc., whereas leaves have β-sitosterol, luteolin, and aphelandrine. It has also been reported to have *p*-methoxy cinnamic acid, linalool, linoleic acid, flavones, luteolin, iridoid glycoside, premnazole, aphelandrine, caryophyllin, premnenol, premnaspirodiene, clerodendrin-A, etc. (Rekha et al 2015).

Identity, Purity, and Strength

Laghu Agnimantha

- Foreign matter: Not more than 2%
- Total ash: Not more than 6%
- Acid-insoluble ash: Not more than 1%
- Alcohol-soluble extractive: Not less than 2%
- Water-soluble extractive: Not less than 5%

(Source: The Ayurvedic Pharmacopeia of India 2001).

Karma (Actions)

In Ayurvedic lexicons and Nighantus, Agnimantha is described as having shothhara (anti-inflammatory), deepan (carminative), jwaraghna (antipyretic), saraka (laxative), medohara (antiobesity), balya (tonic), and thermogenic properties.

- Doshakarma: Kaphavatahara
- Dhatukarma: Medohara
- Malakarma: Saraka

Pharmacological Actions

In vivo and in vitro studies suggested its antibacterial, analgesic, antinociceptive, antiarthritic, anticancer, antitumor, antiinflammatory, hypolipidemic, antioxidant, antiulcer, antiparasitic, gastroprotective, cardiac stimulant, hepatoprotective, central nervous system (CNS) depressant, immunomodulatory, longevity promoting, and neuroprotective effects (Mali 2016).

Indications

In classical literature, roots, stem, and leaves of Agnimantha are reported to be used for the treatment of shotha, pandu, jalodara, vatavyadhi, sthoulya, agnimandhya, adhyaman, arshas, vibandh, sheetpitta, nadishool, sandhivata (arthritis), and jwar (fever).

In ethnomedicine practices, roots of Agnimantha are used in the treatment of cough, asthma, bronchitis, leprosy, skin disorders, anorexia, constipation, diabetes, liver disorders, general debility, anemia, fever, and as a postdelivery tonic for women. Its stem-bark decoction is used as antimalarial. The alkali prepared from the bark ash is used in ascites. Flowers and the whole plant are used for rheumatism, neuralgia, cold, and fever. Leaves are used in the treatment of gonorrhea, cold, fever, flatulence, and vaginal irritation. Decoction of leaves is used for bathing infants, cleaning wounds, and in the treatment of beriberi. Paste of leaves is applied over the bladder to facilitate urination (Mali 2015).

Therapeutic Uses

External Use

1. **Granthi visarpa** (glandular erysipelas): Paste of Vanshpatra and Agnimanth is applied locally to the affected area (C.S.Ci. 21/125).
2. **Arsha** (piles): Avagahan sweda (Sitz bath) with leaf decoction of Agnimanth, Shigru, and Ashmantaka reduces inflammation and pain in arsha (C.S.Ci. 14/45).
3. **Urusthambha** (stiffness of thigh): Regular application of Agnimanth root powder mixed with cow's urine or fomentation with the decoction of Agnimantha and Karanj leaves reduces inflammation in Urusthambha (C.S.Ci. 27/57).

4. **Vyanga** (freckles): Local application of Agnimanth bark paste pounded with aja dugdh (goat's milk) helps in reducing vyanga (G.N. 4/10/101).
5. **Vranashotha** (inflammatory wounds): Regular application of paste prepared with Matulunga, Agnimantha, Devdaru, Sunthi, Ahinsra, and Rasna gives relief in vrana shotha due to vata.

Internal Use

1. **Sheetpitta** (urticaria): Daily intake of Agnimantha root paste with goghrita for 7 days gives relief in sheetpitta, udard, and koth (CD. 51/7).
2. **Vasameha** (type of prameha): Root decoction of Agnimantha and Shinsipa is given daily in vasameha and ikshumeha (S.S.Ci. 11/9).
3. **Sthoulya** (obesity): Consumption of Agnimantha rasa with Shilajit powder helps in reducing weight in obese persons (CD. 36/16).
4. **Udarshotha** (inflammatory diseases of stomach): Oral intake and abhyanga with lukewarm decoction of Agnimantha kshar for 3 days gives relief in udarshotha (G.N. 2/33/69).

Officinal Parts Used

Root, bark, leaves

Dose

Decoction: 50 to 100 mL
Powder: 3 to 6 g

Formulations

Dashmoolarishta, Dashmoolkwath, Agnimanthkasaya, Narayan taila, Dhanvantari ghrita.

Toxicity/Adverse Effect

Not reported yet.

Substitution and Adulteration

Other species of genus *Premna* and *Clerodendrum* are adulterated with Agnimantha.

Points to Ponder

- *Agnimantha is an important ingredient of famous formulation Dashmool.*
- *Botanically laghu Agnimantha is Clerodendrum phlomides L.f. and brihat Agnimantha is Premna integrifolia Linn.*
- *In Ayurvedic Pharmacopeia of India and Database of Medicinal Plants Clerodendrum phlomidis L.f. is described as Agnimantha.*

Suggested Readings

Arya KR, Agarwal SC. Folk therapy for eczema, bone fracture, boils, sores and gingivitis in Taragtal province of Uttaranchal. Ind J Trad Knowl. 2008;7(3):443–445

De Kok R. The genus *Premna* L. (Lamiaceae) in the Flora Malesiana area. Kew Bull. 2013;68:1–30

Harley RM, Atkins S, Budantsev AL, et al. Labiatae. In: Kubitzki K, Kadereit JW, eds. The Families and Genera of Vascular Plants. Flowering Plants, Dicotyledons: Lamiales (except Acanthaceae including Avicenniaceae). Vol. 7. Berlin: Springer; 2004:167–275

Kirtikar KR, Basu BD. Indian Medicinal Plants. 2nd ed. III. Dehradun: International Book Distributors; 1996:1927–1929

Mali PY. Pharmacological potentials of *Premna integrifolia* L. Ancient Sci Life. 2016;35(3):132–142

Mali PY. *Premna integrifolia* L.: A review of its biodiversity, traditional uses and phytochemistry. Ancient Sci Life. 2015:35(1):4–11

Nadkarni KM, Nadkarni AK. Indian Materia Medica. 3rd ed. I. Bombay: Popular Prakashan; 2005:1009–10

Rekha K, Pandey R, Babu KS, Rao JM. A phytochemistry of the genus *Premna*: a review. Int J Pharm Chem Sci. 2015;4(3):317–325

The Ayurvedic Pharmacopeia of India. Part I, Vol. 3., New Delhi: Department of AYUSH, Ministry of Health and Family Welfare, Government of India; 2001:3–4

Warrier PK, Nambiar VP. Indian Medicinal Plants. Madras: Orient Longman; 1997:348–352

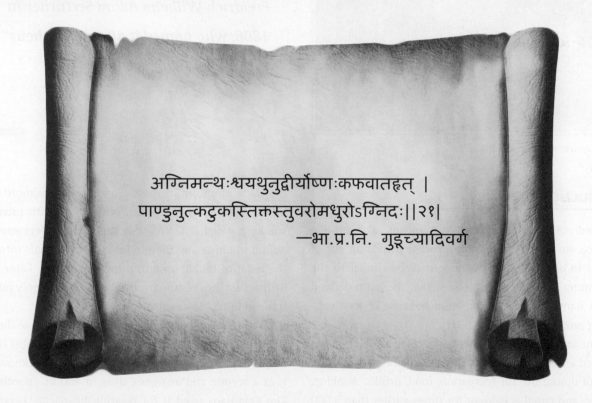

अग्निमन्थःश्वयथुनुद्वीर्योष्णःकफवातहृत् ।
पाण्डुनुत्कटुकस्तिक्तस्तुवरोमधुरोऽग्निदः।।२१।
—भा.प्र.नि. गुड्च्यादिवर्ग

3. Ahiphena [*Papaver somniferum* Linn.]

Family: *Papaveraceae*

Hindi name: *Afeem*

English name: *Opium, Garden poppy, White poppy*

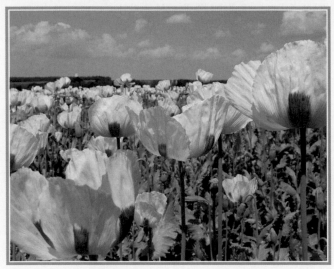

Plant of *Papaver somniferum* Linn.

Morphine, the principal active compound of opium, was isolated by Freidrich Wilhelm Adam Serturner in 1806, who named it after "Morpheus" the Greek God of dreams

Introduction

The word "Ahiphena" in Sanskrit means a foam-like substance. In ancient times, the process of oozing out of exudates in opium fruit was thought to be similar to the foam coming from the mouth of a snake. The plant derived its Latin name *Papaver somniferum* because of its sleep-inducing property (Raymond 2004).

Ahiphena is one of the oldest medicinal plants. It is the most used and abused drug in ethnomedicine practice. The history of opium use for recreation, food, drinks, smoking, medicine, and ritual is evident for times earlier than 5,000 BC. Opium was cultivated first time in Mesopotamia around 3,400 BC. The Sumerian, Assyrian, Egyptian, Indian, Greek, Roman, Persian, Chinese, and Arabian empires all made widespread use of opium in the form of inhalation, suppositories, poultice, hemlock for suicide, sleeping aid, and in surgical procedures. The Sumerians called it the "Joy plant," while the Americans called it as "God's own medicine" (Moraes and Moraes 2003). After the 11th century

the trade of opium increased, and it became more regular by the 17th century when it was mixed with tobacco for smoking, which led to its addiction. Arab traders introduced opium to China and then to India. The Mughals introduced the habit of taking opium to Indian soldiers. Later on, the British East India Company established monopoly on opium trade in India (Ray et al 2015).

In spite of its recreational use, opium is one of the oldest painkillers practiced by human society since ages (Chouvy 2006). Hippocrates (The Father of Medicine) acknowledged it as a styptic and analgesic drug in 460 BC (Booth 1996). The Egyptians used it for treating headache, Persians for inducing anesthesia and treating melancholy, and Chinese for treating migraine, headache, sciatica, and other painful ailments. During the 19th and 20th centuries, in spite of having great medicinal property, opium became the drug of abuse, and due to its illicit use, trade, and trafficking, the world suffered from the biggest addiction. Subsequently, the use, possession, distribution, and trade of opium except for medicine and scientific purpose were prohibited and made illegal. In India, the manufacture, sale, possession, transportation, and purchase of opium is governed by the Narcotics Drugs and Psychotropic Substances Act, 1985.

Since centuries, latex and seeds of poppy have been widely used in folklore, Ayurveda, siddha, homeopathy, and unani medicines for treating diarrhea, cough, insomnia, rheumatism, snake bite, depression, and anxiety. In Ayurvedic literature, Ahiphena was first described in Gadanigraha written by Shodhala in the 12th century (Sharma 1998). In Sharangdhar Samhita, Ahiphena is described as an example of vyavayi dravya (Sh. S. 1/1/19). In Rasatarangani, Ahiphena is the major ingredient of akarkaradi churna which is used as shukra stambhaka drug. There it is described under the category of vyavayi and madakari dravya. Bhavaprakash Nighantu, Raj Nighantu, Dhanvantari Nighantu, and Rasatarangani have categorized it under upavisha. Seeds are used in sweets, condiments, and in medicine too. Poppy seed oil is used as a culinary salad oil, cooking oil, drying oil for use in art, and as a vehicle for various parenteral formulations (Robbers et al 1996; Dewick 1997).

Opium is extensively cultivated worldwide for its major alkaloids: morphine followed by codeine and thebaine. Morphine and its derivatives are CNS depressants and cause analgesia, sedation, and euphoria. Regular use of opium or its derivatives results in intoxication and physical dependence.

Vernacular Names

Arabic: Abunom, Afyiun
Bengali: Pasto, Post
Greek: Agria
Gujarati: Aphina, Khuskhus, Posta
Italian: Papavero, Papavero domestico
Malayalam: Bungapion
Persian: Afiun, Khashkhash, Koknar
Tamil: Abini, Gashagasha, Kasakasa
Urdu: Khuskhus safaid

Synonyms

Aaphuka: Its fully ripened fruit is self-dehiscent in nature.
Khakhustil: Its seeds resemble the seeds of tila.
Khus phal ksheer: Milky exudates of Ahiphena fruit is khus phal ksheer.

Khusbeej: Seeds of Ahiphena are known as khusbeej in market.
Khustil: Its seeds cause paralysis of limbs and other organs.
Tilbhed: Its seeds appear to be a variety of Tila because of morphological similarity.

Classical Categorization

Charak Samhita: Not described
Sushrut Samhita: Not described
Madanpal Nighantu: Abhyadi varga
Kaiyadev Nighantu: Oushadi varga
Raj Nighantu: Pippaliyadi varga
Bhavaprakash Nighantu: Haritakyadi varga

Distribution

The plant is indigenous to warm and temperate regions of Europe and Asia. However, nowadays it is cultivated throughout the world for its alkaloids. In India, it is mostly cultivated in Uttar Pradesh, Madhya Pradesh, Bihar, Rajasthan, Eastern Punjab, Jammu & Kashmir, Sikkim, and Maharashtra up to an altitude of 3,000 m.

Morphology

It is an erect annual herb of 1 to 1.5 m in height. Stem is glabrous and slightly branched.

- **Leaves:** Simple, clasping to the stem by their cordate base, sessile, alternate, ovate-oblong, ash green in color, pinnatifid, irregularly toothed with an acute apex and dentate margin (**Fig. 3.1**).
- **Flowers:** Solitary, terminal, large, scarlet white, purple, or variegated with dark stain at the base (**Fig. 3.2**).
- **Fruits:** Capsulated, glabrous, stalked, up to 4 cm in diameter, globose–sub-globose or ovoid with a round base. The upper part of the fruit has seven- to eight-rayed expanded discs with a hole through which seeds are dispersed. Immature capsule is green in color, which turns brown on maturity (**Fig. 3.3a–c**).
- **Seeds:** Many, white-gray, brown, or black in color, 1 to 2 mm diameter, reniform shape (**Fig. 3.4**). The plant is propagated through seeds.

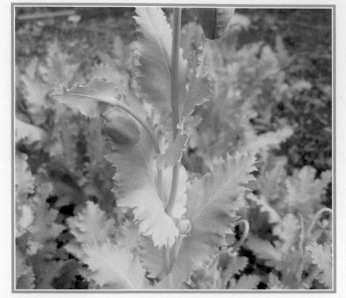

Fig. 3.1 Leaves.

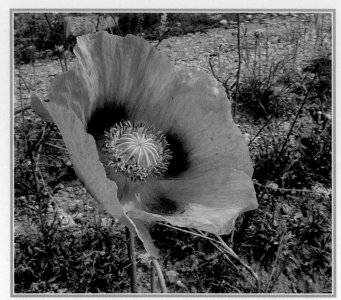

Fig. 3.2 Flower.

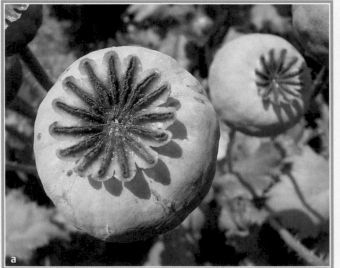

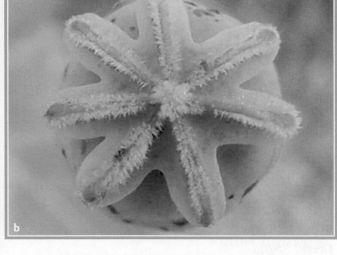

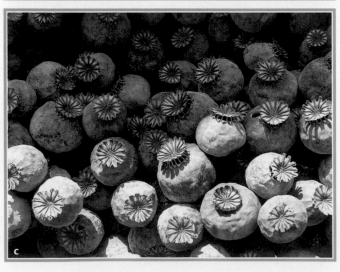

Fig. 3.3 **(a)** Fruits. **(b)** Fruit crowning. **(c)** Dry fruit.

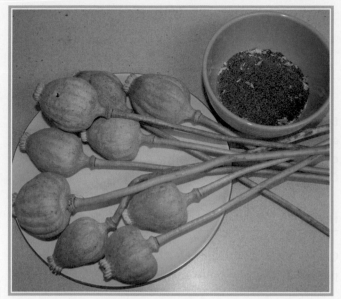

Fig. 3.4 Dry fruit and seeds.

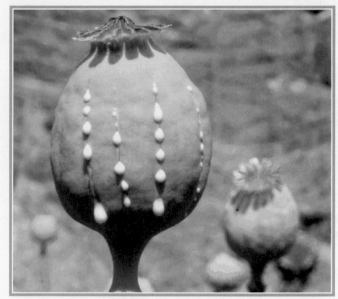

Fig. 3.5 Latex from fruit.

- **Latex:** Milky white when fresh and on drying becomes reddish-brown.

Opium is available in the Indian market as soft, lustrous, homogenous, and shiny masses of various sizes, which on drying changes to hard and brittle, irregular-shaped masses with blackish brown color, strong characteristic odor, and bitter taste (Martindale 1989; **Fig. 3.5**).

Phenology

Flowering time: February to March
Fruiting time: April to August

Collection Time

The ideal time for collecting Ahiphena niryasa is in the month of Magha (January) and Phalguna (February).

Method of Collection

Cultivation and collection of opium in India is done by cultivators under a license issued by the government. The licensed cultivators, on behalf of the government, sow the seeds, lance the capsules, collect the latex, and deliver it to the centers at a price fixed by the government.

Opium is collected from unripe/raw pods with not more than a slight yellow tint. Flowering starts 70 to 80 days after germination of the seeds. After another 8 to 10 days

capsules are ready for lancing. The capsules are lanced three or four times at an interval of 2 to 3 days with a special type of knife known as "Nashtar," which has three to four blades. Lancing is done after midday and exuding latex is allowed to remain on the capsules overnight, during which it coagulates and becomes thick and dark in color. In the morning, usually before sunrise, the coagulated latex, i.e., raw opium is collected from the surface of capsules with a blunt-edged small iron scoop. One acre of harvested crop produces approximately 3 to 5 kg of raw opium (Sharma et al 2001).

Key Characters for Identification

➤ An erect annual evergreen herb of 1 to 1.5 m
➤ Leaves: simple, clasping to the stem, ovate, ash green, pinnatifid
➤ Flowers: terminal, large, scarlet white, purple, or variegated
➤ Fruits: capsulated, sub-globose or ovoid, flat seven- to eight-rayed expanded disc at the top having numerous white-gray reniform seeds

Types

Raj Nighantu has described four varieties of opium:
1. Jaran: Shwet varna—It is used for anna pachan (digestion).

2. Maran: Krishan varna—It causes mrityu (death).
3. Dharan: Peeta varna—It is used for vayastambhan (antiaging).
4. Saran: Karbur varna—It is used for malasaran (removes metabolic waste).

On the basis of trade, three varieties are available in the market:

1. Patna opium
2. Banarasi opium
3. Malva opium—Best quality opium

Botanically, four varieties of *Papaver somniferum* are available:

1. *Papaver somniferum var.album*—Cultivated in India, bears white flowers and white seeds, capsule is egg shaped.
2. *Papaver somniferum var.glabrum*—Native to Turkey, Asia Minor, purple flowers, and purplish black seeds, subglobular capsule.
3. *Papaver somniferum var.nigrum*—Cultivated in Europe, purple flowers, and slate gray seeds (known as maw seeds).
4. *Papaver somniferum var.setigerum*—A wild variety characterized by presence of bristly hairs on peduncle and leaves.

Rasapanchaka

Guna	Laghu, Ruksha, Sukshma, Vyavayi, Vikasi
Rasa	Tikta, Kashaya
Vipaka	Katu, Seeds (Madhur vipaka)
Virya	Ushna
Prabhav	Madaka

Chemical Constituents

Opium is valued for its alkaloid content which varies from 5 to 25%, out of which morphine (7–22%) is the principal one. Opium alkaloids can be classified into the following types:

- Phenanthrene alkaloids: morphine, pseudomorphine, oxymorphine (2–12%), codeine (0.3–4%), thebaine, neopine, and porphyroxine
- Phthalide isoquinoline type: hydrocotarnine, narcotine, oxynarcotine, narcotoline, groscopine, and narceine

- Benzyl isoquinoline type: papaverine, noscapine, laudanine, xanthaline (papaveraldine), laudanosine, and codamine
- Cryptopine type: cryptopine, protoprine
- Unknown constituents: papaveramine, sanguinarine, salutarifine, meconidine, and lanthothine

Besides these it contains acetic acid, meconin acid, lactic acid, sulfuric acid, gum, pectin, resins, albumins, ammonia, calcium, and magnesium salts (Masihuddin et al 2018; Chalise 2015).

Identity, Purity, and Strength

Quality of opium is determined by the amount of morphine present in it, which should not be less than 9.5%.

Karma (Actions)

Nighantus described its latex as grahi (absorbent), dhatu shoshak (dries up cellular tissues), madakrit (induces hallucination), agnivardhaka (increase digestive fire), vaakvardhak (increases power of speech), ruchya (relish), nidrajanak (induces sleep), stambhaka (astringent), vedanastapan (analgesic), muhurmohakaram (induces repeated hallucinations), and punsatvanashnam (anti-fertility), whereas described its seeds as guru, balya, vrishya, kanti, and kaphavardhak.

- Doshakarma: Vata-pitta vardhak, kaphashamaka
- Dhatukarma: Dhatushoshak
- Malakarma: Mala stambhak, shoshak, swedajanan

Pharmacological Actions

Morphine and its derivatives are reported to be analgesic, anti-inflammatory, antipyretic, carminative, decongestant, antitussive, expectorant, demulcent, antispasmodic, muscle relaxant, diuretic, vasodilator, nervine stimulant, aphrodisiac, diaphoretic, abortifacient, antibacterial, hemostatic, euphoric, sedative, hypnotic, deliriant, and tonic (Sharma and Sharma 2017).

Indications

In traditional medicine, Ahiphena niryasa is used for the treatment of all types of shool (painful conditions), krimiroga (worm infestations), pandu (anemia), prameha (diabetes), shwasa (asthma), kasa (cough), pleeharoga (diseases of spleen), atisaar (diarrhea), aamashya-shoth (inflammatory diseases of stomach), vishamjwara (febrile fever), chardi (vomiting), madyapaanjanyashopha (ascites due to alcoholism), pravahika (dysentery), anidra (insomnia), apasmaar (epilepsy), and kampavata (seizures).

Traditionally, seeds are used in insomnia, emaciation, diarrhea, dysentery, and in food preparations like curries, breads, sweets, confectionary, etc. An infusion of the capsules is used as a soothing application for bruises, inflammatory swellings, conjunctivitis, and inflammation of ear, irritant cough, and sleeplessness (Chalise 2015).

Contraindications

As it is a highly addictive narcotic drug, its use is contra-indicated in pregnant women, lactating mothers, aged persons, children, madhumeha, vrikashotha (nephritis), in persons with cold hand and feet, vishuchika, and kasa with copious sputum discharge (Shastri Kashinath 1979). It should be used cautiously in persons suffering from heart, lungs, kidney, and cerebral diseases.

Therapeutic Uses

External Use

1. **Darunaka** (dandruff): Paste of Ahiphena seeds prepared with cow's milk is applied on the scalp to get relief in dandruff (Sharangdhar U.11.19).
2. **Shool** (pain): Its paste is applied externally in painful and inflamed conditions like shirashool, udarshool, sandhishool, arsha, karnashool and netrashotha (Shastri Kashinath 1979).
3. **Kandu** (itching): Topical application of opium powder mixed with sesame oil gives relief in itching, boils, and other skin diseases.

Internal Use

1. **Atisaar** (diarrhea): Opium powder mixed with Kuchla bark powder and madhu is given to cure diarrhea and dysentery (VD. 6/3). Bhaisajyaratnavali also advocated to use Ahiphena niryasa with aja dugdha to cure atisaar (B.R. 7/125).

2. **Shool** (pain): Decoction or tincture of Ahiphena or Ahiphena asava is used for controlling severe painful conditions like cancer, pre- and postsurgery, migraine, headache, sciatica, backache, arthritis, neuralgia, fracture, and duodenal ulcers (R.T. 24/290).
3. **Shushka Kasa** (dry cough): Opium powder is given with honey in dry cough, asthma, bronchitis, and whooping cough.
4. **Vajikaran** (aphrodisiac): Equal quantities of Ahiphena, Akarkara, Jayaphala, Jatipatri, Ela, Lavang, and Kesar powder are mixed together with half amount of Karpur and made into pills with betel leaf juice. One pill is taken daily to prevent premature ejaculation and to get balya, varnya, agnideepan action (Vaidya Lakshmipati Shastri 2015).
5. **Swarbhed** (tonsillitis): Decoction of opium is used daily as gargle in tonsillitis and hoarseness of voice.
6. **Anidra** (insomnia): Daily consumption of kheer prepared with opium seeds relaxes brain and induces sound sleep in hyperactive, sleep-deprived patients.
7. **Pravahika** (dysentery): Ahiphena niryasa is taken with powdered Arkamool twak in pravahika (R.T. 24/264).
8. **Garbhasrava** (threatened abortion): Daily consumption of Pinda Kharjura (date) with Ahiphena prevents threatened abortions (R.T. 24/263).

Officinal Parts Used

Fruit latex and seeds

Dose

Latex: 30 to 120 mg
Seeds: 1 to 5 g

Fatal Dose

Opium: 2 g
Morphine: 0.2 g
Codeine: 0.5 g

Formulations

Ahiphenasava, Nidrodayavati, Akarkarabhadi taila, Vednantaka vati, Karpooradi vati.

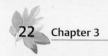

Toxicity/Adverse Effects

Opium is a habit-forming substance; if used for long duration it will cause severe toxic effect on the body. On consumption first it stimulates then depresses and finally paralyzes the nerve centers in brain. It causes euphoria (tandra), digestive impairment, nausea, vomiting, stomach ache, constipation, dry mouth, headache, weakness, anemia, flaccid muscle, infertility, uncoordinated movements, convulsion, insomnia, decreased mental alertness, pin point pupil, palpitation, tachycardia, anxiety, depression (avsada), delirium, respiratory distress (shwasavrodha), coma (sanyasa), and finally death (Sastralu 2011).

Remedial Measures

For detoxification of opium poisoning:

- Intake of Brahati phal swarasa relieves the toxic effects (Sastralu 2011).
- Carry out Aamashya prakshalana by Triphala kwath or potassium permanganate.
- Induce vaman by Reetha water or salted warm water.
- Give heart stimulant drugs like coffee, kasturi, hingu, chandrodaya vati, jaharmohra pisti with honey should in repeated dose.
- Administer antidote Naloxone 0.4 to 0.8 mg i.v. repeated every 5 min till respiration recovers and then every 1 to 3 hours later.

Shodhana (Purification)

Opium powder is dissolved in water, filtered, and heated on mild flame till drying. Then the powder is processed 21 times with Adraka swaras and preserved for further use (Shastri 1979).

Substitution and Adulteration

Opium is adulterated with fresh green parts of plants, ashes, seeds such as linseed, poppy seeds and leguminous seeds, tubers, roots, extracts of poppy, Dhatura, Bhanga, *Lactuca virosa*, *Glycyrrhiza glabra* and *Glaucium flavum* Crantz., gum Arabic, tragacath, salep, aloes, small stones, flowers of *Madhuca longifolia*, Saccharine matter, vegetable oils, ghee, and minute pieces of lead and iron (Sharma et al 2001).

Suggested Readings

Booth M. Opium: A History. New York, NY: St. Martin Press; Chapter 1, 1996:1–40

Chalise U. The poppy plant: phytochemistry & pharmacology. Indo Glob J Pharm Sci 2015;5(1):58–65

Chouvy PA. Afghanistan's opium perspective. China Eurasia Forum Quart 2006;4(1):21–24

Chunekar KC. Bhavaprakash Nighantu of Sri Bhavamisra. Varanasi: Chaukhambha Bharati Academy; 2002:145–147

Dewick PM. Medicinal Plants: A Biosynthetic Approach. New York, NY: John Wiley & Sons; 1997

Masihuddin M, Jafri MA, Siddiqui A, Chaudhary S. Traditional uses, phytochemistry and pharmacological activities of *Papaver somniferum* with special reference of Unani medicine: an updated review. J Drug Deliv Therap 2018;8(5-S):110–114

Moraes F, Moraes D. eds. Opium. Oakland, CA: Romnin Publishing; 2003

Raymond MJ. Isolation and Characterization of Latex-Specific Promoters from *Papaver somniferum* L. Blacksburg, VA: Virginia Polytechnic Institute and State University; 2004

Ray R, Kattimani S, Sharma HK. Opium Abuse and Its Management: Global Scenario. New Delhi: National Drug Dependence Treatment Centre, All India Institute of Medical Sciences; 2015:1–14

Robbers JE, Speedie MK, Tyler VE. Pharmacognosy and Pharmaco Biotechnology. Baltimore, MD: Williams & Wilkins; 1996

Sastralu Nveera Swami. Anupana Manjari. Reprint Edition. Madras: Biblio Bazaar Publication; 2011:32–33

Sharma HL, Sharma KK. Principles of Pharmacology. 3rd ed. New Delhi: Paras Medical Publishers; 2017:502–510

Sharma PC, Yelne MB, Dennis TJ. Data Base on Medicinal Plant used in Ayurveda. Vol. 8. New Delhi: Central Council for Research in Ayurveda and Siddha; 2001:1–10

Sharma PV. Ayurveda ka Vyagyanik Itihaas. Chapter 5; 1998:245

Buckley G. Martindale: The Extra Pharmacopoeia. 29th ed. In: Reynold J, ed. London: Royal Pharmaceutical Society of Great Britain, The Pharmaceutical Press; 1989

Shastri Kashinath. Rasatarangani. 11th edition, Chapter 24. Motilal Banarasidas, 1979:689–701

Vaidya Lakshmipati Shastri. Yogaratnakar. Reprint. Vajikaranyoga. Varanasi: Chaukhamba Prakashan, 2015:495.

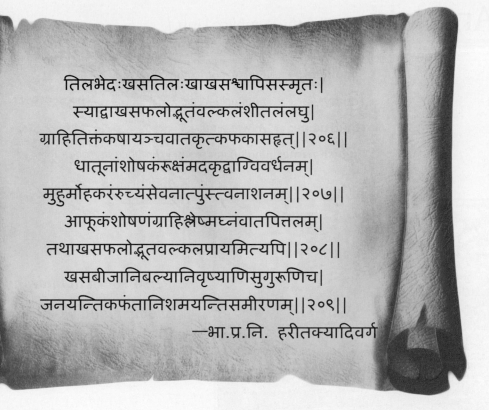

तिलभेदःखसतिलःखाखसश्चापिसस्मृतः।
स्याद्वाखसफलोद्भूतंवल्कलंशीतलंलघु।
ग्राहितिक्तंकषायञ्चवातकृत्कफकासहृत्।।२०६।।
धातूनांशोषकंरूक्षंमदकृद्वाग्निवर्धनम्।
मुहुर्मोहकरंरुच्यंसेवनात्पुंस्त्वनाशनम्।।२०७।।
आफूकंशोषणंग्राहिश्लेष्मघ्नंवातपित्तलम्।
तथाखसफलोद्भूतवल्कलप्रायमित्यपि।।२०८।।
खसबीजानिबल्यानिवृष्याणिसुगुरूणिच।
जनयन्तिकफंतानिशमयन्तिसमीरणम्।।२०९।।

—भा.प्र.नि. हरीतक्यादिवर्ग

4. Amalaki [Phyllanthus emblica Linn.]

Synonyms:	*Emblica officinalis Gaertn.*
Family:	*Euphorbiaceae*
Hindi name:	*Aawla, Amla*
English name:	*Indian gooseberry, Emblica myrobalan*

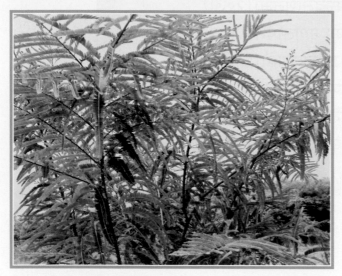

Plant of *Emblica officinalis* Gaertn.

Person born in Bharani Nakshatra should plant, worship, and propagate Amalaki tree in their vicinity so as to attain health, wealth, and prosperity.

Introduction

The word Amalaki means which has the property of removing mala (toxins) from the body. *Phyllanthus* name is originated from the Greek words *Phyllon*, which means a leaf, and *anthos*, which means a flower. The flowering branches give an appearance of pinnate leaves bearing flowers.

Amalaki is a wonder herb and is known as "Divya" and "Amrit" fruit, which literally means fruit of heaven or nectar fruit. It has been considered as a sacred tree in Hindu mythology. It is worshipped as mother earth and is believed to nurture mankind because of its nourishing property.

Kartik Mahatma and Vrat Kaumudi asked their followers to worship this tree. The leaves are offered to Lord Vishnu, Shiva, and Gauri (Onions 1994). It is believed that Lord Vishnu and Goddess Lakshmi reside in this tree. The Amalaki tree is ritually worshipped on Ekadashi (11th day, shukla paksh) in the month of Phalgun (February–March)

to get the blessings of the deity, and the day is celebrated as Amalaki Ekadashi.

It is one of the oldest oriental medicinal plants mentioned in Ayurveda, and is used not only to treat various ailments but also to promote positive health (Amalaki vyasthapananam). Owing to its multiple health benefits, it is known as the "King of Rasayana." It is believed that by using Amalaki, a great sage Chyawan rejuvenated himself and regained his virility. Hence, it is a key ingredient in Triphala and Chyawanprasha. Rajvallabha quoted that if one is willing to get rid of all doshas, then he/she should take Amalaki fruit before, in between, and after food daily. Sushrut considers it as the best fruit among all fruits (S.S.Su. 46/143-44). Charak also highlighted the fact that the properties of Amalaki and Haritaki are same, with the only difference being that they are opposite in virya (C.S.Ci. 1/1/36). Hemadri mentioned that Haritaki is ushna, kashaya, and kaphavataghn, whereas Amalaki is pittakaphaghna in properties. Charak included Amalaki in phalasava (C.S.S. 25/2) and used its powder in the treatment of atisthoulya (C.S.S. 21/23).

Besides its great medicinal value, Amalaki is well known as a rich source of vitamin C and is frequently used in making pickles, curries, preservatives, and jellies. Amalaki juice has the highest concentration of vitamin C (478.56 mg/100 mL) in comparison to other citrus fruits like oranges, lemons, etc. (Jain and Khurdiya 2004).

Vernacular Names

Assamese: Amlaku, Amlakhi, Amlakhu
Bengali: Amla, Dhatri
Chinese: Youganzi
Gujarati: Ambala, Amala
Japanese: Kemloko
Kannada: Nellikayi
Kashmiri: Embali, Amli
Malayalam: Nellikka
Marathi: Anvala, Avalkathi
Oriya: Anala, Ainla
Punjabi: Aula, Amla
Tamil: Nellikkai, Nelli
Telugu: Usirika
Urdu: Amla, Amlaj
Vietnamese: Chu me, Kam lam

Synonyms

Amla: It has the property of removing mala (toxins) from the body.
Amrita: The fruit is as potent as nectar and have rasayana effect.
Amritphala: Its fruit is enriched in rasayana properties.
Dhatri, Dhatriphala: Its fruit nourishes a person like a mother.
Jatiphalrasa: Its fruit juice is beneficial like the Chameli plant.
Kola: The fruit weighs one kola (5 g each).
Sheetphal: Fruit is sheeta in virya.
Shivam: Fruit is beneficial in all ways.
Tishyaphala: It bears fruit in the winter season (in the month of Paush (December)).
Vayastha: The fruit is used to maintain youthfulness.
Vrishya: It has aphrodisiac property.
Vritaphala: The fruit is round in shape.

Classical Categorization

Charak Samhita: Vayasthapana, Virechanopaga, Kasahara, Jwaraghna, Kushtaghna
Sushrut Samhita: Parushakadi, Amalakyadi, Triphala
Ashtang Hridaya: Parushakadi
Dhanvantari Nighantu: Guduchyadi varga
Madanpal Nighantu: Abhyaadi varga
Kaiyadev Nighantu: Oushadi varga
Raj Nighantu: Amraadi varga
Bhavaprakash Nighantu: Haritakyadi varga

Distribution

Amalaki is a native plant of tropical southeastern Asia, Nepal, Pakistan, Bangladesh, Bhutan, Sri Lanka, Malaya, and Myanmar.

It is abundantly distributed in the dry deciduous forests of central and southern India, particularly in the regions of Madhya Pradesh, Gujarat, Rajasthan, Maharashtra, Karnataka, and Andhra Pradesh (Xia et al 1997).

Morphology

A small- to medium-sized deciduous tree of height 8 to 15 m.

- **Leaves:** Simple, many, subsessile, closely set along the branchlets, about 3 mm wide, 1.5 to 2 mm long, linear-oblong, with round base, and obtuse or acute apex; more than 100 leaves are arranged distichously on the branchlets, giving a false appearance of pinnate compound leaves, slightly dark green from the above and light-green from beneath (**Fig. 4.1**).
- **Flowers:** Greenish-yellow, in axillary fascicles on the leaf-bearing branchlets, often on the naked portion below the leaves (**Fig. 4.2**).
- **Fresh fruit:** Globose, 2.5 to 3.5 cm in diameter, fleshy, smooth with six prominent lines, green when tender, changing to light yellowish or red color when mature, with a few dark specks. **Fig. 4.3** shows a fresh fruit, whereas **Fig. 4.4** depicts a dry sample of the fruit.
- **Seeds:** Single, green, and trigonous.
- **Bark:** Thin light-gray bark with exfoliating small, papery, irregular flakes (**Fig. 4.5**).

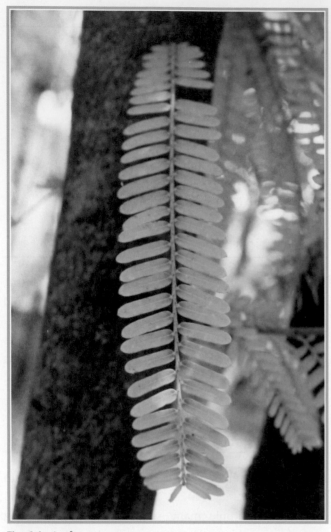

Fig. 4.1 Leaf.

- **Root bark:** Occurs in pieces, 4 to 8 cm long, 2 to 4 cm broad, curved. Outer surface rugged, often scaly without any lenticels, color greenish-sepia to mouse-gray with cracks and fissures, and recurved edges and irregular wrinkles. Fracture fibrous to granular (Sangeetha et al 2010). The plant is propagated through seeds and stem cuttings.

Phenology

Flowering time: March to May
Fruiting time: November to February

Collection Time

Amalaki fruit should be collected in the month of Magha (January) and Phaguna (February) (C.S.Ci. 1/3/3).

Key Characters for Identification

➤ *A medium-sized deciduous tree with thin gray exfoliating bark*
➤ *Leaves: simple, subsessile, distichous opposite, linear shape*
➤ *Flowers: greenish-yellow, in axillary fascicles*
➤ *Fruits: globose, fleshy, smooth with six prominent lines*

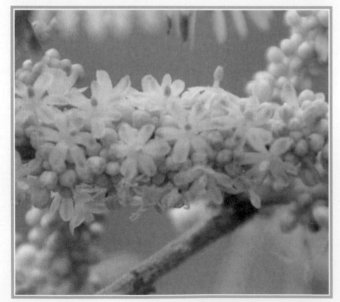

Fig. 4.2 Flowers.

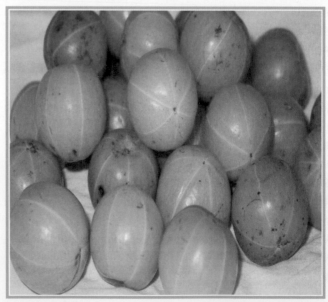

Fig. 4.3 Fresh fruit.

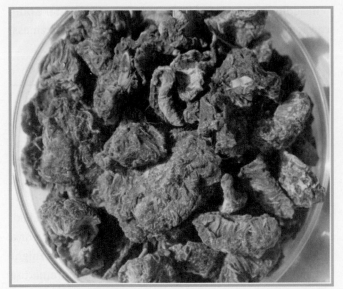

Fig. 4.4 Dry sample of fruit.

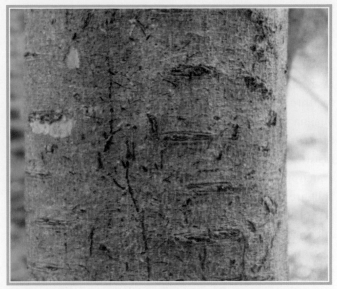

Fig. 4.5 Bark.

Types

Two types of Amalaki are available in the market:

1. Wild (Vanya): Smaller in size, hard and stony seed, less pulpy
2. Cultivated (Gramya): Bigger, fleshy, and smooth

Rasapanchaka

Guna	Guru, Ruksha, Sheeta
Rasa	Panchrasayukta (Amlapradhana) (except lavan)
Vipaka	Madhura
Virya	Sheeta

Chemical Constituents

Its fruit is the richest source of vitamin C (200–900 mg per 100 g of edible portion) (Jain and Akhurdiya 2000), gallic acid, ellagic acid, tannins, minerals, amino acids, fatty acids, glycosides, flavonoids, pectin, various polyphenolic, terpenoids, and alkaloids. Fatty acids reported are linolenic, linoleic, oleic, stearic, palmitic, and myristic acids. D-glucose, D-fructose, D-myo-inositol, D-galacturonic acid, D-arabinosyl, D-rhamnosyl, D-xylosyl, D-glucosyl, D-mannosyl, and D-galactosyl residues are the sugars

reported. Emblicanin A, emblicanin B, pedunculagin, and punigluconin are the major tannins found in the plant. Other reported compounds are quercetin, phyllemblin, arginine, aspartic acid, astragalin, β-carotene, β-sitosterol, chebulagic acid, chebulic acid, chebulaginic acid, chebulinic acid, corilagic acid, corilagin, cysteine, emblicol, gibberellins, glutamic acid, glycine, histidine, isoleucine, kaempferol, leucodelphinidin, methionine, phenylalanine, phyllantidine, phyllemblic acid, riboflavin, rutin, thiamin, and threonine (Habib-ur-Rehman et al 2007; Zhang 2003).

Identity, Purity, and Strength

- Foreign matter: Not more than 2%
- Total Ash: Not more than 7%
- Acid-insoluble ash: Not more than 2%
- Alcohol-soluble extractive: Not less than 40%
- Water-soluble extractive: Not less than 50%
- Moisture content: Not less than 80%

(Source: The Ayurvedic Pharmacopeia of India 1989).

Karma (Actions)

Bhavamishra considered Amalaki fruit similar to Haritaki fruit in properties. In addition, it is param vrishya (highly aphrodisiac), rasayana (rejuvenator) which is especially used in treating rakta pitta (bleeding disorders) and prameha (diabetes). Charak considered it as the best dravya for vyasthapana. In other Ayurvedic treatise and Nighantus, Amalaki fruit is described as stambhaka (astringent), sheeta (coolant), rochana (relish), (digestive), hridya (cardio tonic), bhedan (piercing), sara (laxative), vrishya (aphrodisiac), rasayana, chakshushya (tonic for eyes), kanthya (soothing to throat), keshya (hair tonic), tvachya (skin tonic), bhagna sandhankar (promoting union of fractured bones), dhatuvridhikar (strenthen the tissues), kantikar (imparting lusture to the skin), raktastambhaka (haemostatic), and vranaropaka (wound healer). The roots, bark, and the ripe fruit are reported to be astringent, whereas the unripe fruit is coolant, diuretic, and laxative. Flowers are refrigerant and aperient.

- Doshakarma: Tridoshashamaka, especially Pittashamaka
- Dhatukarma: Rasayana, Sarvadhatuvardhaka
- Malakarma: Malashodhaka

Pharmacological Actions

It has been reported to have antipyretic, antimicrobial, analgesic, anti-inflammatory, antioxidant, antidiabetic, hepatoprotective, adaptogenic, antiulcerogenic, hypolipidemic, diuretic, cardioprotective, antitussive, antiproliferative, anticancerous, immune modulator, and neuroprotective effects (Gaire and Subedi 2015; Bhattacharya et al 1999).

Indications

Traditionally, its fruit is extensively used for the treatment of amlapitta (hyperacidity, peptic ulcer), daha (burning sensation), trishna (thirst), vaman (emesis), prasheetad (scurvy), prameha (diabetes), rakta pitta (hemorrhagic diseases), shrama (fatigue), adhyaman (flatulence), vibandh (constipation), vishtambha (blokage), shopha (inflammation), shosha (emaciation), pandu (anemia), medoroga (obesity), aruchi (distaste), kamala (jaundice), yakritvikara (hepatic disorders), kasa (cough), shwasa (asthma), mukhapaka (stomatitis), pradara (excessive discharge per vagina), akshishotha (inflammatory diseases of eyes), dourbalya (general debility), jwara (fever), kshay (emaciation), udarshool (colic abdominal pain), agnimandhya (decreased digestive fire), atisaar (diarrhea), kushtha (skin diseases), and in eliminating toxins from the body.

In addition, the pulp of the fruit is smeared on snake bite, scorpion sting, and head to alleviate headache and dizziness.

Therapeutic Uses

External Use

1. **Nasagatraktasrava** (epistaxis): Make a paste of fine Amalaki powder fried in ghrita with water or kanji or takra and apply it on the forehead daily. It will control nasal bleeding (VM. 9/30) (SG.3/11/61).
2. **Palitya** (graying of hair): Apply paste of Amalaki, Mandura, and Japa pushpa on hair before bath or, for a week, apply Triphala powder soaked in water overnight for promoting hair growth and preventing premature graying (V.M. 7/91). One can use Amalaki-rich oils and shampoos also.
3. **Vyanga** (freckles): Tender fruits of Amalaki are kept in gomutra for a week and then mixed with aja ksheer to make a paste. The paste is applied on the face to clear off vyanga (AS.U. 37/24).

Internal Use

1. **Rasayana** (rejuvenator): Daily intake of one teaspoonful of Amalaki churna processed 21 times with Amalaki juice twice a day with madhu and mishri increases longevity, imparts youthfulness, enhances immunity, strength, and vigor, improves eye sight, luster, and complexion, and promotes hair growth. Daily eating of one to two fresh Amalaki fruit or 10 to 20 mL fruit juice or Chyawanprasha also gives the same effect (C.S.Ci. 1/107).
2. **Raktapitta** (hemorrhagic diseases): Amalaki swaras or Amalaki churna with madhu and sharkara helps in controlling hemorrhage in Raktapitta (C.S.Ci. 4/57).
3. **Amlapitta** (acidity): Powder prepared from equal quantity of Amalaki, Shatavari, and Sharkara mixed with equal quantity of honey is given with milk or ghee for amlpitta. Around 3 g of Amla powder or 10 mL juice with coconut water twice daily also gives relief in acidity (B.S. Amalpitta Ci. 49).
4. **Prameha** (diabetes): After shodhana of body one should take juice of Amalaki mixed with Haridra and madhu twice daily to prevent and cure prameha (S.S.Ci. 11/8; VM 35/16). Vagbhatta also advocated the use of Nisha Amalaki in prameha (A.H.U. 40/48).

5. **Arsha** (piles): Drinking takra prepared in a vessel pasted with Amalaki churna is an effective remedy for arsha (S.S.Ci. 6/13).

6. **Hikka** (hic-cough): Intake of Amalaki and Kapitha swarasa mixed with Pippali churna and madhu gives relief in hikka (C.S.Ci. 21/132).

7. **Udavarta** (retention of feces, urine, and flatus): Consumption of Amalaki swarasa with water for 3 days gives relief in indigestion, flatulence, and constipation (S.S.U. 55/22).

8. **Raktaatisaar** (bleeding diarrhea): Intake of Amalaki patra swarasa with madhu, ghrita, and dugdha controls bleeding diarrhea (Sh. S.).

9. **Pandu** (anemia): Drinking Amalaki swarasa and Ikshu rasa with madhu daily cures Pandu roga or taking Amalaki powder daily with madhu is beneficial (S.S.U. 44/18, 27).

10. **Vatarakta** (gout): Purana ghrita prepared with Amalaki swarasa is used daily to cure vatarakta (S.S.Ci. 5/12).

11. **Mutrakrkricch** (dysuria): One should take Amalaki juice and Ikshu rasa mixed with madhu to get relief in hematuria and dysuria (B.P.Ci. 35/32).

12. **Hypercholestremia:** Grind dry Amalaki into a fine powder and mix it with sugar candy (mishri). Store this mixture in a glass bottle and take one teaspoonful of this mixture every day empty stomach. This will help maintain the cholesterol level.

13. **Prasheetad** (scurvy): Dry Amalaki powder mixed with an equal quantity of sugar taken in doses of one teaspoon thrice a day with milk provides enough vitamin C to beat scurvy (Singh et al 2011).

14. **Chardi** (vomiting): Intake of a drink prepared by mixing Amalaki fruit, Draksha, Sharkara, madhu four times with water alleviates chardi caused by tridosha (BS. Chardi Ci. /37; B.P.Ci. 17/20).

15. **Pradara** (menorrhagia): Amalaki beej kalka mixed with madhu, sharkara should be taken with water in shweta and rakta pradara. Amalaki churna or rasa can also be used with madhu in pradara (C.S.Ci. 30/117; B.P.Ci. 69/10).

16. **Somaroga** (excessive urination): Fully ripe Kadali, Amalaki swarasa mixed with madhu and sharkara gives relief in somaroga (G.N. 6/1/69).

Officinal Part Used

Fruit

Dose

Juice: 10 to 20 mL
Powder: 3 to 6 g

Formulations

Chyawanprasha, Amalkyadi churna, Dhatri loha, Triphla churna, and Brahma rasayana.

Toxicity/Adverse Effect

No major toxicity has been reported yet. Few phytosterol compounds have been reported to have cytotoxic effect in tumor and nontumor cell lines (Qi et al 2012).

Substitution and Adulteration

None.

Points to Ponder

- *Amalaki is considered as the best rasayana dravya (rejuvenator) and vayasthapana dravya (C.S.Su. 25/40). Thus, the first chapter of Charak chikitsa is named Abhyaamalaki rasayan pada.*
- *Amalaki and Haritaki have same properties but are opposite in virya (C.S.Ci. 1/1/36). Also, Amalaki is best for raktapitta, prameha, vrisya, and rasayan in comparison to Haritaki.*
- *Amalaki fruit is the richest source of vitamin C (200–900 mg per 100 g of edible portion).*

Suggested Readings

Alan O. Siddha medicinal herbs as cosmetic ingredients. SPC, 1994.

Bhattacharya A, Chatterjee A, Ghosal S, Bhattacharya SK. Antioxidant activity of active tannoid principles of *Emblica officinalis* (amla). Indian J Exp Biol 1999;37(7):676–680

Gaire BP, Subedi L. Phytochemistry, pharmacology and medicinal properties of *Phyllanthus emblica* Linn. Chin J Integr Med 2015;1–8

Habib-ur-Rehman, Yasin KA, Choudhary MA, et al. Studies on the chemical constituents of *Phyllanthus emblica Linn*. Nat Prod Res 2007;21(9):775–781

Jain SK, Akhurdiya DS. Anola potential fruit for processing. Delhi Garden Mega 2000;38:50–51

Jain SK, Khurdiya DS. Vitamin C enrichment of fruit juice based ready-to-serve beverages through blending of Indian gooseberry (*Emblica officinalis Gaertn.*) juice. Plant Foods Hum Nutr 2004; 59(2):63–66

Qi WY, Li Y, Hua L, Wang K, Gao K. Cytotoxicity and structure activity relationships of phytosterol from *Phyllanthus emblica*. Fitoterapia 2012;84 C:252–256

Sangeetha N, Mercy S, Kavitha M, Selvaraj D, Kumar RS, Ganesh D. Morphological variation in the Indian gooseberries (*Phyllanthus emblica* and *Phyllanthus indofischeri*) and the chloroplast trn L (UAA) intron as candidate gene for their identification. Plant Genet Resour 2010;8(3):191–197

Singh E, Sharma S, Pareek A, Dwivedi J, Yadav S, Sharma S. Phytochemistry, traditional uses and cancer chemopreventive activity of Amla (*Phyllanthus emblica*): the sustainer. J Appl Pharm Sci 2011;02(01):176–183

The Ayurvedic Pharmacopeia of India. Vol 1, Part I. New Delhi: Department of AYUSH, Ministry of Health and Family Welfare, Government of India; 1989:5–6

Xia Q, Xiao P, Wan L, Kong J. Ethnopharmacology of *Phyllanthus emblica* L. Chin J Chin Mater Med (Chin) 1997;22:515–518, 525,574

Zhang LZ, Zhao WH, Guo YJ, Tu GZ, Lin S, Xin LG. Studies on chemical constituents in fruits of Tibetan medicine *Phyllanthus emblica*. Zhongguo Zhongyao Zazhi 2003;28(10):940–943

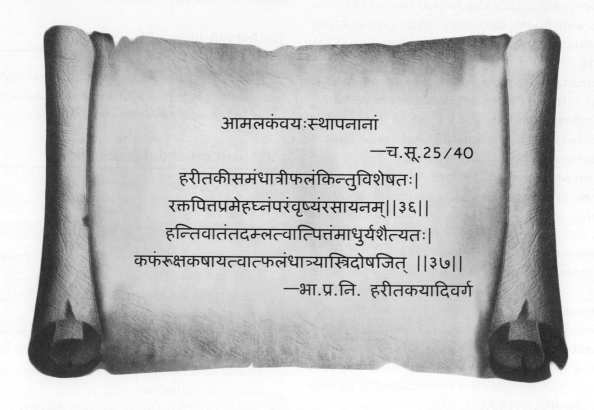

आमलकंवयःस्थापनानां

—च.सू.25/40

हरीतकीसमंधात्रीफलंकिन्तुविशेषतः|

रक्तपित्तप्रमेहघ्नंपरंवृष्यंरसायनम्||३६||

हन्तिवातंतदम्लत्वात्पित्तंमाधुर्यशैत्यतः|

कफंरूक्षकषायत्वात्फलंधात्र्यास्त्रिदोषजित् ||३७||

—भा.प्र.नि. हरीतकयादिवर्ग

5. Apamarga *[Achyranthes aspera Linn.]*

Family: *Amaranthaceae*

Hindi name: *Latjira, Chirchita*

English name: *Prickly chaff flower*

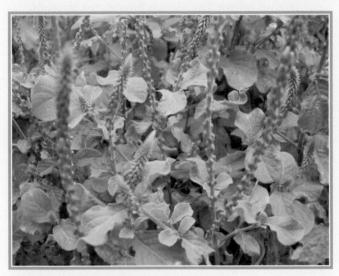

Plant of *Achyranthes aspera* Linn.

In navagraha vatika it should be planted in North direction as it represents the planet Mercury (Budha graha).

Introduction

The word "Apamarga" is derived from *Apamarjana* which means cleansing of all the body channels by expelling out the dosha and hence purifying the body.

Apamarga is a well-known medicinal plant in Ayurvedic, unani, siddha, allopathic, homeopathic, naturopathy, and home remedies (Dhale et al 2013). Charak considered Apamarga beej as the best drug for shirovirecana karma and named a chapter "Apamarga tanduliya" after it (C.S.S. 2/3). It is also stated in phalini dravya and is used as a food supplement in bhasmaka roga (C.S.S. 2/33). Sushrut used it for the treatment of nadivrana, arsha, and as an ingredient of panchgavya ghrita. Besides its medicinal uses, Apamarga roots are tied on the arms and abdomen in fever and to facilitate delivery. It is also used for punsavanasanskara (A.H.Sh. 1/39). Apamarga panchang is crushed and taken internally in pushya nakshatra for punsavana.

The plant is much popular among the masses not only for its therapeutic and nutritive value but also for its religious significance. In navagraha vatika it should be planted in the north direction as it represents the planet Mercury (Budha graha). Its roots are used for samidha in ritual ceremonies (yagna) to pacify the ill effects of Budha graha.

Vernacular Names

Bengali: Apang

Gujarati: Aghedo, Aghede, Angheda

Kannada: Uttarani, Utranigida

Malayalam: Kadaladi

Marathi: Aghada, Aghara

Punjabi: Chichra

Tamil: Nayuruvi, Chirukadaladi

Telugu: Uttareeni, Apamargamu

Urdu: Chirchita

Synonyms

Adhashalya: Its flowers are bent sharply outwards and downwards in an inflorescence.

Dugraha: Its spinous bracteoles and pointed perianth make it difficult to touch.

Kharmanjari: Its inflorescence is rough in touch.

Kinhi: Its touch may produce skin eruptions.

Ksharmadhya: The plant is alkaline in nature and hence a good source of alkali.

Marga: It cleanses the channels of the body.

Markati: The leaves have close apprised hairs beneath.

Mayuraka: The plant has antitoxin properties.

Pratyakpushpa: It has deflexed flowers.

Shavaka: It is used to induce sneezing.

Shikhari: Its flowers are borne at the top of branches (terminal inflorescence).

Classical Categorization

Charak Samhita: Krimighna, Vamanopaga, Shirovirechanopaga

Sushrut Samhita: Arkadi

Ashtang Hridaya: Arkadi

Dhanvantari Nighantu: Guduchyadi varga

Madanpal Nighantu: Abhyaadi varga

Kaiyadev Nighantu: Oushadi varga

Raj Nighantu: Shatavahadi varga

Bhavaprakash Nighantu: Guduchyadi varga

Distribution

The plant is well distributed in India, Sri Lanka, Baluchistan, tropical Asia, Africa, Australia, and America. It is found as wild growth/weed on the roadsides, open spaces, fields, and wastelands throughout India up to an altitude of 2,100 m (Anonymous 2005).

Morphology

It is an annual or perennial erect herb, 1 to 3 feet tall, often with a woody base. Branches are procumbent or erect, striated, pubescent, and stout at the nodes.

- **Leaves:** Simple, opposite, petiolated, lamina variable in shape and size. Shape is ovate-elliptic or obovate-rounded, and size ranges from 1 to 5 inches, apex acute (**Fig. 5.1**).
- **Flowers:** Terminal inflorescence of linear spikes 1 to 1.5 feet (**Fig. 5.2a**). Flowers are numerous, greenish or purple in color, closely deflexed, arranged on rachis, bract, and bracteoles spinescent and persistent (**Fig. 5.2b**).
- **Fruits:** Utricle, oblong, truncate at the apex, and enclosed in hardened perianth (**Fig. 5.3**).
- **Seeds:** Numerous, subcylindrical, rounded at the base, reddish-brown. The plant is propagated by seeds.

Phenology

Flowering time: More or less throughout the year
Fruiting time: More or less throughout the year

Key Characters for Identification

➤ An annual or perennial erect herb with a woody base
➤ Leaves: simple, opposite, and variable in shape and size
➤ Terminal spike inflorescence
➤ Flowers: greenish purple with deflexed arrangement, persistent bract
➤ Fruits: oblong, utricle, enclosed in a hard perianth, deflexedly arranged on pedicel

---

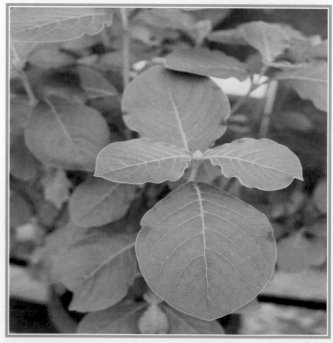

Fig. 5.1 Leaves.

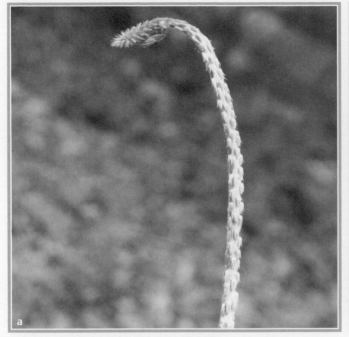

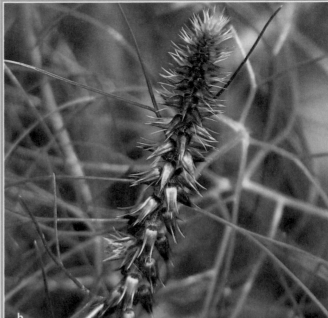

Fig. 5.2 **(a)** Inflorescence of linear spikes. **(b)** Flower.

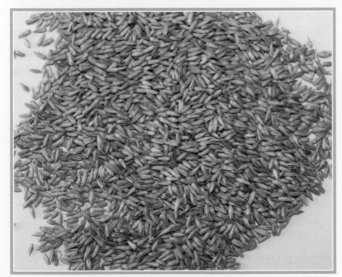

Fig. 5.3 Fruit.

Types

Kaiyadev Nighantu has described its three types:

1. Apamarga
2. Vashir
3. Ramatha (Jal Apamarga)

Bhavprakash Nighantu has described its two types:

1. Apamarga: *Achyranthes aspera* Linn.
2. Rakta Apamarga: *Achyranthes bidentata* Blume

Rasapanchaka

Guna	Laghu, Tikshna, Sar
Rasa	Tikta, Katu
Vipaka	Katu
Virya	Ushna

Chemical Constituents

Different parts of the plant have sterols, alkaloids, saponins, sapogenins, cardiac glycosides, etc. Achyranthine and betaine alkaloid are found in the whole plant; saponin A, B, C, D in seeds and fruits; hentriacontane in fruits; and ecdysone, ecdysterone, and glycosides in roots (Dey 2011).

Identity, Purity, and Strength

- Foreign matter: Not more than 2%
- Total Ash: Not more than 17%
- Acid-insoluble ash: Not more than 5%
- Alcohol-soluble extractive: Not less than 2%
- Water-soluble extractive: Not less than 12%

(Source: The Ayurvedic Pharmacopeia of India 1999).

Karma (Actions)

In Ayurvedic treatise and Nighantus, Apamarga is described as shirovirechana (purification procedures for head), deepan (carminative), pachana (digestive), rochana (relish), medohara (antiobesity), tikshan (stimulant), vamak (emetic), raktasangrahi (hemostatic), krimighna (anthelmintic), sansrana (laxative), chedana (penetrating effect), vatavardhak (vata aggravating), raktapitta (bleeding disorders). Its fruit is madhur in rasa and vipaka, guru (difficult to digest), vatavardhak (aggravate vata dosha), vistambhi (induces constipation), and cures raktapitta. Its root is used for nasya and vaman karma.

Kaiyadev Nighantu has described the properties of three types of Apamarga:

1. Apamarga: Katu, tikta rasa, tikshan, ushna, deepan, sar, pachana, vamak, chedana, medohara, and kaphavatashamaka.
2. Vashira: It is less potent than Apamarga, sheet in virya, visthambhi, and vatavardhak.
3. Ramatha (Jal Apamarga): Katu rasa, shothahara, and kaphavatashamak.
   - Doshakarma: Kaphavatahara
   - Dhatukarma: Rakta, Meda
   - Malakarma: Virechan

Pharmacological Actions

Roots and leaves of the plant are reported to exhibit thermogenic, spermicidal, antiparasitic, hypoglycemic, cancer chemoprotective, hepatoprotective, nephroprotective, antidepressant, expectorant, antiallergic, wound healing, anodyne, depurative, antihelmintic, diuretic, lithotriptic, sudorific, demulcent, hematinic, anti-inflammatory, antiarthritic, and antioxidant properties (Hasan 2014).

Indications

In classical Ayurveda texts whole plant of Apamarga, or its roots, seeds, and kshara, is traditionally used for the treatment of shirashool, arsha, krimi, dadru, kandu, udarshool, apachi, hridyaroga, adhyaman, medoroga, raktaatisaar, ashmari, and vrana. Seeds are used in bhasmakaroga.

The plant is very much popular in folklore and is used by traditional healers in the treatment of asthma, bleeding, facilitating delivery, boils, bronchitis, cold, cough, colic, debility, renal dropsy, dog bite, dysentery, ear diseases, headache, leucoderma, pneumonia, renal complications, scorpion bite, snake bite, and skin diseases (Jain 1991). The juice of the plant is used in ophthalmia and dysentery. The paste made from the roots with buttermilk is taken internally as an antifertility drug (Bhattacharjee and De 1991; Jain et al 2006).

Therapeutic Uses

External Use

1. **Sadhyavrana** (accidental wounds): The paste of Apamarga leaves is locally applied to stop bleeding in sadhyavrana (VM. 16/120; CD. 44/52).
2. **Vrana and Sadhyavrana** (wounds and accidental wounds): Paste prepared by mixing Apamarga, Ashwagandha, Talapatri, Suvarchala, and drugs of kakolyadigana is applied for vrana utsadana (wound elevation). For cleansing of chronic wounds, shodhana taila is prepared with Apamarga, Aragvadha, Nimb, Koshataki, Hartala, and Manahshila (S.S.Su. 37/17, 18, 30).
3. **Yoni shool** (vaginal pain): Application of the paste of roots of Apamarg and Punarnava reduces vaginal pain during puerperium (VM. 13/40).
4. **Shirashool** (headache): Massage the head with Apamarga phal siddha taila. It will remove all types of headache (GN. 3/1/125).

Internal Use

1. **Badhirya** (deafness and tinnitus): Administration of Apamarga kshara taila as ear drops twice daily gives relief in deafness (badhirya) and tinnitus (karnanaad) (VM. 59/24).
2. **Bhasmaka roga** (excessive hunger): Liquid gruel prepared with Apamarga beej, Dugdh, and Godha rasa alleviates excessive hunger (C.S.Su. 2/33).
3. **Arsh** (piles): Apamarga root powder mixed with Madhu and Tandulodaka (rice water) gives relief in arsha (S.S.Ci. 6/13). Apamarga kalka with takra is a good remedy for raktaarsha (SB 4/228). In Vaidyamanorama, decoction of

Apamarga, Nagakesara, Shatavari, and Vasa is given to cure bleeding piles (VM. 5/8).

4. **Visuchika** (cholera): Apamarga root with water is a good remedy for visuchika (B.P.Ci. 6/110).

5. **Sharkara and Ashmari** (urolithiasis): Kshara made by Tila, Apamarga, Kadali, Palasha, and Yava is taken with avi mutra (sheep urine) for the treatment of sharkara and ashmari (A.H.Ci. 11/31). Apamarga root powder taken with Aja dugdh increases urine output in dysuria (VD. 7/4).

6. **Netra roga** (eye diseases): Apamarga root rubbed in copper vessel with rock salt and curd is applied externally on inflammatory eyes diseases (G.N. 3/3/366).

7. **Kashtprasava** (difficult labor): Apamarga root is introduced and kept into vagina for easy induction of labor. Its root paste can also be applied on navel, pelvis, and vulva for the same (G.N. 6/4/23; BS. striroga Ci./233).

8. **Udarshool** (abdominal pain): Ghee cooked with decoction of Apamarga and Pippali paste alleviates abdominal pain (S.Y. ghrta/5).

9. **Kamala, Sotha, and Pandu** (jaundice, inflammations, and anemia): Paste of Apamarga root and Shami is administered with Takra for the treatment of pandu, shotha, and kamala (R.R.S. 19/109).

Officinal Parts Used

Whole plant, root, leaves, seeds

Dose

Juice: 10 to 20 mL
Root powder: 3 to 6 g
Seeds: 3 g
Kshara (alkali): 0.5 to 2 g

Formulations

Apamarga kshara taila, Kapha ketu rasa Apamargadi vati, Mahashankha vati, Agastya haritaki, Apamarga taila, Gulmakalanal rasa, Agnimukha rasa.

Toxicity/Adverse Effect

In high dose it may induce vomiting; otherwise no major side effect has been reported yet.

Substitution and Adulteration

Sometimes Apamarga roots are mixed with similar looking roots of other species of Achyranthes as adulterant.

> **Points to Ponder**
>
> - *Apamarga beej are the best dravya for shirovirechana karma.*
> - *It is extensively used in renal dropsy, skin diseases, asthma, diarrhea, for inducing abortion and facilitating delivery by ethnic people.*
> - *Apamarga is included in the group of ksharshatak and ksharashtaka (Raj Nighantu. mishrakvarga 51, 57).*

Suggested Readings

Anonymous. The Wealth of India-Raw Materials. New Delhi: Council of Scientific & Industrial Research; 2005:55–57

Bhattacharjee SK, De LC. Medicinal Herbs and Flowers. Jaipur: Awishkar Publishers and Distributers; 1991

Dey A. *Achyranthes aspera* L: phytochemical and pharmacological aspects. Int J Pharm Sci 2011;9(2):72–82

Dhale DA, Bhoi S. Pharmacognostic characterization and phytochemical screening of *Achyranthes aspera* Linn. Curr Agric Res J 2013;1(1): 51–57

Gupta AK, Tandon N. eds. Review of Indian Medicinal Plants. Vol. 1. New Delhi: Indian Council of Medical Research; 2004:140–164.

Hasan S. Pharmacological and medicinal uses of *Achyranthes aspera*. Int J Sci Environ Technol 2014;3(1):123–129

Jain JB, Kumane SC, Bhattacharya S. Medicinal flora of Madhya Pradesh and Chhattisgarh: a review. Ind J Trad Knowl 2006;5(2):237–242

Jain SK. Dictionary of Indian Folk Medicine and Ethnobotany. New Delhi: Deep Publications; 1991

The Ayurvedic Pharmacopeia of India. Vol. 2, Part I. New Delhi: Department of AYUSH, Ministry of Health and Family Welfare, Government of India; 1999:7–9

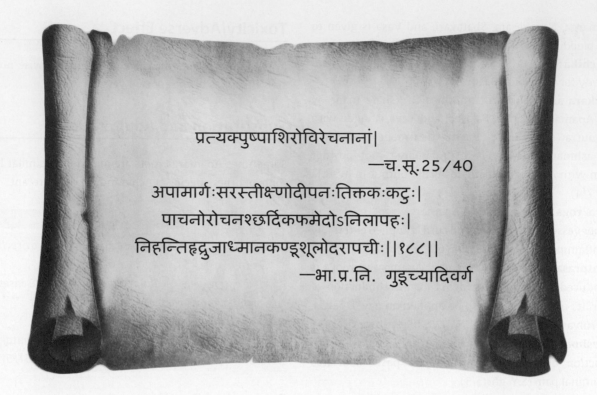

प्रत्यक्पुष्पाशिरोविरेचनानां|

—च.सू.25/40

अपामार्गःसरस्तीक्ष्णोदीपनःतिक्तकःकटुः|

पाचनोरोचनश्छर्दिकफमेदोऽनिलापहः|

निहन्तिहृद्रुजाध्मानकण्डूशूलोदरापचीः||१८८||

—भा.प्र.नि. गुड्ूच्यादिवर्ग

6. Aragvadha *[Cassia fistula Linn.]*

Family: *Fabaceae (Caesalpiniaceae)*

Hindi name: *Amaltas*

English name: *Purging cassia, Indian laburnum, Golden shower, Pudding pipe tree*

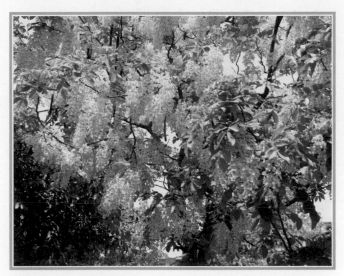

Plant of *Cassia fistula* Linn.

> *The Golden yellow flowers of Aragvadha is the state flower of Kerala and is Thailand's national symbol.*
> *—Royal Thai Government (2001)*

Introduction

The word "Aragvadha" means to kill or to pacify the diseased condition. The Latin name *Cassia* is derived from a Greek word *Kassia* which means fragrance or aroma and fistula means tube, pipe, or reed-like (Datiles and Acevedo-Rodríguez 2017; Orwa et al 2009).

In Vedic literature, its dried branches are used for ritual purposes. The flowers are offered to the lord during the Vishu festival in Kerala.

Aragvadha is a medicinal plant of immense importance. Since ancient times, it has been used in different traditional systems of medicines for treating gastrointestinal disorders, intermittent fever, skin diseases, rheumatism, etc. It is considered as the best drug among mild purgatives and is good for children, elderly, wounded, emaciated, and sensitive people (C.S.Ka.8/5). Charaka named a chapter in its name and considers it as best Kusthaharadravya for external application (C.S.Su. 3/3 & 30). Charaka also included it in phalini dravya (C.S.Su. 1/83). Sushrut uses it as shodhana dravya for vaman, virechan, and basti karma.

Besides its ethnomedicinal use, the wood of the tree is used for fuel, fodder, and timber. The bark yields tannins and dyes. The flowers yield nectar. In folklore, people eat its flowers and unripe pod as a nutritive food. The plant extract is also recommended as a pest and disease control agent (Raja et al 2000).

Vernacular Names

Arabic: Khayarsambhar

Assamese: Sonaroo

Bengali: Bundaralathi, Sondala, Soondali, Sonalu

Gujarati: Garamala, Garamalo

Kannada: Aragvadha, Kakke, Kakke-gida, Kakkernara, Kakkedai, Rajataru

Kashmiri: Kriyangal Phali

Malayalam: Konna, Kritamalam

Marathi: Bahava, Garamala, Amaltas

Oriya: Sunari

Punjabi: Amaltas, Girdnalee

Spanish: Bâtoncasse, Cassedoux, Casseespagnol

Tamil: Sarakonrai, Konnai, Sarakkondi, Sharakkonrai

Telugu: Rela, Kondrakayi, Raelachettu

Thai: Canâfîstulamansa, Chácara, Guaya bacimarrona

Trade name: Indian laburnum

Urdu: Khiyar Shambar

Spanish: canafistola (Honduras), canafistula, canafistula mansa, canapistola, chácara, chorizo, cigarro, guayaba cimarrona

French: baton casse, canéficier, casse doux, casse espagnole, casse fistuleuse, cassie fistuleuse, cassier commun, cytise Indien, douche d'or

Chinese: la chang shu

Bangladesh: bandarlathi, desi asal, shonalu, shondal, sonali, suvarnaka

Bolivia: lluvia de oro

Cuba: cana fistula, cana fistula cimarrona, canafistola, canafistola cimarrona, canafistola exotica, canandonga

Dominican Republic: canafistol, canafistula de purgante, canafistula mansa, canafistula purgante, chácara, guayaba cimarrona

Germany: Fistul-kassie, Kassie, Röhren-, Mannabaum, Indischer, Rohrenkassie

Haiti: baton casse, casse, casse espagnole

Synonyms

Aamha: The fruit pulp is used to pacify Aam.

Arevata: It is a mild and safe purgative.

Arogyasimbhi: Its pods are used to attain a disease-free state.

Chaturangula: Inside the pod the marrow is demarcated at every four-finger distance.

Deerghaphala: The plant has long stick-like fruits.

Jwarantaka: It has antipyretic properties.

Kritamala: Its flowers are arranged on the inflorescence like a garland.

Kusthasudana: It is used to alleviate kushta.

Rajavriksha: It is considered as king of trees because of its beautiful flowers.

Shampaka: After consuming it, dosha pachana occurs properly.

Survarnaka: The plant bears beautiful yellowish golden-colored flowers.

Swarnabhushana: It bears beautiful golden yellow-colored flowers.

Vyadhighata: It is used to alleviate many diseases.

Classical Categorization

Charak Samhita: Kushtaghna, Kandughna, Tiktaskanda, Virechana

Sushrut Samhita: Aragvadhadi, Shyamadi, Adhobhagahara, Shleshmsansamana

Ashtang Hridaya: Aragvadhadi, Shyamadi

Dhanvantari Nighantu: Guduchyadi varga

Madanpal Nighantu: Abhyaadi varga

Kaiyadev Nighantu: Oushadi varga

Raj Nighantu: Prabhadradi varga

Bhavaprakash Nighantu: Haritakyadi varga

Distribution

Cassia fistula L. is a native plant of tropical Asia and is widely cultivated in Africa, South America, China, West Indies, Brazil, etc. Found throughout India in deciduous forests and sub-Himalayan tracts ascending up to an altitude of 1,220 m. Also cultivated in the gardens and avenues for its beautiful yellow flowers (Bhalerao and Kelkar 2012).

Morphology

A medium-sized deciduous tree, 25 to 35 ft in height with straight trunk. Branches are slender and spreading.

- **Leaves:** Pinnately compound leaves, alternate, paripinnate, leaflets four to eight pairs, ovate-oblong in shape, acute apex, bright green (**Fig. 6.1a**), glabrous above, pale beneath, and silvery pubescent beneath when young (**Fig. 6.1b**).
- **Flowers:** Bright yellow in axillary pendulous racemes 30 to 50 cm long, slender, pubescent, and glabrous (**Fig. 6.2a**). Five yellow petals, five sepals, green, the individual flower stalks 3 to 6 cm long. Stamens are 10 and all antheriferous (**Fig. 6.2b**).
- **Pods:** Cylindrical, pendulous, smooth, shining, indehiscent, initially green later turns to dark brown or black, 40 to 60 cm long (**Fig. 6.3a, b**). Internally

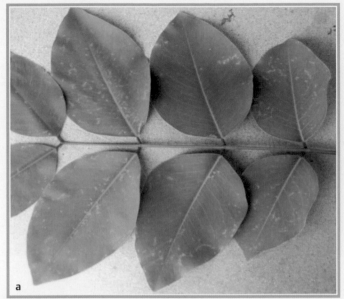
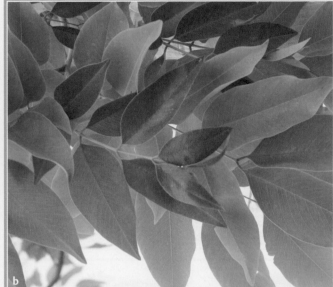

Fig. 6.1 **(a)** Leaves. **(b)** Tender leaves.

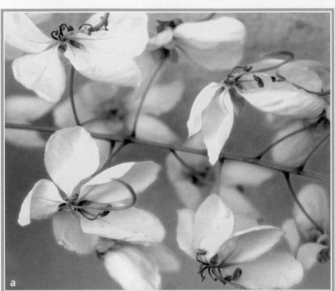
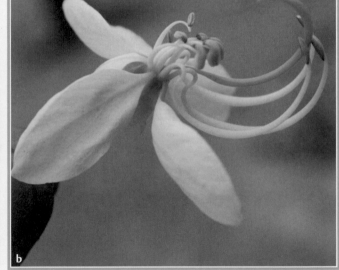

Fig. 6.2 **(a)** Inflorescences. **(b)** Flower.

divided by thin, buff-colored, transverse dissepiments at intervals of about 0.5 cm. Each compartment contains one seed which is immersed in dark-colored sweetish pulp (**Fig. 6.3c**).

- **Seeds:** Biconcave, broadly ovate, light to dark or reddish-brown, with a well-marked raphe (**Fig. 6.4**).
- **Stems bark:** Smooth, 3 to 6 mm thick, externally cream yellow to gray, slightly greenish beneath with lenticular horizontal markings and brownish dots over surface. Externally, bark is rough, dark brown

when old, and internally pale reddish-brown. Fracture fibrous, striations vertical (**Fig. 6.5**).

- **Roots:** Roots are reddish-brown and rough externally with numerous horizontal lenticels (Sharma et al 2001). The plant is propagated by seeds and stump planting.

Phenology

Flowering time: March to June

Fruiting time: November to March

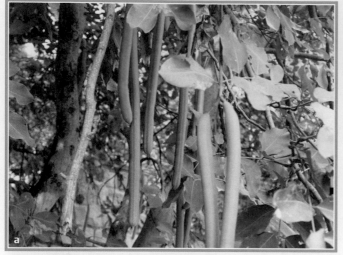

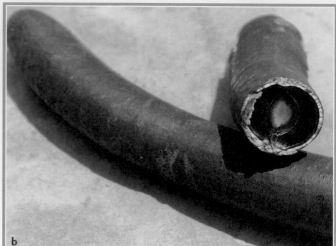

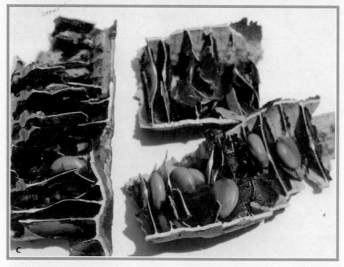

Fig. 6.3 **(a)** Fresh fruits. **(b)** Mature fruits. **(c)** Pulp.

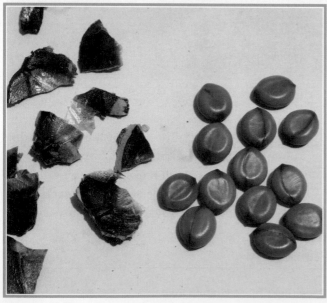

Fig. 6.4 Seeds.

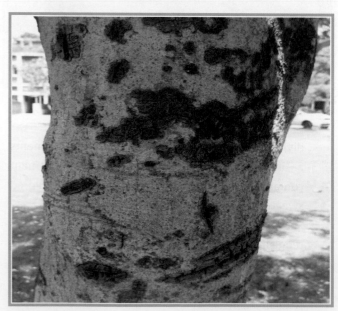

Fig 6.5 Stem bark

Key Characters for Identification

➤ *A medium-sized deciduous tree. Bark cream-yellow externally and reddish-brown internally.*

➤ *Leaves: alternate, pinnate compound, leaflets four to eight pairs, ovate-oblong shape*

➤ *Flowers: bright yellow in axillary pendulous racemes*

➤ *Pods: cylindrical, pendulous, smooth, green to dark brown, black*

Rasapanchaka

Guna	Guru, Mridu, Snigdha
Rasa	Madhura
Vipaka	Madhura
Virya	Sheeta

Chemical Constituents

The plant is rich in phenolic antioxidants, anthraquinones, flavonoids, flavan-3-ol-derivative, alkaloids, terpenoids, saponins, reducing sugar, tannins, and steroids (Ching Kuo et al 2001). The root bark contains tannin, phlobaphenes, oxyanthraquinone, hydroxy methyl anthraquinone, emodin, chrysophanic acid, fistuacacidin, barbaloin, and rhein. Stem bark contains flavnol glycosides, xanthone glycosides, lupeol, beta-sitosterol, and hexacosanol. Flowers contain ceryl alcohol, kaempferol, rhein, and a bianthroquinone glycoside. Leaves contain rhein, rhein glucoside, proteins, and sennosides A and B. The seeds contain anthraquinones, proteins, fat, carbohydrate, and fibers. The fruit pulp contains anthraquinone rhein in free as well as in the form of glycoside. The edible part of the fruit is rich in potassium, calcium, iron and manganese, protein (19.94%), and carbohydrate (26.30%), making it an important source of nutrients and energy (Raghunathan and Mitra 2005; Theeshan et al 2005).

Identity, Purity, and Strength

- Foreign matter: Not more than 2%
- Total ash: Not more than 6%
- Acid-insoluble ash: Not more than 1 %
- Alcohol-soluble extractive: Not less than 15%
- Water-soluble extractive: Not less than 46%

(Source: The Ayurvedic Pharmacopeia of India 1989)

Karma (Actions)

In Ayurvedic lexicon and Nighantus, Aragvadha is described as the best mrudu virechak dravya (laxative drug). Its fruit pulp is sansaran (laxative), rochak (relish), snigdh (unctuousness), and agnivardhak (appetizer), jwaraghna (antipyretics), krimighna (anthelmintic), kushtaghna (antidermatosis), and vranashodhak (wound cleansing) in properties. Its leaves are kapha medovishoshan (dry/absorp kapha and fat), and flowers are madhur (sweet), sheet (cold), kashaya (astringent), tikta (bitter), and grahi (faecal astringent). Fruits are madhur, balya (tonics), and vatapittashamaka (pacify vatapittadosha). Aragvadha phal majja is considered always as a pathya dravya in jwara and is best in purifying/clearing the kostha.

- Doshakarma: Vatapittashamaka, Kaphapittasanshodhaka
- Dhatukarma: Shrotoshodhaka
- Malakarma: Malashodhaka

Besides these properties, the root and stem bark is anthelmintic, purgative, febrifuge, diuretic, depurative, anti-inflammatory, and tonic. The flowers are reported to have demulcent and lubricating effects. The fruit pulp is sweet, cooling with pleasant taste, mild laxative, blood purifier, emollient, anodyne, diuretic, antibacterial, anti-inflammatory, and antipyretic (Ali 2014). Seeds are emetic, cathartic, laxative, carminative, and antipyretic (Markouk et al 2000).

Pharmacological Actions

The plant possesses antibacterial, antidiabetic, antifertility, anti-inflammatory, antioxidant, hepatoprotective, purgative, antitumor, antifungal, antitussive, wound-healing, antitubercular, analgesic, antipyretic, cathartic, antileishmaniatic, hypolipidemic, anti-itching, and antiulcer activities (Ali 2014).

Indications

In Ayurveda classics, the fruit pulp is used in the treatment of gulma (abdominal lump), jwar (fever), udararoga (abdominal diseases), grahani (sprue), krimi (worm infestation), kushta (skin disease), visarpa (erysepalas), prameha (diabetes), shool (colic pain), udavarta (retension of faeces, urine and flatus), hridayaroga (heart disease), vrana (wound), vatavyadhi (neuromuscular disease), mutrakricchta (dysuria), raktapitta (hemorrhage), pandu (anemia), kasa (cough), apasmar (epilepsy) urustambh (stiffness thigh), and visha (poisoning). Its roots are given in vatarakta (gout) and skin diseases like dadru (ring worm), mandal (a skin lesion with circular whitish red elevations).

In other traditional system of medicines like Siddha, Unani, and folklore, the leaves are used in erysipelas, malaria, rheumatism, and ulcers. Paste of leaves mixed with coconut oil is applied over the skin in burn (Patil and Patil 2012). The roots are used for curing adenopathy, intermittent fever especially for black water fever, burning sensations, hemorrhages, wounds, ulcers, heart diseases, urinary tract infections, leprosy, skin diseases, syphilis, and tubercular glands. The powder or decoction of the stem bark is administered in leprosy, jaundice, syphilis, and heart diseases (van Wyk and Wink 2009). The leaves are used externally as emollient; poultice and leaf juice is used for chilblains, skin eruptions, ring worms, eczema, in insect bites, swelling, rheumatism, and facial paralysis (The Ayurvedic Pharmacopoeia of India 1989; Nadkarni 2009). The fruit and fruit pulp is used in cardiac conditions, constipation, fever, flatulence, anorexia, jaundice, abdominal pain, joint pain, arthritis, pruritus, leprosy, eczema, and allied skin infection. Flowers are used in fever, skin diseases, pruritus, burning sensation, dry cough, and bronchitis. The buds are used for biliousness, constipation, fever, leprosy, and skin disease. Ashes from burnt pods mixed with little salt are used with honey which can be taken three to four times to relieve cough. Seed powder is used in amoebiasis, jaundice, biliousness, skin disease, and in swollen throat (Danish et al 2011). In Brazilian herbal medicine, the seeds are used as a laxative and the leaves and/or stem bark are used for pain and inflammation.

Therapeutic Uses

External Use

1. **Dadru, Kitibha** (skin diseases): Young leaves of Aragvadha pounded with Kanji is applied externally in dadru, kitibha Sidhma (VM. 49/9), (BS.kustha Ci. 63).

2. **Vranaprakashalana** (wound washing): Washing the wounds with Aragvadha leaves decoction is beneficial in healing (S.S.Ci. 19/39).

3. **Gandamala** (cervical adenitis): Aragvadhamool rubbed in Tandulodaka is used as nasya or lepa to get relief in gandmala (VM. 41/23).

4. **Updansha** (venereal disease): Decoction prepared with leaves of Karavira, Jati, Aragvadha, Tarkari, and Arka is used for washing the area (S.S.Ci. 19/39), or Aragvadhamool kalka with water can also be applied on the affected area (GN. 44/8/21)

Internal Use

1. **Twakroga** (skin diseases): Leaves of Aragvadha, Kakamachi, and Karanja are pounded with takra and is applied as ointment, after smearing affected part with oil in many skin diseases (C.S.Su. 3/17). Person suffering from skin diseases should use decoction of Aragvadha panchang daily for bathing, washing, and oral consumption (C.S.Ci. 7/97-98).

2. **Kushta** (leprosy/skin disease): Ghee prepared from Aragvadha mool is taken with Khadirsaar decoction twice daily in skin diseases (A.H.Ci. 19/13).

3. **Jwar** (fever): Person suffering from fever can take powdered Aragvadha phal majja with Draksha rasa or godugdh (C.S.Ci. 3/232). An alcoholic extract of the plant is also used to fight the black water fever.

4. **Haridrameha** (type of diabetes): Daily intake of Aragvadha decoction is useful in treating haridrameha (S.S.Ci. 11/09).

5. **Aamvata** (arthritis): One should eat Aragvadha leaves shaka fried in mustard oil to get relief in aamvata (BP. Ci. 26/52).

6. **Kamala** (jaundice): One should take daily Aragvadha, Ikshu rasa, Vidari, Amalaki with Trikatu to alleviate kamala.

7. **Pittoudara** (abdominal disease due hepatic cause): Milk processed with Aragvadha or Trivrit or errand is used as purgative in udarroga caused by pitta dosha (C.S.Ci. 13/70).

8. **Urustambha** (stiffness of thigh): One should consume vegetables cooked with tender leaves of Sunisanaka, Nimb, Arka, Vetasa, Aragvadha, water, and oil without salt in urustambha (C.S.Ci. 27/26).

Officinal Parts Used

Root, leaves, flowers, fruit pulp

Dose

Fruit pulp: 5 to 10 g (purgation dose 10 to 20 g)
Root bark decoction: 50 to 100 mL
Flowers: 5 to 10 g

Formulations

Araghvadharishta, Amaltas gulkand, Kushtarakshas taila, Aragvadhadi kwath, Araghvadhadi taila, Maharasnadi kashaya.

Toxicity/Adverse Effects

No major toxicity is reported. However, in large doses, the leaves and bark can cause vomiting, nausea, abdominal pain, and cramps (Ali 2014).

Substitution and Adulteration

Pods of *Cassia grandis* L. are used as substitute of Aragvadha pods (Sharma et al 2001).

Points to Ponder

- *Aragvadh phal majja is the best mrudu virechak dravya or sransan karma.*
- *For inducing virechana, it is the safest drug for children, old, wounded, emaciated, and sensitive people.*

Suggested Readings

Ali A. *Cassia fistula* linn: a review of phytochemical and pharmacological studies. Int J Pharm Sci Res. 2014;5(6):2125–2130

Bahorun T, Neergheen VS and Aruoma OI. Phytochemical constituents of *Cassia fistula* L. Afr J Biotechnol. 2005;4(13):1530–1540

Bhalerao SA and Kelkar TS. Traditional medicinal uses, phytochemical profile and pharmacological activities of *Cassia fistula* L. Int Res J Biol Sci. 2012;1(5):79–84

Ching Kuo L, Ping Hung L, et al. The chemical constituents from the aril *Cassia fistula* Linn. J Chin Chem Soc. 2001;48:1053–1058

Danish M, Singh P, Mishra G, Srivastava S, Jha KK, Khosa RL. *Cassia fistula* Linn. (Amulthus): an important medicinal plant: a review of its traditional uses, phytochemistry and pharmacological properties. J Nat Prod Plant Resour. 2011;1(1):101–118

Datiles MJ and Acevedo-Rodríguez, P. *Cassia fistula* (Indian laburnum): invasive species compendium. CABI, United Nations. 2017

Markouk M, Bekkouche K, Larhsini M, Bousaid M, Lazrek HB and Jana M. Evaluation of some Moroccan medicinal plant extracts for larvicidal activity. J Ethanopharmacol. 2000;73:293–297

Nadkarni KM. Indian Materia Medica, Vol. 1. Bombay: Bombay Popular Prakashan. 2009:285–286

Orwa C, Mutua A, Kindt R, Jamnadass R, Anthony S. Agroforestree database: a tree reference and selection guide, version 4.0. Kenya: World Agroforestry Centre. 2009

Patil SJ and Patil HM. Ethnomedicinal herbal recopies from Satpura hill ranges of Shirpur Tahsil, Dhule, Maharashtra, India. Res J Recent Sci. 2012;1:333–336

Raghunathan K and Mitra R. Pharmacognosy of indigenous drugs, Vol. 1, 2nd reprint. New Delhi: Central Council for Research in Ayurveda and Siddha. 2005:22–30

Raja N, Albert S, Ignacimuthu S. Effect of solvent residues of *Vitex negundo* Linn. and *Cassia fistula* Linn. on pulse beetle, *Callosobruchus maculates* Fab. and its larval parasitoid, *Dinarmusvagabundus* (Timberlake). Indian J Exp Bot. 2000;38:290–292

Royal Thai Government. ประกาศสำนักนายกรัฐมนตรีเรื่องการกำหนดสัญลักษณ์ประจำชาติ ไทย. Royal Thai Government Gazette. 2001;99D:1

Sharma PC, Yelne MB, Dennis TJ. Database of medicinal plants used in Ayurveda. New Delhi: Central Council of Research in Ayurveda and Siddha, Vol 2. 2001:30

The Ayurvedic Pharmacopeia of India, Part I, Vol. 1. New Delhi: Department of AYUSH, Ministry of Health and Family Welfare, Government of India; 1989:9–10

van Wyk B-E, Wink M. Medicinal plants of the world. Pretoria, South Africa: Briza Publications; 2009:403

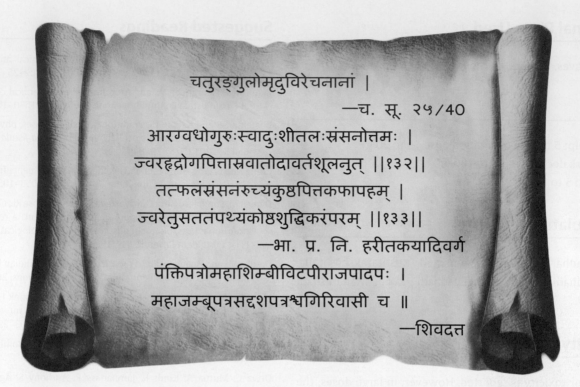

चतुरङ्गुलोमृदुविरेचनानां |

—च. सू. २५/40

आरग्वधोगुरुःस्वादुःशीतलःसंसनोत्तमः |

ज्वरहृद्रोगपित्तासवातोदावर्तशूलनुत् ||१३२||

तत्फलंसंसनंरुच्यंकुष्ठपित्तकफापहम् |

ज्वरेतुसततंपथ्यंकोष्ठशुद्धिकरंपरम् ||१३३||

—भा. प्र. नि. हरीतकयादिवर्ग

पंक्तिपत्रोमहाशिम्बीविटपीराजपादपः |

महाजम्बूपत्रसद्दशपत्रश्चगिरिवासी च ॥

—शिवदत्त

7. Adraka/Shunthi [*Zingiber officinale* Rosc.]

Family:	*Scitamineae*
Hindi name:	*Adrak/Sonth*
English name:	*Ginger*

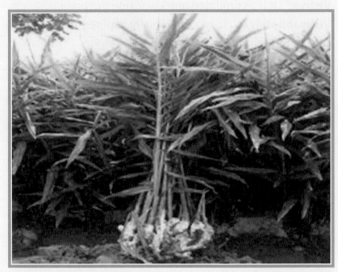

Plant of *Zingiber officinale* Rosc.

Consuming Adraka paste daily with salt before meal on daily basis is always beneficial as it stimulates the digestive fire, increases appetite, and purifies tongue and throat.

Introduction

The word "Adraka" literally means *Aadryati jihva*, i.e., which keeps the tongue moistened by increasing salivation in mouth. Shunthi or Sonth, the dried form of Adraka, dries up the water content of kapha and checks its flow. The Latin name *Zingiber officinale* was given by an English botanist William Roscoe in 1807. The word "Zingiber" is derived from a Sanskrit word *shrungver* denoting "horn-shaped," in reference to the protrusions on the rhizome (Amiril 2006; Awang 1992).

Since ancient times, ginger has been used both as a food and a medicine. The Greek physician, Dioscorides, enlisted ginger as a digestive and an antidote to poisoning. Ginger is mentioned in the Al Qur'an, the Talmud, and the Bible. Records suggest that during the 13th and 14th centuries, ginger became one of the highly valued, traded spices (Abubackar 2011). Ginger was exported from India to the Roman Empire some 2,000 years ago and Arab merchants controlled the ginger trade. Ancient historians equate the ownership of ginger or its trade routes with prosperity in 5,000 BC. Ginger along with cinnamon, galangal, and pepper is buried with the dead in the graves. In 200 AD, ginger became a taxed commodity in Rome, and was first listed as medicine in China.

Both Adraka and Shunthi are indeed very famous medicines in Ayurvedic system for centuries (Grzanna et al 2005). Charak described Shrungvera kanda (tuber of ginger) as the best kanda (tuber) in naturally beneficial food substances (C.S. Su. 25/38). Adraka (fresh ginger) is mentioned in harit varga and the Shunthi (dried ginger) is placed in ahaaryogi varga (C.S.Su. 27/166, 296). Both Adraka and Shrungvera are mentioned in katu skanda (C.S.Vi. 8/142) and Adraka paste is used as a pathya drug in madatyaya due to vata dosha (C.S.Ci. 24/126, 127). In Sushruta Samhita, Adraka and Shunthi are described in shakavarga (S.S.Su. 46/226, 227) and are used in the treatment of udarroga, netrapaka, karnashool, pratishyaya, gulma, madatayaya, and udavrata. In Astanga Hridya, the properties of Shunthi and

Adraka are described in Aushadi varga (A.H.Su. 6/163, 164). Vagbhatta uses Adraka and Shunthi in treating a wide range of ailments like kasa, atisaar, arsha, sotha, pandu, grahni, gulma udarroga, madatyaya, vatavyadhi, granthi, arbuda, shlipada netra, and karna roga. Shunthi is a major content in the group of Trikatu, Chaturushan, Panchkola, Shadushna, Trikarshik, and Chatubhadra (B.P. mishraka varga).

Ginger with its high nutritional value and pungent aroma is used in soft drink manufacturing industry, baking industry, and meat processing industry. Ginger brine is most popular in Japan (Jiang et al 2005). Ginger oil is used as a flavorant in food processing, pharmaceuticals, and also in perfumery. Ginger is extensively used in culinary/kitchen worldwide as a spice in food; in preparing meat; in ginger garlic paste, ginger tea, ginger coffee, and ginger breads; for making cakes, cookies, candies, and syrups; and in refreshing beverages like ginger beer, ginger lemon, ginger honey, and ginger wine (Bag 2018). Hence, it is rightly known as "The Great Medicament" because of its multiple medicinal, ethnomedicinal, and nutritional health benefits.

Vernacular Names

Assamese: Adasuth, Aadar shunth
Bengali: Suntha, Shunthi, Ada
Gujarati: Sunth, Sundh, Suntha
Kannada: Shunthi
Kashmiri: Shonth
Malayalam: Chukku
Marathi: Sunth
Oriya: Shunthi
Punjabi: Sund
Tamil: Sukku, Chukku
Telugu: Sonthi, Sunti
Urdu: Sonth, Zanjabeel
Arab: Zanjibile-yabis
Chinese: Chiang P'i, Kan Chiang, Kiang, Sheng chiang
Japanese: Shokyo
Persian: Zanjabile-khashk
Sinhalese: Velicha-nguru

Synonyms

Avakchatra: Lower leaves of this plant are umbrella shaped.
Kaphaari: It subsides kapha dosha.

Katu: It has pungent taste.
Katubhadra: It is best among pungent drugs.
Katugranthi: Its rhizome is nodular and pungent in taste.
Mahaoushad and Naagar: It is a highly potent and efficacious drug.
Shringaver: Nodular tuberous rhizome of this plant has many germinating buds.
Shoshana: It absorbs watery content.
Ushana: Its rhizome is hot in potency/properties.
Utkata: It has tikshna (sharp) properties.
Vishva: It is assimilated quickly inside the body.
Vishvabhesajya: It is a universally reputed drug used to cure numerous diseases.

Classical Categorization

Charak Samhita: Deepaniya, triptighna, arshoghna, shoolaprasasmana, trishnanigrahan
Sushrut Samhita: Pippalyadi, trikatu
Ashtanga Hridaya: Pippalyadi
Dhanvantari Nighantu: Shatapushpadi varga
Madanpal Nighantu: Shunthyadi varga
Kaiyadev Nighantu: Oushadhi varga
Raj Nighantu: Pippalyadi varga
Bhavaprakash: Haritakyadi varga

Preparation of Shunthi

Soak the fully matured ginger rhizome in water and leave it overnight. Next morning peel off the scaly epidermis with pointed-end bamboo splinters and keep it in sunlight for drying for 8 to 10 days. Soak the dried rhizomes again in a slurry of slaked lime (1 kg of slaked lime in 120 kg of water) for 6 hours followed by sun drying. The process is repeated until the rhizome becomes uniformly white. Finally, dried rhizome has up to 8% to 10% moisture (it should not exceed 12%).

The fully dried rhizomes are stored in air tight containers for future use (Bag 2018).

Distribution

Ginger is indigenous to southern China, from where it spread to the Spice Islands and other parts of Southeast Asia, and subsequently to West Africa and to the Caribbean (Spices: Exotic Flavors & Medicines 2014). Now it is commercially cultivated in nearly every tropical and subtropical country of the world.

In India, it is mainly cultivated in Kerala, Odisha, Karnataka, Andhra Pradesh, Arunachal Pradesh, Sikkim, Uttar Pradesh, West Bengal, and Maharashtra (Khare 2007). India is the largest producer and consumer of ginger, contributing to about 31% of total global production followed by China, Nepal, Indonesia, Nigeria, and Thailand.

Morphology

An aromatic herb with an underground creeping rhizome and erect stem, up to 1 to 1.5 ft in height.

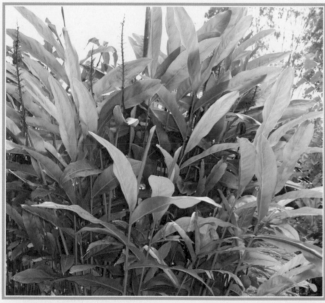

Fig. 7.1 Leaves.

- **Leaves:** Simple, alternate, narrow lanceolate, linear-lanceolate, up to 15 to 30 cm long, acuminate apex, sheathing at the base, and glabrous (**Fig. 7.1**).
- **Flowers:** Inflorescence on a distinct scape, flowers densely arranged in spike, white color flowers with purple streaks, bisexual, irregular, each subtended by a persistent scarious bract. Calyx tubular, shortly three-lobed; corolla bilabiate, tubular below, yellow with purplish spots; stamens three in one whorl, one of which is perfect and the other two unite to form a labellum; filament of perfect stamen short; anther cells contiguous, connective produced into a beak, ovary of three carpels, syncarpous, three-celled, inferior; many ovules on axile placentae, style filiform, lying in a groove of the anther, stigma subglobose (**Fig. 7.2a, b**).
- **Fruit:** Oblong capsule, many seeded, globose shape.
- **Rhizome:** Aromatic, irregular shaped, thick, fibrous, pungent in taste, whitish or buff colored with many nodes and internodes. Externally covered with a papery light brown covering, internally white or cream in color. The odor and taste are characteristic, aromatic, and pungent (**Fig. 7.3a–c**; Kritikar and Basu 2007; Ross 2005).

The plant is propagated through rhizome.

Phenology

Flowering time: September to October

Fruiting time: October to November

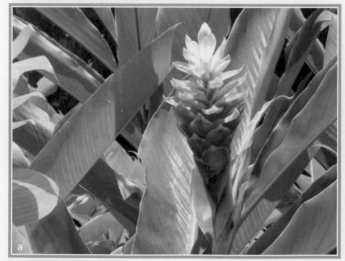

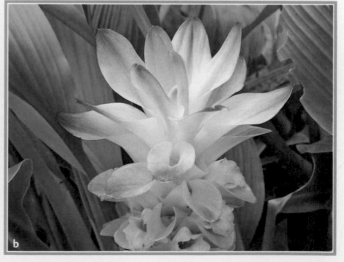

Fig. 7.2 (a, b) Flower.

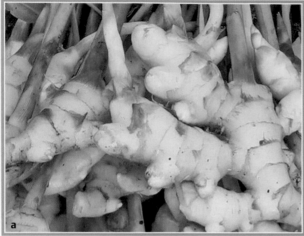
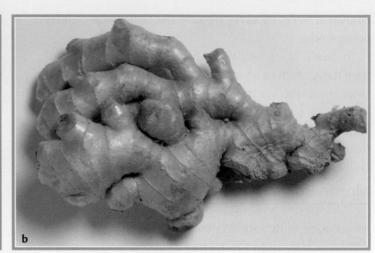
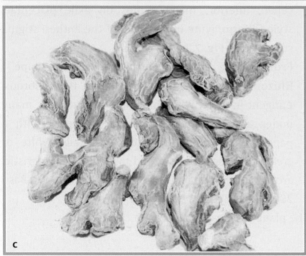

Fig. 7.3 **(a, b)** Fresh ginger. **(c)** Dried ginger.

Key Characters for Identification

➤ An aromatic herb with reduced stem and creeping rhizome
➤ Leaves: simple, glabrous linear-lanceolate, sheathing at the base
➤ Flowers: bisexual, white color with purple streaks in radical spikes
➤ Rhizome: horizontal, buff colored, laterally flat with many sympodial branches, aromatic and pungent

Types

On the basis of trade, different types of Indian ginger are available in the market like Cochin ginger (light brown or yellowish grey), Calicut ginger from Malabar (orange or reddish brown, resembling African ginger), and Kolkata ginger (grayish-brown to grayish-blue; Khare 2007).

Rasapanchaka

Rasapanchaka	Adraka (wet form)	Shunthi (dried form)
Guna	Guru, Ruksha, Tikshan	Laghu, Snigdh
Rasa	Katu	Katu
Vipaka	Katu	Madhur
Virya	Ushna	Ushna
Doshaghanta	Kapha vata hara Pittavardhak	Kapha vata hara Pittashamaka

Chemical Constituents

The fresh and dried rhizome of ginger have been reported to possess gingerols (responsible for pungency of ginger), zingibain (proteolytic enzyme), bisabolene, oleoresins, fibers, starch, volatile oil, essential oil, mucilage, magnesium, calcium, potassium, sulfur, vitamin A, B, and C, protein, diterpenes, and gingerglycolipids A, B, and C (Anonymous 1999). The volatile oil mainly consists of mono and sesquiterpenes; predominantly zingeberene (35%), camphene, β-phellandrene, cineole, curcumene (18%), and farnesene (10%), and geranyl acetate, terphineol, terpenes, borneol, geraniol, limonene, linalool, α-zingiberene (30–70%), β-sesquiphellandrene (15–20%), β-bisabolene (10–15%), and α-farmesene. Oleoresins namely gingerol, shogaol, zingerone, paradols, and zingiberol are present. Essential oil contains mainly zingiberene; smaller amounts of β-sesquiphellandrene, bisabolene, and farnesene; and β-phelladrene, cineol, and citral. Other pungent principles of the rhizomes are gingerdiols, gingerdiacetates, gingerdiones, 6-gingersulfonic acid, gingerenones, etc. In dried ginger, shogaol, a dehydrated product of gingerol, is a predominant pungent constituent (Ghosh et al 2011; Jolad et al 2004; Bao et al 2010).

Fresh ginger contains 80.9% moisture, 2.3% protein, 0.9% fat, 1.2% minerals, 2.4% fibers, 12.3% carbohydrates, lipids (including glycerides, phosphatidic acid, lecithins, and fatty acids), protease, iron, calcium, magnesium, potassium, and phosphorous. It also contains vitamins such as thiamine, riboflavin, niacin, and vitamin C (ICMR Bulletin 2003; Ibrahim et al 2010).

Identity, Purity, and Strength

For Adraka

- Foreign matter: Not more than 0.5%
- Total ash: Not more than 8%
- Acid-insoluble ash: Not more than 1%
- Alcohol-soluble extractive: Not less than 5%
- Water-soluble extractive: Not less than 2%
- Moisture content: Not more than 90%

(Source: The Ayurvedic Pharmacopeia of India 1989)

For Shunthi

- Foreign matter: Not more than 1%
- Total ash: Not more than 6%
- Acid-insoluble ash: Not more than 1.5%
- Alcohol-soluble extractive: Not less than 3%
- Water-soluble extractive: Not less than 10%

(Source: The Ayurvedic Pharmacopeia of India 1989)

Karma (Actions)

Bhavamishra attributed deepana, pachan, rochan, bhedana, grahi, vrishya, swarya, jivah kanth vishodhan (clears throat and tongue) properties to it. Other Ayurvedic lexicons and Nighantus described it as snigdh, sangrahi, swarya, hridya, vrisya, vedanahara, shothahara, mukhashodhak, and vataanulomaka.

- Doshakarma: Kapha vata hara
- Dhatukarma: Dhatu vardhaka, vrishya
- Malakarma: Malabhedana

Pharmacological Actions

Many in vitro and in vivo studies reported its anti-inflammatory, antispasmodic, antimicrobial, antioxidant, diaphoretic, cardioprotective, antinociceptive, expectorant, anticarcinogenic, antiemetic, antithrombotic, antiarthritic, antitussive, hypocholesterolemic, hypolipidemic, antiatherosclerotic, antibacterial, radio protective, antigenotoxic, and mutagenicity effects. It also enhances weight loss and increases bioavailability of many drugs (Agrahari et al 2015).

In vitro research indicates that gingerols and the related shogaols exhibit cardiodepressant activity at low doses and cardiotonic properties at higher doses (Srivastava and Mustafa 1989).

Indications

Shunthi and Adraka swarasa are used traditionally for the treatment of vaman, aanaah, adhyaman, agnimandhya, aruchi, vibanda, gulma, grahani, udarrog, pleeharoga, vishuchika, shoola, shotha, arsha, pandu, hridyaroga, aamvata, sandhivaat, katishool, mukhashodhan, karnashool, shwasa, kasa, hikka, pratishyay, parinaamshool, sheetpitta, shleepada, vataoudar, mukhajadyata, utklesha, jwar, murcha, mutrakricchta, shiroruja, anidra, kantharoga, mukh-akshi gourav, and vrishchikdansa. Due to its wider use in therapeutics, it is known as Vishwa bhesajya.

Contraindications

As Adraka is ushna and tikshna in potency, its use is contraindicated in persons suffering from kustha (skin diseases), daha (burning sensation), vrana (ulcers), jwara (fever), mutrakricchta (dysuria), raktapitta (hemorrhage), in summer and autumn (B.P.N. haritakyadi varga 48). It is to be taken with caution during pregnancy, lactation, or abnormal bleeding and by persons allergic to ginger.

Therapeutic Uses of Adraka (Fresh Ginger)

External Use

1. **Aruchi** (loss of appetite): One should keep Adraka juice mixed with saindhav lavan in mouth as kaval to cure aruchi (anorexia) (B.P.Ci. 1/851).
2. **Murccha** (fainting): One should use snuffing with Adraka juice to regain consciousness in murccha (B.P.Ci. 1/849).
3. **Karnashool** (earache): Instillation of lukewarm Adraka juice with oil, honey, and saindhav lavan relieves pain in karnashool (S.S.Ci. 5/24; S.S.U. 21/18).

Internal Use

1. **Kasa and Shwasa** (cough and asthma): Adraka juice mixed with honey should be taken daily to alleviate shwasa, kasa, pratishyaya, and kapha vikara (B.P.Ci. 14/31; VM 11/10; H.S. 3.12.38).
2. **Agnimandhya** (indigestion): Adraka juice mixed with equal quantity of vinegar is taken to improve digestive fire (A.H.U. 40/55). Intake of Adraka kalka (paste) mixed with lemon juice, sugar, and trijaat powder has hridya action and promotes twice the relish and digestion (SB 4/260).
3. **Shotha** (edema): Intake of Adraka juice with old jaggery along with goat's milk alleviates all types of edema (VM 39/7).
4. **Udararoga** (diseases of abdomen): Milk processed with Adraka juice should be used in udararoga (S.S.Ci. 14/10).
5. **Vrishanagata vata** (aggravated vata in testis): Intake of Adraka juice with proper quantity of oil daily in early morning alleviates vrishanagata vata (SB Vatavyadhi /56).

Therapeutic Uses of Shunthi (Dry Ginger)

External Use

1. **Hikka** (hic-cough): Shunthi powder is given with Guda which is used as nasya in Hikka (CD 12/4; A.H.Ci. 4/46).
2. **Shiro roga** (headache): Nasal inhalation of milk mixed with Shunthi paste gives relief in severe headache of any origin (CD 60/23). Snuffing with Guda Shunthi kalka removes headache (B.P.Ci. 62/33).

Internal Use

1. **Aamvata** (rheumatoid arthritis): Daily intake of Shunthi and Gokshur decoction in the morning gives relief in aamvata, katishool, and stimulates digestion (VM 25/7). Shunthyadi ghrita can also be used for the same condition (VM 39/41, 42, 48; B.P.Ci. 26/80-83). Shunthi kalka impregnated with Eranda mool rasa should be heated in putapaka. The juice thus extracted and mixed with honey is used to allay severe pain of aamvata (SG 2.1.40).
2. **Kasa** (cough): To get relief in this, jaggery mixed with Shunthi and Pippali or Draksha should be taken with ghee and honey (S.S.U. 52/17).
1. **Arsha** (piles): Administration of Pippali and Shunthi powder mixed with equal quantity of Haritaki powder with jaggery cures kaphavataj arsha (VD 5/1). Chitrak and Shunthi mixed with vinegar are also beneficial in arsha (C.S.Ci. 14/68).
2. **Atisara** (diarrhea): Consumption of Shunthi and jaggery mixed with curd, oil, ghee, and milk reduces the frequency of stool and spasmodic pain, improves appetite, and promotes digestion in diarrhea (A.H.Ci. 9/17).
3. **Jwara** (fever): Regular intake of Shunthi, Jiraka, and jaggery with hot water, well-cooked alcohol, or buttermilk checks fever with chill (B.P.Ci. 1/756). Regular intake of milk cooked with Shunthi, Draksha, Kharjura, and mixed with honey, ghee, and sugar allays pipasa and jwara (C.S.Ci. 3/237).
4. **Udarshool** (abdominal pain): In colicky abdominal pain, decoction of Shunthi and Erand mool along with hing and salt gives instant relief (VM 26/7; BS shool Ci/16).
5. **Shotha** (edema): Shunthi powder mixed with equal quantity of jaggery is given with Punarnava decoction to get relief from all types of edema (B.P.Ci. 42/43; AS Ci. 19/3).
6. **Grahani** (sprue): Shunthi and Bilva kalka (paste) taken with masoor yusha (lentil soup) alleviates grahani roga (SG 2/5/28).

7. **Agnimandhya and ajirna** (indigestion): Daily intake of Haritaki and Shunthi with jaggery or saindhav lavan (rock salt) stimulates digestive fire and enhances digestion (B.P.Ci. 6/34).

8. **Hikka** (hic-cough) and **shwasa** (asthma): Powder of Suvarcala, Shunthi, and Bharangi mixed with double quantity of sugar taken with hot water alleviates hikka and shwasa (C.S.Ci. 3/237).

9. **Chhardi** (vomiting) and **vishuchika** (cholera): Decoction of Bilva and Shunthi alleviate chhardi and vishuchika (B.P.Ci 6/112).

10. **Madayatya** (alcoholism): Boiled and cooled water processed with Bala or Prisniparni or Kantakari mixed with Shunthi should be used for drinking in alcoholism (C.S.Ci. 24/166-67).

11. **Vatavyadhi** (neuromuscular diseases): Payasa (rice milk) made with Shunthi and Eranda beej should be consumed in kantishool and gridharsi (B.S. vatavyadhi Ci./592).

Officinal Part Used

Rhizome

Dose

Powder: 1 to 2 g
Juice: 5 to 10 mL

Formulations

Trikatu churna, Adrakapaka, Panchkola phanta, Saubhagya Shunthi khand, Panchasama churna, Samasarkar churna, Rasnadi kwath, and Shunthi sura.

Toxicity/Adverse Effects

Adverse effects, following its consumption, are infrequent and mild, such as heartburn and bad taste in mouth. Routine blood counts, liver, and renal function tests did not provide any evidence of toxicity even after 48 weeks of use (Wigler et al 2003; Black and O'Conner 2008).

Substitution and Adulteration

There are several commercial varieties of ginger, derived from *Z. officinale*. Apart from these, some types are derived from other species. The rhizomes of other species of Zingiberaceae family are sometimes mixed with it. Japanese ginger is obtained from *Z. mioga* Rosc. and Martinique ginger from *Z. zerumbet* Rosc. Ex.Sm. The rhizomes of *Z. casummar* Roxb. are sometimes used as substitute to ginger (Lavekar 2008).

Points to Ponder

- *Ginger was first listed as medicine in China in 200 AD.*
- *India is the largest producer and consumer of ginger, contributing about 31% of total global production.*
- *Adraka is katu vipaka and pitta vardhaka, whereas Shunthi is madhura in vipaka and pittashamaka.*

Suggested Readings

Abubackar ATN. Ginger: a rhizome with high export value. 2011. Available at: http://efy.efymag.com/admin/issuepdf/Ginger_April%2011.pdf

Agrahari P, Panda P, Kumar Verma N, Ullah Khan W, Darbari S. A brief study on *zingiber officinale*: a review. J Drug Discov Therap 2015;3(28):20–27

Amiril NA. Optimization of essential oil extraction from *Zingiber officinale*. A thesis submitted in Faculty of Chemical and Natural Resources Engineering University College of Engineering & Technology Malaysia. 2006:6–9

Anonymous. Indian Herbal Pharmacopoeia. Vol. 2. Indian Drug Manufacturer's Association and Regional Research Laboratory; 1999:163–173

Awang DVC. Ginger. Can Pharm J 1992;125(7):309–311

Bag BB. Ginger processing in India (*Zingiber officinale*): a review. Int J Curr Microbiol Appl Sci 2018;7(4):1639–1651

Bao L, Deng A, Li Z, Du G, Qin H. Chemical constituents of rhizomes of *Zingiber officinale*. Zhongguo Zhongyao Zazhi 2010;35(5):598–601

Black CD, Oconnor PJ. Acute effects of dietary ginger on quadriceps muscle pain during moderate-intensity cycling exercise. Int J Sport Nutr Exerc Metab 2008;18(6):653–664

Ghosh AK, Banerjee S, Mullick HI, Banerjee J. Zingiber officinale: a natural gold. Int J Pharma Bio Sci 2011;2(1):283–294

Ginger: its role in xenobiotic metabolism. ICMR Bull 2003;33(6):57–63

Grzanna R, Lindmark L, Frondoza CG. Ginger: a herbal medicinal product with broad anti-inflammatory actions. J Med Food 2005; 8(2):125–132

Ibrahim TA, Ibo D, Adejare RA. Comparative phytochemical properties of crude ethanolic extracts and physicochemical characteristics of essential oils of *Myristicalfragrans* (nutmeg) seeds and *Zingiber officinale* (ginger) roots. EJEAFChe 2010;9(6):1110–1116

Jiang X, Williams KM, Liauw WS, et al. Effect of ginkgo and ginger on the pharmacokinetics and pharmacodynamics of warfarin in healthy subjects. Br J Clin Pharmacol 2005;59(4):425–32

Jolad SD, Lantz RC, Solyom AM, Chen GJ, Bates RB, Timmermann BN. Fresh organically grown ginger (*Zingiber officinale*): composition and effects on LPS-induced PGE2 production. Phytochemistry 2004;65(13):1937–1954

Joy PP, Thomas J, Mathew S, Skaria BP. Medicinal Plants. Ernakulum: Kerala Agricultural University Aromatic and Medicinal Plants Research Station; 1998

Khare CP. Indian Medicinal Plants: An Illustrated Dictionary. New York, NY: Springer Publications; 2007

Kritikar KR, Basu BD. Indian Medicinal Plants. Vol. 4. 2nd ed. Dehradun: International Book Distributers; 2007

Lavekar GS. Database on Medicinal Plants used in Ayurveda. Vol. 5. New Delhi: CCRAS; Reprint 2008

Ross IA. Medicinal Plants of the World. Vol. 3. New Jersey: Humana Press; 2005

Singh G, Kapoor IPS, Singh P, de Heluani CS, de Lampasona MP, Catalan CAN. Chemistry, antioxidant and antimicrobial investigations on essential oil and oleoresins of *Zingiber officinale*. Food Chem Toxicol 2008;46(10):3295–3302

Spices: exotic flavors & medicines: ginger. Retrieved 2 May 2014

Srivastava KC, Mustafa T. Ginger (*Zingiber officinale*) and rheumatic disorders. Med Hypoth 1989;29(1):25–28

The Ayurvedic Pharmacopeia of India. Part 1, Vol. 2. New Delhi: Department of AYUSH, Ministry of Health and Family Welfare, Government of India; 1999:12–14

The Ayurvedic Pharmacopeia of India. Part I, Vol. 1. New Delhi: Department of AYUSH, Ministry of Health and Family Welfare, Government of India; 1989:103–104

Wigler I, Grotto I, Caspi D, Yaron M. The effects of Zintona EC (a ginger extract) on symptomatic gonarthritis. Osteoarthr Cartil 2003;11(11):783–789

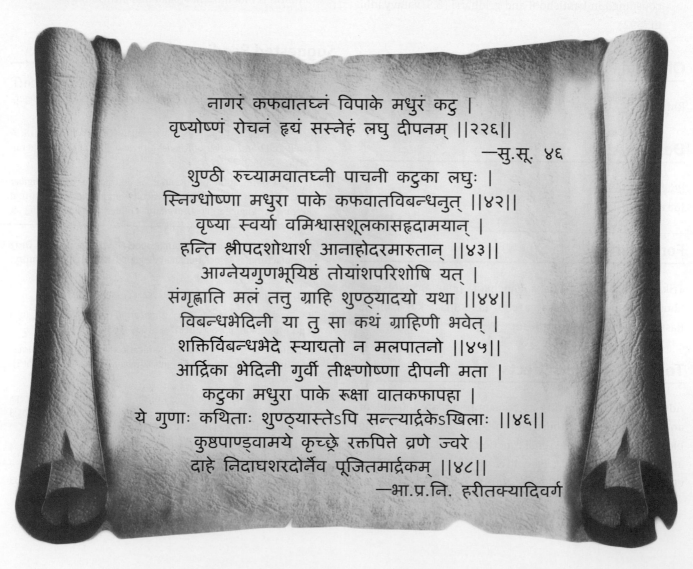

नागरं कफवातघ्नं विपाके मधुरं कटु ।
वृष्योष्णं रोचनं हृद्यं सस्नेहं लघु दीपनम् ॥२२६॥

—सु．सू． ४६

शुण्ठी रुच्यामवातघ्नी पाचनी कटुका लघुः ।
स्निग्धोष्णा मधुरा पाके कफवातविबन्धनुत् ॥४२॥
वृष्या स्वर्या वमिश्वासशूलकासहृदामयान् ।
हन्ति श्रीपदशोथार्श आनाहोदरमारुतान् ॥४३॥
आग्नेयगुणभूयिष्ठं तोयांशपरिशोषि यत् ।
संगृह्णाति मलं तत्तु ग्राहि शुण्ठ्यादयो यथा ॥४४॥
विबन्धभेदिनी या तु सा कथं ग्राहिणी भवेत् ।
शक्तिर्विबन्धभेदे स्याद्धतो न मलपातनो ॥४५॥
आर्द्रिका भेदिनी गुर्वी तीक्ष्णोष्णा दीपनी मता ।
कटुका मधुरा पाके रूक्षा वातकफापहा ।
ये गुणाः कथिताः शुण्ठ्यास्तेऽपि सन्त्याद्रिकेऽखिलाः ॥४६॥
कुष्ठपाण्ड्वामये कृच्छ्रे रक्तपित्ते व्रणे ज्वरे ।
दाहे निदाघशरदोर्नैव पूजितमार्द्रकम् ॥४८॥

—भा．प्र．नि． हरीतक्यादिवर्ग

8. Arjun *[Terminalia arjun W. and A.]*

Family:	*Combretaceae*
Hindi name:	*Arjun*
English name:	*Arjun*

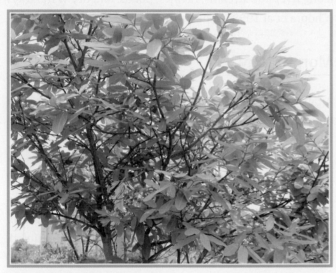

Plant of *Terminalia Arjun* W. and A.

It is believed that Arjun tree should not be planted in the vicinity of residential area (Vrikshayurveda 3/30).

Introduction

The word "Arjun" in Sanskrit means white or bright, which indicates the white and shiny nature of its bark. In the Indian system of medicines, Arjun bark is used as a cardio-protective agent since ages, that is why it is popularly known as the "Guardian of the heart." It is named after the hero of the famous epic "Mahabharata," because of its protective effects.

In Buddhist literature, Arjun is said to have been used as the tree for achieving enlightenment, or Bodhi by the tenth Buddha. Its leaves and flowers are offered to Lord Vishnu and Lord Ganapati on several religious occasions. Raj Nighantu has mentioned this plant as a nakshatra tree. Arjun is associated with Swati nakshatra and it is believed that those born in Swati nakshatra should plant and look after it so as to attain peace and prosperity.

Many references of Arjun are found in Rig Veda and Atharva Veda. In Charak and Sushruta Samhita, description

of Arjun is available, but it hasn't been used as a specific drug for heart diseases. It was Vagbhatta who for the first time mentioned Arjun decoction in the treatment of kaphaja hridayaroga (A.H.Ci. 6/53). Astanga hridya also advocated its use in prameha, mukharoga, asthibhagna, kshudraroga, yoniroga, and visha chikitsa. Vrinda indicated its use in heart diseases for the first time. Later on, it was supported by Chakradutta and Bhavamishra. Shodhala has also praised Arjun in heart diseases. Chakradutta was the first one to use Arjuna Kshirapaka in heart diseases. In Charak Samhita Arjun is used in the treatment of kustha, vrana, prameha, rajayakshma, and yoni roga.

Leaves of Arjun are used as the primary food for the kosi silkworm along with the leaves of Asana, Sala, Kanchnar, Madhuka, Shimshapa, Aswaththa, etc. in sericulture. Bark and heartwood of this plant are used for fuel and also used in timber, tanning, and dyeing industry.

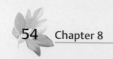

Vernacular Names

Assamese: Arjun, Orjun

Bengali: Arjhan, Arjun

Gujarati: Sadado, Arjun, Sajada

Kannada: Matti, Bilimatti, Neermatti, Mathichakke, Kudare Kivimase

Malayalam: Nirmasuthu, Vellamaruthi, Kellemasuthu, Mattimora, Torematti

Marathi: Arjun, Sadaru

Oriya: Arjun

Punjabi: Arjon

Tamil: Marudam

Telugu: Tela Maddi

Urdu: Arjun

Synonyms

Devshala: It is a potent tree like Shala (*Shorea robusta*).

Dhavala: It has white-colored bark.

Hridyarogaveri: It is useful in heart diseases.

Indradu: Due to its high efficacy, it is well known as the tree of Lord Indra.

Kakubha: It has many spreading branches.

Madhugandhiprasunaka: Its inflorescence has madhu (honey) like aroma.

Nadisarja: It grows in the vicinity of water streams like Sarja tree.

Partha, Dhananjaya: This tree is named after various names of Arjun (the well-known character of the epic Mahabharata).

Shvetavaaha: Its outer stem bark is white in color.

Veervriksha: It is a highly potent drug.

Classical Categorization

Charak Samhita: Udarda prashamana, Kashaya skanda

Sushrut Samhita: Nyagrodhadi, Salasaradi

Ashtanga Hridaya: Nyagrodhadi, Asanadi

Dhanvantari Nighantu: Amradi varga

Madanpal Nighantu: Vatadi varga

Kaiyadev Nighantu: Oushadi varga

Raj Nighantu: Prabhadradi varga

Bhavaprakash: Vatadi varga

Distribution

Arjun tree is abundantly distributed in India, Burma, Mauritius, Sri Lanka, and throughout the sub-Indo-Himalayan tracts of Uttar Pradesh, Punjab, Deccan, South Bihar, Odisha, West Bengal, and Madhya Pradesh, mainly along riverside streams, ravines, ponds, and dry waterways (Chopra et al 1958; Nadkarni 1976).

Morphology

A tall, evergreen deciduous tree of 20 to 25 m height with buttressed trunk and spreading crown with drooping branches.

- **Bark:** Thick, soft, smooth, and whitish cream outside and blood red inside, flakes off in large, flat pieces (**Fig. 8.1a, b**).
- **Leaves:** Simple, subopposite, oblong or elliptical, shortly acute or obtuse apex, short petioled, coriaceous, dull green above and pale brown beneath, presence of two glands at the base on the back side of midrib of leaf (**Fig. 8.2a, b**).
- **Flowers**: Pale yellowish-white color, sessile, bisexual flowers, in short axillary spike or in terminal panicle arrangement (**Fig. 8.3a, b**).
- **Fruits**: Small drupe, ovoid oblong, fibrous woody, smooth skinned with five to seven hard angles or wings that are oblique and curved upwards, initially green in color, blackish brown when mature (**Fig. 8.4a, b**; Ali 1994).

Seeds and stump planting are used for the propagation of this plant.

Phenology

Flowering time: March to June

Fruiting time: September to November

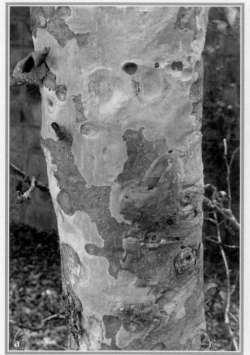

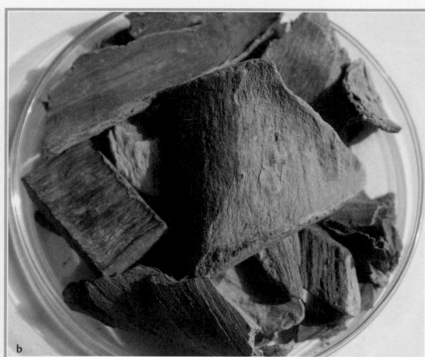

Fig. 8.1 **(a)** Bark. **(b)** Dry sample of bark.

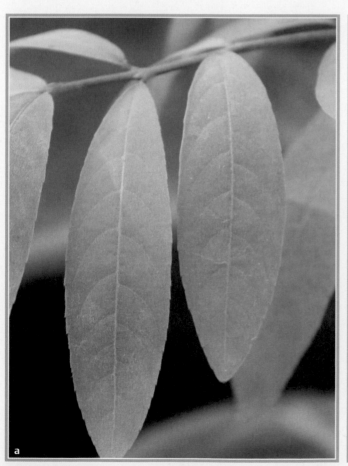

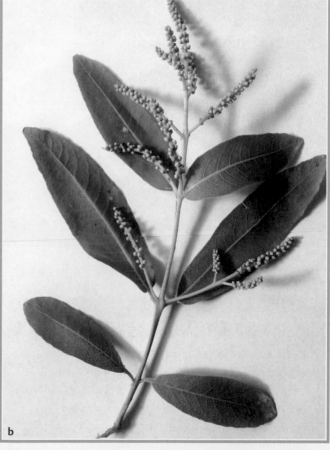

Fig. 8.2 **(a, b)** Leaves.

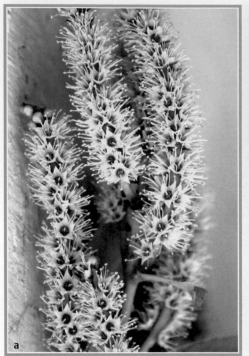

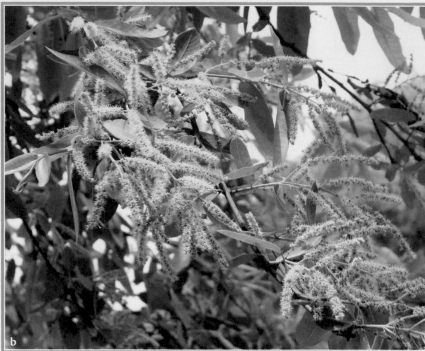

Fig. 8.3 **(a)** Flowers. **(b)** Inflorescences.

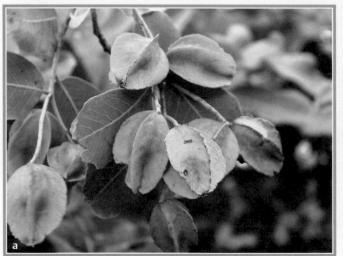

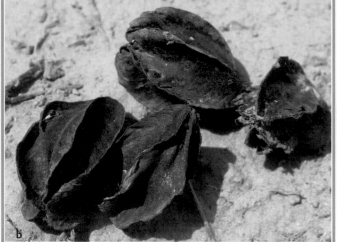

Fig. 8.4 **(a)** Fruit. **(b)** Dry sample of fruit.

Key Characters for Identification

➤ An evergreen deciduous tree. Bark cream is white externally and blood red internally.

➤ Leaves: simple, opposite, coriaceous, oblong, or elliptical shape; two nodes on the back side at the base.

➤ Flowers: pale yellow to white in axillary spikes.

➤ Fruits: drupe, ovoid, woody, with five to seven hard angles or wings.

Rasapanchaka

Guna	Laghu, Ruksha
Rasa	Kashaya
Vipak	Katu
Virya	Sheeta
Prabhava	Hridya

Chemical Constituents

Stem bark contains tannins (pyrocatechols, punicallin, castalagin, casuariin, casuarinin, punicalagin, terchebulin, terflavin c), flavonoids and polyphenols (arjunone, luteolin, baicalein, ethyl gallate, gallic acid, ellagic acid proanthocyanidin, quercetin, catechin, epicatechin, gallocatechin), saponins, triterpenoid (arjunic acid, arjunin, arjunolic acid, arjungenin, terminic acid, terminoltin), glycosides (arjunoside I, II, and IV, arjunetin, arjuno-litin, arjunolone, arjunolitin arjunglucoside IV and V, terminarjunoside I and II, terminoside a, termionic acid), β-sitosterol, calcium, magnesium, aluminum, zinc, copper, silica, amino acids like tryptophan, tyrosine, histidine, and cysteine. Fruit contains triterpenoids and flavonoids such as arjunic acid, arjunone, arachidic stearate, cerasidin, ellagic acid, fridelin, gallic acid, hentriacontane, methyl oleaolate, myristyl oleate, and β-sitisterol. Leaves and seeds are rich in flavanoids and glycosides (Amalraj and Gopi 2016).

Identity, Purity, and Strength

- Foreign matter: Not more than 2%
- Total ash: Not more than 25%
- Acid-insoluble ash: Not more than 1%
- Alcohol-soluble extractive: Not less than 20%
- Water-soluble extractive: Not less than 20%

(Source: The Ayurvedic Pharmacopeia of India 1999)

Karma (Actions)

In classical Ayurveda texts, Arjun bark is described as hridya, stambhak, udardaprasasmana, vranaropaka, vranashodhak, medohara, kantiprada (complexion promoter), asthisand-hanak, vishaghna, and rakta stambhaka dravya.

- Doshakarma: Kapha-pitta shamaka
- Dhatukarma: Medahara, rakta sthambhak, asthisandhanka
- Malakarma: Stambhaka

The bark is astringent, cooling, aphrodisiac, demulcent, cardiotonic, hemostatic, styptic, antidysentric, urinary astringent, expectorant, alexiteric, lithontriptic, and tonic. The fruit is tonic and deobstruent (Sharma et al 2005).

Pharmacological Actions

Arjun showed antioxidant, anti-inflammatory, hypolipid-emic, hemostatic, styptic, antidysentric, antibacterial, expectorant, lithontriptic hypotensive, antiatherogenic, anticarcinogenic, antimutagenic, gastroproductive effect, hypocholesterolemic, antimicrobial, antitumor, antiallergic, antifeedant, antifertility, and anti-HIV activities (Amalraj and Gopi 2016).

Indications

Kshirapaka and decoction of Arjun bark is traditionally used for the treatment of hridya roga, medovriddhi, vrana, kshata, kshaya, visha, asthi bhagna, bhrama, trishna, raktapitta, raktagatavata, daha, prameha, pandu, shwasa, bhasmakroga, mutrakricchta, yoni roga, jeerna jwar, kasa, and grahaniruja. Juice of its fresh leaves is used in karnashoola.

It is also useful in angina, hypertension, hypercholestero-lemia, atherosclerosis, ulcers, urethrorrhea, spermatorrhea, leucorrhea, diabetes, anemia, cardiac disorders, excessive perspiration, fatigue, bronchitis, consumption, intrinsic hemorrhages, tumor, otalgia, dysentery, inflammations, skin diseases like freckles, wound, hemorrhoids, bleeding diarrhea, and cirrhosis of liver (Dwivedi and Udupa 1989).

The traditional claims regarding efficacy of Arjun as a cardioprotective agent are authenticated and documented by many experimental and clinical studies. The plant showed cardioprotective activity by improving the cardiac muscle function and pumping activity of the heart. The saponin glycosides present in the bark are responsible for its inotropic effect, whereas the flavonoids and phenols provide antioxidant activity and vascular strengthening (Kapoor et al 2014; Maulik and Talwar 2012).

Therapeutic Uses

External Use

1. **Vranachhadana:** Arjun leaves are used to tie/cover the wounded area (C.S.Ci. 25/95).
2. **Vyanga** (acne): Regular application of Arjun bark powder or Manjistha with honey prevents acne and other skin diseases (A.H.U. 32/16).

3. **Yoni roga** (gynaecological disorder): Picchu of Shirish, Kakubh decoction is retained inside vagina in yoni roga (A.H.Sh. 2/44).
4. **Arsha** (piles): Decoction of Vasa, Arjun, Yavasa, and Nimba is used for washing the affected part in hemorrhoids (C.S.Ci. 14/214).

Internal Use

1. **Hridyaroga** (heart diseases): Arjun bark ksheerpaka prepared with panchmoola, bala, madhuka, and sarkara is useful in hridyaroga (V.M. 31/8). Powder of Arjun bark and godhuma processed with taila and jaggery consumed with milk combats all types of heart diseases (G.N. 2.26.21).
2. **Asthibhagna** (fracture): One should take Arjun bark powder and godhuma churna with milk and ghee to promote healing of fractured bones (V.M. 46/10). Intake of powdered Arjun bark, laksha, guggul with ghee accelerates union in fractured bones (B.P.Ci. 48/29).
3. **Shukrameha** (spermatorrhea): Decoction prepared with Arjun bark and chandana is useful in shukrameha (S.S.Ci. 11/9).
4. **Grahani** (sprue): Daily consumption of Arjun and Bhringaraj kshar in the morning with butter milk gives relief in pain due to chronic grahani roga (B.S. Grahani Ci. 189).
5. **Raktapitta** (hemorrhage): Arjun bark is soaked in water and is kept overnight. Next morning the water is strained and drunk with honey in raktapitta. Intake of Arjun bark and madhu with milk controls bleeding diarrhea (V.M. 3/41). Consuming hima (cold infusion) prepared with Jambu, Amra, and Arjun daily is useful in arresting bleeding (S.S.U. 45/23).
6. **Puyameha** (gonorrhea/a type of diabetes): Daily intake of Dhava and Arjun bark decoction cures puyameha (H.S. 3.28.7).
7. **Kshayaja kasa** (cough due to consumption): Arjun bark powder processed 21 times with vasa juice is used with honey, ghee, and sugar in kshayaja kasa and raktapitta (B.P.Ci. 12/29).
8. **Hypertension:** Regular intake of one teaspoonful of Arjun bark powder with one cup of milk or water twice daily lowers down high blood pressure and gives symptomatic relief in giddiness, headache, irritability, etc.

Officinal Part Used

Bark

Dose

Bark powder: 3 to 6 g
Decoction: 50 to 100 mL
Kshirapaka (decoction prepared with milk): 5 to 10 g

Formulations

Kakubhadi churna, Prabhakar vati, Arjunksheerpaka, Arjunrishta, Arjun ghrita, Lakshadi guggulu.

Toxicity/Adverse Effects

In different clinical studies, the use of Arjun in an optimum dose of 1 to 2 g showed lesser side effects such as headache, mild gastritis, and constipation. It does not produce any hematological, hepatic, metabolic, and renal toxicity even after more than two years of its administration (Bharani et al 1995).

Substitution and Adulteration

Stem bark of *Lagerstroemia speciosa* (L.) Pers. and other species of *Terminalia* such as *T. alata, T. tomentosa, T. catappa, T. citrina, T. pallid, T. manni, T. paniculata*, etc. are used as an adulterant of Arjun bark (Sharma et al. 2005).

> **Points to Ponder**
>
> - *A pair of knob-like glands on the dorsal (lower) side of the leaf at the junction between the petiole and the lamina.*
> - *Arjun is not included in hridya mahakashaya of Charak Samhita but is considered as the best hridya dravya.*
> - *In heart diseases, it is best to use it in the form of ksheerpaka (Chakradutta).*

Suggested Readings

Ali M. Text Book of Pharmacognosy. 1st ed. New Delhi: CBS Publishers; 1994

Amalraj A, Gopi S. Medicinal properties of *Terminalia arjuna* (Roxb.) Wight & Arn.: a review. J Tradit Complement Med 2016; 7(1): 65–78

Bharani A, Ganguly A, Bhargava KD. Salutary effect of *Terminalia arjuna* in patients with severe refractory heart failure. Int J Cardiol 1995;49(3):191–199

Bhawani G, Kumar A, Murthy KSN, Kumari N. Ganapati Swami Ch. A retrospective study of effect of *Terminalia arjuna* and evidence based standard therapy on echocardiographic parameters in patients of dilated cardiomyopathy. J Pharm Res 2013;6:493–498

Chopra RN, Chopra IC, Handa KL, Kapur LD. *Terminalia arjuna* W&A (Combretaceae): Indigenous Drugs of India. 1st ed. Calcutta: UN Dhur & Sons; 1958:421–424

Dwivedi S, Udupa N. *Terminalia arjuna*: pharmacognosy, phyto-chemistry, pharmacology and clinical use: a review. Fitoterapia 1989;60:413–420

Gyanendra P. Vrikshayurveda of Surpala. 1st ed. Varanasi: Chaukhamba Sanskrit Series Office; 2010:09

Kapoor D, Vijayvergiya R, Dhawan V. *Terminalia arjuna* in coronary artery disease: ethnopharmacology, pre-clinical, clinical & safety evaluation. J Ethnopharmacol 2014;155(2):1029–1045

Maulik SK, Talwar KK. Therapeutic potential of *Terminalia arjuna* in cardiovascular disorders. Am J Cardiovasc Drugs 2012;12(3): 157–163

Nadkarni AK. Indian Materia Medica. 1st ed. Mumbai: Popular Prakashan; 1976

Sharma PC, Yelne MB, Dennis TJ. Database on Medicinal Plants Used in Ayurveda. Vol. 3. New Delhi: CCRAS (The Central Council for Research in Ayurvedic Sciences); 2005:57

Singh N, Kapur KK, Singh SP, Shanker K, Sinha JN, Kohli RP. Mechanism of cardiovascular action of *Terminalia arjuna*. Planta Med 1982; 45(2):102–104

Sumitra M, Manikandan P, Kumar DA, et al. Experimental myocardial necrosis in rats: role of arjunolic acid on platelet aggregation, coagulation and antioxidant status. Mol Cell Biochem 2001; 224(1-2):135–142

The Ayurvedic Pharmacopeia of India. Part I, Vol. New Delhi: Department of AYUSH, Ministry of Health and Family Welfare, Government of India; 1999:17–18

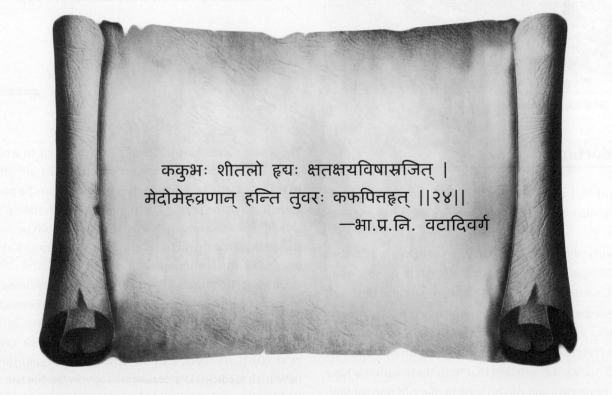

ककुभः शीतलो हृद्यः क्षतक्षयविषास्रजित् ।
मेदोमेहव्रणान् हन्ति तुवरः कफपित्तहृत् ॥२४॥
—भा.प्र.नि. वटादिवर्ग

9. Arkadvaya [*Calotropis procera* Linn. *(Raktarka); Calotropis gigantea* (Linn.) R.Br. *(Shwetarka)*]

Family:	*Asclepiadeaceae*
Hindi name:	*Ark, Akda, Madar, Aak*
English name:	*Gigantic swallow wort, Milkweed, Bowstring hemp*

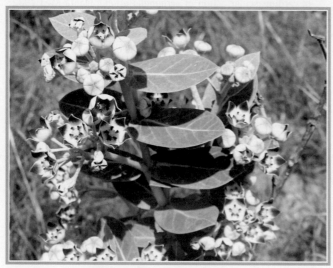

Plant of *Calotropis procera* Linn.

Arka is included in Shadshodhana vriksa and its latex is used for inducing both Vaman and Virechana (C.S.Su. 1/115).

Introduction

The word "Arka" literally means "Sun." The plant is named after the sun because of its hot potency and properties like the sun.

In Ayurvedic classics, the two types of Arka are described as Arkadvaya. These two plants are different species of genus *Calotropis*. These are *Calotropis procera* Linn. and *Calotropis gigantea* (Linn.) R.Br. which are well known as Rakta arka and Shweta arka, respectively. Calotropis with red flowers is known as Arka and the one with white flowers is called Alarka. It is believed that both these varieties have similar properties and can be used in place of one another. Rakta arka is abundantly available, whereas Shweta arka is considered superior in therapeutics.

From Vedic period, Arka is used for worshipping the sun and in performing yagna (a vedic ritual done in front of sacred fire with mantras) in ritual ceremonies.

The flowers and fruits of Shweta arka are used to worship Lord Shiva, whereas the flowers of Rakta arka are offered to Lord Ganesha for worship. It is believed that the plant is beneficial for the persons born in Shravan Nakshatra. They should propagate and look after it so as to attain peace and prosperity. To ward off the ill effects of Surya graha it should be used in ritual ceremonies.

Since ancient times Arka is being used in ethnomedicine to cure common ailments such as fevers, rheumatism, jaundice, intestinal worms, cough, cold, eczema, asthma, wounds, joint pain, elephantiasis, and diarrhea (Verma et al 2010). Its roots, root bark, latex leaves, and flowers have high medicinal value. Charaka advocated the use of its latex and root as an antidote for snake poisoning (C.S.Ci. 1/). Sushruta included it under kshar dravya and used it in the treatment of vrana, vatavyadhi, bhgandara, kustha, granthi, arbuda, vidradhi, shotha, sarpadanstha, and karnashool. In many Rasagrantha, Arka is placed under the category of upvisha.

Research studies also indicated the presence of many toxic principals such as uscharin, calotoxin, calactin, gigantin, and calotropin in it (Shanker 2005). Due to the toxicity of the latex, it is used traditionally to make poison arrow and to induce criminal abortions. The plant also holds a great economic value. Its floss is used to make thread with cotton fiber. The inner bark produces strong fiber called madar which is used in the manufacture of carpets, ropes, sewing threads, and fishing nets. The leaves are used for mulching, green manuring, and for binding sandy soil. Latex is used for removing hair from goat skin to produce "nari leather." Whole plant is used for the production of biofuel through anaerobic fermentation (Gaur et al 2013).

Hence, Calotropis has broad-spectrum use, ranging from therapeutic to poisonous, depending upon the mode of usage and dose.

Vernacular Names

Assamese: Akand, Akan
Bengali: Akanda, Akone
Gujarati: Akado
Kannada: Ekka, Ekkadagida, Ekkegida
Kashmiri: Acka
Malayalam: Erikku, Vellerukku
Marathi: Rui, Akand
Oriya: Arakha, Akondo, Kotuki
Punjabi: Ak
Tamil: Vellerukku,Verukku, Erukkam
Telugu: Jilledu, Mandararamu
Urdu: Madar, Aak

Synonyms of Arka

Arkaparna: Its leaves have tikshna (sharp) property like the sun.
Asphota: Fruits burst themselves when fully mature (self-dehiscent).
Kharjughna: It is a good remedy for itching.
Kshirparna: Its leaves have profuse latex.
Raktapushpa: This plant bears lilac red flowers.
Shukaphala: Fruits of this plant are parrot-shaped.
Tulaphala: The fruit bears coma-shaped seeds like those of cotton.
Vikeerna: It has coma-shaped, scattered seeds.

Synonyms of Alarka

Balarka: It has properties like those of the rising sun.
Ganarupa: The plant has gregarious nature.
Mandara: It is a potent drug for the diseased.
Pratapasa: This is hot and irritant like the sun.
Sadapushpa: This plant bears flowers throughout the year.
Shwetapushpa: This plant has white-colored flowers.
Vasuka: It has potency like the sun.

Classical Categorization

Charak Samhita: Bhedaniya, Vamanopaga, Swedopaga
Sushrut Samhita: Arkadi, Adhobhagahara
Ashtanga Hridaya: Arkadi
Dhanvantari Nighantu: Karviradi varga
Madanpal Nighantu: Abhyadi varga
Kaiyadev Nighantu: Oushadi varga
Raj Nighantu: Karviradi varga
Bhavaprakash: Guduchyadi varga

Distribution

It is found wildly all over India in warm and dry regions of Bihar, Odisha, Punjab, Haryana, Rajasthan, Gujarat, Maharashtra, and from Deccan to Kanyakumari. Commonly found as a weed along the roadside, waste and fallow lands, ruined buildings, pasturelands, riverbanks, etc.; it grows well in coarse, sandy alkaline soil, and doesn't require specific cultivation practices (Sharma et al 2001).

Morphology

Erect (Shwetarka), much branched, bushy (Raktarka), succulent, lactiferous shrub of 1 to 5 m height. Raktarka is larger in size and bushy in comparison to Shwetarka. Latex is present in all plant parts. Branches are somewhat succulent and densely white tomentose (**Fig. 9.1**; Shwetarka).

- **Leaves:** Simple, opposite decussate, subsessile, fleshy, obovate-oblong, with a narrow cordate or often amplexicaul base, smooth pale green above, and cottony below (**Fig. 9.2a, b**).
- **Flowers:** Petal and gynostegium are lilac, purple colored, rosy, or purple tinted in Raktarka (**Fig. 9.3a**);

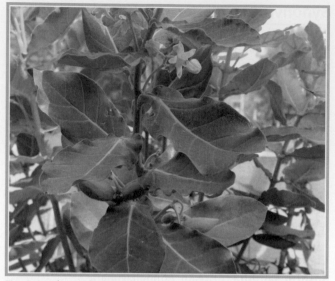

Fig. 9.1   Shwetarka (stem).

however, petals are entirely dull white in Shwetarka (**Fig. 9.3b**), present in lateral or terminal panicles of umbellate cymes. Flower buds are smaller and show a characteristic median depression in white variety, whereas they are straight in purple variety.

- **Fruits:** Fruit of two ovoid follicles; sometimes one follicle is abortive, subglobose to obliquely ovoid, inflated, recurved, 8-9 × 4-5 cm, green in color (**Fig. 9.4**).
- **Seeds:** Brown, broadly ovate, flattened, with white tuft of silky hairs at the pointed end (**Fig. 9.5**).
- **Root:** Rough, fissured longitudinally, corky, soft, externally yellowish-gray, internally white (**Fig. 9.6**) (Gupta and Sharma 2007). It is propagated through seed, root, and shoot cutting.

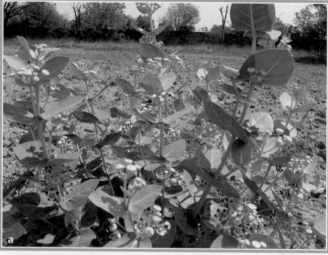

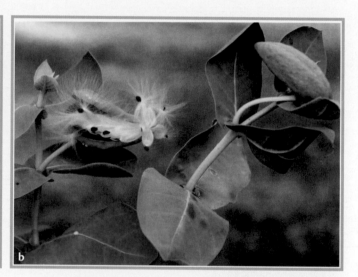

Fig. 9.2   (a, b) Leaves.

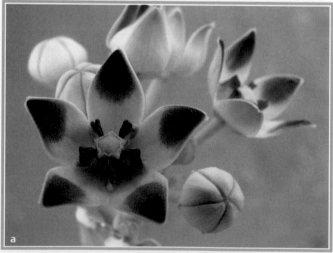

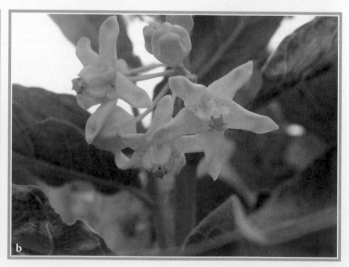

Fig. 9.3   (a) Flowers of Raktarka. **(b)** Flowers of Shwetarka.

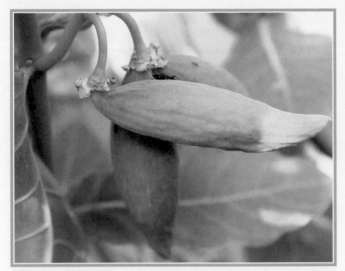

Fig. 9.4 Fruits.

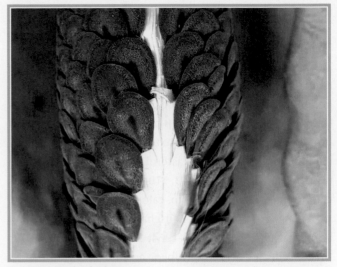

Fig. 9.5 Seeds of Arka.

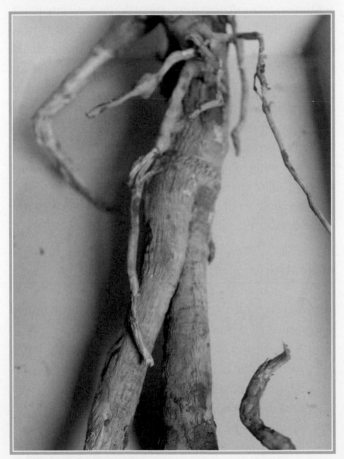

Fig. 9.6 Roots.

Phenology

Fruiting time: Throughout the year
Flowering time: Throughout the year

> ### Key Characters for Identification
>
> ➤ *A branched, succulent, lactiferous shrub*
> ➤ *Leaves: simple, opposite decussate, fleshy, obovate-oblong*
> ➤ *Flowers: lilac, purple, or dull white in terminal panicles of umbellate cymes*
> ➤ *Fruits: follicular, inflated, recurved, subglobose to ovoid shape*

Types

- Charak Samhita: one type—Arka
- Sushruta Samhita: two types—Arka and Alarka
- Abhidhanmanjari, Madanpal: two types—Arka and Alarka
- Dhanwantari Nighantu: two types—Arka and Rajarka
- Bhavaprakash Nighantu: two types—Shuklarka and Raktarka
- Raj Nighantu: four types—Arka, Shuklarka, Rajarka, and Shweta mandara

Rasapanchaka

Guna	Laghu, Ruksha, Teekshna
Rasa	Katu, Tikta, Madhura
Vipaka	Katu
Virya	Ushna

Chemical Constituents

The phytochemicals found in both the species are similar. The whole plant contains usharin, gigantin, calcium oxalate, α- and β-calotropeol, α- and β-amyrin, fatty acids, amino acids, proteases, hydrocarbons, pregnanes, acetates (taraxasteryl acetate, α- and β-amyrin), benzoates (α- and β-amyrin methylbutazone), mixture of tetracyclic triterpene compounds, sterols (taraxasterol, β-sitosterol), giganteol (Murti and Seshadri 1943, 1944, 1945), cardenolides calotropin, calactin, calotoxin, calotropagenin, proceroside, syriogenine, uscharidin, uscharin, uzarigenin, and voruscharin (Kupchan et al 1964; Singh and Rastogi 1972; Brischweiler et al 1969), lupeol acetate B, gigantursenyl acetate A and B (Habib et al 2007; Sen et al 1992), flavonol glycoside, akundarol, frugoside, calotroposides A to G (Crout et al 1963; Perwez and Mohammad 2009). The root contains procerursenyl acetate, proceranol, methyl myrisate, methyl behenate, etc. The root bark has α-amyrin, β-amyrin, lupeol, β-sitosterol, benzoylinesolone, and benzoylisolinelone, and flavanols such as quercetin-3-rutinoside. Leaves possess mudarine (principal active constituent), a bitter resin, and three toxic glycosides calotropin, uscharin and calotoxin. The milky latex contains powerful bacteriolytic enzyme, toxic glycoside calactin, calotropin D I, calotropin D II, calotropin F I, calotropin F II, and nontoxic proteolytic enzyme calotropin (Quazi et al 2013).

Identity, Purity, and Strength

- Foreign matter: Not more than 2%
- Total ash: Not more than 4%
- Acid-insoluble ash: Not more than 1%
- Alcohol-soluble extractive: Not less than 2%
- Water-soluble extractive: Not less than 8%

(Source: The Ayurvedic Pharmacopeia of India 1989)

Karma (Actions)

In Ayurveda classics, Arkadvaya is described as Sara, Kushtaghna, Krimighna, Vishaghna, Deepan, Sothahara, Malashodhak, Bhootaghna, and Medohara.

- Arka mooltwak: Ushna, vamaka, swedan

- Arka pushpa: Madhur, tikta, kusthghna, krimighna, vishaghna, sangrahi
- Alarka pushpa: Vrishya, laghu, deepan, pachan
- Arka ksheer: Tikta, ushna, snigdh, lavan, laghu, shrestha virechan
- Arka kshar: Virekashrastha, kusthaghna
- Doshakarma: Kaphavatashamaka, pittavardhaka
- Dhatukarma: Medohara
- Malakarma: Sarak

Pharmacological Actions

C. procera is reported to have purgative, anthelmintic, anticoagulant, anticancer, antipyretic, analgesic (Sharma et al 2012; Basu and Chaudhuri 1991), antifertility, antitumor, anti-inflammatory, antiarthritic, anticonvulsant, antidiarrheal, antimalarial (Quazi et al 2013) and hypoglycemic activity (Singh et al 2014). Its latex exhibits analgesic, wound-healing with larvicidal activity (Choedon et al 2006). Leaves show potential antioxidant and antibacterial activity.

Root bark, leaves, latex, and ash of *C. gigantea* exhibit hepatoprotective, anticancer, antifertility, antidiarrheal, diuretic, antimicrobial, anthelmintic, and anti-inflammatory activity (Gupta and Sharma 2007).

C. gigantea exhibits anticancer properties due to the presence of cardiac glycosides (Bhat and Sharma 2013).

Indications

In various classical texts different parts of Arka are indicated in many diseases, which are mentioned as follows:

- Arka mool: shotha, vrana, kandu, kustha, krimi, mutrakricchta, medoroga, pleeha, gulma, arsha, udarroga, shakrit krimi
- Arka mooltwak: shwasa and phirangroga
- Alarka pushpa: aruchi, shwasa, kasa, praseka, arsha
- Arka pushpa: kustha, krimi, akhu visha (Rat poison), raktapitta, gulma, shotha
- Arka ksheer: kustha, gulma, udararoga and for inducing vaman and virechan in chronic diseases
- Arka kshar: gulma, udararoga, alarkavisha

Properties of Arka and Its Types in Various Nighantu

Nighantu	Arka	Shwetarka	Rajarka/Alarka	Shweta mandar
Dhanvantari	Katu, ushna, deepan, sar, vatahara	–	Katu, tikta, ushna, medohar, vishaghna, kapha vatahara	–
Kaidev	Tikta, ushna, sar, vatakapha shamak	–	Same as arka	–
Raj	Katu, ushna, vatashamaka, deepan, shothahar	Katu, tikta, ushna, malashodhaka	Katu, tikta, ushna, kapha vata har, medohar, vishaghna	Tikta, atyant ushna, malashodhaka
Madanpal and Bhavaprakash	Sara, kapha vatashamak	Same as Raktarka	–	–

Indications of Arka and Its Types in Various Nighantus

Nighantu	Arka	Shwetarka	Rajarka/Alarka	Shweta mandar
Dhanvantari	Sopha, vrana, kandu, kustha, pleeha, krimi	–	Kustha, vrana, sopha, kandu, visarpa	–
Kaiyadev	Krimi, kustha, vrana, arsha, pleeha, gulma, visha, Graha, rakta vikara	–	Same as arka	–
Raj	Vrana, kandu, kustha, krimi roga	Mutrakricchta, rakta vikara, vrana, sopha, shool	kustha, vrana, sopha, kandu, visarpa	Mutrakricchta, vrana, daruna krimiroga
Madanpal and Bhavaprakash	Kandu, kustha, visha vrana, krimi, gulma, pleeha, arsha, udarroga	Same as Raktarka	–	–

Besides these uses, different parts of Arka are extensively used in folklore. Extract of root is taken orally by tribal women in dysmenorrhea (Showkat 2007). The root powder is mixed with butter and the obtained ointment is applied to rabid dog bites and paralyzed limbs (Sharma and Kumar 2011). The stem is used as a toothbrush in toothache (Jain et al 2007). Dried powdered leaves are dusted over wounds, ulcers, and old sores (Khirstova and Tissot 1995). The paste of leaves and flowers mixed with honey is applied topically in migraine (Maliya 2007). Fresh latex is applied on facial black scars, boils, ear ache, eczema, skin eruptions, inflammatory lesions, painful affections, rheumatism, syphilis, leprosy, edema, piles, toothache, etc. (Kew 1985).

Therapeutic Uses

External Use

1. **Vranaachadana** (covering on wounds): Its leaves are used to cover the wounds as bandage (C.S.Ci. 13).
2. **Arsha** (piles): Dhoopan of Arkamool and Shamipatra is used to reduce inflammation and pain in Arsha (C.S.Ci. 14/49). Paste prepared from Arka ksheer, Snuhi kanda, tender leaves of Katukalabu, Karanj, and Avimutra (goat's urine) is an excellent remedy for Arsha (C.S.Ci. 14/57).
3. **Kustha** (skin diseases): Boil few Arka leaves in water, make a paste, add haridra paste and mustard oil to it.

Applying this poultice on the affected area in kustha, kacchu, pama, and vicharchika gives immediate relief (VM kusthadhikar 136).

4. **Gandmala** (cervical lymphadenitis): Paste prepared by mixing Arka kshar, Japa pushpa, taila, and Laksha rasa applied to the affected part for seven days destroys gandmala (RM 5.30).

5. **Shilipada** (filariasis) and **vriddhiroga** (hernia): A paste is prepared by mixing Arkamulatwak with Kanji. This paste is applied locally on inflamed areas in shilipada and vriddhiroga (V.M. 42.3) (C.D. 40.21).

6. **Danta krimi** (dental caries): Arka ksheer (latex of Arka) or paste prepared by mixing Saptaparna bark and Arka ksheer is filled in the tooth to get relief in caries-induced pain (A.H.U. 22/20).

7. **Vrischikdansa** (scorpion bite)**:** First make a slight cut on the bitten area; after the impure blood wipes out, apply Arka ksheer over the bitten area (G.N.7.5.1. p. 659).

8. **Mukhakrishnata** (black spots on face)**:** Paste prepared by mixing equal amounts of Haridra churna and Arka ksheer when applied daily on face reduces black spots (B.S. Kshudraroga/54).

9. **Karnashool** (earache): Yellow and fully matured leaves of Arka are smeared with ghee and boiled for a few minutes. Then a few drops of extracted juice are instilled in the ear (VM. 59.12 and SG. 3.11.132).

10. **Garbhapata** (abortion): The paste of leaves or Arka ksheer is inserted in the cervix, which causes labor pains and induces abortion.

Internal Use

1. **Pleeharoga** (splenomegaly): Arka leaves are processed with saindhava lavana in fire and a medicine known as Arkalavana is prepared. Daily intake of this powder with Takra cures all types of Udar and Pleeharoga (V.M. 37/43).

2. **Kustha** (skin diseases): Intake of decoction of Nimba, Arka, Alarka, and Saptaparna is beneficial in skin diseases (S.S.Ci. 9/51).

3. **Vishuchika** (cholera): Shade dried root bark of Arka is pounded with Nimbu juice and made into pills. These pills are taken twice a day to alleviate vishuchika caused by kapha and vata (S.B. 4.278).

4. **Shwasa** (asthma): Yava fruits are processed with leaf juice of Arka. Eating these processed yava with honey for a long period gives relief in shwasa (S.S.U. 51/36-37).

5. **Timir roga** (eye disease): Daily intake of milk prepared with boiling Arka seeds in it improves vision loss in timira (B.S.netra 43).

Officinal Parts Used

Root, root bark, leaf, flower, latex

Dose

Root bark: 0.5 to 1 g
Latex: 250 to 750 mg
Flower: 1 to 3 g

Formulations

Arkalavana, Arkadi churna, Arkakolakandadi vati, Arka taila, Arka kshara, Arkeshwara rasa, Arkvati.

Toxicity/Adverse Effects

On topical application, the latex is reported to cause redness, blisters, lesions, and eruptions on skin. If it enters into the eye, it produces sudden dimness or loss of vision with photophobia. Oral intake in large doses will produce mucosal irritation; burning pain in mouth, throat, and stomach followed by salivation, stomatitis, vomiting, diarrhea, dilated pupils, tremors, vertigo, tetanic convulsion, collapse, and death. Sometimes delirium may occur. The fatal period varies from 0.5 to 8 hours (Modi 2007; Dole 2004).

Remedial Measures

1. Oral intake of the Amlika (tamarind) leaf juice or medicated water prepared with Gairika as an antidote.
2. Cow's ghee is given as an antidote for internal use.
3. Milk and ghee are recommended in the diet.
4. Gastric lavage followed with demulcent drink should be administered.
5. Activated charcoal should be administered.
6. Atropine, chloroform, and amyle nitrate are antidotes.
7. Supportive and symptomatic measures are to be followed (Shekar 2014; Namburi 2010).

Substitution and Adulteration

Shwetarka and Raktarka are used as substitutes for one another.

Points to Ponder

- *Calotropis with red flower is known as Arka (C. procera L.) and the one with white flowers is called Alarka (C. gigantea L.).*
- *Arka ksheer is primarily used for kustha, gulma, and udararoga, and is considered as one of the best drugs for virechana karma.*
- *The properties of both Arkas are similar and can be used as a substitute to each other.*

Suggested Readings

Basu A, Chaudhuri AK. Preliminary studies on the antiinflammatory and analgesic activities of *Calotropis procera* root extract. J Ethnopharmacol 1991;31(3):319–324

Bhat KS, Sharma A. Therapeutic potential of cardiac glycosides of *Calotropis gigantea* for breast cancer. Int Res J Pharm 2013;4(6):164–167

Brischweiler F, St6ckel K, Reichstein T. Calotropis- Glykoside, vermutliche Teilstruktur, Glykoside und Aglykone, 321. Helv Chim Acta 1969;52:2276–2303

Choedon T, Mathan G, Arya S, Kumar VL, Kumar V. Anticancer and cytotoxic properties of the latex of *Calotropis procera* in a transgenic mouse model of hepatocellular carcinoma. World J Gastroenterol 2006;12(16):2517–2522

Crout DHG, Curtis RF, Hassall CH. 347. Cardenolides. The constitution of calactinic acid. J Am Chem Soc: Part V 1963;1866–1875

Dole AV. Rasashastra. 1st ed. Varanasi: Chaukhamba Sanskrit Pratishthan; 2004:425–423

Gaur LB, Bornare SS, Chavan AS, et al. Biological activities and medicinal properties of Madar (*Calotropis gigantean R.Br*). Punarna V 2013;1(1):11–19

Gupta AK, Sharma M. Review on Indian medicinal plants. ICMR 2007;5:157–190

Gupta AK, Sharma M. Reviews on Indian Medicinal Plants. Vol.5. New Delhi: Indian Council of Medical Research; 2007:157–190

Habib MR, Nikkon F, Rahman M, Haque ME, Karim MR. Isolation of stigmasterol and β-sitosterol from methanolic extract of root bark of *Calotropis gigantea* (Linn). Pak J Biol Sci 2007;10(22):4174–4176

Jain A, Katewa SS, Galav PK, Nag A. Unrecorded ethnomedicinal uses of biodiversity from Tadgarh Raoli wildlife sanctuary, Rajasthan, India. Yunnan Zhi Wu Yan Jiu 2007;29(3):337–344

Kew F. The Useful Plants of West Tropical Africa. In: Burkill HM, ed., Vol. 1. Families A-D Edition 2. Richmond, England: Royal Botanical Gardens; 1985:219–222

Khirstova P, Tissot M. Soda anthroqinone pulping of *Hibiscus sabdariffa* (Karkadeh) and *C. procera* from Sudan. Bioresour Technol 1995;53:672–677

Kupchan SM, Knox JR, Kelsey JE, Saenzrenauld JA. Calotropin, a cytotoxic principle isolated from Asclepias curassavica L. Science 1964;146(3652):1685–1686

Maliya SD. Traditional fruit and leaf therapy among Tharus and indigenous people of district Bahraich, India. Ethnobotany 2007;19:131–133

Modi PJ. A textbook of Medical Jurisprudence and Toxicology. 23rd ed. First Reprint New Delhi: Lexis Nexis Publication; 2007:467

Murti PBR, Seshadri TR. Chemical composition of *Calotropis gigantea*: Part 1. Wax and resin components of the latex. Proc Indiana Acad Sci 1943;18:145–159

Murti PBR, Seshadri TR. Chemical composition of *Calotropis gigantea*: Part V. Further examination of the latex and root bark. Proc Indiana Acad Sci 1945;21:143–147

Murti PBR, Seshadri TR. Chemical composition of *Calotropis gigantean*. Part II. Wax and resin components of the stem bark. Proc Indiana Acad Sci 1944;21(1):8–18

Namburi R.U.S. Agada Tantra. Varanasi: Chaukhabbha Sanskrit Sansthan; 2010:115

Perwez A, Mohammad A. Phytochemical investigation of *Calotropis procer* roots. Indian J Chem 2009;48B(3):443–446

Quazi S, Mathur K, Arora S. *Calotropis procera*: an overview of its phytochemistry and pharmacology. Ind J Drugs 2013;1(2):63–69

Reddy PS. Rasashastra. 1st ed. Varanasi: Chakhamba Orientalia; 2014:436

Sen S, Sahu NP, Mahato SB. Flavonol glycosides from *Calotropis gigantea*. Phytochemistry 1992;31(8):2919–2921

Shanker A. Hand Book of Poisoning. 2nd ed. Bhalani Publishing House; 2005:736

Sharma H, Kumar Ashwini. Ethnobotanical studies on medicinal plants of Rajasthan (India): A review. J Med Plants Res 2011;5(7):1107–1112.

Sharma PC, Yelna MB, Dennis TJ. Database of Medicinal Plants Used in Ayurveda. Vol. 2. CCRAS; 2001:69

Sharma R, Thakur GS, Sanodiya BS, et al. Therapeutic potential of *Calotropis procera*: a giant milkweed. J Pharm Biol Sci 2012; 4(2):42–57

Singh K, Rao CV, Hussain Z, Pahuja R. Evaluation of in-vivo antioxidant and oral glucose tolerance test of ethanolic extract of *Calotropis gigantea* Linn. against streptozotocin-induced diabetic rats. J Pharmacogn Phytochem 2014;2(5):59–65

The Ayurvedic Pharmacopeia of India. Part I, Vol. 1, 1st ed. New Delhi: Ministry of Health and Family Welfare, Government of India; 1989:8–10

Verma R, Satsangi GP, Shrivastava JN. Ethnomedicinal profile of different plant parts of *Calotropis procera(Ait.)*. R.Br. Ethnobotan Leafl 2010;14:721–742

Singh B, Rastogi RP. Structure of asclepin and some observations on the NMR spectra of Calotropis glycosides. Phytochemistry 1972;11(2):757–762

क्षीरमर्कस्य विशेषे वमने सविरेचने ।

—च. सू. १/115

अर्कद्वयंसरंवातकुष्ठकण्डूविषव्रणान्।
निहन्तिप्लीहगुल्मार्शःश्लेष्मोदरशकृत्कृमीन्।।६१।।
अलर्ककुसुमंवृष्यंलघुदीपनपाचनम्।
अरोचकप्रसेकार्शःकासश्वासनिवारणम्।।६२।।
रक्तार्कपुष्पंमधुरंसतिक्तंकुष्ठक्रिमिघ्नंकफनाशनंच।
अर्शोविषंहन्तिचरक्तपित्तंसंग्राहिगुल्मेश्वयथौहि
तंतत्।।६३।।
क्षीरमर्कस्यतिक्ष्णंस्निग्धंसलवणंलघु।
कुष्ठगुम्लोदरहरं श्रेष्ठमेतद्विरेचनम्।।६४।।

—भा.प्र.नि. गुडूच्यादिवर्ग

10. Ashwagandha *[Withania somnifera (Linn.) Dunal]*

Family:	*Solanaceae*
Hindi name:	*Asgand, Asgandh*
English name:	*Winter cherry*

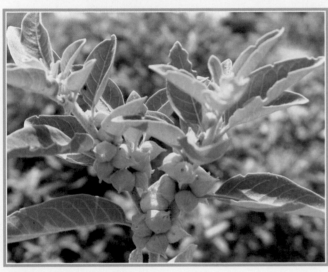

Plant of *Withania somnifera* Linn.

> *It is popularly known as "Indian Ginseng" due to its widespread use in therapeutics.*

Introduction

Aswagandha is a commonly used herb in Indian system of medicine. The root of the plant smells like horse (*ashwa*); hence, it is called Ashwagandha. It provides sexual power to man like a horse. In classical texts of Ayurveda, this plant is named after a horse, for example, Hayahwaya, Vajigandha, Vajinama, etc.

Linnaeus first described this plant as *Physalis somnifera* in 1753. In *Flora of Australia* (Purdie et al 1982:184), it is stated that the genus *Withania* is named after Henry Witham (sic.), an English paleobotanist of the early 19th century. However, the spelling of the name Withania is conserved under the rules of the International Code of Botanical Nomenclature. The species name somnifera means sleep-bearing/sleep-inducer in Latin, which probably refers to its use against stress, anxiety, and insomnia.

Description of Ashwagandha is not found in Vedic literature. It was elaborately described during the Samhita period. Almost all Samhita and chikitsa granthas of Ayurveda have mentioned various therapeutic uses of Aswagandha for external and internal use. Synonyms, properties, and actions are found in all Nighantus.

Vernacular Names

Assamese: Ashvagandha

Bengali: Ashvagandha

Gujarati: Asgandha

Kannada: Angarberu, Hiremaddina-gida

Kashmiri: Asagandh

Malayalam: Amukkuram

Marathi: Asagandha, Askagandha

Oriya: Aswagandha

Punjabi: Asgandh

Sanskrit: Hayagandha, Vajigandha

Tamil: Amukkaramkizangu

Telugu: Pennerugadda

Urdu: Asgand

Synonyms

Aswagandha: It promotes sexual potency like a horse.

Aswakanda: Roots of this plant emit horse-like smell.

Aswavarohaka: It promotes sexual potency like a horse.

Balada: It gives physical strength.

Balya: It provides physical strength.

Gandhapatri: Leaves of this plant also smell like a horse.

Gokarna: Leaves resemble the ear of a cow.

Hayahwaya: It is famous by the name of horse

Kamaroopini: It promotes complexion.

Kanchuka: It retains semen and provides complexion.

Kusthgandhini: It is useful in kustha.

Marutaghni: It cures vatika disorders.

Putrada: It provides male progeny.

Vajigandha: It smells like a horse.

Vajikari: It has aphrodisiac properties.

Vajinama: It is famous by the name of horse.

Vanaja: It grows wildly.

Varada: It acts as a blessing for patients.

Varahakarni: Leaves of this plant resemble the ear of pig.

Vataghni: It pacifies aggravated vata dosha.

Vrisya: It promotes sexual potency like a horse.

Classical Categorization

Charak Samhita: Balya, Brimhaniya, Virechanopaga, Madhura skanda

Sushruta Samhita: Virechanopaga, Urdhwabhaghara dravya

Astanga Sangraha: Madhur skandha

Astanga Hridaya: Madhur varga

Dhanwantari Nighantu: Guduchyadi varga

Madanpal Nighantu: Abhayadi varga

Kaiyadev Nighantu: Oushadhi varga

Raj Nighantu: Shatahwadi varga

Bhavprakash Nighantu: Guduchyadi varga

Distribution

It grows wildly in dry and hot-semiarid climate such as southern Mediterranean region, Canary Islands, and northern Africa to northern India (Iran, Jordan, Sudan, Palestine, Afghanistan, and Egypt; Biswas et al 2015; Kumar et al 2015). It is found throughout the drier part of India both in waste places and in cultivated form in areas of upper Gangetic plain, West Bengal, Bihar, Odisha, Gujarat, Konkan, Deccan, Karnataka, and Coimbatore.

Morphology

It is an erect, evergreen, tomentose shrub of 30 to 150 cm in height. Stem is green and somewhat zigzag in shape, with minute soft hair.

- **Leaves:** Simple, short petiole, alternate, or in subopposite pairs at a node, exstipulate, ovate, acute apex, entire margin, tomentose, and grayish green in color (**Fig. 10.1**).
- **Flowers:** Solitary, greenish yellow arranged in axillary fascicles, sessile, or shortly pedicelled (**Fig. 10.2a, b**).
- **Fruits:** Small globose berries, green when unripe, and orange colored when mature, enclosed in a persistent, light brown–colored membranous calyx (**Fig. 10.3**).
- **Seeds:** Yellow, reniform.
- **Roots:** The fleshy roots are conical and creamish white in color (**Fig. 10.4a**). Dried roots are cylindrical, gradually tapering down. Its outer surface is brownish white and starchy white inside. It can easily break into pieces (**Fig. 10.4b**).

This plant is propagated through seeds.

Phenology

Flowering time: March to April

Fruiting time: Throughout the year

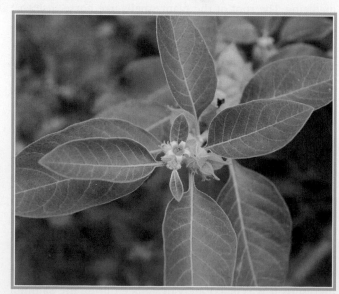

Fig. 10.1 Leaves.

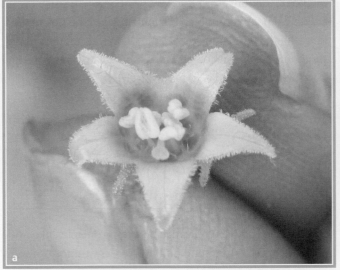

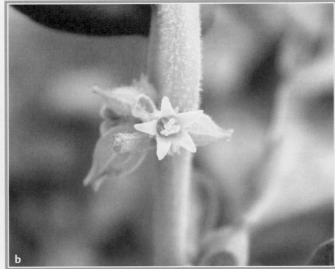

Fig. 10.2 **(a)** Flower. **(b)** Position of flower on the stem.

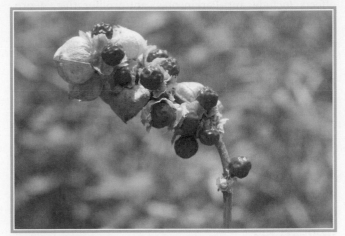

Fig. 10.3 Fruits.

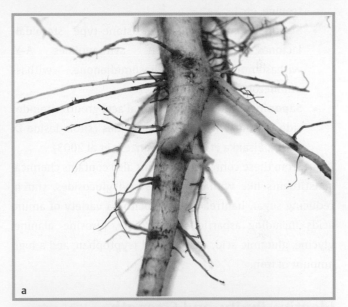

Key Characters for Identification

➤ *Erect, evergreen shrub with 30 to 150 cm height*
➤ *Simple, alternate, short petioled ovate leaf*
➤ *Solitary, greenish yellow color flower*
➤ *Small, globose, orange-red berries covered in a membranous calyx*
➤ *Conical creamy white root*

Types

There are two varieties of Ashwagandha, viz. *Withania somnifera* Dunal and *Withania ashwagandha*. Among both, *W. somnifera* D. is the wild variety, found in forests, and *W. ashwagandha* is the cultivated variety (Vaidya et al 2009).

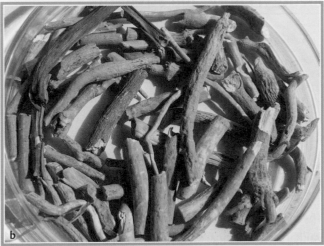

Fig. 10.4 Ashwagandha root. **(a)** Fresh. **(b)** Dried.

A book titled *Unani Dravya Gunadarsha* mentioned that the wild variety of Ashwagandha is used externally in the form of lepa.

Rasapanchaka

Guna	Laghu, Snigdha
Rasa	Madhura, Tikta, Kasaya
Vipaka	Madhura
Virya	Ushna

Chemical Constituents

- **Alkaloids:** ashwagandhine, cuscohygrine, anahygrine, tropine, etc.
- **Steroidal compounds:** ergostane-type steroidallactones, withaferin A, withanolides A-Y, withasomniferin-A, withasomidienone, withasomniferols A-C, withanone, etc.
- **Saponins:** contain an additional acyl group (sitoindoside VII and VIII), and withanolides (sitoindoside IX and X; Elsakka et al 1990; Ganzera et al 2003).

Apart from these contents, the plant also contains chemical constituents like withaniol, acylsteryl glucosides, starch, reducing sugar, hantreacotane, ducitol, a variety of amino acids including aspartic acid, proline, tyrosine, alanine, glycine, glutamic acid, cystine, and tryptophan, and a high amount of iron.

Identity, Purity, and Strength

- Foreign matter: Not more than 2%
- Total ash: Not more than 7%
- Acid-insoluble ash: Not more than 1%
- Alcohol-soluble extractive: Not less than 15% (25%)
- Water-soluble extractive: Nil

(Source: The Ayurvedic Pharmacopeia of India 1989)

Karma (Actions)

The main actions of this drug are balya, brimhniya, rasayana, vajikara, shothaghna, kantiprada, pustikaraka, kanti veerya balaprada, etc.

Other actions are vedanasthapana, mastishkashamaka, deepana, anulomana, shoolaprashmana, krimighna, raktashodhaka, kaphaghna, shwasahara, garbhashayashothahara, yonishoolahara, mootrala, kushthaghna (Sharma et al 2001).

- Doshakarma: Kaphavatashamaka
- Dhatukarma: Balya, brimhaniya, vrisya, and atishukrala
- Malakarma: Mutrala, anulomana

Pharmacological Actions

It is reported to have pharmacological properties like anti-inflammatory, immunomodulatory, antitumor, neuropharmacological, antibiotic, anticancer, chemoprotective, and hepatoprotective (Halder and Ghosh 2015). Other effects include anti-Parkinson's, antiproliferative, neuroprotective, hypoglycemic, and hypolipidemic, antifungal, cardioprotective, antistress, anticatalepsy, antibacterial, anticonvulsant, antimalarial, herbicidal, gamma-aminobutyric acid mimetic activity (Vyas et al 2011), nephroprotective, and nephrocurative (Kushwaha et al 2016), antiaging, antioxidant, hemopoetic, rejuvenating, adaptogenic, tonic, and aphrodisiac.

Most of pharmacological activities of Aswagandha have been attributed to two main withanolides: withaferin A and withanolide D.

Indications

It is indicated in shotha, shopha, kshaya, kshata, daurbalya, vataroga, klaibya, kasa, shwasa, vrana, visha, kandu, switra, and krimi.

It is also useful in galaganda, granthishotha, urustambha, murchchha, bhrama, anidra, udaravikara, raktabharadhikya, raktavikara, shukradaurbalya, pradara, yonishoola, mootraghata, kushtha, balashosha, and shosha (Sharma et al 2001).

It is commonly used in emaciation of children (when given with milk, it is considered as the best tonic for children), and debility from old age, rheumatism, vitiated conditions of vata, leucoderma, constipation, insomnia, nervous breakdown, goiter, etc. (Sharma 1999).

It helps in conditions like chronic fatigue, weakness, dehydration, bone weakness, loose teeth, thirst, impotency, premature ageing, and emaciation (Mishra et al 2000). It is famous to cure impotency and increase sex appeal and fertility when used solitarily or in combination with other medications (Mahdi et al 2011; Sharma et al 2011).

It is used to improve endurance, strength, and general health, and to produce mild sedation. It is also potentially useful in anxiety (Nadkarni 1976). Moreover, it is beneficial in arthritis and other musculoskeletal disorders, stress-induced nervous exhaustion, and hypertension.

Therapeutic Uses

External Use

1. **Granthivisarpa** (type of erysipelas): Warm paste of Aswagandha is applied externally on the affected part (C.S.Ci. 21/123).
2. **Urusthambha** (stiffness of thigh): Aswagandha root powder mixed with honey, mustard oil, and anthill earth, and applied locally as paste in urusthambha (C.S.Ci. 27/50-51).
3. **Kustha** (skin diseases): Paste of roots and bruised leaves are applied to carbuncles, ulcers, and painful swellings (Kritikar and Basu 1935). Paste of root is applied locally to reduce the inflammation at the joints (Bhandari 1970).

Internal Use

1. **Kshaya** (consumption): The powder of Ashwagandha, Tila, and Masha is taken with goat's ghee and honey (SS.U. 41/40).
2. **Balashosha** (emaciation): Ghee processed with one-fourth paste of Aswagandha and 10 times milk is given to emaciated children for promotion of body mass (VM. 67/9).
3. **Rasayana** (rejuvinator): Aswagandha mixed with milk, ghee, and oil taken with warm water for 15 days helps to increase body mass and acts as rasayana (AH.U. 39/158). Mandukparni, Shankhapushpi, Ashwagandha, and Shatavari should be used in order to promote intellect, life span, stability, and strength (AH.U. 39/61).
4. **Shwasa** (asthma): The alkali (ash) of Aswagandha should be taken with honey and ghee (C.S.Ci. 17/117 and AH.Ci. 4/38).
5. **Nidranasha** (insomnia): The powder of Aswagandha mixed with sugar and taken with ghee cures insomnia and brings sleep soon (BS.jaladoshadi. 13).
6. **Bandhatva** (infertility): Milk processed with Aswagandha should be taken with ghee by women in proper time for conception (VM. 14/10; BP Chi 70/26).

7. **Vatavyadhi** (neuromuscular disease): Aswagandha ghrita prepared with the paste and decoction of Aswagandha root, four parts milk, and ghee is given twice daily in all types of vatavyadhi. It also promotes aphrodisiac activity and enhances muscle power (VM. 22/73).

Officinal Parts Used

Root, leaves, fruit

Dose

Powder 3 to 6 g

Formulations

Ashwagandha churna, Ashwagandha ghrita, Brihat Ashwagandha ghrita, Ashwagandharishta, Ashwagandhadi leha, Bala Ashwagandha lakshadi taila, Ashwagandha rasayana, Ashwagandha taila, Madhyamanarayana taila, Brihat Chhagaladyadi ghrita, Saraswata churna, Pramehamihira taila, Nagabala ghrita, Madhusnuhi-rasayana, Trayodashanga guggulu, Phala ghrita, Kasisadi taila.

Toxicity/Adverse Effects

Purified aswagandha extract is nontoxic up to 2,000 mg/kg by weight in rats as shown in acute and subchronic toxicity studies. (at the dosage level of 1,000 mg/kg for 90 days to rats) as per Organisation for Economic Co-operation and Development guidelines (Antony et al 2018).

The activity of *W. somnifera* extract was approximately equal to the *Panax ginseng* extract in a rat model of chronic stress without any side effects (Bhattacharya et al 2003). No adverse events were reported with the use of up to 3 g of *W. somnifera* extract tablets for a period of 1 year in human beings (Kuppurajan et al 1980).

Substitution and Adulteration

Ashwagandha is used as a substitute for Kakoli and Kshirakakoli of Ashtavarga (BPN, Haritakyadivarga/144).

W. somnifera L. Dunal is often adulterated with *W. coagulans* (Bhattacharya et al 1997).

Points to Ponder

- *Aswagandha has balya brimhana, rasayan, and vajikaran properties.*
- *It has aphrodisiac, immunomodulatory, antioxidant, antitumor, antiaging, antistress, rejuvenating, and adaptogenic effects.*
- *It is mainly indicated in male infertility, insomnia, anxiety, and stress, weakness, and arthritis.*

Suggested Readings

Antony B, Benny M, Kuruvilla BT, Gupta NK, Sebastian A, Jacob S. Acute and sub chronic toxicity studies of purified *Withania somnifera* extract in rats. Int J Pharm Sci 2018;10(12):41–46

Bhandari CR. Ashwagandha (*Withania somnifera*) "Vanaushadhi Chandroday" (An Encyclopedia of Indian Herbs), Vol. 1. Varanasi: CS Series of Varanasi Vidyavilas Press; 1970:96–97

Bhattacharya SK, Muruganandam AV. Adaptogenic activity of *Withania somnifera*: an experimental study using a rat model of chronic stress. Pharmacol Biochem Behav 2003;75(3):547–555

Bhattacharya SK, Satyan KS, Chakrabarti A. Effect of Trasina, an Ayurvedic herbal formulation, on pancreatic islet superoxide dismutase activity in hyperglycaemic rats. Ind J Exp Biol 1997; 35(3):297–299

Biswas TK, Pandit S, Jana U. In search of spermatogenetic and virility potential drugs of Ayurvedic leads: a review. Andrology (Los Angel) 2015;04(02):1–4

Davis L, Kuttan G. Immunomodulatory activity of *Withania somnifera*. J Ethnopharmacol 2000; 71(1-2):193–200

Elsakka M, Grigorescu E, Stănescu U, Stănescu U, Dorneanu V. New data referring to chemistry of *Withania somnifera* species. Rev Med Chir Soc Med Nat Iasi 1990;94(2):385–387

Ganzera M, Choudhary MI, Khan IA. Quantitative HPLC analysis of withanolides in *Withania somnifera*. Fitoterapia 2003;74(1-2): 68–76

Halder T, Ghosh B. Phytochemical and pharmacological activity of *Withania somnifera* (L.) Dunal. Int J Econ Plant 2015;2(4):192–196

Kritikar KR, Basu BD. *Withania somnifera*, Indian Medicinal Plants. 2nd ed. IIIrd. Allahabad: Lalit Mohan Basu; 1935:1774–1776

Kumar A, Kumar R, Rahman MS, et al. Phytoremedial effect of *Withania somnifera* against arsenic-induced testicular toxicity in Charles Foster rats. Avicenna J Phytomed 2015;5(4):355–364

Kuppurajan K, Rajagopalan SS, Sitoraman R, et al. Effect of Ashwagandha (*Withania somnifera* Dunal) on the process of ageing on human volunteers. J Res Ayurv Siddha 1980;1(2):247–258

Kushwaha V, Sharma M, Vishwakarma P, Saini M, Saxena K. Biochemical assessment of nephroprotective and nephrocurative activity of *Withania somnifera* on gentamicin induced nephrotoxicity in experimental rats. Int J Res Med Sci 2016;4(1):298–302

Mahdi AA, Shukla KK, Ahmad MK. *Withania somnifera* improves semen quality in stress-related male fertility. Evid Based Complement Alternat Med 2011;ArticleID576962, 9 pages

Mishra LC, Singh BB, Dagenais S. Scientific basis for the therapeutic use of *Withania somnifera* (ashwagandha): a review. Altern Med Rev 2000;5(4):334–346

Nadkarni KM. Indian Materia Medica. Bombay: Popular Prakashan Limited; 1976:1291

Purdie RW, Symon DE, Haegi L. Solanaceae. Flora of Australia 1982; 29:184

Sharma PC, Yelne MB, Dennis TJ. Database Medicinal Plants used in Ayurveda, Vol. 3. New Delhi: CCRAS; 2001:88–130

Sharma PV. Ashwagandha, Dravyaguna Vijana. Varanasi: Chaukhambha Vishwabharti; 1999:763–765

Sharma V, Sharma S, Pracheta, Paliwal R. *Withania somnifera*: a rejuvenating Ayurvedic medicinal herb for the treatment of various human ailments. Int J Pharm Tech Res 2011;3(1):187–192

The Ayurvedic Pharmacopeia of India. Part I, Vol. 1. New Delhi: Department of AYUSH, Ministry of Health and Family Welfare, Government of India; 1989:15–16

Vaidya BG, Adarsha N. Adarsha Nighantu. Vol. 2, Reprint. Varanasi: Chaukhambha Bharati Academy; 2009:134

Vyas VK, Bhandari P, Patidar R. A comprehensive review on *Withania somnifera* Dunal. J Nat Rem 2011;11(1):1–13

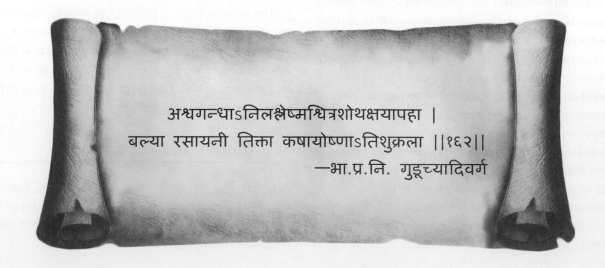

अश्वगन्धाऽनिलश्लेष्मश्चित्रशोथक्षयापहा ।
बल्या रसायनी तिक्ता कषायोष्णाऽतिशुक्रला ॥१६२॥
—भा.प्र.नि. गुडूच्यादिवर्ग

11. Ashok [*Saraca asoca* (Roxb.), De.wild]

Family:	*Fabaceae*
Hindi Name:	*Sita Ashok*
English Name:	*Ashok*

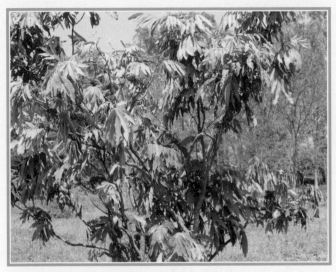
Plant of *Saraca asoca* (Roxb.), De.wild

To protect children from grief and sorrow, married women in North East India eat the flower buds of Ashok on the "Ashok Shasthi day."

Introduction

The word "Ashok" means "without sorrow," which gives no grief or which is capable of relieving the sorrow of people.

Ashok tree occupies a privileged place in classical Indian texts, folk medicine, and in sociocultural traditions since thousands of years. It is considered as one of the most legendary and sacred trees of India. It is considered as a symbol of love and is dedicated to Kamadeva (God of Love). It is believed that Gautama Siddhartha, founder of Buddhism, was born under the Ashok tree (Pradhan et al 2009). In Hindu mythology, Ashok tree is worshipped in Chaitra and is mentioned in the Ramayana in reference to the Ashok vatika where Sitaji lived during her exile period. Tribal women wear root pieces of Ashok as herbal rosary for mental tranquility (Singh et al 2015).

Ancient texts of Ayurveda, unani, siddha, and other systems of medicine clearly highlighted the use of Ashok in gynecological disorders along with many other health benefits. Charak described it as vedanasthapaka and stambhaka dravya. Sushruta used it in uterine disorders, fever, neurological complaints, snake bites, disease of the eye, and wounds. Vagbhatta mentioned the use of seeds in the treatment of cough. Chakradatta prescribed Ashok bark in excessive bleeding and seeds in urinary obstruction. *Gadanigraha* and Yogaratnakara advocated the use of Ashok bark in menorrhagia. Shaligram Nighantu cited its use to improve skin complexion as well as in treatment of abdominal pain, piles, abdominal complications, burning sensation, tumors, etc. (Biswas and Debnath 1972). Bhaisajya Ratnavali described its two popular formulations, i.e., Ashokghrita and Ashokarista. Ashok twak is also mentioned as an ingredient of muktadhyaavleha, pradarari rasa, and lakshmanaloha, and is prescribed in rakta pradar, shweta pradar, yonishool, kukshishool, bastishool, mutraroga, raktaatisaar, raktapitta, and raktarsha (B.R. 66/100-114).

Due to the extensive folklore and ethnomedicinal uses, the plant is becoming rarer in its natural habitat and is currently listed as a "globally vulnerable" species by the IUCN 2013.

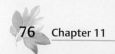
Vernacular Names

Assamese: Ashok
Bengali: Ashok
Gujarati: Ashok
Kannada: Ashokdamara, Ashokmara, Kankelimara, Akshth
Kashmiri: Ashok
Malayalam: Asokam
Marathi: Ashok, Jasundi
Oriya: Ashok, osoko
Punjabi: Asok
Tamil: Asogam, Asogu, Asokam
Telugu: Ashokpatta, Asokamu, Vanjulamu
Burmese: Thawgabo, Thawka
Sinhalese: Diyaratmal, Diyeratembela
Thai: Sokanam

Synonyms

Gandhapushpa: This plant has fragrant flowers.
Hemapushpa: Flowers are golden-yellow in color.
Kankeli: It gives pleasant feeling and has a krimighna action.
Madhupushpa: It bears flowers in spring season.
Pindapushpa: Flowers are borne in dense clusters.
Stripriya: It is useful in gynecological disorders.
Tamrapallava: Young leaves of this plant are copper colored.
Vanjula: It possesses sheet guna.

Classical Categorization

Charak Samhita: Vedanasthapana, Kasaya skanda
Sushrut Samhita: Rodhradi
Ashtanga Hridaya: Rodhradi
Dhanvantari Nighantu: Amradi varga
Kaiyadev Nighantu: Oushadhi varga
Raj Nighantu: Karaviradi varga
Bhavaprakash: Pushpa varga

Distribution

It is found throughout India up to an altitude of 750 m, especially in the foothills of central and eastern Himalayas, Western Ghats, Kerala, Bengal, and whole southern region. It is also cultivated in many gardens because of its decorative orange red flowers and evergreen beautiful foliage. It has become quite scarce in several areas and nowadays is reported to be a threatened species (Warrier et al 2000).

Morphology

A medium-sized evergreen tree of 6 to 8 m height with beautiful red flowers and copper-colored tender leaves.

- **Stem bark:** Dark brown or gray in color, and rough and uneven due to the presence of lenticels. Bark channeled, smooth with circular lenticels and transversely ridged, sometimes cracked. Fracture splinting exposing striated surface, a thin whitish and continuous layer is seen beneath the cork layer (**Fig. 11.1**).
- **Leaves:** Paripinnate compound leaves with four to six pairs of oblong or lanceolate-shaped leaflets, leaflets cork-like at the base, stipules short, intrapetiolar, and completely united (**Fig. 11.2**).
- **Flowers:** Polygamous apetalous, orange or orange-yellow, eventually turning vermillion, fragrant, found in dense axillary corymbs, bract small, deciduous, and calyx petaloid (**Fig. 11.3**).
- **Fruit:** Pods flat, linear-oblong, leathery, 10 to 25 cm long. Seeds four to eight, ellipsoid-oblong, compressed (**Fig. 11.4**).
- **Dried stem bark:** Channeled, outer surface is rusty brown, rough with warty protuberances and exfoliations (**Fig. 11.5**). Lenticels are conspicuous

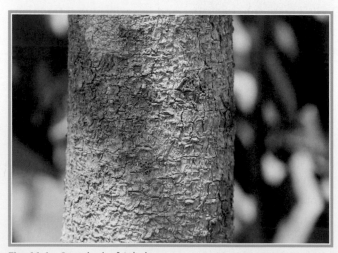

Fig. 11.1 Stem bark of Ashok.

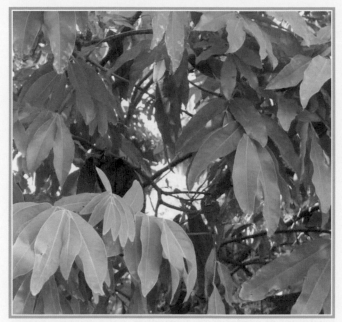

Fig. 11.2 Leaves.

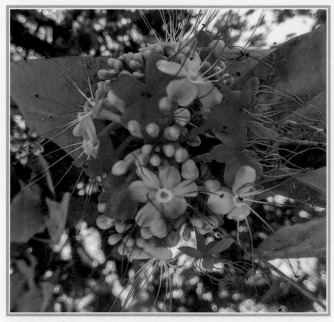

Fig. 11.3 Flowers.

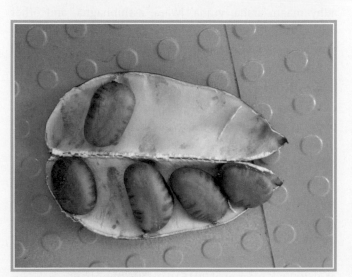

Fig. 11.4 Fruits with seeds.

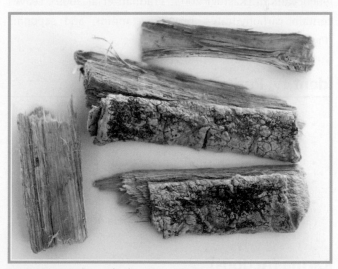

Fig. 11.5 Dried stem bark.

along with transverse and longitudinal cracks. The inner surface of the bark is reddish brown in color. The fracture is short and fibrous with indistinct odor and astringent taste (Ali et al 2008).

The plant is propagated by seeds.

Phenology

Flowering time: February to April

Fruiting time: May to July

Key Characters for Identification

➤ *A medium-sized evergreen tree. Bark is rough, rusty brown*

➤ *Leaves: paripinnate, leaflets four to six pairs, oblong to lanceolate*

➤ *Flowers: orange or orange-yellow in dense axillary corymbs*

➤ *Pods: flat, leathery, linear-oblong shaped*

Rasapanchaka

Guna	Laghu, Ruksha
Rasa	Kashaya, Tikta
Vipaka	Katu
Virya	Sheeta

Chemical Constituents

Bark contains tannins, catechin, epicatechin, catechol, glucosides, procynidine, leucopelargonidin, leucocyanidin esters, and primary alcohols. Flowers have β-sitosterol, quercetin, apigenin, gallic acid and kaempferol, pelargonidin-3, 5-diglucoside, cyanidin-3, 5-diglucoside, leucocyanidin, and gallic acid. Seeds and pods contain oleic, linoleic, palmitic and stearic acids, catechol, epicatechol, and leucocyanidin (Rastogi 2003; Pradhan et al 2009). Leaves contain carbohydrates, proteins, tannins, and saponins (Pradhan et al 2010).

Identity, Purity, and Strength

- Foreign matter: Not more than 2%
- Total ash: Not more than 11%
- Acid-insoluble ash: Not more than 1%
- Alcohol-soluble extractive: Not less than 15%
- Water-soluble extractive: Not less than 11%
(Source: The Ayurvedic Pharmacopeia of India 1989)

Karma (Actions)

In Ayurveda classics Ashok bark is described as stambhana (astringent), varnya, vishaghna, vranashodhaka, vranaropaka, hridya, krimighna, sandhaniya, sheet, snigdh, artavajanan, shonitsthapana, sothahara sugandhik dravya.
- Doshakarma: Kaphapittashamaka
- Dhatukarma: Raktasthambhak, artavasangrahniya (Sharma 2001)
- Malakarma: Stambhaka

Pharmacological Actions

The bark and flowers are reported to have antiestrogenic, anti-inflammatory, anti-implantation, antioxidant, spasmogenic, antitumor, oxytocic, antiprogestational, anti-menorrhagia, CNS depressant, analgesic and antipyretic, antimicrobial, anticancer (Pradhan et al 2009; Preeti et al 2012), anthelmintic (Sarojini et al 2011), larvicidal (Mathew et al 2009), and antiulcer activity (Maruthappan et al 2010). It also acts as a uterine stimulant, stomachic, febrifuge, blood purifier, refrigerant, and demulcent. Flowers are uterine tonic and seeds are diuretic.

Indications

In Ayurveda text, the bark of the plant is used in the treatment of pradar roga, ashrigdhar, daha, trishna, apachi, shotha, krimi, gulma, visha, udarshool, atisaar, prameha, adhyamaan, arsha, vrana, jwara, asthibhagna, and other diseases of pitta and rakta.

It is a very popular medicine in folklore for gynecological disorders, and the traditional healers used its bark as an emmenagogue in the treatment of uterine hemorrhage, dysmenorrhea, menorrhagia, leucorrhoea, amenorrhea, uterine fibroid, endometriosis, premenstrual syndrome, and threatened abortion (Mitra et al 1999). It also has stimulating effect on endometrium and the ovarian tissue. The extract of Ashok flower is useful in hemorrhoid, diabetes, cancer, and hemorrhagic dysentery and in uterine infections. Seeds are used for treating bone fracture, strangury, and vesicle calculi. Dried root is used in paralysis, hemiplegia, visceral numbness, and in healing broken bones and skin (Pradhan et al 2009; Kauser et al 2016).

Therapeutic Uses

External Use

1. **Mental peace:** For attaining mental peace and relaxation people are advised to take bath under the shade of Ashok tree or wear the herbal Maalaa (garland) using root pieces of Sita Ashok.

2. **Kushta** (skin diseases): Paste of roots and flowers is useful in freckles, discoloration, inflammations, ulcers, eczema, psoriasis, dermatitis, pruritis, scabies, tinea pedis, and skin diseases (Pradhan et al 2009).

Internal Use

1. **Ashrigdhara** (menorrhagia): Decoction of Ashok bark is taken with milk daily to control excessive bleeding during menstruation (C.D. 63.5).
2. **Mutraghaat** (urinary obstruction): Ashok seed powder with water is used in mutraghaat and ashmari (CD 33/12).
3. **Vatavyadhi** (neuromuscular diseases): Daily intake of Ashokghrita is prescribed in vatavyadhi (S.S.Ci. 4/27).
4. **Kasa** (cough): One should use ghrita processed with Ashok seeds, Vidang, Rasanjana, and Padmaka in kasa (A.H.Ci. 3/10).
5. **Prameha** (diabetes): Dried flower powder of Ashok is taken with milk or honey, and its bark decoction is taken twice a day for the treatment of prameha (Jayakumar et al 2010).
6. **Gynecological disorders:** To prevent themselves from gynecological disorders, the folk women of Chhattisgarh boil the bark of Ashok in cow's milk and consume it after adding sugar once a day for three days and repeat the course after three months (Pradhan et al 2009).
7. **Asthibhagna** (fracture): Bark decoction (40–80 mL) of Ashok is an effective remedy in treating bone fractures, rickets, delayed bone consolidation, and calcium deficiency (Pradhan et al 2009).
8. **Adhyaman** (gastralgia): Juice of its leaves mixed with cumin seed is used to cure gastralgia.

Officinal Parts Used

Bark, flowers, seeds

Dose

Bark decoction: 50 to 100 mL
Seed powder: 3 to 6 g
Flower powder: 3 to 6 g

Formulations

Ashokrishta, Ashok ghrita, Pradarari rasa, Kasisadi taila, Madhukadyavaleha, Devadarvyarishta, and Mahamarichyadi taila.

Toxicity/Adverse Effects

Toxicological evaluation of *Saraca indica* bark extracts indicates no toxicity or mortality (Yadav et al 2015).

Substitution and Adulteration

The barks of Kasthadaru (*Polyalthia longifolia* Benth. & Hook.), *Tecoma undulata*, *Bauhinia variegata* L., *Trema orientalis* L., *Afanamexis polystakis*, and *Sicalpinea pulchirena* are often adulterated with Ashok bark (Sharma 2001).

> **Points to Ponder**
> - *It is the drug of choice for gynecological disorders.*
> - *Due to its large-scale use and extensive destruction of natural habitat, Ashok is enlisted in vulnerable species.*

Suggested Readings

Ali M. Pharmacognosy. New Delhi: CBS Publishers & Distributors; 2008:668–669

Biswas TK, Debnath PK. Aśoka (Saraca indica Linn): a cultural and scientific evaluation. Indian J Hist Sci 1972;7(2):99–114

http://www.iucnredlist.org/apps/redlist/deta ils/34623/0

Jayakumar G, Ajthab*ai MD, Sreede*vi S, Vishwanathan PK, Rameshkumar B. Ethnobotanical survey of the plants used in the treatment of diabetes. Indian J Tradit Knowl 2010;9(1):100–104

Kauser AS, Hasan A, Parrey SA, Ahmad W. Ethnobotanical, phytochemical and pharmacological properties of Saraca asoca bark: a review. Eur J Pharm Med Res 2016;3(6):274–279

Maruthappan V, Sakthi Shree K. Anti-ulcer activity of aqueous suspension of Saraca indica flower against gastric ulcers in albino rats. J Pharm Res 2010;3(1):17–20

Mathew N, Anitha MG, Bala TS, Sivakumar SM, Narmadha R, Kalyanasundaram M. Larvicidal activity of Saraca indica, Nyctanthes arbor-tristis, and Clitoria ternatea extracts against three mosquito vector species. Parasitol Res 2009;104(5):1017–1025

Mitra SK, Gopumadhavan S, Venkatarganna MV, Sharma DNK, Anturlikar SI. Uterine tonic activity of U-3107 (Evecare): a herbal preparation in rats. Indian J Pharmacol 1999;31:200–203

Pradhan P, Joseph L, George M, Kaushik N, Chulet R. Pharmacognostic, phytochemical & quantitative investigation of *Saraca asoca* leaves. J Pharm Res 2010;3(1):776–780

Pradhan P, Joseph L, Gupta V, et al. *Saraca asoca* (Ashoka): a review. J Chem Pharm Res 2009;1(1):62–71

Preeti B, Bharti A, Sharma A, Singh V. A review on *Saraca indica* plant. Int Res J Pharm 2012;3(4):80–84

Rastogi VD. Pharmacognosy & Phytochemistry. Nashik: Career Publication; 2003:269–270

Sarojini *N, Manjari S*A, Kanti CC. Phytochemical screening and anthelmintic activity study of Saraca indica leaves extracts. Int Res J Pharm 2011;2(5):194–197

*Shar*ma PC, Yelna MB, Dennis TJ. Database of medicinal plants used in Ayurveda. CCRAS;2001;3:76

Sharma PV. Dravyaguna Vigyan, Vol. II. Varanasi: Chaukhambha Bharti Academy; 2001:618

Singh S, Krishna TH Anantha, Kamalraj Subban, Kuria*kose Gini C,* Valayil Jinu Mathew, Jayabaskaran Chelliah. Phytomedicinal importance of Saraca asoca (Ashoka): an exciting past, an emerging present and a promising future. Curr Sci 2015;109(10):1790–1825

The Ayurvedic Pharmacopoeia of India. Part I, Vol. 1. New Delhi: Department of AYUSH, Ministry of Family and Welfare of India, Government of India; 1989:Appendices

Warrier PK, Nambier VPK, Ganpathy PM. Some Important Medicinal Plants of the Western Ghats India: A Profile. New Delhi: International Development Research Centre; 2000:345–359

Yadav NK, Sain KS, Hussain Z, Omer A, Sharma C, Gayen R, Singh P, Arya KR, Singh RK. *Saraca indica* bark extract shows in vitro antioxidant, anti-breast cancer activity and does not exhibit toxicological effects. Oxidat Med Cell Longevity 2015;1–15

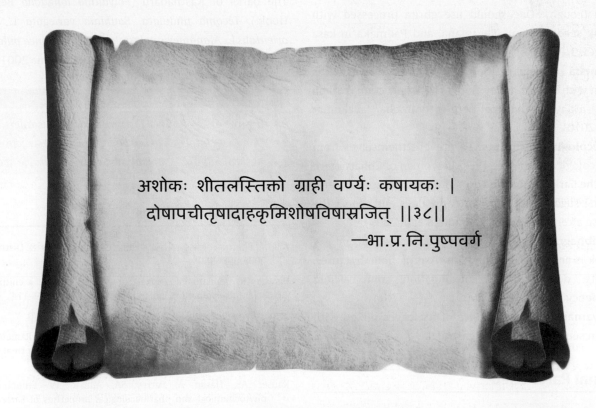

अशोकः शीतलस्तिक्तो ग्राही वर्ण्यः कषायकः |
दोषापचीतृषादाहकृमिशोषविषास्रजित् ||३८||

—भा.प्र.नि.पुष्पवर्ग

12. Ativisha [Aconitum heterophyllum Wall. Cat.]

Family:	*Ranunculaceae*
Hindi name:	*Atees*
English name:	*Indian Atees, Asian Monkshood*

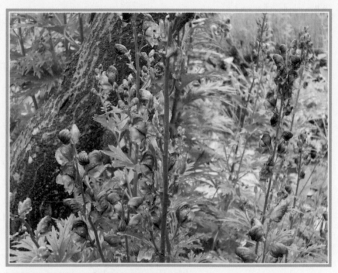

Plant of *Aconitum heterophyllum* Wall. Cat.

> *Most of the Aconitum species are highly toxic in nature and are known as devil's helmet, Queen of all poisons, or blue rocket.*

Introduction

The word "Ativisha" is derived from the phrase *Atikrantam visham*, which means to pacify the effect of visha (poison), though it belongs to the genus of poisonous plants.

There are about 300 species of Aconitum all over the world out of which only 24 species are found in India such as *A. napellus* Linn., *A. chasmanthum* Stapf. ex. Holmes, *A. ferox* Wall. ex Ser., *A. palmatum* D. Don, and *A. heterophyllum Wall.* ex Royle (Chopra and Chopra 2006). Most of the Aconitum species are toxic in nature but some are nonpoisonous too.

Ativisha is described in Vedas as *Ativishwa*, which means it can cure all the diseases of the world (vishwa). It is also mentioned in vidhiricha and its decoction is considered as the best drug for pralapa (Gopesh 2007). Charaka considered Ativisha as the best deepana, pachana, sangrahi, sarvadoshahar dravya (C.S.S. 25/40). Sushruta used it in the treatment of vriddhi, updansha, mudhgarbha, vrana, jwar, atisaar, mukharoga, and udavrat. It is also included in the group of trikarshika and chaturbhadra (D.N. Mishrakadi varga /7-8). In classical texts, Ativisha is categorized as an abhava dravya, and Musta is suggested as the pratinidhi dravya (substitute) for it (B. P. N. prastavana /165). Due to habitat loss, illegal collection, and marketing in wild, the species is under severe threat of extinction and is included in the critically endangered appendices of the Convention of International Trade in Endangered Species (CITES).

As it is an endangered species, the director general of foreign trade prohibits the export of Aconitum species of plants, plant portions, and their derivatives and extracts obtained from the wild (Zoo rules 1992). Cultivation has been undertaken in Chamoli, Pithoragarh, Milam (Munsiyari), Deoban (Chakrata), Uttarkashi, and Berinaag areas in Uttarakhand as a resource augmentation effort (Nautiyal and Nautiyal 2004; Srivastava et al 2010).

Its roots are easily infested by insects so these are kept in powdered lime to protect it from infestation. Traditionally, it is used as an antidote to poisoning (Khare 2008).

Vernacular Names

Assamese: Aatich
Bengali: Ataicha
Gujarati: Ativishni kali, Ativikhani kali
Kannada: Ativisha, Athihage
Kashmiri: Kath
Malayalam: Atividayam, Ativitayam
Marathi: Ativisha
Oriya: Atushi
Punjabi: Atisa, Atees
Tamil: Atividayam
Telugu: Ativasa
Urdu: Atees

Synonyms

Aruna: Its rhizome is reddish brown in color.
Atisaaraghni: It is used to alleviate atisaar (diarrhea).
Bhangura: Rhizome of this plant is in fragile nature.
Ghunavallabha: Rhizome gets infested by insects easily.
Kashmira: It grows in high altitude region like Kashmir.
Pittavallabha: It alleviates disorders of pitta.
Prativisha: It is an antidote for many poisons.
Shishubhaishajya: It is a popular remedy of the diseases of children.
Shringi: Its rhizome is horn shaped.
Shuklakanda: It has white colored tuber or rhizome.
Visha: It is assimilated quickly in the body like poison.
Vishva: It spreads to the minutest channel in the body.

Classical Categorization

Charak Samhita: Lekhniya, Arshoghna, Tikta Skanda
Sushrut Samhita: Pippalayadi, Vachadi, Mustadi
Ashtanga Hridaya: Pippalayadi, Vachadi, Mustadi
Dhanvantari Nighantu: Guduchyadi varga
Madanpal Nighantu: Abhyadi varga
Kaiyadev Nighantu: Oushadhi varga
Raj Nighantu: Pippalayadi varga
Bhavaprakash: Haritakyadi varga

Distribution

It is commonly found in alpine and subalpine zones of Himalayas from Indus to Kumaon at an altitude of 6,000 to 15,000 ft.

This species is endemic to Himalayan region of India, Pakistan, and Nepal. In India, the wild population has been recorded in Jammu and Kashmir, Himachal Pradesh, and Uttarakhand (Jabeen et al 2011).

Morphology

It is an erect herb of 2 to 4 ft height. Stem is green, round, erect, simple or branched, and surrounded with leaves of different shapes and sizes, glabrous below, and crispo-pubescent in the upper part.

- **Leaves**: Simple, alternate, heteromorphous (variously shaped). Basal leaves have long petiole (12 cm), lamina orbicular, ovate or cordate in shape, five partite up to middle with further divisions ending into crenate margin. Upper leaves are small, short petiolate, ovate or elongate, dentate margin, and amplexicaul (clasping the stem) (**Fig. 12.1**).
- **Flowers:** Inflorescence terminal raceme or few flowered panicle, bluish- or violet-colored petals, uppermost petal boat-shaped, shortly beaked, many stamen, ovary of five carpels (**Fig. 12.2a, b**).

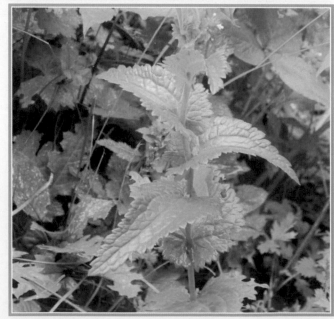

Fig. 12.1 Leaves.

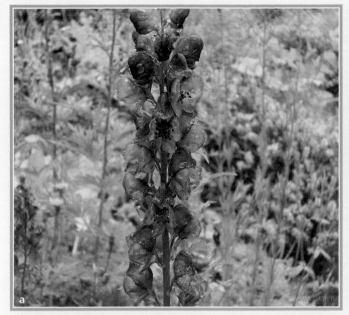
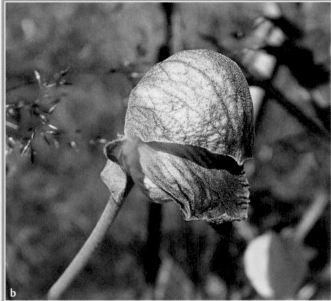

Fig. 12.2 **(a)** Inflorescence. **(b)** Flowers.

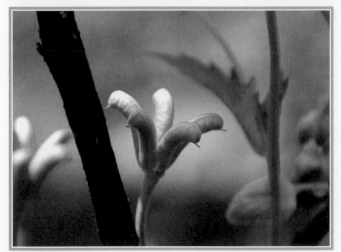
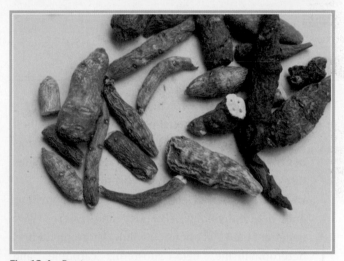

Fig. 12.3 Fruits.

Fig. 12.4 Roots.

- **Fruits:** Follicular fruit, soft hairy, linear-oblong, 16 to 18 mm long with many black brown color seeds (**Fig. 12.3**).
- **Roots:** Biennial, paired with old (mother root) and new roots (daughter root), and tuberous. New root is cylindrical or conical in shape, 1 to 1.5 inch long, ½ inch broad, outer surface is thin and whitish gray, internally white and starchy, on fracture four black spots are visible centrally. Old root is brownish white and shrinked (**Fig. 12.4**).

The roots procured from 2-year-old plants with fully developed tubers are used for medicinal purpose. This plant is propagated through tuber.

Phenology

Flowering time: August to September
Fruiting time: May to September

Key Characters for Identification

➤ *An erect to branched herb of 2 to 4 ft*
➤ *Leaves: simple, alternate, heteromorphous*
➤ *A terminal raceme inflorescence of bluish-violet flowers*
➤ *Roots: biennial, tuberous, paired with old and new roots*

Types

- Vagbhatta: two types—Ativisha, Visa
- Dhanvantari Nighantu: two types—Ativisha (Suklakanda), Prativisha (Shyamkanda)
- Priya Nighantu: two types—Sweta and Aruna
- Raj Nighantu: three types—Shukla, Rakta, Krisna
- Nighantu Ratnakar: three types—Shukla, Krishna, Aruna
- Sodhala Nighantu: four types—Sweta, Rakta, Krishna, Peeta.

Rasapanchaka

Guna	Laghu, Ruksha
Rasa	Katu, Tikta
Vipaka	Katu
Virya	Ushna

Chemical Constituents

The constituents of its tuber include the following:
- Diterpene alkaloids: Atisine (major alkaloid, first isolated by Broughton), hetisine, heteratisine, benzoylheteratisine (Jacob and Craig 1942), atidine, dihydroatisine, hetidine, and hetisone.
- Lactone alkaloids: Heterophyllisine, heterophylline, and heterophyllidine (Pelletier and Aneja 1967; Pelletier et al 1968), heterophylline, heterophyllidine, heterophyllisine, beta sitosterol, carotene, and atisenol (diterpenoid lactone) (Pelletier et al 1982).

The other constituents present in the plant are tannic acid, starch, fat, mixture of fatty acids and their glycerides, carbohydrates, etc.

Identity, Purity, and Strength

- Foreign matter: Not more than 2%
- Total ash: Not more than 4%
- Acid-insoluble ash: Not more than 1%
- Alcohol-soluble extractive: Not less than 6%
- Water-soluble extractive: Not less than 24%

(Source: The Ayurvedic Pharmacopeia of India 1989)

Karma (Actions)

Charaka attributed deepan (appetizer), pachana (digestive), sangrahik (absorbent), krimighna (anthelmintic), vrishya (aphrodisiac), balya (strength promoting), vishaghn (antidote), and visham jwaraghna (antipyretic).
- Doshakarma: Kapha pittahara
- Dhatukarma: Balya, vrishya
- Malakarma: Sangrahi

Pharmacological Actions

The plant is reported to exhibit antidiarrheal, expectorant, diuretic, tonic, hepatoprotective, antipyretic, analgesic, anti-inflammatory, antioxidant, alexipharmic, anodyne, anti-atrabilious, antiflatulent, antiperiodic, antiphlegmatic, and carminative activities (Ukani et al 1996; Shyaula 2012).

Indications

In therapeutics, it is used for the treatment of aamatisara (diarrhea), jwaratisara, sangrahani (sprue), chhardi (vomiting), kasa (cough), krimiroga (worm infestation), balaroga (pediatric disease), mushikavisha (rat poisoning), mutrakricchta (dysuria), udarshool (abdominal pain), apachan (indigestion), agnimandhya (loss of appetite), raktapitta (hemorrhagic diseases), jeerna jwar (fever), arsha (piles), grahni, pittaoudar, peenasa (nasal discharge), kustha (skin diseases), and urustambha (filariasis).

Homeopathy designates this herb as a main drug for neuralgia and used it in rheumatism, hysteria, and nervous pain as an analgesic and nerve sedative (Ukani et al 1996).

Therapeutic Uses

External Use

Paste of leaves mixed with rock salt is applied locally in headache. The seeds crumpled in honey are applied locally on throat and in tonsillitis. Smoke inhalation of root powder is beneficial in headache, especially migraine (Buddhadev et al 2017).

Internal Use

1. **Aamatisara** (diarrhea): Daily intake of liquid gruel processed with Ativisha, Sunthi, and Amladravya (C.S.Su. 2/22) or intake of avaleha preparation with Ativisha, Bilva, Mochrasa, Lodhra, Dhatakipushpa, and Amrabeej checks diarrhea (B.P.Ci. 2/148).
2. **Grahani** (sprue): The decoction made of Ativisha, Sunthi, and Musta is administered orally to destroy the ama in grahani (C.S.Ci. 15/98).
3. **Balaroga** (pediatric disease): Ativisha powder alone with honey or in combination with Karkatshringi and Pippali powder is given in cough, fever, cold, vomiting, and abdominal pain in children (A.H.U. 2/57 and VM. 66/10).
4. **Musikavisa** (rat bite poisoning): Oral administration of Ativisha root paste with honey in the morning is an effective remedy in rat bite poisoning (S.S.Ka. 7/39).
5. **Udarroga** (abdominal diseases): Three parts of Ankola mixed with one part of Ativisha powder is given with rice water to cure all abdominal diseases (BS. Grahni Ci. 167).
6. **Visa roga** (poisoning): Ghee prepared with Ativisha and cow's milk is used orally or as nasal drops in case of acute poisoning. The ghee may also be processed with Sveta and Madayantika (S.S.Ka. 1/64.7.
7. **Jvaratisara** (fever with diarrhea): Shunthi, Kutaja, Musta, Guduchi, and Ativisha are given orally in the form of decoction in diarrhea associated with fever.

Officinal Part Used

Tuberous root/Rhizome

Dose

Powder: 1 to 3 g

Formulations

Balachaturbhadra churna, Balasanjeevani churna, Ativisha avaleha, Shringyadi churna, Ativishadi churna, Pusyanuga churna, Mahavishagarbha taila, Devdarvyadi kwatha, Sunishanaka changeri ghrita, Bala Taila, Panchatiktaghrita guggulu, Amritarishta, Chaturbhadravaleha, Rodhrasava, Chandraprabha vati, and Kutajaghana vati.

Toxicity/Adverse Effects

Ativisha when given in a dose of 4 to 6 g causes symptoms like dryness of mouth, tremors, etc. (Yelne et al 2005).

Substitution and Adulteration

Roots of *Aconitum kashmericum* Stapf. Ex Coventry are sold in the market in the name of Kala Atisa. Its roots are adulterated with roots of *Asparagus racemosus* Willd., *Asparagua gonocladus* Baker, *Delphinium denudatum* Wall ex Hook (Yelne et al 2005).

> **Points to Ponder**
>
> - *Ativisha is a well-known drug for diseases of children and is hence named as Shishubhaisajya.*
> - *For medicinal use, the tubers of at least 2-year-old plants must be collected.*
> - *Due to loss of habitat and overexploitation, the plant is kept under critically endangered species.*

Suggested Readings

Buddhadev SG, Buddhadev SS. A complete review on *Ativisha–Aconitum heterophyllum*. Pharma Sci Monitor 2017;8(1):111–114

Chopra RN, Chopra IC. Chopra's Indigenous Drugs of India. Kolkata: Academic Publishers; 2006:52–61

Gopesh GP. Sudhanidhi Vanoushadhiratnakara Anka, Part 1. 3rd ed. Aligarh: Sudhanidhi Office Vijaygarh; 2007:99

http://www.spicesmedicinalherbs.com/aconitum-heterophyllum. html, 2016

Jabeen N, Rehman S, Bhat KA, Khuroo MA, Shawl AS. Quantitative determination of aconitine in *Aconitum chasmanthum* and *Aconitum heterophyllum* from Kashmir Himalayas using HPLC. J Pharm Res 2011;4(8):2471–2473

Jacobs WA, Craig LC. The aconite alkaloids Ix: the isolation of two new alkaloids from *Aconitum heterophyllum*, heteratisine and hetisine. J Biol Chem 1942;143:605–609

Jacobs WA, Craig LC. The aconite alkaloids VIII: on atisine. J Biol Chem 1942;143:589–603

Khare CP. Indian Medicinal Plants: An Illustrated Dictionary. New York, NY: Springer Science & Business Media; 2008

Nautiyal MC, Nautiyal BP. Agrotechniques for High Altitude Medicinal and Aromatic Plants. Dehra Dun: Bishen Singh Mahendra Pal Singh; 2004:30

Pelletier SW, Aneja R, Gopinath KW. The alkaloids of *Aconitum heterophyllum* wall: isolation and characterization. Phytochemistry 1968;7(4):625–635

Pelletier SW, Aneja R. The diterpene alkaloids: three new diterpene lactone alkaloids from *Aconitum heterophyllum* wall. Tetrahedron Lett 1967;6:557–562

Pelletier SW, Ateya AMM, Finer-Moore J, Mody NV, Schramm LC. Atisenol: a new ent-atisene diterpenoid lactone from *Aconitum heterophyllum.* J Nat Prod 1982;45:779–781

Shyaula SL. Phytochemicals, traditional uses and processing of aconitum species in Nepal. Nepal J Sci Technol 2012;12:171–178

Srivastava N, Sharma V, Kamal B, Jadon VS. Aconitum: need for sustainable exploitation (with special reference to Uttarakhand). Int J Green Pharm 2010;4(4):220–228

The Ayurvedic Pharmacopeia of India. Part I, Vol. 1. New Delhi: Department of AYUSH, Ministry of Health & Family Welfare, Government of India; 1989:22

Ukani MD, Mehta NK, Nanavati DD. *Aconitum heterophyllum* (ativisha) in Ayurveda. Anc Sci Life 1996;16(2):166–171

Yelne MB, Dennis TJ, Chaudhari BG, Billore KV. Database of Medicinal Plants Used in Ayurveda, Vol. 7. New Delhi: Central Council for Research in Ayurveda & Siddha, Department of AYUSH, Ministry of Health & Family Welfare, Government of India; 2005:39–51

Zoo rules 1992 notification. Available from: http://www. envfor.nic.in/legis/ wildlife/wildlife9.html

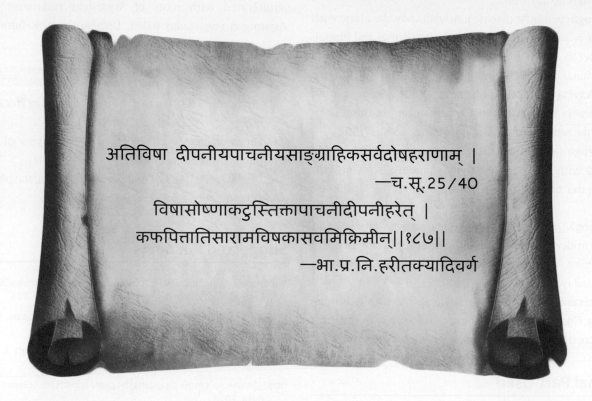

अतिविषा दीपनीयपाचनीयसाङ्ग्राहिकसर्वदोषहराणाम् |

—च.सू. 25/40

विषासोष्णाकटुस्तिक्तापाचनीदीपनीहरेत् |

कफपित्तातिसारामविषकासवमिक्रिमीन्||१८७||

—भा.प्र.नि.हरीतक्यादिवर्ग

13. Atibala [*Abutilon indicum* Linn.]

Family: *Malvaceae*

Hindi name: *Kanghi, Kakahi*

English name: *Indian mallow , Country mallow*

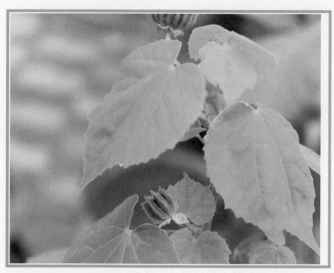

Plant of *Abutilon indicum* Linn.

Leaves of Atibala are used as a food in piles by Siddha physicians.

Introduction

The plants Bala and Atibala are collectively known as Bala dvaya. The plant Atibala is bigger in size compared to Bala. It also provides more physical strength than Bala; hence, it is called Atibala. The properties and actions of Bala and Atibala are almost similar.

Atibala (*Abutilon indicum* Linn.) is an erect, woody, shrubby plant. It is widely distributed in tropical and sub-tropical countries. In Kerala, *Urena lobate* is considered as a source for Atibala, but most commonly, *Abutilon indicum* Linn. is used as Atibala.

Vernacular Names

Arabian: Masthul Gola
Assamese: Jayavandha, Jayapateri
Bengali: Petari, Jhapi, Badela
Farsi: Darakhtashaan

Gujarati: Khapat, Dabali, Kamsaki
Kannada: Tutti, Shrimudrigida, Mudragida, Turube
Kashmiri: Kath
Malayalam: Vellula, Uram, Katuvan, Urubam, Urabam, Vankuruntott, Oorpam, Tutti
Marathi: Mudra, Chakrabhendi, Petari
Oriya: Pedipidika
Punjabi: Kangi, Kangibooti
Tamil: Perum Tutti, Paniyara Hutti, thuthi,
Telugu: Tutturu Benda, Duvvenakaya, Duvvena Kayalu

Synonyms

Atibala: It provides more physical strength than Bala.
Kanktika: Fruit of Atibala resembles a comb.
Petarika: Its fruit resembles a basket.
Pittapuspika: It bears yellow flower.
Rishyaprokta: It grows wildly.
Saha: It gives physical strength.

Varshapuspika: It blossoms in rainy season.

Vatyapuspi: Flowers of this plant resembles the flowers of Vatyaa (Bala).

Vrushyagandhika: It is an effective aphrodisiac drug.

Vrushya: It is a potent aphrodisiac drug.

Classical Categorization

Charak Samhita: Balya, Brimhaniya, Madhur Skand

Sushrut Samhita: Vatashamshamana, Madhur Skand

Dhanwantari Nighantu: Guduchyadi varga

Madanpal Nighantu: Abhayadi

Kaiyadev Nighantu: Oshadhi varga

Raj Nighantu: Shatahwadi varga

Bhavaprakash: Guduchyadi varga

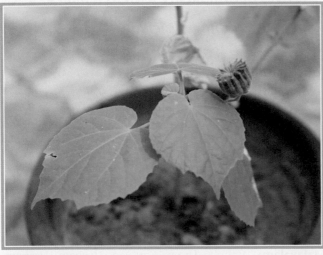

Fig. 13.1 Leaves.

Distribution

The plant is found in India, Sri Lanka, topical regions of America, and Malaysia (Anonymous 1985). It is found as a weed in sub-Himalayan tracts, hilly regions up to 1,200 m, and hotter parts of India.

Morphology

Erect annual herb or perennial shrub of 1 to 3 m height. The stems are stout, branched, 1 to 2 m tall, pubescent.

- **Leaves:** Cordate, ovate, acuminate, toothed, rarely subtrilobate and 9 by 5 cm, grayish green, both surface studded with soft hairs, petioles 3.8 to 7.5 cm long (**Fig. 13.1**).
- **Flowers:** Yellow, peduncle joined above the middle, stipules is 9 mm long; pedicels are often 2.5 to 5 mm long, axillary, solitary, calyx is 12.8 mm long, divided in middle, lobes ovate, apiculate, and corolla is 2.5 cm in diameter, yellow, and opens in the evening (**Fig. 13.2a, b**).
- **Fruits:** A globose schizocarp (capsule), green when young, later black, mericarps 15 to 20, conspicuous and horizontally spreading beaks, stellate hairy; seeds are three per cell (**Fig. 13.3a, b**).
- **Seeds:** Reniform, tubercled, or minutely stellate-hairy, 3 to 5 mm, black or dark brown.
- **Root:** Smooth, cylindrical, and yellow in color.

The plant is propagated through seeds (Kirtikar and Basu 1994; Prajapati et al 2003; Chopra et al 1956; Nadakarni 1995).

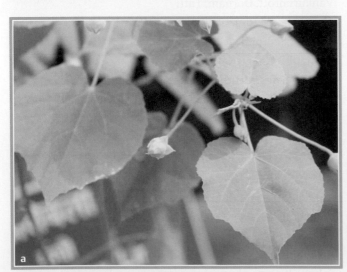
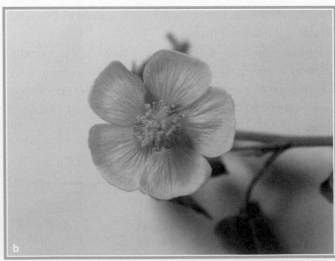

Fig. 13.2 **(a)** Flower buds. **(b)** Flower.

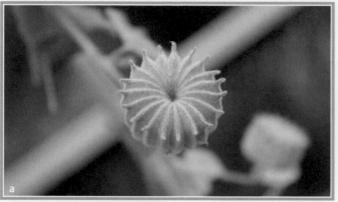
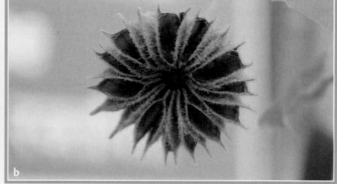

Fig. 13.3 **(a)** Young fruit. **(b)** Mature fruit.

Phenology

Flowering time: February to June

Fruiting time: Almost throughout the year

Key Characters for Identification

➤ *Erect annual herb or perennial shrub of 1 to 3 m height*

➤ *Leaves: cordate, ovate, acuminate, toothed, 9 by 5 cm, soft hairs on both surface, long petiole*

➤ *Flowers: yellow color*

➤ *Fruits: capsule, densely pubescent, with conspicuous and horizontally spreading beaks*

➤ *Seeds: small reniform, minutely stellate-hairy, black or dark brown*

➤ *Roots: smooth, cylindrical and yellow*

Types

It is found in two types:

1. Small-sized Atibala: *Abutilum indicum*
2. Big size: *Abutilum hirtum* G.Don. It is bigger than *A. indicum*. It has hairy branches and pedicle (Sharma 2009).

Rasapanchaka

Guna	Guru, Snigdh
Rasa	Madhura
Vipaka	Madhura
Virya	Sheeta

Chemical Constituents

Its leaves are rich in mucilage, aminoacids, tannins, gallic acid, glucose, sesquiterpene alkaloids, flavonoids, sterols, triterpenoids, saponins, cardiac glycosides, and asparagine, whereas its roots contain many fatty acids such as linoleic, oleic, and stearic.

Identity, Purity, and Strength

- Foreign matter: Not more than 2%
- Total Ash: Not more than 8%
- Acid-insoluble ash: Not more than 3%
- Alcohol-soluble extractive: Not less than 3%
- Water-soluble extractive: Not less than 9%

(Source: The Ayurvedic Pharmacopoeia of India 1989)

Karma (Actions)

Atibala is described as balya (strength promoting), vrishya (aphrodisiac), sangrahi (absorbent), brimhana (increases weight), vedanasthapana (analgesic), shothahara (reduces inflammation), and mutral (diuretic).

- Doshakarma: Vatapittashamak
- Dhatukarma: Balya, brimhana
- Malakarma: Grahi

Pharmacological Actions

It possesses diuretic, antioxidant, hypoglycemic, larvicidal, antidiabetic, antiulcer, lipid lowering, anticonvulsant, wound healing, analgesic, antiestrogenic, antiarthritic, antidiarrheal, immunomodulatory, anti-inflammatory, antimycotic, antimalarial, hepatoprotective, and antiasthmatic activities (Sharma et al 2013; Gautam et al 2013).

Indications

Bhavaprakash Nighantu has described Bala chatushtya under one group. So its properties and indications are same as Bala. It is used in raktapitta (bleeding disorders), vatarakta (gout), and Meha (diabetes; The Ayurvedic Pharmacopoeia of India 1989).

The roots of the plant are considered as demulcent and diuretic. Its root is used in fever, chest infection, gonorrhea, hematuria, strangury leprosy, dry cough, bronchitis, gout, polyuria, uterine hemorrhagic discharge, urinary discharge, and urethritis (Giri et al 2009). Root infusion is given to cure fever, dry cough, and bronchitis (Gautam et al 2013).

The leaves are found to be good for ulcer and as a fomentation to painful parts of the body. The decoction of the leaves is used in toothache, tender gums, lumbago, and ear-ache. It is used in eye wash and mouth washes (Prakshanth et al 2006; Mohapatra and Sahoo 2008). Leaves are used to treat ulcer, inflammation, rheumatism, syphilis of penis, piles, pain in legs, uterus displacement, inflammation of bladder, catarrhal bilious diarrhea, bronchitis, gonorrhea, and fever (Kaladhar 2012).

The bark is used as febrifuge, anthelmintic, and alexiteric, astringent, diuretic, aphrodisiac, and laxative (Singh et al 2002).

The seeds are used in chest problem, bronchitis, piles, laxative, expectorant, chronic cystitis, gleet, and gonorrhea (The Ayurvedic Pharmacopoeia of India 1989; Kumar and Gali 2011).

Therapeutic Uses

External Use

1. **Mudhagarbha** (obstructed labour): Oil cooked with Atibala etc. (like bala taila) is applied in case of mudhagarbha (S.S.Ci. 15/44-45).
2. **Updansha** (syphilis): The paste of leaves and seeds is applied externally to penis to cure syphilis (Jain et al 2004; Kaushik et al 2009; Lakshmayya et al 2003).

3. **Dantshool** (toothache and tender gums): The decoction of its leaves should be used for gargles in toothache and tender gums.

Internal Use

1. **Prameha** (diabetes): Root decoction or seed powder of Atibala should be taken with milk and sugar to control diabetes.
2. **Mutrakricchta** (dysuria): Root decoction of Atibala alleviates all types of dysuria (CD 32.33 BPChi. 35/40).
3. **Mutragata vyadhi** (urinary obstruction): Its leaves decoction or seed powder gives relief in dysuria, gonorrhea, and other urinary disorders whereas root decoction should be used in hematuria.
4. **Rakt pradar** (menometrorrhagia): Atibala root powder mixed with sugar and honey is effective in controlling excessive bleeding in raktapradar (BP.Ci. 68/13).
5. **Rasayana** (rejuvinator): It is used as Rasayana (C.S.Ci. 1.2.12 and S.S.Ci. 27/10).
6. **Arsha** (piles): Root decoction is given twice a day for 2 weeks in bleeding piles.

Officinal Parts Used

Whole plant, roots, seeds, and leaves

Dose

Decoction: 50 to 100 mL
Powder: 3 to 6 g

Formulations

Bala taila, Narayan taila, Mahanarayan taila, and Atibala rasayana.

Toxicity/Adverse Effects

Not reported yet.

Substitution and Adulteration

Bala and Atibala are used as substitutes of each other.

Suggested Readings

Anonymous. The Wealth of India: A Dictionary of Indian Raw Materials, Vol. I. New Delhi: CSIR; 1985:20–23

Chopra RN, Nair SL, Chopra IC. Glossary of Indian Medicinal Plants. New Delhi: CSIR; 1956:2

Giri RK, Kaungo SK, Patro VJ, Das S, Sahoo DE. Lipid lowering activity *Abutilon indicum* (L) leaf extract in rats. J Pharm Res 2009;2(11):1725–1727

Jain A, Katewa SS, Chaudhary BL, Galav P. Folk herbal medicines used in birth control and sexual diseases by tribals of southern Rajasthan, India. J Ethnopharmacol 2004;90(1):171–177

Kaladhar DSVGK. Traditional and Ayurvedic Medicinal Plants from India: Practices and Treatment for Human Diseases. Germany: Lap Lambert Academic Publishing; 2012:176

Kaushik P, Kaushik D, Khokra S, Choudhary B. *Abutilon indicum* (Atibala): Ethano-botany, phytochemistry and pharmacology: a review. Int J Pharm Clin Res 2009;1(1):4–9

Kirtikar KR, Basu BD. Indian Medicinal Plants. 2nd ed., Vol. I. Delhi: Periodical Expert Book Agency; 1994:314–317

Kumar GG, Gali V. Phytochemical screening of *Abutilon muticum* (Del. ex DC.) and *Celosia argentea* Linn. Int J Pharm Bio Sci 2011;2(3):463–467

Kumar VP, Chauhan NS, Padh H, Rajani M. Search for antibacterial and antifungal agents from selected Indian medicinal plants. J Ethnopharmacol 2006;107(2):182–188

Lakshmayya, Nelluri NR, Kumar P, Agarwal NK, Shivaraj GT, Ramachandra SS. Phytochemical and pharmacological evaluation of leaves of Abutilon indicum. Indian J Tradit Knowl 2003;2(1):79–83

Mohapatra SP, Sahoo HP. An ethno-medico-botanical study of Bolangir, Orissa, India: native plant remedies against gynaecological diseases. Ethnobotan Leafl 2008;12:846–850

Nadakarni AK. Indian Materia Medica. Bombay: Popular Prakashan (Pvt) Ltd.; 1995:8–9

Prajapati ND, Purohit SS, Sharma AK, Kumar TA. Handbook of Medicinal Plants. Jodhpur: AGROBIOS (India); 2003:3

Prakshanth V, Neelam S, Padh H, Rajani M. Search for antibacterial and antifungal agents from selected Indian medicinal plants. J Ethnopharmacol 2006;107:182–188

Sharma A, Sharma RA, Singh H. Phytochemical and pharmacological profile of Abutilon indicum L. sweet: a review. Int J Pharm Sci Rev Res, May–Jun 2013;20(1):120–127

Sharma PV. Dravyaguna Vigyan. Vol. 2. Varanasi: Chaukhambha Bharati Academy, Reprint; 2009:737

Singh AK, Raghubanshi AS, Singh JS. Medical ethnobotany of the tribals of Sonaghati of Sonbhadra district, Uttar Pradesh, India. J Ethnopharmacol 2002;81(1):31–41

The Ayurvedic Pharmacopoeia of India. Part I, Vol. 1. New Delhi: Department of AYUSH, Ministry of Health & Family Welfare, Government of India; 1989:25–28

Vadnere G, Pathan A, Kulkarni B, Kumar SA. Abutilon indicum Linn: a phytopharmacological review. Int J Res Pharm Chem 2013;3(1):153–156)

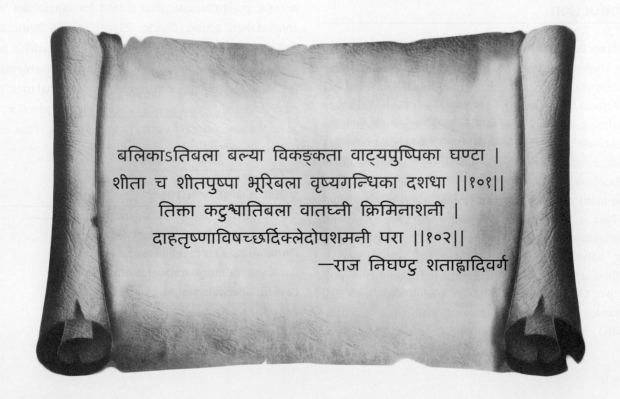

बलिकाऽतिबला बल्या विकङ्कता वाट्यपुष्पिका घण्टा |
शीता च शीतपुष्पा भूरिबला वृष्यगन्धिका दशधा ||१०१||
तिक्ता कटुश्चातिबला वातघ्नी क्रिमिनाशनी |
दाहतृष्णाविषच्छर्दिक्लेदोपशमनी परा ||१०२||
—राज निघण्टु शताह्वादिवर्ग

14. Bala *[Sida cordifolia Linn.]*

Family:	*Malvaceae*
Hindi name:	*Kharenti, Barial, Barriar, Khareti, Kungyi*
English name:	*Country mallow*

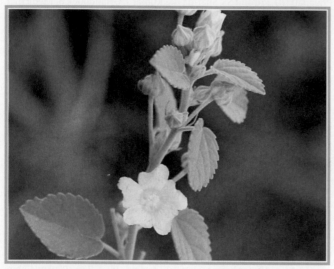

Plant of *Sida cordifolia* Linn.

Bala is best for sangrahika, balya, and vatahara action (C.S.Su. 25/40).

Introduction

The plants Bala and Atibala are collectively known as Bala dvaya. These two types of bala dvaya are described by Charak and Sushruta, whereas Vagbhatta mentioned Bala traya, i.e., Bala, Atibala, and Nagbala. In Bhavprakash Nighantu's Bala chatushtaya, i.e., four types of Bala are described, which are Bala, Atibala, Mahabala, and Nagbala. Acharya Priyavrata Sharma mentioned five types of bala, i.e., Bala chatushtaya plus Rajabala.

The plant provides physical strength, and so it is called Bala. Bala is described as rasayan, vishaghna, balya, and pramehaghna in Vedic literature. Charak described Bala under balya, brumhaniya dashaimani, while Sushrut described both Bala and Atibala in madhur skandha.

As per Charak Samhita, Bala is mainly used as balya, brimhana, ojabardhaka, rasayana, nadibalya, vedana-sthapana, shothahara, vatashamak, hridya, jvaraghna, sukrala, prajasthapana. Bala is best for sangrahika, balya, and vatahara action (Cha.Su. 25/40). Several formulations and recipes such as baladi pralepa, baladi pradeha, baladi yavagu, baladi yapana basti, and baladi ghrita are mentioned in Charak Samhita for both external and internal uses. These medicines are used in a wide range of clinical practices such as vatavyadhi, vatarakta, raktapitta, raktarsha, vrana, ardita, pakshaghata, grahani, pradar, and shotha.

Vernacular Names

Bengal: Bala, Barila, Brela, Svetberela
Cambodia: Kantrangbai sa
Canarese: Chittuharalu, Hettutli
Ceylon: Chevakanpudu
Fanti: Kumpa
Gujarati: Baladana, Kharati

Hausa: Maikafu

Katagum: Kardafi

Konkan: Ko birsir bhaiji, Muttava

La Reunion: Mauv

Malay: Kelulutputih

Malayalam: Katturam

Marathi: Chikana, Khiranti

Mundari: Marang lupa arabi, huring mindilata

Oriya: Badiananla, Bisvokopasi

Pore Bandar: Bala, Baldana, Balnochotvo

Punjabi: Kharent, Kowar, Simak

Sinhalese: Hinadona

Tamil: Arivalmanani pupundu, Nilatutti

Telugu: Antisa, Chirubenda, Muttavapulagamu

Synonyms

Bala: The plant promotes physical strength.

Baladhya: It gives tenacity and strength.

Bhadrodani: Seeds are like audana (cereals).

Kharayastika: The plants have hairy and rough stem.

Odanahwaya: Seeds are like audana (cereals).

Pitapuspi: Flowers are yellow in color.

Shitapaki: Fruits are ripe in the winter.

Vatya: The stem of the plant have strong fibers.

Vatyalaka: This plant grows in the field.

Vatyalika: This plant grows in the field.

Vinaya: The plant is used for promoting strength.

Classical Categorization

Charak Samhita: Balya, Brimhaniya, Prajasthapana, Madhur skanda

Sushrut Samhita: Kakolyadi, Sursadi, Vata shansamana

Dhanwantari Nighantu: Guduchyadi varga

Madanpal Nighantu: Abhayadi

Kaiyadev Nighantu: Oshadhi varga

Raj Nighantu: Shatahwadi varga

Bhavaprakash: Guduchyadi varga

Distribution

Sida cordifolia is widely distributed along with other species throughout the tropical and subtropical plains all over India and Sri Lanka up to an altitude of 1,050 m (Jain et al 2011; Kanth and Diwan 1999).

Morphology

It is an erect, annual herb or under shrub of 0.75 to 1.5 m height.

- **Leaves:** simple, alternate, 2.5 to 7 cm long and 2.5 to 5 cm broad, with seven to nine veins, cordate, oblong, ovate-oblong, serrated margin, obtuse or subacute apex, hairy on both surface, long petiole (**Fig. 14.1**).
- **Flowers:** solitary, axillary, small, yellow or yellowish-white with a pair of awns on each carpel (**Fig. 14.2**).

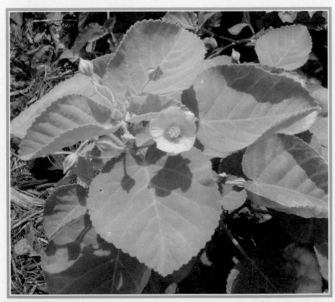

Fig. 14.1   Leaves.

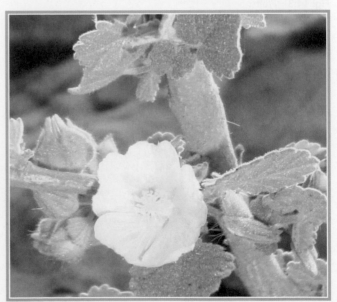

Fig. 14.2   Flowers.

- **Fruits:** schizocarp, sub-discoid, and of the size of moong dal (lentils), 6 to 8 mm in diameter with many seeds (**Fig. 14.3**).
- **Seeds:** small, smooth, trigonous, dusky black in color. Its seeds are popularly known as **beejband** (**Fig. 14.4**).
- **Stem:** stout, strong, and minutely hairy (**Fig. 14.5**).
- **Roots**: 5 to 15 cm, stout and grayish yellow outer surface.

It is propagated by seed.

Phenology

Flowering time: August to December

Fruiting time: October to January (Pole et al 2006)

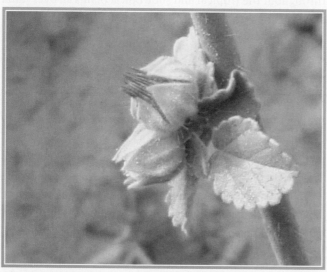

Fig. 14.3 Fruits.

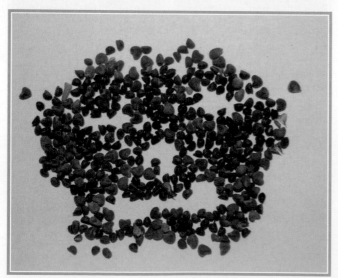

Fig. 14.4 Seeds.

Key Characters for Identification

➤ Erect, annual herb or under shrub of 1 to 1.5 ft height
➤ Stout and strong stem
➤ 2.5 to 7 cm long and 2.5 to 5 cm broad leaves, with seven to nine veins
➤ Small, yellow, or white in color flowers, solitary and axillaries.
➤ Moong-sized fruits, 6 to 8 mm in diameter
➤ Small, grayish black in color and smooth seeds

Rasapanchaka

Guna	Guru, Snigdh
Rasa	Madhura
Vipaka	Madhura
Virya	Sheeta

Chemical Constituents

Phytochemical screening revealed the presence of ephedrine, pseudoephedrine, quinazolines (vasicine, vasicinol), cryptoleptins, phytosterols (stearic and hexacosanoic acids, sterculic, malvalic, and fumaric acid), flavonoids, saponins, aspargine, N-methyl tryptophan in *S. cordifolia* (Ghosal et al 1975; Ranajit et al 2008; Singh 2006).

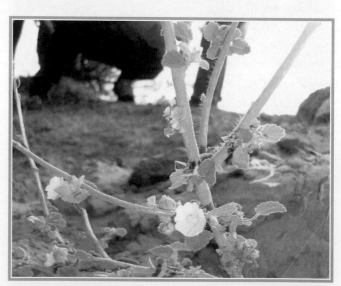

Fig. 14.5 Stem of Bala.

Types

1. Bhavaprakash Nighantu: four types—Bala, Atibala, Mahabala, Nagabala
2. Dhanwantari Nighantu: five types—Bala, Atibala, Mahabala, Nagabala. Rajbala

Karma (Actions)

The main actions of this plant are balya (strength promoting), brumhana (weight promoting), ojovardhaka (increases oja), vatahara (pacify vata), vedanasthapana (anodyne), shotahara (anti-inflammatory), grahi (absorbent), hrudya (cardio tonic), shukrala (spermatogenic), prajasthapana (procreanta), mutrala (diuretic), and jvaraghna (antipyretic).

The plant is an alternative tonic, astringent, emollient, aphrodisiac, etc. Bark is considered as cooling, seeds are aphrodisiac and roots have cooling, astringent, stomachic, tonic, aromatic, bitter, and diuretic properties (Singh and Navneet 2018).

- Doshakarma: Vatapitta shamaka
- Dhatukarma: Balya, brimhana, shukrala
- Malakarma: Mutrala

Pharmacological Actions

The pharmacological screening of Bala shows to have central nervous system activity along with analgesic, anti-inflammatory, hypotensive, hepatoprotective, antibacterial, antifungal, adaptogenic, anti-Parkinsonism, wound healing, antihyper triglyceridemic, hypoglycemic, antioxidant, blood-coagulant, antifertility, antihelmintic, hypolipidemic, antipyretic, antirheumatism, antiulcerogenic, antidiabetic, nephroprotective, antistress, anticancer, cytotoxic, and antinociceptive properties (Ajeet et al 2018).

Indications

Bala is a popular drug used in traditional practices for enhancing physical strength and lustre. It is useful in the treatment of rakta vikara (bleeding disorders), respiratory disorders, kshaya (emaciation), mutra atisara (diarrhea), mutrakricchta (dysuria), prameha (diabetes), pradar (leucorrhea), vrana (wounds/ulcers), pakshaghat (paralysis), shirashool, sciatica, and kshat (traumatic injuries). It is also useful in asthma, cough, tuberculosis, fever, colic, rheumatism, arthritis, cardiac irregularities, and nervous system disorders.

Bala is used for galaganda (goiter), pakhaghata (hemiplegia), swarabheda (tonsillitis), murdhagarbha (obstructed labor), etc. as per Sushrut Samhita. Vagbhatta advised to use Bala in rajayakshma (consumption), vatarakta, swarabheda, etc. Other indications are antravriddhi, garbhadharana (Chakradutta), atisara (Bhavprakash), bahusosa (atrophy of arm), avabahuka, shlipada urograha (distress in chest), and in unmad (insanity) (Bangasena).

This plant is tonic, astringent, emollient, aphrodisiac, and useful in treatment of respiratory system–related troubles (Agharkar 1991).

Decoction of Bala root and ginger is given in intermittent fever with cold shivering fits. Root juice is also used to promote healing of wounds. Bark of this plant is useful in blood, throat, urinary system–related troubles, piles, phthisis, insanity, etc. Powder of the root and bark is given with milk and sugar for frequent micturition. Oil prepared from the decoction of root bark mixed with milk and sesame oil is used in diseases of the nervous system, facial paralysis, and sciatica (Singh 2006).

Therapeutic Uses

External Use

3. **Vatavyadhi** (neuromuscular diseases): The medicated oil of Bala is massaged to alleviate pain and swelling in vatik disorders.
4. **Kshaya** (muscular weakness): Regular massage of Candanbalalaksadi taila (oil prepared with Bala root, Chandan and Laksha, and other drugs) is beneficial in kshaya (muscular weakness), vatik disorders, neuritis, backache and joint pain, kasa, shwasa, raktapitta, weakness, etc. (B.R. 14/304-311).
5. **Vrana and Akshi roga** (wounds and eye diseases): Paste of leaves is applied locally for wound dressing and in eye diseases.

Internal Use

1. **Vatavyadhi** (neuromuscular diseases): Bala taila is used in vatavyadhi (C.S.Ci. 28/148-156). Bala root decoction

is given twice daily or is massaged with Bala siddha taila to give relief in paralysis, facial palsy, cervical spondylosis, sciatica, arthritis, headache, and other neuralgic pain. Bala taila can also be used for giving basti (enema) in hemiplegia (S.S.Ci. 5/19).

2. **Kshaya** (emaciation): Bala root paste processed with 10 times milk is used daily with honey for the treatment of kshaya.

3. **Vatarakta** (gout): Sahasrapaka or shatapaka Bala taila (C.S.Ci. 29/119-120, AH.Ci. 22/45-46) is used as bath, dipping, enema, and diet in vatarakta (S.S.Ci. 5/12).

4. **Raktapradar** (menometrorrhagia): Bala root powder is mixed with honey and taken with milk (VM. 63/10).

5. **Rasayana** (rejuvinator): Bala rasayan is used for rasayana purpose (S.S.Ci. 27/10).

6. **Rakta arsha** (bleeding piles): Liquid gruel prepared with parched paddy and processed with Bala and Prishniparni alleviate bleeding piles (C.S.Ci. 14/199).

7. **Atisaar** (diarrhea): Milk cooked with Bala and Shunthi is given in morning and after that jaggery and oil is taken (BP.Ci. 2/111).

8. **Raktapitta** (bleeding disorders): Cow's milk cooked with Bala or Gokshur is useful (C.S.Ci. 21/79).

9. **Mutrakrichha** (dysuria): Daily intake of Bala root processed with milk heals up the ulcers and wounds of urinary tract and cures dysuria and hematuria.

10. **Rajyakshma** (tuberculosis): Root decoction of Bala is given with honey and ghee to promote the healing of lung tissue and cavitation in tuberculosis.

11. **Jwar** (fever with cold): Decoction of Bala root and ginger gives relief in intermittent fever with cold shivering, cough, nasal congestion, bronchitis, and asthma.

12. **Shwetpradar** (leucorrhea): Powder of Bala root bark along with milk and sugar is given daily to prevent frequent micturition, leucorrhea, and gonorrhea.

Officinal Parts Used

Root and seeds

Dose

Powder: 3 to 6 g
Decoction: 40 to 80 mL

Formulations

Baladyarishta, Baladighrita, Satapakikshirabala, Bala curna/swarasa, Baladikwatha, Maashabaladikwath, Baladyaghrita, Dashmoolarishta, Narayan taila, Mahanarayan taila, Ksheerbala taila, Chandanbalalaxadi taila, Dhanvantaram taila, Bala taila.

Toxicity/Adverse Effects

The aqueous extract of *S. cordifolia* was tested for toxic effect on viability of PC12 cell line with no signs of toxicity (Auddy et al 2003). A further toxicity study on *S. cordifolia* was conducted in mice and was found to be very low, approximately 3 g/kg p.o. (Franzotti et al 2000; Medeiros et al 2006). The LD50 of the hydroalcoholic extract of the leaves was determined in mice to be 2.639 g/kg with 90% confidence limits of 2.0683 to 3.67 g/kg, when administered intraperitoneally. Administration of doses up to 5.0 g/kg was found not lethal to the animals.

Substitution and Adulteration

S. rhombifolia, *S. cordata*, *S. spinosa*, and *S. alba* are frequently used as adulterant for *S. cordifolia*.

> **Points to Ponder**
> - *Baladwaya includes Bala and Atibala.*
> - *Balatraya is of three types: Bala, Atibala, and Nagbala.*
> - *Bala chatushtaya can be of four types, namely, Bala, Atibala, Nagbala, and Mahabala.*
> - *Panchabala is of five types: the types listed under Bala chatushtaya plus Rajabala.*
> - *Seed of Bala is known as beejabanda.*
> - *Bala is best for sangrahika, balya, and vatahara actions (Cha.Su. 25/40).*

Suggested Readings

Agharkar SP. Medicinal Plants of Bombay Presidency. Jodhpur, India: Pbl. Scientific Publishers; 1991:194–195

Ajithabai MD, Sunitha Rani SP, Jayakumar G. Review on the species of *Sida* for the preparation of Nayopayam kashayam. Int J Res Rev Pharm Appl Sci 2012;2(2):173–195

Anonymous. Wealth of India. New Delhi: CSIR-NISCAIR; 1952–2006

Auddy B, Ferreira M, Blasina F, et al. Screening of antioxidant activity of three Indian medicinal plants, traditionally used for the management of neurodegenerative diseases. J Ethnopharmacol 2003;84(2-3):131–138

Franzotti EM, Santos CV, Rodrigues HM, Mourão RH, Andrade MR, Antoniolli AR. Anti-inflammatory, analgesic activity and acute toxicity of Sida cordifolia L. (Malva-branca). J Ethnopharmacol 2000;72(1-2):273–277

Ghosal S, Chauhan RRPS, Mehta R. Alkaloids of Sida cordifolia. Phytochemistry 1975;14:830–832

Jain A, Choubey S, Singour PK, Rajak H, Pawar RS. Sida cordifolia (Linn): an overview. J Appl Pharm Sci 2011;1(02):23–31

Kanth VR, Diwan PV. Analgesic, antiinflammatory and hypoglycaemic activities of Sida cordifolia. Phytother Res 1999; 13(1):75–77

Kumar RS, Mishra SH. Anti-inflammatory and hepatoprotective activities of Sida cordifolia Linn. Ind J Pharmacol 1997;29:110–116

Medeiros IA, Santos MRV, Nascimento NMS, Duarte JC. Cardiovascular effects of Sida cordifolia leaves extract in rats. Fitoterapia 2006;77(1):19–27

Pole S. Ayurvedic Medicine. Elsevier Health Sciences; 2006:137

Ranajit KS, Sutradhar AKM, Matior R, Mesbah UA, Sitesh CB. Bioactive flavones of Sida cordifolia. Phytochem Lett 2008;1(4):179–182

Sharma PV. Dravya GunaVignana, Vol. II. Varanasi: Chaukhambha Bharati Academy; 2001:735

Singh A, Navneet. A review: traditional, ethnomedicinal utilization, pharmacological properties and phytochemistry of Barleria prionitis Linn. Int J Pharm Sci Rev Res 2017;44(2):19–26

Singh A, Navneet. Ethnobotanical, pharmacological benefits and phytochemistry of Sida cordifolia (Linn.): a review. Int J Pharm Clin Res 2018;10(1):16–21

Singh AP. Bala (Sida cordifolia L.): is it a safe herbal drug? Ethanobot Leafl 2006;10:336–342

Chopra RN, Nayar SL. Glossary Indian Med: Plants. New Delhi: PID; 1956:227

Nadkami KM. The Indian Materia Medica. Vol. 1, 2nd ed. Mumbai: Popular Prakashan; 1954:1137

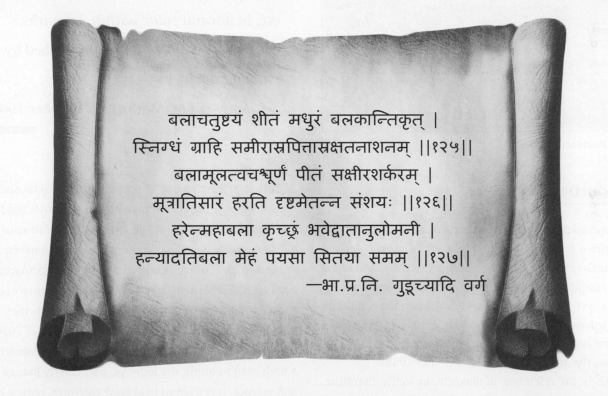

बलाचतुष्टयं शीतं मधुरं बलकान्तिकृत् |
स्निग्धं ग्राहि समीरास्रपित्तासृक्षतनाशनम् ||१२५||
बलामूलत्वचश्चूर्णं पीतं सक्षीरशर्करम् |
मूत्रातिसारं हरति दृष्टमेतन्न संशयः ||१२६||
हरेन्महाबला कृच्छ्रं भवेद्वातानुलोमनी |
हन्यादतिबला मेहं पयसा सितया समम् ||१२७||
—भा.प्र.नि. गुडूच्यादि वर्ग

15. Bakuchi [*Psoralea corylifolia* Linn.]

Family: *Fabaceae*

Hindi name: *Babchi, Somraji, Babachi, Bavanchiyan, Bhavaj, Bakuci, Bemchi*

English name: *Psoralea seed, Malaya tea, Babchi seeds, Scurf-pea, Fountain bush, West Indian Satinwood*

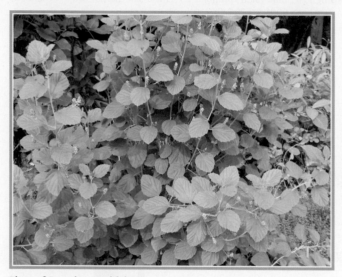

Plant of *Psoralea corylifolia* Linn.

> *Oil Bowchi (oil psoralea) discovered by D. N. Basu in School of Tropical Medicine, Calcutta, changes white skin, gray hair, rough, scaly, discolored skin, nails, hairs, etc. to normal color within 3 months, and that is well tried and prescribed by eminent doctors*
> *—Sunday Times, Madras, 27 October 1940*

Introduction

It is a reputed drug to treat kusta (skin diseases) successfully, and hence it is called Bakuchi. The word *Psoralea* is derived from the Greek word *psoraleos* meaning "scabby" and refers to the appearance given to the plants by the small glands which cover them; *corylifolia* comes from the similarity of the leaves to those of Corylus, a genus of trees in the northern regions and common in Sweden, the home of Linnaeus, the author of the species (Miller 1988).

There is no reference of Bakuchi in Vedic literature. Various synonyms like Avalguja, Somaraji, etc. are found in Agnipuran (Pandey 1997) and many uses of Bakuchi in skin diseases are mentioned in Garuna purana (Sankshipta Garuna Purana). The use of Bakuchi seeds is described in many Rasagrantha for various purposes like Abhrak Marana, Parada bandhan, khotnirmana, parada nirvikarana, and marana.

This is considered as a prime drug for skin diseases, especially for vitiligo (shwetakustha). The plant is used both internally and externally. The external application of seed oil is extremely beneficial in numerous skin ailments.

Its medicinal usage is reported in Indian Pharmaceutical Codex, Chinese, British, and the American pharmacopoeias, and in different traditional systems of medicines such as Ayurveda, unani, and siddha (Shilandra et al 2010). *P. corylifolia* L., or *Bu Gu Zhi* in traditional Chinese medicine, is a herb used to tonify the kidneys, particularly kidney yang and essence. It is used to heal bone fractures, reduce lower back and knee pain, impotency, bed wetting, hair loss, and vitiligo (Cheng 2001).

Seeds are used to make perfumed oil (Nadkarni 1976). The ethanolic extract has been used as a food additive for the preservation of some processed foods or pickles in Japan (Qiao et al 2007).

Vernacular Names

Arabic: Loelab el abid, Mahalep

Assamese: Habucha

Bangla: Buckidana

Bengali: Bavachi, Hakuch, Latakasturi, Kakuch, Barachi, Bakuchi

Chinese: Ku Tzu, Pu Ku Chih, Bu Ku Zhi, Cot Chu

German: Bawchan

Gujarati: Babchi, Bavacha, Babichi, Bawchi

Kannad: Somaraji, Bavanchigida, Karbekhiga

Kashmiri: Babchi

Malayalam: Karkokil, Karkokilari, Kaurkoalari

Marathi: Babachi, Bavachya, Bavachi, Bavanchi

Nepalese: Bakuchi

Oriya: Bakuchi

Persian: Waghchi, Vabkuchi, Ba bakhi

Punjabi: Babchi

Sinhalese: Bodi-ata

Tamil: Karpokarishi, Karpuva-arishi, Karpuvanshi, Kaarboka-arisi, Karpogalarisi

Telugu: Bavanchalu, Bavanchi-vittulu, Bogi-vittulu, Karu-bogi, Kala-ginja

Urdu: Babechi

Synonyms

Avalguja: The appearance of fruit of this plant is somewhat ugly.

Bakuchi: It is a reputed drug for treatment of kusta (skin diseases).

Kalameshi: The plant survives for long periods and has black fruits.

Krishnaphala: It has blackish brown fruits.

Kushthaghni: It cures kusta.

Malayu: It is effective in switra (vitiligo).

Putiphali: Fruits have foul smell.

Shashilekha: Seeds have white streak.

Somaraji: Seeds have white streak.

Suparnika: The plant bears beautiful leaves.

Switraghni: It is effective in treating switra (vitiligo).

Classical Categorization

Charak Samhita: Tikta skanda
Susruta Samhita: Katu varga

Astanga Sangraha: Shaka varga
Astanga Hridaya: Shaka varga
Dhanwantari Nighantu: Guduchyadi varga
Madanpal Nighantu: Abhayadi varga
Kaiyadev Nighantu: Oshadhi varga
Raj Nighantu: Shatahwadi varga
Bhavaprakash: Haritakyadi varga

Distribution

P. corylifolia is native to India and Sri Lanka. The plant grows in tropical and subtropical regions of the world including Southern Africa, China (Krishnamurthi 1969). It grows throughout the plains of India, especially in the semi-arid regions of Rajasthan and Eastern districts of Punjab, adjoining Uttar Pradesh.

Morphology

It is a small, erect, annual herb growing up to 60 to 120 cm in height with longitudinally striated stems and branches.

- **Leaves:** Simple, alternate, long petiole, ovate to round, obtuse-mucronate apex, serrated margin, clothed with white hairs on both surfaces, covered with numerous black dots, main nerves 5, originating from base (**Fig. 15.1**).
- **Flowers**: Dense, bluish-purple, axillary, 10 to 30 flowered racemes (**Fig. 15.2**).
- **Fruits:** Pod is small, 5 mm long, ovoid/sub-globular, single seeded, indehiscent, slightly compressed, closely pitted, black, beaked without hairs (**Fig. 15.3a, b**).
- **Seeds:** Oblong ovoid or bean shaped, flattened, dark brownish black, 2 to 4 mm long, 2 to 3 mm broad, and 1 to 1.5 mm thick, hard, smooth, exalbuminous with straw-colored testa, an agreeable aromatic odor and taste (**Fig. 15.4**; Rajpal 2005).
- **Roots:** Cylindrical root with many secondary roots, tapering (**Fig. 15.5**).

This plant is propagated by seed germination. However, seed germination percentage is very low (5–7%) because of hard seed coat (Chand and Sahrawat 2002).

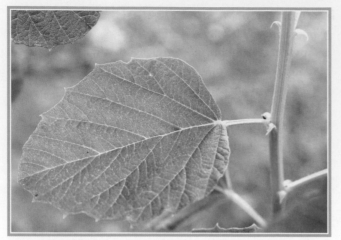

Fig. 15.1 Leaf.

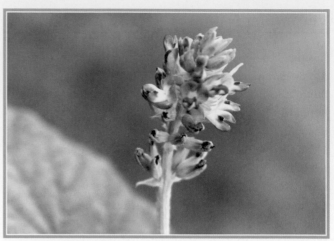

Fig. 15.2 Flower.

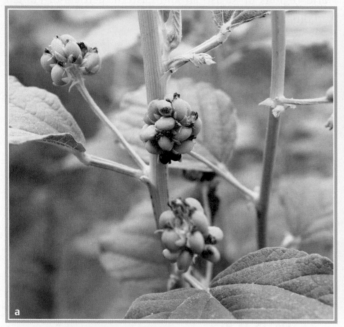

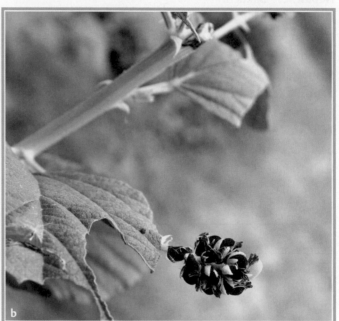

Fig. 15.3 (a) Fruit. (b) Mature fruit.

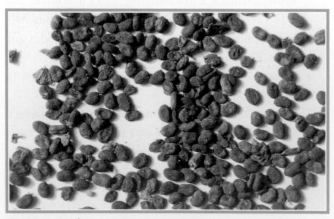

Fig. 15.4 Seeds.

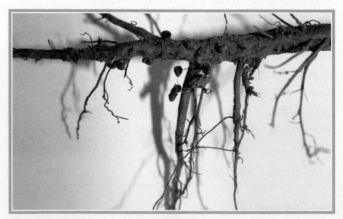

Fig. 15.5 Roots.

Phenology

Flowering time: August to December
Fruiting time: November to February

Key Characters for Identification

➤ Erect annual herb, 60 to 120 cm in height
➤ Leaf: simple, alternate, ovate- to round, mucronate apex, clothed with white hairs on both surfaces and black dots
➤ Flower: bluish-purple, axillary, 10 to 30 flowered racemes
➤ Fruit: single-seeded, small, 5-mm long, black pod
➤ The most distinctive feature is the occurrence of minute brown glands which are immersed in surface tissue on all parts of the plant

Rasapanchaka

Rasa	Tikta, Madhur
Guna	Laghu, Ruksha
Vipaka	Katu
Virya	Ushna (Shaka-Sheeta veerya)
Prabhava	Switrakushthanashaka

Chemical Constituents

Phytochemical studies indicated that flavonoids, coumarins, and meroterpenes are the main components of *P. corylifolia* and most of these components are present in the seeds or fruits.

- **Flavonoids:** corylifolean, corylifolin, corylifolinin, bakuchicin, bavachin, isobavachin, bavachinin, bavachalcone, isobavachalcone, 7-O-methyl bavachin, bavachromanol, corylin, corylidin, corylinal, 4-O-methyl bavachalcone, neobavaisoflavone, bavachromene, neobavachalcone are flavonoids isolated from the seeds of *P. corylifolia* (Szliszka et al 2011; Khushboo et al 2010).
- **Coumarins**: psoralidin, psoralen, isopsoralen, and angelicin
- **Meroterpenes**: bakuchiol and 3-hydroxybakuchiol (Zhao et al 2005).

Identity, Purity, and Strength

- Foreign matter: Not more than 2%
- Total ash: Not more than 8%
- Acid-insoluble ash: Not more than 2%
- Alcohol-soluble extractive: Not less than 13%
- Water-soluble extractive: Not less than 11%

(Source: The Ayurvedic Pharmacopoeia of India 2003)

Karma (Actions)

This plant has many actions such as kushthaghna (anti-dermatosis), jantughna (antibacterial), vranashodhana (wound purifiers), vranaropana (wound healer), keshya (hair tonic), nadibalya (provide nervine strength), deepana (stomachics), pachana (digestant), anulomana (laxative), krimighna (ant helmintics), yakridottejaka (liver stimulant), hridayottejaka (cardiac stimulant), shothahara (anti-inflammatory), kaphaghna, pramehaghna (antidiabetic), and vajikara (aphrodisiac) (Kapoor 2001; Sharma et al 2001).

- Doshakarma: Vatakaphashamaka
- Dhatukarma: Vajikara, kusthaghna
- Malakarma: Anulomana

Pharmacological Actions

The extracts and active components of *P. corylifolia* demonstrated multiple biological activities, including estrogenic, antitumor, antioxidant, antimicrobial, antidepressant, anti-inflammatory, osteoblastic, and hepatoprotective activities (Zhang et al 2016).

Other pharmacological actions like skin-related problem/leukoderma, anti-inflammatory, antiaging, anticarcinogenic, pesticidal activity, anthelmintic effect, estrogenic, bone density, and osteoblastic proliferation are also reported.

Indications

It is useful in mahakushtha (major skin ailments), kshudrakushtha (minor skin diseases), switra (leucoderma), khalitya (alopecia), vrana (wounds), nadidaurbalya (nervine weakness), agnimandya (decreased digestive fire), amadosha (undigested food), vibandha (constipation), krimi (worms), arsha (piles), kasa (cough), shwasa (asthma), pandu (anemia), hritshaithilya (cardiac weakness), hritshotha (cardiomegaly), klaibya (infertility), twaka roga (skin diseases), and jeerna jwara (chronic fever).

It is useful to treat a variety of skin problems, such as leukoderma, skin rashes, infections, and is regarded as a very ancient remedy for leukoderma; it has been tried extensively not only by the practitioners of the Indian medicine but also by the followers of the Western system (Chopra and Chopra 1958).

The powder is used by vaidyas internally and externally in the form of paste and ointment for leprosy and leukoderma (Panda 2000; Nadkarni 1976). Oil helps to fight against vitiligo. It also alleviates several skin diseases like tinea versicolor, scabies, ringworm, psoriasis, boils, and skin eruptions.

This plant has blood-purifying properties. It is used to treat itching red papules, itching eruptions, extensive eczema with thickened dermis, ringworm, rough and discolored dermatosis, dermatosis with fissures, and scabies (Khare 2004). It has shown to improve the color of skin, hair, and nails.

Seeds are sweet, bitter, acrid, and astringent. They impart vigor and vitality, and improve digestive power and receptive power of mind (Joshi 2000). Seeds are given in scorpion sting and snake bite. Seeds are useful in bilious disorders (Panda 2000; Kapoor 2001).

The root is useful in treating the caries of the teeth. It is used to promote bone calcification, making it useful for treating osteoporosis and bone fractures (Krishnamurthi 1969; Joshi 2000). Leaves are used to alleviate diarrhea (Krishnamurthi 1969). Fruit is bitter, helps to prevent vomiting, cures difficulty in micturition, used in treating piles, bronchitis, and anemia, and improves complexion (Joshi 2000). The fruits are believed to have aphrodisiac properties and can be applied to the genital organs, as a tonic.

P. corylifolia has been also widely used for cardiovascular diseases, nephritis, osteoporosis, and cancer (Zhang et al 2016).

Contraindications

It should not be prescribed to the patients suffering from liver diseases, lupus erythematosus, hydro porphyria, or other diseases associated with light sensitivity.

Therapeutic Uses

External Use

1. **Keshpatan** (hair fall): Regular application of Bakuchi oil on hair twice a week prevents hair fall, baldness, dandruff, and graying of hair.
2. **Kustha** (skin diseases): The seed powder is used externally in scabies, ulcers, skin diseases, vitiligo, leukoderma, eczema, leprosy, and psoriasis (Pathak and Acharya 2018). In chronic skin diseases, a mixture of Bakuchi and Karanja oil is commonly used with vaseline. Scabies, psoriasis, ringworm, and tinea versicolor are treated successfully with Bakuchi (Xiong et al 2003).
3. **Scorpion sting and snake bite**: The paste of its seeds is applied locally in scorpion sting and snake bite.

Internal Use

1. **Shwetakustha** (Leukoderma): (a) Decoction of Khadir and Aamalaki is given with Bakuchi seed powder regularly, keeping the patient on wholesome diet to alleviate vitiligo (SG. 2.2.137). Bakuchi oil also can be applied on the affected parts. (b) Bakuchi seeds 160 g with Haratal 40 g pounded with cow's urine are given to restore normal color in vitiligo (VM. 51/33).
2. **Psoriasis:** One gram of purified Bakuchi seed powder mixed with Aamalaki powder and Guduchi satva is given with water twice daily in psoriasis, eczema, dermatitis, and skin eruptions. For these conditions, local application of paste prepared by mixing Bakuchi seed powder, coconut oil, and Karpura is also used.
3. **Kustha** (skin diseases): Tuvarak, Bhallatak, Bakuchi, root of Chitrak, and Shilajatu are given as per rasayana process to cure kusta (AH.Ci. 19/53). Paste prepared by mixing Bakuchi seed powder and ginger juice is applied locally on the affected area for the treatment of severe and chronic kusta (BP.Ci. 54/53).
4. **Rasayana** (rejuvinator): Bakuchi rasayana (AS.U. 49/145-155), Somaraji rasayana (AH.U. 39/107-110), and Swetaavalgujaphala rasayana (S.S.Ci. 28/3) are given for rasayana purpose.
5. **Visha** (poisoning): Gruel cooked with Bakuchi is useful in poisoning (C.S.Ci. 2/24).
6. **Krimidanta** (dental caries): Roots of Bijapura and Bakuchi in equal quantity are pounded and made into

pills. The pill is kept under the teeth. It relieves pain in dental caries (BS.Danta 98-99).

7. **Shlipada** (filaria): Decoction of Bakuchi destroys filaria (GN. 4.2.38).

8. **Kamala** (jaundice): Around 2 g of seed powder mixed with 10 mL Punarnava root juice is used to treat jaundice and other liver diseases.

9. **Varna** (wound): Paste of Bakuchi leaves is applied locally to check the bleeding in wound (VD. 16.119).

10. **Badhirya** (deafness): Powder of Bakuchi and Mushali is given in the treatment of deafness (BS.Karna 85).

Officinal Parts Used

Seeds, seed oil, roots, and leaves are used for medicinal purposes (Khare 2004), but seeds are most commonly used (Khushboo et al 2010).

Dose

Seed powder: 1 to 3 g
Oil: applied externally
Tincture: 3 to 15 mL/day

Formulations

Sashishekara vati, Brihatsomaraji taila, Somaraji taila, Avalgujadi lepa, Somaraji ghrita, Sarvaanga sunder rasa, Khadirasava Kanakarishta, Khadirarishta, Bhihatmanjishthadi kwatha, Savarnakar lepa Pathyadi lepa, Daradadi lepa. Grahdhumadi lepa, Panchnimba churna Pashupati churna, Bhallatakadya churna, Mahaneel taila, Mahaneel ghrita, Astang ghrita, Maheshwar ghrita, Chandrashakaladi vatak, Triphala gutika, Shashilekha vati, Khadir vati, Vidangadi pindi, and Vidangadi vatika.

Toxicity/Adverse Effects

An overdose of the seed powder may cause hrllāsa (nausea), chhardi (vomiting), avasāda (depression), shirahshoola (headache), and virechana (Sharma 2013).

A mixture of psoralen, isopsoralen, and imperatorin caused hypertrophy of liver, kidney, and spleen in rats at a daily dose of 2.5 mg/75 g for 60 days (Sharma et al 2001).

Long-term therapy has been found to affect eyes, liver, and immune system (Rajpal 2005).

Treatment of Adverse Effects

Emptying stomach by aspiration and lavage may treat overdose of the drug. The patient should be kept in a dark room for a minimum of 12 hours (Rajpal 2005).

Precautions

It should be used with caution in pregnancy. Milk, ghee, and butter should be consumed in the diet during Bakuchi regimen. It is advised to avoid spicy diet, salt, and late night sleep. Seed oil should be avoided on eyes and it should be mixed with coconut oil before application because it is thermogenic (Seth 2005).

Purification of Bakuchi

It is recommended to dip Bakuchi seeds into the cow's urine or juice of ginger (Adrak Swaras) for 7 days (Sharma 2013).

Substitution and Adulteration

Chakramarda (*Cassia tora* Linn. of Caesalpiniaceae family) has been indicated as the substitute of Bakuchi (Laxmipati 2013).

> **Points to Ponder**
>
> - *Bakuchi is considered as a prime drug for vitiligo (swetakusta).*
> - *Bakuchi is widely famous since ages for its magical effects against several skin diseases, such as psoriasis, leukoderma, and leprosy.*

Suggested Readings

Chand S, Sahrawat AK. Somatic embriogenesis and plant regeneration from root segments of *Psoralea corylifolia* L.: an endangered medicinal plant. In Vitro Cell Dev Biol 2002;38:33

Cheng X. Easy Comprehension of Traditional Chinese Medicine: Chinese Materia Medica. Beijing: Canadian Institute of Traditional Chinese Medicine; 2001:343

Chopra RN, Chopra IC. Indigenous Drugs of India. 2nd ed. Kolkata: Academic Publishers; 1958:391–394

Joshi SG. Medicinal Plants. New Delhi: Oxford and IBH Publishing Co. Pvt. Ltd; 2000:206–207

Kapoor LD. Handbook of Ayurvedic Medicinal Plants. Boca Raton, FL: CRC Press; 2001:274–275

Khare CP. Encyclopedia of Indian Medicinal Plants. New York, NY: Springer-Verlag; 2004:384–386

Khushboo PS, Jadhav VM, Kadam VJ, Sathe NS. *Psoralea corylifolia* Linn.: Kushtanashini. Pharmacogn Rev 2010;4(7):69–76

Kiritikar KR, Basu BD. Indian Medicinal Plants. Vol. I. 2nd ed. Dehradun: International Book Distributors; 2008:717–721

Krishnamurthi A. The Wealth of India: Raw Material. Vol. VIII. 1969

Laxmipati S. Yogratnakara. Bhrahmasankar Shashtri, editor. Varanasi: Chaukhamba Prakashana; 2013.

Miller GA, Morris M. Plants of Dhofar. Oman: Office of the Adviser for Conservation of the Environment, Diwan of Royal Court, Sultanate of Oman:1988:174–175

Mishra S. Rasatrangani. Kashinath Shastri, editor. Varanasi: Motilal Banarasidas; 2000:161

Mookerjee B. Rasa Jala Nidhi. Vol. 3. Varanasi: Chaukhambha Publishers; 1999:301

Nadkarni KM. Indian Materia Medica. Vol. 1. Mumbai: Popular Prakashan Pvt. Ltd; 1976:1019–1022

Panda H. Herbs, Cultivation and Medicinal Uses. New Delhi: National Institute of Industrial Research; 2000:479–481

Pandey V. Agni Purana ki Ayurvediya Anusandhanatmaka Samiksha. 1st ed. Delhi: Shree Satguru Publications; 1997:101

Pathak J, Acharya R. Bākucī (*Psoralea corylifolia* Linn.) and its classical āyurvedic and ethnomedicinal uses: a critical review. Int J Res Ayurveda Pharm 2018;9(4):129–135

Qiao CF, Han QB, Song JZ, et al. Chemical fingerprint and quantitative analysis of fructus psoraleae by high-performance liquid chromatography. J Sep Sci 2007;30(6):813–818

Rajpal V. Standardization of Botanicals. Vol. 2. New Delhi: Eastern Publishers; 2005:284–95

Rasendrachudamani S, Bajpai RD, editor. Varanasi: Chaukhamba Krishnadas Academy; 2004:15

Sah P, Agrawal D, Garg SP. Isolation and identification of furocoumarins from the seeds of *Psoralea corylifolia* L. Indian J Pharm Sci 2006;68(6):768–771

Sankshipta Garuna Purana. Achara Kanda. Gorakhpur: Kalyan Karyalaya, Patralaya, Geeta Press; 1867:267, 268

Seth A. The Herbs of Ayurveda. 1st ed. Vol. 4. Gujarat: Hi Scan Pvt. Ltd; 2005:950

Shanker Dutta Gauda. Shanker Nighantu. Chaukhamba Subharti Prakashan; 2002:185

Sharma PC, Yelne MB, Dennis TJ. Database on Medicinal Plants Used in Ayurveda. Vol. 2. New Delhi: Central Council for Research in Ayurveda and Siddha; 2001:89–93

Sharma PV. Dravya Guna Vigyan. Vol. II. Chaukhamba Bharti Academy. Reprint 2013:177, 178

Sharma PV. Namarupaviygyana. Varanasi: Chawkhamba Visvabharati Oriental publishers; 2015:138

Shilandra KU, Yadav AS, Sharma AK, Rai AK, Raghuwanshi DK, Badkhane Y. The botany, chemistry, pharmacological and therapeutic application of *Psoralea corylifolia* Linn.: a review. Int J Phytomed 2010;2(2):100–107

Szliszka E, Skaba D, Czuba ZP, Krol W. Inhibition of inflammatory mediators by neobavaisoflavone in activated RAW264.7 macrophages. Molecules 2011;16(5):3701–3712

The Ayurvedic Pharmacopoeia of India. E-book. Part 1. Vol. 1. New Delhi: Department of AYUSH, Ministry of Health and Family Welfare, Government of India; 2003:25

Tripathi I, ed. Rasarnava Nama Rasatantra. Varanasi: Chaukhamba Sanskrit Series; 2010:221, 279, 280, 281

Xiong Z, Wang D, Xu Y, Li F. Osteoblastic differentiation bioassay and its application to investigating the activity of fractions and compounds from *Psoralea corylifolia* L. Pharmazie 2003;58(12):925–928

Yashodhara. Rasa Prakasha Sudhakara. Siddhinanda Mishra, editor. Varanasi: Chaukhamba Orientalia; 2013:209, 216, 218

Zhang X, Zhao W, Wang Y, Lu J, Chen X. The chemical constituents and bioactivities of *Psoralea corylifolia* Linn.: a review. Am J Chin Med 2016;44(1):35–60

Zhao L, Huang C, Shan Z, Xiang B, Mei L. Fingerprint analysis of *Psoralea corylifolia* L. by HPLC and LC-MS. J Chromatogr B Analyt Technol Biomed Life Sci 2005;821(1):67–74

Vagbhatta. Rasaratnasammuchaya. Ambika Dutta Shastri, editor. New Delhi: Amar Bharti Sansthan; 2012:112

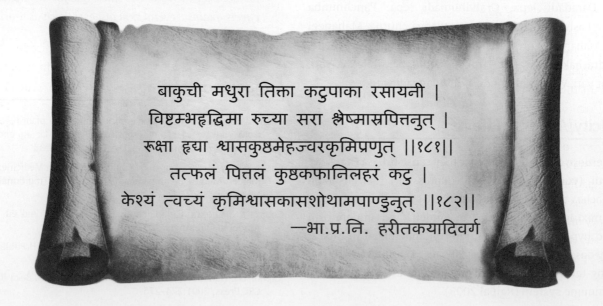

बाकुची मधुरा तिक्ता कटुपाका रसायनी |
विष्टम्भहृद्दिमा रुच्या सरा श्लेष्मास्रपित्तनुत् |
रूक्षा हृद्या श्वासकुष्ठमेहज्वरकृमिप्रणुत् ||१८१||
तत्फलं पित्तलं कुष्ठकफानिलहरं कटु |
केश्यं त्वच्यं कृमिश्वासकासशोथामपाण्डुनुत् ||१८२||
—भा.प्र.नि. हरीतकयादिवर्ग

16. Bhallataka [Semecarpus anacardium Linn. F.]

Family:	*Anacardiaceae*
Hindi name:	*Bhilawa (bhilv), Bhela (bhel), Bhelwa, Bhilwa*
English name:	*Marking nut, Marsh nut, Oriental cashew nut*

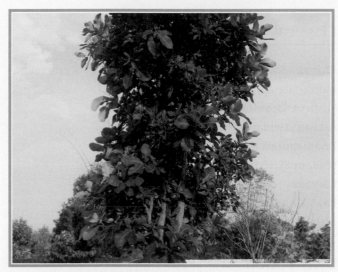

Plant of *Semecarpus anacardium* Linn. F.

The availability of tree of Bhallataka indicates fear (Bhaya) (Vrikshaayurveda 21/323).

Introduction

Bhallataka (*Semecarpus anacardium* Linn. F.) is a medium-to large-sized tree with many medicinal properties. The word "Semecarpus" is derived from Greek word simeion meaning marking or tracing, and carpus meaning nut. Anacardium means like cardium. *Semecarpus anacardium* means "heart-shaped marking nut." The literal meaning of the term "Bhallataka" is sharp-like spear which produces blisters on touch.

Bhallataka is acclaimed as a drug of choice in the treatment of piles of vata and kapha types. Acharya Charak stated that there is no kaphaj vyadhi or vibandh (constipation) which cannot be cured by Bhallataka. *Semecarpus anacardium* is classified in Ayurveda under the category of toxic plants (Sharma 1975). It is extremely hot and sharp in its attributes; it should be used with caution. It has also got the potential to produce allergic manifestations such as dermatitis, blisters, and swelling on direct contact with skin. Hence, it is advised to use this medicinal plant after proper purification. Individuals showing allergic reactions to it should stop and avoid the usage of Bhallataka.

The fruit pericarp is used by dhobis as marking ink for cotton clothes, and hence it is known as the marking nut. Dhanvantari nighantu and Rasatarangani mentioned it in upavisha varga whereas Charak kept it under rasayana drugs. Acharya Charak has considered its fruit as teekshna (piercing), paki (corrosive), agnisama (properties like fire), medhya, and agnivardhak. Raj Nighantu stated that fully ripe Bhallataka fruits which sink in water are considered best and should be used in therapeutics.

Bhallataka is used for hair care in traditional system of medicines. It is used for dyeing and promoting hair growth in folk medicine (Gaur 1991; Semalty et al 2008).

In Charak Samhita, ten different types of Bhallataka preparations are mentioned in rasayana chapter, namely, Bhallataka sarpi, Bhallataka kshir, Bhallataka kshoudra, Bhallataka guda, Bhallataka yusha, Bhallataka taila,

Bhallataka patala, Bhallataka saktu, Bhallataka lavan, and Bhallataka tarpan.

Thousand Bhallataka nuts are used during the schedule of one therapeutic course of vardhamana prayoga (gradually increasing the numbers of nuts) as per Sushrut Samhita and Astanga Hridaya.

Vernacular Names

Arabic: Habb al fahm, Habb al qalb

Assamese: Bhelaguti

Bengali: Bhela (bhela), Bhelatuki

Danish: Ostindisk elefantlus

Dutch: Malakkanoot, Oostindische acajounoot, Oost-Indische olifantsluis

French: Anacarde d'Orient, Noix à marquer, Noix des marais

German: Anakardien-Herznub, Malakkanub Elefantenlausbaum, Ostindische Elefantenlaus

Greek: Semekarpos anakardion

Gujarati: Bhilamu

Kannada: Bhallataka, Bhallika, Goddugeru, Karigeri

Italian: Anacardio orientale

Japanese: Anakarudiumu orientaare, Anakarudiumu orientaru, Makingunatto, Makingunattsu

Malayalam: Alakkuceru (alakkuceru), Chera

Marathi: Bibba, Bibha

Nepalese: Kaag bhalaayo

Oriya: Bhollataki

Portuguese: Anacárdio oriental

Punjabi: Bhilawa

Russian: Semekarpus Anakardii

Spanish: Anacardio oriental

Tamil: Erimugi (erimuki)

Telugu: Nallajeedi

Synonyms

Agnika: It produces burning like fire.

Agnimukhi: Fruits are seated on a fleshy orange cap.

Arushkar: The juice of the fruit produces blisters on touch.

Arushka: The juice of the fruit produces blisters on touch.

Bhallataka: It produces blisters due its tikshna guna.

Bhalli: A tree with irritant sap of the bark.

Bhedan: It is useful in tumor due to its tikshna action.

Bhutaghni: The drugs kill organisms or drive away the evil spirit.

Dhanurbeeja: Fruits are obliquely ovoid.

Krimighna: The drugs kill worm.

Ranjaka: It is used as blackening agent.

Shophkrit: The juice of the fruit produces blisters and swelling on touch.

Tailabeeja: The nuts are oily or having oil.

Vatari: It cures vatika disorder.

Veeravriksh: It is a highly potent drug.

Classical Categorization

Charak Samhita: Deepaniya, Bhedaniya, Kushtaghna, Mutrasangrahniya

Sushrut Samhita: Nyagrodhadi, Mustadi

Astanga Hridaya: Mustadi

Dhanwantari Nighantu: Chandanadi varga

Madanpal Nighantu: Abhayadi varga

Kaiyadev Nighantu: Oshadhi varga

Raj Nighantu: Amradi varga

Bhavaprakash: Haritakyadi varga

Distribution

It is a moderate-sized deciduous tree found in the outer Himalayas and hotter parts of India up to 3,500 ft height. The plant is found in abundance in Assam, Bihar, Bengal, and Odisha, Chittagong, central India, and western peninsula of East Archipelago, Northern Australia. (Kirtikar and Basu 1975).

Morphology

It is a medium-to-large size deciduous tree of about 15 to 25 m height.

- **Bark:** Gray and exfoliates regularly in small irregular flakes and exudes a red irritant resin on incising, which blackens on exposure (**Fig. 16.1**).
- **Leaves:** Simple, alternate, 8 to 12 inch long, 3 to 4 inch wide, obovate-oblong shape, rounded apex, leathery in texture, glabrous above, and pubescent beneath (**Fig. 16.2a, b**).
- **Flowers:** Greenish-white, fascicled in pubescent panicles (**Fig. 16.3a, b**).

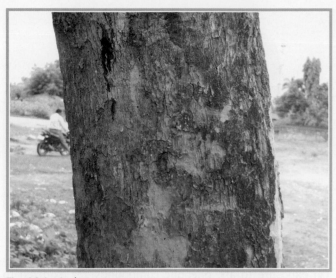

Fig. 16.1 Bark.

- **Fruits:** Obliquely ovoid or oblong drupes, 2.5 to 4 cm long, compressed, shining black when ripe, seated on a fleshy orange-colored receptacle (**Fig. 16.4a, b**). Milky exudate secretes from unripe fruits, which becomes black on ripening (Bhitre et al 2008). The seed inside the black fruit, known as godambi, is edible when properly prepared. The plant is propagated through seeds.

Phenology

Flowering time: July to August
Fruiting time: October to December

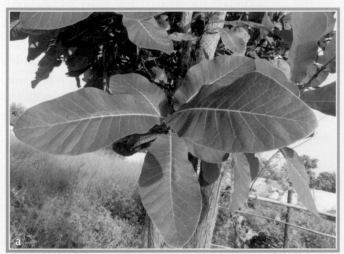

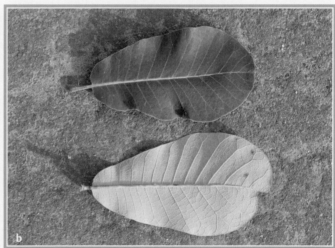

Fig. 16.2 **(a)** Leaves. **(b)** Dorsal and ventral sides of leaves.

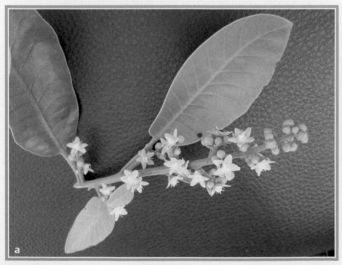

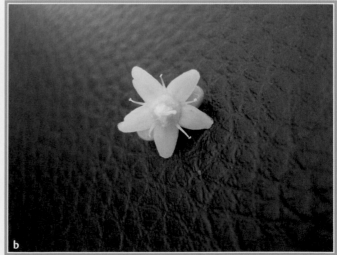

Fig. 16.3 **(a)** Inflorescence. **(b)** Flower.

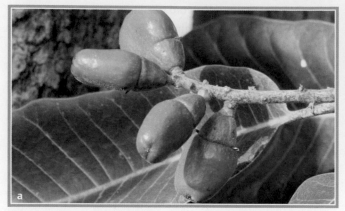
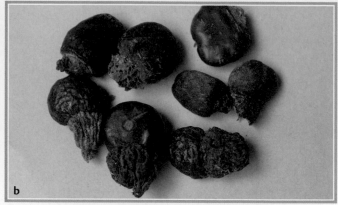

Fig. 16.4 **(a)** Fresh fruit. **(b)** Mature fruit.

Key Characters for Identification

➤ *Medium-to-large size deciduous tree of about 15 to 25 m tall*

➤ *Bark: gray, small irregularly flakes, exudates red resin that turns to black later on*

➤ *Leaf: simple alternate, 8 to 12 inch long and 3 to 4 inch wide, obovate-oblong shape, rounded apex*

➤ *Flowers: greenish white, fascicled in pubescent panicles*

➤ *Fruits: oblong drupe seated on a fleshy receptacle, shining black when ripe*

Rasapanchaka

Guna	Laghu, Snigdha, Tikshna
Rasa	Kashaya, Madhur
Vipaka	Madhur
Virya	Ushna
Fruit pulp	Madhur, vrusya, brimhana, vatapittahara
Vrinta	Madhur, pittaghna, kesya, agni vardhak

Chemical Constituents

The most important components of *Semecarpus anacardium* Linn. are bhilwanols, phenolic compounds, biflavonoids, sterols, and glycosides.

An alkaloid, Bhilwanol, has been isolated from oil and seeds. Bhilwanol from fruits was shown to be a mixture of cis and trans isomers of ursuhenol. Oil from nuts, bhilavinol, contains a mixture of phenolic compounds mainly of 1,2-dihydroxy-3 (pentadecadienyl-8, 11) benzene and 1,2dihydroxy-3 (pentadecadienyl-8', 11')-benzene. On exposure to air, phenolic compounds get oxidized to quinones.

Nut shells contain the biflavonoids: biflavones A, C, A1, A2, tetrahydrorobustaflavone, B (tetrahydromentoflavone), jeediflavanone, semecarpuflavan, and gulluflavone.

Other components isolated are anacardic acid, cardol, catechol, fixed oil, semecarpetin, anacardol, anacardoside, and semecarpol. The kernel oil contains oleic acid, 60.6%; linoleic acid, 17.1%; palmitic acid, 16%; stearic acid, 3.8%; and arachidic acid, 1.4% (Jain and Sharma 2013).

Identity, Purity, and Strength

- Foreign matter: Not more than 1%
- Total ash: Not more than 4%
- Acid-insoluble ash: Not more than 0.5%
- Alcohol-soluble extractive: Not less than 11%
- Water-soluble extractive: Not less than 5%

(Source: The Ayurvedic Pharmacopoeia of India 1999)

Karma (Actions)

The actions of Bhallataka are deepan (appetizer), pachan (digestive), bhedan (purgative), medhya (brain tonic), chhedan (expectorant), shitaprasaman (calefacient), kushtaghna (antidermatosis), mutrasangahaniya (urinary astringent), shukral (spermatogenic) jwaraghna (antipyretic), swadajanana (diaphoretic), hridya (cardio tonic), brimhana (weight promoting), etc.

- Doshakarma: Kaphavata hara
- Dhatukarma: Shukral
- Malakarma: Bhedan

Pharmacological Actions

The pharmacological properties of Bhallataka are reported as antiatherogenic, anti-inflammatory, CNS activity, antimicrobial, antibacterial, hypoglycemic, anti-carcinogenic, antispermatogenic, ache inhibitory, antirheumatic, anthelmintic activity (Pallavi et al 2015).

Indications

It is used in kaphavata diseases, kushta (skin diseases), arsha (piles), vrana (wounds), udara (abdominal diseases), grahani (sprue), gulma (abdominal lump), shopha (swelling), anaha (abdominal distention), jwara (fever), krimi (worm infestation), sweta kushta (leucoderma), shwasa (asthma), vibandha (constipation), shool (pain).

Contraindications

Bhallataka's use is contraindicated in
- Children, old age, pregnant women, and individuals of pitta constitution
- Pittaj vyadhi, hemorrhagic diseases, diarrhea, and nephritis
- Summer season

Therapeutic Uses

External Use

1. **Inflammation** (shotha): One to two drops of Bhallataka oil mixed with butter is applied locally as ointment in rheumatism, neuritis, chronic skin diseases, goiter, tumors, cystic swellings, and in piles.
2. **As depilatory:** Bhallataka oil and Snuhi latex is applied together for depilatory action (SB.Ci. 1/106).
3. **Varnyaprasadana** (For restoring normal color): Bhallataka oil is applied locally on wound scar to regain the normal complexion (S.S.Ci. 1/90-93).
4. **Visha anjana** (counter collyrium): If collyrium is poisoned (vishayukta anjana), the flowers of Bhallataka are rubbed in milk which is used as counter-collyrium (S.S.Ka. 1/69-71).

Internal Use

1. **Arsha** (piles): (a) Bhallataka and bark of Kutaj is considered as best drug for dry and bleeding piles, respectively. Buttermilk is wholesome in all types of piles in all seasons (AH.Ci. 8/62 and AH.U. 40/49). (b) A saturating drink of buttermilk with Bhallataka, Sunthi, and Chitraka can also be taken (C.S.Ci. 14/70). (c) Bhallataka kalpa and Bhallataka taila (S.S.Ci. 6/17-18) is useful in piles.
2. **Kushta** (skin diseases): (a) Intake of ghrita processed with Bhallataka, Haritaki, and Vidang is an effective remedy to cure skin diseases originated due to aggravated kapha. Local application of oil of Bhallataka or Tuvraka is also beneficial (S.S.Ci. 9/7). (b) Food and ghee prepared with Bhallataka, Triphala, and Nimba should be used (C.S.Ci. 7/82). (c) Tuvarak, Bhallataka, Bakuchi, root of Chitrak, and Shilajatu are given as per rasayana process to cure kushta (AH.Ci. 19/53).
3. **Pleehodara** (splenomegaly): Daily intake of Bhallataka, Haritaki, Jeeraka mixed with jaggery is used to cure splenomegaly (VM. 37/45). Tablet prepared with equal quantity of Bhallataka, Haritaki, Til, and jaggery should be given to cure plleharoga, pandu, jwra, kasa, and shwasa (Rasatarangini. 24/483).
4. **Shweta kustha** (Vitiligo): Bhallataka fruits should be crushed and kept overnight in cow's urine and then dried; repeat the same for three times. Then pound with latex of Snuhi and apply the paste on the affected area (AH.Ci. 20/11).
5. **Jwara (fever):** Bhallataka should be given with jaggery to prevent jwara (AH.Ci. 1/154).
6. **Vrishya** (aphrodisiac): Medicated milk prepared with Bhallataka nuts should be consumed daily for aphrodisiac purpose (AS.U. 50/29).
7. **Rasayana** (rejuvinator): Bhallataka rasayana (C.S.Ci. 1.2.13-19 and AH.Ci. 39/66-83) and Bhallataka vardhaman (VM. 69.23-27) are given for rasayana purposes.
8. **Krimi** (worm infestation): Oral consumption of Bhallataka taila mixed with half quantity of Vidang churna helps in expulsion of worms (GN. 2.6.39).
9. **Urustambha** (filariasis): Paste of Pippali, Pippalimool, and Bhallataka fruit with honey gives relief in urustambha (VM. 5-10; RM. 22.1).
10. **Shwasa and Kasa** (asthma and cough): Tablet prepared from equal quantity of Bhallataka powder, Haritaki

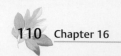

powder, Til powder, and jaggery is given to cure shwasa and kasa (Rasatarangini 24/483).

Officinal Parts Used

Fruit and oil

Dose

Oil: 10 to 20 drops
Ksheerpaka: 1 to 2 g
Paste: 3 to 6 g

The dose of Bhallataka should be decided with due consideration of physical strength, habitat, time or season, and body constitution (prakriti) of the patients and decide 1 rati (123 mg) to 3 rati of purified bhallataka (Rasatarangini 24/482).

Formulations

Bhallataka taila, Bhallataka ghrita, Amrita Bhallataka, Bhallataka guda, Chincha Bhallataka, Bhallataka avaleha, Sanjivani vati, Bhallataka rasayana, Kankayan vati, Bhallataka lavana, Bhallatakadi modak, Bhallataka lepa.

Toxicity/Adverse Effects

If the milky juice exudate from Bhallataka fruit comes in contact with the skin, it causes severe daha (burning sensation), itching all over the body, blisters, vrana (ulcers), skin rashes, shopha (inflammation), atisaar (diarrhea), and hematuria. Hence, it should be used after proper purification (shodhana).

Treatment/Remedial Measures

Treatment is symptomatic. Wash the exposed area with water and apply antidote or ointments. If consumed orally, first cleanse the stomach by consuming warm water and then give milk, ice to suck, and 10 mg morphine for pain.

Antidote

Coconut and coconut oil, Til, Rala ointment, ghee, paste of Dhanyak leaves, juice of Amlika leaves (Imli), and lead lotion are used as antidote of Bhallataka poisoning. Bibhitaka fruit

decoction or powder is also used as specific antidote in Bhallataka toxicity.

Pathya and Apathya

Pathya: Person should consume ghee, milk, and rice in large quantity during intake of Bhallataka. Because it is hot in nature, it is best to use it in the winter season.

Apathya: Exposure to sun and heat, excessive sex, consumption of meat and salt, exercise, Kullatha, curd, shukta, and oil massage should be avoided during the administration of Bhallataka. The use of Bhallataka should be restricted in summer season (AH.U. 39/83).

Shodhana (Method of Purification)

Mature and fully ripe fruits that sink in water are selected for Shodhana. Fruits are then put into a bag containing coarse brick powder with which they are rubbed carefully. When the brick powder becomes wet with oil, the fruit skin is peeled off. The fruits are then washed with hot water, dried, and kept for further use. Before performing shodhana (purification), a person should apply coconut oil on face, hand, legs, and other exposed body parts to avoid the side effects.

Substitution and Adulteration

Bhallataka fruit is substituted by heartwood of Rakta Chandan (Pterocarpus santalinus Linn. of Fabaceae family) or by root bark of Chitrak (Plumbago zeylanica Linn. of Plumbaginaceae family; Bhavamishra 2010).

Points to Ponder

- *Bhallataka is effective in Kaphaja vyadhi and Vibandha (C.S.Ci. 1/2/19 and AH.U. 39/82).*
- *Bhallataka is best for arsha (AH.U. 40/49).*
- *Charak has mentioned 10 preparations of Bhallataka in rasayan chapter (C.S.Ci. 1/2/16).*
- *Acharya Sushruta and Vagbhatta advised to take total 1,000 bhallataka nuts in vardhaman yoga.*
- *Rakta Chandan and Chitrak mool are the substitute drugs for Bhallataka.*
- *Bhallataka should be used after purification with brick powder; otherwise, it may cause severe daha, vrana, shotha, and visarpa.*

Suggested Readings

Bhavmishra. Bhavprakash Nighantu: Commentary by KC Chunekar. In GS Pandey, ed. Varanasi: Choukhambha Bharati Academy; 2010:960

Bhitre MJ, Patil S, Kataria M, Anwikar S, Kadri H. Antiinflammatory activity of the fruits of *Semecarpus anacardium*. Linn Asian J Chem 2008;20:2047–2050

Chopra RN. Indigenous Drugs of India. 2nd ed. Calcutta: Academic Publishers; 1982:407–409

Dr. Ananta Ram Sharma, Sushrut Samhita of Sushrut. Reprint ed. Varanasi: Chaukhambha Surabharati Prakashan; chikitstasthana 6/17, Arshachikista adhyay, 2010:231

Gaur RD. Flora and Fauna of Garhwal Himalaya. Srinagar Garhwal: Trans Media; 1991:315–316

Jain P, Sharma HP. A potential ethnomedicinal plant: *Semecarpus anacardium* Linn.: a review. Int J Res Pharm Chem: IJRPC 2013; 3(3):554–572

Khare CP. Encyclopedia of Indian Medicinal Plants. New Delhi: Springer; 1982:419–421

Kirtikar KR, Basu BD. Indian Medicinal Plants. Vol. 3. Dehradun, India: International Booksellers and Publishers; 1975:667

Matthai TP, Date A. Renal cortical necrosis following exposure to sap of the marking-nut tree (*Semecarpus anacardium*). Am J Trop Med Hyg 1979;28(4):773–774

Mishra B, Nighantu B. Commentary by K.C. Chunekar and edited by G.S. Pandey. Varanasi: Choukhambha Bharati Academy; 2010:960

Niteshwar K. Text Book of Dravyaguna. Varanasi: Chaukhambha Surbharti Prakashan

Pallavi AD, Charandas Tumram A, Dashrath Lambat R, Shirish Suryawanshi S. Therapeutic significance of *Semecarpus anacardium* Linn: a review. Int J Res Ayurveda Pharma 2015;6(4)

Pande G. Vrikshaayurveda of Surapal. 1st ed. Varanasi: Chaukhamba Sanskrit Series Office; 2010:102

Semalty M, Semalty A, Joshi GP, Rawat MS. Herbal hair growth promotion strategies for alopecia. Ind Drugs 2008;45:689–700

Sharma S. Rastarangini, by P. Kashinath Shastri, commentary by Shri Haridatta Shastri. Varanasi: Motilal Banarsidas; 1975:670

Shukla Acharya V, Tripathy RD. Charak Samhita of Agnivash. Reprint ed. Delhi: Chaukhambha Sanskrit Pratishtan; chikitstasthan1/2–16, rasayan adhyay, pranakamiya pada, 2009:24

The Ayurvedic Pharmacopoeia of India. Part 1. Vol. 2. New Delhi: Ministry of Health of Family Welfare, Government of India; 1999:19

Tripathi B. Astanga Hridaya of Vagbhatta. Reprint ed. Delhi: Chaukhambha Sanskrit Prakashan; uttarasthan 39/66–71, rasayanavidhi adhyay, 2011:1191

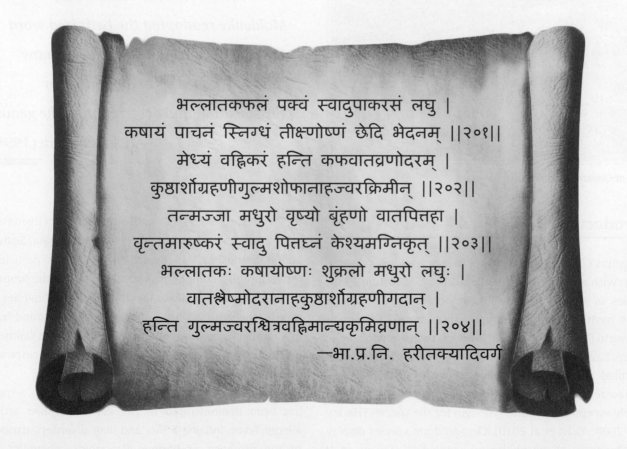

भल्लातकफलं पक्वं स्वादुपाकरसं लघु |
कषायं पाचनं स्निग्धं तीक्ष्णोष्णं छेदि भेदनम् ||२०१||
मेध्यं वह्निकरं हन्ति कफवातव्रणोदरम् |
कुष्ठार्शोग्रहणीगुल्मशोफानाहज्वरक्रिमीन् ||२०२||
तन्मज्जा मधुरो वृष्यो बृंहणो वातपित्तहा |
वृन्तमारुष्करं स्वादु पित्तघ्नं केश्यमग्निकृत् ||२०३||
भल्लातकः कषायोष्णः शुक्लो मधुरो लघुः |
वातश्लेष्मोदरानाहकुष्ठार्शोग्रहणीगदान् |
हन्ति गुल्मज्वरश्चित्रवह्निमान्द्यकृमिव्रणान् ||२०४||
—भा.प्र.नि. हरीतक्यादिवर्ग

17. Bharangi [*Clerodendrum serratum* Spreng.]

Family: *Verbenaceae (recently placed in Lamiaceae)*

Hindi name: *Bharangi, Babhneti*

English name: *Blue glory, Beetle killer*

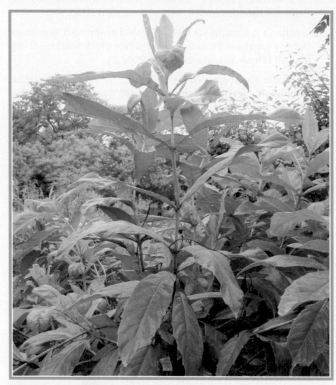

Plant of *Clerodendrum serratum* Spreng.

> *The genus Clerodendrum was first described by Linnacus in 1753 based on the species Clerodendrum infortunatum from India and later Adanson changed the Latinized form "Clerodendrum" to its Greek form "Clerodendron" in 1763. After almost two centuries, Moldenke readopted the Latinized word "Clerodendrum" in 1942 which is now commonly used by taxonomists for classification and description of the genus.*
> —Hsiao and Lin (1995)

Introduction

The genus *Clerodendrum* of Verbenaceae family is a diverse genus with about 560 (Moldenke 1971) to 580 (Munir 1989) species of small trees, shrubs, or occasionally perennial herbs, mostly found in the tropics and subtropics region of the world (Verdcourt 1992). However, recent phylogenetic studies have reported that genus *Clerodendrum* traditionally classified in Verbenaceae has now been included in Lamiaceae, and *Rotheca serrata* (L.) Steane & Mabb. is widely accepted scientific synonym for the species (Harley et al 2004; Yuan et al 2010). *Clerodendrum* species display a high degree of morphological, cytological (Steane et al 1997), and chemical variations.

The term "Bharangi" indicates its effectiveness in respiratory tract disorders like kasa and shwasa. Sushruta and Bhavamishra had described this plant particularly for respiratory complaints viz. cold, bronchitis, bronchial asthma, and tuberculosis as it effectively liquefies the mucus (Nighantu 2005; Chunekar 2013). Roots and leaves of Bharangi have great medicinal value and are claimed to be useful in pain, inflammation, rheumatism, respiratory disorders, and fever especially in malarial fever.

Therapeutic potential of roots and leaves of *C. serratum* has been demonstrated in the conditions like asthma, allergy, fever, inflammation, and liver disorders attributed to the presence of various flavonoids, phenolics, and saponins present in the drug. Ethnomedicinal reports have also advocated *C. serratum* as one of the potential traditional medicines in India claimed for the treatment of asthma, inflammation, wounds, snake bite, liver diseases, fever, and headache.

Natural population of the plant species is diminishing owing to habitat destruction, overexploitation, along with poor seed setting and germination. As *C. serratum* is categorized under nearly threatened species by IUCN (International Union for the Conservation of Nature and Natural Resources; Singh and Singh 2009; Kumari et al 2012), effective preventive measures must be taken to preserve natural populations of this plant in India.

Vernacular Names

Bengali: Bamun Hatee, Baman hatee, Bhuijam
Gujarati: Bharangee
Kannada: Gantubarangee
Malayalam: Cheruteku
Marathi: Bharangee, Bharang
Oriya: Chinds
Punjabi: Bhadangee
Tamil: Cheruteku
Telugu: Ganttubrarangee
Urdu: Bharangi, Baharangi

Synonyms

Angaarvalli: A plant grows wild.
Bhangura: The wood breaks easily.
Bharangi: It alleviates disease like kasa.
Bhramarapriya/Bhrungaja: The flowers attract bees.
Bhrugubhava: It is originated from sage in Himalayas.
Brahmani: The stems are thin and branchless.
Brahmanyashtika: The stems are thin and without branches.
Hinjika: The plant is beautiful.
Kharapuspa: The flowers are rough.
Kharashaka: The leaves are rough.
Padma: Flowers resemble lotus flowers.
Phanji: The stick of this plant is useful.
Suroopa: The plant is beautiful.
Varshabarbaraka: The plant sprouts in Varsha ritu.
Vatari: It is useful in vatik disorders.

Classical Categorization

Charak Samhita: Krimighna, Purish sangrahaniya
Sushrut Samhita: Pippalyadi, Arkadi
Ashtanga Sangraha: Pippalyadi
Ashtanga Hridaya: Arkadi, Surasadi
Dhanwantari Nighantu: Guduchyadi varga
Madanpal Nighantu: Abhayadi varga
Kaiyadev Nighantu: Oushadhi varga
Raj Nighantu: Pippalyadi varga
Bhavaprakash: Haritakyadi varga

Distribution

Clerodendrum serratum Linn. is found more or less throughout India, in forests up to 1,500 m altitude. It is reported to be rare and endangered in Gujarat (Kiritikar and Basu 1999). In India, it is specially found in Karnataka (Koppa, Manipal, Mudbidri), Tamil Nadu, forests of Kerala, Konkan region of Maharashtra.

Morphology

It is a perennial, woody shrub of 1 to 2 m of height.

- **Stem**: Woody, not much branched, bluntly quadrangular, and younger parts are glabrous.
- **Leaves:** Simple, or in whorl of three at node, subsessile, obovate to oblong shape, 4 to 10 inches long, shortly acuminate, base cuneate, serrated margin, thick, and coriaceous. Leaves are attached with sharp, pulpy, and oily thorns (**Fig. 17.1**).

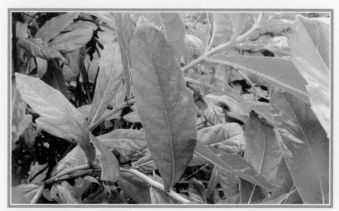

Fig. 17.1 Leaves.

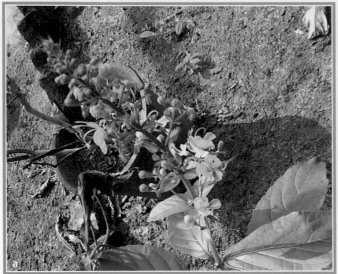

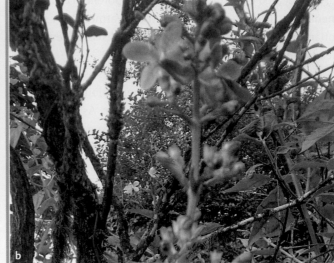

Fig. 17.2 (a) Inflorescence. **(b)** Flower.

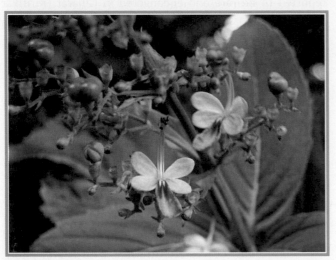

Fig. 17.3 Fruits.

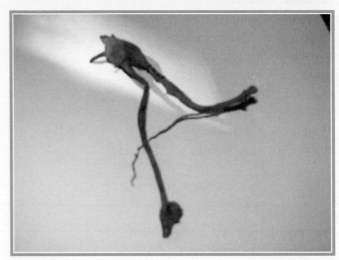

Fig. 17.4 Root.

- **Flowers:** Numerous, slightly fragrant, pale blue to purple in color, in terminal inflorescence of 8 to 10 inches, pubescent, dichotomous cymes with a pair of acute bracts at each branching and a flower in the fork. They are bisexual, zygomorphic, rarely sub-actinomorphic, and bracteolate or not. Corolla with a slender tube, five lobes, spreading; stamens epipetalous, four or two, free; one anther or two-celled usually dehiscing longitudinally; disc persistent. Ovary superior, two-celled and each cell is two-ovuled; and style subterminal and gynobasic (**Fig. 17.2a, b**).
- **Fruits:** Four-lobed purple drupe with 5 to 14 mm length and 5 to 8 mm width and usually separating into pyrenes at maturity, appears in group, obovoid shape, somewhat succulent, and purple black color on ripening, four-seeded (**Fig. 17.3**).
- **Seeds:** Oblong with little or no endosperm.
- **Root:** Mature root hard, woody, up to 5 cm thick, cylindrical, outer surface light brown with lenticels (**Fig. 17.4**).

The plant is propagated through seeds and stem cutting.

Phenology

Flowering time: August to September

Fruiting time: October to December

Rasapanchaka

Guna	Laghu, Ruksha
Rasa	Katu, Tikta, Kashaya
Vipaka	Katu
Virya	Ushna

Chemical Constituents

Major chemical constituents present in the root and leaves of Bharangi are carbohydrates, phenols, terpenes, flavonoids, and steroids. Its roots have D-mannitol, hispidulin (flavonoids), cleroflavones, apigenin, glucuronides, scutellarin, acteoside, verbascoside, uncinatone γ & β-sitosterol, saponnins, oleanic acid, ferulic acid, arabinose, and urosolic acid.

Identity, Purity, and Strength

- Foreign matter: Not more than 2%
- Total ash: Not more than 11%
- Acid-insoluble ash: Not more than 1%
- Alcohol-soluble extractive: Not less than 6%
- Water-soluble extractive: Not less than 12%
(Source: The Ayurvedic Pharmacopeia of India 2001)

Karma (Actions)

The actions of Bharangi are as deepana (carminative), pachana (digestive), ruchya (improves taste), Vatahara (pacify vata), Kaphahara (pacify kapha), Swasahara (antiasthmatic).

- Doshakarma: Kapha vatahara
- Dhatukarma: Raktashodhan
- Malakarma: Shwedajanana

Pharmacological Actions

Various pharmacological actions of Bharangi are bronchodilator, antiallergic, antiasthmatic, antibacterial, wound-healing, antiulcer, anticarcinogenic, anti-inflammatory, antioxidant, antiangiogenic, and vasorelaxant activities (Kumar and Nishteswar 2013; Sharma and Gupta 2013).

Recent reports have focused on evaluating the antiasthmatic, anti-inflammatory, hepatoprotective, anticancer, antioxidant, and antibacterial activities of mostly roots and leaves of the plant, which can be explained by the presence of various flavonoids, phenolics, and saponins in roots.

Indications

It is useful in the treatment of shwasa, hikka, apasmara, gandamala, galaganda, kuranda, vataja kasa, bradhana, vata rogas, rajayakshma, shopha, vrana, krimi rogas, daha, gulma, rakta dosha (bleeding disorders), shotha (inflammation), kasa (chronic cough), shwasa (asthma), peenasa (coryza), and jwara (fever).

Sushruta used it in the management of apasmara whereas Shodhala in vrana ropana. Roots are reported to be used clinically for the treatment of bronchitis, asthma, fever, blood diseases, tumors, inflammations, burning sensation, epilepsy, malaria, ulcer, and wounds (Vidya et al 2007). Roots and leaf extracts of *C. serratum* have been used for the treatment of rheumatism, asthma, and other inflammatory diseases (Hazekamp et al 2001).

The root juice with ginger is used to relieve bronchospasms in asthma and reduce the attacks of dyspnea while the root powder is given along with sugar or as jam in hic-cough.

The decoction of root is extremely effective in edema over body, especially due to kapha, and is used in worm infestations while decoction of sesame seeds (tila) mixed with ghee, jaggery, *C. serratum* root powder, and Trikatu powder is used as the best remedy for amenorrhea and uterine tumor (Sharma et al 2002). The root paste has been applied on the forehead to alleviate headache. The leaves are used in fever and burning sensation and are boiled in oil or butter for external applications in ophthalmia and cephalalgia.

It is reported in clinical study that the efficacy of Bharangyadi yoga (30 mL bd with honey for 30 days in 30 clinically diagnosed bronchial asthmatic patients) and its nebulizer (2.5 mL bd for 15 days in 30 clinically diagnosed bronchial asthmatic patients) has been successfully evaluated for the management of chronic persistent asthma as well as acute attack of asthma (Kajaria et al 2012).

Therapeutic Uses

External Use

1. **Gandmala** (cervical lymphadinitic): Bharangi root paste with rice water is applied locally in gandmala (goiter), galagand (cervical adenitis), kurand (scrotal enlargement) (CD.41.24, RM.17.1).
2. **Kshataj vrana** (accidental wounds): Root of Bharangi pounded with water applied locally in accidental wound (GN. 4.4.56).

Internal Use

1. **Shwasa** (asthma): (a) Paste of Bharangi and Shunthi or Maricha and Yavakshara is taken with the decoction of Devadaru, Chitrak, Aspota, and Murva (C.S.Ci. 17/110). (b) Bharangi should be taken with honey and ghee (S.S.U. 51/39). (c) Bharangi and Shunthi should be taken with hot water or with sugar and sauvarchala in asthma and hic-cough (VM. 12.9).
2. **Kasa** (chronic cough): Ghee prepared with Bharangi paste, four times curd, and double quantity of Brihati decoction is an excellent remedy for vatik kasa (BS.Kasa.17).
3. **Visha** (poisoning): Root of Bandhuka, Bharangi, and black Tulsi should be taken as nasya in case of poison located in head (C.S.Ci. 23/181).
4. **Madaatya** (alcoholism): Bath is taken with water boiled with Bharangi (S.S.U. 47/36).

5. **Jwara** (fever): Decoction of Bharangi, Shunthi, or Vacha is used twice daily in kaphaj jwara. Its leaves are eaten as vegetable in malaria.
6. **Shotha** (inflammation): Regular consumption of Bharangi decoction is recommended in shotha.

Officinal Parts Used

Root and leaves

Dose

Powder: 3 to 6 g
Decoction: 40 to 80 mL

Formulations

Bharangi guda, Bharangi avleha, Bharangyadi kwath, Bharangi sura, Ayaskriti, Kanakasava, Dashamoolarista, Rasnadi kvatha churna, Dhanvantara ghrita, Maha vatagajankusa rasa.

Toxicity/Adverse Effects

Not clinically reported yet but spermatotoxic effect reported in rats.

Spermatotoxic Activity

Methanolic extract of *C. serratum* at dose 100, 300, and 500 mg/kg shows significant spermatotoxic activity in male Albino rats. The *C. serratum* treatment results in impairment of male fertility in the rat by both spermatogenesis and cauda epididymal spermatozoa (Sarathchandiran et al 2014).

Substitution and Adulteration

Talisa patra (*Abies webbiana* Lindl is used as substitute of Bharangi. *Clerodendrum indicum* (Linn.) Kuntze and *Premna herbacea* Roxn. are also famous in the name of Bharangi.

Bark of *Picrasma quassioides* Ben. and *Gardenia turgida* Roxb are sold in the name of Bharangi in Indian market (Sharma 2009).

Points to Ponder

- *Bharangi is a prime drug for kasa and shwasa.*
- *Many species of Clerodendrum are found in India in the name of Bharangi.*
- *Talisa patra is used as substitute for Bharangi.*

Suggested Readings

Chunekar KC. Bhavaprakasha Nighantu. Revised ed. Varanasi: Chaukhamba Bharati Academy; 2013:98–99

Hazekamp A, Verpoorte R, Panthong A. Isolation of a bronchodilator flavonoid from the Thai medicinal plant *Clerodendrum petasites*. J Ethnopharmacol 2001;78(1):45–49

Hsiao JY, Lin MI. A chemotaxonomic study of essential oil from the leaves of genus *Clerodendrum* (Verbenaceae) native to Taiwan. Bot Bull Acad Sin 1995;36:247–251

Kajaria D, Tripathi JS, Pandey BI. Antimicrobial and antiinflamatory effect of an indigenous Ayurvedic drug: Bharangyadi. Sci Int J Pharm Sci 2012;1:479–483

Kiritikar KR, Basu BD. Indian Medicinal Plants, Vol. III. 2nd ed. Dehradun: International Book Distributors; 1999:1948

Kumari P, Joshi GC, Tiwari IM. Biodiversity status, distribution and use pattern of some ethno medicinal plants. Int J Conserv Sci 2012;3:309–318

Kumar P, Nishteswar K. Phytochemical and pharmacological profiles of *Clerodendrum serratum* Linn. (Bharngi): a review. Int J Res Ayurveda Pharm 2013;4(2):276–278

Moldenke HN. A Fifth Summary of Verbenaceae, Avicenniaceae, Stillbaceae, Dicrastylidaceae, Nymphoremaceae, Nyctanthaceae, and Eriocaneaceae of the World as to Valid Taxa, Geographic Distribution and Synonym, Vol. 1. New Jersey: BrawnBrumðeld Inc.;1971:312–314

Munir AA. A taxonomic revision of the genus *Clerodendrum* L. (Verbenaceae) in Australia. J Adel Bot Gard 1989;11:101–173

Nadkarni KM, Nadkarni AK, Chopra RN. Indian Materia Medica, Vol. 1. Mumbai: Popular Prakashan;1954:354

Sarathchandiran I, Kadalmani B, Navaneethakrishnan S. Evaluation of *Clerodendrum serratum* in male Albino rats. Int J Biol Pharmaceut Res 2014;5(1):16–21

Sharma M, Gupta A. Preliminary phytochemical investigation of methanolic root extract of *Clerodendrum serratum*: anticancer activity and histopathological study of stomach mucosa of Wistar rats in ethnol-induced ulcer. J Pharm Res Opinion 2013;1(7):202–208

Sharma PC, Yelne MB, Dennis TJ. Data Base on Medicinal Plants Used in Ayurveda, Vol. I. New Delhi: Ministry of Health and Family Welfare, Government of India; 2002:74

Sharma PV. Dravyaguna Vigyan Vol. II. Varanasi: Chaukhambha Bharati Academy;2009:298–300

Singh NR, Singh MS. Wild medicinal plants of Manipur included in the red list. Asian Agrihist 2009;13:221–225

The Ayurvedic Pharmacopoeia of India. Part I, Vol. 3. 1st ed. New Delhi: Ministry of Health and Family Welfare, Government of India; 2001:25

Verdcourt B. Flora of Tropical East Africa: Verbenaceae. Netherlands: Brookfield; 1992

Vidya SM, Krishna V, Manjunatha BK, Mankani KL, Ahmed M, Singh SD. Evaluation of hepatoprotective activity of *Clerodendrum serratum* L. Indian J Exp Biol 2007;45(6):538–542

Yuan YW, Mabberley DJ, Steane DA, Olmstead RG. Further disintegration and redefination of Clerodendrum (Lamiaceae): implication for the understanding of the evolution of an intriguing breeding strategy. Taxon 2010;59:125–133

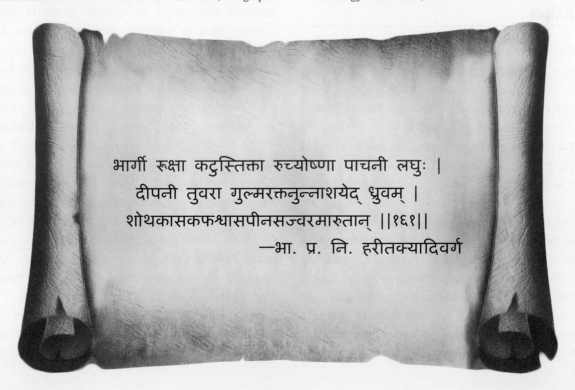

भार्गी रूक्षा कटुस्तिक्ता रुच्योष्णा पाचनी लघुः |
दीपनी तुवरा गुल्मरक्तनुन्नाशयेद् ध्रुवम् |
शोथकासकफश्वासपीनसज्वरमारुतान् ||१६१||
—भा. प्र. नि. हरीतक्यादिवर्ग

18. Bhringaraj [*Eclipta alba* Hassk]

Family: *Asteraceae*

Hindi name: *Bhangra, Bhamgra, Mochakand, Babri*

English name: *False Daisy, Trailing Eclipta*

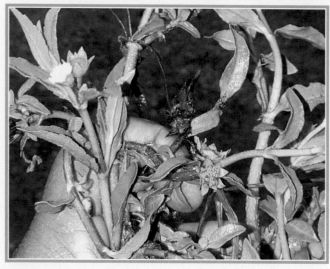

Plant of *Eclipta alba* Hassak

It is popularly known as "king of hairs" and is used in indigenous system of medicine.

Introduction

Eclipta alba (L.), commonly known as False Daisy and Bhringaraj, is a medicinal plant belonging to the family Asteraceae. The genus name comes from a Greek word "Eclipta" meaning "deficient," with reference to the absence of the bristles and awns on the fruits. The specific epithet *alba* means "white," which refers to the color of the flowers. It shines like a hornet and therefore is called Bhringaraj. *Eclipta prostrate* Linn. is the synonym of *Eclipta alba* (L.).

Bhringaraj is a well-known drug from the ancient period. In Atharva Veda, Maharishi Sayana has mentioned it in the treatment of kushta and palita. Acharya Charaka has mentioned this drug at various instances such as Kaphaj kasa chikitsa (C.S.Ci. 18/117), Raktapittanashaka yoga, and Krimihar dravya (C.S.Ci. 4/68, V. 7/21). Acharya Sushruta advised to use Bhringaraj in khalitya and palitya, and also proved its keshya activity (S.S.Ci. 25/28-32; Ka. 8/54).

Sushruta also stated its vishahar property and use in diseases such as nadivrana, ashmari, shwasa, kasa, and vataj swarabheda (S.S.Ci. 7/24, 17/42). Harita opined to use Bhringaraj in the form of lepa in indralupta and kushtaroga (H.S. 43/6-7). It is used for the purification of shilajatu as per Sharangadhar Samhita (Sa.S.M. 12/86). Bhavmishra also mentioned that Bhringaraj is used in khalitya, palitya (B.P.M. 62/4-5, 18), shiroroga, and urdhvajatrugataroga (B.P.M. 63/39), and as an ingredient in various formulations in the form of lepa and oil. Vangasen used "Keshraj" term for Bhringaraj in the treatment of aamatisar and raktatisar and also used the word Markav for the treatment of yonishool. As per Chakradutt, it is also used in shodhan, maran, and bhasma vidhi of the abhrak (C.D. 20/93-98). Almost all Samhitas and Nighantus advocated the use of Bhringaraj in khalitya and palitya.

The whole plant and parts of the plant are used by folk medicinal practitioners and tribal medicinal practitioners of the Indian subcontinent for the treatment of hair loss and graying of hair, liver disorders (including jaundice), gastrointestinal disorders, respiratory tract disorders (including asthma), fever, skin disorders, spleen enlargement, and cuts and wounds. Ethnomedicinal uses of the plant have been reported from Bangladesh, India, Nepal, and Pakistan.

Vernacular Names

Arabic: Kadim-el-bint

Assamese: Bhrngaraja

Bengali: Bheemraja, Kesuriya, Kesari, Kesuti, Keshwri

Gujarati: Bhangra, Kaluganthi, Dodhak, Kalobhangro

Kannada: Garagada, Soppu

Malayalam: Kannunni, Kayyonni

Marathi: Maka, Bhringuraja

Oriya: Kesara, Kesarda

Punjabi: Bhangra

Santhal: Lal Kesari

Sindhi: Tik

Tamil: Kaikesi, Garuga, Kayanthakara

Telugu: Guntakalagara, Guntagalagara

Urdu: Bhangra

Synonyms

Angaraka: It looks like fire.

Arangaka: Plant with colorless (white) flower.

Bhring: It blackens hair like hornet due to rasayana property.

Bhring: The plant is attracted by bees and wasps.

Bhringar: It stabilizes rasadi dhatu, hair, and ojus.

Bhringaraja: The plant is attracted by bees and wasps.

Bhringarenu: Pollen grains are transferred through bees and wasps.

Bhringraj: It shines like hornet.

Keshraj: It is a potent drug for hair.

Keshranjan: It colors the hair.

Kuntal Vardhan: It helps to grow hair in quantity and quality.

Maarkar: It prevents whitening of hair.

Markar: It turns white hairs into black.

Markav: It kills the disease like baldness and cures white hair.

Markava: It cures hair-related problems and prevents premature graying of hairs.

Pankajata: It grows in marshy watery place.

Pantang: It promotes blackening of hairs.

Pitripriya: Its flowers are used in death rituals.

Ravipriya: The plants prefer sunlight.

Suryavarta: It grows in the direction of sun.

Classical Categorization

Charak Samhita: not mentioned in any Mahakashaya/gana

Sushrut Samhita: not mentioned in any varga

Astanga Sangraha: not mentioned in any varga

Astanga Hridaya: not mentioned in any varga

Dhanwantari Nighantu: Karavveradi varga

Madanpal Nighantu: Abhayadi varga

Kaiyadev Nighantu: Oshadhi varga

Raj Nighantu: Shatahwadi varga

Bhavaprakash: Guduchyadi varga

Distribution

It grows as a common weed throughout India, ascending to 1,800 m in the Himalayas, upper Gangetic plains, and in Chota Nagpur, Bihar, Odisha, Punjab, and Western and Southern part of India (Sharma et al 2001).

This herb is found throughout India near moist water sources like river bank, ponds, canals, marshy places, and water reservoir.

Morphology

It is an erect or prostrate herb that grows up to 40 cm high.

- **Stem:** Herbaceous, branched, occasionally rooting at nodes, cylindrical or flat, rough due to oppressed white hair, node distinct, greenish, occasionally brownish (**Fig. 18.1**).
- **Leaves**: Simple, opposite, sessile, lanceolate-oblong, 2 to 8 cm length, 1.2 to 2.3 cm width, and strigose with oppressed hair on both the sides (**Fig. 18.2**).
- **Flowers:** Small, white colored, axillary with peduncled rayed heads, receptacle flat. Ray florets female, white, ligulate, as long as involucral bracts. Disc flowers are bisexual, tubular, and greenish-yellow. Corolla is often

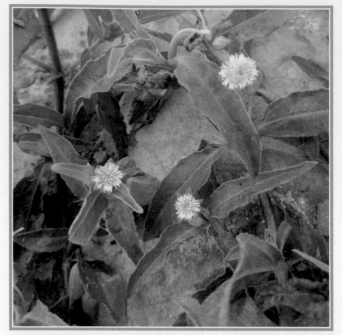

Fig. 18.1 Stem.

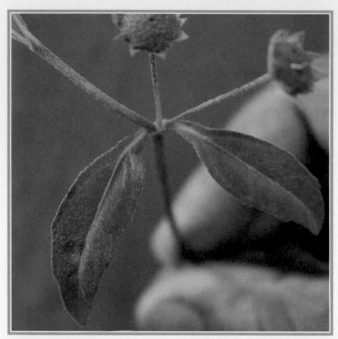

Fig. 18.2 Leaves.

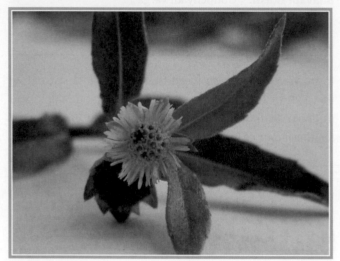

Fig. 18.3 Flower.

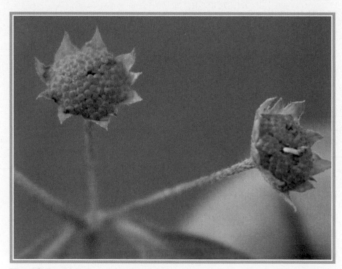

Fig. 18.4 Fruit.

four toothed. Stamens are five, filament epipetalous, free, anther united into a tube with base obtuse. Pistil is bicarpellary. Ovary is inferior and unilocular with one basal ovule (**Fig. 18.3**).

- **Fruits**: Achene type, single seeded, cuneate, brown color with a narrow wing, covered with warts (**Fig. 18.4**).
- **Seeds**: Small, dark brown, and hairy.
- **Root**: Cylindrical, grayish, white-colored tap root with many secondary branches (**Fig. 18.5**).

Cultivation of the drug Bhringaraj is not needed as it is a very common weed of the rainy season growing gregariously on waste places. It is easily propagated by seeds. Vegetative propagation of *Eclipta alba* was tried by stem cuttings.

Phenology

Flowering time: August to September

Fruiting time: Up to November

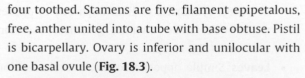

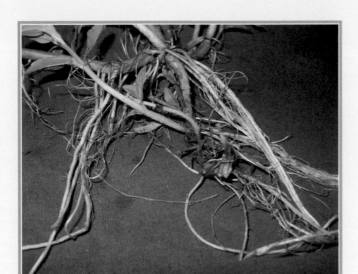

Fig. 18.5 Root.

Key Characters for Identification

➤ An erect or prostrate herb found in wet marshy land
➤ Leaves: Simple, opposite, lanceolate-oblong, 2 to 8 cm length attached with greenish or brownish stem
➤ Flowers: small and white flower, axillary with peduncled rayed heads
➤ Fruits: Achene type single seeded brown color fruit with a narrow wing

Types

Raj Nighantu has described its three varieties on the basis of flower color.
- Shwet Bhringaraj: *Eclipta alba*
- Peet Bhringaraj: *Weddelia chinensis*—It bears yellow flower
- Neel Bhringaraj

Bhavprakash Nighantu and Adarsh Nighantu mentioned two types of Bhringaraj: Shwet and Pita Bhringaraj.

Rasapanchaka

Guna	Ruksha, Tikshan
Rasa	Katu, Tikta
Vipaka	Katu
Virya	Ushna

Chemical Constituents

Eclipta alba (L.) contains a wide range of active principles which includes coumestans, alkaloids, flavonoids, glycosides, and triterpenoids. The leaves contain stigmasterol, β-terthienylmethanol, wedelolactone, demethylwedelolactone, and demethylwedelolactone-7-glucoside. The roots give hentriacontanol and heptacosanol (Chopra et al 1955).

The roots contain polyacetylene-substituted thiophene. The aerial part contains phytosterol, β-amyrin in the *n*-hexane extract and luteolin-7-glucoside, β-glucoside of phytosterol, a glucoside of a triterpenic acid, and wedelolactone. The polypeptides isolated from the plant yield cystine, glutamic acid, phenyl alanine, tyrosine, and methionine on hydrolysis. Nicotine and nicotinic acid occur in this plant (Everitt et al 2007).

Identity, Purity, and Strength

- Foreign matter: Not more than 2%
- Total ash: Not more than 22%
- Acid-insoluble ash: Not more than 11%
- Alcohol-soluble extractive: Not less than 5%
- Water-soluble extractive: Not less than 15%

(Source: The Ayurvedic Pharmacopeia of India 1999)

Karma (Actions)

Bhringaraj is keshya (hair tonic), twachya (skin tonic), dantya (strengthen tooth), rasayana (rejuvenator), balya (strength promoting), chakshushya (eye tonic). It also has amahara, vishahara (anti-poison), shothahara (anti-inflammatory), deepan (appetizer), pachan (digestive), yakrituttejak (hepatic stimulant), and medhya (intellect promoter) properties.
- Doshakarma: Kaphavatahara
- Dhatukarma: Rasayana, twachya, balya
- Malakarma: Kesya

Pharmacological Actions

Several studies prove that Bhringaraj possesses hepatoprotective, analgesic, anti-inflammatory, antimicrobial, antibacterial, antifungal, antimalarial, antihyperglycemic, antioxidant, hypolipidemic, neuropharmacological, hair promoting, proteolytic, osteoblast differentiation, immuno-modulatory, anticancer activities (Bhalerao et al 2013).

Other pharmacological properties reported are anti-venom, antihemorrhagic, diuretic, wound healing, and hemostatic properties.

Indications

It is used in the treatment of kushta (skin diseases), shotha (inflammatory disease), as rasayana (for rejuvenation), krimi (worm infestation), kasa (cough), shwasa (asthma), pandu (anemia), danta roga (diseases of teeth), netra roga (eye diseases), shiro roga (diseases of head), etc. (Chunekar 2002). Bhringaraj has been used for generations in traditional medicine for promoting hair growth.

Some tribes of Odisha use paste and pill prepared with Bhringaraj and black pepper in fever and jaundice (Sahu et al 2013). Tribes of Tripura state of India use 5 to 10 mL of leaf juice daily for hepatic disorder (Das et al 2012). Leaf extract of Bhringaraj is applied to remove dandruff and also make hair silky and shiny by people from Uttar Pradesh (Kumar et al 2012). Leaves and flowers are used for the treatment of urinary problems, jaundice, asthma, and cough by the local practitioners of Mount Abu in Rajasthan, India (Gautam and Batra 2012).

In the Caribbean, the juice is taken for asthma, bronchitis; dizziness, vertigo, blurred vision, skin problems (Khare 2004). The root is used as an emetic and purgative (Williamson 2002). Plant juice is applied externally in cuts and wounds by traditional healers and local people of Arghakhanchi District, Nepal (Panthi and Singh 2013). Whole plant is used to ensure fetal development and facilitate childbirth in Anyi-Ndenye pregnant women of Eastern Coted'Ivoire, Africa (Malan and Neuba 2011). It is used as antivenom against snakebite in China and Brazil (Mors and Wagner 1991).

Therapeutic Uses

External Use

1. **Twacharoga** (skin disease): Paste of leaves of Mehendi, Murva, and Bhringaraj is applied externally in skin disease, burn, ulcers, and wounds.

2. **Upadansha** (soft chancre): Bhringaraj juice is used to wash the wound of venereal disease (GN. 4.8.13).

3. **Varahadamstra:** Powder of Haridra and Bhringaraj is applied locally in varahadamstra (BP.Ci. 61/113).

Internal Use

1. **Palitya** (graying of hair): Medicated oil prepared with juice of Bhringaraj, milk, and madhuka is used as nasya daily in the treatment of khalitya and palitya (C.S.Ci. 26/267).

2. **Kamala** (hepatitis and jaundice): Bhringaraj powder with Purnarnava decoction is used daily in jaundice, hepatitis, hepato-splenomegaly, anemia, indigestion, and anorexia.

3. **Rasayana** (for rejuvenation): Bhringaraj juice is taken daily for a period of one month. During this period patient should take milk only. It helps to provide strength and vigor and also attain 100 years of life span (A.H.U. 39/163).

4. **Amlapitta** (acidity): Regular use of Haritaki powder and Bhringaraj mixed with jaggery prevents vomiting caused by hyperacidity in amalpitta (CD. 52/12).

5. **Shwasa and Kasa** (asthma and cough): Daily consumption of juice of Kasamard, Bhringaraj, horse dung, Vartaka, Tulsi mixed with honey gives relief in kasa and shwasa (C.S.Ci. 18/117). Oil cooked with Haritaki and Bhringaraj alleviates cough and asthma (K.S.K. 16/11).

6. **Shvitra** (vitiligo): Bhringaraj is fried with oil in an iron vessel and this is given to vitiligo patient with milk which is processed with Bijaka (AH.Ci. 20/8).

7. **Garbh sthapaka** (establishment of fetus): Regular intake of Bhringaraj juice mixed with equal quantity of milk helps in maintaining pregnancy and prevents habitual abortion (VD. 13/20).

8. **Naktandhya** (night blindness): Intake of fish eggs cooked with Bhringaraj for a week, keeping the patient on wholesome diet, cures night blindness (CD. 59.172). Til oil and Bibhitaki oil cooked with Bhringaraj juice and decoction of asana in an iron vessel is used as snuff. It improves eye sight (AH.U. 13/46).

9. **Yonishoola** (vaginal pain): Paste of root of Bilwa and Bhringaraj is taken with wine. It reduces pain in vagina (BS.Striroga.249).

10. **Suryavarta** (a type of headache): Equal quantity of Bhringaraj juice and milk is heated in the sunlight and is used as snuff. It provides relief from suryavarta (a type of headache; BP.Ci. 62/50).

Officinal Parts Used

Whole plant, roots, seeds, and seed oil.

Dose

Juice: 5 to 10 mL (Williamson 2002; Sharma et al 2001).

Formulations

Bhringaraj asava, Bhringaraj ghrita, Bhringaraj churna, Shadbindu taila, Bhringaraj taila, Mahabhringaraj taila, Nilibhringyadi taila, Soothshekhar rasa, Tekaraja marica, Bhringamalakadi taila, Mahavatavidhwansana rasa, Nilikadya taila, Anandabhairava rasa, Bhringarajasava, and Tekaraja marica.

Toxicity/Adverse Effects

It is reported that the alcoholic extract of *Eclipta alba* shows no signs of toxicity in rats and mice and the minimum lethal dose was found to be greater than 2.0 g/kg when given orally and intraperitoneally in mice (Singh et al 1993).

Substitution and Adulteration

Pitta Bhringaraj (*Wedelia chinensis*) is used as substitute of *Eclipta alba* (Rakesh and Sapanrao 2015).

> **Points to Ponder**
>
> - *Bhringaraj is considered as best hair tonic.*
> - *It is mainly used for blackening of hair and growth, khalitya, palitya, liver disease, and for rasayan purpose.*

Suggested Readings

Banshidhar DR, Sawant BS. Current scenario of adulterants and substitutes of medicinal plants: a review. J Pharm Scient Innov 2015;4(5)

Bhalerao S, et al. Eclipta alba (L.): an overview. Int J Bioassays 2013;02(11):1443–1447

Chopra RN, Nayar SL, Chopra IC, et al. Glossary of Indian Medicinal plants. New Delhi: CSIR; 1955

Chunekar KC. Bhavprakash Nighantu of Bhavmishra. Varanasi: Chaukhambha Bharati Academy; 2002:429–430

Das S, Choudhury MD, Mandal SC, Talukdar AD. Traditional knowledge of ethnomedicinal hepatoprotective plants used by certain ethnic communities of Tripura state. Ind J Fund Appl Life Sci 2012;2(1):84–97

Dubey RB, Sapanrao B. Sawant: current scenario of adulterant and substitutions of medicinal plants: a review. J Pharm Sci Innov 2015;4(5):247–250

Everitt JH, Lonard RL, Little CR. Weeds in South Texas and Northern Mexico, Lubbock: Texas Tech University Press; 2007

Gautam A, Batra A. Ethnomedicinal plant product used by the local traditional practitioners in Mount Abu. World J Pharm Sci 2012; 1(1):10–18

Khare CP. Encyclopedia of Indian Medicinal Plants. New York: Springer-Verlag; 2004:197–198

Kumar A, Agarwal S, Singh A, Deepak D. Medico-botanical study of some weeds growing in Moradabad District of Western Uttar Pradesh in India. Ind J Sci Res 2012;3(1):107–111

Malan DF, Neuba DFR. Traditional practices and medicinal plants use during pregnancy by Anyi-Ndenye women (Eastern Côte d'Ivoire). Afr J Reprod Health 2011;15(1):85–93

Mors WB, Wagner H. Plants active against snake bite. Econ Med Plant Res 1991;5:353–373

Panthi M, Singh AG. Ethnobotany of Arghakhanchi District, Nepal: Plants Used in Dermatological and Cosmetic Disorders. Int J Appl Sci Biotechnol 2013;1(2):27–32

Sahu CR, Nayak RK, Dhal NK. Traditional herbal remedies for various diseases used by tribals of Boudh District, Odisha, India for sustainable development. Int J Herbal Med 2013;1(1):12–20

Sharma PC, Yelne MB, Denn TJ. Database on Medicinal Plants Used in Ayurveda. Vol. 2. New Delhi: Central Council for Research in Ayurveda and Siddna; 2001:112

Singh B, Saxena K, Chandan B, Agarwal S, Bhatia MS, Anand KK. Hepatoprotective effect of ethanolic extract of *Eclipta alba* on experimental liver damage. Phytother Res 1993;7:154–158

The Ayurvedic Pharmacopoeia of India. Part I, 1st ed. Vol. II. New Delhi: Ministry of Health of Family Welfare, Government of India; 1999:21–22

Tripathi I. Raj Nighantu of Pandit Narahari. Varanasi: Chaukhambha Krishnadas Academy; 2006:89

Williamson EM. Major Herbs of Ayurveda. China: Churchill Livingstone; 2002:126–128

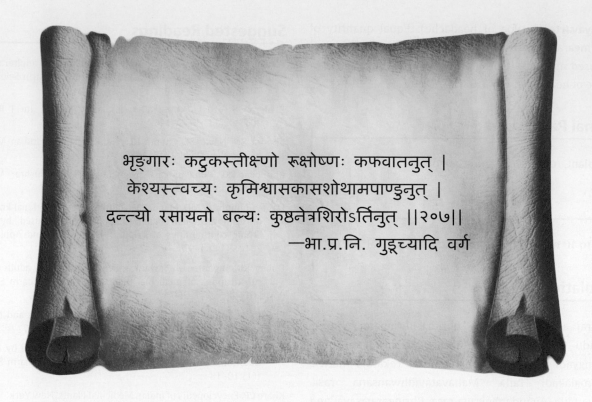

भृङ्गारः कटुकस्तीक्ष्णो रूक्षोष्णः कफवातनुत् ।
केश्यस्त्वच्यः कृमिश्वासकासशोथामपाण्डुनुत् ।
दन्त्यो रसायनो बल्यः कुष्ठनेत्रशिरोऽर्तिनुत् ।।२०७।।
—भा.प्र.नि. गुडूच्यादि वर्ग

19. Bibhitaki [*Terminalia bellirica* (Gaertn.) Roxb.]

Family:	*Combretaceae*
Hindi name:	*Baheda, Bahera*
English name:	*Belleric myrobalan, Bedda nut tree*

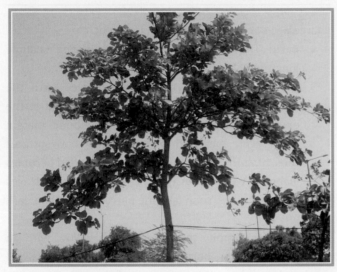

Plant of *Terminalia bellirica* (Gaertn.) Roxb.

Mythologically it is believed to be inhabited by demons (bhutabhasa) and it's a prime cause of dispute (kalidruma) among people sitting under it.

Introduction

The word "Bibhitaki" means one that takes away the fear of disease. It is rightly said for this drug as its fruit is widely used in traditional system of medicines for the treatment of a number of ailments.

The generic name "terminalia" comes from Latin word *terminus* or *terminalis* (ending) and refers to the habit of the leaves being crowded or borne on the tips of the shoots.

In Charak Samhita, Bibhitaki fruits are mentioned as having qualities to alleviate many diseases, and bestow longevity, intellectual power, and strength. There are several "rasayan medicines" like fourth Amalaka rasayan which has been described in the Charak Samhita, in which Bibhitaki is used as an ingredient.

The nuts of the tree are rounded but with five flatter sides. These nuts are likely used as dice in the epic Mahabharata and in Rig-Veda book 10 hymn 34. A handful of nuts would be cast on a gaming board and the players would have to call whether an odd or even number of nuts had been thrown (Bennett et al 1999). In the Nala, King Rituparna demonstrated his ability to count large numbers instantaneously by counting the number of nuts on an entire bough of a tree (Nala and Damayanti 2011).

Bibhitaki is one of the ingredients of an important Ayurvedic medicine "Triphala" available in the Indian market for the treatment of dyspepsia, diarrhea, dysentery, inflammation of the small intestine biliousness, flatulence, liver disease, and leprosy (Sharma et al 2005).

Vernacular Names

Assamese: Bhomora, Bhomra, Bhaira
Burmese: Thitsein
French: Myrobalan beleric
Gujarati: Bahedam, Beheda
Javanese: Jaha sapi, jaha kebo
Kannada: Shanti, Shantikayi, Tare, Tarekayi

Lao (Sino-Tibetan): Nam kieng dam, haen-ton

Malay: Jelawai, mentalun, simar kulihap

Malayalam: Tanni, Tannikai

Marathi: Beheda

Oriya: Beheda, Bhara

Tamil: Thanakkai, Tanri, tanrikkai, Tani

Telugu: Tannikkaya, Vibhitakami, Tani

Thai: Haen-khao, samo-phiphek

Vietnamese: b[af]ng n[uw][ows]c, simar kulihap, b[oo]ng d[ee]u, heen, mung tr[awf]ng

Synonyms

Aksha: Each fruit is one karsha. In ancient times it was used as dice (aksha).

Bahedaka: Commonly known as baheda/bahedaka.

Bahuveerya: It has broad actions.

Bhutavasa: It is regarded as abode of demon.

Bibhedaka: Maintains health by curing or alleviating diseases.

Bibhitaki: It removes the fear of suffering or disease.

Kalidruma: It is regarded as abode of kali (quarrel).

Karshaphala: Weight of each fruit is one karsha (12 g).

Kasaghna: It particularly cures cough.

Samvartaka: Maintains health by curing or alleviating diseases.

Taila phala: Seed kernel is oily.

Tusa: Maintains health by curing or alleviating diseases.

Vasant: It blooms in spring.

Vindhyajata: It grows mostly in Vindhya area.

Classical Categorization

Charak Samhita: Jwaraghna, Virechanopaga

Sushrut Samhita: Triphala, Mustadi, Muskakadi, Parushadi

Ashtang Hridya: Mustadi, Muskakadi, Parushadi

Dhanvantari Nighantu: Guduchyadi varga

Madanpal: Abhyadi varga

Kaiyadev: Oushadhi varga

Raj Nighantu: Amraradi varga

Bhavaprakash: Haritakyadi varga

Distribution

The plant is native to Bangladesh, Bhutan, Cambodia, China, Indonesia, Laos, Malaysia, Nepal, Pakistan, Sri Lanka, Thailand, and Vietnam. It is mostly found in monsoon forests, mixed deciduous forests, or dry deciduous dipterocarp forests, associated with teak (Tectona grandis) (Orwa et al 2009).

It is wild throughout the Indian subcontinent, Sri Lanka, and SE Asia, up to 1,200 m in elevation and is abundantly available in Madhya Pradesh, Uttar Pradesh, Maharashtra, and Punjab (Kirtikar and Basu 1935; Warrier et al 1996).

Morphology

A large deciduous tree 20 to 30 m in height.

- **Bark:** Thick brownish gray bark having shallow longitudinal fissures (**Fig. 19.1**).
- **Leaves:** Simple, alternate, long petioled with the dimension of 4–24 cm x 2–11 cm, crowded at the extremities of the branches broadly elliptic, margin entire, acute apex, midrib prominent on both surfaces (**Fig. 19.2a**). It is pubescent when young and becomes glabrous with maturity (**Fig. 19.2b**). Young leaves are copper-red, soon become parrot green, then dark green.
- **Flowers:** Simple, solitary, greenish yellow with an offensive odor, borne in axillary spikes generally 3 to 15 cm long. Upper flowers of the spike are male. Lower flowers are bisexual (**Fig. 19.3a, b**).

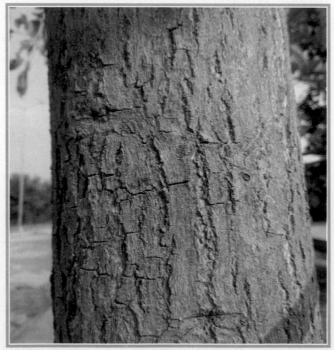

Fig. 19.1 Bark.

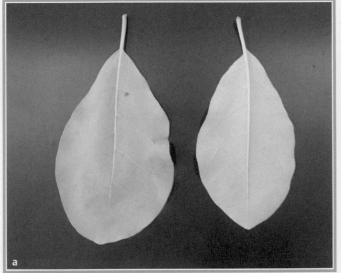
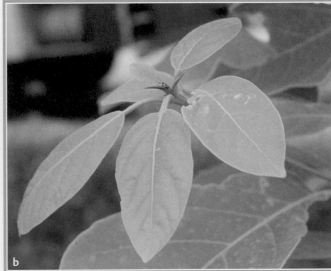

Fig.19.2 **(a)** Dorsal and ventral view of leaves. **(b)** Leaves in bunch.

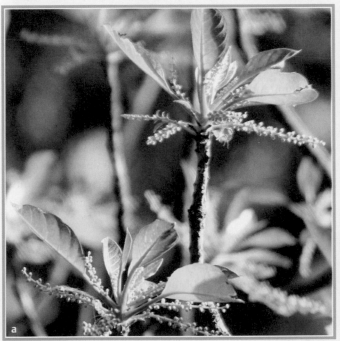
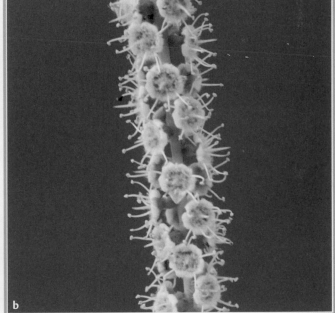

Fig.19.3 **(a)** Flowers in axillary spike. **(b)** Flower.

- **Fruit**: Spherical to ovoid drupe, 1.5 to 2.5 in. in diameter, tapering toward both the ends with a stony nut. Fresh ripe fruits are slightly silvery with whitish shiny pubescent surface (**Fig. 19.4a**). Mature fruits are gray or grayish brown with slightly wrinkled appearance (**Fig. 19.4b**). Rind of fruit shows variation in thickness from 3 to 5 mm (Singh 2011; Nadkarni 2002).

The plant is propagated through seeds, root, or shoot cutting and stump planting.

Phenology

Flowering time: March to May

Fruiting time: December to February

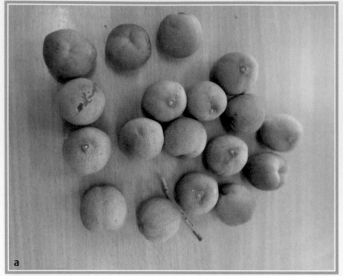
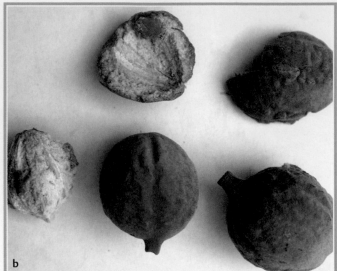

Fig 19.4 **(a)** Fresh fruits. **(b)** Dry mature fruit.

Key Characters for Identification

➤ *Moderate size deciduous tree.*
➤ *Leaves: simple, obovate, crowded at the extremities/ ends of the branches*
➤ *Flowers: greenish yellow in axillary spikes*
➤ *Fruits: ovoid, 1.5 to 2.5 in. in diameter, light brown, pubescent surface, hard single seeded*

Rasapanchaka

Guna	Ruksha, Laghu
Rasa	Kashaya
Vipaka	Madhura (Katu vipak and Dhanwantari Nighantu)
Virya	Ushna

Chemical Constituents

The principal phytoconstituents are beta-sitosterol, gallic acid, ellagic acid, ethyl gallate, galloyl glucose, chebulagic acid. Four lignans including termilignan, thannilignan, hydroxy-3′,4′-(methylenedioxy) flavan, and anolignan-B have been found (Singh 2006).

Fruit contains terpenoids (belleric acid and chebulagic acid), saponin (bellericoside and bellericanin) (Meena

et al 2010; Sharma 2012), and tannins (23.60–37.36%), which are composed of chebulinic acid, chebulagic acid, 1,3,6-trigalloylglucose and 1,2,3,4,6-pentagalloylglucose, corilagin, and glucogallin (Saxena et al 2013; Gangadhar et al 2011).

Seeds contain alkaloids, coumarin, flavone, glycosides (D-glucose, fructose, sucrose, galactose, and mannose) (Kadian et al 2014). Bark contains beta-sitosterol, tannins, ellagic acid, gallic acid, and catechol. Its oil contains palmitic, oleic, and linoleic acids such as major fatty acids.

Identity, Purity, and Strength

- Foreign matter: Not more than 2%
- Total ash: Not more than 7%
- Acid-insoluble ash: Not more than 1%
- Alcohol-soluble extractive: Not less than 8%
- Water-soluble extractive: Not less than 35%

(Source: The Ayurvedic Pharmacopeia of India 1989)

Karma (Actions)

Bibhitaki produces actions like bhedan, kasaghna, kesya, keshvridhikar, chakshusya, krimighna, and sara.

Other actions of Bibhitaki are shothahara (anti-inflammatory), vedanasthapana (anodyne), raktastambhana (hemostatic), krishnikarana (used for blackening), deepana (appetizer), anulomana (laxative), rechana (purgative), grahi (absorbent), trishnanigrahana (antithirst), chhardi-nigrahana (antiemetic), vajikarana (aphrodisiac), jwaraghna (antipyretics), and dhatuvardhaka (nourishment to all dhatus; Sharma et al 2005).

Phala majja is laghu, kashaya, kaphavatahara, madakarak, and is used in trishna and chardi.

Fruit is used as laxative, astringent, anthelmintic, and antipyretic. It is also said to cleanse the blood and voice and promote hair growth. Gum of the bark is demulcent and purgative.

- Doshakarma: Tridoshashamaka, especially kaphapittashamaka
- Dhatukarma: Rasayana, dhatuvardhaka
- Malakarma: Bhedan, sara

Pharmacological Actions

It is reported to have analgesic, antidiarrheal, antihypertensive effect, antisalmonella, antispasmodic, and bronchodilatory properties, antimicrobial, antioxidant, wound-healing, immunological, immune response in vitro, hepatoprotective, antibiofilm, anticancer, β-lactamase inhibitor, antiulcer, antithrombotic, thrombolytic, antipyretic, antimutagenic activities (Deb et al 2016).

Indications

It is used in kasa (cough), shwasa (asthma), sweta kustha (vitiligo), krimi (worm infestation), swarabheda (hoarseness of voice), netraroga (eye diseases), mukharoga (mouth diseases), palitya (premature graying of hair), shotha (edema), granthi visarpa (erysipelas), vrana (wound), atisara (diarrhea), pravahika (dysentery), dantaroga, pratishyaya, hridyaroga (heart diseases), netrabhishyanda (conjunctivitis), vatavyadhi (neuromuscular diseases), anidra (insomnia), adhmana (abdominal distention), trishna (thirst), chhardi (vomiting), arsha (piles), vibandha (constipation), raktanishthivana (hemoptysis), ashmari (urinary calculus), klaibya (impotency), jwara (fever), samanya daurbalya (weakness), etc.

Fruits are useful in treatment of hepatitis, bronchitis, asthma, dyspepsia, piles, diarrhea, coughs, hoarseness of voice, eye diseases, scorpion-sting, and are also used as a hair tonic (Singh 2011; Rastogi and Mehrotra 2004). Decoction of the green fruit is used for cough. Pulp of the fruit is useful in dysenteric-diarrhea, dropsy, piles, and leprosy. Half ripe fruit is used as purgative. Kernel of the fruit is narcotic. Inhabitants of Khagrachari in Bangladesh use fruits in menstrual disorder. Seed oil is used in rheumatism. Kernel oil has purgative action and its prolonged use is well tolerated in mice (Ghani 2003).

Contraindications

Vataprakopa (Malik et al 2012).

Therapeutic Uses

External Use

1. **Shotha** (edema): Paste of Bibhitaka fruit alleviates burning sensation and pain in all types of edema (C.S.Ci. 12/71.)
2. **Granthi Visarpa** (erysepalas): Hot paste of Bibhitaka is applied locally (C.S.Ci. 12/124).
3. **Sweta kustha** (vitiligo): Ash of black snake mixed with Bibhitaka oil is applied locally. It removes all types of vitiligo (S.S.Ci. 19/18; AH.Ci. 20/12).

Internal Use

1. **Kasa and Shwasa** (cough and asthma): Only Bibhitaki is sufficient to cure all types of cough and asthma (AH.Ci. 3/173). Bibhitaki powder 10 g is taken with honey after meal which alleviates cough and dyspnea (CD. 12/18; RM 11.5).
2. **Vrana ropana** (wound healing): Apply paste prepared with Bibhitaki powder in water regularly to heal up chronic wounds, ulcers, cut, minor injuries, and bruises.
3. **Atisaar** (diarrhea): Burnt Bibhitaki fruit mixed with salt checks severe type of diarrhea (BS.Atisara 173).
4. **Dant roga** (dental disorders): Bibhitaki fruit is broken into pieces and boil the pieces in a cup of water. Cool this infusion and use it as a mouthwash daily in bad odor, mouth ulcer, pyorrhea, and tooth ache.
5. **Palitya** (premature graying of hair): The oil obtained from the seed and pulp is applied regularly for promoting hair growth, preventing premature graying, and making them black.
6. **Netra roga** (eye diseases): Decoction of the dry fruit is used for eye wash in conjunctivitis and eye infections.

Til oil, Bibhitaki oil, and Bhringaraj juice and decoction of Asana are cooked together in an iron vessel and taken as snuff. It improves eye sight (AH.U. 13/46).

7. **Hridya** (as cardio tonic): Bibhitaka, Aswagandha, and jaggery are pounded together and taken with hot water. It alleviates vata from heart (BS. Vatavyadhi 60).

Officinal Parts Used

Fruit, seed, bark

Dose

Powder: 3 to 6 g

Formulations

Triphala churna, Triphala ghrita, Phalatrikadi kvatha, Talishadi churna, Lavangadivati.

Toxicity/Adverse Effects

Acute and chronic toxicity studies of *Terminalia bellerica* dried fruits reveal no signs of toxicity such as general behavior changes, morbidity, mortality, changes on gross appearance, or histopathological changes of the internal organs of rats (Sireeratawong et al 2010). Subacute toxicity study of ethanolic extract of *T. bellerica* also didn't suggest any change in general behaviors, mortality, weight gain, hematological, and histological parameters (Thanabhorn et al 2009).

No data found for toxicity.

Substitution and Adulteration

The bark of *T. bellerica* is used as adulterant of bark of *Terminalia arjuna*. The fruit of *T. bellerica* is reported to be used as a substitute in tanning industry for *Terminalia chebula* (Dubey et al 2015).

Points to Ponder

- *Bibhitaka is ushna veerya but sheeta sparsha. Its fruit pulp is madakari (BPN).*
- *It removes the dosha of rasa, rakta, mamsa meda dhatu (C.S.Su. 27/148).*

Suggested Readings

Bennett D. Randomness. Boston: Harvard University Press; 1999:24

Deb A, Barua S, Das B. Pharmacological activities of Baheda (*Terminalia bellerica*): a review. J Pharmacogn Phytochem 2016;5(1):194–197

Deborah B. Randomness. Boston: Harvard University Press; 1999:24

Dubey RB, Sapanrao B. Sawant: current scenario of adulterant and substitutions of medicinal plants: a review. J Pharm Sci Innov 2015;4(5):247–250

Dubey RB, Sawant BS. Current scenario of adulterants and substitutes of medicinal plants: a review. J Pharm Sci Innov 2015;4(5):247–250

Gangadhar M, Patil B, Yadav S, and Sinde D. Isolation and characterization of gallic acid from Terminalia belerica and its effect on carbohydrate regulatory system in vitro. Int J Res Ayur Pharm 2011;2:559–562

Ghani A. Medicinal Plants of Bangladesh with Chemical Constituents and Uses. 2nd ed. Dhaka, Ramna: Asiatic Society of Bangladesh; 2003:184

Indian Herbal Pharmacopoeia Revised New Edition. Mumbai: Indian Drug Manufacturer's Association; 2002:429–438

Kadian R, Parle M, Yadav M. Therapeutic potential and phyto-pharmacology of *Terminalia bellerica*. World J Pharm Pharm Sci 2014;3(10):804–819

Kirtikar KR, Basu BD. *Terminalia chebula*: Indian Med Plant 1935;1:1020–1023

Mallik J, Das P, Karon B, Das S. A review on phytochemistry and pharmacological activity of *Terminalia bellerica*. Int J Drug Formul Res 2012;3(6):1–5

Meena AK, Yadav A, Singh U, et al. Evaluation of physiochemical parameters on the fruit of *Terminalia bellerica* Roxb. Int J Pharm Pharm Sci 2010;2:97–99

Meshram G, Patil B, Yadav S, Sinde D. Isolation and characterization of gallic acid from *Terminalia bellerica* and its effect on carbohydrate regulatory system in vitro. Int J Res Ayurveda Pharm 2011;2(2):559–562

Nadkarni KM. Indian Materia Medica. Mumbai: Ramdas Bhatkal for Popular Prakashan Pvt. Ltd.; 2002;01:202–205

Nala and Damayanti 5: Nala Learns the Science of Numbers: Math or Magic. Retrieved February 12, 2011. Agroforestry Database 4.0 (Orwa et al 2009)

Orwa C, Mutua A, Kindt R, Jamnadass R, Simons A. 2009. Agroforestree Database: a tree reference and selection guide version 4.0. Available at: http://www.worldagroforestry.org/af/treedb/

Panunto W, Jaijoy K, Lerdvuthisopon N, et al. Acute and chronic toxicity studies of the water extract from dried fruits of *Terminalia chebula* Rezt. in rats. Int J Appl Res Nat Prod 2010;3(4):3643

Rastogi RP, Mehrotra BN. Compendium of Medicinal Plants. New Delhi: Central Drug Research Institute (CDRI) and Lucknow: National Institute of Communication and Information Resources; 2004:406

Row JR, Murty PS. Chemical examination of *Terminalia bellerica* Roxb. Indian J Chem 1970;8:1047–1048

Saxena V, Mishra G, Saxena A, Vishwakarma KK. A comparative study on quantitative estimation of tannins in *Terminalia chebula*, *Terminalia bellerica*, *Terminalia arjuna*, and *Saraca indica* using spectrophotometer. Asian J Pharm Clin Res 2013;6(3):148–149

Sharma PC, Yelne MB, Dennis TJ. Database on Medicinal Plants Used in Ayurveda. 3rd ed. New Delhi: Central Council for Research in Ayurveda and Siddha; 2005:282–284

Sharma PV. Charaka Samhita. Varanasi: Chaukhamba Orientalia; 1998

Sharma S. Chemical investigations of *Terminalia bellerica*. Acta Chim Pharm Ind 2012;2:132–133

Singh A. Medicinal Plants of the World. New Delhi: Mohan Primlani for Oxford and IBH Co. Pvt; 2006

Singh AS. Herbalism Phytochemistry and Ethanopharmacology. Science Publishers; 2011:357–361

Sireeratawong S, Jaijoy K, Panunto W, et al. Acute and chronic toxicity studies of the water extract from dried fruits of Terminalia bellirica (Gaertn.) Roxb. in Spargue-Dawley rats. Afr J Tradit Complement Altern Med 2013;10(2):223–231

The Ayurvedic Pharmacopoeia of India. Part I, Vol. 1. New Delhi: Department of AYUSH, Ministry of Health & Family Welfare, Government of India; 1989:25–28

Thanabhorn S, Jaijoy K, Thamaree S, Ingkaninam K. Acute and subacute toxicities of the ethanol extract of fruit of *Terminalia bellerica*. J Pharm Sci 2009

Warrier PK, Nambiar VPK, Ramankutty C. Indian Medicinal Plants: A Compendium of 500 Species. Hyderabad: Orient Longman; 1996:258

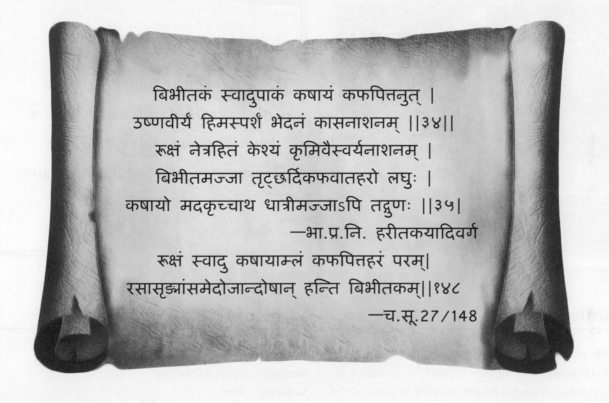

बिभीतकं स्वादुपाकं कषायं कफपित्तनुत् |
उष्णवीर्यं हिमस्पर्शं भेदनं कासनाशनम् ||३४||
रूक्षं नेत्रहितं केश्यं कृमिवैस्वर्यनाशनम् |
बिभीतमज्जा तृट्छर्दिकफवातहरो लघुः |
कषायो मदकृच्चाथ धात्रीमज्जाऽपि तद्गुणः ||३५|
—भा.प्र.नि. हरीतकयादिवर्ग
रूक्षं स्वादु कषायाम्लं कफपित्तहरं परम्|
रसासृङ्मांसमेदोजान्दोषान् हन्ति बिभीतकम्||१४८
—च.सू.27/148

20. Bijak/Vijaysar *[Pterocarpus marsupium Roxb.]*

Family:	*Fabaceae*
Hindi name:	*Bijasal, Vijaysar, Bija*
English name:	*Indian Kino tree*

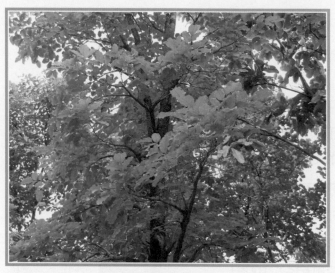

Plant of *Pterocarpus marsupium* Roxb.

The beakers made from heartwood of Bijak are filled with water and are allowed to stand overnight to give "Beeja wood water" for medicinal use.

Introduction

Pterocarpus marsupium Roxb. is commonly called Indian kino tree (English) and Bijasal (Hindi). It is native to India, Nepal, and Sri Lanka, where it exists in parts of the Western Ghats. Traditionally, the plant material has been used as a cooling for external application in headache, inflammations, as antipyretic, anthelminthic, aphrodisiac, mental aberrations, and ulcers. The bark is used for the treatment of stomachache, cholera, dysentery, urinary complaints, tongue diseases, and toothache (Dharshan et al 2014). The heartwood and bark of *P. marsupium* are known for their antidiabetic activity (Mishra et al 2013).

Each mature tree yields approximately 500 kg of dry heartwood after 10 to 15 years. Thus, an estimated yield of 750 to 800 quintals/hectare is obtained. Due to the exploitation of the tree for its timber and medicinal bark, its population is decreasing in the wild, and thus, it has been listed in the red data book (Ramya et al 2008).

Vernacular Names

Assamese: Aajar
Bengali: Piyasala, Pitasala
Gujarati: Biyo
Kannada: Bijasara, Asanamara, Honne mara
Kashmiri: Lal Chandeur
Malayalam: Venga
Marathi: Bibala
Oriya: Piashala
Punjabi: Chandanlal, Channanlal
Tamil: Vengai
Telugu: Yegi, Vegisa
Urdu: Bijasar

Synonyms

Asana: It alleviates disease like prameha.

Bandhukpushpa: This plant bears flowers like Bandhuka.

Bijaka: Heartwood of this plant is used for medicinal purpose.

Karsya: It removes obesity.

Mahasarja: This is a big plant resembling Sarja.

Neelaniryasa: Its exudate is blue in color.

Peetashalak: This is a big plant resembling Shala.

Peetsaar: The heartwood is yellow.

Peevara: It has thick stem.

Priyaka: It makes the physique charming.

Sarjaka: This is a big plant resembling Sarja.

Sugandhi: The flowers have good fragrance.

Tishya: It blossoms in winter.

Classical Categorization

Charak Samhita: Udarda prasashmana

Sushrut Samhita: Salasaradi gana

Astanga Sangraha: Asanadi gana

Dhanwantari Nighantu: Amradi varga

Madanpal Nighantu: Vatadi varga

Kaiyadev Nighantu: Oshadhi varga

Raj Nighantu: Prabhadradi varga

Bhavaprakash: Vatadi varga

Distribution

P. marsupium is growing in defoliate and evergreen jungles of Southern, Western, and Central regions of India. It is native to India, Sri Lanka, and Nepal. In India, it is found in Gujarat, Bihar, West Bengal, Orissa, Uttar Pradesh, Western Ghats, Kerala, Karnataka, and Madhya Pradesh. Generally, it is found on hills or undulating lands or rocky grounds up to a height of 150 to 1100 meter. The usual rainfall in its habitat ranges from 750 to 2000 mm and maximum temperature ranges from 35°C to 48°C and minimum from 0°C to 18°C. It favors well-drained sandy and sedimentary soil to loamy soil. The species is adequate light loving and the young seedlings are frost-tender (Anonymous 1959; Kundu and Schmidt 2015; Dharshan et al 2014).

Morphology

It is a medium- to large-sized deciduous tree of about 15 to 30 m height. Stem bark is thick, dark brown to gray in color, with vertical cracks, exfoliating in thin flakes (**Fig. 20.1**). On injury, a reddish brown gummy exudate comes out from the bark which is known as Malabar Kino.

- **Leaves:** Alternate, compound, imparipinnate, leaflets are five to seven, coriaceous, oblong, obtuse, emarginated or even bilobed at the apex, and glabrous on both surfaces. The petioles are round, smooth, and waved from leaflet to leaflet, 5 or 6 inches long, and there are no stipules (**Fig. 20.2**).

- **Flowers:** Flowers are 1.5 cm long, white with a minor yellow tinge in terminal and lateral panicles. Stamens are 10, united near the base, but soon dividing into two parcels of 5 each; anthers are globose and two-lobed. Ovary is oblong, pedicelled, hairy, generally two-celled; cells are transverse and one-seeded. Style is ascending (**Fig. 20.3**).

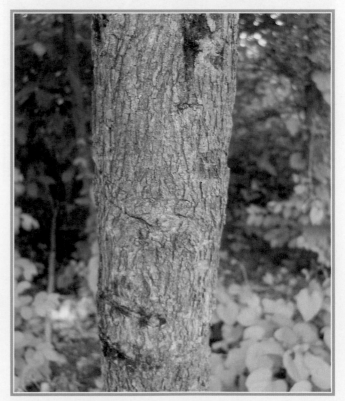

Fig. 20.1 Stem bark.

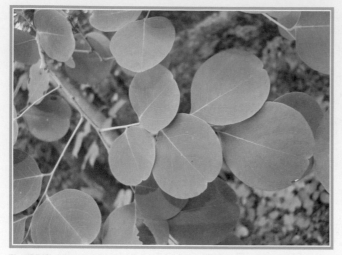

Fig. 20.2 Leaves.

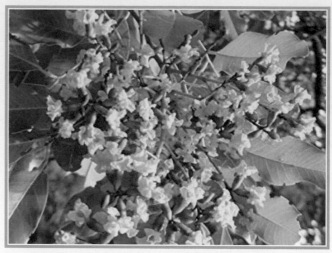

Fig. 20.3 Flower.

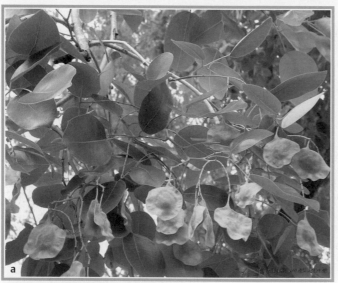

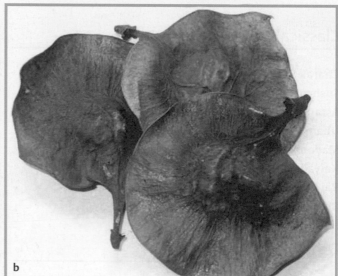

Fig. 20. 4 (a) Fresh fruit. (b) Dry fruit.

- **Fruits:** The legume, which is borne on a long petiole, is three-fourths orbicular, flat, winged, indehiscent pod of about 5 cm in diameter, surrounded with a waved, veiny, downy, membranous wing, swelled, rugose, woody in the center, where the seed is lodged without any opening (**Fig. 20.4a, b**).
- **Seeds:** Single-seeded, convex, bony, and reniform.
- **Heartwood:** It consists of irregular pieces of variable size and thickness. It is golden yellowish brown in color with darker streaks.

The plant is propagated through seed (The Ayurvedic Pharmacopoeia of India 1989; Warier 1995; Manish et al 2009; Rajpal 2005; Yadav and Sardesai 2002).

Phenology

Flowering time: March to June
Fruiting time: March to June

Key Characters for Identification

➤ It is a medium-sized deciduous tree of about 15 to 30 m height.

➤ Stem bark is thick, dark brown to gray color, with vertical cracks. On injury, a reddish brown gummy exudate comes out from the bark.

➤ Leaves: Imparipinnate compound, leaflets are five to seven, oblong, obtuse, emarginated, or even bilobed at the apex.

➤ Flowers: white with a minor yellow tinge flower in terminal and lateral panicles.

➤ Fruits: Three-fourths orbicular, flat, winged, indehiscent pod, 5 cm in diameter, surrounded with a waved, veiny, downy, membranous wing.

➤ Heartwood: Irregular pieces of variable size and thickness, golden yellowish brown color with darker streaks.

Rasapanchaka

Guna	Laghu, Ruksha
Rasa	Kashaya, Tikta
Vipaka	Katu
Virya	Sheet

Chemical Constituents

Literature survey indicated the presence of flavonoids, alkaloids, resin, fixed oil, saponin, tannin, mucilage, isoflavon glycosides, and polyphenol compounds in various parts of the plant.

Early research revealed that the plant P. marsupium is a very rich source of flavonoids and polyphenolic compounds. All the active phytoconstituents of P. marsupium were thermostable. It contains pterostilbene (45%), alkaloids (0.4%), tannins (5%), and protein (Tiwari et al 2015).

The primary phytoconstituents were liquiritigenin, isoliquiritigenin, pterostilbene, pterosupin, epicatechin, catechin, kinotannic acid, kinoin, kino red, β-eudesmol, carsupin, marsupial, marsupinol, pentosan, and p-hydroxy-benzaldehyde (Badkhane et al 2010; Katiyar et al 2016).

Aqueous extract of the heartwood of P. marsupium contains five new flavonoid C-glucosides, namely, 6-hydroxy-2-(4-hydroxybenzyl)-benzofuran-7-C-β-D-glucopyranoside, 3-(α-methoxy-4-hydroxybenzylidene)-6-hydroxybenzo-2(3H)-furanone-7-C-β-Dglucopyranoside, 2-hydroxy-2-phydroxybenzyl-3(2H)-6-hydroxybenzofuranone-7-C-β-D-glucopyranoside, 8-(C-β-D glucopyranosyl)-7,3',4'-trihydroxyflavone, and 1,2-bis(2,4-dihydroxy,3-C-glucopyranosyl) (Maurya et al 2004).

Identity, Purity, and Strength

- Foreign matter: Not more than 2%
- Total ash: Not more than 2%
- Acid-insoluble ash: Not more than 0.5%
- Alcohol-soluble extractive: Not less than 7%
- Water-soluble extractive: Not less than 5%

(Source: The Ayurvedic Pharmacopeia of India 1989)

Karma (Actions)

Bhavaprakash Nighantu has mentioned its heartwood as twachya (skin tonic), keshya (hair tonic), rasayana (rejuvenator). Other actions are kusthaghna (antidermatosis), krimighna (anthelminthic), raktashodhaka (blood purifier), medohara (antiobesity).

- Doshakarma: Kaphapitta shamak
- Dhatukarma: Rasayana, raktashodhak
- Malakarma: Mutrasangrahaniya

Pharmacological Actions

The pharmacological actions are antidiabetic, antifungal, antihyperlipidemic, analgesic, antibacterial, anticancer, anticataract, anti-inflammatory, antioxidant, aphrodisiac, cardiotonic, antidiarrheal, hepatoprotective (Katiyar et al 2016).

Other actions reported are CNS activity, antimicrobial, hypoglycemic, cytotoxic, antiproliferative, cox-2 inhibition, anti-hyperinsulinemic, anti-hypertriglyceridemic, and anticataract activity (Gairola et al 2010).

It is a drug that is believed to have some unique features such as beta-cell protective and regenerative properties apart from blood glucose reduction (WHO 1980; Chakravarthy et al 1981).

Indications

Since time immemorial Vijaysar has been used as a prime drug for the treatment of diabetes. To control blood sugar level, diabetic patients drink water kept in wooden glasses or vessels made out of the heartwood of Vijaysar.

Charaka has used its heartwood and bark in skin diseases, and its niryasa (exudate) for shirovirechana. It is used for the treatment of kushta (skin diseases), raktapitta (bleeding disorders such as nasal bleeding, heavy periods, etc.), prameha (diabetes), visarp (erysipelas), shiwitra (leucoderma), guda krimi (helminthiasis) as per Bhavprakash Nighantu.

The bark and resin decoction of Bijak is astringent and used for the treatment of severe diarrhea, dysentery, tumors of the gland, urethral discharges, ringworm of the scalp and chronic ulcers, abortifacient (Basu et al 1975).

The heartwood is astringent, bitter acrid, anti-inflammatory, anthelmintic, anodyne (Kirtikar 1987). It is good for elephantiasis, leucoderma, diarrhea, rectalgia, cough, and grayness of hair (Mankani et al 2005). It is safe and effective in wounds, fever, stomachache, diabetes, jaundice, and antiulcer (Jung et al 2006).

Various parts of this plant are used for various diseases like leaves for boils, sores, skin diseases, and stomach pain; flowers for fever; Gum Kino for diarrhea, dysentery, and leucorrhea, and bark as astringent and for toothache (The Ayurvedic Pharmacopoeia of India 1989; Pullaiah 1999).

Therapeutic Uses

External Use

Upadamsha (soft chancre): Decoction of khadir and bijak taken orally as well as an external application of paste of Khadir, Bijak, and Guggul or triphala destroys all types of upadamsha (BS.Upadamsha.24).

Internal Use

1. **Prameha** (diabetes): Decoction of Vijaysar or plants of Salasaradi gana is used in the treatment of prameha, kustha, pandu, and elevated kapha and meda (Su.Su. 38/9).
2. **Kushta** (skin disease): Khadir and Bijaka are drugs of choice for kushta (Su.Chi. 6/39).
3. **Sthoulya** (obesity): Intake of decoction of Bijaka mixed with honey in the morning helps in reducing excessive weight in obesity (VD. 12/30).
4. **Shleepada** (filariasis): Intake of paste of heartwood of Khadira, Asana, and Shala with cow's urine mixed with honey alleviates filariasis (GN. 4.2.42).
5. **Netrya** (for improving vision): Sesamum oil, Bibhitaka taila, Bhringaraj swaras, and asana kwath all cooked together in iron vessel is used as Nasya for improving eye sight (AH.U. 13/46).
6. **Raktapitta** (bleeding disorders): Alkali of Madhuka and Asana is used to prevent bleeding in Raktapitta (Cha.Chi. 4/94).
7. **Pandu** (anemia): Bijakarishta is prescribed in anemia (AS.Chi. 18/13).
8. **Sweta kusta** (vitiligo): Bhringaraj cooked with oil in an iron pan and taken orally followed by intake of milk cooked with bijaka alleviates vitiligo (AH.Chi. 20/8).

Officinal Parts Used

Heartwood, gum, bark

Dose

Decoction: 50 to 100 mL
Powder: 3 to 6 g
Gum: 1 to 3 g

Formulations

Bijakarishta, Vijaysar kwath, Mahakhadir ghrita, Asana manjishtadi taila, Narasimha rasayan, Asana vilwadi taila.

Toxicity/Adverse Effects

It is not advised during constipation because of its astringent property (The Ayurvedic Pharmacopoeia of India 1989). As the herbal treatment for diabetes is given for a longer duration, so the genotoxic assessment of Vijaysar was done using both somatic and germ cells. The results indicated that the extract was not genotoxic (Mahnaz et al 2010).

(-)-Epicatechin isolated from Vijaysar was studied for its action on CNS of frog, rat, and mice. The results did not show any toxic effects on heart. Even higher doses of (-)-epicatechin exhibited no untoward effects (Chakravarthy and Gode 1985).

A study group of ICMR investigated the antidiabetic activity of Vijaysar at multicenter level and found that the blood glucose level got significantly decreased without any side effects (ICMR 1998).

Substitution and Adulteration

Terminalia tomentosa is often used as substitute of Bijak. Dried juice of *Butea monosperma* trunk is called Bengal kino and is used as adulterant and substitute of Indian kino (Rakesh et al 2015).

Points to Ponder

- *Asana and Vijaysar are the important synonyms of Bijaka.*
- *Bijaka is mainly used in prameha, kushta, swetakushta and sthoulya.*
- *Bijaka is commonly known as Indian kino tree.*
- *Heartwood and gum of this plant are used for medicinal purpose.*

Suggested Readings

Anonymous. The Wealth of India: Raw Materials. New Delhi: Council of Scientific and Industrial Research; 1959

Badkhane Y, Yadav AS, Sharma AK, et al. *Pterocarpus marsupium* Roxb.: biological activities and medicinal properties. Int J Adv Pharm Sci 2010;1(4):350–357

Basu K. Indian Medicinal Plant. 2nd ed. Delhi: Dehradun Jayed Press; 1975:828

Chakravarthy BK, Gode KD. Isolation of (-)-epicatechin from *Pterocarpus marsupium* and its pharmacological actions. Planta Med 1985;51(1):56–59

Chakravarthy BK, Gupta S, Gambhir SS, Gode KD. The prophylactic action of (-)-epicatechin against alloxan induced diabetes in rats. Life Sci 1981;29(20):2043–2047

Devgun M, Nanda A. Ansari SH. *Pterocarpus marsupium*: a comprehensive review. Phytochemistry 2009;3(6):359–363

Dharshan S, Veerashekar T, Kuppast IJ, Raghu JD. A review on *Pterocarpus marsupium*. Int J of Uni Phar Bio Sci 2014;3(6):32–41

Dubey RB, Sawant BS. Current scenario of adulterants and substitutes of medicinal plants: a review. J Pharm Sci Innov 2015;4(5):247–250

Gairola S, Gupta V, Singh B, Maithani M, Bansal P. Phytochemistry and pharmacological activities of *Pterocarpus marsupium*: a review. Int Res J Pharm 2010;1(1):100–104

ICMR Study Group. Flexible dose open trial of Vijayasar in cases of newly-diagnosed non-insulin-dependent diabetes mellitus. Indian Council of Medical Research (ICMR), Collaborating Centres, New Delhi. Indian J Med Res 1998;108:24–29

Jung M, Park M, Lee HC, Kang YH, Kang ES, Kim SK. Antidiabetic agents from medicinal plants. Curr Med Chem 2006;13(10):1203–1218

Katiyar D, Singh V, Ali M. Phytochemical and pharmacological profile of *Pterocarpus marsupium*: a review. Pharma Innov 2016;5(4):31–39

Kirtikar B. Indian Medicinal Plants. 2nd ed. Vol. I. New Delhi: Materia Medica; 1987:826–827

Kundu M, Schmidt LH. *Pterocarpus marsupium* Roxb.: Seed Leaflet. Mandla Road, Jabalpur India. 2015;482021:163

Mahnaz M, Swapnil S, Devasagayam G, Saroj S. J Comp Int Med 2010;7(1):14

Mankani KL, Krishna V, Manjunatha BK, et al. Evaluation of hepatoprotective activity of stem bark of *Pterocarpus marsupium* Roxb. Indian J Pharmacol 2005;37(3):165–168

Maurya R, Singh R, Deepak M, Handa SS, Yadav PP, Mishra PK. Constituents of *Pterocarpus marsupium*: an ayurvedic crude drug. Phytochemistry 2004;65(7):915–920

Mishra A, Srivastava R, Srivastava SP, et al. Antidiabetic activity of heart wood of *Pterocarpus marsupium* Roxb. and analysis of phytoconstituents. Indian J Exp Biol 2013;51(5):363–374

Pullaiah T. Medicinal Plants of Andhra Pradesh. New Delhi, Regency Publications; 1999:63

Quality Standards of Indian Medicinal Plants, Medicinal Plants Unit. New Delhi: Indian Council of Medical Research; 2008; 6:205

Rajpal V. Standardization of Botanicals, Testing and Extraction Methods of Medicinal Herbs. New Delhi: Eastern Publisher; 2005;1: 296–306

Ramya S, Kalayansundaram M, Kalaivani T, Jayakumararaj R. Phytochemical screening and antibacterial activity of leaf extracts of *Pterocarpus marsupium* Roxb. Ethnobotan Leafl 2008;12:1029–1034

Roxb M. Int J Universal Pharm Biosci 2014;3(6):32–41

The Ayurvedic Pharmacopeia of India. Department of AYUSH, Ministry of Health and Family Welfare, Government of India; 1989:15–17

The Ayurvedic Pharmacopeia of India. Part I. Vol. 1. Department of Indian System of Medicine & Homeopathy, The Controller of Publications, Ministry of Health and Family Welfare, Government of India; 1989:12–13

The Ayurvedic Pharmacopoeia of India. 1st ed. New Delhi: Department of Indian System of Medicine & Homeopathy, Ministry of Health and Family Welfare, Government of India; 2001:12–13

Tiwari M, Sharma M, Khare HN. Chemical constituents and medicinal uses of *Pterocarpus marsupium* Roxb. Flora Fauna 2015;21(1): 55–59

Warier PK. Indian Medicinal Plants: A Compendium of 500 Species. Vol. 3. Delhi: University Press (India) Private Limited; 1995:280

WHO. Second Report of the WHO Expert Committee on Diabetes Mellitus. Geneva: World Health Organization; 1980:58–67

Yadav SR, Sardesai MM. Flora of Kolhapur District. 2002, 87

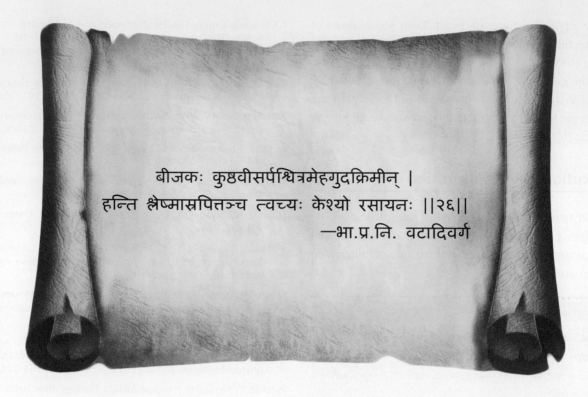

बीजकः कुष्ठवीसर्पश्चित्रमेहगुदक्रिमीन् ।
हन्ति श्रैष्मास्त्रपितञ्च त्वच्यः केश्यो रसायनः ॥२६॥
—भा.प्र.नि. वटादिवर्ग

21. Bilva [Aegle marmelos (Linn.) Corr.]

Family:	*Rutaceae*
Hindi name:	*Bael, Bel, Sriphal*
English name:	*Bengal quince, Apple Wood, Bael tree*

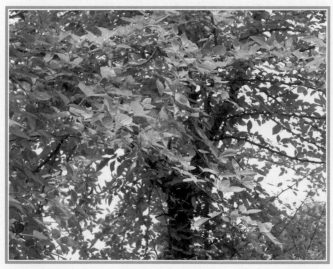

Plant of *Eagle marmelos* (Linn.) Corr.

> *The trifoliate leaf of Bel tree is symbolic of Trikal (Brahma, Vishnu, and Mahesh), three eyes of Lord Shiva, Trishakti (volition, action, and knowledge), three lingas, and three syllables of Omkar (Dutta et al 2014).*

Introduction

Bael is considered as one of the sacred trees of Hindus. Earliest evidence of religious importance of Bael appears in Shri Shuktam of Rig Veda which reveres this plant as the residence of Goddess Lakshmi, the deity of wealth and prosperity (The Astrological Magazine, Vol. 92). Bael trees are considered an incarnation of Goddess Parvati (The Handbook of Tibetan Buddhist Symbols). Bael trees can be usually seen near the Hindu temples and in home gardens of Hindus. It is believed that Hindu deity Lord Shiva is fond of Bael tree and its leaves and fruits still play a major role in his worship (Lim 2012). It is also referred to as "Shivadruma" because its leaves are offered to Hindu gods, Shiva and Parvati. The word "bilva" (Bel tree) is usually used as bilva-patra (leaf of Bel). It is a sacred tree having sacrificial importance. The leaves of this sacred tree are generally trifoliate. This trifoliate leaf is symbolic of Trikal (Brahma, Vishnu, and Mahesh), three eyes of Lord Shiva,

Trishakti (volition, action, and knowledge), three lingas, and three syllables of Omkar (Dutta et al 2014).

In the traditional practice of the Hindu and Buddhist religions by people of the Newar culture of Nepal, the Bael tree is part of a fertility ritual for girls, which is known as the "Bel bibaaha." Girls are "married" to the Bael fruit; as long as the fruit is kept safe and never cracks, the girl can never become widowed, even if her human husband dies. This is seen to be protection against the social disdain suffered by widows in the Newar community (Gutschow et al 2008).

Apart from religious importance, the plant Bilva has a wide range of medicinal potentials. All parts of this tree, viz., root, leaf, trunk, fruit, and seed, are used for curing human ailments. There is a thorough description of Bilva in Vedas, Samhitas, Nighantus, and other classical literature of Ayurveda and religious scriptures. It is used to cure many different diseases like atisara (diarrhea), pravahika (dysentery), arsha (piles), grahani (sprue), agnimandya (loss of appetite), gulma (andominal lump), kasa (cough), shwasa (asthma), parshwashula (pain in lateral side of andomen), halimaka (a type of liver disease), etc. Root of Bilva is one of the components of Brihat panchmool and dashmool and its patra (leaf) is included under panchpallava.

British pharmacopoeia has included *A. marmelos* fruit because of its effectiveness against diarrhea and dysentery (Chopra 1982). Moreover, Chopra (1982) has appropriately stated that "no drug has been longer and better known, nor more appreciated by the inhabitants of India than the Bael fruit."

Vernacular Names

Assamese: Bael, Vael
Bengali: Bela, Bilva
Gujarati: Bill, Bilum, Bilvaphal
Kannada: Bilva
Kashmiri: Bel
Malayalam: Koovalam
Marathi: Bel, Baela
Oriya: Bela
Punjabi: Bil
Tamil: Vilvam
Telugu: Maredu
Urdu: Bel

Synonyms

Bilva: It is useful in bowel ailment particularly in diarrhea and dysentery.
Gandhagarbha: Pulp of fruit has a peculiar smell.
Gandhapatra: Leaves are aromatic.
Goharitaki: Useful in veterinary practices like Haritaki for abdominal complaint.
Granthila: Branches are nodular.
Hridyagandha: Fruits are beautiful with pleasant aroma.
Kantaki: It is a thorny tree.
Karkata: Fruit is covered with hard rind.
Kuchama: Fruits are globose.
Mahakapittha: The fruit are similar to the fruits of Katittha but larger in size. Mahaphala: Fruit of Bilva is big.
Maloora: It is useful in bowel ailment.
Putimaruta: It has carminative action.
Sadaphala: The plant bears fruits throughout the year.
Shailoosha: It grows even in hilly area.

Shalatu: Unripe fruits are of therapeutic use.
Shandilya: It is wholesome and cures diseases.
Shivesta: It is offered to Lord Shiva as it is favorite to him.
Shrigandhaphala: Pulp of fruit has a peculiar smell.
Shreevasa: Goddess Lakshmi lives there.
Shriphala: It bears beautiful fruit with pleasant aroma.
Tripatra: It has trifoliate leaves.
Vatasara: It has carminative action and relieves flatulence from abdomen.

Classical Categorization

Charak Samhita: Shothahara, Arshoghna, Asthapanopaga, Anuvasanopaga
Sushrut Samhita: Varunadi, Ambashtadi, Brihat panchamool
Astanga Sangraha: Ambashtadi, Brihat panchamool
Astanga Hridaya: Varunadi, Ambashtadi, Mahapanchmool.
Dhanwantari Nighantu: Guduchyadi varga
Madanpal Nighantu: Abhayadi varga
Kaiyadev Nighantu: Aushadhi varga
Raj Nighantu: Amradi varga, Dharanyadi, Mishrakadi.
Bhavaprakash Nighantu: Guduchyadi varga, Amradiphalavarga.

Distribution

A. marmelos is a subtropical plant and grows up to an altitude of 1,200 m above sea level. It grows well in the dry forests on hilly and plain areas. It is a widely distributed plant and found in India, Ceylon, China, Nepal, Sri Lanka, Myanmar, Pakistan, Bangladesh, Nepal, and Vietnam. In India it is found in sub-Himalayan tracts from Jhelum eastwards to West Bengal, in central and south India. It is extensively planted near Hindu temples for its leaves and wood which is used for worship. It is found almost in all the states of India (Sekar et al 2011). It is also grown in Egyptian gardens in Surinam and Trinidad (Sukhdev 1975).

Morphology

It is a slow-growing, medium-sized tree, 12 to 15 m tall. The stem is short, thick, soft, flaking bark, and spreading, sometimes spiny branches (**Fig. 21.1**), the lower ones

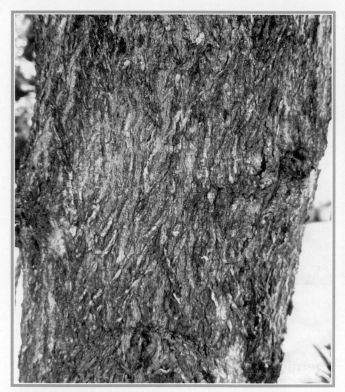

Fig. 21.1 Stem.

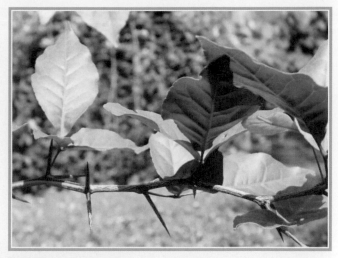

Fig. 21.2 Spines.

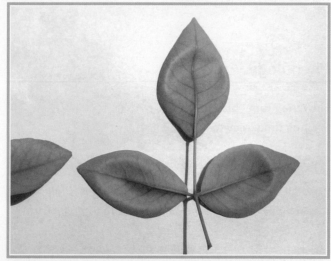

Fig. 21.3 Leaves.

drooping. There are sharp, axial one-inch long spines on this tree (**Fig. 21.2**).

- **Leaves:** Leaves are composed of three to five leaflets in it. The leaflets are oval or lancet shaped, 4 to 10 cm long, 2 to 5 cm wide. The lateral leaflets are without petiole and the terminal one has a long one. The petiole is 1 to 2.5 inch long. Mature leaves emit a peculiar fragrance when bruised (**Fig. 21.3**).

- **Flowers:** Found in cluster of four to seven along the young branchlets, with four recurved, fleshy petals. The flowers are greenish white in color with a peculiar fragrant (**Fig. 21.4**).

- **Fruits:** Spherical or oval in shape with a diameter of 2 to 6 inches. Shell is thin, hard, and woody in nature. It is greenish when unripe and it turns into yellowish color after ripening. The pulp of the fruit has 8 to 15 segments. The pulp is yellow, soft, pasty, sweet, resinous, and fragrant (**Fig. 21.5a, b**).

- **Seeds:** The small seeds are embedded in the pulp. It is hard, flattened-oblong, bearing woolly hairs, and each enclosed in a sac of adhesive, transparent mucilage that solidifies on drying (Lambole et al 2010; Sharma et al 2007).

The plant is propagated through seeds, root, or stem cutting.

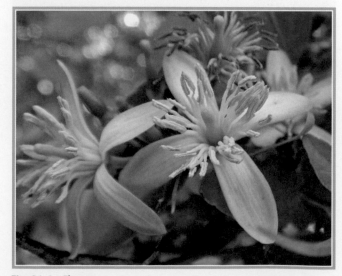

Fig. 21.4 Flowers.

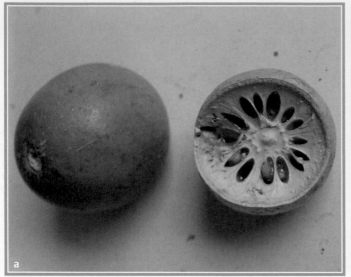
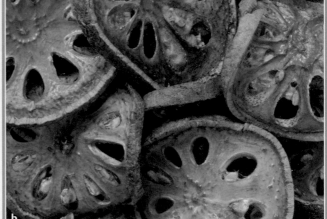

Fig. 21.5 **(a)** Fruit. **(b)** Fruit pulp.

Phenology

Flowering time: May to June

Fruiting time: May to June

Key Characters for Identification

➤ Bilva is a medium-sized tree, 12 to 15 meters tall
➤ Stem: Short, thick, soft, flaking bark that spread with sharp spines
➤ Leaves: Three to five leaflets, oval or lancet shaped
➤ Flowers: Found in cluster, greenish white with a peculiar fragrant
➤ Fruits: Spherical or oval, 2 to 6 inches in diameter; shell is thin, hard, and woody, greenish when unripe and yellowish after ripening
➤ Seeds: Embedded in yellow soft pulp, hard, flattened-oblong, bearing woolly hairs

Rasapanchaka

Guna	Laghu, Ruksha
Rasa	Tikta, Kasaya
Vipaka	Katu
Virya	Ushna

Chemical Constituents

Various chemical constituents like alkaloids, coumarins, and steroids have been isolated and identified from different parts of the tree.

- Alkaloids: aeglin, aegelenine, dictamine, fragrine ($C13H11O3N$), o-methylhalfordinine, isopentenylhalfordinol, N-2-[4-(3′, 3′-dimethylallyloxy) phenyl] ethyl cinnamide, N-2-hydroxy-2-[4(3′, 3′-dimethylallyloxy) phenyl] ethyl cinnamide, N-2-hydroxy-(4-hydroxyphenyl) ethyl cinnamide, O-(3, 3-dimethylallyl) halofordinol, N-2-ethoxy-2-(4-methoxy phenyl) ethyl cinnamide, N-2-methoxy-2-[4(3′, 3¢dimethylallyloxy) phenyl] ethylcinnamide, N-2-methoxy-2-(4-methoxy-phenyl)-ethylcinnamide (Manandhar et al 1978; Tuticorin et al 1983).
- Coumarins: marmelosin, marmesin, imperatorin, marmin, alloimperatorin, methyl ether, xanthotoxol, scopoletin, scoparone, umbelliferone, psoralen, and marmelid. Marmenol, a 7-geranyloxycoumarin [7-(2, 6-dihydroxy-7-methoxy-7-methyl-3-Octaenyloxy) coumarins] (Farooq 2005).
- Polysaccharides: galactose, arabinose, uronic acid, and L-rhamanose are obtained on hydrolysis. Seed oil is composed of palmitic, stearic, oleic, linoleic, and linolenic acid (Basak et al 1982).

- Tannins: Tannin content is maximum in the Bilva fruit in the month of January. There is as much as 9% tannin in the pulp of wild fruits, less in cultivated type. Tannin is also present in leaves as skimmianine.

The pale color of the fruit is because of the presence of carotenoids. There is a small amount of ascorbic acid, sitosterol, crude fibers, tannins, α-amyrin, and carotenoids, and crude proteins are also present. The roots contain psoralen, xanthotoxin scopoletin, and also compounds like praealtin D, trans-cinnamic acid, 4-methoxy benzoic acid, betulunic acid, and montanin (Ali et al 2004). Bael tree also possesses a large number of bioactive compounds in its various parts.

Identity, Purity, and Strength

- Total ash: Not more than 4%
- Acid-insoluble ash: Not more than 1%
- Alcohol-soluble extractive: Not less than 6%
- Water-soluble extractive: Not less than 50%

(Source: The Ayurvedic Pharmacopeia of India 1989)

Karma (Actions)

Balya, deepana, grahi, pacana, pittakrit, vatakaphahara, pakwa phala-madhur, guru, visthambhi, vidhahi.

The actions of different parts of Bilva are as under:

- Apakva phala (baala phala): Samgrahi (astringent), deepana (appetizer), pacana (digestive), aamanashana (cure indigestion), ruchya (relish), hridya (cardiotonic), kaphavatahara (pacify vatakapha)
- Pakva phala (mature fruit): Durjara (difficult to digest), pootimaruta (foul smell), vidahi (burning/gastric irritation), vishtambh (stasis of food), agnisada kara (reduce digestive power), dahakara (burning sensation), vrishya (aphrodisiac), grahi (astringent), shukrala (spermatopoetic), sugandhi (fragnance), adhmanakara (causes distension)
- Apakwa phalamajja (pulp of immature fruit): Grahi (astringent), aamanashana (cure indigestion)
- Patra (leaves): Aamanashana, grahi, rochana, hridya, vatahara
- Kanda (stem): Amanashana, hridya, ruchya, deepana
- Moola (root): Mutral (diuretics)
- Doshakarma: Vatakaphahara

- Dhatukarma: Balya
- Malakarma: Grahi

Pharmacological Actions

The plant has antidiarrheal, antiulcer, antioxidant, antimalarial, antidiabetic, anti-inflammatory, antibacterial, histamine receptor antagonism, antifungal, antiviral, radioprotective, anticancer, antihyperlipidemic, hepatoprotective, and wound-healing properties (Dutta et al 2014; Patel et al 2012).

Indications

All parts of the plants are used to cure many different diseases such as atisara (diarrhea), pravahika (dysentery), arsha (piles), grahani (sprue), agnimandya (loss of appetite), gulma (abdominal lump), kasa (cough), shwasa (asthma), parshwashula (pain in lateral side of abdomen), and halimaka (a type of liver disease).

Indication of various parts of Bilva is given below:

- Apakva phala (tender fruit): Shoola (colic), grahnidosha (irritable bowel syndrome), atisara (diarrhea)
- Apakwaphalamajja (pulp of tender fruit): Shoola (colic), grahanidoshahara (IBS)
- Moola (root): Chhardi (vomiting), mutrakrichha (dysuria), shwasa (asthma), kasa (cough), hikka (hic-cough), kshaya (debility), jwar (fever), atisara (fever), shoola (colic), raktapitta (internal hemorrhoea)
- Patra (leaves): Kasa (cough)
- Pushpa (flower): Atisara (diarrhea), trishna (thirst), chhardi (vomiting)

Therapeutic Uses

External Use

1. **Inflammation:** A hot poultice of the leaves is applied in ophthalmia or severe inflammation of conjunctiva with acute bronchitis and inflammation of other body parts (Kurian 1992).
2. **Rheumatic pain:** Leaf paste of *A. marmelos* is applied for rheumatic pain (Orwa et al 2009).

3. **Bone fracture**: Paste of leaves are mixed with butter, applied over fractured area, and bound in bone fracture (Reddy 2003).

Internal Use

1. **Atisara** (diarrhea):
   (a) One gets rid of diarrhea after taking Pippali with honey or buttermilk with Chitrak or tender fruit of Bilva (C.S.Ci. 19/113).
   (b) Tender fruit of Bilva is taken with liquid jaggery, honey, and oil to cure diarrhea with blood. It controls the disease immediately (S.S.Ci. 40/119).
   (c) Fruit pulp of Bilva and Madhuka is mixed with sugar and honey and is taken with rice water which checks diarrhea caused by pitta and rakta (S.S.Ci. 40/127).
   (d) Intake of Bilva and jaggery checks diarrhea with blood, removes pain due to ama (a type of toxin) and constipation, and alleviate bowel diseases (VM. 3/40; BP/2/57).
   (e) Decoction of Bilva and Amra seed mixed with honey and sugar checks vomiting and diarrhea (VM. 3/30).
2. **Arsha** (hemorrhoids):
   (a) Powder of equal parts of fruit pulp of Bilva, Shunthi, Ajwain, and Citraka root is given in a dose of 3 g with Takra (butter milk) twice a day in nonbleeding piles. After massaging the affected area, it is advised to sit in the warm decoction of Bilva or butter milk (C.S.Ci. 14/47).
   (b) Saturating drink of butter milk should be given with Bilva and Kapittha or Shunthi and bida or Bhallatak or Yavani (AH.Ci. 8/35).
3. **Pravahika** (dysentery): Khada (one type of dietary preparation) prepared with tender fruit of Bilva, equal quantity of sesame paste, supernatant layer of sour curd, and ghee checks dysentery (C.S.Ci. 19/34).
4. **Otalgia**: Pouring lukewarm oil prepared with Bilva roots daily into the ear gives relief in earache and deafness (S.S.U. 21/35; see also VM 59/27 and SG 2/9/171).
5. **Nausea and vomiting**:
   (a) Cold decoction of Bilva or Guduchi added with honey or Murva with rice water should be taken in three types of vomiting (VM. 15/15, see also BS.Chhardi 3, SG. 2.2.85, BP.Ci. 17/25).

   (b) Decoction of Bilva and Shunthi checks vomiting and visuchika (BP.Ci. 6/112).
6. **Jaundice:** Intake of Bilva leave juice mixed with Trikatu alleviates jaundice (C.S.Ci. 16/59).
7. **Udarroga** (abdominal disease): Oil mixed with alkali of Bilva should be given in pain of sides caused due to vata, stiffness, and cardiac distress (AH.Ch. 15/45).
8. **Grahani roga** (sprue): Paste of tender fruit of Bilva mixed with Shunthi powder and jaggery keeping the patient on the diet of butter milk alleviates severe grahani roga (VM. 4/10).
9. **Edema:** Juice of Bilva leaves mixed with maricha is useful in edema caused by the following three doshas: constipation, piles, and jaundice (VM. 39/9).
10. **Jwara** (fever): Milk cooked with Erand root or tender fruit of Bilva gives relief from fever (C.S.Ci. 3/235).

Officinal Parts Used

Root, bark, fruit pulp, leaves, seeds

Dose

Fruit pulp: 3 to 6 g
Juice: 10 to 20 mL

Formulations

Dashmoolarishta, Amritarishta, Brihat gangadhara churna, Bilvapanchaka Kvatha, Bilvadi churna, Bilvadi ghrita, Bilva taila, Bilvadi Leha, Agasthya haritaki leha, Pusyanuga choorna, Mahanarayan taila, Vatsakadi kwat.

Toxicity/Adverse Effects

A. marmelos has been used for centuries in India not only for its dietary purposes, but also for its various medicinal properties (Sudharameshwari and Radhika 2006). Hence, it is generally considered safe and few studies have been carried out with respect to its toxicity. Nevertheless, aqueous extract of *A. marmelos* fruit has been reported to be nonmutagenic to *S. typhimurium* strain TA 100 in the Ames assay (Kruawan and Kangsadalampai 2006).

It is reported from various studies that hydroalcoholic extract of fruit and leaves of *A. marmelos* is nontoxic, and there were no remarkable changes noticed in histopathological studies when administered intraperitoneally at different doses like 6 g/kg body weight in mice (Jagetia et al 2004a), 250 mg/kg body weight for 30 days (Jagetia et al 2004b), and doses of 50 to 90 and 100 mg/kg body weight for 14 consecutive days to male and female Wistar rats (Veerappan et al 2007). Collectively, these data demonstrate that the extracts of the leaves and fruits of *A. marmelos* have a high margin of drug safety.

Substitution and Adulteration

Bel fruits are occasionally substituted with wood apple (*Feronia limonia* Linn.) and mangosten (*Garcinia mangostana* Linn.; Sharma et al 2005).

Points to Ponder

- *Bilva is one of the components of Brihat panchamool and Dashamool.*
- *Bilva is sangrahika, deepaniya, vatakaphashamak.*
- *It is mainly used in atisara, pravahika, arsha, grahani, agnimandya, gulma, kasa, shwasa, parshwashula, halimaka.*

Suggested Readings

Ali MS, Pervez MK. Marmenol: a 7-geranyloxycoumarin from the leaves of *Aegle marmelos* Corr. Nat Prod Res 2004;18(2):141–146

Bakhru HK. Foods That Heals. Orient Paperbacks. 1995:28–30

Basak RK, Mandal PK, Mukherjee AK. Investigation on the structure of a hemicellulose fraction isolated from the trunk of young Bael (*Aegle marmelos*) tree. Carbohydr Res 1982;104(2):309–317

Chopra R. Indigenous Drugs of India. Calcutta: Academic Publishers; 1982

Dutta A, Neeta L, Musarrat N, Ghosh A, Rupa V. Ethnological and ethnomedicinal importance of *Aegle marmelos* (L.) Corr (Bael) among indigenous people of India. Am J Ethnomed 2014;1(5):290–312

Farooq S. 555 Medicinal Plants: Field and Laboratory Manual. Dehradun: International Book Distributors; 2005:40–42

Gutschow N, Axel M, Christian B. The Girl's Hindu Marriage to the Bel Fruit: Ihi and The Girl's Buddhist Marriage to the Bel Fruit: Ihi. Growing Up-Hindu And Buddhist Initiation Ritual among Newar Children in Bhaktapur, Nepal. Wiesbaden, GER: Otto Harrassowitz Verlag; 2008:93–173

Jagetia GC, Venkatesh P, Baliga MS. Evaluation of the radioprotective effect of bael leaf (*Aegle marmelos*) extract in mice. Int J Radiat Biol 2004;80(4):281–290

Jagetia GC, Venkatesh P, Baliga MS. Fruit extract of *Aegle marmelos* protects mice against radiation-induced lethality. Integr Cancer Ther 2004;3(4):323–332

Jain SM, Ishii K. Micropropagation of Woody Trees and Fruits, Volume 75 of Forestry Sciences. Springer Science & Business Media; 2012

Korkina LG, Afanas'ev IB. Antioxidant and chelating properties of flavonoids. Adv Pharmacol 1997;38:151–163

Kruawan K, Kangsadalampai K. Antioxidant activity, phenolic compound contents and antimutagenic activity of some water extract of herbs. Thai J Pharma Sci 2006;30:1–47

Kurian JC. Plants That Heals. Oriental Publishing House; 1992:26–27

Lambole VB, Murti K, Kumar U, Sandipkumar PB, Gajera V. Phytopharmacological properties of Aegle marmelos as a potential medicinal tree: an overview. Int J Pharm Sci Rev Res 2010;5:67–72

Lim TK. Edible Medicinal and Non-Medicinal Plants. Vol. 4. Springer Science & Business Media; 2012:613

Manandhar MD, Shoeb A, Kapil RS, Popli SP. New alkaloids from *Aegle marmelos*. Phytochemistry 1978;17:1814–1815

Orwa C, Mutua A, Kindt R, Jamnadass R, Simons A. Agroforestree Database: a tree reference and selection guide. Version 4.0. Available at: http://www.worldagroforestry.org/af/treedb/

Panda H. Medicinal Plants Cultivation and Their Uses. Delhi: National Institute of Industrial Research; 2002:159

Patel PK, Sahu J, Sahu L, Prajapati NK, Dubey BK. *Aegle marmelos*: a review on its medicinal properties. Int J Pharm Phytopharm Res 2012;1(5):332–341

Peg S. Spiritual Gardening: Creating Sacred Space Outdoors. Novato, CA: New World Library; 2003

Reddy VR. Plants in Ethno Veterinary Practices in Anantapur District, Andhra Pradesh: Ethnobotany and Medicinal Plants of Indian Subcontinent. Jodhpur: Scientific Publishers (India); 2003:356

Sekar DK, Kumar G, Karthik L, Bhaskara Rao KV. A review on pharmacological and phytochemical properties of *Aegle marmelos* (L.). Corr Serr (Rutaceae). Asian J Plant Sci Res 2011;1(2):8–17

Sharma PC, Bhatia V, Bansal N, Sharma A. A review on Bael tree. Nat Prod Radiance 2007;6(2):171–178

Sharma PC, Yelne MB, Dennis TJ, Joshi A, Prabhune YS. Database of Medicinal Plants Used in Ayurveda and Siddha, Vol. 1. New Delhi: CCRAS; 2005

Sudharameshwari K, Radhika J. Antibacterial screening of *Aegle marmelos*, *Lawsonia inermis* and *Albizzia libbeck*. Afr J Tradit Complement Altern Med 2006;4(2):199–204

Sukhdev AR. A selection of prime Ayurvedic plant drugs: ancient-modern concordance, Anamaya Publicatons. Br J Surg 1975;62:542–552

The Astrological Magazine. Vol. 92. Raman Publications; 2003:48

The Ayurvedic Pharmacopoeia of India. Part I, Vol. 1. New Delhi: Department of AYUSH, Ministry of Health & Family Welfare, Government of India; 1989:25–28

Tuticorin RG, Manakkal SP. Some alkaloids from Aeglemarmelos. Phytochemistry 1983;22:755–757

Veerappan A, Miyazaki S, Kadarkaraisamy M, Ranganathan D. Acute and subacute toxicity studies of *Aegle marmelos* Correa: an Indian medicinal plant. Phytomedicine 2007;14:209–215

Govindachari TR, Premila MS. Some alkaloids from *Aegle marmelos*. Phytochemistry 1983;22(3):755–757

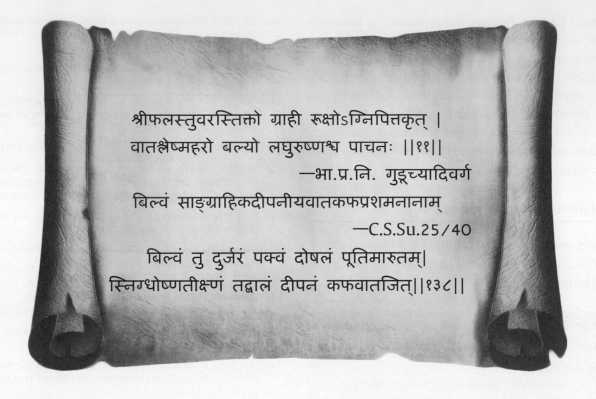

श्रीफलस्तुवरस्तिको ग्राही रूक्षोऽग्निपित्तकृत् |
वातश्लेष्महरो बल्यो लघुरुष्णश्च पाचनः ||११||
—भा.प्र.नि. गुडूच्यादिवर्ग
बिल्वं साङ्ग्राहिकदीपनीयवातकफप्रशमनानाम्
—C.S.Su.25/40
बिल्वं तु दुर्जरं पक्वं दोषलं पूतिमारुतम्|
स्निग्धोष्णतीक्ष्णं तद्वालं दीपनं कफवातजित्||१३८||

22. Brahmi *[Bacopa monnieri (L.) Pennell]*

Family: *Scrophulariaceae/Plantaginaceae*

Hindi name: *Brahmi, Jalnim, Manduka parni, Barambhi, Adha birni*

English name: *Thyme-leaved gratiola, Water hyssop*

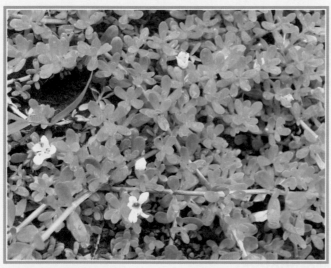

Plant of *Bacopa monnieri* L.

It was found that aged people were able to acquire, store, and retain their memory over time by consuming Brahmi as a supplement. (Calabrese et al 2008; Morgan and Stevens 2010).

Introduction

Bacopa monnieri is one of the traditional medicinal plants in Ayurveda medicine, where it is also called Brahmi, a name derived from Brahma, the creator God of the Hindu Pantheon.

Centella asiatica and *Bacopa monnieri* is widely known as Brahmi. However, these plants are distinctly different. The name Brahmi is assigned to *B. monnieri* whereas "Mandukaparni," often confused with Brahmi, refers to *C. asiatica*. Brahmi is largely treasured as a revitalizing herb that has been used by Ayurvedic medical practitioners for almost 3,000 years. The herb has been mentioned in several Ayurvedic treatises including Charaka Samhita, Sushruta Samhita, Astanga Hridaya, and almost in all Nighantus. Acharya Vagbhatta in Uttara sthana quoted Brahmi as the best remedy for apasmara (epilepsy). It has many medicinal potentials like medhya (intellect), ayushya (longevity),

rasayana (rejuvenation), hridhya (heart), balya (strength, especially mind), jivaniya (life energy), nidrajanana (sleep), etc. Over the centuries, the role of Brahmi in the treatment of kustha (leprosy/skin disorder), pandu (anemia), meha (diabetes), asra vikara (blood disorders), kasa (cough), visa (poison), sopha (edema), jwara (fever), unmada (insanity), and manasavikara (mental disorders) has been well described.

Brahmi is a well-known nootropic herb and its uses in neurological and psychiatric disorders are well recognized. Its efficacy and safety are supported by research and thousands of years of knowledge and experience.

It is one of the highly demanded medicinal plants. According to the National Medicinal Plants Board report, the annual market demand for Brahmi (*B. monnieri*) was around 1,000 tones in year 2000, which increased many folds due to its potential uses in Ayurvedic medicine to treat variety of diseases (Tripathi et al 2012).

Vernacular Names

Arabic: Zarazab, farfakh

Assamese: Brahmi

Bengali: Brahmi sak, Jalanimba, Vdhabini, Birmi

Bombay: Bama

Chinese: Pa-Chi-Tlien, jia ma chi xian

French: Petite bacopa

German: Kleine fettblatt

Gujarati: Neerbrahmi, Bamanevari, baam

Hebrew: Psheta srua

Japanese: bakopa

Kannada: Nirubrahmi, Valabrahmi, Ondelaga, Manduka-parni, Kiru brahmi, Neeruppi gida, Jala brahmi

Konkan: Brahmi

Malay: Bremi

Malayalam: Bhahmi, Nirbrahmi, barna

Marathi: Jalnim, Brahmi, Birami, Nirbrahmi, ghola

Nepalese: Medha giree

Oriya: Brahmi

Persian: Jaranab

Polish: bakopa drobnolistna

Punjabi: Brahmibuti,

Sanskrit: Sarasvata, Kapotavanka, Aindri, Brahmi, Jalasaya, Matyaksi,

Tamil: Nirabrahmi, Brahmi vazhukkai, Nir pirami, Piramiye pundu, Vivitam campirani, ahaznda poozndu

Telugu: Sambarenu, Sambrani, Chettu, Neeri, Sambraani mokka, Sambraani aaku

Thai: Phrommi

Urdu: Brahmi, Jalanim, Nirabrahmi

Vietnamese: rau dang bien

Synonyms

Bharati: It is an indigenous plant.

Brahmi: It promotes memory and intellect.

Divyateja: It provides divine complexion.

Jalashaya: It grows in marshy area and is considered as aquatic plant.

Lavani/Vara: It beautifies hair and helps in hair growth.

Munibhi: This plant is used by sages.

Saraswati: It improves intellect like Goddess Saraswati.

Smarani: It improves memory power.

Somavalli: A creeper grows in marshy area.

Somya: It is a pleasant looking herb.

Suswara: It is used to improve voice.

Vaidhatri: It is considered as good as a mother.

Vayastha: It improves longevity.

Classical Categorization

Charaka Samhita: Prajasthapana

Sushruta Samhita: Veeratharvadi gana

Dhanwantari Nighantu: Karaveeradi varga

Madanpal Nighantu: Abhayadi varga

Kaiyadev Nighantu: Aushadha Varga

Raj Nighantu: Parpatadi varga

Bhavaprakash: Guduchyadi varga

Distribution

It commonly grows in wet, damp, and marshy areas throughout India, Nepal, Sri Lanka, China, Taiwan, Viet Nam, Florida and other southern states of the United States (Daniel 2005; Warrier et al 1996; Khare 2003).

Morphology

A prostrate or creeping, succulent, annual herb rooting at the nodes with numerous ascending branches, 20 cm or more long.

- **Stem:** Thin, green or purplish green, about 1 to 2 mm thick, soft, nodes and internodes prominent, glabrous, slightly bitter taste (**Fig. 22.1**).
- **Leaves:** Simple, oppositely decussate, obovate-oblong or spatulate, 8 to 15 mm long and 4 mm wide, slightly bitter in taste, fleshy, entire margin, sessile or short petioled (**Fig. 22.2**).
- **Flowers:** Small, solitary, axillary, white, purple, pink or pale violet in color, five petaled, pedicels 6 to 30 mm long, bracteoles shorter than pedicels (**Fig. 22.3**).
- **Fruits:** Fruits are capsules up to 5 mm long, ovoid, glabrous, and sharp at apex.
- **Root:** Thin, wiry, small, branched, and creamish-yellow in color (**Fig. 22.4**) (Khare et al 2003; Trivedi et al 2011).

This plant is propagated through seeds and stem cutting.

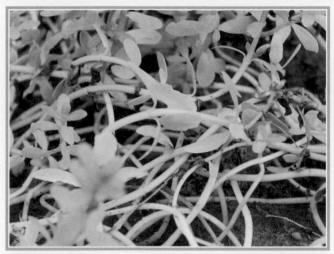

Fig 22.1 Stem of Brahmi.

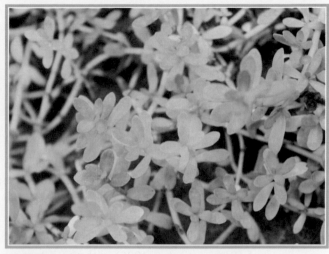

Fig 22.2 Leaves.

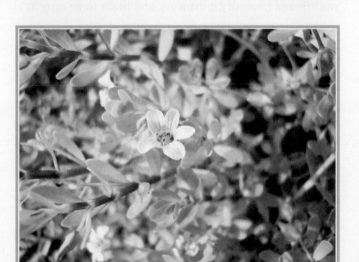

Fig 22.3 Flower.

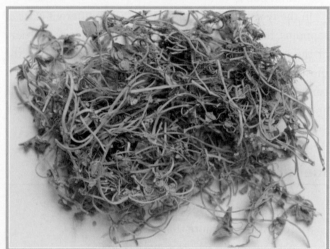

Fig 22.4 Dry sample of Brahmi.

Phenology

Flowering time: April to June
Fruiting time: June to December

Key Characters for Identification

➤ It is a prostrate or creeping, succulent, annual herb,
  near about 20 cm long
➤ Leaves: simple, oppositely decussate, obovate-oblong
  or spatulate, entire, 8 to 15 mm by 4 mm, slightly bitter
➤ Flowers: small, solitary, axillary, white, purple, pink or
  pale violet color with five petals
➤ Fruit: small glabrous capsule

Rasapanchaka

Guna	Laghu, Sara
Rasa	Tikta, Kasaya, Madhura
Vipaka	Madhura
Virya	Sheeta
Prabhava	Medhya

Chemical Constituents

A number of chemical compounds have been isolated from *B. monnieri* which are mentioned as under:

- Alkaloids: Hydrocotyline, brahmine, and herpestine
- Glycosides: Asiaticoside and thanakunicide
- Flavonoids: Apigenin and luteonin
- Saponins: D-mannitol, acid A, monnierin [C51H82O213H2O], bacoside A [C41H68O134H2O], and bacoside B [C41H68O135H2O]). Saponins are considered to be the major active constituents of the plant. However, the main active chemical constituents of *Bacopa* are the dammarane-type triterpenoid saponins (Saraswati et al 1996) with the aglycones (jujubogenin and pseudojujubogenin) (Deepak and Amit 2004)

In the recent past, bacopasides I–XII, a different class of saponins, have been identified as an important constituent of the herbal extract (Rauf et al 2013). Bacoside A is the most studied and potent constituent of *Bacopa*, which is composed of bacoside A3, bacopasaponin C, bacopaside II, and bacopaside X (Srivastava et al 2012; Deepak et al 2013; Singh et al 2014).

Identity, Purity, and Strength

- Foreign matter: Not more than 2%
- Total ash: Not more than 18%
- Acid-insoluble ash: Not more than 6%
- Alcohol-soluble extractive: Not less than 6%
- Water-soluble extractive: Not less than 15%

(Source: The Ayurvedic Pharmacopeia of India 1989)

Karma (Actions)

Medhya, smrutiprada, rasayana, svarya, vatahara, vishahara, ayusya, matiprada, prajasthapana, mohahara, deepan.

- Doshakarma: Vatapittashamaka
- Dhatukarma: Rasayana
- Malakarma: Sara, Anulomana

Pharmacological Actions

Its actions include memory enhancement, antidepressant, anxiolytic, antiparkinson, anticonvulsant, antioxidant, anti-inflammatory and analgesic, antimicrobial, endocrine, antistroke, neuroprotective, ameliorating cognitive dysfunction, increasing cerebral blood flow, enhancing the activity of antioxidant enzymes and intracellular signaling pathways, reducing blood pressure, hepatoprotective, antifertility, antiaddiction, antistress, antiulcer, anticancer, etc.

Indications

It is used in kusta (skin disease), jvara (fever), shopha (swelling), pandu (anemia), prameha (diabetes), manasavikara (psychological problems), visha (poison), sotha (inflammation), kasa (cough).

The plant is a well-known medhya (intellect promoting), smritiprada (memory enhancer), and brain tonic drug. It is useful in epilepsy, insanity, Alzheimer disease, Parkinson diseases, amentia, anxiety, neuralgia, inflammation, ulcers, ascites, asthma, bronchitis, skin diseases, and hoarseness of voice, fever, and general debility.

Recently, the acute effects of Brahmi (320 and 640 mg doses) on stress and mood swings generated by multitasking were demonstrated in a double-blind, placebo-controlled clinical trial involving 17 healthy volunteers (Benson et al 2014). Brahmi supplementation reduced stress as observed by reduction in cortisol levels and alleviated mood in these participants.

Therapeutic Uses

External Use

Cough: Poultice made of boiled plant is placed on the chest in acute bronchitis and chronic coughs of children.

Internal Use

1. **Anxiety and stress:** Regular intake of Brahmi juice (1–2 tsf) with 1 tsf ghee and half tsf honey gives smooth and calming effect, relieves from stress anxiety, and increases the learning performance and mental ability of children.
2. **Memory enhancer:** Brahmi, Mandukaparni, Triphala, Chitrak, Vacha, Satapuspa, Shatavari, Danti, Nagabala, and Trivrit—any one of these drugs should be taken with honey and ghee for improving intellect (KS.P. 5).

3. **Hypertension:** 1 tsf of Brahmi juice with half spoon of honey helps in lowering blood pressure.

4. **Insanity:** Brahmi juice with Kustha powder is taken with honey to cure insanity (VM. 20/3; also SG. 2.1.18).

5. **Epilepsy:**

    (a) Old ghee processed with Brahmi juice, Vacha, Kustha, and Shankhapuspi alleviates insanity, epilepsy, inauspiciousness, and sinful conditions (C.S.Ci. 10/25).

    (b) Brahmi juice is considered as best remedy for epilepsy (AH.U. 40/51).

    (c) Panchagavya ghrita mixed with Brahmi swaras should be used for the treatment of epilepsy. In addition to this, Shankhapuspi and other intellect promoter rasayan medicines should also be taken (C.S.Ci. 10/62).

    (d) Brahmi ghrita (VM. 21/56).

6. **Pox**: Brahmi juice mixed with honey is given in pox (VM. 56/2).

7. **As rasayan** Brahmi rasayan (Su.S.Ci. 28/5-6).

Officinal Part Used

Whole plant

Dose

Juice: 10 to 20 mL
Powder: 5 to 10 g

Formulations

Brahmi ghrita, Brahmi taila, Brahmi rasayana, Brahmi Vati Saraswatarishta, Brahmiprash. Ratnagiri Rasa, Saraswat churna, Smutisagar Rasa, Mahapaishachaka gritha, Aindri / andri rasayana, Indrokta rasayana, Astamangala Ghrta.

Toxicity/Adverse Effects

Therapeutic doses of Bacopa are not associated with any known side effects, and Bacopa has been used safely in Ayurvedic medicine for several hundred years.

The clinical studies have confirmed the safety of the bacosides in healthy male volunteers at single (20–30 mg)

as well as multiple (100–200 mg) doses on daily basis for 4 weeks. These were well tolerated without any adverse effects (Singh et al 1997).

Neither alcoholic (17 g/kg) nor aqueous extract (5 g/kg) of Bacopa administered orally to rats resulted in gross behavioral changes (Martis et al 1992). Aqueous extracts of *B. monnieri* may have reversible adverse effects on spermatogenesis, sperm count, and fertility in male mice (Singh et al 2009).

The most commonly reported adverse side effects of *B. monnieri* in humans are nausea, increased intestinal motility, and gastrointestinal upset (Kishore et al 2005; Ryan et al 2008).

Substitution and Adulteration

Brahmi is often substituted and confused with *C. asiatica* (Linn.) Urban, as both the plants possess the same vernacular name Brahmi (Sharma et al 2005).

> **Points to Ponder**
>
> - *Brahmi is an important medhya drug.*
> - *Although Brahmi and Mandukparni are two different plants, both plants have some same synonyms.*
> - *Brahmi is B. monneri and Mandukparni is C. asiatica.*
> - *It is considered as the best remedy for apasmara according to Astanga Hridaya.*

Suggested Readings

Benson S, Downey LA, Stough C, Wetherell M, Zangara A, Scholey A. An acute, double-blind, placebo-controlled cross-over study of 320 mg and 640 mg doses of *Bacopa monnieri* (CDRI 08) on multitasking stress reactivity and mood. Phytother Res 2014;28(4):551–559 10.1002/ptr.5029

Calabrese C, Gregory WL, Leo M, Kraemer D, Bone K, Oken B. Effects of a standardized *Bacopa monnieri* extract on cognitive performance, anxiety, and depression in the elderly: a randomized, double-blind, placebo-controlled trial. J Altern Complement Med 2008; 14(6):707–713 10.1089/acm.2008.0018

Daniel M. Medicinal Plants: Chemistry and Properties. Enfield: Science Publishers; 2005:225

Deepak M, Amit A. The need for establishing identities of 'bacoside A and B', the putative major bioactive saponins of Indian medicinal plant *Bacopa monnieri*. Phytomedicine 2004;11(2-3):264–268

Garai S, Mahato SB, Ohtani K, Yamasaki K. Dammarane-type triterpenoid saponins from *Bacopa monniera*. Phytochemistry 1996;42(3):815–820

Khare CP. Indian Herbal Remedies: Rational Western Therapy, Ayurvedic, and Other Traditional Usage, Botany. Berlin Heidelberg: Springer-Verlag; 2003:89

Kirtikar KR, Basu BD. Indian Medicinal plants with Illustrations. Revised by Blatter E, Caius JF, Mhaskar KS, 2nd ed. Oriental Enterprises. 2001:1724

Kishore K, Singh M. Effect of bacosides, alcoholic extract of *Bacopa monniera* Linn. (brahmi), on experimental amnesia in mice. Indian J Exp Biol 2005;43(7):640–645

Martis G, Rao A, Karanth KS. Neuropharmacological activity of *Herpestis monniera*. Fitoterapia 1992;63:399–404

Morgan A, Stevens J. Does *Bacopa monnieri* improve memory performance in older persons? Results of a randomized, placebo-controlled, double-blind trial. J Altern Complement Med 2010;16(7):753–759 10.1089/acm.2009.0342

Philippine Medicinal Plants (PMP). *Bacopa monnieri* (Linn.) Wettst, 2014

Rauf K, Subhan F, Al-Othman AM, Khan I, Zarrelli A, Shah MR. Preclinical profile of bacopasides from *Bacopa monnieri* (BM) as an emerging class of therapeutics for management of chronic pains. Curr Med Chem 2013;20(8):1028–1037 10.2174/0929867311320080006

Ryan J, Croft K, Mori T, et al. An examination of the effects of the antioxidant Pycnogenol on cognitive performance, serum lipid profile, endocrinological and oxidative stress biomarkers in an elderly population. J Psychopharmacol 2008;22(5):553–562

Sharma PC, Yelne MB, Dennis TJ, Assisted by Joshi A, Prabhune YS. Database of Medicinal Plants Used in Ayurveda and Sidhha. Vol. 1. New Delhi: CCRAS; 2005

Singh A, Singh SK. Evaluation of antifertility potential of Brahmi in male mouse. Contraception 2009;79(1):71–79

Singh HK, Dharwan BN. Neuropsychopharmacological effects of the Ayurvedic nootropic *Bacopa monniera* Linn (Brahmi). Indian J Pharmacol 1997;29(5):S359–S365

Singh R, Ramakrishna R, Bhateria M, Bhatta RS. In vitro evaluation of *Bacopa monniera* extract and individual constituents on human recombinant monoamine oxidase enzymes. Phytother Res 2014;28(9):1419–1422 10.1002/ptr.5116

The Ayurvedic Pharmacopoeia of India. Part 1, Vol. II. 1st ed. Reprint. New Delhi: Department of Indian Science of Medicine and Homeopathy, Controller of Publication Civil Lines, Ministry of Health and Family Welfare, Government of India; 1999

Tripathi N, Chouhan DS, Saini N, Tiwari S. Assessment of genetic variations among highly endangered medicinal plant *Bacopa monnieri* (L.) from central India using RAPD and ISSR analysis. 3 Biotech 2012;2(4):327–336

Trivedi Manisha N, Khemani A, Vachhni Urmila D, Shah Charmi P, Santani DD. Comparative pharmacognostic and phytochemical investigation of two plant species valued as Medhya Rasayanas. Int J Appl Biol Pharm Technol 2011;2:28–36

Warrier PK, Nambiar VPK, Ramankutty C, Ramankutty R, Nair V. Indian Medicinal Plants: A Compendium of 500 Species. Orient Blackswan, University of Michigan; 1996:238

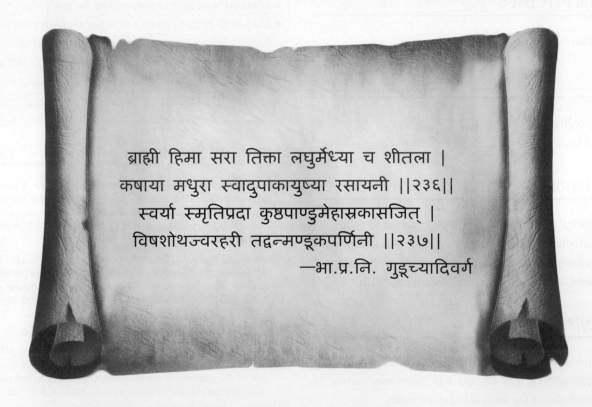

ब्राह्मी हिमा सरा तिक्ता लघुर्मेध्या च शीतला |
कषाया मधुरा स्वादुपाकायुष्या रसायनी ||२३६||
स्वर्या स्मृतिप्रदा कुष्ठपाण्डुमेहास्रकासजित् |
विषशोथज्वरहरी तद्वन्मण्डूकपर्णिनी ||२३७||
—भा.प्र.नि. गुड्ूच्यादिवर्ग

23. Brihat Ela *[Ammomum subulatum Roxb.]*

Family: *Scitamineae (Zingiberaceae)*

Hindi name: *Badi ilayachi*

English name: *Greater cardamom, Nepal cardamom*

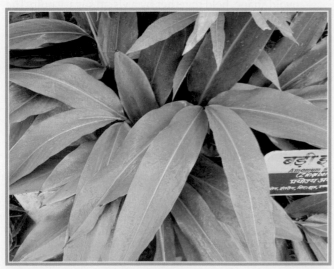

Plant of *Ammomum subulatum* Roxb.

India is the largest producer of Brihat Ela and Sikkim is the largest producer state.

Introduction

Ela dvay includes Shukshm Ela (*Elletaria cardamomum* Maton) and Brihat Ela (*Ammomum subulatum* Roxb.) (For more detail, refer to Chapter : Shukshm Ela).

Properties of Brihat Ela are very much similar to small cardamom and it is often substituted as a spice or as an ingredient of chewing preparations. Seeds and fruits of Brihat Ela are added to cooked food items as spices by the general population on a daily basis. It can play a preventive role in the occurrence of gastrointestinal disorders and respiratory problems. It increases palatability, adds flavor, and maintains good health (Rahmatullah et al 2009).

Vernacular Names

Bengali: Bara elachi, Baro elach

Gujarati: Moti elaichi, Moto elachi

Kannada: Dodda yalakki

Malayalam: Chandrabala, Paeraelam, Peri elav

Marathi: Mote velldode, Moto eldori

Oriya: Bada alaicha

Tamil: Periya aelakkaai, Periyayelam

Telugu: Adavi elakkay, Peddayelakkaylu, Pedda elakkay, Peddayelaki

Synonyms

Sthoolaila: It is the bigger variety of Ela.

Bhadraila: Its fruit is highly efficacious or useful.

Prithvika: The plant bears fruits on the stem just above the ground.

Sthoola: It is bigger in size and shape in comparison to Shukshm Ela.

Brihadaila: This variety of Ela is bigger in size.

Bahula: The fruit contains many seeds.

Triputa: The fruit has three surfaces.

Chandrabala: The seeds' aroma resembles the aroma of karpura.

Nishkuti: The seeds lie within a covering and are taken out before use.

Classical Categorization

Dhanwantari Nighantu: Shatapuspadi varga
Kaiyadev Nighantu: Aushadhi varga
Madanpal Nighantu: Karpuradi varga
Raj Nighantu: Pippalyadi varga
Bhavprakash Nighantu: Karpuradi varga

Distribution

The plant is indigenous to Central and Eastern Himalaya, Nepal, Bhutan, and North-East India. It is mainly cultivated in swampy, moist, shady regions of West Bengal, Sikkim, Assam, Uttarakhand, and Karnataka (Sharma et al 2000; Bisht et al 2010).

Morphology

Tall, evergreen perennial herbs, with leafy stems, up to 2.5 m height. The plant consists of underground creeping rhizomes with several erect leafy shoots and panicles. The plant gets mature during the third year of its growth.

- **Leaves:** Aromatic, linear-lanceolate, 30 to 60 cm long, bright green with sheathing leaf base, glabrous on both side, acuminate apex.

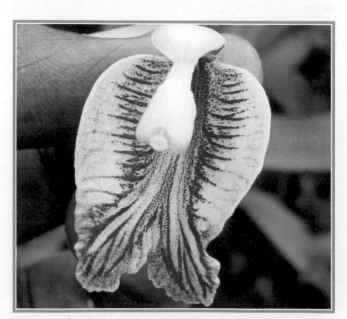

Fig. 23.1 Flower.

- **Flowers:** White with red streaks in between, globose in short peduncle spikes borne on long panicles that emerge directly from the rootstock. The peduncle bears 40 to 50 flower buds in an acropetal sequence (**Fig. 23.1**).
- **Fruits**: Trilocular, dark red-brown capsules, 2.5 cm long, oval to globose, anterioposteriorly flattened, embraced by fleshy receptacle, pericarp fleshy, rough, and indehiscent (**Fig. 23.2**).
- **Seeds:** 40 to 50 in number, aromatic, black color, ovoid shape, held together by a viscid sugary pulp. The plant is propagated through seeds and by divisions of rhizomes (Rao et al 1993).

Phenology

Flowering time: April to May
Fruiting time: October to November

Key Characters for Identification
➤ A tall evergreen perennial herb with branched creeping rhizome
➤ Leaves: aromatic, linear-lanceolate, about 30 to 60 cm long
➤ Flowers: white with red streaks, arises in short peduncle spikes
➤ Fruits: trilocular, oval-globose shape, dark red brown color
➤ Seeds: 40 to 50, aromatic, black color, lies in viscid sugary pulp

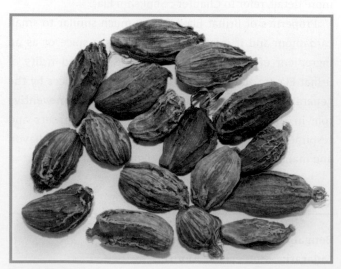

Fig. 23.2 Fruits.

Rasapanchaka

Guna	Laghu, Ruksha
Rasa	Katu, Tikta
Vipaka	Katu
Virya	Ushna

Chemical Constituents

The fruit contains essential oil, protein, starch, crude fibers, cyaniding-3-glucoside, cyaniding-3,5-diglucoside, and pinenes. The major constituents of essential oil are 1,8-cineole (65–80%), terpenyl acetate, limonene, sabinene, terpenes, pinenes and cardamonin, alpinetin, flavanone, glycosides, petunidin, aurone glycoside, subulin, chalcone, leucocyanidin, protocatechualdehyde, diphenyl picrylhydrazyl, α-terpineol, α-pinene, β-pinene, and bisabolene (Gupta 2004).

Karma (Actions)

Brihat Ela is tikshna (pungent), rochan (relish), deepan (appetizer), vishghna (antidote), mukhashodhan (mouth cleanser), and mastaka shodhani (brain purifier).

- Doshakarma: Shleshmpittahara
- Dhatukarma: Deepan
- Malakarma: Malashodhaka

Pharmacological Actions

The seeds of greater cardamom are reported as analgesic, anti-inflammatory, antimicrobial, germicidal, hypolipidemic, antioxidant, cardio-adaptogen, diuretic, antidiabetic, and hepatoprotective in properties (Kumar et al 2012).

Indications

Brihat Ela is prescribed in the treatment of kandu, kasa, shwasa, trishna, hrillasa, visha, bastiroga, shukrashmri, vaman, shiroroga, hridyaroga, vrana, and kanthruja.

In Ayurveda it is commonly used for dyspepsia, cough, nausea, vomiting, and itching.

It is also used as a preventive as well as curative drug for throat troubles, inflamed eyelids, lung congestion, pulmonary tuberculosis and digestive disorders (Verma et al 2010; Wealth of India 1985).The decoction of the seeds is useful as a gargle in infections of the teeth and gums while the pericarp is useful in headache and stomatitis (Shukla et al 2010). Seeds and fruits were found to be useful in prevention of hyperlipidemia (Joshi and Joshi 2007).

Therapeutic Uses

External Use

1. **Raktapravartana:** For letting out blood in venesection, powder of Ela, Karpura, Kustha, Tagar, and Patha mixed with lavan and taila should be rubbed on the wound (S.S.U. 14/35).
2. **Mukhapaka** (stomatitis): Regular use of Ela seed decoction as a gargle prevents stomatitis, bad breath, and pyorrhea.
3. **Timira** (vision defect): Ela powder dipped in aja mutra for three days is used as anjana (collyrium) in timira, krimi, and pilla roga (C.S.Ci. 26/249).

Internal Use

1. **Hridya roga** (heart disease): Intake of powder of Shukshm Ela and pippalimool with ghrita prevents hridyaroga (B.S.hridyarog/28).
2. **Mutrakricchta** (dysuria): Intake of Shukshm Ela churna with Amalaki swarasa daily increases urine output in dysuria (S.S.U. 58/41) or intake of Ela with curd water is also beneficial (GN. 2/27/44).
3. **Mutraghat** (urinary obstruction): Intake of Ela beej and Sunthi with Dadima juice gives relief in mutraghat (VM. 33/7).
4. **Chardi** (vomiting): Eladi churna gives relief in nausea and vomiting (CD. 15/23).
5. **Pratishyay** (common cold): Tea prepared by mixing Ela powder, Tulsi, Marich, and Adraka should be taken twice daily to get relief in common cold, asthma, throat infections, fever, pulmonary tuberculosis, and liver congestions. Or one can take 250- to 500-mg Ela powder with honey twice daily.
6. **Cigarette de-addiction:** Eating few seeds of Ela daily helps in easing cigarette addiction (Peter 2001).

7. **Malaria:** Jeerak seeds and Brihat Ela are powdered and a mixture is prepared. Daily intake of this mixture is prescribed in the treatment of malaria (Thakur et al 1989).

8. **Visha** (poisoning): Local and oral intake of Ela seeds or paste is used as an antidote to snake bite and scorpion sting (Bisht et al 2010).

Officinal Part Used

Seeds

Dose

Seed powder: 1 to 3 g

Formulations

Eladi churna, Anantadya ghrita, Eladi gutika, Sitopaladi churna, Avipattikar churna, Eladi ghrita, Eladi mantha, Kushmandavleha, Chandanadi vati.

Toxicity/Adverse Effect

Not reported yet.

Substitution and Adulteration

Both the drugs are used as substitutes of each other.

Suggested Readings

Anonymous. Wealth of India: A Dictionary of Indian Raw Materials and Industrial Research. Revised ed.; 2006:226–229

Gupta AK, Sharma M. Reviews on Indian Medicinal Plants. Vol. 2. New Delhi: Indian Council of Medical Research; 2004:215–219

Joshi SC, Joshi V. Effect of *Ammomum subulatum* on oxidative stress and atherosclerosis in cholesterol fed rabbits. Pharmacology 2007; 1:451–463

Kumar G, Chauhan B, Ali M. *Ammomum subulatum* Roxb: An overview in all aspects. Int Res J Pharm 2012;3(7):96–99

Rahmatullah M, Noman A, Hossan MS, et al. A survey of medicinal plants in two areas of Dinajpir district, Bangladesh including plants which can be used as functional foods. Americ-Euras J Sustain Agric 2009;3(4):862–876

Rao YS, Gupta U, Kumar A, Naidu R. A note on large cardamom (*Ammomum subulatum* Roxb.) germplasm collection. J Spices Aromat Crops 1993;2(1 & 2):77–80

Sharma E, Sharma R, Singh KK, Sharma G. A boon for mountain populations: large cardamom farming in the Sikkim Himalaya. Mountain Res Res Dev 2000;20(2):108–111

Shukla SH, Mistry HA, Patel VG, Jogi BV. Pharmacognostical, preliminary phytochemical studies and analgesic activity of *Ammomum subulatum* Roxb. Pharma Sci Monitor 2010;1(1):90–102

Verma SK, Rajeevan V, Bordia A, Jain V. Greater cardamom (*Ammomum subulatum* Roxb.): a cardio-adaptogen against physical stress. J Herb Med Toxicol 2010;4(2):55–58

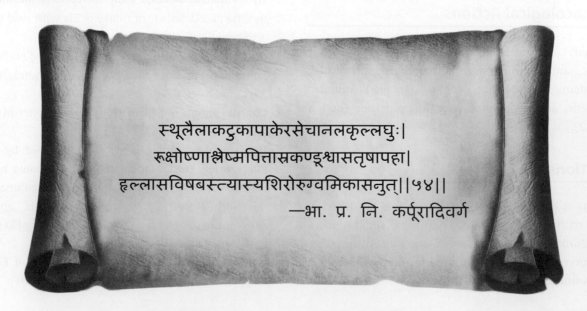

स्थूलैलाकटुकापाकेरसेचानलकृल्लघुः।
रूक्षोष्णाक्ष्लेष्मपित्तास्रकण्डूश्वासतृषापहा।
हृल्लासविषबस्त्यास्यशिरोरुग्वमिकासनुत्॥५४॥
—भा. प्र. नि. कर्पूरादिवर्ग

24. Brihati [*Solanum indicum* Linn.]

Family:	*Solanaceae*
Hindi name:	*Badi Kateri*
English name:	*Indian Night shade, poison berry*

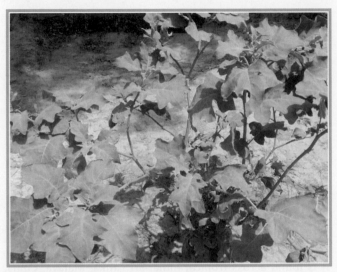

Plant of *Solanum indicum* Linn.

The pregnant women should take white Brihati root by right nostril for male progeny and by left nostril for female child.

—BS, Streeroga.153

Introduction

Brihati and Kantakari are considered as Brihati dwaya in Ayurveda. Brihati is bigger in size as compared to Kantakari and that's why it is called Brihati or Mahati. Kaiyadev Nighantu has mentioned 11 types of Brihati with their properties and actions. Likewise, Dhanwantari Nighantu mentioned four types of Brihati, and Raj Nighantu described three types of Brihati with the properties and actions of each variety.

Brihati is an important medicinal plant in Indian systems of medicine such as Ayurveda, Siddha, and Unani. It is an important ingredient of dashamoola (a group of ten root drugs) group of plants used in Ayurveda and Siddha system of medicine and is used in vitiated conditions of vata, pita, and kapha, and cures vomiting, heart diseases, poisonous affections, skin diseases, ulcers, difficult breathing, abdominal pain, cough, and dyspepsia. Roots are bitter and pungent. It removes bad taste in the mouth and helps to restore normal taste (Iyer and Kolammal 1960).

Sushruta has placed it under the group of laghupanchmool, which is therapeutically used as balya, brimhaniya, and grahi. Charaka has used Brahati dway in asmari bhedana whereas in yogatarangani its root is applied externally for indralupta. Bhavaprakash Nighantu has mentioned Brihati in guduchyadi varga. Its root are sangrahi, hridya (cardiotonic), pachaka (digestive), ruchya, kanthya, aasya vairasya, nashaka (removes foul smell in mouth), and is used in the treatment of kushta (skin diseases), jwara (fever), shwasa (bronchial asthma), shool (colic pain), kasa (cough), aruchi (loss of appetite), shotha (inflammation), and agnimandhya.

Vernacular Names

Assamese: Tilabhakuri
Bengali: Byakud
Betsileo: Roingivy, Voapo
Betsimisaraka: Ankivy

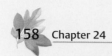
Canarese: Badane, Gulla, Habbagulla, Kachi, Kadusonde, Kamanja, Kempugulla

Central Provinces: Ringni

Chinese: Houang K'iue

Gujarati: Mhotiringni, Motaringni, Ubhibhoringni, Vadaringni

Hova: Angivibe, Angivy, Hery, Voangivy, Voampo, Voampoa

Kannada: Kirugullia, Heggulla, Gulla, Kirigulla, Sonde, Vayase

Kumaon: Bhnbhatta

La Reunion: Bringelllier marron

Las Bela: Didi

Lepcha: Kadombee

Malayalam: Cheru Vazhuthina, Putirichunda

Marathi: Dorli, Chichuriti, Dorale

Mundari: Hanjeddaru, Huringhanjeddaru

Nepali: Hihi

Northwestern Provinces: Kantangkari

Oriya: Dengabheji

Persian: Badengawejangali, Ustargar

Punjabi: Kandyari, Kandiarivaddi

Sinhalese: Tibbatu

Tamil: Chiru vazhuthalai, Papparamulli, Mullamkatti

Telugu: Tella Mulaka, Adaviyuchinta, Chittimulaga, Challamulaga, Kakimachi, Nallamulaka, Tellamulaka

Urdu: Kateli

Synonyms

Brihati: It is bigger in size as compared to Kantakari.

Dushpradharshani: It is difficult to touch due to excessive thorns in the plants.

Hinguli: This term refers to the color of its fruits resembling that of Hingula.

Kantalu/Kantaki: The plant bears spine.

Kshudrabhantaki: The fruit resembles bhantaki brinjal but is smaller in size.

Kuli: Fruits are in cluster.

Mahati: It is respected by the physicians. Brihati and Mahati means bigger.

Mahoushtri: A bigger variety of brihatidwaya.

Pittatandula: It has yellow seeds.

Rashtrika: Easily available throughout the country.

Singhi: It improves the voice like the roar of a lion and cures kasadi disease.

Sthulakantaki: It has a strong thorn.

Vanabrintaki: It grows wildly.

Vartaki: The plants resemble the small variety of brinjal/ available in many geographical areas.

Classical Categorization

Charak Samhita: Kanthya, Hikkanigrahan, Shothhara, Angamardaprasaman

Sushruta Samhita: Vidarigandhadi, Varunadi, Brahatyadi, Laghu Panchmool

Astanga Sangraha: Shirovirechanopayogi gana, Vidaryadi gana

Astanga Hridaya: Shakavarga, Vataghna gana, Vidaryadi gana

Dhanwantari Nighantu: Guduchyadi varga

Madanpal Nighantu: Abhayadi varga

Kaiyadev Nighantu: Aushadhi varga

Raj Nighantu: Shatahwadi varga

Bhavaprakash: Guduchyadi varga

Distribution

It is found across tropical India, Sri Lanka, Malaya, China, and Philippines. In India, it is distributed all over the tropical parts in waste lands, roadsides, etc., from sea level to about 2,000 feet (Kirtikar and Basu 1991; Sivarajan and Balachandran 1994).

Morphology

It is an erect, perennial, much branched, prickly undershrub of 1 to 2 m height.

- **Stems:** much branched, very prickly, and bearing compressed, stout, often recurved prickles (**Fig. 24.1**).
- **Leaves:** simple, alternate, stellate hairy beneath, ovate shape, 5 to 15 cm length, 2.5 to 8 cm width, cordate-truncate base, subacute apex, pinnafid or lobed margin, petiole 2 to 4 cm long, midrib covered with hard pointed spines both on upper and under surface of leaves (**Fig. 24.2**).
- **Flowers:** axillary, in bunches, blue purple or white in color in corymbose cymes, five petals (**Fig. 24.3a, b**).
- **Fruits:** globose berries of 1.5 cm diameter, occur in axillary bunches, unripe green, turning to yellow

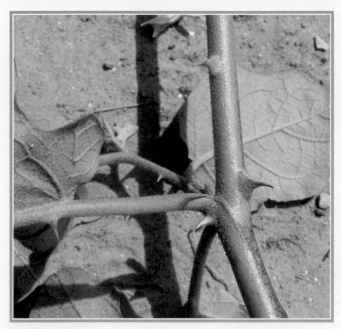

Fig. 24.1 Stem.

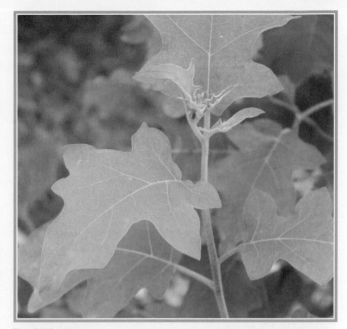

Fig. 24.2 Leaves.

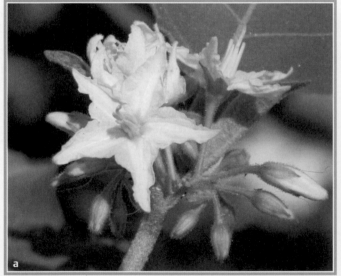

Fig. 24.3 **(a)** White flower. **(b)** Blue flower.

on maturity, black on drying, with many flat and minutely pitted seeds (**Fig. 24.4**).

- **Root:** well-developed, long, ribbed, woody, cylindrical, pale yellowish-brown, 1 to 2.5 cm in diameter, a number of secondary roots and their branches present, surface rough due to the presence of longitudinal striations and root scars, fracture, short, and splintery; no distinct odor and taste (The Ayurvedic Pharmacopeia of India 2001; Kirtikar and Basu 1975; The Wealth of India 1988).

This plant is propagated through seeds, and stem cutting.

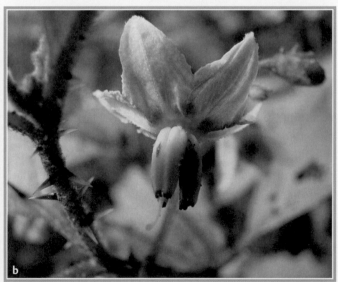

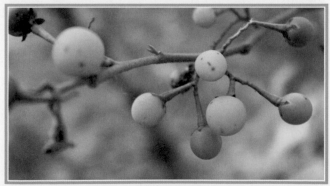

Fig. 24.4 Fruits.

Phenology

Flowering time: March to April

Fruiting time: May to October

Key Characters for Identification

➤ Erect, perennial, much branched, prickly undershrub of 1 to 2 m height.

➤ Leaves: simple, alternate, stellate hairy beneath, ovate, 5 to 15 cm length, 2.5 to 8 cm width, spine on both surfaces.

➤ Flowers: blue purple or white color in corymbose cymes.

➤ Fruits: globose berries, 1.5 cm diameter, in axillary bunches, initially green, turning to yellow on maturity.

➤ Root: long, ribbed, woody, cylindrical, pale yellowish-brown.

Types

In classical texts of Ayurveda, Brihati and Kantakari are considered as Brihati dwaya. But as per Acharya Priyavrat Sharma and Prof. K.C. Chunekar, Brihati is of two types according to the color of its flowers: Neela puspi Brihati (*Solanum indicum*) and sweta puspi brihati (*Solanum torvum*). Dalhan described brihatidwaya as per the size of the fruit: smaller fruit and bigger fruit. Types of Brihati according to different Nighantus is as under:

- Dhanvantari Nighantu: four types—Brihati, Lakshmana, Kasaghni, Vrintaki
- Kaiyadeva Nighantu: eleven types—Brihati, Simhi, Kantakari, Nidigdhika, Valli brihati, Vriksha Brihati, Shweta, Alabuphala, Amlabrihati, Jalaja, Sthula Brihati
- Bhavaprakasha Nighantu: one type—Brihati
- Raj Nighantu: three types—Brihati, Sarpatanu, Sweta Brihati

Rasapanchaka

Guna	Laghu, Ruksha
Rasa	Katu, Tikta
Vipaka	Katu
Virya	Ushna

Chemical Constituents

Various phytoconstituents like phytosterols, steroidal glycosides, steroidal glycoalkaloids, flavonoids, and fatty acid have been reported from the plants (Maurya 2014).

The fruits of the *S. indicum* have 8% crude fiber, 40.67% total carbohydrate, 23.47% crude protein, 5.26% crude fat, and caloric value of 303.9 in wet weight basis. Apart from this, alkaloids (0.2–1.8% in fruits and 0.32% in leaves), polyphenols (7.02 mg/g), and saponins are also found (Aberoumand 2012).

Out of all constituents, steroidal glycosides and steroidal glycoalkaloids are most commonly found in the plants (Khare 2004). *S. indicum* contains most common steroidal alkaloids/glycoalkaloids, viz. solasodine, solanidine, solasonine, solamargine, and solanine (Maurya 2014; Khare 2004; Syu-Wan et al 2001).

Apart from steroidal alkaloids, other constituents like carotene, carpesterol, solanocarpone, diosgenin, β-sitosterol, lanosterol, solavetivone, solafuranone, scopoletin N-(ptranscoumaroyl) tyramine, N-trans-feruloyltyramine, and indiosides are also reported in the plant (Gupta et al 2010; Aberoumand 2012; Maurya and Manika 2013; Syu-Wan 2001).

Identity, Purity, and Strength

- Foreign matter: Not more than 2%
- Total ash: Not more than 6.5%
- Acid-insoluble ash: Not more than 1%
- Alcohol-soluble extractive: Not less than 3%
- Water-soluble extractive: Not less than 4%

(Source: The Ayurvedic Pharmacopeia of India 1999)

Karma (Actions)

- Deepana (appetizer), pachana (digestive), rochan (relish), grahi (absorbent), hridya (cardio tonic)
- Doshakarma: Vatakapha shamaka
- Dhatukarma: Sukrarechaka
- Malakarma: Grahi, mutrala

Pharmacological Actions

Its actions include hepatoprotective, anthelmintic, antioxidant, antimicrobial, anti-inflammatory, antibacterial, antiplasmodial, anticancer, laxative, cardiotonic, CNS depressant, antihypertensive (Jayanthy et al 2016; Sharma et al 2017).

Indications

Kasa (cough), shwasa (asthma), hridroga (cardiac disease), kushta (skin disease), jvara (fever), shola (colic pain), shotha (inflammation), agnimandya (loss of appetite), arochak (loss of appetite), amadosha, aasyavairasya (tastelessness).

The roots are useful in vitiated conditions of vata and kapha, odontalgia, dyspepsia, flatulence, colic, verminosis, diarrhea, leprosy, strangury, cough, asthma, fever, skin diseases, respiratory and cardiac disorders, ulcers and poisonous affections (Iyer and Kolammal 1960; Sivarajan and Balachandran 1994; Warrier et al 1996). The root is employed in difficult parturition and in tooth ache. It is also used in fever, worm infestation, and colic. It is regarded as expectorant, which is useful in cough and catarrhal affections. It is prescribed in the case of dysuria and inchuria (Kirtikar and Basu 1991). The root and the fruit are prescribed in snake bites and scorpion sting (Sharma 1996).

Therapeutic Uses

External Use

1. **Khalitya** (alopecia): The fruit juice of Brihati mixed with honey and applied locally to inhibit alopecia (VM. 57.76; GN. 3.1.78; SG. 3.11.21).
2. **Khalitya** (alopecia): Fruit and root of gunja are pounded with the juice of brihati fruits and rubbed with Datura fruit. It stops alopecia (VM. 57.77).

Internal Use

1. **Aruchi** (anorexia): Brihati fruits are cooked and mixed with spices and then consumed with curd to increase appetite (VD. 4.4).
2. **Jwar** (fever): Powder of Brihati fruit, Pippali, and Shunthi is used as nasya to prevent sneezing and regain consciousness in fever (GN. 2.1.400).
3. **Grahaniroga** (sprue): Brihati fruit powder with buttermilk is taken daily to treat indigestion and grahani (SG. 2.5.28).

4. **Kasa** (cough): Steam boiled Brihati fruit is processed with ghee & is taken with saindhav lavan to control excessive cough and enhance digestion.(K.Ki.8.62)
5. **Punsavan sanskar** (conception): Pregnant women should take white Brihati root by right nostril for male progeny and by left nostril for female child (BS, Streeroga. 153).
6. **Bal roga** (pediatric diseases): The child who vomits breast milk frequently should be given fruit juice of Brihati and Kantakari mixed with Panchkola, honey, and ghee (AH.U. 2.58).
7. **Arsha** (piles): Brihati fruit boiled with alkaline water of Kosataki and fried with ghee is given with jaggery followed by intake of butter milk to control piles. It destroys hemorrhoid within a week (VM. 5.14-15).

Officinal Parts Used

Root, stem, fruit

Dose

Decoction: 50 to 100 mL
Powder: 3 to 6 g

Formulations

Brihatyadikwath, Dashmularishta, Dashamulakwatha

Toxicity

Preliminary phytochemical screening and pharmacological evaluation of the dried fruit extract of *S. indicum* L. on experimental animal models for a variety of ailments, viz. pain, fever, inflammation, and CNS complication was carried out (Deb et al 2014). The acute toxicity study as per OECD Guideline 423 revealed the drug to be safe till a dose of 2,000 mg/kg. Adult Wistar albino rats (180–200 g) of either sex was used for the study and subdivided into four groups.

Substitution and Adulteration

Different species of Solanum like *Solanum torvum* Swartz, *S. melongena* Linn., *S. incanum* Linn. of Solanaceae family are used as or sold as Brihati in Indian market.

Points to Ponder

- *Brihati and Kantakari are considered as Brihati dwaya.*
- *Brihati is included under laghu panchmool and dashmool.*
- *It is mainly indicated in kasa, shwasa, hikka, shotha, and hridroga.*

Suggested Readings

Aberoumand A. Protein, fat, calories, minerals, phytic acid and phenolic in some plant foods based diet. 2012

Aberoumand A. Screening of phytochemical compounds and toxic proteinaceous protease inhibitor in some lesser-known food based plants and their effects and potential applications in food. Int J Food Sci Nutr Eng 2012;2(3):16–20

Deb PK, Ghosh R, Chakraverty R, Debnath R, Lakshman Das L, Tejendra Bhakta T. Phytochemical and pharmacological evaluation of fruits of *Sola numindi* cum Linn. Int J Pharm Sci Rev Res 2014;25(2)

Gupta AK, Tandon N, Sharma M, eds. Quality Standards of Indian Medicinal Plants. Indian Council of Medical Research, Vol. 7. 2010:242–253

Iyer KN, Kolammal M. Pharmacognosy of Ayurvedic Drugs. Trivandrum: Department of Pharmacognosy, Government Ayurveda College; 1960:I (4):99

Jayanthy A, Maurya A, Verma SC, et al. A brief review on pharmacognosy, phytochemistry and therapeutic potential of *Solanum indium* L. used in Indian systems of medicine. Asian J Res Chem 2016;9(3): 127–132

Khare CP. Encyclopedia of Indian Medicinal plants. New York, NY: Springer; 2004

Khare CP. Indian Medicinal Plants: An Illustrated Dictionary. First Indian Reprint. New Delhi: Springer (India) Pvt. Ltd; 2007

Kirtikar KR, Basu BD. Indian Medicinal Plants. 2nd ed. Vol. II. Dehradun: International Book Publication Distribution; 1975:1755–1757

Kirtikar KR, Basu BD. Indian Medicinal Plants. Vol. I. Dehradun: Bishen Singh Mahendra Pal Singh; 1991

Maurya A, Manika N, Verma RK, Singh SC, Srivastava SK. Simple and reliable methods for the determination of three steroidal glycosides in the eight species of *Solanum* by reversed-phase HPLC coupled with diode array detection. Phytochem Anal 2013;24: 87–92

Maurya A. Chemical investigation and development of validated analytical methods for some selected medicinal plants. PhD Thesis. Dr. R. M. L. Avadh University, Faizabad, India. 2014

Sarin YK. Illustrated Manual of Herbal Drugs Used in Ayurveda. New Delhi: Council of Industrial and Indian Council of Medical Research; 1996

Sharma PV. Classical Uses of Medicinal Plants. Varanasi: Chaukhambha Visvabharati; 1996

Sharma V, Hem K, Seth A, Maurya SK. *Solanum indicum* Linn.: An ethnopharmacological, phytochemical and pharmacological review. Curr Res J Pharma Allied Sci 2017;1(2):1–9

Sivarajan VV, Balachandran I. Ayurvedic Drugs and Their Plant Sources. New Delhi: Oxford and IBH; 1994

Sukhdev. A Selection of Prime Ayurvedic Plant Drugs Ancient: Modern Concordance. New Delhi: Anamaya Publishers; 2006

Syu WJ, Don MJ, Lee GH, Sun CM. Cytotoxic and novel compounds from *Solanum indicum*. J Nat Prod 2001;64(9):1232–1233

The Ayurvedic Pharmacopoeia of India. Part 1, Vol. II. New Delhi, Department of I. S. M. & H. (AYUSH), Ministry of Health and Family Welfare, , Government of India; 2001:27

The Ayurvedic Pharmacopoeia of India. Part I, Vol. II. New Delhi: Department of AYUSH, Ministry of Health and Family Welfare, Government of India; 1999:28

The Wealth of India, Raw Materials Vol. IX (Rh-So). New Delhi: Council of Scientific and Industrial Research; 1988

Vaidya BCV. Some Controversial Drugs in Indian medicine. Varanasi: Chaukhamba Orientalia; 1982

Warrier PK, Nambiar VPK, Ramankutty C. Indian Medicinal Plants: A Compendium of 500 Species, Vol. 5. Orient Longman Ltd; 1996

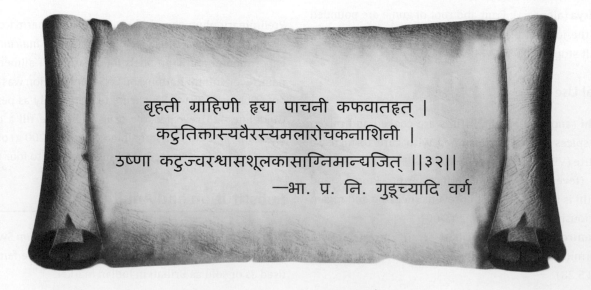

बृहती ग्राहिणी हृद्या पाचनी कफवातहृत् ।
कटुतिक्तास्यवैरस्यमलारोचकनाशिनी ।
उष्णा कटुज्वरश्वासशूलकासाग्निमान्द्यजित् ॥३२॥
—भा. प्र. नि. गुडूच्यादि वर्ग

25. Chandana Shwet [*Santalum album* Linn.]

Family: Santalaceae

Hindi name: Safed Chandan

English name: White Sandalwood

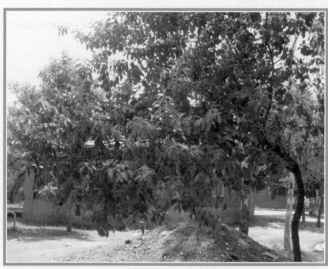

Plant of *Santalum album* Linn.

Chandana which is bitter in taste, yellow color on rubbing, red color on fracture, externally white colored, and the one with tubercles and cavities is the best one.

Introduction

There are two types of Chandan which is known as Chandan dvaya. It includes Shwet Chandan and Rakt Chandan.

The word "Chandana" literally means the one which gives cooling, soothing, or pleasing effect. The specific epithet *album* refers to the white color of the heartwood. Among all the tikta dravya Chandana is considered as the best sheetal dravya (D.N chandanadi varga/ 3).

Since time immemorial sandal wood is being used to worship Lord Vishnu and Goddess Lakshmi in spiritual practices, rituals, yagna, lepa, etc. Its paste is applied on the forehead to attain peace and to bring the devotee close to God. The Egyptians used it for embalming the dead and in ritual burning whereas the European physician used it first as a medicine (Ghani 2007; Sindhu et al 2010).

Ancient Ayurveda texts Charak and Sushrut considered Chandana as best drug for giving pleasure, relaxation, peace, and cooling effect (C.S.Su. 25/40). Its lepa is recommended in greeshma and vasant ritu (S.S.Su. 6/25). Sushrut uses its lepa for samyaka dagdh, agnikarma, pitta vidriddhi (S.S.Su. 12/23) and vranaropana. Sharagdhara Samhita states that for preparing churna, sneha, asava, leha one should use Shwet Chandana and for making kashaya and lepa Rakt Chandana should be used (Sh.S. 1/53). So many varieties of Chandana are described in Nighantu kaal but Shwet Chandana (*Santalum album* Linn.) and Rakt Chandana (*Pterocarpus santalinus* Linn. F.) varieties are taken from Chandana dvaya.

Nowadays sandalwood oil is being extensively used in perfumes, cosmetics, room fresheners, deodorants, creams, body lotions, soaps, aromatic candles, incense sticks, and as a flavor component in food items. The outer hardwood is used to make beads, malas, and carved statues. The seeds and bark are used in paint and tanning industry, respectively. Being the second most expensive wood in the world it is designated as the *Royal tree* (Fox 2000). It is estimated that about 10 mL oil is extracted from 1 kg of sandalwood.

In recent years Shwet Chandana is categorized under vulnerable species by the International Union for the Conservation of Nature (IUCN; Asian Regional Workshop 1998). It is threatened because of overexploitation and loss of its natural habitat. In India exportation of sandalwood is strictly banned. In Southern India especially in Karnataka and Andhra Pradesh all sandalwood trees greater than a specified width is the property of state government. Hence, rules and regulations for production, cutting, and maintenance of sandalwood tree are under strict monitoring of the government (Sindhu et al 2010).

Vernacular Names

Arabic: Sandal abyaz
Assam: Sandale Avyaj
Bengali: Chandan, Sadachandan
Gujarati: Sukhad, Suket
Kannada: Shrigandhamara, Shrigandha, Chand
Kashmiri: Safed chandan
Malayalam: Chandanam, Malayajam
Marathi: Chandan, Gandhachakoda
Persian: Sandal Suped
Punjabi: Chandan, Chandal, Sufed Sandal
Sindhi: Sukhad
Tamil: Chandana maram, Sandanam, Ingam
Telugu: Gandhapu Chekka, Manchi Gandham, Tella Chandanam, Sriganda
Unani: Santalon
Urdu: Safed Sandal

Synonyms

Bhadrashri: The heartwood pieces are beautiful and beneficial.
Chandradhruti: Heartwood gives cooling and pleasing effect like moon.
Gandharaja: The wood is best among all aromatic drugs.
Gandhsaar: The heartwood is aromatic in nature.
Malyaja: The plant grows abundantly in Malaya region (part of Western Ghats).
Shishira: It is sheet in touch and virya.
Shrikhanda: The heartwood pieces are used for worshipping Goddess Lakshmi.
Tailaparnik: Leaves are lustrous/oily in appearance.

Classical Categorization

Charak Samhita: Dahaprasmana, Angamardprasmana, Trishnanigrahan, Kandughna, Varnya, Vishaghna
Sushrut Samhita: Salasaradi, Sarivadi, Patoladi, Priyangvadi, Guduchyadi
Ashtang Hridaya: Asanadi, Sarivadi, Patoladi, Priyangvadi, Guduchyadi
Dhanvantari Nighantu: Chandanadi varga
Madanpal Nighantu: Karpuradi varga
Kaiyadev Nighantu: Oushadi varga
Raj Nighantu: Chandanadi varga
Bhavaprakash Nighantu: Karpuradi varga

Distribution

Chandana plant is distributed in the peninsular India, Malaysia, Australia, New Zealand, Sri Lanka, and Pakistan.

In India it is available in Southern India, especially in Karnataka and Tamil Nadu, and also in Kerala Andhra Pradesh, Madhya Pradesh, Orissa, Maharashtra, Gujarat, Rajasthan, Uttar Pradesh, Bihar, and Bengal. It generally grows at altitudes of 2,000 to 3,000 feet. The important Chandana-producing regions in Karnataka are Mysore, Dharwar, Shimoga, Chikmaglur, Tumkur, Hassan, Mercara, Bangalore, and scattered areas of Kolar. In Tamil Nadu it is chiefly available in Coimbatore, Nilgiri, Salem, Vellore, Trinuleveli, and Tiruchchirappalli (Anonymous 2003).

Morphology

A medium-sized evergreen tree reaching up to a height of 18 to 20 m. The tree is semi-root parasite and overall appears shiny with slender drooping branches.

- **Leaves:** Simple, opposite, shiny, glabrous, ovate, or elliptic to lanceolate shape, 2 to 3 inch long, 1 to 2 inch width, subacute apex, and entire margin (**Fig. 24.1**).
- **Flowers:** Bisexual, reddish-brown in color in terminal or axillary paniculate cymes, unscented, and occurs in clusters (**Fig. 24.2**). The tree starts blooming after 7 years. Initially, young flowers are white which later on turns into purple reddish-brown.
- **Fruits:** Obovoid or globose drupe with a thin fleshy coat, 1 to 1.5 cm in diameter, green when unripe and turns into purple black on maturity, crowned with a

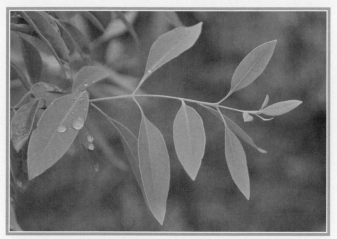

Fig. 24.1 Leaves of Chandan.

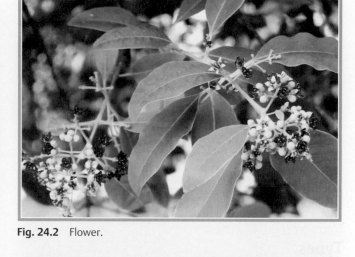

Fig. 24.2 Flower.

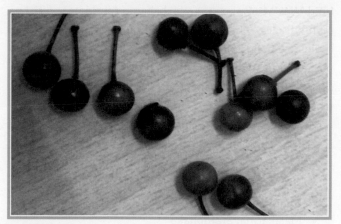

Fig. 24.3 Fruit.

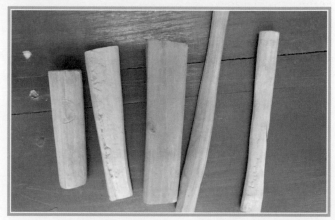

Fig. 24.4 Heartwood.

annular scary rings of fallen perianth, and endocarp is woody which encloses a hard, globose, solitary seed (**Fig. 24.3**).

- **Heartwood:** Aromatic, light, yellowish-brown when fresh and turns brown to reddish-brown on exposure (**Fig. 24.4**). The heartwood starts developing aroma after about 10 years of growth.
- **Bark:** Brownish-black to dark gray, rough with short vertical cracks, and sapwood is white and odorless (**Fig. 24.5**).

The plant is propagated through seeds. The plant is an obligate semiroot parasite which hosts on Karanj, Lantana, and Cassia species.

Phenology

Flowering time: June to December
Fruiting time: October to January

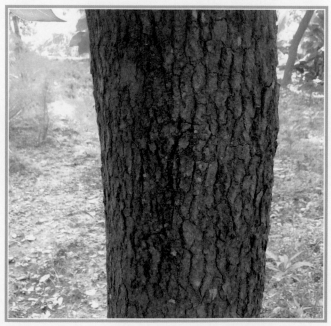

Fig. 24.5 Bark.

Key Characters for Identification

➤ A medium-sized evergreen tree which is an obligate semiroot parasite
➤ Leaves are opposite, shiny, ovate, or elliptic to lanceolate in shape
➤ Flowers are unscented, borne in clusters, purple to reddish-brown in color
➤ Fruits are globose, single-seeded drupe, 1 to 1.5 cm in diameter
➤ Heartwood is highly aromatic, light, yellowish-brown when fresh

Types

- Dhanvantari Nighantu: five types—Chandana, Rakta Chandana, Kuchandana, Kaleyak, Barbarik
- Kaiyadeva Nighantu: three types—Rakt, Peeta, and Pandu
- Raj Nighantu: seven types—Bet, Sukaddi, Rakta Chandana, Kaleyak, Kuchandana, Barbarik, Harichandana
- Bhavaprakash Nighantu: four types—Chandana, Rakta chandana, Kuchandana (patrang), Kaleyak (peeta chandana)

Rasapanchaka

Guna	Laghu, Ruksha
Rasa	Tikta, Madhura
Vipaka	Katu
Virya	Sheet

Chemical Constituents

Heart wood contains 2% to 6% of volatile oil, resins, and tannic acids whereas 90% of the volatile oil consists of sesquiterpene alcohol, α-santalol, and β-santalol. Other constituents are bergamotols, lanceol, nuciferol, bisabolol, α- and β-santalenes, santene, santenol, tetra-santenol, santalic acid, santalal, santenone, bergamotenes, α-, β-, and γ-curcumenes, β-bisabolene, and organic acids (Adams et al 1975; Demole et al 1976; Kumar et al 2015).

Identity, Purity, and Strength

- Foreign matter: Not more than 1%
- Total ash: Not more than 1%
- Acid-insoluble ash: Not more than 0.2%
- Alcohol-soluble extractive: Not less than 8%
- Water-soluble extractive: Not less than 1%
- Volatile oil: Not less than 1.5%

(Source: The Ayurvedic Pharmacopeia of India 2001)

Karma (Actions)

Ayurvedic texts described Chandana as sheetal (cooling), aahladana (pleasing to mind, relaxant), varnya (improves complexion), vishahara (antidote), vrishya (aphrodisiac), hridya (cardiotonic), dahaprasasmana (relief from burning sensation), rakta prasadana (blood purifier), angamardprasasmana (antifatigue), chardighna (antiemetic), shramhara (antifatigue), jwarghna (antipyretic), krimighna (anthelmintic), sugandhi (deodorant), santaaphar, and kantida in action. Sandalwood oil is coolant, emollient, antibacterial, antiseptic, disinfectant, expectorant, and diuretic in properties.

- Doshakarma: Shleshmpittahara
- Dhatukarma: Rakta prasadana, Vrishya, Aahladana
- Malakarma: Stambhaka

Pharmacological Actions

Research studies have reported that the heartwood and oil possess hepatoprotective, antiherpetic activities, anticancerous, antihypertensive, sedative, insecticidal, antibacterial, antiviral, antifungal, antioxidant, analgesic, anti-inflammatory, antipyretic, antiulcer, memory enhancer, antianginal, antihyperglycemic, antihyperlipidemic, cardioprotective, and neuroprotective activities (Kumar et al 2015; Sindhu et al 2010).

Indications

Heartwood and oil is extensively used in the treatment of shram (fatigue), shosh (emaciation), visha (poison), trishna (excessive thirst), raktapitta (bleeding disorders), daha (burning sensation), antradaha (acidity), bhranti (giddiness), vaman (emesis), jwar (fever), krimi (bacterial infections), mukharoga (diseases of oral cavity), raktavikara (bleeding disorders), hikka (hic-cough), raktasrava (internal hemorrhage), raktarsha (piles), prameha (diabetes), ashrigdhar (uterine bleeding), and sheetpitta (urticaria).

Sandalwood oil is used for the treatment of urinary tract infection, dysuria, hematuria, varicose veins, filariasis, small pox, pruritis, itching, psoriasis, palpitations, sunstroke, purulent ulcers, gonorrhea, syphilis, cystitis, purulent cough, headache, insomnia, nervous tension, and skin diseases.

Therapeutic Uses

External Use

1. **Visha** (poisoning): Application of Chandana paste over the cardiac region gives relief in poisoning (S.S.Ka. 1/36).
2. **Hikka** (hic-cough): Chandana mixed with Nari ksheer is used as nasya to control hikka (C.S.Ci. 17/131).
3. **Nabhipaka** (inflamed umbilicus): In nabhipaka the navel region should be dusted with powder of Chandana bark (B.P.Ci. 71/180).
4. **Netraroga** (eye diseases): Eyes should be washed with milk processed with Chandana (A.H.U. 9/18).

Internal Use

1. **Rakta atisaar** (bleeding diarrhea): Chandana powder taken with madhu and sharkara along with tandulodaka gives relief from daha, raktaatisaar, trishna, and prameha (C.S.Ci. 19/86; A.H.Ci. 9/92).
2. **Chardi** (vomiting): Chandan powder taken with Amalaki juice or with mudga yusha prevents all types of vomiting (C.S.Ci. 20/32; S.S.U. 49/33).
3. **Pradara** (menorrhagia): Chandana powder should be taken with milk mixed with ghrita, sharkara, and madhu daily to cure raktpradara, shwetpradar, and ashrigdhar (G.N. 6/1/42).
4. **Jwar** (fever): Chandana kashaya with madhu sharkara or Chandanasava is used twice daily in jwar associated with aggravated pitta (S.S.Ci. 5/8).
5. **Prameha** (diabetes): Decoction of Manjistha and Chandan should be taken daily in manjisthmeha and decoction of Arjuna and Chandan is useful in shukrameh (S.S.Ci. 11/9).

6. **Rakta pitta** (bleeding disorders): Ushir, Kaliyaka, Lodhra, etc. with equal quantity of Chandana and sharkara is given with tandulodaka to arrest internal bleeding (C.S.Ci. 04 /73); one can take Chandan, Madhuka, and Lodhra powder in equal quantity with madhu sharkara to check bleeding (S.S.U. 45/25).
7. **Amalpitta** (acidity): Chandana powder with Amalaki and Madhuyashti powder is used to control acidity, sour belching, and indigestion.
8. **Visarpa** (erysipelas): Chandana Utpala decoction should be taken daily to prevent visarpa (A.H.Ci.18/4).
9. **Shitapitta** (urticaria): Chandana powder mixed with Guduchi swarasa should be used to cure shitapitta (VM. 11/22).
10. **Masurika** (small pox): Hilmochika rasa mixed with Shwet Chandana kalka should be taken in initial phase of Masurika (B.P.Ci. 60/35).
11. **Ushnavata** (gonorrhea): Cold infusion of Chandana powder with tandulodaka and sharkara should be used daily in hematuria and gonorrhea (VM. 33/10).
12. **Trishna** (thirst): To control excessive thirst one should take Chandana powder with coconut water.

Officinal Parts Used

Oil and heartwood

Dose

Powder: 1 to 3 g
Oil: 5 to 10 drops

Formulations

Chandanasava, Chandanadi kwath, Chandanadi vati, Chandanadi churna

Toxicity/Adverse Effect

No major toxicity has yet been reported.

Substitution and Adulteration

- Adulterant: The wood of *Erythroxylum monogynum* Roxb. is perfumed with sandalwood oil and used as an adulterant. Sandalwood oil is often adulterated with castor oil and cedar oil.

- Substitute: The heartwood of *Mansonia gagei* J.R. Drumm, *Pterocarpus santalinus L.* (Rakt Chandan), and other species of Santalum are used as substitutes of Shwet Chandana (Sharma et al 2001). Bhavaprakasha advocated the use of Karpura in the absence of Shwet Chandana, and if Karpura is unavailable, use Rakt Chandana (Bhavmishra 2010).

Points to Ponder

- *Among all tikta dravya, Chandana is the best sheetal dravya.*
- *Shwet Chandana is widely used in the treatment of bleeding disorders, urinary tract infection, purulent non-healing ulcers, skin diseases, and poisoning.*

Suggested Readings

Adams DR, Bhatnagar SP, Cookson RC. Sesquiterpenes of *Santalum album* and *Santalum spicatum*. Phytochemistry 1975;14(5/6):1459–1460

Anonymous. The Wealth of India. Vol. 9. New Delhi: Council of Science and Industrial Research; 2003:208–211

Asian Regional Workshop. *Santalum album*. IUCN Red List of Threatened Species. Version 2006. International Union for Conservation of Nature; 1998

Bhavmishra. Bhavprakash Nighantu, Commentary by K.C. Chunekar and Edited by G.S. Pandey. Varanasi: Choukhambha Bharati Academy; 2010:960

Demole E, Demole C, Enggist P. A chemical investigation of the volatile constituents of East Indian Sandalwood Oil (*Santalum album* L.). Helv Chim Acta 1976;59:737–747

Fox JE. Sandalwood: the royal tree. Biologist (London) 2000;47(1): 31–34

Ghani N. Khazainul Advia. New Delhi: Aijaz Publishing House; 2007: 932–933

Kumar R, Anjum N, Tripathi YC. Phytochemistry and pharmacology of *Santalum album* L.: a review. World J Pharm Res 2015; 4(10):1842–1876

Sharma PC, Yelne MB, Dennis TJ. Database on Medicinal Plants Used in Ayurveda, Vol. 3. New Delhi: CCRAS; 2005;3:184–205

Sindhu RK, Upma, Kumar A, Arora S. *Santalum album* Linn: a review on morphology, phytochemistry and pharmacological aspects. Int J Pharm Tech Res 2010;2(1):914–919

The Ayurvedic Pharmacopeia of India. Part I, Vol. 3. New Delhi: Department of AYUSH, Ministry of Health and Family Welfare, Government of India; 2001:209

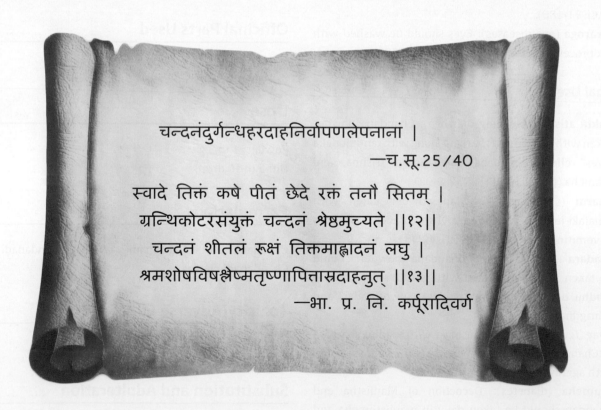

चन्दनंदुर्गन्धहरदाहनिर्वापणलेपनानां |

—च.सू.25/40

स्वादे तिक्तं कषे पीतं छेदे रक्तं तनौ सितम् |
ग्रन्थिकोटरसंयुक्तं चन्दनं श्रेष्ठमुच्यते ||१२||
चन्दनं शीतलं रूक्षं तिक्तमाह्लादनं लघु |
श्रमशोषविषश्लेष्मतृष्णापित्तासृदाहनुत् ||१३||

—भा. प्र. नि. कर्पूरादिवर्ग

26. Chitraka [*Plumbago zeylanica* Linn.*]*

Family: *Pumbaginaceae*

Hindi name: *Cheeta, Chitrak*

English name: *Ceylon leadwort, Doctorbush*

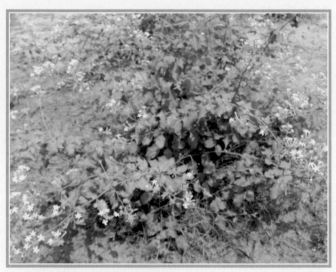

Plant of *Plunbago zeylanica* Linn.

Red variety of Chitraka is considered as rasayan, kustaghn, and is used for increasing body weight, in rasakarma, and lohavedhana

—R.N.pippalyadi/47

Introduction

The word Chitraka means spotted, which is compared with the spotted appearance of a leopard. The plant is compared with a leopard in terms of its sharpness and tearing nature. The genus name *Plumbago* is derived from a Latin word *plumbum* which means lead (Gogte 2009), because of its ability to cure lead palsy or ability to produce lead colored spots on skin (Kishore 2012). That is why it is also known as leadwort.

Chitraka has a long history of its usage as a drug that increases the digestive fire. Charak stated Chitraka mool as best deepan pachan dravya and best for the treatment of guda roga, sotha, arsha, and shool (C.S.S. 25/40). It is also included in shoolaghni and vataanulomani yavagu, moolasava (C.S.S. 25/49), and shaka varga (C.S.S. 26/106). Sushrut used Chitraka for preparation of tikshna kshar and

as prativaap dravya in kshar. Chitraka shaka is laghu and kaphasophahara in properties (S.S.Su. 46/239). Sushrut and Vagabhatt described it as rasayana dravya similar to that of Bakuchi and Pippali rasayana, respectively (S.S.Ci. 28/3; A.H.U. 39/62-65). Sharangdhar samhita described it as the best deepana pachana dravya (Sh.S. 1/4/1). Raj nighantu named rakta Chitraka as Kalaha. Chitraka is one of the ingredients in trimada, panchkola, and shadushna (Murthy 1998).

The roots and leaves are used in veterinary medicines for treating ailments like flatulence, edema, and intestinal worms (Deshmukh et al 2011). Tribal people in Assam use its root for family planning, birth control, permanent sterilization, and for inducing abortions (Tiwari et al 1982).

Botanically three varieties of Chitraka are available in India, i.e., *Plumbago zeylanica* Linn. with white flowers, *Plumbago rosea* Linn. with red flowers, and *Plumbago capensis* Thunk with blue flowers (Sastry 2014).

Vernacular Names

Assamese: Agiyachit, Agnachit
Bengali: Chita
Gujarati: Chitrakmula
Kannada: Chitramula, Vahni, Bilichitramoola
Kashmiri: Chitra, Shatranja
Malayalam: Vellakeduveli, Thumpokkoduveli
Marathi: Chitraka
Oriya: Chitamula, Chitoparu
Punjabi: Chitra
Tamil: Chitramoolam, Kodiveli
Telugu: Chitramulam
Urdu: Sheetraj

Synonyms

Agni: It has fiery hot nature like fire.
Agnika: It is similar to fire in properties and virya.
Analanama: It is named after fire.
Daruna: It is extremely hot in property.
Dipaka: It stimulates digestive fire.
Jaran: It promotes digestion of food.
Pathi: It is sharp like the teeth of wild animals.
Ushana: It is hot in pungency and virya.
Vyala: It has sharpness and tearing effect like wild animals (leopard, etc.).

Classical Categorization

Charak Samhita: Lekhaniya, Bhedaniya, Deepaniya, Shoolprashamana, Triptighna, Arshoghna

Sushrut Samhita: Pippalyadi, Amalakyadi, Mustadi, Mushkakadi, Aragvadhadi, Varunadi
Ashtang Hridaya: Pippalyadi, Mustadi, Aragvadhadi, Varunadi
Dhanvantari Nighantu: Shatpushpadi varga
Madanpal Nighantu: Sunthyadi varga
Kaiyadev Nighantu: Oushadi varga
Raj Nighantu: Pippalayadi varga
Bhavaprakash Nighantu: Haritakyadi varga

Distribution

Chitraka is a native plant of South Asia and is available in tropical and subtropical countries of the world. It is distributed throughout India, mainly in West Bengal, Maharashtra, Madhya Pradesh, Uttar Pradesh, Bihar, Rajasthan, and some parts of South India both in wild and cultivated state.

Morphology

A perennial, subscandent shrub, 60 to 120 cm high with woody, spreading, green striated branches.

- **Leaves:** Simple, alternate, about 8 cm long and 3 cm broad, ovate shape, acute apex, glabrous, entire, short red petiole, amplexicaul at the base, and often dilated into stipule like auricles (**Fig. 26.1**).
- **Flowers:** White, bracteate, often branched, glandular in long terminal spikes, 10 to 30 cm long, bisexual. Calyx densely covered with stalked, sticky glands. Corolla are white, slender, and tubular. Stamen are free and five. Ovary is superior (**Fig. 26.2**).

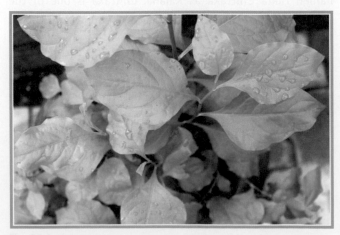

Fig. 26.1 Leaves.

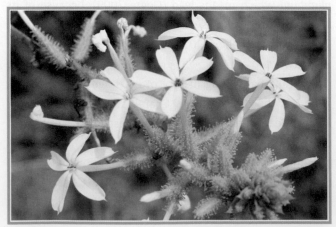

Fig. 26.2 Flower.

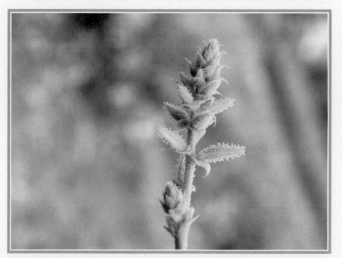

Fig. 26.3 Fruit.

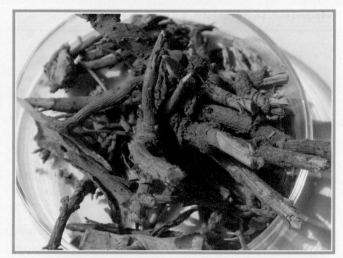

Fig. 26.4 Root.

- **Fruits:** Oblong capsules, pointed, contained in viscid, glandular, persistent calyx (**Fig. 26.3**). Seeds oblong and purple colored.
- **Roots:** Cylindrical, stout, irregularly bent, light yellow colored when fresh, reddish-brown when dry, found in the form of tough pieces, slightly branched with or without secondary roots, uniform and smooth texture, strong and characteristic odor with acrid and bitter taste (**Fig. 26.4**). Bark is thin and brown colored (Kapoor 1990). The plant is propagated through seeds and stem cuttings.

Phenology

Flowering time: September to November
Fruiting time: October to January

Key Characters for Identification
➤ *A perennial sub-scandent shrub with striated branches*
➤ *Leaves: simple, alternate, ovate, amplexicaul at the base*
➤ *Flowers: white, bracteate, in terminal spikes*
➤ *Fruit: oblong contained in viscid persistent calyx*
➤ *Roots: stout, cylindrical, reddish-brown when dried*

Types

- Vagabhatt: three types—Peeta, Sita (white), Asita (black)

- Yogaratnasamuccayam: three types—Krishn, Shwet, Rakt (AVS, 1995)
- Bhavaprakash: three types—Shwet, Rakt, Neel

Rasapanchaka

Guna	Laghu, Ruksha, Tikshna
Rasa	Katu
Vipaka	Katu
Virya	Ushna

Chemical Constituents

The major compounds isolated from Chitraka plant are naphthoquinones, flavonoids, terpenes, and sterols. The root bark of Chitraka has plumbagin, 3-chloroplumbagin, 3,3-biplumbagin, binaphthoquinone, and four other pigments identified as isozeylanone, zeylanone, elliptinone, and droserone (Satyavati 1987; Kapoor 1990). Two plumbagic acid glucosides, five naphthaquinones (plumbagin, chitranone, maritinone, elliptinone, and isoshinanolone), and five coumarins (seselin, methoxyseselin, suberosine, xanthyletin, and xanthoxyletin) were isolated from the roots (Lin et al 2003). Leaves contain plumbagin, chitanone. Stem has plumbagin, zeylanone, isozeylanone, sitosterol, stigmasterol, campesterol, and dihydroflavinol-plumbaginol. Fruits contains plumbagin, glucopyranoside, and sitosterol.

Identity, Purity, and Strength

- Foreign matter: Not more than 3%
- Total ash: Not more than 3%
- Acid-insoluble ash: Not more than 1%
- Alcohol-soluble extractive: Not less than 12%
- Water-soluble extractive: Not less than 12%

(Source: The Ayurvedic Pharmacopeia of India 1989)

Karma (Actions)

In Ayurveda classics Chitraka is described as deepana (appetizer), pachana (digestive), lekhana (scrapping), bhedana (purgative), triptighna (antithirst), grahi (absorbent), arshoghna (antihemorrhoid), shothahar (antiinflammatory), pittasarak (chlagogue purgative), krimighna (anthelmintic), kusthaghna (antidermatosis), shoolhara (analgesic), swedajanan (diaphoretic), kanthya (promotes voice), raktapitta prakopaka (aggravate rakta & pitta dosha), jwaraghna (antipyretic), garbhashya sankochaka (uterine astringent), katupaushtika (bitter tonic), and rasayana (rejuvinator).

- Doshakarma: Vatakaphashamaka, Pittavardhaka
- Dhatukarma: Rasayana
- Malakarma: Bhedana, Swedajanan

The root is a well-known abortifacient and vesicant. Tincture of root bark is used as a sudorific and antiperiodic. Leaves are caustic, vesicant, and aphrodisiac (The Wealth of India 1948; Nadkarni 1999).

Pharmacological Actions

The root and root bark of Chitraka are stimulant, and have expectorant, laxative, digestive, carminative, analgesic, anti-inflammatory, anthelmintic, antimalarial, antiarthritic, antioxidant, antibacterial, antifungal, anticarcinogenic, antiallergic, rejuvenator, wound-healing activity, antifertility, antihyperglycemic, hypolipidemic, and antiatherosclerotic properties (Chaudhari and Chaudhari 2015; Gani et al 2013).

Indications

In classical texts Chitraka is used for the treatment of shotha (inflammations), udar roga (diseases of abdomen),

arsha (piles), grahani (sprue), krimi (worm infestation), kandu (pruritus), agnimandya (loss of appetite), ajirna (indigestion), gulma (abdominal tumor), atisaar (diarrhea), gudashotha (rectal inflammation), kasa (cough), jeerna pratishyay (cold), swarabheda (hoarseness of voice), medoroga (obesity), prasutivikara (diseases of puerperium), rajorodha (amenorrhea), makkalasula, vishamajvar, jirnajvara (chronic fever), ksaya (emaciation), panduroga (anemia), pliharoga (splenomegaly), shlipada (filariasis), vrana (wounds), and shivitra (vitiligo).

In ethnic practice Chitraka is also used in the treatment of rheumatism, laryngitis, scabies, disease of spleen, joint pain, muscular pain, hepatomegaly, dysentery, leucoderma, malaria, toxic swelling, and furunculous scabies. In Africa it is also used in influenza and black water fever (Tyagi and Menghani 2014).

Therapeutic Uses

External Use

1. **Shotha** (inflammation): Application of warm paste of Chitraka and Devadaru pounded with gomutra reduces swelling (VM. 42/5).
2. **Shlipada** (filariasis): Application of Chitraka or Devadaru paste is beneficial (CD. 42/5).
3. **Vrana vidarana:** For tearing of wounds and abscesses, paste prepared with Chirbilva, Bhallataka, Danti, Chitraka, Karavira, and excrete of pigeon, heron, and vulture is applied locally (S.S.U. 37.10).

Internal Use

1. **Grahni and udar roga** (sprue): Chitraka ghrita 1 tea spoonful twice daily is given in grahani and udar roga (CD. 4/43) (C.S.Ci. 13/116) (VM. 37/28).
2. **Arsha** (piles): Paste of Chitraka mool twak is applied within a jar and curd or buttermilk is prepared in that jar. Daily consumption of curd or buttermilk is recommended in arsha (C.S.Ci. 14/76) (VM. 5/18). Daily intake of powdered Chitraka root and Sunthi mixed with sour gruel or guda or gomutra is the best remedy for arsha (A.H.Ci. 8/61) (RM. 19/7).
3. **Atisaar** (diarrhea): After eating Pippali with madhu, if one drinks buttermilk pounded with Chitraka, it gives relief in diarrhea (C.S.Ci. 19/113).

4. **Kasa and pratishyay** (cough and cold): Chitrakadi leha (C.S.Ci. 18/56, 57) and Chitraka haritaki (VM. 60/26-28) are best remedy for kasa and pratishyay.

5. **Medoroga** (obesity): Intake of Chitraka root powder with madhu followed by wholesome diet is useful in medoroga (B.S. medoroga Ci./22).

6. **Shivitra** (vitiligo): Cow's urine mixed with Chitraka root powder, Trikatu and madhu is kept in a jar of ghrita for 15 days. Taking this ghrita daily reduces white spots of shivitra (S.S.Ci. 9/39).

7. **Kustha** (skin diseases): Intake of Chitraka paste with gomutra daily for a month alleviates kustha (S.S.Ci. 9/45).

8. **Swarabheda** (hoarseness of voice): Aja ghrita processed with yavakshar, Ajmoda, Chitraka and Amalaki or Devadaru and Chitraka with madhu is useful in swarbheda (S.S.U. 53/11).

9. **Prameha** (diabetes): Chitraka decoction is useful in siktameha (S.S.Ci. 11/9).

10. **Pandu roga** (anemia): Root powder of Bala and Chitraka should be taken with warm water in pandu roga (S.S.U. 44/26).

Officinal Part Used

Root

Dose

Powder: 1 to 2 g

Formulations

Chitrakadi vati, Chitrakadi gutika, Panchkola churna, Chitrakadi lepa, Punarnava mandur, Yograaj guggulu, Vyoshadi gutika, Aryogyovardhini vati, Chitraka haritaki, Chitrakadhya ghrita, Chandraprabha vati, Agnitundivati, Abhayarista, Ajamodadi churna, Shaddharan yoga.

Toxicity/Adverse Effects

Plumbagin the main active constituent of Chitraka is a powerful irritant. Topical application of Chitraka root or any other part produces redness and blisters. If taken internally in large doses, it produces abdominal colicky pain, increased perspiration, redness and itching of skin, dilated pupils, feeble pulse, gasping respiration, hypotonia, myotonia, collapse, and death (Modi 2005). Topical application of plant extract shows moderate irritation (Teshome et al 2008).

- Shodhana: For purification, pieces of Rakta Chitraka moola are soaked in lime water, washed and dried under the sun (Shastri 1979).
- Antidote: Sheeta Snighda, Pittashamaka preparations should be used like Ghrita, Dugdh, Navneet, ushira, chandana, etc. (Shastri 1979).

Substitution and Adulteration

In common practice, roots of other species of *Plumbago* are adulterated with Chitraka roots and kshar of Danti or Apamarga is used as substitute drugs (B.P.N. prastavana/ 149).

> **Points to Ponder**
>
> - *It is the best dravya for deepana (appetizer) and pachana (digestive) karma.*
> - *It is a drug of choice for digestive complaints, piles, cough, edema, and obesity.*
> - *Rakta chitraka is used as a rasayana dravya.*

Suggested Readings

Arya Vaidya Sala, ed. Indian Medicinal plants: A Compendium of 500 Species. Vol. 4. Orient Longman Ltd; 1995:321–326

Chaudhari SS, Chaudhari GS. A review on *Plumbago zeylanica* Linn.: A divine medicinal plant. Int J Pharm Sci Rev Res 2015;30(2): 119–127

Deshmukh RR, Rathod VN, Pardeshi VN. Ethnoveterinary medicine from Jalna district of Maharashtra State. Indian J Tradit Knowl 2011;10(2):344–348

Ganesan K, Banu GS. Ethnomedical and pharmacological potentials of *Plumbago zeylanica* L.: a review. Am J Phytomed Clin Therap 2013;1(3):313–337

Gogte VM. Ayurvedic Pharmacology and Therapeutic Uses of Medicinal Plants (Dravyagunavignyan). Translation by the academic team of Bharatiya Vidya Bhavan's SPARC. New Delhi: Chaukhambha Publication; 2009:370–372

Kapoor LD. Handbook of Ayurvedic Medicinal Plants. London: CRC Press; 1990

Kishore N, Mishra BB, Tiwari VK, Tripathi V. An account of phytochemicals from *Plumbago zeylanica* (Family: Plumbaginaceae): A natural gift to human being. Chron Young Sci 2012;3(3):178–198

Lin LC, Yang LL, Chou CJ. Cytotoxic naphthoquinones and plumbagic acid glucosides from Plumbago zeylanica. Phytochemistry 2003;62(4):619–622

Modi's Medical Jurisprudence and Toxicology. 23rd ed. Lexis Nexis Butter Worths; 2005:143

Murthy KR. Srikantha (Translator), Bhāvaprakāśa of Bhāvamiśra. Vol. I. Varanasi: Krishnadas Academy; 1998:169–170

Nadakarni AK, Nadakarni KR. Indian-Materia Medica. Bombay: Popular Prakashan; 1999:564

Sastry JLN. Dravyaguna vijñāna. Vol. II. Varanasi: Chaukhambha, Orientalia; 2014:314–317

Satyavati GV, Gupta AK, Tondon N. Medicinal Plants of India. 1st ed. Vol. 2. New Delhi: Indian Council of Medical Research; 1987

Shastri K. Rasatarangani. 11th ed. Chapter 24. New Delhi: Motilal Banarsidas; 1979:575

Teshome K, Gebre-Mariam T, Asres K, Perry F, Engidawork E. Toxicity studies on dermal application of plant extract of *Plumbago zeylanica* used in Ethiopian traditional medicine. J Ethnopharmacol 2008;117(2):236–248

The Ayurvedic Pharmacopeia of India. Part I, Vol. 1. New Delhi: Department of AYUSH, Ministry of Health and Family Welfare, Government of India; 1989:5–6

The Wealth of India. A Dictionary of Raw Material and Industrial Products. Raw Material Series, Vol. I–IX. New Delhi: Publication and Information Directorate, CSIR; 1948

Tiwari KC, Majumder R, Bhattacharjee S. Folklore information from Assam for family planning and birth control. Int J Crude Drug Res 1982;20(3):133–137

Tyagi R, Menghani E. A review on *Plumabgo zeylanica*: a compelling herb. Int J Pharm Sci Res 2014;5(4):119–126

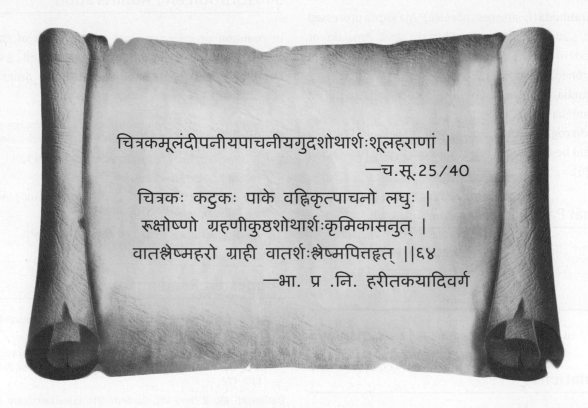

चित्रकमूलंदीपनीयपाचनीयगुदशोथार्शःशूलहराणां |

—च.सू. 25/40

चित्रकः कटुकः पाके वह्निकृत्पाचनो लघुः |

रूक्षोष्णो ग्रहणीकुष्ठशोथार्शःकृमिकासनुत् |

वातश्लेष्महरो ग्राही वातर्शःश्लेष्मपित्तहत् ||६४

—भा. प्र .नि. हरीतकयादिवर्ग

27. Dadima *[Punica granatum Linn.]*

Family: *Punicaceae*

Hindi name: *Anar*

English name: *Pomegranate tree*

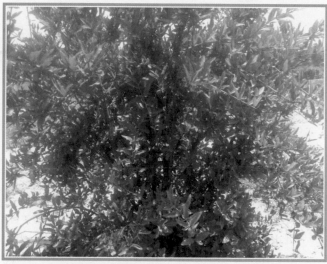

Plant of *Punica granatum* Linn.

> *In Hindu mythology Dadima fruit is considered as a symbol of prosperity, fertility, and good luck.*

Introduction

The genus *Punica* was derived from a roman word "carthage" pertaining to Carthaginian apple and "granatus" which means filled with seeds. So *Punica granatus* refers to an apple-like fruit filled with seeds (Jurenka 2008).

Since centuries, Dadima fruit has been appreciated in different cultures (Langley 2000). In Hindu mythology, it is believed to be related with goddess Earth and Lord Ganesha. It was praised in the Bible as a sacred fruit conferring the powers of fertility, abundance, and good luck (Jurenka 2008). In holy Quran, it is believed that Dadima fruit grows in the garden of paradise (Rahimi et al 2012). In Buddhism, it is considered to be one of the three sacred fruits symbolizing the essence of favorable influences. In Greek mythology, it represents life, prosperity, regeneration, and marriage. Islamic legend believed that each Dadima fruit contains one seed that has come down from paradise (Bhandari 2012).

Dadima fruit or its fruit juice is being used as a part of healthy diet in Indian homes since ages. Ayurveda has described the fruit in phala varga. Sushrut considered Dadima as best amla (sour) dravya (S.S.Su. 46/336) whereas Charak used it as a content of pachani, grahini, and yavagu (C.S.Su. 2/19). Since 1550 BC, Dadima is a well-known fruit for its medicinal use in different countries. The Romans used its root for treating tapeworm infestation (Langley 2000), and Indians used it in diabetes (Saxena and Vikram 2004).

Dadima is also used as a coloring agent in textile dyestuff (Adeel et al 2009) and as a flavoring agent for making juice, jelly, and grenadine.

Vernacular Names

Assamese: Dalim
Bengali: Dadima, Dalimgach, Dalim
Gujarati: Dadam, Dadam phala

Kannada: Dalimba, Dalimbe haonu
Malayalam: Mathalam, Dadiman
Marathi: Dalimba
Oriya: Dalimba
Punjabi: Anar
Tamil: Madulam Pazham
Telugu: Dadimbakaya, Dadimma
Urdu: Anar

Synonyms

Karak: The seeds are uniformly scattered inside the fruit.
Lohitpushpak: The plant bears red flowers.
Dantbeej: The shapes of the seeds are like teeth.
Raktbeej: The seeds are red in color.
Phalshadava: The fruit is madhura amla in taste, like a food preparation shadava.
Shukeshta: The fruits are favorite fruits of parrots.
Valkalphal: The fruit is covered with a thick rind.
Vritaphal: Fruits are round in shape.

Classical Categorization

Charak Samhita: Hridya, Chardinigrahana, Shramhara
Sushrut Samhita: Parushakadi
Ashtang Hridaya: Parushakadi
Dhanvantari Nighantu: Shatpushpadi varga
Madanpal Nighantu: Phal varga
Kaiyadev Nighantu: Oushadi varga
Raj Nighantu: Amraadi varga
Bhavaprakash Nighantu: Phal varga

Distribution

Dadima is a native plant of Iran, Afghanistan, and Baluchistan. It grows wild throughout the warm arid regions of Southeast Asia. Kandahar in Afghanistan is famous for its high-quality pomegranate. Found throughout India both in cultivated and wild form up to an altitude of 1,000 to 3,000 feet.

Morphology

It is a large deciduous glabrous shrub or a small tree of 1.5 to 5 m. Branchlets often spinescent. Bark is smooth, turns grey as the tree ages, and peels off in small flakes.

- **Leaves:** Simple, glossy, opposite, short petiole, lamina elliptical to lanceolate, entire to wavy margin, glabrous bright green surface (**Fig. 27.1**).
- **Flowers:** Solitary, axillary, scarlet, or blood red to orange colored, pedicellate, thick, coriaceous, calyx tubular, and funnel-shaped, petals five to seven, inferior ovary (**Fig. 27.2**).
- **Fruit:** A large balausta, globose-shaped, 5 to 12 cm in diameter, with a thick red, yellow coriaceous rind. The rind is crowned with a persistent calyx along with withered stamens. It contains numerous seeds separated by white, membranous pericarp (**Fig. 27.3**).
- **Seeds:** Embedded in a white, spongy pulp and surrounded by water-laden pulp (aril) ranging in color from white to deep red. They appear hard, angular, with an astringent taste. The plant is propagated through seeds and stem cuttings (**Fig. 27.4**).

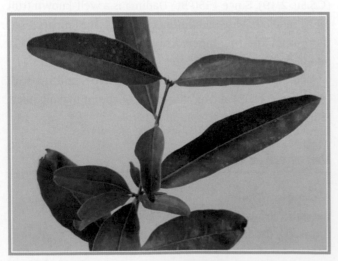

Fig. 27.1 Leaves.

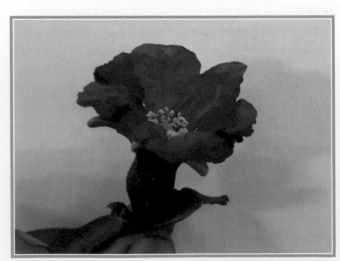

Fig. 27.2 Flower.

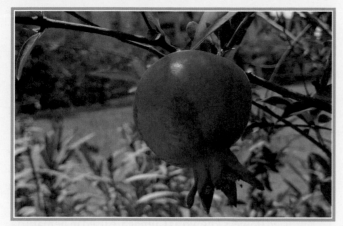

Fig. 27.3 Fruit.

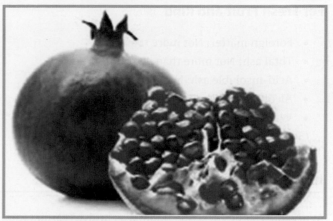

Fig. 27.4 Seed.

Phenology

Flowering time: Throughout year, particularly from March to July

Fruiting time: Throughout year, particularly from March to July

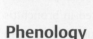

Key Characters for Identification

➤ *A large deciduous shrub or a small tree*
➤ *Leaves: simple, glossy, opposite, and lance shaped*
➤ *Flowers: scarlet or blood red to orange colored, solitary, and funnel shaped*
➤ *Fruit: globose with thick red rind crowned with persistent calyx*
➤ *Seeds: numerous, angular embedded in red white spongy pulp*

Types

Dhanvantari and Raj Nighantu: two types, i.e., Swadu and Amla

Bhavaprakash and Kaiyadev Nighantu: three types, i.e., Swadu, Swadu-amla, and Amla

Rasapanchaka

Guna	Laghu, Snigdh
Rasa	Madhura, Amla, Kashaya
Vipaka	Madhur
Virya	Ushna

Chemical Constituents

Fruit juice contains anthocyanins, procynadine, glucose, ellagic acid, gallic acid, caffeic acid, catechin, quercetin, vitamin C, vitamin E, coenzyme Q10, lipoic acid, rutin, amino acids, and numerous minerals particularly iron (Vroegrijk et al 2011). The pericarp and rind primarily contain ellagitannins (punicalin, punicalagin, and punicafolin), tannic acid, flavones, flavonone, anthocynidin, quercetin, polysaccharides, gum, and minerals like potassium, nitrogen, calcium, magnesium, phosphorus, sodium, etc. (Viuda-Martos et al 2010). Leaves have tannins, flavones, glycosides, luteolin, and apigenin. Flowers have gallic acid, ursolic acid, triterpenoids (maslinic and asiatic acid). Seeds have sugars, vitamin C, sitosterol, ursolic acid, protein, fat, mineral, nicotinic acid, pectin, riboflavin, thiamine, aspartic, citric, ellagic, gallic, malic acids, glutamine, isoquercetin, estrogenic flavones, and punicic acid. The root and bark have ellagitannins, numerous piperidine alkaloids, punicalin, and punicalagin (Jurenka 2008; Prakash and Prakash 2011).

Identity, Purity, and Strength

For Seed

- Foreign matter: Not more than 2%
- Total ash: Not more than 4%
- Acid-insoluble ash: Not more than 0.5%
- Alcohol-soluble extractive: Not less than 20%
- Water-soluble extractive: Not less than 35%

(Source: The Ayurvedic Pharmacopeia of India 1999)

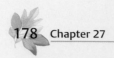

For Fresh Fruit and Rind

- Foreign matter: Not more than 2%
- Total ash: Not more than 4%
- Acid-insoluble ash: Not more than 0.4%
- Alcohol-soluble extractive: Not less than 9%
- Water-soluble extractive: Not less than 20%

(Source: The Ayurvedic Pharmacopeia of India 2004)

Karma (Actions)

Ayurvedic classics describe Dadima as hridya (cardiotonic), grahi (absorbent), balya (strength promoting), chardighna (antiemetic), medhya (brain tonic), pittahara (pacify pitta), rochana (relish), mukhagandhahara (removes foul smell from mouth), shramahara (antifatigue), jwaraghna (antipyretic), shukrala (spematogenic), and tarpaka (nutritive). Bhavaprakash has described the properties of three types of Dadima as follows:

- Swadu: hridya, kanthya, tarpaka, grahi, medhya, balya
- Swadu-amla: deepan, rochan
- Amla: pittavardhaka, aamhara
- Doshakarma: Swadu is tridoshghna, Swadu-amla is vatapitta hara, and Amla variety is rakta pittavardhaka
- Dhatukarma: Balya, tarpaka
- Malakarma: Stambhaka

The fresh Dadima juice is considered to be refrigerant, the rind is astringent, seeds are stomachic, pulp is cardiac tonic and stomachic in properties (Anonymous 1969; Chopra et al 1956; Satyavati et al 1987).

Pharmacological Actions

Several in vivo and in vitro studies suggested that its fruit juice and rind exhibit antioxidant (Gil et al 2000), antimicrobial, antifungal, anthelmintic (Naz et al 2007), antihypertensive (Mohan et al 2010; Asgary et al 2017), antiproliferative (Malik and Mukhtar 2006), aphrodisiac, antidiarrheal, antipyretic, anti-inflammatory (Rasheed et al 2009), anticancerous (Panth et al 2017), antiaging, hemostatic, diuretic, expectorant, hepatoprotective, anti-diabetic (Vroegrijk et al 2011), cardioprotective (Arun et al 2017), anti-angiogenesis activities. Besides, inhibitory effect on motility, cell cycle arrest, apoptosis, stimulation of cell differentiation, antimutagenic, and inhibitory effects on

vital enzymes such as COX, LOX, CYP450 are also caused by this plant (Rahimi et al 2012).

Indications

In traditional system of medicines Dadima phal and phal twak are used as a remedy for daha (burning sensation), trishna (thirst), jwara (fever), hridya roga (heart diseases), aruchi (dyspepsia), atisaar (diarrhea), raktapitta (bleeding disorders), kasa (cough), krimi (helminthes), kantha roga (throat infection), and mukha durgandhya (foul breath).

The dried flowers known as Gulnar are used in hematuria, hemorrhoids, hemoptysis, and dysentery. The powdered flower buds and green leaves paste are used in bronchitis and conjunctivitis, respectively (Anonymous 1969; Chopra et al 1956). Seeds are used to treat vaginal discharge and wound while root barks are used to expel out intestinal worms (Amin 1991).

Dadima juice and seed oil not only are used as a potential nutritional supplement but also are known for its preventive role in cancer, heart diseases (Schubert et al 1999), AIDS (Lee and Watson 1998), menopausal syndrome, Alzheimer disease (Hartman et al 2006), ultraviolet-induced skin damage (Kasai et al 2006), and dental plaques (Menezes et al 2006). The presence of phytoestrogenic compounds in pomegranate seed oil and juice paves the way for its use as an alternative to hormone replacement therapy in postmenopausal women. The fruit is being recommended as an immunity enhancer and food supplement in the treatment of acquired immune deficiency syndrome (HIV/AIDS) due to the presence of diverse bioflavonoids.

Therapeutic Uses

External Use

1. **Nasagatraktapitta** (epistaxis): Snuffing with Dadima flower or Durva swarasa or Amra asthi and Palandu checks bleeding in epistaxis (VM. 9/32).
2. **Vyanga** (freckles): Fresh Dadima twak mixed with aja dugdh (goat's milk) is applied on face daily to prevent acne (A.S.U. 37/24).
3. **Upadansha** (soft chancre): Vrishna region is dusted with powder of Bandhuka leaves and Dadima twak in upadansha (B.P.Ci. 51/26).

Internal Use

1. **Atisaar** (diarrhea): Decoction of Dadima and Kutaja bark mixed with honey is used to check bleeding in diarrhea and dysentery (VM. 3/39) (VJ. 2/13). Paste of flower bud with honey also controls diarrhea (SB. 4/147).

2. **Rakta arsha** (bleeding piles): Daily consumption of Dadima phal twak decoction (A.H.Ci. 8/103) or Dadima phal twak with Chandana and Sunthi is helpful in curing raktaarsha (C.S.Ci. 14/185).

3. **Rakta Pitta** (hemorrhage): Oral intake of Dadima pushpa rasa or Amra pushpa or Durva rasa prevents internal and external hemorrhage (A.H.Ci. 2/41).

4. **Pandu** (anemia): One teaspoonful of Dadimadya ghrita twice daily should be administered in pandu roga (C.S.Ci. 16/45-46).

5. **Madatyya** (alcoholism): To quench the thirst of alcohol one should drink Dadima swarasa or decoction of laghu panchmool (A.H.Ci. 7/16).

6. **Aruchi** (anorexia): Intake of Yusha mixed with Dadima juice is a wholesome diet in aruchi (VM. 56/29).

7. **Trishna** (excessive thirst): Daily intake of leha prepared with Dadima seed, Jeerak, Nagkeshar churna with sugar and honey prevents excessive thirst (B.S.balroga/53).

8. **Visarpa** (erysipelas): Sour mantha prepared by adding Dadima, Amalaki, Parushaka, Mrudvika, Kharjura sweetened with madhu sharkara should be taken with lukewarm water (C.S.Ci. 21/108-109).

9. **Puyameha** (gonorrhea): Cold infusion Dadima phal twak madwixed with sugar should be taken daily in the morning (SB. 4/811).

Officinal Parts Used

Fruit, pericarp, root

Dose

Fruit juice: 20 to 40 mL
Decoction: 40 to 80 mL
Powder: 3 to 6 g

Formulations

Dadimashtaka churna, Dadimadi ghrtam, Dadimadi churna, Hingvadi gutika, Hinguvacadi churna, Bhaskara lavan, Dadimavaleha.

Toxicity/Adverse Effects

Histopathological, preclinical, and clinical studies do not report any toxicities or adverse effects on consuming pomegranate juice and its constituents even at conventional doses (Vidal et al 2003; Cerdá et al 2003; Heber et al 2007).

Substitution and Adulteration

None.

> ### Points to Ponder
>
> - *Dadima fruit is madhura and amla in rasa while its rind is predominantly kashaya in rasa.*
> - *Its fruit juice is a well-known nutrition supplement, cardioprotective, anticancerous, immunity enhancer, and antioxidant drug.*

Suggested Readings

Adeel S, Ali S, Bhatti IA, Zsila F. Dyeing of cotton fabric using pomegranate (*Punica granatum*) aqueous extract. Asian J Chem 2009;21(5):3493–3499

Amin GR. Iranian Traditional Medicinal Plants. Tehran, Iran: Farhang Publications; 1991

Anonymous. The Wealth of India: A Dictionary of Indian Raw Material & Industrial Products. Vol. VIII: (Ph-Re). New Delhi: Publication & Information Directorate, CSIR, Reprint 2009; 1969:317–324

Arun KB, Jayamurthy P, Anusha CV, Mahesh SK, Nisha P. Studies on activity guided fractionation of pomegranate peel extracts and its effect on antidiabetic and cardiovascular protection properties. J Food Process Preserv 2017;41(1):e13108

Asgary S, Keshvari M, Sahebkar A, Sarrafzadegan N. Pomegranate consumption and blood pressure: a review. Curr Pharm Des 2017;23(7):1042–1050

Bhandari PR. Pomegranate (*Punica granatum* L.): ancient seeds for modern cure? Review of potential therapeutic applications. Int J Nutr Pharmacol Neurolog Dis 2012;2(3):171–184

Cerdá B, Cerón JJ, Tomás-Barberán FA, Espín JC. Repeated oral administration of high doses of the pomegranate ellagitannin punicalagin to rats for 37 days is not toxic. J Agric Food Chem 2003;51(11):3493–3501

Chopra RN, Nayar SL, Chopra IC. Glossary of Indian Medicinal Plants. New Delhi: CSIR; 1956:46

Gil MI, Tomás-Barberán FA, Hess-Pierce B, Holcroft DM, Kader AA. Antioxidant activity of pomegranate juice and its relationship with phenolic composition and processing. J Agric Food Chem 2000;48(10):4581–4589

Hartman RE, Shah A, Fagan AM, et al. Pomegranate juice decreases amyloid load and improves behavior in a mouse model of Alzheimer's disease. Neurobiol Dis 2006;24(3):506–515

Heber D, Seeram NP, Wyatt H, Henning SM, Zhang Y, Ogden LG, et al. Safety and antioxidant activity of a pomegranate ellagitannin-enriched polyphenol dietary supplement in overweight individuals with increased waist size. J Agric Food Chem 2007;55:10050–54

Jurenka JS. Therapeutic applications of pomegranate (*Punica granatum* L.): a review. Altern Med Rev 2008;13(2):128–144

Kasai K, Yoshimura M, Koga T, Arii M, Kawasaki S. Effects of oral administration of ellagic acid-rich pomegranate extract on ultraviolet-induced pigmentation in the human skin. J Nutr Sci Vitaminol (Tokyo) 2006;52(5):383–388

Langley P. Why a pomegranate? BMJ 2000;321(7269):1153–1154

Lee J, Watson R. Pomegranate: a role in health promotion and AIDS. In: Watson R, ed. Nutrition Food and AIDS. Boca Raton, FL: CRC Press; 1998:179–192

Malik A, Mukhtar H. Prostate cancer prevention through pomegranate fruit. Cell Cycle 2006;5(4):371–373

Menezes SM, Cordeiro LN, Viana GS. *Punica granatum* (pomegranate) extract is active against dental plaque. J Herb Pharmacother 2006;6(2):79–92

Mohan M, Waghulde H, Kasture S. Effect of pomegranate juice on angiotensin II-induced hypertension in diabetic Wistar rats. Phytother Res 2010;24(Suppl 2):S196–S203

Naz S, Siddiqi R, Ahmad S, Rasool SA, Sayeed SA. Antibacterial activity directed isolation of compounds from *Punica granatum*. J Food Sci 2007;72(9):M341–M345

Panth N, Manandhar B, Paudel KR. Anticancer activity of *Punica granatum* (pomegranate): a review. Phytother Res 2017;31(4):568–578

Prakash CVS, Prakash I. Bioactive chemical constituents from pomegranate (*Punica granatum*) juice, seed and peel: a review. Int J Res Chem Environ 2011;1(1):1–18

Rahimi HR, Arastoo M, Ostad SN. A comprehensive review of *Punica granatum* (pomegranate) properties in toxicological, pharmacological, cellular and molecular biology researches. Iran J Pharm Res 2012;11(2):385–400

Rasheed Z, Akhtar N, Anbazhagan AN, Ramamurthy S, Shukla M, Haqqi TM. Polyphenol-rich pomegranate fruit extract (POMx) suppresses PMACI-induced expression of pro-inflammatory cytokines by inhibiting the activation of MAP Kinases and NF-kappaB in human KU812 cells. J Inflamm (Lond) 2009;6:1

Satyavati GV, Gupta AK, Tandon N. Medicinal Plants of India. New Delhi: Indian Council of Medical Research; 1987: Vol. 2:539–540

Saxena A, Vikram NK. Role of selected Indian plants in management of type 2 diabetes: a review. J Altern Complement Med 2004;10(2):369–378

Schubert SY, Lansky EP, Neeman I. Antioxidant and eicosanoid enzyme inhibition properties of pomegranate seed oil and fermented juice flavonoids. J Ethnopharmacol 1999;66(1):11–17

Vidal A, Fallarero A, Peña BR, et al. Studies on the toxicity of *Punica granatum* L. (Punicaceae) whole fruit extracts. J Ethnopharmacol 2003;89(2-3):295–300

Viuda-Martos M, Fernández-López J, Pérez-Álvarez JA. Pomegranate and its many functional components as related to human health: a review. Compr Rev Food Sci Food Saf 2010;9(6):635–654

Vroegrijk IOCM, van Diepen JA, van den Berg S, et al. Pomegranate seed oil, a rich source of punicic acid, prevents diet-induced obesity and insulin resistance in mice. Food Chem Toxicol 2011;49(6):1426–1430

The Ayurvedic Pharmacopeia of India. Part I, Vol. 2. New Delhi: Department of AYUSH, Ministry of Health and Family Welfare, Government of India; 1999:33

The Ayurvedic Pharmacopeia of India. Part I, Vol. 4. New Delhi: Department of AYUSH, Ministry of Health and Family Welfare, Government of India; 2004:23, 23

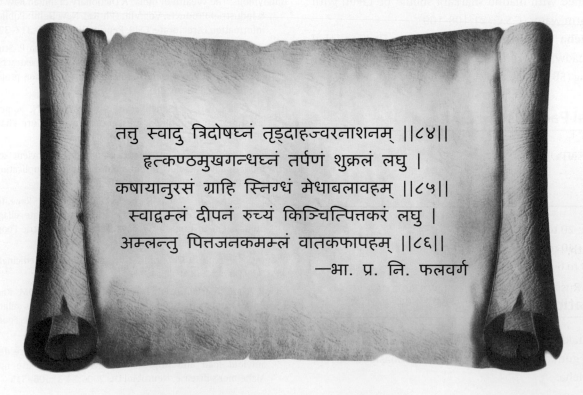

तत्तु स्वादु त्रिदोषघ्नं तृड्दाहज्वरनाशनम् ॥८४॥
हृत्कण्ठमुखगन्धघ्नं तर्पणं शुक्रलं लघु ।
कषायानुरसं ग्राहि स्निग्धं मेधाबलावहम् ॥८५॥
स्वाद्वम्लं दीपनं रुच्यं किञ्चित्पित्तकरं लघु ।
अम्लन्तु पित्तजनकमम्लं वातकफापहम् ॥८६॥
—भा. प्र. नि. फलवर्ग

28. Daru Haridra *[Berberis aristata DC.]*

Family:	*Berberidaceae*
Hindi name:	*Daruhaldi, Darhald*
English name:	*Indian berberry, tree turmeric*

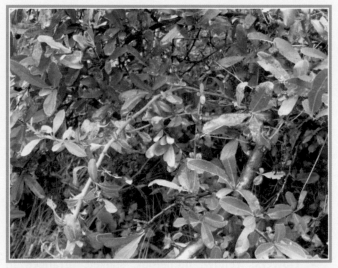

Plant of *Berberis aristata* DC.

> *The root, root bark, and lower part of the Daruharidra stem is boiled in water, strained and evaporated till a semi-solid mass is obtained. This mass is known as Rasanjana or rasauth.*

Introduction

The name "Daruharidra" suggests that the wood of this plant resembles the color of Haridra, i.e., yellow color. In ancient Ayurveda literature, both the drugs (Haridra and Daruharidra) have been mentioned together as Haridra dvay, which suggests that its properties are analogous to that of Haridra.

Daruharidra is being used as a popular remedy for diseases of upper clavicular region since time immemorial. Charak, Sushrut, Astang, Vrinda madhav all advocated the use of Daruharidra or Rasanjana in diseases of eyes, ears, mouth, etc. The ancient Egyptians used it to prevent plagues. Europeans used it to treat liver and gallbladder ailments. Russians used it for inflammations, high blood pressure, and abnormal uterine bleeding. In the Unani system of medicine, it is used in leprosy. The Tibetan people used its decoction in piles and gastric disorders, and the plant is known as *Kershuen* there (Chauhan et al 1978/79).

In Uttaranchal's tribal region, the plant is used to treat fish poison and snake and scorpion sting (Mittre 1981; Jain and Suri 1979/80).

The fully ripe, juicy fruits are eaten by local inhabitants often as dessert and nutrient supplement in their diet. The roots can also be used for making alcoholic drink, dyeing clothes, and tanning leather.

Vernacular Names

Bengali: Daruharidra
Gujarati: Daruharidra, Daruhuladur
Himachali: Rasont, Kashmal
Kannada: Maradarishana, Maradarishina, Daruhaladi
Malayalam: Maramannal, Maramanjal
Marathi: Daruhalad
Nepal: Chitra, Chutro
Oriya: Daruharidra, Daruhalidi
Punjabi: Sumlu, Simlu, Kasmal

Tamil: Gangeti, Varatiu manjal
Telugu: Manupasupu
Urdu: Darhald

Synonyms

Darunisha: Its stem has similar actions like nisha (haridra).
Darvi: The wood is used as medicine in therapeutics.
Kaleyaka: It is similar to peetchandana.
Kantakateri: The plant bears many spines on leaves.
Panchampacha: It helps digestion and improves liver functions.
Parjanya: The plant bears fruits in rainy season.
Peetadaru: The wood is yellow in color.
Peetadru: The plant has yellow-colored wood and flowers.

Classical Categorization

Charak Samhita: Lekhaniya, Arshoghna, Kandughna
Sushrut Samhita: Haridradi, Mustaadi, Lakshadi
Ashtang Hridaya: Haridradi, Mustadi, Shirovirechan
Dhanvantari Nighantu: Guduchyadi varga
Madanpal Nighantu: Abhyadi varga
Kaiyadev Nighantu: Oushadi varga
Raj Nighantu: Pippalayadi varga
Bhavaprakash Nighantu: Haritakyadi varga

Distribution

It is distributed in temperate and sub-tropical regions of Asia (India, Nepal, Tibet, Sri Lanka, etc.), Europe, and America. In India, the plant is native to the whole region of Himalaya mountains at an elevation of 2,000 to 3,500 m, and it also grows in Nilgiri mountains of Southern India.

Morphology

It is an erect, glabrous, spinescent shrub, 3 to 6 m in height, with a thick woody yellow root covered with a thin brittle bark.

- **Stem:** Cylindrical, with scars of the lateral branching, some lenticels and longitudinal fine wrinkles on the external surface, internally yellow with a distinct central pith (**Fig. 28.1a, b**).
- **Leaves:** Simple in tufts of five to eight, obovate or elliptic, leathery, sessile, about 5 cm long and 2 cm wide, subacute to obtuse apex, entire or spinous-toothed margin, base gradually narrowed, with prominent reticulate nerves, glossy dark green above, glossy pale green beneath (**Fig. 28.2**).
- **Flowers:** Yellow, numerous, stalked, arranged in drooping corymbose racemes (**Fig. 28.3**).
- **Fruits:** Smooth berries, globose to ovoid shape, unripe green which turns aconite violet on maturity.

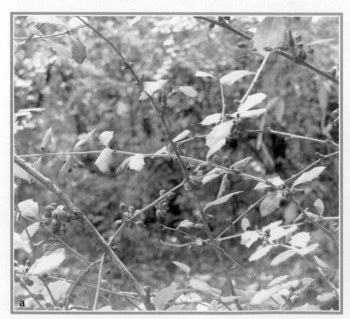
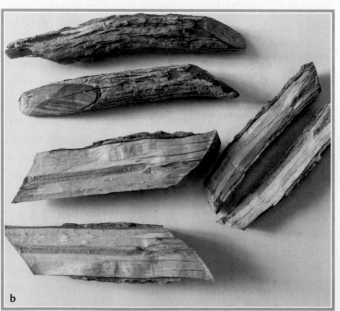

Fig. 28.1 **(a)** Stem. **(b)** Dry stem.

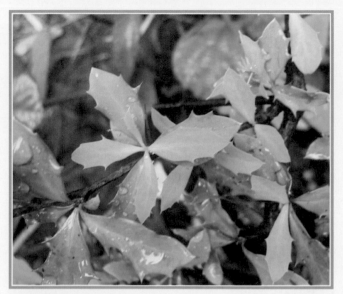

Fig. 28.2 Leaves.

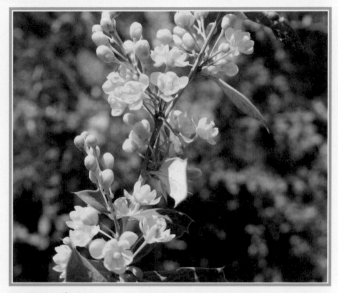

Fig. 28.3 Flowers.

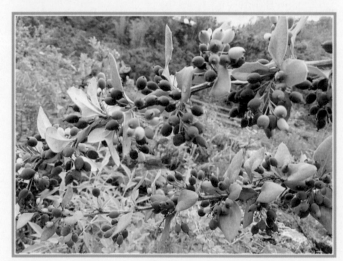

Fig. 28.4 Fruit.

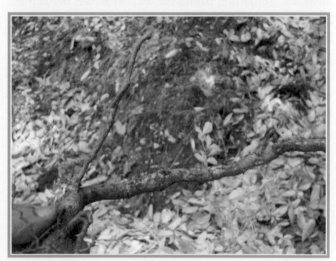

Fig. 28.5 Root.

The fruits are popularly known as Jharishka. Seeds are two to five in number (**Fig. 28.4**).

- **Root:** Cylindrical, thick, woody yellowish-brown, more or less knotty, and covered by a thin brittle bark. Bark is internally pale brown, rough, furrowed, fracture hard, odorless, and bitter in taste (**Fig. 28.5**).

The plant is propagated by seeds (Srivastava et al 2001; Chopra et al 1958).

Phenology

Flowering time: March to April

Fruiting time: May to July

- Collection time: Stem bark should be collected in vasanta ritu.

Key Characters for Identification

➤ *An erect, glabrous, spinescent shrub of about 3 to 6 m.*

➤ *Leaves in tufts of five to eight, obovate, sessile with spinous-toothed margin.*

➤ *Flowers: numerous, yellow in corymbose racemes.*

➤ *Fruits: globose to ovoid berries that turn aconite violet on maturity.*

➤ *Roots: thick, cylindrical, knotted internally yellowish-brown.*

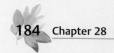

Types

None

Rasapanchaka

Guna	Laghu, Ruksha
Rasa	Tikta, Rasanjana (katu)
Vipaka	Katu
Virya	Ushna

Chemical Constituents

Root and stem of Daruharidra contain a large number of alkaloids. Berberine, palmatine, oxyberberine, berbamine, aromoline, karachine, oxycanthine, taxilamine, epiberberine, dehydrocaroline, jatrorhizine, columbamine, karachine, dihyrokarachine, oxyberberine, pakistanine, 1-O methyl pakistanine, pseudopalmatine chloride, and pseudoberberine chloride are the major alkaloids reported from the plant (Bhakuni et al 1968 ; Chakarvarti et al 1950).

Identity, Purity, and Strength

For Stem

- Foreign matter: Not more than 2%
- Total ash: Not more than 14%
- Acid-insoluble ash: Not more than 5%
- Alcohol-soluble extractive: Not less than 6%
- Water-soluble extractive: Not less than 8%
  (Source: The Ayurvedic Pharmacopeia of India 2001)

Karma (Actions)

Ayurvedic classics described it as shothaghna (reduce swelling), jwaraghna (antipyretics), vishaghna (antidotes), varnya (complexion promoter), vranaropana (wound healing), vranashodhana (cleansing of wound), chakshushya (beneficial for eyes), deepan (appetizer), grahi (astringent), pittasaraka, swedajanan, raktashodhaka (blood purifier).

Rasanjana: Rasayana (rejuvenation), chhedana (antitussive), vishaghna (antidotes), raktastambhaka (hemostatic).

- Phal: Rochana (relish), trishnanigrahan (antithirst)
- Doshakarma: Kaphapitta shamaka
- Dhatukarma: Chakshushya, vishaghna
- Malakarma: Swedajanan, pittasaraka

Pharmacological Actions

Studies have revealed that the plant contains antimicrobial, hepatoprotective, immunomodulatory, antipyretic, antidiabetic, antidepressant, antioxidant, anticancerous, cardiovascular (Mitra et al 2011), antihyperglycemic (Singh and Kakkar 2009), antiamoebic (Sohni et al 1995), and wound-healing properties.

Indications

Pharmacopeias and Nighantus indicated Daruharidra in karnaroga (ear disease), netraroga (eye disease), mukharoga (diseases of mouth), kantharoga (diseases of throat), shotha (inflammations), kandu (pruritus), vrana (wounds), visarpa (erysipelas), meha (diabetes), pradar (leucorrhea), arsha (piles), kushta (skin diseases), kapha abhishyandi (conjunctivitis), jeerna jwar (chronic fever), updansha (soft chancre), kamala (jaundice), yakrita vikara (liver diseases), pleehavridhi (splenomegaly), mukhapaka (stomatitis), gandmala (cystic swellings), bhagandar (fistula), and daurbalya (general debility).

Rasanjan is a special type of preparation prepared from Daruharidra. It is used in raktapitta (bleeding disorders), vrana (wound), vranashotha (inflammation), visham jwar (intermittent fever), hikka (hic-cough), shwasa (asthma), visha (poisoning). In folklore, rasauth (rasanjana) is used in infections of eyelids and chronic ophthalmia, ulcers, periodic fever, diarrhea, jaundice, and skin diseases. Its watery solution is also used for washing piles, oriental sores, and glandular swellings (Anonymous 1988).

Therapeutic Uses

External Use

1. **Netraroga** (eye disease): Decoction of Daruharidra mixed with madhu (A.H.U. 16/8) or milk processed with Daruharidra and little saindhav lavan should be used for washing the inflamed eyes (S.S.U. 9/23). In anjannamika

(sty), the paste of rasanjana and trikatu is rubbed and applied locally (SG. 3/11/49).

2. **Pratishyay** (rhinitis/common cold): Dhumapana with the sticks of Daruharidra, Ingudi, Danti, Kinhi, and Tulsi is used (VM. 60/16).

3. **Visha** (poisoning): In case of poisoning, paste of Haridra and Daruharidra is applied locally on the affected part (G.N. 7/1/11).

4. **Updansha** (soft chancre): Paste of Rasanjana, Shirish, and Haritaki mixed with madhu should be applied (SG. 3/11/107).

Internal Use

1. **Mukhroga** (mouth disease): The dried extract of Daruharidra, i.e., rasanjana mixed with madhu and gairika is effective in mukhpaka, nadiroga, and vrana (A.H.U. 22/105) (VM. 58/81).

2. **Kushta** (skin disease): Bark decoction of Daruharidra, Khadira, and Nimba is used to alleviate kushta (A.H.Ci. 19/37) or decoction of Daruharidra and rasanjana is used in all forms like oral intake, for bathing, rubbing, dusting, ghrita, and tailapaka in kushta (C.S.Ci. 7/98).

3. **Shwetpradar** (leucorrhea): Decoction of Daruharidra mixed with madhu should be used followed by tandulodaka in shwetpradar (G.N. 6/1/24).

4. **Prameha** (diabetes): Daily intake of Darvi and Amalaki juice mixed with madhu alleviates all prameha (VD. 7/20).

5. **Kamala** (jaundice): Persons suffering from kamala roga should take cooled decoction of Triphala, Guduchi, and Darvi with madhu daily in the morning (C.S.Ci. 16/63).

6. **Vriddhi** (scrotal edema): Intake of Darvi paste with gomutra is recommended in kaphaja vriddhi roga (A.H.Ci. 13/33) (VM. 40/5).

7. **Mutrakricchta** (dysuria): Daruharidra with Amalaki swarasa mixed with madhu should be used in mutrakricchta due to aggravated pitta (C.S.Ci. 26/53).

Officinal Parts Used

Stem, root, fruit

Dose

Decoction: 50 to 100 mL
Rasanjana (crude extract): 1 to 3 g
Fruit: 5 to 10 g

Formulations

Bhringraj taila, Ashwagandharistha, Khadiradi gutika, Khadirarista, Triphala ghrita, Jatyadi taila.

Substitution and Adulteration:

Other species of Berberis, such as *B. asiatica, B. lycium, B. chitria,* are used as its substitute and adulterants. *Curcuma longa* (Haridra) is sometimes used as substitute. In South India and Sri Lanka, *Coscinium fenestratum* Colebr. is known and used as Daruharidra. Sometimes Haridra is used as its substitute (Sharma et al 2000; Balasubramani and Venkatasubramanian 2011).

> **Points to Ponder**
>
> - *The properties of Haridra and Daruharidra are analogous to each other and can be used in place of each other.*
> - *Rasanjana (crude extract of daruharidra) is specially used for inflammatory eye diseases and indolent ulcers.*

Suggested Readings

Anonymous. *The Wealth of India: Raw Materials*, Vol. 2B. New Delhi: Public Information Department, Council of Scientific & Industrial Research; 1988:114–118

Balasubramani SP, Venkatasubramanian P. Molecular identification and development of nuclear DNA its sequence based marker to distinguish *Coscinium fenestratum* gaertn. (Menispermaceae) from its adulterants. Curr Trends Biotechnol Pharm 2011;5:1163–1172

Bhakuni DS, Shoheb A, Popali SP. Medicinal plants: chemical constituent of *Berberis aristata*. Ind J Chem 1968;6(2):123

Chakarvarti KK, Dhar DC, Siddhiqui S. Alkaloidal constituent of the bark of *Berberis aristata*. J Scientific Industrial Res 1950;9b(7):161–164

Chauhan NS, Uniyal MR, Sannad BN. A preliminary study of the indigenous drug used at Tibetan medical centre, Dharamshala (H.P.). Nagarjuna 22; 1978/79:190–193

Chopra RN, Chopra IC, Handa KL, Kapoor LD. Indigenous drugs of India. Kolkata: UN Dhur and Sons; 1958:503

Jain N, Suri RK. Insecticidal, insect repellent and pesticidal plants of DehraDun. Nagarjuna 23; 1979/80:177–181

Kant BT, Biswapati M. Plant medicines of Indian origin for wound healing activity:a review. Int J Low Extremity Wounds 2003;2: 25–39

Mitra MP , Das S, Das S, Das KM. Phyto-pharmacology of *Berberis aristata* DC: a review. J Drug Deliv Ther 2011;1(2):46–50

Mittre V. Wild plants in Indian folk life: a historical perspective. In Jain SK (ed), Glimpses of Indian Ethnobotany. New Delhi: Oxford & IBH Publ. Co.; 1981:37–58

Sharma PC, Yelne MB, Dennis TJ. Database on Medicinal Plants Used in Ayurveda, Vol.1. New Delhi: CCRAS; 2000:121

Singh J, Kakkar P. Antihyperglycaemic and antioxidant effect of *Berberis aristata* root extracts and its role in regulating carbohydrate metabolism in diabetic rats. J Ethnopharmacology 2009;123: 22–26

Sohni YR, Kaimal P, Bhatt RM. The antiamoebic effect of a crude drug formulation of herbal extracts against *Entamoeba histolytica n vitro* and *in vivo*. J Ethnopharmacology 1995;45:43–52

Srivastava SK, Khatoon S, Rawat AK, Mahrotra S, Pushpangandan P. Pharmacognostical evaluation of the root of *Berberis aristata* DC. Nat Prod Sci 2001;7:102–106

The Ayurvedic Pharmacopeia of India. Part I, Vol. 2. New Delhi: Department of AYUSH, Ministry of Health and Family Welfare, Government of India; 2001:35

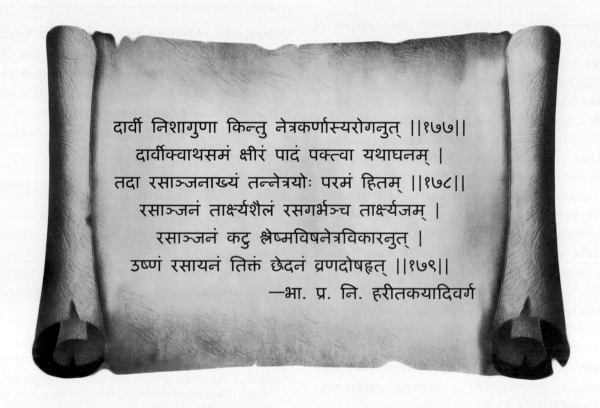

दार्वी निशागुणा किन्तु नेत्रकर्णास्यरोगनुत् ||१७७||
दार्वीक्वाथसमं क्षीरं पादं पक्त्वा यथाघनम् |
तदा रसाञ्जनाख्यं तन्नेत्रयोः परमं हितम् ||१७८||
रसाञ्जनं ताक्ष्यशैलं रसगर्भञ्च ताक्ष्यजम् |
रसाञ्जनं कटु श्लेष्मविषनेत्रविकारनुत् |
उष्णं रसायनं तिक्तं छेदनं व्रणदोषहृत् ||१७९||
—भा. प्र. नि. हरीतकयादिवर्ग

29. Devadaru *[Cedrus deodara (Roxb.) Loud]*

FFamily: *Pinaceae*

Hindi name: *Deodar, Diyar*

English name: *Himalayan Cedar, True Cedar*

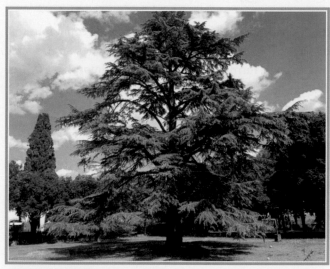

Plant of *Cedrus deodara* (Roxb.) Loud

> *Devadaru is crowned as the state tree of Himachal Pradesh and national tree of Pakistan.*

Introduction

The Sanskrit word "Devadaru" is derived from the phrase *Devanam daru iti* which means the wood of God. *Deva* means a divine deity and *Daru* cognate with the word *durum* meaning tree or wood. The name suggested that the tree is worshiped as a divine tree since ages. The generic name *Cedrus* is derived from Latin word "cedar" suggesting that the wood is having aroma like cedar tree.

Devadaru has great religious significance as the deodar forests were the favorite abode or living places of ancient Indian sages to perform meditation. Historically, its wood has been used for landscaping and construction of religious temples. In *Atharva veda* it is described by the name *Bhadra* and in *Kalpasutra* by *Daru*. It is also described in Shaunik Atharveda samhita, Paraskar grahsutra, Kaushik sutra, Patanjal mahabhapya, Ramayan, and Mahabharat (Singh. In Egyptian, Sumerian, and Tibetan culture, Devadaru oil is used as a preservative for embalming mummies. Charak has

advocated the use of Devadaru in hikka, shwasa, atisaar, and arsha for fumigation. Sushrut mainly used it for cleansing, healing (S.S.Su. 37/26), and fumigation (S.S.Su. 37/21) of nonhealing ulcers and wounds.

Devadaru is an economically important wood, as it is an ideal wood for making furniture, houseboats, instruments, storage rooms, or storage boxes for meat, food grains, etc. Its oil is used in cosmetics, soaps, perfumes, aromatherapy, incense sticks, insect repellant sprays, floor polishes, in herbal pesticides, insecticides, and as clearing oil in microscopes. The oldest Devadaru tree is of 745 years with 900 rings (Yadav and Bhattacharyya 1992).

Vernacular Names

Assamese: Shajar tuljeen
Bengali: Devdaroo
French: Cedre de l'himalaya
German: Himalaja-zeder

Gujarati: Devdar, Teliyo devdar

Italian: Cedro dell'Himalaia

Kannada: Deevdar, Bhadradaaru, Daevadaaru, Gunduguragi

Kashmiri: Dadar, Dar, Deodar, Diar

Malayalam: Devtaram, Devadaram

Marathi: Devdar, Telya dedaroo

Punjabi: Diyar, Dewdar

Spanish: Cedro del himalaya, Cedro de la India

Tamil: Devdaroo, Tevadaram, Tevadari

Telugu: Devdari chettu, Devdaree

Tibetan: Than sin, than-sin

Urdu: Deodar, Burada

Synonyms

Daru: It is the general term used for wood or tree.

Darubhadra: Its wood is considered as best among all the woods.

Darvendra: It is considered as the king of trees like Lord Indra the king of gods.

Druklim: Gum exudates from its stem.

Indradaru: The tree is favorite tree of Lord Indra.

Klim: Its wood is light in weight.

Mastdaru: The wood is highly efficacious.

Shakrapadapa: The tree is considered as the tree of Lord Indra.

Suravah: It is believed that God resides in this tree and it is the wood of God.

Surbhuruh: The wood is aromatic in nature.

Classical Categorization

Charak Samhita: Stanyashodhana, Anuvasanopaga, Katu skanda

Sushrut Samhita: Eladi, Vachadi, Vatasansamana

Ashtang Hridaya: Eladi, Rodhradi, Vidaryadi, Vataghna gana

Dhanvantari Nighantu: Guduchyadi varga

Madanpal Nighantu: Abhyadi varga

Kaiyadev Nighantu: Oushadi varga

Raj Nighantu: Chandanadi varga

Bhavaprakash Nighantu: Karpuradi varga

Distribution

Devadaru is the native plant of Western Himalayas, Eastern Afghanistan, Northern Pakistan, North East India, Tibet, and Nepal.

In India it is distributed from Kumoun to Sikkim up to an altitude of 1,000 to 3,600 m, especially in Himachal Pradesh, Uttarakhand, and Jammu and Kashmir.

Morphology

It is a beautiful, large, evergreen, long-living coniferous tree of 160 to 180 feet height or more. Branches spread with black, rough, furrowed bark. Shoots are dimorphic. The tree can live up to 600 years.

- **Leaves:** Triquetrous, acicular (needle shape), silver or silvery-green, sharp, 3 to 5 cm long closely arranged with pointed tips. Spirally arranged on larger branches and appears in bunches on younger branches (**Fig. 29.1**). It is a monoecious plant, i.e., male and female cones appear on separate branches of same tree or on separate trees. Cones are solitary and present at the end of branchlets.

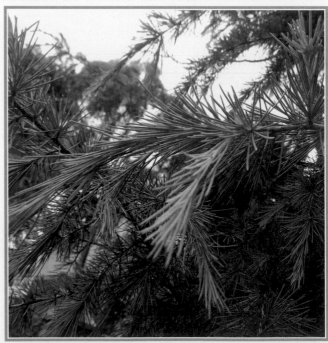

Fig. 29.1 Leaves.

- **Fruits:** Male cones are numerous, erect, solitary, pale green to yellowish-green with purplish tinge, oblong, ovoid cylindrical at the end of leaf, bearing branchlets (**Fig. 29.2a**), whereas female cones are barrel shaped, glaucous green, borne singly at the tip of dwarf shoots (**Fig. 29.2b**). Each cone is composed of imbricating thin, woody, placental scales, arranged spirally on a woody central axis. Each scale has a pair of pale brown winged seeds. Unripe cones are green, shiny, aromatic, whereas dried cones are brownish-black, hard, and woody (**Fig. 29.3a**). About 13 months are required from flowering to fruiting.

- **Heartwood:** Light, fragrant, strong, oily, yellowish-brown, and turning brown black on exposure. The oil is known as kanol oil. The plant is propagated through seeds (**Fig. 29.3b**).

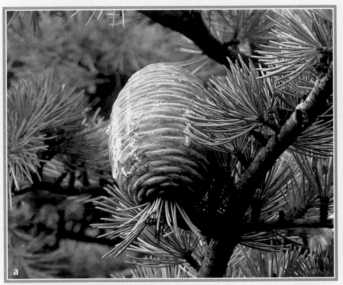

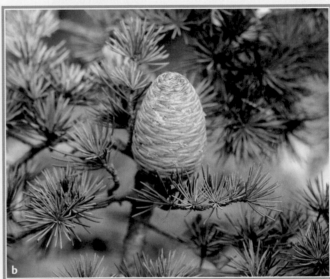

Fig.29.2 **(a)** Male cone. **(b)** Female cone.

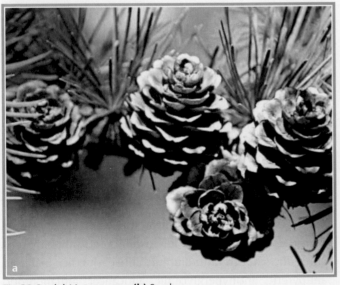

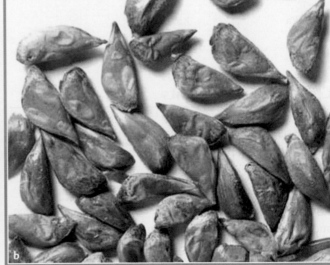

Fig 29.3 **(a)** Mature cone. **(b)** Seeds.

Phenology

Flowering time: September to October

Fruiting time: April to September

> **Key Characters for Identification**
>
> ➤ *A beautiful, evergreen, long-living coniferous tree of about 80 m*
> ➤ *Leaves: triquetrous, acicular, sharp pointed, silver green colored*
> ➤ *Male cones are numerous erect, oblong ovoid, pale to yellowish-green*
> ➤ *Female cones are barrel shaped and glaucous green*
> ➤ *Heartwood is light, aromatic, oily, and blackish-brown*

Types

- Raj Nighantu has described two types of Devadaru:
- Snigdhdaru
- Kasthadaru

Rasapanchaka

Guna	Laghu, Snigdh
Rasa	Tikta
Vipaka	Katu
Virya	Ushna

Chemical Constituents

The essential oil of Devadaru is reported to contain sequesterpenes I, II, III, α-himachalene, and β-himachalene (Gulati 1977), isohemacolon, deodarone, atlantone, isohimachalone, α-hemacolon (13%), β-hemacolon (43%), α-pinene, β-pinene, myrcene, cis-atlantone, α-atlantone, and sesquiterpene alcohols himachalol, allohimachalol, hemadarol, isocentdarol, centdarol (Kar et al 1975). It also contains α-terpineol, linalool, limonene, anethole, caryophyllene, and eugenol. The dried heartwood has matairesinol, nortrachelogenin, dibenzylbutyrolactollignan, wikstromal, benzylbutyrolactol, cedeodarin, dihydro-myricetin, cedrin, and cedrinoside (Agarwal et al 1980).

The leaves have dodecanoic acid, ethyl laurate, ethyl stearate, oleonolic acid, β-sitosterol, shickimic acid, methyl coniferin, ferulic acid, and β-glucoside.

Identity, Purity, and Strength

- Foreign matter: Not more than 1 %
- Total ash: Not more than 2 %
- Acid-insoluble ash: Not more than 1 %
- Alcohol-soluble extractive: Not less than 7 %
- Water-soluble extractive: Not less than 1.5 %

(Source: The Ayurvedic Pharmacopeia of India 2004)

Karma (Actions)

In Ayurvedic classics Devadaru is described as sugandhi (aromatic), krimighna (anthelmintic), kusthaghna (anti-dermatosis), vranashodhak (purifies wound), vranaropaka (wound healing), stanyashodhana (galacto purifier), vatahara (pacify vata), bhootaghna (antibacterial), shothahara (anti-inflammatory), vedanasthapana (anodyne), deepan (stomachics), hridyottejaka (cardiac stimulant), raktaprasadana (blood purifier), kaphanis-saraka (expectorant), shleshmaputihara (removes foul smell of phelgam), hikkanighrahana (antihic-cough), garbhashayashodhana (uterine purifier), and jwaraghna (antipyretic).

- Doshakarma: Vata kaphahara
- Dhatukarma: Stanyashodhana, Raktaprasadana, Vrana ropaka
- Malakarma: Mutral (diuretic), Swedal (diaphoretic)

Kanol oil is antiseptic, depurative, analgesic, diaphoretic, insecticidal, and diuretic in properties. Bark is astringent and leaves are thermogenic.

Pharmacological Actions

Several in vivo and in vitro studies have suggested that the heartwood and oil exhibit anti-inflammatory, antiseptic, expectorant, diuretic, antispasmodic, analgesic, antipyretic, antihyperglycemic, anticancer, antiapoptotic, antitubercular, immunomodulator, anxiolytic, anticon-vulsant, insecticidal antifungal, antibacterial, wound-healing, antiulcer, antiallergic, and antimalarial properties (Gupta et al 2011; Sharma et al 2018; Chaudhary et al 2011).

Indications

Various parts of the plant are used in the traditional system of medicines for the treatment of hikka (hic-cough), peenasa (rhinitis), kasa (cough), shwasa (asthma), vibandh (constipation), arsha (piles), adhyamaan (abdominal distension), shoth (edema), aamdosha (indigestion, tandra (giddiness), jwar (fever), prameha (diabetes), kandu (pruritus), krimi (worm infestation), kustha (skin diseases), raktadosha (bleeding disorders), sutikarog (puerperial diseases), and dustavrana (chronic wounds).

All parts of this plant are useful in curing diseases like inflammation, insomnia, cough, fever, urinary discharges, itching, tuberculosis, ophthalmic disorders, mental disorders, diseases of the skin and blood. The leaves are useful in inflammatory diseases and tubercular glands. The heartwood decoction is used in diabetes, cephalgia, arthritis, ascites, neuralgic pain, palsy, and insomnia.

Kanol oil is used in curing skin diseases, wounds, chronic nonhealing purulent ulcers, urogenital diseases, tuberculosis, joint pain, hair loss, and in nervous tensions (Sharma et al 2016).

Therapeutic Uses

External Use

1. **Shleepada** (filariasis): External application of paste of deodar and Chitraka is effective in shleepada (CD. 42/5).
2. **Galganda** (goitre): Paste of deodar and Vishala is effective in the treatment of gandmala of kaphaj origin (VM. 41/3).
3. **Vrana** (wounds): External application of Devadaru oil or paste of Devadaru and Sunthi enhances the healing power in wound and ulcers. Fumigation with Saral, Sarjrasa, Shriveshtaka, and Devadaru is also helpful (S.S.U. 39/204).
4. **Karnashool** (earache): One or two drops of lukewarm Dipika taila (prepared with Kushta, Devadaru, and Saral) should be instilled in ear to get relief in earache (S.S.U. 21/22).

Internal Use

1. **Kasa** (cough): Oil extracted from Devadaru wood added with Trikatu and Yavakshara should be given with honey in chronic cough (A.H.Ci. 3/40).

2. **Jwar** (fever): Devadaru decoction is recommended in fever associated with thirst (S.S.U. 39/204).
3. **Shotha** (edema): To reduce any type of edema, either Devadaru kwath mixed with Sunthi (S.S.Ci.23/12) or milk boiled with Devadaru, Punarnava, and Sunthi should be used daily (VM. 39/15).
4. **Vatarakta** (gout) and **Aamavaat**: Devdarvadi kwath is used twice daily to get relief in arthritis, gout, gonorrhea, syphilis, etc.
5. **Vatavyadhi** (neuromuscular disorders): Oral consumption of Devadaru and Sunthi powder reduces pain in vattik hridya roga. Devdarvadi kwath should be used in the treatment of vatavyadhi (BP.Ci. 24/22; B.S.vatavyadhi 61).
6. **Krimi** (worms): Oil of Devadaru or Saral is used to expel worms in krimi roga (A.H.Ci. 20/32).
7. **Kushta** (skin diseases): Oral intake of Devadaru oil and ghrita followed by diet of shali rice and dugdha cures all the skin diseases (RH/19/13).

Officinal Parts Used

Heartwood, oil, leaves

Dose

Powder: 3 to 6 g
Oil: 10 to 40 drops
Decoction: 50 to 100 mL

Formulations

Devdarvadi kwath, Devdarvadi churna, Devdarvaristha, Anu taila, Chandraparbha vati, Khadiraristha, Dashmoolarista, Mritasanjivanisura, Mahavishagarbha taila, Pradarantaka lauha.

Toxicity/Adverse Effects

Safety profile study showed nontoxic, nonirritant effect in rabbit and sheep and no alteration in blood urea nitrogen and blood glucose level (Mall et al 1985; Tandon et al 1989).

Substitution and Adulteration

In some parts of Uttarakhand *Pinus* species such as *P. excelsa* Wall. and *P. longifolia* Roxb. are used as substitute of Devadaru (Sharma et al 2001).

Points to Ponder

- *It is a high-altitude plant native to Western Himalayas.*
- *Devadaru is a renowned drug for dustavrana shodhana, vrana ropana, vatavyadhi, shotha, hikka, penasa, karnaroga, and kustha.*
- *Kanol oil is a potent antiseptic, depurative, diaphoretic, and insecticide.*

Suggested Readings

Agarwal PK, Agarwal SK, Rastogi RP. Dihyroflavonols from *Cedrus deodara*. Phytochemistry 1980;19:893–898

Chaudhary AK, Ahmad S, Mazumder A. *Cedrus deodara* (Roxb.) Loud.: a review on its ethnobotany, phytochemical and pharmacological profile. Pharmacogn J 2011;3(23):12–17

Gulati BC. Cultivation and utilization of aromatic plant. In: Atal CK, Kapur BM, et al. Jammu-Tawi, India: Regional Research Laboratory; 1977;640–652

Gupta S, Walia A, Malan R. Phytochemistry and pharmacology of *Cedrus deodera*: an overview. Int J Pharm Sci Res 2011;2(8):2010–2020

Kar K, Puri VN, Patnaik GK, et al. Spasmolytic constituents of *Cedrus deodara* (Roxb.) Loud: pharmacological evaluation of himachalol. J Pharm Sci 1975;64(2):258–262

Mall HV, Asthana A, Dubey NK, Dixit SN. Toxicity of cedar wood oil against some dermatophytes. Indian Drugs 1985;22(6):296

Sharma A, Parashar B, Vatsa E, Chandel S, Sharma S. World J Pharm Pharm Sci 2016;5(8):1618–1628

Sharma A, Prashar B, Arora P. *Cedrus deodara*: a medicinal herb. Der Pharma Chem 2018;10(4):6–10

Sharma PC, Yelne MB, Dennis TJ. Database on Medicinal Plants Used in Ayurveda. Vol. 7. New Delhi: Central Council for Research in Ayurveda and Siddha, Department of AYUSH, Ministry of Health and Family Welfare, Government of India; 2001:

Singh LP, Kamlesh T, Yadav RB, Yadav KN. Devadaru (*Cedrus deodara* (roxb.) Loud.): a critical review on the medicinal plant. Int J Ayur Pharma Res 2014;2(1):1–10

Tondon SK, Singh S, Gupta S, Chandra S, Jawahar L. Subacute dermal toxicity study of *Cedrus deodara* wood essential oil. Indian Vet J 1989;66(11):1088

The Ayurvedic Pharmacopeia of India. Part I, Vol. 4. New Delhi: Department of AYUSH, Ministry of Health and Family Welfare, Government of India; 2004:28

Yadav RR, Bhattacharyya A. A 745-year chronology of *Cedrus deodara* from Western Himalaya, India. Dendrochronologia 1992;10:53–61

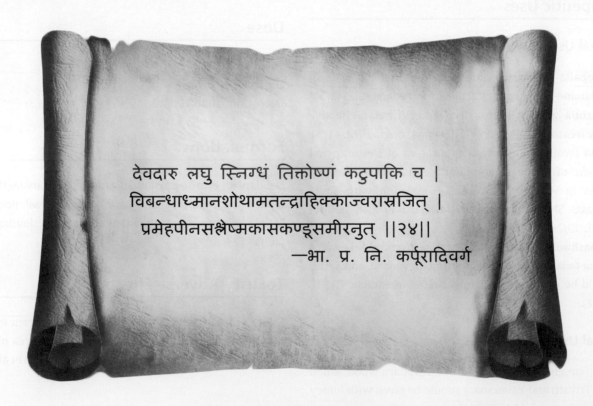

देवदारु लघु स्निग्धं तिक्तोष्णं कटुपाकि च ।
विबन्धाध्मानशोथामतन्द्राहिक्काज्वरास्रजित् ।
प्रमेहपीनसश्लेष्मकासकण्डूसमीरनुत् ॥२४॥
—भा. प्र. नि. कर्पूरादिवर्ग

30. Dhataki *[Woodfordia fruticosa* Linn. (Kurz)]

Family:	*Lythraceae*
Hindi name:	*Dhay, Dhay ke phool*
English name:	*Fire flame bush, Shiranji tea*

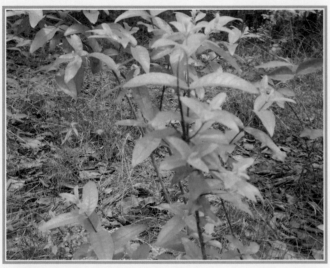

Plant of *Woodfordia fruticosa* Linn. (Kurz).

Dhataki is a well-known drug used in the preparation of asava and aristha.

Introduction

The word "Dhataki" in Sanskrit literally means which strengthens all the dhatu of the body and provides nourishment. The generic name of the plant honors a botanist E. James Alexander Woodford who for the first time successfully grew this plant to flowers (Graham 1995). The specie name *fruticosa* is derived from a Latin word "frutex" which means a shrub. It has two main species, namely, *W. fruticosa* and *W. uniflora* which are distributed in Asia and Africa, respectively. Though the plant is endemic to India, it is enlisted in the lower risk or least concern category of International Union for the Conservation of Nature (IUCN) Red List of Threatened Species.

In ancient texts Dhataki is a well-known drug used in the preparation of asava and aristha. It is used as prakshepa dravya in many classical formulations. Charak has kept it in pushpa asavayoni (C.S.Su 25/49). Kaiyadev nighantu has described its shaka as pathya in atisaar (K.D.N. 1074).

Yogaratnakara has described its flowers as substitute drug for Yashtimadhu. Besides, this is the plant that is much more popular in traditional folklore medicines and is used by tribal people for wound healing, dysmenorrhea, dysentery, diabetes fever, hemoptysis, rheumatism, and as disinfectant (Jeyaprakash et al 2011; Xavier et al 2012). The infusion of its flowers and leaves is used as a herbal tea.

Leaves are also used for enhancing milk production in livestock (Salave and Reddy 2012). The red pigment extracted from the flowers is used in perfumes, leather, and textile industries (Das et al 2007; Gaur 2008).

Vernacular Names

Assamese: Dhaiphool
Bengali: Dhaiphul, Dhai, Dawai
Farsi: Dhaava
Gujarati: Dhavadi, Dhavani
Kannada: Dhataki, Tamrapushpi

Kashmiri: Kath

Malayalam: Tattiripuvu, Tatire

Marathi: Dhayati, Dhavati, Dhalas

Nepali: Dhangera

Oriya: Dhaiphula, Dhatuki, Dhobo, Jaliko

Persian: Gule dhawa

Punjabi: Dhavi, Phul Dhava

Tamil: Kattati, Kattathi, Kattattipoo, Dhatari Jargi

Telugu: Aarl Puruvu, Sireenji

Urdu: Dhawa ke phool

Synonyms

Bahupushpi: The plant bears flowers profusely.

Dhatupushpi: The flower color resembles the color of ochre metal.

Kunjara: Nectar-rich flowers are regularly visited by insects for pollination.

Madahetu: The flowers are used in initiation of fermentation.

Madavaasini: The flowers are used to ferment alcoholic beverages (asava, aristha).

Parvatiya: The plant grows abundantly in hilly regions.

Subhiksha: The plant occurs abundantly.

Tamrapushpi: The flowers are coppery red in color.

Vahinjwala: The flowers are fire-red in color resembling the fire flame.

Classical Categorization

Charak Samhita: Sandhaniya, Purisha sangrahniya, Mutra viranjaniya

Sushrut Samhita: Priyangvadi, Ambashthadi

Ashtang Hridaya: Priyangvadi, Ambashthadi

Dhanvantari Nighantu: Chandanadi varga

Madanpal Nighantu: Abhyadi varga

Kaiyadev Nighantu: Oushadi varga

Raj Nighantu: Pippaliyadi varga

Bhavaprakash Nighantu: Haritakyadi varga

Distribution

The plant is distributed in countries of South East and East Asia like India, Sri Lanka, Pakistan, China, Japan, Malaysia, Indonesia, and in tropical Africa. It is found everywhere in lower mountainous regions of North and Eastern India up to an altitude of 1,500 to 3,000 ft. It is abundantly found in forest regions of Uttarakhand, Assam, Sikkim, Mizoram, West Bengal, and Gangetic plains (Kirtikar and Basu 1935).

Morphology

It is a much branched, deciduous shrub of about 3 to 5 m with long arching branches and fluted stem. Bark is smooth, cinnamon brown-colored, and peels off in fibers. Young shoots are terete and pubescent.

- **Leaves:** Simple, sessile, opposite to subopposite, ovate to lanceolate, 4 to 6 inches long, 2 to 3 inch width, entire margin, acute apex, subcoriaceous, upper surface smooth, pubescent, dark green, lower surface pubescent, glabrous, light green (**Fig. 30.1**).

- **Flowers:** Bright red, numerous, small about 1 to 2 cm long, occurs in dense paniculate-cymose clusters of 2 to 15 flowers, axillary, glabrous, ridged, bright red when fresh but fades on drying, six petals, superior ovary, style filiform, longer than ovary and stamen. Calyx long, tubular, striated, and covered with glandular dots (**Fig. 30.2–30.4**).

- **Fruits:** Small, ellipsoidal capsule, membranous, enclosed within the calyx tube, irregularly dehiscent. Seeds are numerous, minute, brown, obovoid shape, smooth, and shiny. The plant is propagated through seeds (Khare 2004; Sharma et al 2001).

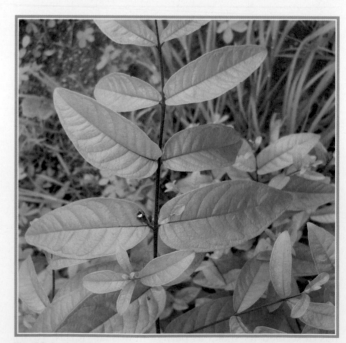

Fig. 30.1 Leaves.

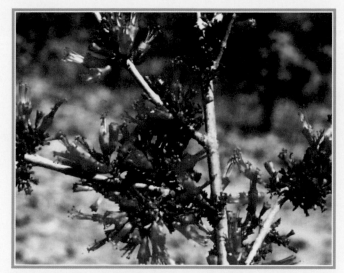

Fig. 30.2 Inflorescence.

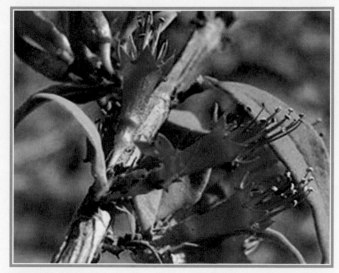

Fig. 30.3 Flower.

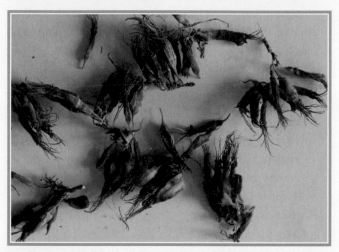

Fig. 30.4 Dry flower.

Phenology

Flowering time: April to June

Fruiting time: May to June

Key Characters for Identification

➤ *A branched deciduous shrub with fluted stem and brown bark*

➤ *Leaves simple, sessile, subopposite, ovate to lanceolate shape*

➤ *Flowers bright red, numerous occurs in dense cluster of 2 to 15*

➤ *Fruits small, ellipsoidal capsule with small brown, shiny seeds*

Rasapanchaka

Guna	Laghu, Ruksha
Rasa	Katu, Kashaya
Vipaka	Katu
Virya	Sheeta

Chemical Constituents

Major chemical compounds found in the leaves, flowers, and stem of Dhataki are tannins, woodfordins A, B, C D, E, F, G, H, I (Yoshida et al 1992), tellimagrandin, gemin D, heterophyllin A, oenothein B, steroids (hecogenin, meso-inositol), octacosanol, β-sitosterol, triterpenoids (lupeol, betulin, betulinic acid, urosolic acid), phenolic compounds (bergenin, gallic acid, ellagic acid), a naphthaquinone pigment lawsone and anthocyanidin pigment cyanidin 3,5-diglucoside. The flavonoid constituents include six quercetin glycosides, three myricetin glycosides, and kaempferol (Chauhan et al 1979; Dan and Dan 1984; Desai et al 1971; Nair et al 1976).

Identity, Purity, and Strength

- Foreign matter: Not more than 2%
- Total ash: Not more than 10%
- Acid-insoluble ash: Not more than 1%
- Alcohol-soluble extractive: Not less than 7%

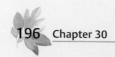

- Water-soluble extractive: Not less than 28%
(Source: The Ayurvedic Pharmacopeia of India 1989)

Karma (Actions)

Ayurvedic classics describe it as a drug possessing madakrita (induces delerium), vishaghna (antidote), garbhasthapaka (maintains pregnancy), sangrahik (astringent), krimighna (anthelmintic), raktasravarodhaka (hemostatic), vrana-shodhaka (wound purifier), and vrana ropaka (wound healer) properties.

- Doshakarma: Kapha pitta shamaka
- Dhatukarma: Vranaropaka, garbhasthapaka
- Malakarma: Malasangrahi

Pharmacological Actions

Its flowers have also been reported to have antibacterial, antimicrobial, anti-inflammatory, antifertility, antiulcer, antioxidant, DNA topoisomerase inhibitor, antihyperglycemic, hepatoprotective, cardioprotective, immunomodulatory, antitumor (Muvel et al 2014), anthelminthic (Kumar et al 2016), antipsoriatic (Srivastava et al 2016), and antiasthmatic activities (Murali et al 2006).

Indications

In traditional medicines it is widely prescribed in the treatment of trishna (thirst), jwar (fever), raktaatisar (diarrhea), raktapitta (internal hemorrhage), raktarsha (bleeding piles), visha (poisoning), krimi (worm infestation), kushta (skin disease), visarp (erysepalas), pravahika (dysentery), shwet pradar (leucorrhea), ashrigdhar (menorrhagia), vrana, asthibhagna (fracture), balroga (diseases of children), balgraha (evil spirits affecting children), yonivyapada (diseases related to female genital organs), abhishyandi (channel blocker), agnidadha (burn), karna roga (ear diseases), mukharoga (diseases of mouth), prameha (diabetes), urustambha (stiffness of thigh), and vidridhi (abscess).

Tribal people in Chhattisgarh use its dried flowers' powder in otorrhea and fresh flowers to arrest bleeding in wounds and cuts (Oudhia 2003). Leaves of dhataki are used as a folk medicine in India and Nepal for fever. Tribals in Beed district of Maharashtra used its flowers as antidiabetic agent. Flower-based preparation is a popular remedy for infertility (Das et al 2007).

Therapeutic Uses

External Use

1. **Svrana bhagna** (fracture with wound): The wounded area at the fracture site is dusted with the powders of Lodhra, Priyangu, Dhataki, Katphala, and Lajjalu to prevent bleeding and to enhance healing. Panchvalkal kwath mixed with Dhataki, Lodhra, and Badar can also be used for wound cleansing (C.S.Ci. 25/66-67).
2. **Netrabhishyandi** (conjunctivitis): Churna or swarasa of Chandana and Dhataki mixed with breast milk is used as collyrium in pittaja netrabhishyandi (S.S.U. 10/9).
3. **Kushta** (skin diseases): Paste prepared with Lodhra, Dhataki, Indrayava, Karanj, and Malti pushpa should be applied locally as ointment in kushta (C.S.Ci. 7/95).

Internal Use

1. **Rakta pitta** (hemorrhage): Powder of dried flowers in curdled milk is used in treating bleeding disorders, hemorrhage, thirst, diarrhea and dysentery, poisoning, piles, and burning sensation. Paste of Dhataki flowers with coconut oil gives relief in burns.
2. **Garbhajanan** (for conception): So as to conceive one should consume Nilotphala and Dhataki pushpa with madhu every morning in season (G.N. 6/5/9).
3. **Atisaar** (diarrhea): Dhataki pushpa mixed with Badar leaves, Kapitha juice, Lodhra twak, and madhu when consumed daily with curd reduces the frequency of stool in diarrhea and dysentery (B.P.Ci. 2/120). Intake of liquid gruel processed with Dhataki decoction and Sunthi added with Dadima is useful in jwar, atisaar, and shool (B.S.atisaar/318).
4. **Shwet pradar** (leucorrhea): Intake of Dhataki powder with honey checks white discharge in shweta pradar (VM. 63/4). In rakta pradar, Dhataki powder is used with rice water.
5. **Prameha** (diabetes): To restore normal color of urine and to combat thirst, Dhataki flower decoction is used in diabetes.
6. **Prolapse:** Decoction of Dhataki pushpa is used in uttarbasti for treating vaginal and anal prolapse. Dhataki

pushpa avleha is also given in menstrual pain and menorrhagia.

Officinal Part Used

Flowers

Dose

Powder: 1 to 3 g

Formulations

Pushyanuga churna, Dhatkayadi churna, Ashokaristha, Dhatkayadi taila, Laghugangadhara churna, Kutajashtaka churna, Arvindasava.

Toxicity/Adverse Effect

Not reported yet.

Substitution and Adulteration

Dhataki pushpa is used as the substitute of Yashtimadhu (B.P./158).

> ### Points to Ponder
>
> - *Dhataki pushpa is an important constituent for initiation of fermentation in asava and aristha.*
> - *Dhataki pushpa is well known for the treatment of diarrhea, ulcers, wounds, menorrhagia, fever, prolapse, and bleeding disorders in folk medicines.*

Suggested Readings

Charters ML. Fruticosa: California Plant Names: Latin and Greek Meanings and Derivations. A Dictionary of Botanical and Biographical Etymology. Available at: http://www.calflora.net/botanicalnames/pageF.html. Accessed on November 21, 2013

Chauhan JS, Srivastava SK, Srivastava SD. Chemical constituents of the flowers of *Woodfordia fruticosa* Linn. J Indian Chem Soc 1979;56:1041

Dan S, Dan SS. Chemical examination of the leaves of *Woodfordia fruticosa*. J Indian Chem Soc 1984;61:726–727

Das PK, Goswami S, Chinniah A, et al. Woodfordia fruticosa: traditional uses and recent findings. J Ethnopharmacol 2007;110(2):189–199

Desai HK, Gawad DH, Govindachari TR, et al. Chemical investigation of some Indian plants. VI. Indian J Chem 1971;9:611–613

Gaur RD. Traditional dye yielding plants of Uttarakhand, India. Nat Prod Radiance 2008;7(2):154–165

Graham SA. Systematics of *Woodfordia* (Lythraceae). Syst Bot 1995; 20(4):482–502

Jeyaprakash K, Ayyanar M, Geetha KN, Sekar T. Traditional uses of medicinal plants among the tribal people in Theni District (Western Ghats), Southern India. Asian Pac J Trop Biomed 2011; 1(1):S20–S25

Khare CP. Encyclopedia of Indian Medicinal Plants: Rational Western Therapy, Ayurvedic and Other Traditional Usage, Botany. Berlin: Springer; 2004:483–484

Kirtikar KR, Basu BD. Indian Medicinal Plants, Parts 1–3. Allahabad: L.M. Publications, Allahabad; 1935

Kumar D, Sharma M, Sorout A, Saroha K, Verma S. *Woodfordia fruticosa* Kurz.: a review on its botany, chemistry and biological activities. J Pharmacogn Phytochem 2016;5(3):293–298

Murali PM, Rajasekaran S, Krishnarajasekar OR, et al. Plant-based formulation for bronchial asthma: a controlled clinical trial to compare its efficacy with oral salbutamol and theophylline. Respiration 2006;73(4):457–463

Nair AGR, Kotiyal JP, Ramesh P, Subramanian SS. Polyphenols of the flowers and leaves of *Woodfordia fruticosa*. Indian J Pharm 1976;38(4):110–111

Oudhia P. Interaction with the Herb Collectors of Gandai Region, Chhatisgarh, MP, India; 2003

Salave AP, Reddy PG. Documentation of traditional knowledge on fodder uses by the native Inhabitants in Beed District (M.S.) India. Life Sci Leafl 2012;9:24–34

Sharma PC, Yelne MB, Dennis TJ. Database on Medicinal Plants Used in Ayurveda. Vol. 3. New Delhi: Central Council for Research in Ayurveda and Siddha, Department of AYUSH, Ministry of Health and Family Welfare, Government of India; 2001:206–216

Srivastava AK, Nagar HK, Chandel HS, Ranawat MS. Antipsoriatic activity of ethanolic extract of *Woodfordia fruticosa* (L.) Kurz flowers in a novel *in vivo* screening model. Indian J Pharmacol 2016;48(5):531–536

The Ayurvedic Pharmacopeia of India. Part I, Vol. 1. New Delhi: Department of AYUSH, Ministry of Health and Family Welfare, Government of India; 1989:44

Uday M, Kishor D, Ajay R. A pharmacognostic and pharmacological overview on *Woodfordia fruticosa* Kurz. Scholars Acad J Pharm 2014;3(5):418–422

Xavier F, Arun VR, Rose F. Ethnopharmacological studies on the medicinal plants used by tribal inhabitants of Meenagadi region in Wayanadu district of Kerala, South India. Int J Med Plant Res 2012;1:58–62

Yoshida T, Chou T, Nitta A, Okuda T. Tannins and related polyphenols of Lythraceous plants. III. Hydrolyzable tannin oligomers with macrocyclic structures, and accompanying tannins from *Woodfordia fruticosa* Kurz. Chem Pharm Bull (Tokyo) 1992;40(8): 2023–2030

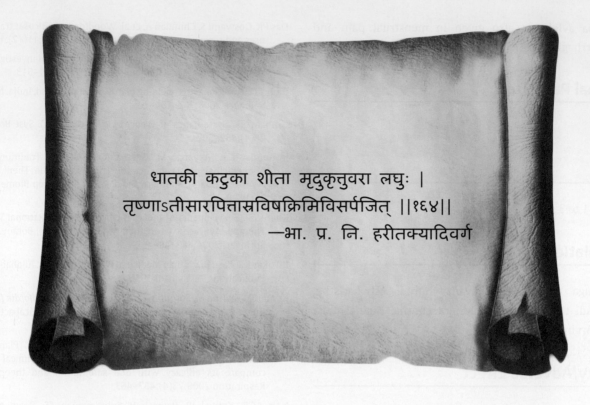

धातकी कटुका शीता मृदुकृतुवरा लघुः |
तृष्णाऽतीसारपित्तास्त्रविषक्रिमिविसर्पजित् ||१६४||
—भा. प्र. नि. हरीतक्यादिवर्ग

31. Durva *[Cynodon dactylon Linn. Pers.]*

Family:	*Poaceae*
Hindi name:	*Doob, Dhub*
English name:	*Couch grass, Bermuda grass, Creeping Cynodon, Bahama grass, Devil's grass, Dog's teeth grass*

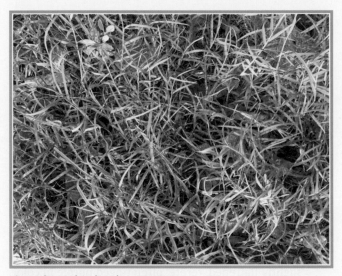

Plant of *Cynodon dactylon* Linn. Pers.

> *Durva is originally from the savannas of Africa and is known as Bermuda grass in the United States because it was introduced there from the Bermuda Island.*

Introduction

The word "Durva" in Sanskrit means which is cut or eaten by animals. The generic name is derived from a Greek word *kuon*, meaning dog, and *odous*, meaning a tooth referring to the sharp teeth of the glumes, while the specific name is derived from *daktulos*, meaning a finger, which refers to its digitate inflorescence (Paul et al 2012).

Durva is considered as the most sacred herb (next to Tulsi) by the Hindus. It is a symbol of purity, prosperity, and fertility. In many parts of India, a ceremony known as Durva ashtami is celebrated in bhadrapada, Krishna ashtami (September–October), in which Durva is offered to Lord Ganesha. Its leaves are used extensively to worship Lord Ganesha on Ganesh Chaturthi and in many other rituals. Hindus believe that Lord Brahma resides in its roots, Lord Vishnu in the middle part, and Lord Shiva at the tip. It is also among the ten auspicious herbs that constitute the group dashapushpa (Sindhu et al 2009).

Charak mentioned Durva in varnya mahakashaya (drugs under complexion promoter group) under the name of Sita and Lata, which Chakrapani has considered as shwet and shyama Durva, respectively (C.S.Su. 4/8). Sushrut has used Durva as paste in pittasopha, as anupana for katu dravya (S.S.Su. 46/432) in a yoga for medha budhi bala vardhanam (S.S.Sh. 10/69-70), and in the treatment of shukrameha. Sushrut also used shatvirya and sahastravirya in mutraghatva and vrana chikitsa. Dalhana considered sahastravirya as shwet Durva and shatvirya as neel Durva or Shatavari. Durva as a whole is of immense medicinal value and has ample use both externally and internally in therapeutics.

The plant invades other habitat easily and becomes hard to eradicate. Due to its weedy nature, it is often known as Devil's grass. It also plays an important role in soil conservation, provides good grazing grass for cattle, and is used in fermentation process to make beer soup (Raghunathan and Mitra 1982).

Vernacular Names

Bengali: Durva, Dub, Dubla, Durba, Doorva, Neel Doorva
French: Chiendent pied-de-poule, Cynodon dactyle
German: Bermudagras, Hundezahngras
Gujarati: Khadodhro, Lilidhro, Dhro, Dhrokad, Gharo
Italian: Gramina
Kannada: Garike Hullu, Kudigarike, Kudigarikai
Malayalam: Koruka Pullu
Marathi: Doorva, Hariyalee, Harlee, Karala
Portuguese: Capim-Bermuda
Punjabi: Dubada, Daurva, Dun, Dubra, Khabbal, Tilla, Talla, Dhub
Spanish: Grama rastrera, Zacate de Bermuda
Swedish: Hundtandsgräs
Tamil: Aruvam Pullu, Hariali, Muyalphul, Arugam Pullu
Telugu: Garika, Pacchgaddi, Ghericha, Garicagaddi, Gerike, Harvali
Urdu: Doob Ghas, Doob

Synonyms

Golomi: It bears linear-shaped leaves that resemble cow's hairs.
Shatvirya: The plant is efficacious in hundreds of ailments.
Shahastravirya: The plant is used to cure thousands of diseases.
Shatavalli: The plant bears hundreds of roots.
Shatparvika: It has many nodes and internodes.
Bhargavi: It is the favorite plant of sage Bhargava
Ananta: It spreads extensively over the ground
Ruha: It regenerates easily by stem cutting and spreads fast on the ground
Pratanika: The plant spreads out extensively

Classical Categorization

Charak Samhita: Varnya, Prajasthapana
Sushrut Samhita: Pittasansamana
Ashtang Hridaya: Pittanashak gana
Dhanvantari Nighantu: Karviradi varga
Madanpal Nighantu: Abhyadi varga
Kaiyadev Nighantu: Oushadi varga
Raj Nighantu: Shalmalyadi varga
Bhavaprakash Nighantu: Guduchyadi varga

Distribution

Durva is a native plant of Africa and is now widely distributed throughout the world in temperate and subtropical regions. Throughout India it is available as a weed in open wastelands, lawns, parks, residential houses, etc.

Morphology

It is a prostrate, creeping, glabrous, highly branched perennial stoloniferous herb with rhizomes rooting at every node.

- **Stem:** Creeping, erect, branched, 20 to 30 cm long, slightly flattened, terete, often tinged purple in color. In winter it becomes dormant and turns brown colored (**Fig. 31.1**).
- **Leaves:** Gray green, narrow, linear, about 2 to 15 cm long, 4 mm broad, soft, smooth, distichous at the base, flat to slightly keeled, edges rough, tip sharp, ligule with ring of hairs or membrane (**Fig. 31.2**).
- **Flowers:** Inflorescence terminal spikes, green or purplish, 2 to 5 cm long, flowers spikelet with one perfect floret. Spikelets are arranged in two alternating

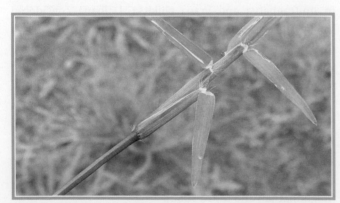

Fig. 31.1 Stem.

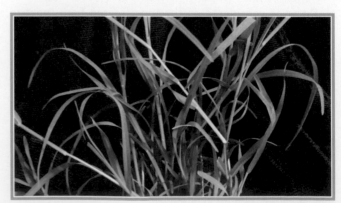

Fig. 31.2 Leaves.

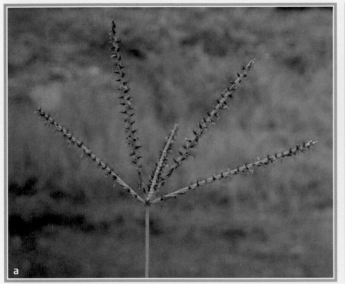
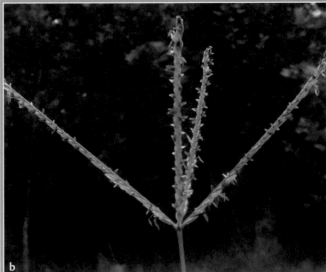

Fig. 31.3 **(a)** Inflorescence. **(b)** Flowers.

series on the rachis. Two glume, lower glume smaller than the upper one (**Fig. 31.3a, b**).

- **Fruits:** Grains, oblong, about 1 cm long, laterally compressed. Seed ovoid, yellow to red in color. The plant is propagated by stem and root cuttings.
- **Roots:** Thread like thin, pale white roots, cylindrical and tapering root (**Fig. 31.4**; Billore et al 2004).

Phenology

Flowering time: Throughout the year
Fruiting time: Throughout the year

Key Characters for Identification

➤ It is a perennial, branched prostrate herb rooting at every node
➤ Leaves: linear, greenish-gray distichous at the base
➤ Flowers: green or purple inflorescence of terminal spikes
➤ Fruits are laterally compressed oblong grains

Types

Dhanvantari and Bhavaprakash Nighantu have described its three varieties:

- Shwet Durva
- Neel Durva
- Ganda Durva

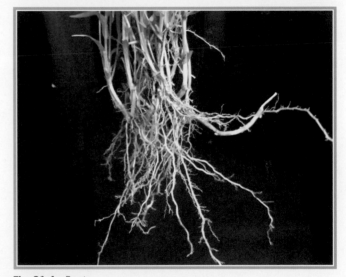

Fig. 31.4 Roots.

Rasapanchaka

Guna	Laghu
Rasa	Tikta, Madhur, Kashaya
Vipaka	Madhur
Virya	Sheeta

Chemical Constituents

The whole plant mainly contains proteins, carbohydrate, β-sitosterol, carotene, oxides of calcium, magnesium, phosphorous, potassium, alkaloid-ergonovine and ergono-vinine, cyanogenic hyperoside, cyanogenic glucoside (triglochinin), triterpenoids, methoxy propionic acid, phytol benzoic acid, vitamin C, arundoin, friedelin, selenium, *p*-coumaric, vanilic, furfural, *p*-hydroxybenzoic, *o*-hydroxyphenyl acetic acids, furfuryl alcohol, phenyl acetaldehyde, acetic acid, β-ionone, lignin and palmitic acid. The aerial parts contain tritriacontane esters, eicosanoic, docosanoic acids, hexadecanal, hexadecanoic acid, flavones (apigenin, luteolin), flavone glycosides orientin, vitexin, and iso-vitexin (Paranjpe 2001; Asthana et al 2012).

Identity, Purity, and Strength

For Root

- Foreign matter: Not more than 2%
- Total ash: Not more than 7%
- Acid-insoluble ash: Not more than 3%
- Alcohol-soluble extractive: Not less than 1%
- Water-soluble extractive: Not less than 5%

(Source: The Ayurvedic Pharmacopeia of India 2001)

For the Whole Plant

- Foreign matter: Not more than 2%
- Total ash: Not more than 9%
- Acid-insoluble ash: Not more than 4.5%
- Alcohol-soluble extractive: Not less than 3%
- Water-soluble extractive: Not less than 9.5%

(Source: The Ayurvedic Pharmacopeia of India 2004)

Karma (Actions)

In traditional system of medicine it is considered as jeevaniya (nutrient), varnya (improves complexion), prajasthapana (procreants), jwarghna, raktaprasadani, rochak, raktapittahara, shramhara, vranaropana, dahaprasamana, raktashodhaka, chardighna, triptida, vishaghna, and raktastambhaka.

- Doshakarma: Kapha pitta hara
- Dhatukarma: Jeevaniya, raktastambhaka
- Malakarma: Mutral

Pharmacological Actions

The plant also shows biological activities like antibacterial, analgesic, antipyretic, antioxidant, chemopreventive, anti-inflammatory, diuretic, antidiabetic, immunomodulator, hepatoprotective, antiulcer, hyperglycemic, antiarrhythmic, wound healing, CNS depressant, anticonvulsant, and cardio-protective (Al-Snafi 2016; Das et al 2013).

Indications

In Ayurveda classics Durva is used for the treatment of rakta shrava (hemorrhages), visarp (erysipelas), jwar (fever), shotha (inflammation), vicharchika (scabies), trishna (thirst), daha (burning sensation), twak amaya (skin diseases), kandu (itching), aruchi (dyspepsia), vaman (emesis), murcha (fainting), grahabadha, raktapitta (bleeding disorders), rakta atisaar (diarrhea with blood), rajyakshma (tuberculosis), hematuria (urinary bleeding), vrana (ulcers), shirashool (headache), and for garbhasthapana (to maintain pregnancy).

Durva is a popular folk remedy for calculus, dropsy, hemorrhage, urogenital disorders, cough, headache, sores, cancer, carbuncles, convulsions, cramps, diarrhea, dysentery, epilepsy, piles, leucoderma, hypertension, hysteria, tumors, measles, rubella, snakebite, warts, wounds, weak vision, and dandruff. The expressed juice of plant is applied to cuts and wounds to arrest bleeding in day-to-day practice. Its juice or paste mixed with honey is used in epistaxis. Oral administration of its juice with honey two to three times a day is an effective remedy of menorrhagia. Its decoction mixed with sugar is useful in treating urinary retention (Chopra et al 1999; Rajakumar and Shivanna 2009; Saikia et al 2006).

Therapeutic Uses

External Use

1. **Shitapitta** (urticaria): External application of Durva paste with Haridra gives relief in eczema, urticaria, scabies, ringworm, erysipelas, and infections (VM. 52/6).

Oil cooked with Durva swaras can also be used for the same (VM. 51/135).

2. **Nasagata raktapitta** (epistaxis): Fresh juice of Durva installed as nasal drops prevents ·nasal bleeding in epistaxis (C.S.Ci. 5/).

3. **Raktarsha** (bleeding piles): Local application of ointment of ghrita cooked with Durva and washed hundred or thousand times checks bleeding in arsha (C.S.Ci. 14/219).

Internal Use

1. **Raktapitta** (internal hemorrhage): One should take Durva swarasa, Vata patra, and white variety of Girikarnika mixed with honey (S.S.U. 45/20).

2. **Vrana** (wound/ulcers): Oil prepared with Durva swaras and kalka of Darvi twak is good remedy for non-healing ulcers and wounds (C.S.Ci. 25/93; VM. 45/28).

3. **Chardi** (vomiting): Durva swaras when taken with Tandulodaka checks vomiting (G.N. 2/14/30).

4. **Amalpitta**: Daily intake of 1 to 2 tsf Durva swaras mixed with mishri or coconut water gives tremendous relief in sour belching, hyperacidity, and burning sensation.

5. **Garbhasthapaka:** Daily consumption of Durva swarasa with dugdh or ghrita is prescribed to check uterine bleeding, strengthen uterus, prevent abortions, and to augment fetal growth (C.S.Sh. 8/20).

Officinal Parts Used

Whole plant and root

Dose

Juice: 10 to 20 mL

Formulations

Durvadhya ghrita, Durvadi kwath, Durvadi taila.

Toxicity/Adverse Effects

The study of the toxicity of Durva's aqueous extracts was found safe and no mortality was reported up to a dose of 4,000 mg/kg in rats (Garg and Paliwal 2011).

Substitution and Adulteration

None.

Points to Ponder

- *Durva is an easily available, economical, and a highly potential home remedy to cure multiple ailments.*
- *It is a renowned medicine for maintaining pregnancy, treating bleeding disorders, skin diseases, thirst, wound, and urinary tract infections.*

Suggested Readings

Al-Snafi AE. Chemical constituents and pharmacological effects of *Cynodon dactylon:* a review. IOSR J Pharm 2016;6(7):17–31

Ashokkumar K, Selvaraj K, Muthukrishnan SD. *Cynodon dactylon* [L.] Pers.: an updated review of its phytochemistry and pharmacology. J Med Plants Res 2013;7(48):3477–3483

Asthana A, Kumar A, Gangwar S, Dora J. Pharmacological perspectives of *Cynodon dactylon.* Res J Pharm Biol Chem Sci 2012;3(2):1135–1147

Billore KV, Yelne MB, Dennis TJ, Chaudhari BG. Database on Medicinal Plants Used in Ayurveda, Vol. 6. New Delhi: Central Council for Research in Ayurveda and Siddha; 2004:38–54

Chopra RN, Nayar SL, Chopra IC. Council of Scientific and Industrial Research (CSIR). 1st ed. New Delhi: Council of Scientific and Industrial Research (CSIR); 1999:88–89

Das M, Shama S, Chandra S. Overview of *Cynodon dactylon* (doob grass) in modern medicine as antidiabetic herb. J Drug Deliv Ther 2013;3(6):117–120

Garg VK, Paliwal SK. Anti-inflammatory activity of aqueous extract of *Cynodon dactylon.* Int J Pharmacol 2011;7(3):1–6

Paranjpe P. Durva in Indian Medicinal Plants: Forgotten Healers. 1st ed. Delhi: Chaukhambha Sanskrit Pratishtan; 2001:75–76

Paul R, Mandal A, Kumar Dutta A. An updated overview on *Cynodon dactylon*(L.). Pers. Int J Res Ayurv Pharm 2012;3(1):11–14

Raghunathan K, Mitra R. Pharmacognosy of Indigenous Drugs, Vol. 1. New Delhi: Central Council for Research in Ayurveda and Siddha; 1982:41–50

Rajakumar N, Shivanna MB. Ethno-medicinal application of plants in the eastern region of Shimoga District, Karnataka, India. J Ethnopharmacol 2009;126(1):64–73

Saikia AP, Ryakala VK, Sharma P, Goswami P, Bora U. Ethnobotany of medicinal plants used by Assamese people for various skin ailments and cosmetics. J Ethnopharmacol 2006;106(2):149–157

Sindhu G, Ratheesh M, Shyni GL, Helen A. Inhibitory effects of *Cynodon dactylon* L. on inflammation and oxidative stress in adjuvant treated rats. Immunopharmacol Immunotoxicol 2009;31(4):647–653

The Ayurvedic Pharmacopeia of India. Part I, Vol. 3. New Delhi: Department of AYUSH, Ministry of Health and Family Welfare, Government of India; 2001:47

The Ayurvedic Pharmacopeia of India. Part I, Vol. 4. New Delhi: Department of AYUSH, Ministry of Health and Family Welfare, Government of India; 2004:34

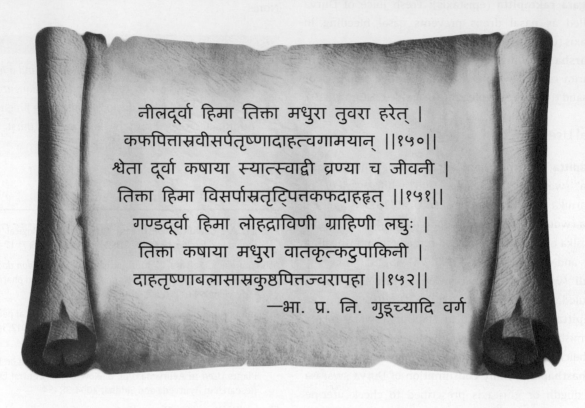

नीलदूर्वा हिमा तिक्ता मधुरा तुवरा हरेत् |
कफपित्तास्रवीसर्पतृष्णादाहत्वगामयान् ||१५०||
श्वेता दूर्वा कषाया स्यात्स्वाद्वी व्रण्या च जीवनी |
तिक्ता हिमा विसर्पास्रतृट्पित्तकफदाहहृत् ||१५१||
गण्डदूर्वा हिमा लोहद्राविणी ग्राहिणी लघुः |
तिक्ता कषाया मधुरा वातकृत्कटुपाकिनी |
दाहतृष्णाबलासास्रकुष्ठपित्तज्वरापहा ||१५२||

—भा. प्र. नि. गुडूच्यादि वर्ग

32. Ela [Elletaria cardamomum Maton]

Family: *Scitamineae*

Hindi name: *Choti ilayachi*

English name: *Lesser Cardamom, Gujarat Cardamom, True Cardamom*

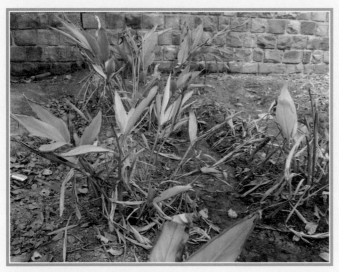

Plant of *Elettaria cardamom* Maton.

> In India, cardamom grows naturally in abundance on a mountain range of southern part of Western Ghats, located in southeast Kerala and southwest Tamil Nadu. Due to extensive plantation of cardamom, the area is known as Cardamom hills or Yela mala.

Introduction

Ela dvay includes Shukshm Ela (*Elleteria cardamomum* Maton) and Brihat Ela (*Amomum subulatum* Roxb.). (For more details, refer to Chapter 23: Brihat Ela.)

The word Ela in Sanskrit means the one that energizes the body. The generic name is derived from a Tamil word *elattari*, which means the seed of *Elam* (cardamom) (Mahindru 1982).

Ela is well known for its medicinal and culinary use since centuries. After saffron and vanilla, it is the third most expensive and widely used spice of the world. Ancient Greek and Egyptians used it for medicinal purposes, rituals, embalming the dead, and as a flavoring ingredient in tea and coffee. Ela seeds are chewed by people to cleanse their teeth and to freshen their breath (Ajarem and Ahmad 1991). The Arabians used it in preparing their traditional coffee called "Gahwa," which is offered to guests as a symbol of their hospitality. The Greeks and Romans used it in perfumes, food, and medicines. In South Asia and South East Asia, it is an ingredient in betel nut chewing.

Besides being an important dietary constituent, it has immense pharmacological benefits too. Ela is mentioned in Atharva Veda for bathing in a specific Nakshtara (Sastry 2014). In Matsya purana, it is described as a constituent of antivenom drug. Sushruta includes it in the group of drugs used for rubbing the skin during bloodletting whereas Charak used it in the treatment of respiratory diseases. It is used as an awaap or prakshepa dravya (additive) in many classical formulations and in preparation of basti (C.S.Si. 10/15). Vagabhatta has quoted Ela as an anupana dravya for Virechana yogas (A.H.Ka. 2/62). It is included in the famous groups of medicine called trijaat and chaturjaat. In classical texts of Ayurveda, two types of Ela, i.e., Sukshma and Brihat are described but the properties and actions of both types are similar. Owing to its versatile health benefits, it is rightly known as the "Queen of Spices."

The dried seeds are used as a flavoring agent in tea, coffee, cakes, curries, confectionaries, custards, meat products, wines, and liqueurs (Ebru et al 2013). The seed oil is used in aromatherapy, perfumes, cosmetics, and fumigation.

Vernacular Names

Arabian: Qaqilah, Hel, Hel-bava, Shoshmir
Assamese: Sarooplaachi
Bengali: Chota elaich, Ilachi
Gujarati: Elchi, Elachi, Elayachi
Kannada: Elakki, Sanna yalakki,Yerakki
Kashmiri: Kath, Aalbuduaal
Malayalam: Elam, Chittelam, Elathari, Yelam
Marathi: Velloda, Lahanveldoda, Velchi
Oriya: Chotaa leicha, Alaicha
Persian: Kakilahe – khurd
Punjabi: Illachi, Chhoti Lachi, Elchi
Sinhalese: Enasal
Tamil: Siruelam, Yellakai, Elam, Ellakay
Telugu: Chinne elakulu, Sanna elakulu, Elaki chettu, Ellaay, Vittula
Urdu: Heel Khurd

Synonyms

Sukshma: It is the smaller variety of Ela and is smaller in size.
Upkunchika: It is sukshma in property and gets easily distributed in the body.
Tutha: It pacifies doshas or gives relief in painful condition or roga.
Korangi: It grows in Koranga desha.
Dravadi: It grows abundantly in southern India.
Truti: It pacifies kapha dosha.

Classical Categorization

Charak Samhita: Shwashara, Angamardaprashmana, Shirovirechanopaga, Katuskanda
Sushrut Samhita: Eladi
Ashtang Hridaya: Eladi, Anjanadi, Vatsakadi, Trijataka, Chaturjataka
Dhanvantari Nighantu: Shatpushpadi varga
Madanpal Nighantu: Karpuradi varga
Kaiyadev Nighantu: Oushadi varga

Raj Nighantu: Pippalyadi varga
Bhavaprakash Nighantu: Karpuradi varga

Distribution

The plant is indigenous to India, Pakistan, Burma, and Sri Lanka. In India, it is mainly found in evergreen forests of Kerala, Karnataka, and Tamil Nadu. It is a shade loving plant cultivated at an altitude of 600 to 1,200 m. It is cultivated in Western ghats, especially in Mysore, Kurg, Travancore, Cochin, Venaad, Kanara, Gujarat, etc. Guatemala is the largest producer and exporter of cardamom.

Morphology

It is an evergreen perennial herb, with subterranean aromatic root stock. Branches are about 2 to 4 m high.

- **Leaves:** Alternate, subsessile, aromatic, elliptical lanceolate, with sheathing leaf base, bright green color (**Fig. 32.1**).
- **Flowers:** White with violet streaks in between, arise in many panicles, arise directly from vegetative shoots, upright first but become prostrate later. Stamen single with bilobed anthers, pistil is trilocular, style is filliform terminating in a cup-shaped stigma located slightly above the anther. The inner surface of the stigmatic cup is lined with a viscous exudates (**Fig. 32.2**).

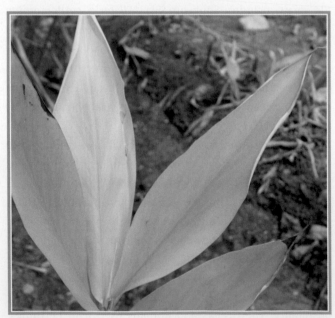

Fig. 32.1 Leaves.

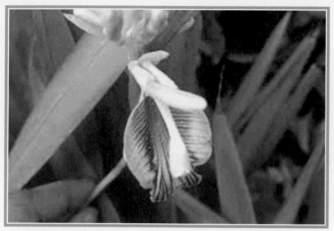

Fig. 32.2 Flower.

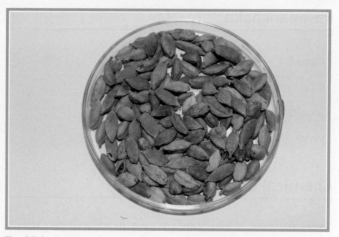

Fig. 32.3 Fruits.

- **Fruit:** Trilocular capsule, subglobose-oblong shape, marked with fine vertical ribs, greenish-yellow capsules, about 0.5 inch long (**Fig. 32.3**).
- **Seeds:** 15 to 20 per capsule, aromatic, brownish-black colored, ovoid, covered with a thin mucilaginous membrane.
- **Rhizomes:** Rhizomes are like creepers, branched with several erect leafy shoots and panicles (**Fig. 32.4**).

The plant is propagated through seeds and by divisions of rhizomes (Warrier and Nambiar 1994; Madhusoodan et al 2002).

Phenology

Flowering time: June to August
Fruiting time: October to November

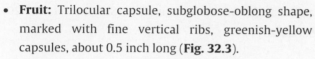

Key Characters for Identification

➤ *An evergreen perennial herb of 2–4 m height*
➤ *Leaves: bright green, aromatic, elliptical–lanceolateFlowers: white with violet streaks, arise from the vegetative shoots*
➤ *Fruits: trilocular, oblong shape, greenish-yellow.*
➤ *Seeds: blackish-brown, 15–20 per capsule, aromatic.*

Types

Two types of Ela are described by Nighantus, which are as follows:

- Sukshma Ela (*Elletaria cardamomum* Maton)
- Brihat Ela (*Amomum subulatum* Roxb.)

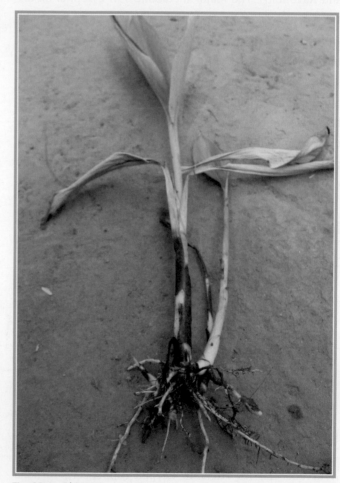

Fig. 32.4 Rhizomes.

The three most popular cultivated varieties of Ela are as follows (Ali 2008):

- Mysore variety: with erect panicles
- Malabar variety: with prostrate panicles
- Vazhukka variety: with semierect panicles

Rasapanchaka

Guna	Laghu, Ruksha
Rasa	Katu, Tikta
Vipaka	Katu
Virya	Sheeta

Chemical Constituents

Seeds of lesser cardamom are rich in volatile oil, which contains phenols, alkaloids, terpernoids, anthocyanins, and flavonoids. The major metabolites in essential oil are 1,8-cineole (50%), linalool, sabinene, myrcene, germaniol, alpha-phellandrene, terpinene, cymene, terpenolene, terpinyl acetate, limonene, α-terpineol, α-pinene, β-pinene, cardamonin, geraniol, geranyl acetate, aurone glycoside, pyrogallol acid, gallic acids, protocatechouic acid, catechin, caffeic acid subulin, alpinetin, leucocyanidin, diphenylpicrylhydrazyl, and bisabolene. The other components are starch, protein, waxes, and sterols (Amma et al 2010; Badei et al 1991).

Identity, Purity, and Strength

- Foreign matter: Nil
- Total ash: Not more than 6%
- Acid-insoluble ash: Not more than 4%
- Alcohol-soluble extractive: Not less than 2%
- Water-soluble extractive: Not less than 10%
- Volatile oil: Not less than 4%

(Source: The Ayurvedic Pharmacopeia of India 1989)

Karma (Actions)

Ayurveda classics attribute deepan (appetizer), rochana (relish), sugandhi (aromatic/fragrance), chardinigrahan (antiemetic), trishna nigrahan (antithirst), kanthya (voice promoter/beneficial for throat), hridya (cardio tonic), garbhavishodhani (uterine cleansing), asyavairasyanashini (cures tastelessness of mouth), anulomana (laxative), mutrajanan (diuretics), and balya (tonic) properties to it.

The essential oil is stimulant, aromatic, expectorant, deodorant, analgesic, anti-inflammatory, antimicrobial, germicidal, diuretic, wound healer, and hypnotic.

- Doshakarma: Tridoshashamaka
- Dhatukarma: Uttejaka, durgandhnashak, balya
- Malakarma: Mutral, anulomana

Pharmacological Actions

Research studies demonstrated that Ela possesses antioxidant, anticancer, anti-inflammatory, analgesic, antispasmodic, antibacterial, antifungal, antiproliferative, antidiabetic, antiviral, antihypertensive, anticonvulsant, and gastroprotective activities (Sharma et al 2011; Sarkar 2011).

Indications

Ela seeds are prescribed for the treatment of mukha-durgandha (halitosis), mutrakricchta (dysuria), chardi (vomiting) kasa (cough), shwasa (asthma), kshaya (consumption), arsha (piles), aruchi (dyspepsia), trishna (thirst), daha (burning sensation), ajeerna (indigestion), udar shool (abdominal pain), visha (poisoning), nausea (hrillasa), kandu (pruritis), dysnea (bronchitis), yakshma (tuberculosis), hriddaurbalya (cardiac debility), bhram (giddiness), and netraroga (eye diseases).

Therapeutic Uses

External Use

1. **Raktapravartana**: For letting out blood in venesection, powder of Ela, Karpura, Kushta, Tagar, and Patha mixed with lavan and taila should be rubbed on the wound (S.S.U. 14/35).
2. **Mukhapaka** (stomatitis): Regular use of Ela seed decoction as a gargle prevents stomatitis, bad breath, and pyorrhea.
3. **Timira** (vision defect): Ela powder dipped in aja mutra for three days is used as anjana (collyrium) in timira, krimi, and pilla roga (C.S.Ci. 26/249).

Internal Use

1. **Hridya roga** (heart disease): Intake of powder of Shukshm ela and pippalimool with ghrita prevents hridyaroga (B.S. hridyarog/28).
2. **Mutrakricchta** (dysuria): Intake of Shukshm ela churna with Amalaki swarasa daily increases urine output in dysuria (S.S.U. 58/41) or intake of Ela with curd water is also beneficial (GN. 2/27/44).
3. **Mutraghat** (suppression of urine): Intake of Ela beej and Shunthi with Dadima juice gives relief in mutraghat (VM. 33/7).
4. **Chardi** (vomiting): Eladi churna gives relief in nausea and vomiting (CD. 15/23).
5. **Pratishyay** (rhinitis/common cold): Tea prepared by mixing Ela powder, Tulsi, Marich, and Adraka should be taken twice daily to get relief in common cold, asthma, throat infections, fever, pulmonary tuberculosis, and liver congestions. Or one can take 250 to 500 mg Ela powder with honey twice daily.
6. **Cigarette de-addiction:** Eating few seeds of Ela daily helps in easing cigarette addiction (Peter 2001).
7. **Malaria:** Jeerak seeds and Brihat Ela are powdered and a mixture is prepared. Daily intake of this mixture is prescribed in the treatment of malaria (Thakur et al 1989).
8. **Visha** (poisoning): Local and oral intake of Ela seeds or paste is used as an antidote to snake bite and scorpion sting (Bisht et al 2010).

Officinal Part Used

Seeds

Dose

Seed powder: 1 to 3 g

Formulations

Eladi churna, Anantadya ghrita, Eladi gutika, Sitopaladi churna, Avipattikar churna, Eladi ghrita, Eladi mantha, Kushmandavleha, Chandanadi vati.

Toxicity/Adverse Effects

Some of the constituents of Ela are found to be mutagenic in bacterial strains and carcinogenic in rodent model (Balaji and Chempakam 2008). However, no such study on human participants was conducted.

Substitution and Adulteration

Brihat Ela is used as substitute drug for Sukshma Ela and vice versa, whereas other species of Amomum like *A. kepulaga, A. korarima, A. aromaticum*, etc., are common adulterants (Padhi et al 2008).

> **Points to Ponder**
>
> - *It is a native plant of Western Ghats.*
> - *It is well known in medicines for the treatment of halitosis, vomiting, cough, asthma, tuberculosis, poisoning, and dysuria.*

Suggested Readings

Ajarem JS, Ahmad M. Effect of perinatal exposure of cardamom (*Elettaria cadrdamomum*) on the post-natal development and social behaviour of mice offspring. J King Saud Univ Sci 1991;4(2):34–57

Ali M. Cultivation of Medicinal Plants: Pharmacognosy (Pharmacognosy and Plant Cultivation). 1st ed. New Delhi: CBS publication; 2008: 644–645

Amma KPAP, Rani MP, Sasidharan I, Nisha VNP. Chemical composition, flavonoid-phenolic contents and radical scavenging activity of four major varieties of cardamom. Int J Biol Med Res 2010;1(3):20–24

Badei AZM, Morsi HHH, El-Akel ATM. Chemical composition and antioxidant properties of cardamom essential oil. Bulletin of the Faculty of Agriculture University of Cairo 42; 1991:199–215

Balaji S, Chempakam B. Mutagenicity and carcinogenicity prediction of compounds from cardamom (*Elettaria cardamom* Maton). Ethnobot Leafl 2008;12:682–689

Bisht VK, Purohit V, Negi JS, Bhandari AK. Introduction and advancement in cultivation of large cardamom (*Amomum subulatum* Roxb.) in Uttarakhand, India. Res J Agric Sci 2010;1(3):205–208

Madhusoodanan KJ, Kumar P, Ravindran PN, Ravindran PN, Madhusoodanan KJ. Botany, Crop Improvement and Biotechnology of Cardamom, Cardamom: The Genus Elettaria. London: Taylor & Francis; 2002:12–68

Mahindru SN. Spices in Indian Life. New Delhi: Sultanchand & Sons; 1982

Padhi MM, Joseph GVR, Selvarajan S, Yelne MB, Mangal AK, Raman Ganapathi K, Sharma PC, Dennis TJ. Database on Medicinal Plants Used in Ayurveda and Siddha, Vol. 5. New Delhi: Central Council for Research in Ayurveda and Siddha, Department of AYUSH, Ministry of Health & Family Welfare; 2008:391–395

Peter KV. Handbook of Herbs and Spices. Abington, Cambridge, England: Woodhead Publishing Limited; 2001:132

Sarkar PR. Yaogic Treatment and Natural Remedies. Purulia, West Bengal: AMPS Publication; 2011:105

Sastry JLN. Illustrated Dravyaguna Vigyana. Vol. 2. Varanasi: Chaukhamba Orientalia; 2014:527

Savan EK, Küçükbay FZ. Essential oil composition of *Elettaria cardamomum* Maton. J Appl Biol Sci 2013;7(3):42–45

Sharma S, Sharma J, Kaur G. Therapeutic uses of *Elettaria cardomum*. Int J Drug Formul Res 2011;2(6):102–108

Thakur RS, Puri HS, Hussain A. Major medicinal plants of India. Lucknow: CIMAP; 1989:154

The Ayurvedic Pharmacopeia of India, Part 1, Vol 1. New Delhi: Department of AYUSH, Ministry of Health and Family Welfare, Government of India; 1989:137

Warrier PK, Nambiar VPK, Ramankutty. Indian Medicinal Plants: A Compendium of 500 Species. Vol. 2. Orient Longman Ltd; 1994:360

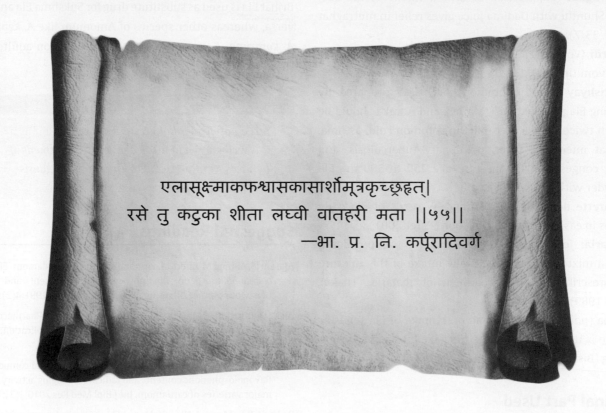

एलासूक्ष्माकफश्वासकासार्शोमूत्रकृच्छ्रहत्।
रसे तु कटुका शीता लघ्वी वातहरी मता ॥५५॥
—भा. प्र. नि. कर्पूरादिवर्ग

33. Eranda [*Ricinus communis* Linn.]

Family:	*Euphorbiaceae*
Hindi name:	*Arand, Arandi*
English name:	*Castor oil*

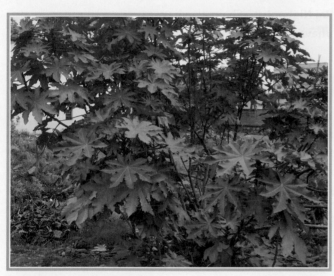

Plant of *Ricinus communis* Linn.

> *Ricin and Ricinine are the main toxic principles of Eranda seeds. If the seed is swallowed without chewing (without damaging seed coat), it passes out the digestive tract harmlessly but if chewed, broken, and then ingested it will cause intoxication.*

Introduction

The Sanskrit word "Eranda" means having the property of dispelling diseases. The generic name "Castor" is derived from the North American beaver (*Castor canadensis*) and the brightest double star in Gemini constellation. Castor was apparently coined by English traders who confused it with the oil of vitex agnus–castus, which the Spanish and Portuguese in Jamaica called agno–casto. Ricinus is the Latin word for ticks, especially the sheep ticks of Mediterranean because the mottled body of the sheep ticks resembles the castor bean seed (Laxmikanta Ladda and Kamthane 2014).

Historically the plant, especially its seeds and oil are used in different aspects of life. Its oil has long been used as an inexpensive fuel for lightening oil lamps. It is popularly known as the palm of Christ because of its immense medicinal use. The seed oil has been used as a powerful laxative for centuries, and it is evident long back in classical Ayurveda texts. Sushrut described Eranda taila as the best among all the laxative oils (S.S.Su. 44/3). Charak mentioned Eranda mool as the best vatahara and aphrodisiac drug (C.S.Su. 25/40). Charaka and Vagabhatt used Eranda patra for swedana karma and described the meat cooked in eranda taila as sanskara viruddh dravya (C.S.Su. 26/84). It is an important constituent of madhyam panchmool (A.H.Su. 6/169) and an ingredient of brahmarasayana (C.S.Ci. 1/1/43). Vagabhatt used it first time for the treatment of night blindness whereas Sushrut described it as adhobhagadoshhara (S.S.Su. 45/114). Raj Nighantu has described another variety of Eranda, namely, sthula Eranda and considered it as superior in rasa, virya, and vipaka (R.N.shalmalyadi varga/59).

The treated castor oil can also be used in paints, enamels, varnishes, oiled fabrics, linoleum, patent leather, flypaper, typewriting, printing inks, greases, as special lubricant, as softening agent for gelatin, as a vehicle for parenteral administration of steroidal hormone (Bhakta and Das 2015). The plant as a whole is used as excellent feed for cattle and for biofuel/biodiesel production. Castor cakes are used as biomanure in agriculture. The dried leaves are used as insect repellant and in making insecticides.

Vernacular Names

Arab: Khirva

Assamese: Eda, Era

Bengali: Bherenda

Gujarati: Erandio, Erando, Divelio, Diveli

Kannada: Haralu, Oudala gida

Kashmiri: Aran, Banangir

Malayalam: Avanakku

Marathi: Erand Erandi

Oriya: Jada, Gaba

Persian: Bedanjir

Punjabi: Arind, Aneru

Sindhi: Ayrun-kukri, Heran

Tamil: Amanakku, Kottaimuttu, Amanakam ceti, Sittamunuk

Telugu: Amudapu veru, Erandamu, Amudamu, Kottei

Urdu: Bedanjir, Arand

Synonyms

Aamand: It is a beautiful plant.

Chitra: The seeds are variously colored.

Chitrabeej: Its seeds are mottled in appearance.

Deerghdanda: Its leaves have long petiole.

Gandharvhasta: It has palmate-shaped leaves.

Hastiparnaka: The plant has large-sized leaves.

Panchangula: The plant bears palmate-lobed leaves.

Shoolshatru: The plant is a good remedy for pain.

Snehaprada: Its seeds yield oil.

Urubuka: It pacifies aggravated vata.

Uttanpatraka: The leaves are arranged on the stem facing upwards.

Vardhmaan: The growth of the plant is fast.

Vatari: The plant is a highly potent remedy for vatika disorders.

Vyadambaka: It stimulates downward displacement of mala.

Classical Categorization

Charak Samhita: Bhedaniya, Angamardaprashmana, Swedopaga, Madhurskanda

Sushrut Samhita: Vidarigandhadi, Adhobhaghara, Vatasanshamana

Ashtang Hridaya: Vidarigandhadi

Dhanvantari Nighantu: Guduchyadi varga

Madanpal Nighantu: Abhyadi varga

Kaiyadev Nighantu: Oushadi varga

Raj Nighantu: Shalmalyadi varga

Bhavaprakash Nighantu: Guduchyadi varga

Distribution

Eranda is a native plant of Africa and is now cultivated in many tropical and subtropical countries of the world. In India it is both cultivated and found wild up to an elevation of 2,000 m. It has become naturalized as weed throughout India especially in wastelands, open gardens, roadside, barren land, etc.

Morphology

An evergreen, perennial, bushy, soft woody, small tree reaching up to 3 m in height. The stem is hollow, erect, and grayish-green in color when tender, and later on, the stem changes to brownish-red color.

- **Leaves:** Alternate, long petiolate, broad, palmate-lobed with 5 to 11 serrated lobes, nearly orbicular, lobes membranous, oblong to linear, acute or acuminate apex. Presence of 2 prominent glands at the top of the petiole. Upper surface of leaves is green whereas lower surface is whitish-gray (**Fig. 33.1**).
- **Flowers:** Monoecious, greenish-yellow, in terminal paniculate racemes with crowded male flowers on the upper half of the inflorescence and female flower at the basal half. Styles three, short, or long spreading, often very large and brightly or lightly colored, entire, bifid, or bipartite. Stigmas are feathery (**Fig. 33.2**).
- **Fruit:** Globose, 1 to 2 cm long, explosively dehiscent, splitting into three two-valve cocci, when young green, covered with fleshy prickles, three seeded (**Fig. 33.3a, b**).

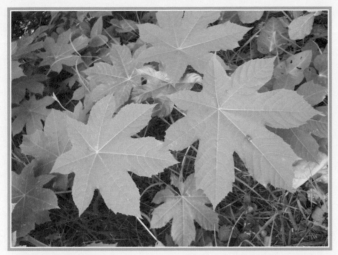

Fig. 33.1 Leaves.

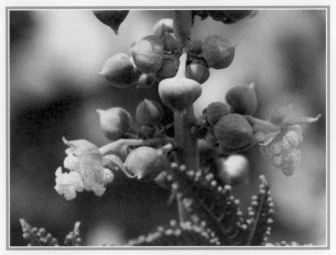

Fig. 33.2 Flowers.

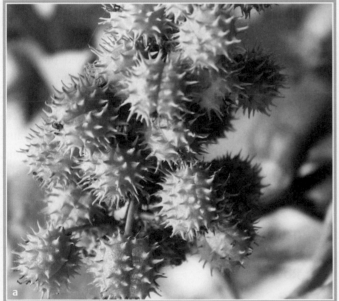

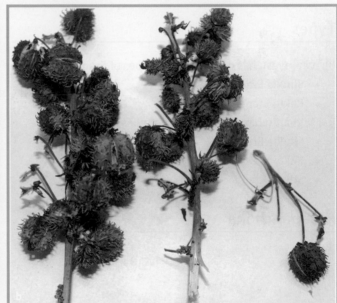

Fig. 33.3 **(a)** Young fruits. **(b)** Dry fruit.

- **Seeds:** Oblong-ovoid with smooth hard variously colored mottled testa, a white caruncle at the top enclosing an oily endosperm. Embryo thin, with flat broad cotyledons (**Fig. 33.4**).
- **Roots:** Profusely branched, light, outer surface yellowish-brown, rough, and wrinkled. Odorless, taste acrid, and fracture granular. The plant is propagated through seeds (**Fig. 33.5**).

Phenology

Flowering time: More or less throughout the year
Fruiting time: More or less throughout the year

Key Characters for Identification

➤ It is an evergreen, perennial, bushy, semi-woody, small tree of about 3 m
➤ Leaves: alternate, orbicular, palmately lobed with 5 to 11 serrated lobes
➤ Flowers: greenish-yellow, monoecious, in terminal paniculate racemes
➤ Fruits: globose, 1 to 2 cm long, covered with fleshy prickles
➤ Seeds: oblong-ovoid with mottled testa and a caruncle at the top

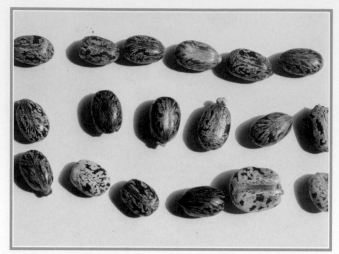

Fig. 33.4 Seeds.

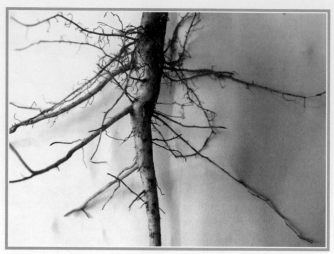

Fig. 33.5 Roots.

Types

Bhavaprakash has described two types of Eranda:

- Shukla Eranda
- Rakta Eranda

Raj Nighantu has described three types of Eranda:

- Shukla Eranda
- Rakta Eranda
- Sthula Eranda

Rasapanchaka

Guna	Guru, Shukshm, Tikshna, Snigdha
Rasa	Madhura
Vipaka	Madhura
Virya	Ushna

Chemical Constituents

The Eranda roots contain indole-3-acetic acid, germanicol, triterpene, gallotannins, and inorganic minerals like sodium, potassium, nitrate, chloride, iron, manganese, carbonates, etc. Its leaves have alkaloid (ricinine, N-dimethyl ricinine), monoterpenoids (1,8-cineole, camphor, α-pinene), sesquiterpenoid (β-caryophyllene), phenolic compounds (gallic acid, quercetin, gentisic acid, rutin, epicatechin, ellagic acid), disaccharide glycoside, flavonoids (kaempferol-3-O-beta-rutinoside and kaempferol-3-O-beta-D-xylopyranoside), and tannins.

Flowers have apigenin, chlorogenin, rutin, coumarin, and hyperoside.

The seeds and fruits contain 45% of fixed oil, which has glycosides of ricinoleic, isoricinoleic, stearic, dihydroxystearic acids, lipases, and an alkaloid ricinine (pericarp). The seeds also contain three toxic proteins ricin A, B, and C and one ricinus agglutinin. Castor oil contains palmitic, stearic, arachidic, hexadecenoic, oleic, linoleic, linolenic, ricinoleic, and dihydroxy stearic acids (Bhakta and Das 2015; Jena and Gupta 2012).

Identity, Purity, and Strength

For Root

- Foreign matter: Not more than 2%
- Total ash: Not more than 8%
- Acid-insoluble ash: Not more than 1%
- Alcohol-soluble extractive: Not less than 3%
- Water-soluble extractive: Not less than 9%

(Source: The Ayurvedic Pharmacopeia of India 1989)

For Seed

- Foreign matter: Not more than 2%
- Total ash: Not more than 4%
- Acid-insoluble ash: Not more than 1%
- Alcohol-soluble extractive: Not less than 36%
- Water-soluble extractive: Not less than 6%
- Fixed oil: Not less than 37%

(Source: The Ayurvedic Pharmacopeia of India 2004)

Karma (Actions)

In Ayurveda texts Erandayugma is described as having virechan (purgative), bhedana (drastic purgative), krimighna (anthelmintic), kusthghna (antileprotic), shoolghna (antispasmodic), shothaghna (edema reducing), vrishya (aphrodisiac), deepan (appetizer), mutral (diuretic), shrotoshodhan (channel clearing), bastishodhana (bladder purifier), vishaghna (antidote), swedopaga and jwaraghna (antipyretic) properties. Eranda patra is vataghna, krimighna, and pittaraktaprakopaka. Eranda pushpa is vataghna, kaphapitta vinashak, mutradoshhara, and raktpittaprakopaka. Erandaphal has deepan, atyaushna, krimighna, shoolghna, and phal majja (fruit pulp) is bhedana (laxative) properties. Eranda taila has suksham, snehana, tvachya, virechak, shrotoshodhana, vyasthapana, yoni-shukra vishodhana, medhya, balya, kantivardhaka, arogyaprada, and shothahara properties.

- Doshakarma: Kapha vata shamaka
- Dhatukarma: Balya, Vrishya
- Malakarma: Virechana

Pharmacological Actions

The plant is reported to possess antioxidant, anti-implantation, anti-inflammatory, antidiabetic, analgesic, antitumor, larvicidal, antinociceptive, antiasthmatic, anti-microbial, antifungal, antidiabetic, free radical scavenging, antifertility, cytotoxic, antihistaminic, immunomodulatory, hepatoprotective, wound healing, lipolytic, antiulcer, and bone regeneration activities (Gupta and Singh 2015).

Indications

In classical Ayurveda texts both types of Eranda are used in therapeutics. Eranda root is prescribed in the treatment of shotha (edema), shool (pain), katishool (backache), vibandh (constipation), basti roga (diseases of bladder), shirashool (headache), udarroga, gridharsi (sciatica), jwar (fever), braghna (hernia), shwasa (asthma), parshvashool (pleurisy), vatavikara, anaah (flatulence), udavarta (abdominal distension), kasa (cough), kustha (skin diseases), aamdosha (malabsorption syndrome), yonivyapada (diseases of female gentalia), meha (diabetes), medoroga (obesity), netraroga (eye diseases). Eranda patra and pallava are used in treatment of krimi (worms), mutrakricchta (dysuria), gulma, bastiroga, vriddhi (prolapse), and shool. Eranda phal is used in gulma, udarshool, yakrit, pleeha, udarroga, and arsha. Eranda taila is used in the treatment of vibandh, aamvata (arthritis), katishool, kampa (tremor), sandhivata, vatavikara, karnaroga, and twakroga.

In traditional folklore practice its mool kwath or mool kalka is used in toothache and dental caries. Leaves are used in the form of a poultice or fomentation on sores, boils, and swellings. In children leaves coated with oil and warmed are applied over the abdomen to give relief in flatulence. Fresh juice of the leaves is used as an emetic in opium poisoning. Leaves are considered as galactagogue and are applied as poultice over the breasts or taken internally in the form of juice for enhancing milk production. It is also applied externally as emollient in seborrheic dermatitis and other skin infections (Anonymous 2005; Nadkarni 1954).

Contraindications

- During pregnancy because it induces uterine contractions.
- In persons suffering from kidney infections or intestinal infections like appendicitis, enteritis, and peritonitis.

Therapeutic Uses

External Use

1. **Aamvata** (rheumatoid arthritis): Fomentation of the affected joint with Eranda kwath gives relief in pain and inflammation (B.P.Ci. 26/28).
2. **Vranaachadana** (covering of wound): Vrana caused by aggravated vata should be covered with the leaves of Eranda, Bhurja, Putik, Ashwabala, and Kashmari (S.S.Ci. 1/113).
3. **Arsha** (hemorrhoid): Fomentation of the affected part with decoction of Vasa, Erand, Bilva patra is beneficial in arsha (C.S.Ci. 14/44).
4. **Vatarakta** (gout): In case of pain due to gout, local application of Erand beeja, kalka pounded with milk is recommended (C.S.Ci. 29/140).
5. **Karnashool** (earache): Lukewarm Erandadi taila should be instilled in earache (B.S.karnaroga/38).

Internal Use

1. **Vibanda** (constipation): Oral intake of Eranda oil mixed with double quantity of Triphala kwath or milk gives instant relief in constipation (Sh.S. 3/4/20).

2. **Aamvata** (rheumatoid arthritis): Paste of Sunthi mixed with root decoction of Eranda should be cooked in a closed container. The juice extracted is used in aamvata with honey (Sh.S. 2/1/40-41). Regular intake of Haritaki mixed with Eranda taila gives relief in arthritic pain.

3. **Udar shool** (abdominal pain): Intake of Eranda taila mixed with Yashtimadhu kwath alleviates paittika shool and gulma (CD. 26/32). Decoction of Eranda, Methika, and gud pacifies all types of abdominal pain (SB. 4/507).

4. **Gulma** (abdominal lump): Castor oil mixed with Madhya or dugdha is prescribed in vatika gulma (C.S.Ci. 5/92).

5. **Shotha** (edema): Consumption of Eranda taila with gomutra or godugdh subsides edema (Ka.S. 342).

6. **Vatavyadhi** (neuromuscular disease): In vata disorders patralavan is prescribed. It is prepared by fresh leaves of Eranda, Muskaka, Karanj, Vasa, Putika, Aragvadh, Chitrak mixed with lavan and pounded in a mortar, then kept in a pot smeared with ghrita. The pot is pasted with cow dung and then put in fire (S.S.Ci. 4/30).

7. **Gridharsi** (sciatica): Payasa prepared with purified Eranda seeds and milk is a very good remedy for gridharsi and katishool (VM. 22/50).

8. **Yonishool** (pain in vagina): Cotton swab impregnated with castor oil should be put into the vagina to get relief in pain (GN. 6/6/8).

9. **Udarroga** (abdominal diseases): Eranda taila mixed with Dashmool or Triphala kwath added with gomutra alleviates vatoudar, shotha, and shool (VM. 38/2).

10. **Atisaar** (diarrhea): Daily intake of milk cooked with Eranda mool or unripe Bilva fruits is beneficial in atisaar (A.H.Ci. 9/38; C.S.Ci. 19/48).

11. **Kasa** (cough): Erand patra kshar mixed with trikatu, gud, and taila gives relief in kasa (C.S.Ci. 18/172).

12. **Medovriddhi** (obesity): One should take Eranda patra kshar with hingu followed by manda in diet in medovriddhi (B.P.Ci. 39/21).

13. **Garbhajanan** (promotes conception): For having conception, one should take Eranda beeja and matulunga pounded with ghrita (GN. 6/5/4).

Officinal Parts Used

Root, leaves, seed, oil

Dose

Root paste: 10 to 20 g
Decoction: 40 to 80 mL
Seed oil: 5 to 15 mL
Seeds: 2 to 6 seeds

Formulations

Eranda saptaka kwath, Eranda paka, Gandharva hasta taila, Vatari guggulu, Aamvatari rasa, Saindhavadi taila, Vishvadi kwath, Shoolgajendera taila, Mashabaladi kwath churna.

Toxicity/Adverse Effects

Long-term use of Eranda taila can cause colic abdominal pain, dehydration, electrolytic imbalance, reduction in nutrient absorption because of its purgative action (Sharma et al 2005).

Accidental or suicidal intoxications by ingestion of Eranda seeds may result in abdominal pain, vomiting, diarrhea with or without blood, muscular pain, cramps in the limbs, circulatory collapse, dyspnea, and dehydration (Worbs et al 2011).

Fatal dose: 6 to 20 seeds.

Substitution and Adulteration

Eranda taila is often adulterated with rosin oil, blown oil, groundnut oil, mahua, coconut oil, cotton seed oil, and poppy seed oil (Sharma et al 2005).

> *Points to Ponder*
>
> - *Eranda oil is the best among all the vegetable oil for inducing purgation.*
> - *Eranda moola is best for vrisya and vatahara actions.*
> - *It is a well-known drug for the treatment of vibandha, shotha, shool, vatavyadhi, aamvata, gulma, udarroga, vriddhi, bastiroga, and mutrakrichhta.*

Suggested Readings

Anonymous. Pharmacognosy of Indigenous Drugs. New Delhi: Central Council for Research in Ayurveda and Siddha,Vol. 1, reprint 2005; 1972

Bhakta S, Das SK. In praise of the medicinal plant *Ricinus communis* L.: a review. Glob J Res Med Plants Indig Med 2015;4(5):95–105

Gupta N, Singh AK. A review on *Ricinus communis* Linn. Int Ayur Med J 2015;3(2):492–495

Jena J, Gupta A. *Ricinus communis* Linn: a phytopharmacological review. Int J Pharm Pharm Sci 2012;4(4):25–29

Laxmikanta Ladda P, Kamthane RB. *Ricinus communis* (castor): an overview. Int J Res Pharmacol Pharmacotherap 2014;3(2):136–144

Manoj K. A review on phytochemical constituents and pharmacological activities of *Ricinus communis* L. plant. Int J Pharmacogn Phytochem Res 2017;9(4):466–472

Nadkarni KM. Indian Materia Medica, Vol. 1. 2nd ed.; 1927, 1954:1065–1070

Sharma PC, Yelne MB, Dennis TJ. Database on Medicinal Plants Used in Ayurveda, Vol. 4, CCRAS. New Delhi: Reprint Ed. 2005; 2005: 122–126

Worbs S, Köhler K, Pauly D, et al. *Ricinus communis* intoxications in human and veterinary medicine: a summary of real cases. Toxins (Basel) 2011;3:1332–1372

The Ayurvedic Pharmacopeia of India. Part I, Vol. 1. New Delhi: Department of AYUSH, Ministry of Health and Family Welfare, Government of India; 1989:46

The Ayurvedic Pharmacopeia of India. Part I, Vol. 3. New Delhi: Department of AYUSH, Ministry of Health and Family Welfare, Government of India; 2004:52

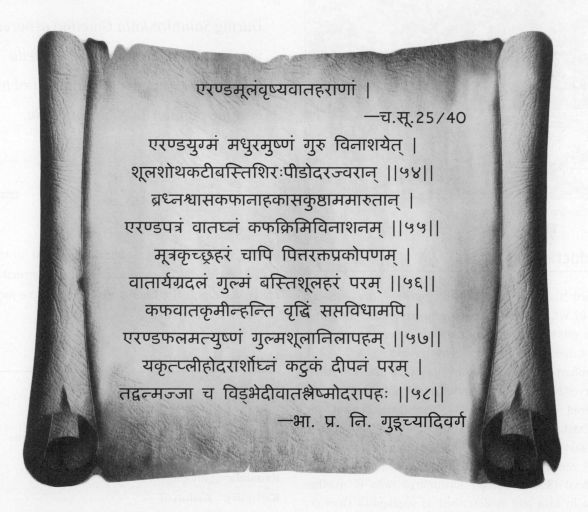

एरण्डमूलंवृष्यवातहराणां |

—च.सू. 25/40

एरण्डयुग्मं मधुरमुष्णं गुरु विनाशयेत् |

शूलशोथकटीबस्तिशिरःपीडोदरज्वरान् ||५४||

ब्रध्नश्वासकफानाहकासकुष्ठाममारुतान् |

एरण्डपत्रं वातघ्नं कफक्रिमिविनाशनम् ||५५||

मूत्रकृच्छ्रहरं चापि पित्तरक्तप्रकोपणम् |

वातार्यग्रदलं गुल्मं बस्तिशूलहरं परम् ||५६||

कफवातकृमीन्हन्ति वृद्धिं सप्तविधामपि |

एरण्डफलमत्युष्णं गुल्मशूलानिलापहम् ||५७||

यकृत्प्लीहोदरार्शोघ्नं कटुकं दीपनं परम् |

तद्वन्मज्जा च विड्भेदीवातश्लेष्मोदरापहः ||५८||

—भा. प्र. नि. गुडूच्यादिवर्ग

34. Gambhari [*Gmelina arborea* Roxb.]

Family:	*Verbenaceae*
Hindi name:	*Gambhar*
English name:	*Cashmeri tree, Coomb teak, Candhar Tree*

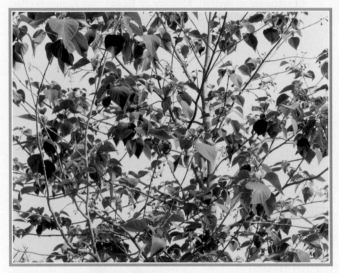

Plant of *Gmelina arborea* Roxb.

During Samhita kala Gmelina arborea was named kashmarya in Ayurveda scriptures, whereas the name Gambhari became popular in Nighantu kala.

Introduction

The word "Gambhari" is derived from the phrase *ga gati bibhati iti*, which means the one who grows fast. The genus *Gmelina* gets its name in honor of famous German naturalist George Gmelin and *arborea* means tree-like.

Gambhari is mentioned in almost all the scriptures of Ayurveda due to its versatile medicinal value. Charak considered Gambhari fruit as best raktasangrahi and raktapittashamka dravya (C.S.Su. 25/40) and included it in phalaasava yoni (C.S.Su. 25/50) and phal varga (C.S.Su. 27/135). Sushrut has described it as a content of Brihat panchmool (S.S.Su. 38/68). Kashmarya taila is madhur kashaya in rasa and is described as kaphapitta shamaka (S.S.Su. 45/121) whereas in phal varga its fruit is described as madhur, snigdh, and raktapittahara (S.S.Su. 46/184).

Besides its medicinal value the timber of Gambhari is used extensively in constructions, furniture, artificial limb, picture frames, handles of agricultural tools, carom boards, carriages, sports material, musical instruments, instrument boxes, thermometer scales, papermaking, and matchwood industry. Leaves are used as cattle fodder and silkworm food.

Vernacular Names

Assamese: Gamari
Bengali: Gambhar, Gamar
Burma: Kyunboc, Kywonpho, Yamanai, Yemene
Gujarati: Shivan
Kannada: Shivanigida, Shivani
Kashmiri: Kashmari
Malayalam: Kumizhu, Kumpil, Kumil, Kumbil, Kumilu
Marathi: Shivan, Shewan
Nepal: Gambari, Khamari
Oriya: Gambhari, Bodhroparnni
Punjabi: Gumhar, Kumhar

Tamil: Kumishan, Kumizhan, Perumkumbil, Komizh-pazham, Perunkurmizh

Telugu: Peggummudu, Peggummadi, Gummadi, Gumaditeku

Urdu: Gambhari

Synonyms

Bhadraparni: Its leaves are beautiful and beneficial.

Hira: Its fruits are used as rasayana.

Kashmari: The plant looks beautiful.

Kashmiri: Grows in places like Kashmir.

Krishnavrinta: The leaves have blackish petiole.

Madhurasa: Its fruits and flowers are madhura rasa pradhana.

Mahakusumika: It bears large flowers.

Peetarohini: Its bark is yellowish-brown in color.

Sarvatobhadra: Each parts of the plant have medicinal value.

Shriparni: The plant has beautiful leaves.

Classical Categorization

Charak Samhita: Shothara, Dahaprashmana, Virechanopaga

Sushrut Samhita: Sarivadi, Brihat panchmool

Ashtang Hridaya: Sarivadi

Dhanvantari Nighantu: Guduchyadi varga

Madanpal Nighantu: Abhyadi varga

Kaiyadev Nighantu: Oushadi varga

Raj Nighantu: Prabhadradi varga

Bhavaprakash Nighantu: Guduchyadi varga

Distribution

It is found throughout greater part of India, Western Ghats, foothills of North-West Himalaya to Chittagong, and throughout Deccan Peninsula.

Morphology

A moderate-sized deciduous tree of about 18 to 20 m height.

- **Bark:** Yellowish-gray, corky lenticellate, exfoliating in thin flakes. Young parts densely velvety and tomentose (**Fig. 34.1**).

- **Leaves:** Simple, opposite, petiolate, 10 to 25 cm long, 5 to 18 cm width, broadly ovate or cordate in shape, acuminate apex, glabrous above when mature, fulvous tomentose beneath (**Fig. 34.2a, b**).
- **Flowers:** Orange–yellow or brownish-yellow in color, in terminal panicles of three-flowered cymes and appears when the tree is more or less leafless. Calyx 5 mm long, broadly campanulate, densely fulvous-hairy. Corolla brownish-yellow, densely hairy outside, five-lobed with upper and lower lips (**Fig. 34.3**).
- **Fruits:** Fleshy, ovoid, or oblong drupes, 2 to 5 cm long, unripe fruit is green in color and it becomes orange-yellow or black when mature. One or two seeded (**Fig. 34.4**).
- **Roots:** Cylindrical, covered by thin yellowish-gray bark, externa l surface rugged due to the presence of vertical cracks, ridges, fissures, and numerous lenticels (**Fig. 34.5**). The plant is propagated by its seeds.

Phenology

Flowering time: February to April

Fruiting time: May to July

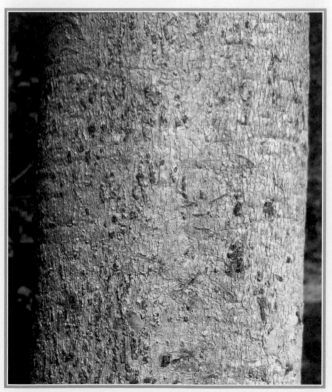

Fig. 34.1 Bark.

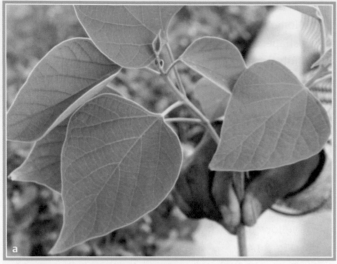

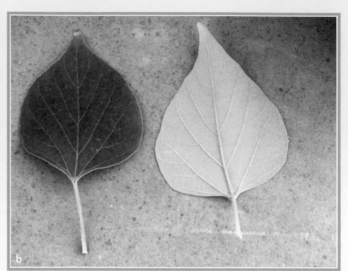

Fig. 34.2 **(a)** Leaves. **(b)** Dorsal and ventral view.

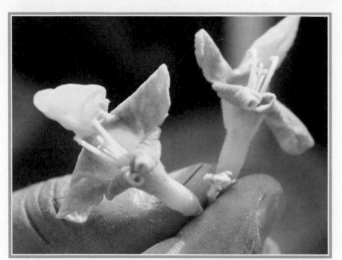

Fig. 34.3 Flower.

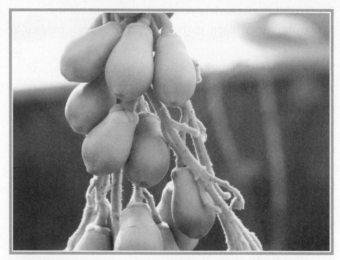

Fig. 34.4 Young fruits.

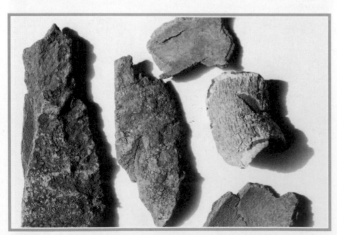

Fig. 34.5 Root bark.

Key Characters for Identification

➤ *A moderate-sized deciduous tree of about 18 to 20 m*
➤ *Leaves: simple, ovate-cordate shape, glabrous above tomentose beneath*
➤ *Flowers: orange–yellow in terminal panicles of three-flowered cymes*
➤ *Fruits: fleshy, ovoid, or oblong drupes*
➤ *Roots: cylindrical with thin yellowish-gray bark*

Types

Not mentioned.

Rasapanchaka

Rasapanchaka	Roots	Fruits
Guna	Guru	Guru, Snigdh
Rasa	Tikta, Katu, Kashaya	Madhur, Amla, Kashaya
Vipaka	Madhur	Madhur
Virya	Ushna	Sheet

Chemical Constituents

The plant is rich in gmelofuran, sesquiterpenes, cerylalcohol, hentriacontanol-1, α– and β-sitosterol, *n*-octacosanol, gmelinol, apiosylskimmin. The root contains cluytylferulate, *n*-octacosanol, gmelinol, arboreol, 2-0-methyl arboreal, 2-0-ethylarboreol, isoarboreol, gmelanone, β-sitosterol, paulownin, 6″-bromoisoarboreol, 4-hydroxysesamin, 4,8-dihydroxysesamin, gummadiol, 4-epigummadiol-4-0-glucoside, gmelanone, palmitic, oleic, linoleic acids, stigmasterol, stigmastanol, campesterol, butulinol. Its leaves have luteolin, apigenin, quercetin, hentriacontanol, β-sitosterol, quercetogenin, and other flavones. The fruits contain butyric, tartaric acids, saccharine substances and little tannin, β-sitosterol, ceryl alcohol, gmelinol, arborone, arboreal, luteolin, apigenin, quercetin, hentriacontanol, and quercetogenin (Sharma et al 2001).

Identity, Purity, and Strength

For Root Bark

- Foreign matter: Not more than 2%
- Total ash: Not more than 5%
- Acid-insoluble ash: Not more than 0.3%
- Alcohol-soluble extractive: Not less than 7%
- Water-soluble extractive: Not less than 20%

(Source: The Ayurvedic Pharmacopeia of India 1989)

For Fruit Foreign matter: Not more than 1%

- Total ash: Not more than 6%
- Acid-insoluble ash: Not more than 0.4%
- Alcohol-soluble extractive: Not less than 8%
- Water-soluble extractive: Not less than 25%

(Source: The Ayurvedic Pharmacopeia of India 2001)

Karma (Actions)

In Ayurvedic literature it is recommended to use roots, flowers, fruits, leaves of Gambhari therapeutically. These parts exhibit multiple actions which are as follows:

Roots: Deepan (appetizer), pachan (digestive), krimighna (anthelmintic), bhedana (purgative), stanyajanan (galactogogue), shothahara (anti-inflammatory), vishaghna (antidote), vedanasthapana (anodyne), jwaraghna (antipyretic)

Fruits: Sheetal (coolant), snehana (oleation), raktasangrahi (blood astringent), hridya (cardio tonic), keshya (hair tonic), rasayana (rejuvinator), vrishya (aphrodisiac), medhya (intellect promoting), brihmaniya (weight promoting), balya (strength promoting), sandhaniya (union promoter), mutral (diuretic), trishnanigrahan (antithirst), dahaprashamana (refrigerant), garbhasthapaka (maintain pregnancy), raktapittanashak (pacify diseases of rakta)

- Flowers: Balya, vrishya, sangrahi
- Doshakarma: Tridoshashamaka
- Dhatukarma: Balya, rasayana, vrishya
- Malakarma: Mruduvirechaka, mutral

Pharmacological Actions

In vivo and in vitro studies on Gambhari exhibit antioxidant, anthelmintic, antimicrobial, analgesic, antipyretic, antidiabetic, diuretic, cardioprotective, hepatoprotective, antiepileptic, anticancer, immunomodulatory, insecticidal, antiulcer, and hypoglycemic activities (Arora et al 2017; Kaswala et al 2012).

Indications

In classical texts Gambhari roots are recommended to be used in the treatment of shotha, shool, jwar, brahm (giddiness), vatavikara, vibandh, mutaavrodha, arsha, hridyaroga, visha, daha, aamdosha, trishna, agnimandhya, and adhyaman. Its fruits are used in daha (burning sensation), raktapitta, trishna, kshat, kshaya, mutraghat (difficult urination), vatarakta, sosha (emaciation), dourbalya, twak vikara, palitya, raktatisara, raktaarsha, mutrakricchta, shitapitta, puyameha, garbhpata, sarpavisha, vrishchik visha. Its flowers are used in raktapitta and ashrigdhar. The paste and juice of its leaves are applied on headache and foul-smelling ulcers.

Therapeutic Uses

External Use

1. **Pilatya:** Taila prepared with Gambhari is taken as nasya to control graying of hairs (Sh.S. 3/8/46).
2. **Vatarakta:** Application of Gambhari and Madhuka paste or Siddh taila is beneficial in vatarakta (S.S.Ci. 5/12).

Internal Use

1. **Raktapitta** (bleeding disorders): Pakwa fruits of Udumbar, Kashmarya, Haritaki, Kharjura, and Draksha each taken separately with madhu control hemorrhage (CD. 9/25). Flowers of Kovidara, Kashmarya, and Shalmali taken as vegetable daily is useful in raktapitta (C.S.Ci. 4/39).
2. **Jwar** (fever): Cold decoction of Kashmarya mixed with sharkara pacifies trishna and daha in pittaj jwar (S.S.U. 39/80).
3. **Raktaarsha** (bleeding piles): Khada (a dietary preparation) prepared with Kashmarya, Amalaki, Karburdar, amla fruits, Grinjanaka, Shalmali, Kshirini, Chukrika, Nyaygrodh shung, and Kovidara pushpa with supernatant fatty layer of curd should be given in rakta arsha (C.S.Ci. 14/203).
4. **Rakta atisaar** (diarrhea associated with blood): Intake of yusha prepared with Kashmarya phal, added with sharkara and amla controls bleeding diarrhea (A.H.Ci. 9/84).
5. **Trishna** (thirst): Kashmarya and sharkara should be taken to control excessive thirst (VM. 16/9).
6. **Garbhshosh and Balshosh** (fetal atrophy): Daily intake of milk cooked with sharkara, Kashmarya, and Mulethi stimulate growth in atrophy of fetus during pregnancy (C.S.Ci. 28/95).
7. **Pandu** (anemia): Kashmarya fruit is dipped in the tepid decoction of Danti and then pressed. The extracted juice is taken in pandu roga (A.H.Ci. 16/6).
8. **Sitapitta** (urticaria): In sitapitta fully ripe and dried Gambhari fruits are cooked in godugdh and is taken with dugdh followed by wholesome diet (RM. 8/12; CD. 51/12).
9. **Angulivestha** (whitlow): Wrapping the infected finger with seven tender leaves of Gambhari helps in curing the disease (B.P.Ci. 61/77).
10. **Stanyajanan** (galactogogue): Regular intake of root powder of Gambhari and Mulethi with sugar and honey increases milk production in lactating mother (A.H.Sa. 2/57).

Officinal Parts Used

Root, bark, leaf, flower, fruit

Dose

Root bark decoction: 50 to 100 mL
Fruit powder: 1 to 3 g

Formulations

Dashamoolarishta, Shriparnyadi kvatha, Shriparni taila, Brihat panchamoolyadi kvatha, Kashmaryadi sheeta kashaya, Dashamoolaharitaki, Dashamoola ghrita, Dhanvantara ghrita, Arvindasava.

Toxicity/Adverse Effects

Acute and subacute toxicity study of fruit powder showed no mortality, behavioral, hematological, biochemical, and histological changes (Ashalatha and Sankh 2014).

Substitution and Adulteration

Gmelina asiatica Linn. roots are used as substitute to Gambhari. However if Drakshaphal is not available Gambhari phal is used in its place (B.P. prastavana/159).

Points to Ponder

- *Gambhari root is an important ingredient in famous anti-inflammatory formulation Dashmool.*
- *Charak considered Gambhari fruit as best raktasangrahi and raktapittashamka dravya (C.S.Su. 25/40)*
- *Its root is ushna virya whereas its fruits are sheet virya.*
- *Its fruits are drug of choice for raktapitta, daha, trishna, mutrakricchta, and dourbalya.*

Suggested Readings

Arora C, Tamrakar V. *Gmelina arborea*: chemical constituents, pharmacological activities and applications. Int J Phytomed 2017;9(4):528–542

Ashalatha M, Sankh K. Toxicity study of Gambhari phala churna. Int Ayur Med J 2014;2(6):959–963

Kaswala R, Patel V, Chakraborty M, Kamath JV. Phytochemical and pharmacological profile of *Gmelina arborea*: an overview. Int Res J Pharm 2012;3(2):61–64

Sharma PC, Yelne MB, Dennis TJ. Database on Medicinal Plants Used in Ayurveda. Vol. 3. New Delhi: CCRAS, Reprint 2005; 2001:217–221

The Ayurvedic Pharmacopeia of India. Part I, Vol. 1. New Delhi: Department of AYUSH, Ministry of Health and Family Welfare, Government of India; 1989:48

The Ayurvedic Pharmacopeia of India. Part I, Vol. 2. New Delhi: Department of AYUSH, Ministry of Health and Family Welfare, Government of India; 2001:45

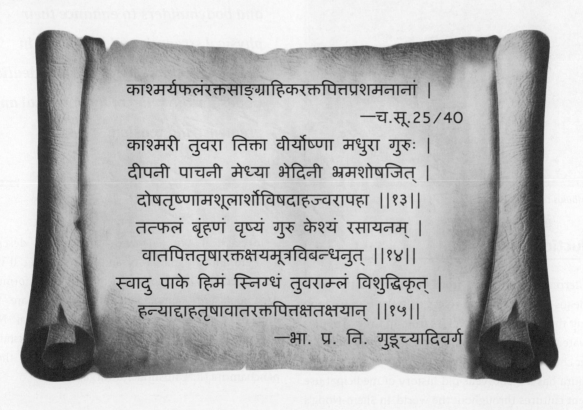

काश्मर्यफलंरक्तसाङ्ग्राहिकरक्तपित्तप्रशमनानां |

—च.सू.25/40

काश्मरी तुवरा तिक्ता वीर्योष्णा मधुरा गुरुः |
दीपनी पाचनी मेध्या भेदिनी भ्रमशोषजित् |
दोषतृष्णामशूलार्शोविषदाहज्वरापहा ||१३||
तत्फलं बृंहणं वृष्यं गुरु केश्यं रसायनम् |
वातपित्ततृषारक्तक्षयमूत्रविबन्धनुत् ||१४||
स्वादु पाके हिमं स्निग्धं तुवराम्लं विशुद्धिकृत् |
हन्याद्दाहतृषावातरक्तपित्तक्षतक्षयान् ||१५||

—भा. प्र. नि. गुडूच्यादिवर्ग

35. Gokshura *[Tribulus terrestris Linn.]*

Family: *Zygophyllaceae*

Hindi name: *Gokhuru*

English name: *Small caltrops, Puncture vine, Cow hage, Goat's head, devil's thorn*

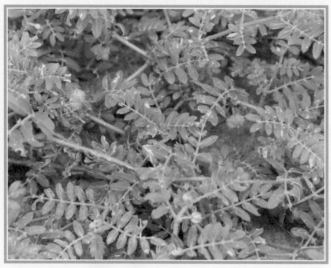

Plant of *Tribulus terrestris* Linn.

> *The herb is widely used by athletes and bodybuilders to enhance their physical strength and is enlisted in the Australian Register of Therapeutic Goods for the relief of menopausal and premenstrual tension.*

Introduction

Tribulus terrestris is derived from *Tribulus* a Latin word which means caltrop. Caltrop refers to spiky iron weapon suggesting the spinous nature of its fruit. In Greek *Tribulus* means water chestnut, suggesting the shape of its fruit like the water chestnut.

Gokshura has a 5,000-year-old history of medicinal use in different cultures throughout the world. In Shem-Nong's Chinese Pharmacopoeia it is described as a valuable drug to detoxify liver and kidney, for treatment of abdominal distention, mastitis, acute conjunctivitis, pruritis, infertility, sexual dysfunction, headache, and vertigo (Chinese Pharmacopoeia Commission 2015). In Bulgarian folk medicine it is recommended for blood purification and for treating piles and infertility. In South Africa it is used as a tonic and for treating diarrhea, throat, and eye infections. In folk medicine of Turkey it is used in colic pains, hypertension, and hypercholesterolemia (Arcasoy et al 1998).

In classical Ayurveda texts Gokshura is described as a potent anti-inflammatory and diuretic drug. It is one of the ingredients of famous anti-inflammatory formulations, dashmool and kantakapanchmool, which are used in urogenital diseases (S.S.Su. 38/66, 73). Raj Nighantu attributed rasayana properties to Brihat Gokshura (R.N. shatvahadi varga/43). It is also included in the group panchamrita (R.N. mishrakadi varga/30).

Vernacular Names

Assamese: Gokshura, Gukhurkata

Bengali: Gokshura, Gokhri

Gujarati: Be tha gokharu, Nana gokharu, Mithogokharu

Kannada: Sannanaggilu, Neggilamullu, Neggilu

Kashmiri: Michirkand, Pakhda

Malayalam: Nerinjil

Marathi: Sarate, Gokharu

Oriya: Gukhura, Gokhyura

Punjabi: Bhakhra, Gokhru
Tamil: Nerinjil, Nerunjil, Nerinci
Telugu: Palleruveru, Palleru Kayalu
Urdu: Khar-e-Khasak Khurd

Synonyms

Chandruma: Its leaves resemble those of Bengal gram leaves.
Gokantak: The fruit is armed with spines which injure the grazing animals.
Ikshugandhika: The root smells like sugarcane.
Kshurak: Its spines are sharp like the hood of the animals.
Palankasha: The sharp spines cause injury to the tissues.
Swadranstha: The plant bears sharp spines like the canine teeth of dog.
Swadukantaka: The fruit is madhura rasa pradhana.
Swadvi: The predominant rasa in it is madhur.
Trikantaka: The fruit is armed with spines.
Vanshringataka: The fruit resembles water chestnut and occurs wildly.

Classical Categorization

Charak Samhita: Krimighna, Shothahara, Mutravirechaniya
Sushrut Samhita: Vidarigandhadi, Veertarvadi, Laghu Panchmool
Ashtang Hridaya: Vidaryadi gana
Dhanvantari Nighantu: Guduchyadi varga
Madanpal Nighantu: Abhyadi varga

Kaiyadev Nighantu: Oushadi varga
Raj Nighantu: Shatvahadi varga
Bhavaprakash Nighantu: Guduchyadi varga

Distribution

Gokshura is widely distributed in warm regions of Europe, Asia, America, Africa, and Australia. It grows almost in every part of India as a common weed. They are wildly available in pasture land, fields, wastelands, and gardens, and on roadsides in dry warm, sandy regions of Rajasthan, Gujarat, Haryana, and Punjab.

Morphology

It is a perennial, prostrate, much branched, summer annual herb, densely covered with minute silky hair. Stems are often 30 to 70 cm long simple or freely branched, prostrate forming flat patches.

- **Leaves:** Pinnately compound, opposite, paripinnate, leaflets five to eight pairs, up to 8 cm long, subequal, oblong to linear-oblong, mucronate apex, pubescent on both surfaces (**Fig. 35.**1).
- **Flowers:** Solitary, axillary, five petals, lemon yellow to white yellow.
- Flowers often consist stamens and an ovary that has five cells, style short, and stout (**Fig. 35.2**).
- **Fruits:** A depressed schizocarp, globose, hairy, spinous, or tuberculate unripe green, fully mature yellowish-brown, each having five woody spinous cocci and each coccus has four pointed rigid spines.

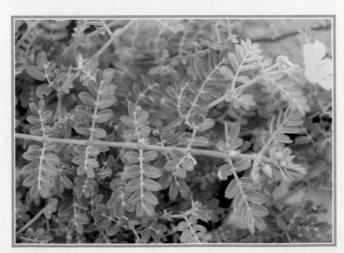

Fig. 35.1 Leaves.

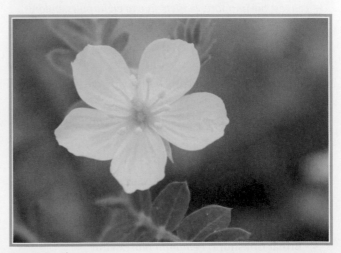

Fig. 35.2 Flower.

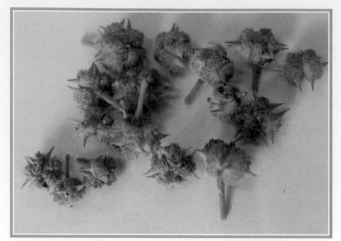

Fig. 35.3   Fruits.

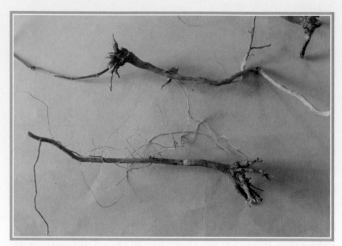

Fig. 35.4   Roots.

Out of which two are long and two are short. Larger spines are directed toward the apex and the smaller ones are directed downward (**Fig. 35.3**). Each coccus has many seeds. Fruits often cling to clothes and bodies of animals and humans.

- **Root:** Slender, fibrous, cylindrical, and light brown in color (**Fig. 35.4**). The plant is propagated by seeds (Jayanthy et al 2013).

Phenology

Flowering time: April to August
Fruiting time: April to August

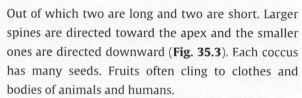

Key Characters for Identification

➤ *A creeping, branched, annual herb with silky hairs*
➤ *Leaves: paripinnate, leaflets five to eight pairs, oblong to linear-oblong shape*
➤ *Flowers: solitary, axillary, pentapetalous, lemon yellow colored*
➤ *Fruit: a globose schizocarp, hairy with five woody spinous cocci*
➤ *Roots are fibrous, cylindrical, and light brown in color*

Types

Two types of Gokshura are described by Bhavaprakash Nighantu:

- Brihat Gokshura: *Pedalium murex* Linn
- Laghu Gokshura: *Tribulus terrestris* Linn

Rasapanchaka

Guna	Guru, Snigdh
Rasa	Madhur
Vipaka	Madhur
Virya	Sheeta

Chemical Constituents

The plant is reported to have steroidal glycoside, steroidal saponin, flavonoids, alkaloids, lignanamides, and cinammic acid amides. The fruits have steroidal saponins terrestrosins A, B, C, D, and E, diosgenin, desgalactotigonis, gitonin, F-gitonis, desglucolanatigoneis, gitnin, hecogenins neotigogenin, chlorogenin, spirostanol, furostanol, protodioscin, yamogenin, gitogenin, rutin, and rahmnose. The stem contains starch, fructose sucrose, *p*-carboline alkaloids (norharman, harman, harmol, harmine, 3-hydroxymethyl-norharman, harmalol, harmaline, tetrahydroharman, and amides [terrestriamide, tribulusamides A and B]). The leaves contain moisture, protein, calcium, phosphorous, iron, vitamin C, and saponins (diosgenin, gitogenin, chlorogenin spirostanol, furostanol). The root contains alkaloid (Harman, harmol), flavonoids (kaempferol, quercetin), campsterol, β-sitosterol, stigmasterol, neotegogenin resins, nitrate, and fixed oils. Other constituents include fatty acids, polysaccharides, protein, tannins, amino acids and calcium, potassium salts (Xu et al 2001; Zafar and Nasa 1987; Wang et al 1997; Wu et al 1999).

Identity, Purity, and Strength

For Root

- Foreign matter: Not more than 2%
- Total ash: Not more than 13%
- Acid-insoluble ash: Not more than 3%
- Alcohol-soluble extractive: Not less than 4%
- Water-soluble extractive: Not less than 10%

(Source: The Ayurvedic Pharmacopeia of India 1989)

Karma (Actions)

Various Nighantus have described it as swadu (sweet), balkrit (strength promoting), bastishodhana (urinary depurative), mutral (diuretic), brihmaniya (body mass increasing), deepana (appetizer), vrishya (aphrodisiac), pushtikar (nutritive), ashmarbhedana (lithontriptic), hridya (cardioprotective), vedanasthapana (analgesic), anulomana (laxative), raktapittashamaka (pacify rakta and pitta), shothahara (swelling reducing), kaphanissaraka (anti-tussive), garbhasthapana (promote fertility), vajikaran (aphrodisiac).

- Doshakarma: Vata pitta shamaka
- Dhatukarma: Rasayana, Balya, Vrishya
- Malakarma: Mutral, Anulomana

Pharmacological Actions

Gokshura is reported to exhibit antiurolithic, diuretic, aphrodisiac, immunomodulatory, cardioprotective, hepato-protective, antidiabetic, antioxidant, anti-inflammatory, antibacterial, antiaging, memory enhancer, antitumor, antimicrobial, hypolipidemic, anticancer, anti-infertility, antispasmodic, neuroprotective, antifatigue, anthelmintic, larvicidal, anticarious, and absorption enhancer activities (Zhu et al 2017; Sivapalan 2016; Li et al 2002).

Indications

In Ayurveda classics Gokshura is reported to be used in the treatment of mutrakricchta (dysuria), daha (burning sensation), ashmari (renal calculi), prameha (diabetes), shwasa (asthma), kasa (cough), arsha (piles), shool (pain), hridya roga (cardiac diseases), and disorders caused by aggravated vata.

In other traditional systems of medicines the plant and fruits are used in the treatment of spermatorrhea, impotence, infertility, sexual dysfunction, phosphaturia, gonorrhea, gleet, chronic cystitis, incontinence, gout, menstrual disorders, morbid leucorrhea, postpartum hemorrhage, skin diseases, eye trouble, edema, abdominal distention, ulcerative stomatitis, typhoid fever, and general debility (Nadkarni and Nadkarni 2000; Gehlot and Bohra 2000; Selvam 2008).

Therapeutic Uses

External Use

Keshvardhan: Application of paste prepared with Gokshura and Tila pushpa mixed with madhu, ghrita in the root hairs promotes hair growth (Sh.S. 3/11/22).

Internal Use

1. **Ashmari** (calculus): Roots of Gokshura, Kokilaksha, Eranda, and Brahati dvay pounded together with dugdh and dissolved in madhur dahi help to dissolve calculus (C.S.Ci. 26/62). Seed powder of trikantaka mixed with madhu and taken with avi dugdh for a week breaks the calculus (S.S.Ci. 7/19; VM. 34/28).
2. **Mutrakricchta** (dysuria): Decoction of Gokshura seeds mixed with Yavakshara is given in dysuria, gravel, and calculus (VM. 32/16; B.P.Ci. 35/33). Decoction of Gokshura panchang mixed with madhu sarkara is administered in dysuria (B.S.mutraghat Ci/30). In nephritis and cystitis when the urine becomes alkaline and purulent, its root decoction is given with Shilajeet.
3. **Rakta pitta** (mutramarggat raktasrava): Intake of milk cooked with Shatavri, Gokshura, and four parni (i.e., shalaparni, prishanparni, mugdaparni, mashaparni) checks hematuria (C.S.Ci. 4/85).
4. **Shosha** (consumption): Powder of Gokshura fruit and Ashwagandha mixed with madhu when taken with milk alleviates cough and consumption (RM. 12/3).
5. **Aamvaat** (arthritis): Regular use of decoction of Sunthi and Gokshura in the morning digests aam, and reduces pain and inflammation in arthritis and backache (CD. 25/9).
6. **Vajikarana** (aphrodisiac): Powder of Gokshura, Ikshuraka, Shatavari, Kapikacchu, Nagbala, and Atibala

taken with milk every night cures infertility and acts as a good aphrodisiac (VM. 70/14).

7. **Rasayana** (rejuvinator): Intake of Gokshura powder pounded with Gokshura swarasa with dugdh followed by diet of shali rice and milk gives rasayana effect (A.H.U. 39/56).

Officinal Parts Used

Whole plant, roots, fruit

Dose

Powder: 3 to 6 g
Decoction: 40 to 100 mL

Formulations

Gokhuradi guggulu, Dashmoolarishta, Gokshuradi churna, Trikantakadi ghrita, Trikantakadi churna, Sahcharadi taila, Abhyarishta, Ashmarihara kashaya, Dashmool kwath.

Toxicity/Adverse Effects

Acute toxicity studies of *Tribulus terrestris* showed no behavioral changes, toxicological signs, or mortality in animals (Abudayyak et al 2015).

Substitution and Adulteration

Laghu Gokshura is often substituted with Brihat Gokshura (*Pedalium murex* Linn.) and the fruits of *Acanthospermum hispidum* DC. is mixed with Gokshura, because of close resemblance of the individual cocci (Sharma et al 2005).

Points to Ponder

- *Laghu Gokshura is traditionally known for antiurolithiatic, diuretic, and aphrodisiac properties whereas Brihat Gokshura for its rasayana properties.*
- *It is a renowned drug for dysuria, calculus, infertility, debility, and edema.*

Suggested Readings

Abudayyak M, Jannuzzi AT, Özhan G, Alpertunga B. Investigation on the toxic potential of *Tribulus terrestris* in vitro. Pharm Biol 2015;53(4):469–476

Arcasoy HB, Erenmemisoglu A, Tekol Y, Kurucu S, Kartal M. Effect of *Tribulus terrestris* L. saponin mixture on some smooth muscle preparations: a preliminary study. Boll Chim Farm 1998;137(11):473–475

Chinese Pharmacopoeia Commission. Chinese Pharmacopoeia. Vol. I. Beijing: China Medical Science Press; 2015:352

Gehlot D, Bohra A. Toxic effect of various plant parts extracts on the causal organism of typhoid fever. Curr Sci 2000;78(7): 780–781

Georgiev P, Dimitrov M, Vitanov S. The effect of the preparation Tribestan on the plasma concentration of testosterone and spermatgenesis of lambs and rams. Vet Sb 1988;3:20–22

Jayanthy A, Deepak M, Remashree AB. Pharmacognostic characterization and comparison of fruits of *Tribulus terrestris* L. and *Pedalium murex* L. IJHM 2013;1(4):29–34

Li M, Qu W, Wang Y, Wan H. Hypoglycemic effect of saponin from *Tribulus terrestris*. Zhong Yao Cai 2002;25(6):420–422

Nadkarni KM, Nadkarni AK. Indian Materia Medica-2. 3rd ed. Bombay: Popular Prakasan; 2000:1229–1232

Selvam ABD. Inventory of vegetable crude drug samples housed in Botanical Survey of India, Howrah. Pharmacogn Rev 2008;2(3): 61–94

Sharma PC, Yelne MB, Dennis TJ. Database on Medicinal Plants Used in Ayurveda, Vol. 3. New Delhi: CCRAS. Reprint 2005; 2005:229–234

Sivapalan R. Biological and pharmacological studies of *Tribulus terrestris* Linn.: a review. Int J Multidiscipl Res Dev 2016;3(1):257–265

The Ayurvedic Pharmacopeia of India. Part I, Vol. 1. New Delhi: Department of AYUSH, Ministry of Health and Family Welfare, Government of India; 1989:50

Wang Y, Ohtani K, Kasai R, Yamasaki K. Steroidal saponins from fruits of *Tribuliis terrestris*. Phytochemistry 1997;45:811–817

Wu TS, Shi LS, Kuo SC. Alkaloids and other constituents from *Tribulus terrestris*. Phytochemistry 1999;50(8):1411–1415

Xu YJ, Xie SX, Zhao HF, Han D, Xu TH, Xu DM. Studies on the chemical constituents from *Tribulus terrestris*. Yao Xue Xue Bao 2001;36(10):750–753

Zafar R, Nasa AK. Quercentin and kaempferol from the fruits and stem of *Tribulus terrestris*. Indian J Nat Prod 1987;3:17–18

Zhu W, Du Y, Meng H, Dong Y, Li L. A review of traditional pharmacological uses, phytochemistry, and pharmacological activities of *Tribulus terrestris*. Chem Cent J 2017;11(60):1–5

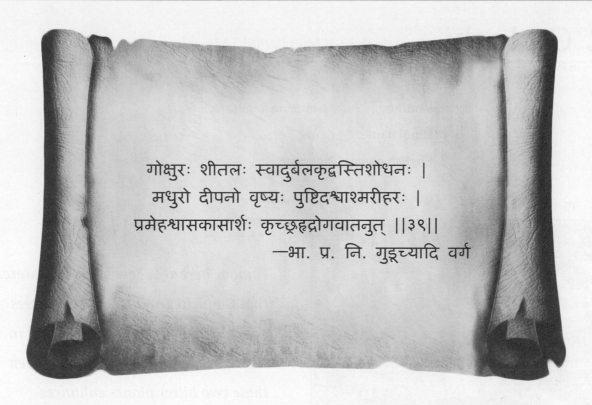

गोक्षुरः शीतलः स्वादुर्बलकृद्वस्तिशोधनः |
मधुरो दीपनो वृष्यः पुष्टिदश्चाश्मरीहरः |
प्रमेहश्वासकासार्शः कृच्छ्रहृद्रोगवातनुत् ||३९||
—भा. प्र. नि. गुडूच्यादि वर्ग

36. Guduchi [Tinospora cordifolia [Willd.] Miers]

Family: *Menispermaceae (moon seed)*

Hindi name: *Giloy*

English name: *Tinospora*

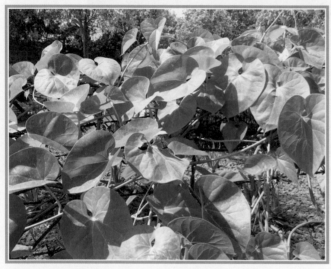

Plant of *Tinospora cordifolia* (Willd.) Miers.

> *Famous herbalist Sebastian Pole states that Guduchi growing on Neem trees are said to be more bitter and best in therapeutics, as the synergy between these two bitter plants enhances its efficacy.*

Introduction

The term "Guduchi" is derived from the phrase *gud rakshane*, which means the one who protects us from diseases. *Cordifolia* refers to the cordate shape of the leaves.

Guduchi is considered as a divine herb owing to its multifaceted health benefits. In Hindu mythology, it is believed to have been originated from nectar (elixir, *amrita*). A myth about the origin of Guduchi is that during the war between Lord Rama and Ravana, when the army of monkeys started dying, Lord Indra dispensed amrit among them. While distributing amrit, some of its drops fell on the ground and Guduchi plant originated from that (B.P.N). Hence, to ensure long and healthy life, our ancestors advised to plant Guduchi sapling in everyone's house.

Ayurveda classics have praised this versatile herb since ages. Charak Samhita considered Guduchi as the best sangrahi, vatahara, deepaniya, shlesm-shonita vibandh shamak dravya (C.S.S. 25/40) and described it as one of the medhya rasayana (C.S.Ci. 1/3/30). In Sushrut Samhita, it is mentioned in tikta patra shaka varga under the name of vatsadini, while in Ashtang Hridaya it is considered as best drug for the treatment of vatarakta (A.H.U. 40/59). Sharangdhar Samhita recommended the use of Guduchi in fresh state (Sh.S. 1/1/45-47). Guduchi is included in the group of panchtikta (Rasatarangani 2/18), vallipanchmool (S.S.Su. 38/72), and chatubhadra (R.N. mishrakadi/17).

Vernacular Names

Assamese: Siddhilata, Amaralata
Bengali: Gulancha
Gujarati: Galac, Garo
Kannada: Amrutaballi
Kashmiri: Amrita, Gilo
Malayalam: Chittamrutu
Marathi: Gulvel
Oriya: Guluchi

Punjabi: Gilo
Tamil: Seendal, Seendilkodi
Telugu: Thippateega
Urdu: Gilo

Synonyms

Amrita: It means the plant never dies and has properties like nectar, i.e., which provides immortality.

Amritvallari: The climber never dies and regenerates easily.

Bhishakpriya: The plant is popular in therapeutics.

Chakralakshanika: Transverse section of stem shows the configuration of spoke of a wheel.

Chandrahasa: The seeds are semilunar in shape.

Chinnarooha: The plant regenerates from stem cutting.

Devnirmita: The plant is formed by deity.

Jwarnashini: It is efficacious in fever.

Kandodbhava: The plant is regenerated from stem.

Kundlini: The plant ascends by coiling its stem around a support.

Madhuparni: The leaves contain viscid juice like honey.

Rasayani: The plant has rejuvenating property.

Soma: It promotes strength and vitality.

Tantrika: The coiled stem appears like a rope.

Vatsadani: Its leaves are eaten by calves.

Vishaghni: It has the properties to counteract poison.

Vyastha: It has antiaging properties, i.e., keeps one eternally young.

Classical Categorization

Charak Samhita: Sandhaniya, Triptighna, Stanyashodhana, Snehopaga, Trishna nigrahan, Mutravirechaniya, Daha prashman, Vyasthapana.

Sushrut Samhita: Araghvadhadi, Shyamadi, Patoladi, Kakolyadi, Guduchyadi, Valli panchmool.

Ashtang Hridaya: Guduchyadi, Patoladi, Araghvadhadi

Dhanvantari Nighantu: Guduchyadi varga

Madanpal Nighantu: Abhyadi varga

Kaiyadev Nighantu: Oushadi varga

Raj Nighantu: Guduchyadi varga

Bhavaprakash Nighantu: Guduchyadi varga

Distribution

This plant is indigenous to India, Sri Lanka, and Myanmar. It is distributed throughout the tropical regions of India up to an elevation of 1,200 m. It is a fairly common plant of deciduous and dry forest, growing over hedges and trees.

Morphology

It is a perennial, deciduous, woody, dextrorotatory climber. This herb is often seen growing upon Neem and Mango trees.

- **Fresh stem:** Green, mucilaginous, soft, succulent, glabrous, terete, sparsely lenticellate and often producing filliform aerial roots from branches. Bark warty, creamish-white when green and gray when mature (**Fig. 36.1a, b**).
- **Dried stem:** Cylindrical, slender, slightly twisted shape, 6 to 12 cm in diameter with rough surface due to longitudinal fissures of cracks along with rows of lenticels. Outer bark is thin and papery brown to grayish in color. Lenticels are circular and prominent. Transverse cut section shows a wheel-like structure, a characteristic feature of menispermaceae family (**Fig. 36.2**).
- **Leaves:** Simple, alternate, long petiolate up to 15 cm, lamina broadly ovate-cordate 10 to 20 cm long, 8 to 15 cm broad, seven-nerved and deeply cordate at the base, membranous, pubescent above whitish tomentose beneath, acute to acuminate apex, margin entire, reticulate venation. The leaves when seen in bulk look intensely green but over mature leaves are yellowish-green to yellow color. Leaves are bitter and have an indistinct odor (**Fig. 36.3**).
- **Flowers:** Male and female flowers occur on separate plants (dioceious/unisexual plant) and appear when plant is leafless. Flowering is axillary raceme type. Male flowers are small, yellow or green in color, and occur in clusters. Female flowers are usually solitary and are green (**Fig. 36.4**).
- **Fruit:** Aggregate of one to three, ovoid, smooth, drupaceous, equal to the size of a large pea, unripe green and turns red when fully ripe (**Fig. 36.5a, b**). The plant is propagated by stem cutting and seeds.

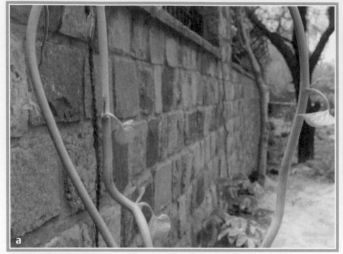

Fig. 36.1 **(a)** Young stem. **(b)** Mature stem.

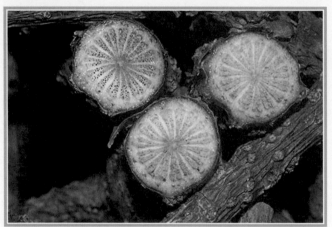

Fig. 36.2 T.S. of stem.

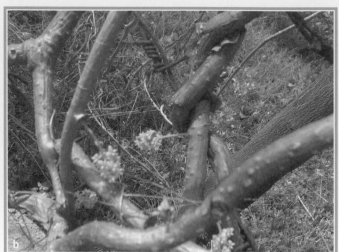

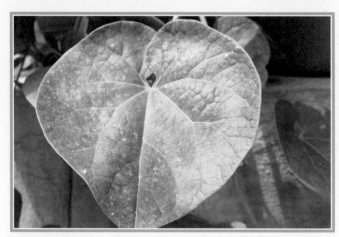

Fig. 36.3 Leaf.

Phenology

Flowering time: May to June

Fruiting time: August to December

> ### Key Characters for Identification
>
> ➤ *It is a perennial deciduous dextrorotatory climber.*
> ➤ *Stem: green, mucilaginous, soft, succulent produces aerial roots. Dried stem is cylindrical, light, lenticellate, and peels off.*
> ➤ *Leaves: simple, alternate, cordate shape, with a long petiole.*
> ➤ *Flowers: small yellowish-green, dioecious in axillary raceme.*
> ➤ *Fruits: drupe, aggregate of one to three, oval shape, red on ripening.*

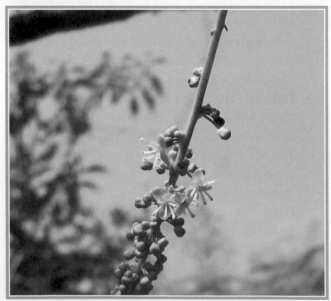

Fig. 36.4 Flower.

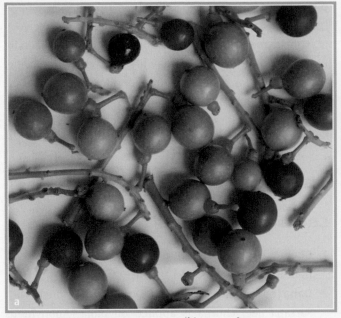 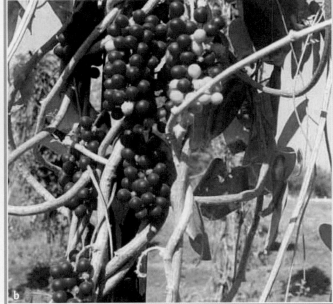

Fig. 36.5 **(a)** Fruits in various stages. **(b)** Mature fruits.

Types

Dhanvantari and Rajanighantu have described two types of Guduchi:

- Guduchi
- Kandodbhav Guduchi

Rasapanchaka

Guna	Laghu, Snigdha
Rasa	Tikta, Katu, Kasaya
Vipaka	Madhura
Virya	Ushna
Prabhava	Tridoshahara

Chemical Constituents

The stem is rich in sesquiterpene tinocordifolin alkaloids (berberine, choline, magnoflorine, palmatine, tembetarine magnoflorine, tinosporin, tetrahydropalmatine, isocolumbin), glycosides (furanoid diterpene glucoside, tinocordiside, tinocordifolioside, cordioside, cordifolioside A, B, syringin, syringin-apiosylglycoside, palmatosides C, F, cordifoliside A, B, C, D, E), lactones (clerodane derivatives, tinosporon, tinosporides, jateorine, columbin), and steroids (sitosterols, hydroxy ecdysone, ecdysterone, makisterone, giloinsterol). Other compounds are jatrorrhizine, tinosporidine, cordifol, cordifelone, giloin, giloinin, and tinosporic acid (Khatun et al 2016; Promila et al 2017).

Identity, Purity, and Strength

- Foreign matter: Not more than 2%
- Total ash: Not more than 16%
- Acid-insoluble ash: Not more than 3%
- Alcohol-soluble extractive: Not less than 3%
- Water-soluble extractive: Not less than 11%
- Moisture content (in fresh drug): Not less than 75%

(Source: The Ayurvedic Pharmacopeia of India 1989)

Karma (Actions)

In Ayurvedic treatise and Nighantus, Guduchi stem is described as sangrahi (absorbent), hridya (cardio tonic), balya (strength promoting), agnideepak (appetizer), rasayana (rejuvinator), ayushya (longevity), medhya (intellect promoting), and jwaraghna (antipyretic) in karma. Guduchi satva (starch from stems) is laghu, madhura, pathya, deepan, cakshushya (beneficial for eyes), dhatuvardhak (enhances all dhatu), vyasthapana (promotes longevity). Guduchi swaras (juice from fresh plant) is guru, tikta, kashaya, ushna, and tridoshshamaka (Sharma

1982). Guduchi patra shaka is laghu, katu, tikta, kashaya rasa, madhura vipaka, ushna virya, tridoshaghna, pathya, chakshushya, deepan, vyasthapana, medhya, balya, grahi in properties (Sharma 1979). Kandodbhava Guduchi is katu, ushna virya, sannipatah, vishaghna, jwarbhootaghna, and valli palitya nashini (Tripathi 2003; Sharma 1982).

- Doshakarma: Tridoshashamaka
- Dhatukarma: Rasayana, ayushya, balya
- Malakarma: Mutral

Pharmacological Actions

The stem is reported to possess antiperiodic, antipyretic, hepatoprotective, analgesic, antispasmodic, anti-inflammatory, adaptogenic, antioxidant, antidiabetic, anti-allergic, diuretic, hypoglycemic, antibacterial digestive, carminative, cardiotonic, neuroprotective, expectorant, aphrodisiac, antileprotic, antitumor, anti-HIV, antiosteo-porotic, and immunomodulatory properties (Singh et al 2003; Tiwari et al 2018).

Indications

Traditionally, Guduchi stem is used in the treatment of jwar (chronic intermittent fever), trishna (thirst), daha (burning sensation), kushta, kandu, visarp (skin diseases) krimi, chardi, vatarakta (gout), pandu (anemia), kamala (jaundice), prameha (diabetes), bhram, kasa, aam, raktaarsha, amlapitta (hyperacidity). Guduchi satva is useful in acid peptic diseases, jeernajwar, vatarakta, pandu, kamala, prameha (diabetes), aruchi (anorexia), shwasa (asthma), kasa (cough), hikka (hic-cough), daha (burning sensation), arsha (piles), mutrakricchta (dysuria), pradar (menorrhagia), and somaroga. Guduchi swaras is used in jwar (fever), kushta (leprosy), krimi (worm infestation), raktarsha (bleeding piles).

Guduchi patra shaka is used in the treatment of vatarakta (gout), trishna (thirst), daha (burning sensation), prameha (diabetes), kushta (skin diseases), pandu (anemia), kamala (jaundice), etc. Dhanvantari and Madanpal Nighantu have described the use of Guduchi with specific anupaan (vehicle) to alleviate vibandh (constipation), aamvaat (rheumatoid arthritis), vatarakta (gout), and diseases of vata, pitta, kapha. Guduchi is given with ghee, sugar, honey, jaggery, eranda taila (castor oil), and shunthi (ginger) to treat vata, pitta, kapha diseases, vibandha (constipation), vatarakta (gout), and aamvaat (rheumatoid arthritis), respectively.

Tribals and ethnic groups in different regions of India use Guduchi in their day-to-day life as food and medicine. They use it for treating ailments like periodic fever, jaundice, diarrhea, dysentery, cancer, fracture, skin diseases, leucorrhea, cough, asthma, general debility, and earache (Sinha et al 2004).

Traditional Uses

External Use

1. **Bhagna** (fracture): Paste of whole plant is applied on fractures and rheumatoid arthritis.
2. **Daha** (burning sensation): Paste or juice of Guduchi with Sarsapa beej churna is applied on daha (Anonymous 1999).

Internal Use

1. **Visham jwar** (intermittent fever): Decoction of Guduchi, Nimba, and Amalaki mixed with madhu is beneficial in visham jwar (S.S.U. 39/213). Taking Guduchi swaras daily gives relief in visham jwar (intermittent fever) (C.S.Ci. 3/299).
2. **Jeerna jwar:** In all types of jeerna jwar (chronic fever), Guduchi swaras mixed with pippali and honey is given (B.P.Ci. 1/818). Cold infusion (hima) of Guduchi gives relief in jeerna jwar (Sh.S. 2/2/46).
3. **Dengue fever:** 1 tsf of fresh giloy stem juice, 1 tsf of aloe vera pulp and half tsf papaya leaf juice taken with water increases platelet count in dengue patient.
4. **Rasayana** (immunity enhancer/rejuvenator): Daily intake of Guduchi swaras enhances body immunity and acts as an adaptogen. It expels out toxins from the body and rejuvenates it at tissue level (C.S.Ci. 1.3/30).
5. **Cancer:** Daily intake of 4 tsf Guduchi swaras or 1 g of Giloy satva before and after chemotherapy helps in reducing the side effects of chemotherapy in cancer patients.
6. **Kamala** (jaundice): Daily intake of Guduchi swaras mixed with honey in the morning cures jaundice (C.S.Ci. 16/63). Paste of Guduchi leaves taken with takra as anupana is used to cure jaundice (BS.pandu/70).

7. **Vatarakta** (gout): Decoction made up of Guduchi stem, Eranda mool, and Vasa mool taken with Eranda taila twice daily cures vatarakta (gout) (Sh.S. 2/2/150). Oil prepared with Guduchi, til taila, and milk is used to treat vatarakta (C.S.Ci. 29/121). By using Guduchi swaras, kalka, and kwath regularly, one becomes free from vatarakta (VM. 23/10) (B.P.Ci. 29/41).
8. **Prameha** (diabetes): Guduchi swaras mixed with honey is taken twice daily in all types of prameha (A.H.Ci. 12/6).
9. **Amlapitta** (hyperacidity): Decoction of Guduchi, Neem, Patola leaves, and Triphala or Giloy satva with honey gives relief in acid peptic diseases, dyspepsia, and burning sensation (B.P.Ci. 10/16).
10. **Netra roga:** In all types of eye disorders, decoction of Guduchi and Triphala mixed with pippali and madhu is beneficial (Sh.S. 2/2/150).
11. **Kushta** (skin diseases): Intake of Guduchi swaras as per one's capacity followed by diet of rice, moong, yusha, and ghrita gives relief in skin diseases (G.Ni. 2/36/83).
12. **Chardi:** Cold infusion (hima) of Guduchi mixed with madhu checks vomiting caused by three doshas (B.P.Ci. 17/21).
13. **Shlipada** (filariasis): Consumption of Guduchi swaras with til taila daily helps in reducing inflammation in shlipada (CD. 42/16).
14. **Raktapradar** (menometrorrhagia): Daily intake of Guduchi swaras or vasa swaras gives relief in raktapradar (G.N. 6/1/10).
15. **Stanyashodhana** (detoxification of breast milk): For detoxification of breast milk, decoction of Guduchi and Saptaparna with Shunthi is recommended daily (C.S.Ci. 30/261).

Officinal Parts Used

Stem, root, leaves

Dose

Powder: 2 to 4 g
Powder: 3 to 6 g
Decoction: 50 to 100 mL
Satva: 1 to 2 g with honey

Formulations

Guduchyadi churna, Amritarishta, Sansamani Vati, Guduchi satva, Guduchi ghrita, Amrita guggulu, Amritashtaka kwath, Panchnimba churna, Kantakari avleha.

Toxicity/Adverse Effect

No adverse reactions or toxicity of Guduchi have been noted. However, there is little information about its toxicology in humans (Anonymous 2003).

Substitution and Adulteration

Guduchi is substituted or adulterated with other species of Tinospora, i.e., *T. malabarica, T. crispa,* and *T. sinensis.* The extract of Guduchi (Guduchi satva) is adulterated with powder, flour of potato, sweet potato, arrow root, and banana powder (Sharma et al 2005).

> *Points to Ponder*
> - *Guduchi is the most renowned immunomodulator, rejuvenator, adaptogen, and antioxidant drug in Ayurveda.*
> - *Charak Samhita considered Guduchi as the best sangrahi, vatahara, deepaniya, shlesm-shonita vibandh shamak dravya (C.S.S. 25/40).*
> - *Guduchi swaras is used as medhya rasayan.*
> - *It is the drug of choice in treatment of vatarakta, jwar, amalpitta, kamala, daha, prameha, vyasthapana, and for enhancing immunity.*

Suggested Readings

Anonymous. An Appraisal of Tribal folk Medicines. New Delhi: CCRAS; 1999:24

Anonymous. Quality Standards of Indian Medicinal Plants, Vol. 1. New Delhi: ICMR; 2003:212

Hazera K, Suman K, Kazi MM, Mohiuddin A. Guduchi (*Tinospora cordifolia* (Willd)), a traditional Indian herb and its medicinal importance: an Ayurvedic approach with contemporary view. Int J Ayur Herb Med 2016;6(4):2260–2267

Promila S, Sushila S, Devi P. Pharmacological potential of Tinospora cordifolia (Willd.) Miers ex hook. & Thoms. (Giloy): A review. J Pharmacogn Phytochem 2017;6(6):1644–1647

Sharma PC, Yelne MB, Dennis TJ. Database on Medicinal Plants Used in Ayurveda, Vol. 3. New Delhi: CCRAS; 2005, Reprint 2005:256

Sharma PV. Dhanwantari Nighantu (Hindi). 1st ed. 1982, Varanasi: Chowkhamba Oriental;1982, Guduchyadi varga, shloka no. 5 & 8, Reprint 2008:16

Sharma PV. Kaiyadev Nighantu. 1st ed. Varanasi, Delhi: Chowkhamba Oriental;1979, Oushadi varga, shloka no.11, Reprint 2009:5

Singh SS, Pandey SC, Srivastava S, Gupta VS, Patro B, Ghosh AC. Chemistry and Medicinal Properties of *Tinospora cordifolia* (Guduchi). Ind J Pharmacol 2003;35:83–91

Sinha K, Mishra NP, Singh J, Khanuja SPS. *Tinospora cordifolia* (Guduchi):

A reservoir plant for therapeutic application—a review. Ind J Tradit Knowl 2004;3(3):257–270

The Ayurvedic Pharmacopeia of India, Part I, Vol. 1. New Delhi: Department of AYUSH, Ministry of Health and Family Welfare, Government of India; 1989:54

Tiwari P, Nayak P, Prusty SK, Sahu PK. Phytochemistry and pharmacology of *Tinospora cordifolia*: A review. System Rev Pharm 2018;9(1):70–78

Tripathi I. Raja Nighantu of Pt. Narhari. 3rd ed. Varanasi: Chowkhamba Krishnadas Academy, Oriental Publisher; 2003, Guduchyadi varga, shloka no. 18:31

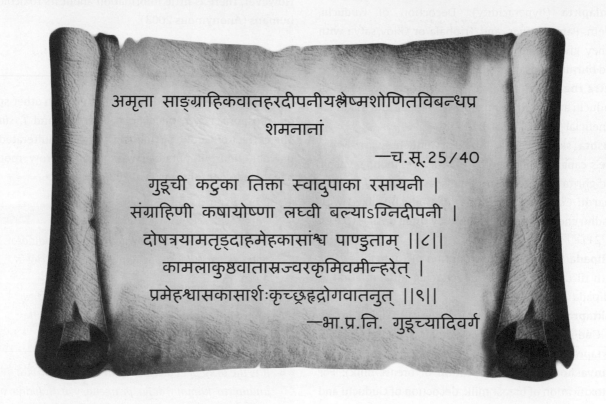

अमृता साङ्ग्राहिकवातहरदीपनीयश्लेष्मशोणितविबन्धप्रशमनानां

—च.सू. 25/40

गुडूची कटुका तिक्ता स्वादुपाका रसायनी ।
संग्राहिणी कषायोष्णा लघ्वी बल्याऽग्निदीपनी ।
दोषत्रयामतृड्दाहमेहकासांश्च पाण्डुताम् ॥८॥
कामलाकुष्ठवातास्रज्वरकृमिवमीन्हरेत् ।
प्रमेहश्वासकासार्शःकृच्छ्रहृद्रोगवातनुत् ॥९॥

—भा.प्र.नि. गुडूच्यादिवर्ग

37. Guggulu *[Commiphora mukul (Hook ex stocks)]*

Family:	*Burseraceae*
Hindi name:	*Guggal, Gugal*
English name:	*Indian bedellium tree, Hill mango*

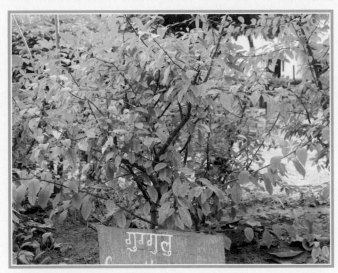

Plant of *Commiphora mukul* (Hook ex stocks).

> *The best method for enhancing the production of oleo gum resin in Guggulu is tapping technique. For this, a plant that is over 5 years old with a basal diameter greater than 7.5 cm is best suitable.*
>
> **—Bhatt et al 1989**

Introduction

The word "Guggulu" is derived from the phrase "gudti rakshyati vatarogata iti Guggulu," which means the one having the potential of protecting from vata roga is Guggulu. Mythologically, it is believed that Guggulu was evolved as nectar during Devasur Sangrama by Lord Vishnu *to* replenish the lost bala, shourya, and tejas of Devtas (Astang Sangraha 2005).

Guggulu has a wide range of uses in traditional medicine and is considered as the best analgesic and anti-inflammatory drug in Ayurveda. In Atharva Veda, it is mentioned that fumigating the area with Guggulu prevents spreading of yakshma and other diseases (19/381/1). Sayana also described it as a well-known dravya for dhupana karma. During samhita period, the internal use of Guggulu increased tremendously. Charak described it as dhupan dravya in kaumar paricharya (C.S.Sa. 8/61) and in treatment of vishamjwar (C.S.Ci. 3/107), as an ingredient in prayogik dhumpana varti (C.S.Su. 5/21) and as pradeh kalpa in twak roga (C.S.Su. 3/4). Astanga Sangraha used it as dhupana dravya in balaroga chikitsa (A.S.U. 4/13). Sharangdhar quoted it as examples of drugs used for rasayana karma (Sh. purva khand 4/13, p. 34). Kaiyadev classified different colored Guggulu in terms of their doshaghanta like Krishna varna Guggulu is best for rakta-pitta dosh, pingal varna Guggulu is best for kapha-pitta dosh, and shweta varna Guggulu is best for vata-pitta dosh (Sharma and Sharma 2006). In Rasagranthas, it is used as a reducing agent for metals and minerals and thus included in dravaka gana and mitra panchaka gana (Shastri kashinath 1979). It is also used for the treatment of diseases of cattle.

Vernacular Names

Arabic: Aflatan, Moql, Mukulearabi
Assamese: Guggul
Bengali: Guggula, Guggal

Gujarati: Gugal, Guggal, Gugar

Kannada: Kanthagana, Guggala, Mahishaksha guggulu, Guggulugida, Guggulu

Kashmiri: Guggul Dhoop, Kanth Gan

Malayalam: Gulgulu, Guggulu

Marathi: Guggul, Mahishaksh

Oriya: Guggulu

Persian: Boejahudan

Punjabi: Guggal

Sindhi: Gugal, Guggul, Mukul, Ranghanturb

Singhlese: Gugula, Jatayu, Javayu, Ratadummula

Tamil: Mahisaksi, Guggalu, Gukkal

Telugu: Makishakshi guggulu, Guggipannu

Urdu: Muqil (Shihappu)

Synonyms

Devadhupa: Incenses prepared from its resin are used in worshipping God.

Kananiryasa: The exudate is crystalline in nature.

Kaushika: The gum resin is produced from the cells of this plant.

Kumbholukhalaka: The exudate is produced inside the cavities in tree.

Mahishaksha: The color of gum resin resembles the color of the eyes of a buffalo.

Marudeshya: The plant grows naturally in sandy arid regions.

Palankasha: The exudate is used to scrape away the excessive fat.

Pura: Its exudate is highly potent in action.

Rakshoha: Its resin is antiseptic and is used in fumigation.

Ulukhala: The exudate is produced and collected inside the cavities of the tree.

Classical Categorization

Charak Samhita: Sangyasthapana

Sushrut Samhita: Eladi

Ashtang Hridaya: Eladi

Dhanvantari Nighantu: Chandanadi varga

Madanpal Nighantu: Karpuradi varga

Kaiyadev Nighantu: Oushadi varga

Raj Nighantu: Chandanadi varga

Bhavaprakash Nighantu: Guduchyadi varga

Distribution

Guggulu is a native plant of northern Africa and central Asia. In India, it is mostly found in arid rocky places of Rajasthan, Gujarat, Haryana, Madhya Pradesh, and Karnataka.

Morphology

A small tree or shrub with spinescent branches reaching up to a height of 7 to 8 feet. Young branches are aromatic and brownish-red in color. Plant exists in three forms, i.e., male, female, and bisexual.

- **Bark:** It is characterized by the presence of silvery paper-like brownish bark which peels off regularly, and below it the stem is green (**Fig. 37.1**).
- **Leaves:** Trifoliate in which the terminal leaflet is biggest and lateral leaflets are less than half the size of the terminal one, alternate, rhomboid-ovate shape, serrated margin, and reddish-brown petiole (**Fig. 37.2**).
- **Flowers:** Small, brownish-red in fascicles of two to three, pedicels are very short. Calyx is glandular, hairy, and campanulate. Petals are brownish-red,

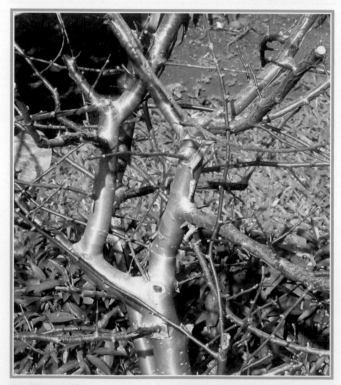

Fig. 37.1 Bark.

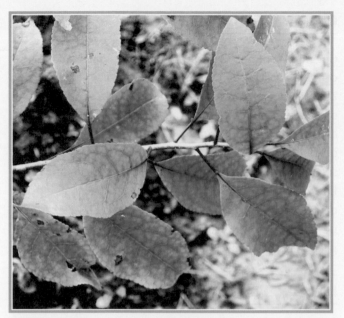

Fig. 37.2 Leaves.

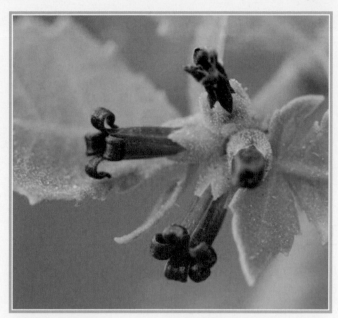

Fig. 37.3 Flowers.

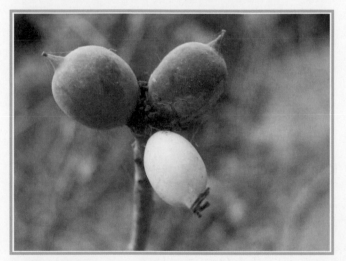

Fig. 37.4 Fruits.

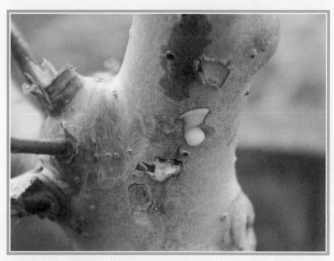

Fig. 37.5 Exudate.

broadly linear, nearly thrice the length of the calyx, reflexed at the apex. Stamens are eight to ten in number, alternatively long and short, half the length of the petals. Ovary oblong-ovoid, attenuated into the style (**Fig. 37.3**).

- **Fruits:** Small, oval shape drupes, red when ripe, easily splits into two (**Fig. 37.4**).
- **Exudate:** Obtained from the oleo resin ducts in the bark; when fresh, the resin is pale yellow to brown, and aromatic. After collection, it is opaque, aromatic, reddish-brown, dusty surface, mixed with sand,

consists of irregular roundish masses of varying sizes (Kirtikar and Basu 2012; **Fig. 37.5**). Best resin is the one that is thick, aromatic, burns completely in fire, melts easily in sun heat, and turns milky white when dissolved in water (Sharma and Sharma 2006). The plant is propagated by seeds and stem cuttings.

Phenology

Flowering time: March to April
Fruiting time: May to June

Key Characters for Identification

➤ A small tree of about 7 to 8 feet, green stem covered with silver papery bark.

➤ Leaves trifoliate, ovate, serrated with reddish-brown petiole.

➤ Flowers small, red brown in fascicles of two or three.

➤ Fruits small, oval drupes turn red on maturity.

➤ Exudate oleo gum resin, aromatic pale yellow to brown colored.

Types

In Atharva Veda, two types—Sindhuj and Samudraj—are described.

Bhavaprakash and Kaiyadev Nighantu have described five types of Guggulu:

Types	Color resembles with	Prescribed for
Mahishaksh	honey bee or anjan (black)	Elephants
Mahanil	Neelvarna (blue)	Elephants
Kumud	Kumud pushpa (white)	Horses
Padma	Manikya (red ruby)	Horses
Hiranya	Gold	Humans

Commercially, two varieties are available:

- Bhesha Guggulu (Mahishaksh)—dark green to yellow in color, found in Gujarat
- Kana Guggulu (Hiranya)—reddish-yellow in color, found in Rajasthan

(Source: Singh 1969)

Rasapanchaka

Guna	Laghu, Ruksha, Tikshna, Vishad, Shukshma, Sara (old Guggulu); Snigdha, Pichchhil (fresh Guggulu)
Rasa	Tikta, Katu, Kashaya
Vipaka	Katu
Virya	Ushna

Chemical Constituents

Guggulu contains volatile oil, resin, gum, and bitter compounds. The oleo gum resin contains guggulsterones Z & E, guggulusterols I, II, III, cholesterol, mucolol, α camphorene, cembrene, allylcembrol, ferulic acids, aminoacids, guggulligans I, II, β-sitosterol, sesamin. The other compounds reported are myrcene, polymyrcene, sugar, aldobiouronic acid, myricyl alcohol, caryophyllene flavonoids, viz. quercetin, quercetin-3-0-α-L arabinoside, quercetin-3-0-α-D-galactoside, quercetin-3-0-β-L rhamnoside, quercetin-3-0-β-D glucuronide, ellagic acid, pelargonidin, and pregnenones I, II, III (Sangolgi et al 2017).

Identity, Purity, and Strength

For Exudate

- Foreign matter: Not more than 4%
- Total ash: Not more than 5%
- Acid-insoluble ash: Not more than 2 %
- Alcohol-soluble extractive: Not less than 2%
- Water-soluble extractive: Not less than 53%
- Volatile oil: Not less than 1%

(Source: The Ayurvedic Pharmacopeia of India 1989)

Karma (Actions)

In traditional Ayurvedic system of medicine, Guggulu niryasa is described as sangyasthapana, bhagnasandhankar, swarya, krimighna, kushtaghna, shothahara, hridya, gandmalanashaka, vedanasthapana, deepan, sheetaprashamana vranashodhana, vranaropana, varnya, nadibalya, anulomana, pittasaraka, yakridottejaka, raktaprasadana, bhootghna, medhya kaphadurgandhahara, ashmaribhedana, and mutral. However, fresh and old Guggulus have different properties which are as follows:

Fresh Guggulu

Snigdh, picchila, kanchansankashya, looks like pakwajambuphal (ripen Jambu fruit), sugandhi (aromatic), balya (strength promoting), brihmaniya (weight promoting), rasayana (rejuvinator), vrishya (aphrodisiac), artavajanana (emmnogogoe), uttejaka (stimulant).

Old Guggulu

Sushka, durgandhi (bad odor), lekhana (scrapping), medohara (antiobesity), shukranashana (destroy semen), and devoid of natural color and potency.

Guggulu shaka is guru, ruksha guna, madhur, katu in rasa and sheet virya, produces constipation, kapha vata prakopaka, and induces easy flow of urine and feces.

- Doshakarma: Tridoshashamaka
- Dhatukarma: Rasayana
- Malakarma: Anuloman, mutral

Pharmacological Actions

The gum resin of Guggulu has reported to exhibit anti-inflammatory, antiproliferative, anticancer, antimicrobial, hypolipidemic, antidiabetic, antiarthritic, anthelmintic, antioxidant, cardioprotective, neuroprotective, anodyne, antiseptic, aphrodisiac, liver stimulant, antispasmodic, diuretic properties and is considered as general tonic (Shishodia et al 2008).

Indications

Guggulu niryasa is used in the treatment of vata vyadhi, gridhrasi (sciatica), ardita (facial paralysis), pakshghata (hemiplegia), nadishool (neuralgic pains), amavata (arthritis), sandhivata, vatarakta (gout), medoroga (obesity), prameha (diabetes), sopha (swelling), gandmala (scrofula), kushta (skin diseases), shweta kushta (leucoderma), krimi (worm infestations), arsha (hemorrhoids), apachi, granthi, durgandhyuktavrana, agnimandya, vibandha, hridroga, hridyavarodha (atherosclerosis), pandu (anemia), klaibya (infertility), mutrashmari (renal calculus), kshaya (emaciation), bhootvikara, kasa, shwasa, pleeha, shlipada, puyameha, yonivyapada, and vrana.

Contraindications:

During the administration of Guggulu, intake of amla dravya, tikshna dravya, ajirna bhojan, vyavaya, shrama, atapa sevan, madya, and rosha should be avoided (Chunekar 2006).

Therapeutic Uses

External Use

1. **Shwasa** (asthma): Shallaki, Guggulu, Agaru, and Padmaka mixed with ghrita are used for fumigation in shwasa roga (A.H.Ci. 4/14).
2. **Karnadourgandhya** (fetid ear): Dhupana with Guggulu niryasa is beneficial in fetid ear (S.S.U. 21/53) (VM. 59/43).
3. **Vrana** (wounds): Decoction of Guggulu and Triphala is used for washing of vrana, kushta, nadi, and bhagandar (G.N. 4/3/73-74).

Internal Use

1. **Sthoulya** (obesity): Regular use of Rasanjana, Brihat panchmool, Guggulu, Shilajatu, and Agnimantha is beneficial in sthoulya (A.H.U. 14/23).
2. **Aamvaat** (rheumatoid arthritis): 50 mL of decoction prepared with Guggulu, Guduchi, Shunti, and Gokshura is given twice daily in rheumatoid arthritis, osteoarthritis, joint pain, stiff joints, muscular pain, and backache.
3. **Vatarakta** (gout): Regular use of Shilajatu, Guggulu, and madhu is beneficial in vatarakta (C.S.Ci. 29/159).
4. **Shotha** (swelling): Persons suffering from edema should use Guggulu with gomutra (S.S.Ci. 23/12) (A.H.Ci. 19/3) or decoction of Guggulu, Punarnava, Devadaru, and Shunti (VM. 39/8).
5. **Vatavyadhi** (neuromuscular diseases): Using Silajatu and Guggulu with dugdha alleviates vatavyadhi (C.S.Ci. 28/241).
6. **Gridharsi** (sciatica): Pills made up of Rasna and Guggulu pounded with ghrita is used in gridharsi (CD. 22/50).
7. **Urustambha** (filariasis): Intake of Guggulu with gomutra is a good remedy for urustambha (S.S.Ci. 5/35).
8. **Udarroga** (abdominal disease): Use of Shilajatu, gomutra, Guggulu, Triphala, and Snuhi ksheer alleviates all types of udarroga (VM. 37/9).
9. **Vidridhi** (abscess): In vata dominance, vidridhi Guggulu or Eranda taila should be used (VM. 43/4).
10. **Bhagandar** (fistula in ano): Intake of Guggulu and Vidanga mixed decoction of Triphala and Khadira destroys bhagandar (GN. 4.7.27).

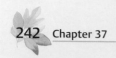

Officinal Part Used

Niryasa (Oleo gum resin)

Dose

Powder: 2 to 4 g

Formulations

Yograj guggulu, Kaishore guggulu, Triphala guggulu, Gokshuradi guggulu, Trayodashang guggulu, Lakshadi guggulu, Vyoshadi guggulu, Vatari guggulu, Singhnada guggulu, Kanchnar guggulu, Saptavinshati guggulu, Punarnavadi guggulu, Chandraprabha vati.

Toxicity/Adverse Effect

If taken in inappropriate dose, it can cause liver and lung damage and over dose can cause vertigo, dryness in mouth, impotence, debility, muscle wasting (Sharma et al 2001). Long-term and higher dose administration of Guggulu may lead to side effects like timira (cataract), mukhshosh (dryness of mouth), klaivayta (impotency), karshya (emaciation), moha (delusion), shamal shithil bhava (diarrhea), deha rukshta (dryness of body) (Astang Sangraha 2005; Sharma 2004).

Purification Methods

Traditionally, Guggulu is purified by keeping in triphala kvatha for 3 hours in dola yantra and then fried with ghee. According to Bhaisajyaratnavali, decoction of Guduchi, Triphala, and godugdh is used for its purification.

Substitution and Adulteration

Guggulu is adulterated with the gums resin of *Boswellia serrata* Roxb. (salai Guggulu), *Hymenodictyon excelsum* (Roxb.) Wall., *Commiphora myrrha (bol)*, *Commiphora roxburghii* (Arn) Engl., *Sterculia urens* Roxb., *Butea monosperma* Kurz., *Acacia nilotica* Willd., *Moringa oliefera* Lamk., *Acacia senegal* Willd., and *Acacia catechu* Willd.

However, salai Guggulu is the most common adulterant (Dhar et al 2011).

> **Points to Ponder**
>
> - *Guggulu is one of the best rewarding herbs for vata roga.*
> - *Nav Guggulu is snigdh, sugandhi, brihmaniya, vrisya whereas purana Guggulu is shushk, durgandhi, lekhana.*
> - *It is remarkably used to lower down blood cholesterol level.*

Suggested Readings

Astanga Sangraha, Uttara Tantra, 49/158, Hindi Vyakhya, Atrideva Gupt. Varanasi: Chokhambha Krushnadas Academy; Reprint 2005

Bandeppa S, Ganapathi R, and Praveen S. Concept of guggulu (*Commiphora mukul* linn.): a review. Int J Curr Med Pharm Res 2017;3(6):1836–1844

Bhatt JR, Nair MNB, Mohanram HY. Enhancement of oleogum resin production in *Commiphora wightii* by improved tapping technique. Curr Sci 1989;58:349–354

Chunekar KC. Bhavaprakasha Nighantu of Bhavmishra. Varanasi: Chaukhambha Bharti Academy; Reprint edition 2006, karpuradi varga:205

Dhar BP, Agrawala DK, Gaur SK, and Babu DR. Biology, Cultivation and Conservation of *Guggulu*. Paper presented at National Workshop on Conservation and Utilization of *Commiphora wightii* (Guggal), CCRAS, on 15–16th September 2011, Gandhinagar, Gujarat.

Kashinath S. Rasatarangani of Shri Sadanand Sharma, 11th ed. Motilal Banarshi Das Publication; 1979:18

Kirtikar KR and Basu BD. Indian Medicinal Plants, Vol. 1, edited, enlarged and mostly rewritten by E. Blatter, J.F. Caius and K.S. Mhaskar. Dehradun: International Book Distributor; 2012:526–527.

Sharma PC, Yelne MB, Dennis TJ. Database on Medicinal Plants Used in Ayurveda, Vol. 2. New Delhi: CCRAS; 2001:217–221

Sharma PV. Priya Nighantu. Varanasi: Chaukhamba Surbharati Prakashan; 2004:20

Sharma PV and Sharma GP. Kaiyadev Nighantu (pathyaapathya vibodhaka), 2nd ed. Varanasi: Chaukhambha Orientalia; 2006: 260–263.

Shishodia S, Kuzhuvelil BHR, Dass S, Ramawat KG, Aggarwal BB. The guggul for chronic diseases: ancient medicine, modern targets. Anticancer Res 2008;28:3647–3664

Singh R. Vanoushadi Nidarshika, Hindi Samiti Granthmala. Lucknow; 1969:128–129

The Ayurvedic Pharmacopeia of India. Part I, Vol. 1. New Delhi: Department of AYUSH, Ministry of Health and Family Welfare, Government of India; 1989:56–57

स नवो बृंहणो वृष्यः पुराणस्त्वतिलेखनः ||३८||

स्निग्धः काञ्चनसंकाशः पक्वजम्बूफलोपमः |

नूतनो गुग्गुलुः प्रोक्तः सुगन्धिर्यस्तु पिच्छिलः ||३९||

शुष्को दुर्गन्धकश्चैव त्यक्तप्रकृतिवर्णकः |

पुराणः स तु विज्ञेयो गुग्गुलुर्वीर्यवर्जितः ||४०||

— भा.प्र.नि. कर्पूरादिवर्ग

गुग्गुलुर्विशदस्तिक्तो वीर्योष्णः पित्तलः सरः |

कषायः कटुकः पाके कटू रूक्षो लघुः परः ||३५||

भग्नसन्धानकृद्दृष्यः सूक्ष्मः स्वर्यो रसायनः |

दीपनः पिच्छिलो बल्यः कफवातव्रणापचीः ||३६||

मेदोमेहाश्मवातांश्च क्लेदकुष्ठाममारुतान् |

पिडकाग्रन्थिशोफार्शोगण्डमालाकृमीञ्जयेत् |

— भा.प्र.नि. कर्पूरादिवर्ग

38. Haridra [Curcuma longa Linn.]

Family: *Scitaminae*

Hindi name: *Haldi*

English name: *Turmeric, Indian saffron*

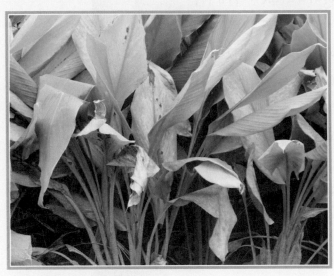

Plant of *Curcuma longa* Linn.

> *Erode city of Tamil Nadu is known as "Yellow City" or "Turmeric City" because it is the world's largest producer and most important trading center of turmeric in Asia followed by Sangli of Maharashtra.*

Introduction

The Latin name *curcuma* is derived from the word *kurkum* which is used for saffron because of its use as a coloring agent in food. It has been known as poor man's saffron because it offers a less-expensive alternative of saffron as a yellow coloring agent. It forms an integral part of Indian cuisine, socioritual practices, and religious ceremonies. In Hindu weddings, brides rub turmeric on their bodies for glowing skin. Newborn babies are also rubbed with haldi on their forehead for good luck. It is customary to use Haridra rhizome in yagnas and pujas.

Besides being an integral component of diet, Haridra has a long-documented history of its use as a medicine. It is a general practice in Indian homes to use Haridra powder with lukewarm milk in traumatic injuries as a healing agent. Womenfolk apply turmeric paste before bathing. In Chinese, medicine it is believed to be blood and Qi (vital energy) stimulant, a pain killer, and is used in the treatment of flatulence, ringworm, hepatitis, and chest pain (Burnham, 1993; Chang and But, 1987). The Hawaiians used it for prevention and treatment of sinus infections, ear infections, and gastrointestinal ulcers. Vrinda Madhav used Haridra pounded with kanji (rice porridge) to prevent diseases caused by change in place (VD. 1/16). Charak kept it in tikta skanda and shirovirechana gana (C.S.Vi. 8/143, 151). Sushrut placed it in vata and kapha sansaman varga. In rasagranthas, it is used for shodhana and maran of drugs.

Haridra is an approved food additive in the United States. All over the world it is used as preservative, coloring agent in food and pharmaceuticals, veterinary medicine, cosmetics, and dyeing agents.

Vernacular Names

Arabic: Kurkum, Zarsud, Aurukesafur

Assamese: Haldhi, Haladhi

Bengali: Halud, Haldi

Chinese: Iyu-chin
Dutch: Geelwortel
Gujarati: Haldar
Indonesia: Kunyit
Kannada: Arishina
Kashmiri: Ledar, Ladhir
Malayalam: Manjal
Malaysia: Temukunyit
Marathi: Halad
Oriya: Haladi
Portuguese: acafrao da India
Punjabi: Haldi, Haldar
Tamil: Manjal
Telugu: Pasupu, Pampi
Urdu: Haldi

Synonyms

Gauri: It is used to improve skin complexion.

Hatvilasini: It draws attention due to its bright color.

Kanchani: The color of dried rhizome resembles the color of gold.

Krimighni: Its rhizome exhibit antimicrobial properties.

Lomasmulika: The rhizome is hairy in nature.

Mangalya: It is used abundantly in all auspicious/religious functions.

Mehaghni: It has antidiabetic action.

Nisha: Like the moon light it has the property to illuminate darkness.

Ranjani: It is used for dyeing clothes etc.

Varnavilasini: It has vrana prasadana action.

Varvarini: It is best drug for enhancing complexion.

Vishaghni: The plant has antitoxin action.

Yoshitpriya: It is very much popular among womenfolk as a cosmetic drug.

Classical Categorization

Charak Samhita: Lekhaniya, Vishaghna, Kushtaghna, Kandughna

Sushrut Samhita: Haridradi, Vachadi, Mustadi, Lakshadi, Vallipanchmool, Shleshmsanshamana

Ashtang Hridaya: Haridradi, Mustadi

Dhanvantari Nighantu: Guduchyadi varga

Madanpal Nighantu: Abhyadi varga

Kaiyadev Nighantu: Oushadi varga
Raj Nighantu: Pippalayadi varga
Bhavaprakash Nighantu: Haritakyadi varga

Distribution

Haridra is a native drug of South East Asia and is mostly cultivated in India, Bangladesh, China, Thailand, Malaysia, Indonesia, and Philippines. In India it is abundantly cultivated in Andhra Pradesh, Tamil Nadu, Maharashtra, Karnataka, Orissa, Punjab, West Bengal, and Kerala. India is the largest producer, consumer, and exporter of Haridra in the world and has the highest diversity of curcuma species.

Morphology

An aromatic perennial herb with short stem and tufts of erect leaves arising from the rhizome, reaching up to a height of 1 to 2 feet.

- **Leaves:** Simple, oblong-lanceolate, apex caudate-acuminate, base tapering, glabrous, glossy, smooth surface, bright green in color which turns yellow when mature (**Fig. 38.1**).

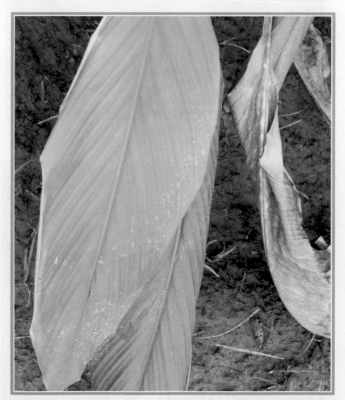

Fig. 28.1 Leaves.

- **Flowers:** White to pale yellow in bracteates, strobiliform spikes arising from the center of the leafy shoot, corolla white, flowering bracts pale green (**Fig. 38.2**).
- **Rhizomes:** Highly aromatic, yellowish-orange internally and yellowish to yellowish-brown externally with root scars and remnants of leaf bases, ovate, oblong, pyriform, or cylindrical in shape, fracture horny, fractured surface orange to reddish-brown (**Fig. 38.3a, b**) The plant is propagated by its rhizome (Nadkarni 1976).

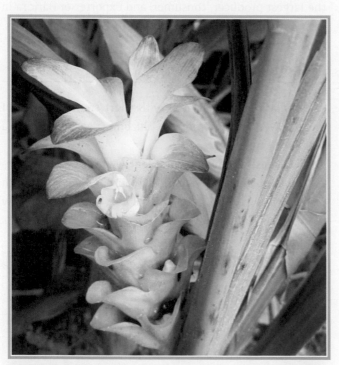

Fig. 28.2 Flower.

Phenology

Flowering time: October to December
Fruiting time: October to December

Key Characters for Identification

➤ An aromatic perennial herb of 1 to 2 feet.
➤ Leaves: Oblong-lanceolate, glossy, bright green, yellow on maturity
➤ Flowers: White to pale yellow in strobiliform spikes
➤ Rhizome: Ovate to oblong, aromatic, yellowish-orange internally and yellowish-brown externally with root scars and remnants of leaf bases

Types

Bhavaprakasha has described four varieties of Haridra:
- Haridra (*Curcuma longa* Linn.)
- Vanyaharidra (*Curcuma aromatic* Salisb.)
- Aamragandhi haridra (*Curcuma amada* Roxb.)
- Daruharidra (*Berberis aristata* DC.)

Rasapanchaka

Guna	Laghu, Ruksha
Rasa	Tikta, Katu
Vipaka	Katu
Virya	Ushna

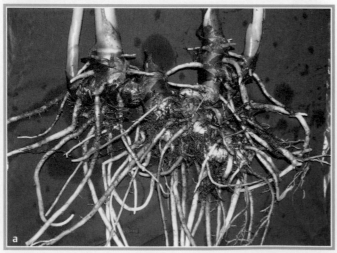

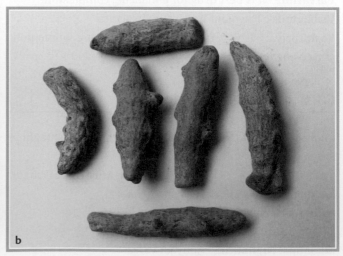

Fig. 28.3 **(a)** Fresh rhizome. **(b)** Dry rhizome.

Chemical Constituents

The main constituents are a group of compounds called curcuminoids, which include curcumin (comprising curcumin I [94%], curcumin II [6%], and curcumin III [0.3%]), diferuloylmethane, demethoxycurcumin (12%), dihydrocurcumin, and bisdemethoxycurcumin (Maiti et al 2007), volatile oils, terpenoids (eugenol, geraniol, limonene), sesquiterpenes (α curcumene, curlone, curcumenol, turmerone, termerol, zingiberin), fatty acids (linoleic acid, palmatic, oleic acid, stearic acid), β-sitosterol, stigmasterol, gitoxigenin sugar, protein, minerals, resins, and essential oil. The essential oil contains α-phellandrene, sabinene, cineol, camphene, pinene, limonene, borneol, zingiberene, curcumenone, and sesquiterpenes (Kapoor 1990; Shiyou Li et al 2011; Rastogi and Mehrotra 2001).

Identity, Purity, and Strength

For Rhizome

- Foreign matter: Not more than 2%
- Total ash: Not more than 9%
- Acid-insoluble ash: Not more than 1%
- Alcohol-soluble extractive: Not less than 8%
- Water-soluble extractive: Not less than 12%
- Volatile oil: Not less than 4%

(Source: The Ayurvedic Pharmacopeia of India 1989)

Karma (Actions)

Ayurvedic classics described Haridra as varnya (complexion promoter), shothaghna (anti-inflammatory), jwaraghna (antipyretic), vishaghna (antidote to poisoning), krimighna (anthelmintic), kandughna (antipruritis), vishodhani (purifier), hikkanigrahana (antihic-cough), vedanasthapana (analgesic), raktaprasadana (blood purifier), raktastambhana (hemostatic), vranashodhan-ropana (purify and heal up wound), anulomana (laxative), ruchivardhaka (taste enhancer), pittarechaka, mutrasangrahaniya (urinary astringent), mutravirajaniya (corrective of urinary pigment).

- Doshakarma: Kaphapittashamak
- Dhatukarma: Varnya, Raktashodhaka
- Malakarma: Anulomana

Pharmacological Actions

The rhizomes is reported to have antiseptic, germicidal, antioxidant, hepatoprotective, analgesic, anti-inflammatory, antispasmodic, antihistaminic, anticarcinogenic, antitumor, antineoplastic, immunosuppressive, neuroprotective, antiparasitic, antifungal, antiviral, antidiabetic, hypocholesteremic, carminative, anthelmintic, nephroprotective, diuretic, expectorant, hematinic, styptic, antiperiodic, and antitoxin properties (Ammon and Wahl 1991; Ramsewak et al 2000; Aggarwal et al 2003).

Indications

Meha (diabetes), kandu (itching), kushta (skin diseases), krimi (worms infestation), vrana (wound), peenasa (rhinitis), aruchi (anorexia), pandu (anemia), kamala (jaundice), apachi, visha (poison), shotha (inflammation), vatarakta (gout), daha (burning), vibandha (constipation), kasa (cough), shwasa (asthma) pratishyaya (running nose), shukrameha (a variety of diabetes), sheetpitta (urticaria). Bhavaprakash has described amragandhi haridra as sarvkanduvinashini (alleviate all types of allergy) and vanyaharidra as kushtavatarakta nashak (cures leprosy and gout).

In traditional medicine, Haridra mixed with slaked lime is a well-known household remedy for sprains and swellings caused by injury (Ammon and Wahl 1991). Women, in folklore, use fresh Haridra paste and Sunthi with honey and milk twice daily after childbirth. To facilitate healing of lacerated birth canal, poultice of Haridra is applied to the perineum. Powdered turmeric when taken with boiled milk is helpful in respiratory ailment, and roasted turmeric is used in dysentery for children. Turmeric is also used in the treatment of dental diseases and to alleviate the hallucinatory effects of hashish, and other psychotropic drugs (MacGregor 2006; Pandeya 2005).

Therapeutic Uses

External Use

1. **Kamala** (jaundice): Haridra, Gairika, and Amalaki should be applied as anjana in kamala (A.H.Ci. 16/44).

2. **Visarpa** (erysipelas): Paste prepared with Haridra and Bhringraj root pounded with cold water is applied topically in visarpa (VM. 57/97).

3. **Arsha (piles):** Paste of Haridra and Snuhi ksheer or paste of gopitta, Pippali and Haridra is applied externally in piles (C.S.Ci. 14/52).

4. **Shwasa** (asthma): Inhalation of smoke by burning wick made up of Haridra patra, Eranda mool, laksha, manashila, hartal, Devadaru, and Jatamansi is useful in shwasa roga (C.S.Ci. 17/77).

5. **Vyanga** (freckles): Paste of Haridra and Rakta chandana pounded with buffalo's milk is applied on dark spots in vyanga (RRS. 24/45).

Internal Use

1. **Prameha** (polyuric disorders/diabetes): Haridra powder mixed with madhu should be used with fresh Amalaki juice daily in the morning to cure different types of prameha (A.H.Ci. 12/5) (A.S.Ci. 14/5) (C.S.Ci. 6/26) (S.S.Ci. 11/8).

2. **Pandu** (anemia): One should use leha prepared by mixing Haridra, Triphala, madhu, and ghrita in pandu roga (S.S.U. 44/17).

3. **Kushta** (skin diseases): Daily intake of Haridra powder with gomutra for a month freed a person from any type of kushta (S.S.Ci. 9/45) (BS.Ci. 6/46).

4. **Kshudraroga** (minor skin diseases): Haridra kalka mixed with gomutra should be taken in minor skin ailments like pama, kandu, etc. (VM. 51/41).

5. **Vatarakta** (gout): Decoction of Haridra and Amrita mixed with madhu is used in kapha predominant vatarakta (B.P.Ci. 29/79).

6. **Trishna** (excessive thirst): To combat excessive thirst, water processed with Haridra and mixed with madhu sharkara should be used (A.H.Ci. 6/42).

7. **Visha** (poisoning): Intake of ghrita prepared with kalka of haridra, Nakuli, and Jati is efficacious in poisoning (A.H.U. 40/127).

8. **Shlipada** (filariasis): Intake of Haridra and guda with gomutra destroys shlipada (B.P.Ci. 45/14).

9. **Ashmari** (urinary calculus): Intake of Haridra and guda in equal quantity with kanji helps in flushing away gravels in ashmari (B.S.ashmari./45).

10. **Kasa** (cough): In shushk kasa Haridra powder impregnated with Vasa juice should be taken with fatty layer of milk (S.B. 4/333).

Officinal Part Used

Rhizome

Dose

Powder: 1 to 3 g
Juice: 10 to 20 mL

Formulations

Haridrakhand, Rajniyadi churna, Panchnimbadi churna.

Toxicity/Adverse Effect

No significant toxicity has been reported following acute or chronic administration of turmeric extracts at standard doses. However, at very high doses (100 mg/kg body weight), curcumin may be ulcerogenic in animals, although there have been no reports of this in humans (Commandeur and Vermeulen 1996; Soleimani et al 2018).

Substitution and Adulteration

Haridra is rarely adulterated or substituted. Sometimes it is mixed with other species of *curcuma*. Bhavaprakash samhita has described Haridra as a substitute for Daruharidra (BP.S./155) (Sharma et al 2000).

Points to Ponder

- *Haridra forms an integral component of Indian cuisine.*
- *It is used as household remedy for cuts, bruises, wounds, ulcers, improving complexion, and in other skin infections.*
- *It is a well-known anti-inflammatory, anticancerous, antidiabetic, antioxidant, and antihistaminic drug.*

Suggested Readings

Aggarwal BB, Kumar A, Bharti AC. Anti-cancer potential of Curcumin: preclinical and clinical studies. Anticancer Res 2003; 231:363–398

Ammon HP, Wahl MA. Pharmacology of Curcuma longa. Planta Medica 1991;57:1–7

Chang HM, But PP. Pharmacology and applications of Chinese Materia Medica. Singapore: World Scientific Publishing; 1987:936–939

Commandeur JNM, Vermeulen NPE. Cytotoxicity and cytoprotective activities of natural compounds: the case of curcumin. Xenobiotica 1996;26:667–680

Kapoor LD. Handbook of Ayurvedic Medicinal Plants. Boca Raton, FL: CRC Press; 1990:185

MacGregor H. Out of the Spice Box, into the Lab: Turmeric, an Indian Staple, has Long had Medicinal Uses. Now the West is Taking Notice. Los Angeles, CA: Los Angeles Times; 2006

Maiti K, Mukherjee K, Gantait A, Saha BP, Mukherjee PK. Curcumin-phospholipid complex: preparation, therapeutic evaluation and pharmacokinetic study in rats. Int J Pharm 2007;330:155–163

Nadkarni. Curcuma longa. In: Nadkarni KM (ed.), Indian Materia Medica. Bombay: Popular Prakashan Publishing Company; 1976:414–416

Pandeya N. Old wives tales: modern miracles turmeric as traditional medicine in India. Trees Life J 2005;1:3

Ramsewak RS, DeWitt DL, Nair MG. Cytotoxicity, antioxidant and anti-inflammatory activities of curcumins I-III from Curcuma longa. Phytomedicine 2000;7(4):303–308

Rastogi RP, Mehrotra BN. Compendium of Indian Medicinal Plants, Vol. 3. New Delhi: Central Drug Research Institute, Lucknow & National Institute of Science Communication & Information Resources; 2001:220–221

Sharma PC, Yelne MB, Dennis TJ. Database on Medicinal Plants Used in Ayurveda, Vol. 1. New Delhi: CCRAS; 2000:217–221

Shiyou Li et al. Chemical composition and product quality control to Turmeric (Curcuma longa Linn.), pharmaceutical crops; 2011;2: 28–54

Soleimani V, Sahebkar A, Hosseinzadeh H. Turmeric (Curcuma longa) and its major constituent (curcumin) as nontoxic and safe substances. Rev Phytother Res 2018;32:985–995

The Ayurvedic Pharmacopeia of India. Part I, Vol. 1. New Delhi: Department of AYUSH, Ministry of Health and Family Welfare, Government of India; 1989:61

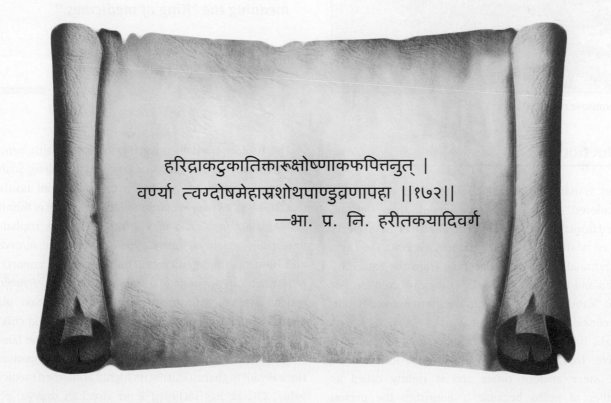

हरिद्राकटुकातिक्तारूक्षोष्णाकफपित्तनुत् |
वर्ण्या त्वग्दोषमेहास्रशोथपाण्डुव्रणापहा ||१७२||
—भा. प्र. नि. हरीतकयादिवर्ग

39. Haritaki *[Terminalia chebula [Gaertn.] Retz.]*

Family: *Combretaceae*

Hindi name: *Harad*

English name: *Chebulic myrobalan, Black myrobalan, Ink tree*

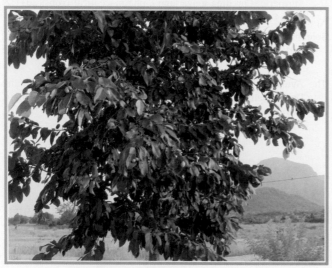

Tree of *Terminalia chebula* (Gaertn.) Retz.

In Tibetan medicine, Haritaki is known as A-ru-ra and praised with the adjective Sman-mchog-rgyal-pa meaning the "King of medicines."

Introduction

The plant is named Haritaki because of its dark green, yellow-colored fruits. It is considered that Haritaki originated from the abode of Lord Shiva and has the property to drive away all diseases (D.N. guduchyadi/208). The Latin name "terminalia" means proceeding from the extremity at the end and the word "chebula" is the distorted form of the word "Kabul" (Gogte 2000). In regard to market, Kabuli harad is considered as best variety.

Haritaki has been used in traditional medicine as a preventive, therapeutic remedy against various human ailments since ancient times and is rightly called as the mother of herbs because it nourishes the person as a mother. There is a mythological belief that during Samudra manthan, when Lord Indra was drinking nectar, few drops of it fell on earth and Haritaki plant originated from those nectar drops. That is why it possesses immense medicinal potency.

The fruit of Haritaki possesses diverse health benefits and is considered as a rasayana (rejuvenator) drug. Sushrut has considered it as the best fruit among all laxatives (S.S.Su. 44/3). Its fruit in combination with fruits of Bibhitaki and Amalaki in a ratio of 1:2:4 is known as triphala, a universally acclaimed formulation used in Unani, Ayurveda, and Homeopathic medicines. The therapeutic importance of Haritaki can be judged by the fact that many Ayurvedic lexicon started with the description of Haritaki plant. Charak Samhita has named a chapter in rasayana chikitsa "Abhayamalakiyarasayanapada" after Haritaki. The famous drug lexicon Bhavaprakasha Nighantu is also known as Haritakyadi Nighantu stating its highly acclaimed medicinal value. Charak has included it in virechan dravya, phala asava yoni, to alleviate santarpana roga (C.S.Su. 23/35), as pathya dravya, as sanshodhana dravya, and rasayana dravya (C.S.Ci. 1/1/29-34). Sushrut described it in phala varga (S.S.Su. 46/199). Vagabhatta has mentioned it as best drug to subside deranged vata kapha dosha (A.H.U. 40/48).

Kaiyadeva has documented the properties of prasashta and aprasashta Haritaki (K.D./233-34). Raj Nighantu has considered it as a yogavahi drug (R.N.amradi varga /216). Bhavaprakash has described different methods of using Haritaki to attain different actions. When it is chewed, it enhances digestive fire; when used after rubbing, it acts as malashodhana (cleanses toxins); when used after boiling, it acts as sangrahi (absorbent); and when it is used after frying, it becomes tridoshashamaka (pacify tridoshas). When Haritaki is taken with food, it enhances buddhi, bala, and indriya, and pacifies tridoshas and dispels out mala, mutra, and other toxins. When it is taken after food, it readily cures digestive disorders and pacifies diseases of vatu, pitta, and kapha. To pacify vata disorders, Haritaki should be used with ghrita (ghee), in pitta disorders with sharkara (sugar), in kapha disorders with lavana (salt), and in all other diseases with guda (B.P.N. 1/30-33).

Vernacular Names

Arabian: Halilah, Halilaje-asfar
Assamese: Shilikha, Karitaki
Bengali: Haritaki
Gujarati: Hirdo, Himaja, Pulo-harda
Kannada: Alalekai, Harra, Karakkayi
Kashmiri: Halela
Malayalam: Katukka
Marathi: Hirda, Hirda-phula, Harda, Hireda
Oriya: Harida, Horitoli, Harira
Persian: Halilah, Halilahe-siyah
Punjabi: Halela, Harar, Hurh, Har
Santhal: Rola, Hadra
Sindhi: Har
Tamil: Kadukkay
Telugu: Karaka, Karakkaya
Urdu: Haejarad

Synonyms

Abhaya: Its daily intake removes the fear of being diseased.
Amogha: It is an unfailing remedy for diseased condition.
Amrita: The plant bears rasayana properties.
Avyatha: It is a potent remedy for pain or makes the body disease-free.

Chetaki: It promotes the health of mind and soul.
Haimavati: It grows in Himalayan region also.
Kayastha: It promotes body health.
Panchbhadrika: Its fruit has five rasa.
Pathya: Its fruit is beneficial for everyone and it cleanses all the body channels.
Putana: It eliminates impurities and purifies the body.
Rohini: It regenerates tissues and enhances wound-healing activity.
Shiva: It shows salutary effect on the body.
Vayastha: It exhibits antiaging effect and thus helps in maintaining youthfulness.

Classical Categorization

Charak Samhita: Jwaraghna, Arshoghna, Kushtaghna, Kasahara, Hikkanigrahana, Virechanopaga, Prajasthapana, Vayasthapana
Sushrut Samhita: Amalakyadi, Mustadi, Mushkakadi, Vachadi, Parushakyadi
Ashtang Hridaya: Parushakyadi, Mushkakadi, Vachadi, Virechan
Dhanvantari Nighantu: Guduchyadi varga
Madanpal Nighantu: Abhyadi varga
Kaiyadev Nighantu: Oushadi varga
Raj Nighantu: Amraadi varga
Bhavaprakash Nighantu: Haritakyadi varga

Distribution

Haritaki is abundantly distributed throughout India, especially in deciduous forest of West Bengal, Tamil Nadu, Bihar, Orissa, Haryana, Punjab, Rajasthan, Madhya Pradesh, Maharashtra, Western Ghats, and Southern India up to an altitude of 3,000 ft.

Morphology

A large deciduous tree of about 15 to 25 m height, with a cylindrical trunk, rounded crown, and spreading branches. The bark is dark brown with longitudinal cracks (**Fig. 39.1**).

- **Leaves:** Simple, alternate, short petioled, ovate, or elliptic with a pair of large glands on both sides of midrib on the upper surface of leaf, glabrous, tomentose beneath (**Fig. 39.2a, b**).

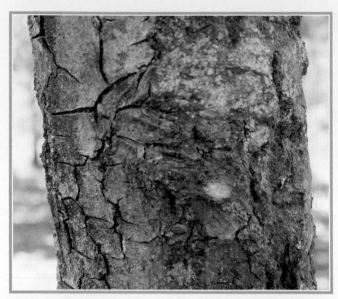

Fig. 39.1 Bark.

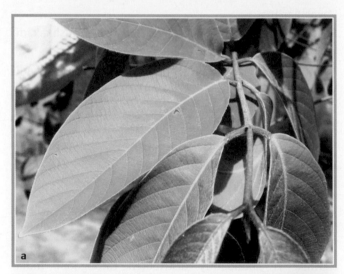

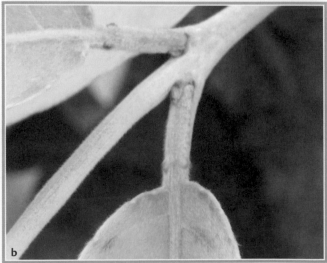

Fig. 39.2 (a) Leaves. (b) Glands on upper surface of leaf.

- **Flowers:** Monoecious inflorescence, dull white to yellow, with a strong unpleasant odor, borne in terminal spikes or short panicles (**Fig. 39.**3).
- **Fruits:** Ellipsoidal, obovoid, or ovoid drupes, smooth, 3 to 5 cm long, initially green changes to yellow to orange-brown on maturity, sometimes tinged with red or black, dried fruit is black, wrinkled shiny surface, hard, five-ribbed longitudinally (**Fig. 39.4a, b**).
- **Seeds:** Single, hard, and pale yellow. The plant is propagated by seeds and stem cuttings.

Phenology

Flowering time: March to May
Fruiting time: October to February

Key Characters for Identification

➤ A large deciduous tree of about 15 to 25 m height.
➤ Leaves are simple, alternate, tomentose, ovate, or elliptic with a pair of large glands at the top of the petiole.
➤ Flowers yellowish-white in terminal spike inflorescence.
➤ Fruits obovoid or ovoid drupes, smooth, unripe green, yellow–orange on maturity and dried black color, five-ribbed.

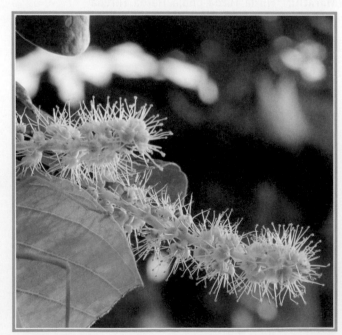

Fig. 39.3 Flowers.

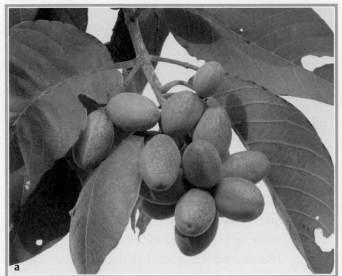 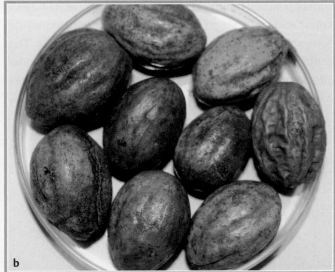

Fig. 39.4 **(a)** Fruits. **(b)** Dried fruit.

Types

Kaiyadeva: three types: Jalaja (aquatic origin), Vanaja (terrestrial/wild origin), and Parvatiya (mountainous origin).

Bhavaprakash and Raj Nighantu has classified Haritaki into seven types.

Sr. No.	Name	Shape of fruit	Place of origin	Disease in which it is used
1.	Vijaya	Alabu vritta	Vindahya parvata	Sarva roga
2.	Rohini	Vritta	Pratyeka desh	Vranaropana
3.	Putana	Asthimati shukshma	Sindhu desh	Pralepanartha
4.	Amrita	Masal	Champay	For Shodhana
5.	Abhya	Panchrekha	Champay	Akshiroga
6.	Jeevanti	Swarna varni	Saurashtra	Sarva roga
7.	Chetaki	Tri rekha	Himalaya	For churna

Rasapanchaka

Guna	Laghu, Ruksha
Rasa	Kashaya, Tikta, Madhura, Katu, Amla (Panchrasa alavana)
Vipaka	Madhura
Virya	Ushna
Prabhava	Rasayana

The fruit of Haritaki contains five rasas in different parts of the fruit as follows:

- Majja (fruit pulp): Madhura rasa
- Snayu (ridges) : Amla rasa
- Vrinta (stalk) : Tikta rasa
- Twak (outer covering): Katu rasa
- Asthi (seed): Kashaya

Chemical Constituents

Haritaki fruit contains anthraquinone glycoside, tannin, chebulagic acid, chebulic acid, chebupentol, chebulanin, corilagin, neochebulinic acid, ellagic acid, gallic acid (1.21%), tannic acid, punicalagin, quercetin, arjunolic acid, sennoside A, succinic acid, β-sitosterol, vitamin C, and proteins. The fruit kernel has arachidic, behenic, linoleic, oleic, palmitic, and stearic acid. The flowers contain chebulin and leaves have terflavins B, C, and D, punicalagin, and punicalatin (Evans 1996; Mammen et al 2012).

Identity, Purity, and Strength

- Foreign matter: Not more than 1 %
- Total ash: Not more than 5%
- Acid-insoluble ash: Not more than 5%
- Alcohol-soluble extractive: Not less than 40%
- Water-soluble extractive: Not less than 60%
  (Source: The Ayurvedic Pharmacopeia of India 1989)

Karma (Actions)

Ayurvedic classics have attributed rechana (laxative), lekhana (scraping), medhya (intellect promoter), netrya (beneficial for vision), deepan (appetizer), pachana (digestive), vataanulomaka (carminative), hridya (cardiotonic), indriyaprasadana (pleasant for sense organ), ayushya (healthy long life), brihmaniya (bulk promoting), vayasthapana (antiaging), rasayana (rejuvenating), bala–budhi–smriti vardhaka (promotes physical strength, intellect power, and memory enhancer), shothahara (reduce swelling), grahi (astringent), vedanahara (analgesic), vranashodhan-ropana (wound cleansing and healing). properties to it.

- Doshakarma:Tridoshashamaka, especially Vatashamaka
- Dhatukarma: Rasayana
- Malakarma: Vataanulomana, Rechana

Characteristics of Best Quality Haritaki

नवा स्निग्धा घना वृत्ता गुर्वी क्षिसा च याऽम्भसि ।
निमज्जेत्सा प्रशस्ता च कथिताऽतिगुणप्रदा ||२५||
—B. P. N. Haritakyadi

It should be new (fresh), snigdha (smooth), ghana (bulky), vrita (ovoid shape), guru (heavy), drown when dipped in water and weigh about two karsh, i.e., equal to the weight of two Bibhitaki fruit (approx. 20 g). This type of Haritaki is considered as best for medicinal usage.

Pharmacological Actions

The fruit has multiple pharmacological and medicinal activities such as astringent, laxative, digestive, carminative, anthelmintic, antiulcer, antispasmodic, antioxidant, antimicrobial, antiviral, antiseptic, anti-inflammatory, anticancerous, antiaging, aphrodisiac, diuretic, purgative, radioprotective, antidiabetic, hepatoprotective, cardio-protective, blood purifier, cytoprotective, antiarthritic, hypolipidemic, adaptogenic, immunomodulator, and wound-healing activity (Anwesa et al 2013).

Indications

Haritaki fruit singly or in combination with triphala is used in vibandha, (constipation), vrana (wounds/ulcers), arsha (hemorrhoids), krimi (worm infestation), shotha (inflammations), kushta (skin diseases), kandu, prameha (diabetes), agnimandhya (anorexia), ajeerna (indigestion), adhyaman (flatulence), kamala (jaundice), yakritapleeha vridhi (hepato-splenomegaly), pandu (anemia), shwasa (asthma), kasa (cough), tamaka shwasa (asthma), swarbheda (tonsillitis), mutrakricchta (dysuria), ashmari, mutraghata, shiroroga, abhishyandi (conjunctivitis), vaman (vomiting), atisara (diarrhea), grahani (irritable bowel syndrome [IBS]), gulma, visham jwara (intermittent fevers), hridya daurbalya (cardiac debility), shlipada (filariasis), medoroga (obesity), gandmala (glandular swelling), shool, aamvata (rheumatoid arthritis), chipa (whitlow), darunaka (dandruff), bradhna (inguinal hernia), vriddhi (scrotal enlargement), vatarakta (gout), amalpitta (acidity), visarpa, and daurbalya (general debility).

For the purpose of rasayana, Haritaki is taken along with different vehicles in different seasons. This regimen is called as Ritu Haritaki. It is as follows:

सिंधूत्थशर्कराशुण्ठीकणामधुगुडैः क्रमात् ।
वर्षादिष्वभया प्राश्या रसायनगुणैषिणा ||३१||

Ritu (seasons)	Vehicle with which Haritaki is taken
Varsha (rainy season)	Saindhava lavan (rock salt)
Sharad (autumn)	Sharkara (sugar)
Hemant (early winter)	Shunthi (dried ginger)
Shishir (late winter)	Pippali (long pepper)
Vasant (spring)	Madhu (honey)
Greeshma (summer)	Guda (jaggery)

Contraindications

Trishna (thirst), mukhashosha (dryness in oral cavity), hanustambha (lock jaw), galgraha (stiffness of neck), navajwara (acute fever), ksheen (emaciated), garbhini (pregnant), vridha (elderly) (D.N./207), adhvya (after long walk)) atikhinna (severe emaciation), bala varjita (weak person), ruksha (dry/rough), krisha (weak), langhana karshita (after fast), pittaadhikya (pitta dominant person), and raktamokshan (after blood letting) (B.P.N./35).

Therapeutic Uses

External Use

1. **Jwara** (fever): Leha (linctus) prepared with Haritaki, ghrita, madhu, taila cures all types of fever (C.S.Ci.3/233).
2. **Mukhvrana** (mouth ulcers): Haritaki fruit is broken into pieces and boiled in a cup of water. This infusion is cooled and used to rinse the mouth, two to three times a day for a week. It will heal the ulcers completely. Or take few pieces of Haritaki fruit and chew it four to five times a day in mouth ulcers and tonsillitis.
3. **Netraroga** (eye disease): Haritaki and ghrita processed with Tuvaraka should be applied in pakshmakopa (S.S.U. 16/8). Triphala decoction is used for washing eyes in conjunctivitis, eye infections, chronic purulent wounds, diabetic ulcers, and bed sores.

Internal Use

1. **Agnimandhya, Ajeerna** (loss of appetite, indigestion): Haritaki powder taken regularly with Shunthi or Jaggery or saindhava lavan initiates digestive fire and gives relief in indigestion (VM. 6/8). Trisama (powder of Haritaki, Pippali, and Shunthi in equal quantity) also gives the same effect (BS.ajeerna/19).
2. **Vibandha** (constipation): One teaspoonful of Haritaki powder or Triphala powder should be taken at night, after food with lukewarm water daily to treat chronic constipation.
3. **Arsha** (piles): A sitz bath with two tablespoons of Haritaki or Triphala powder, in half a bucket of water, for 10 minutes, before bath, is useful in reducing the swelling and pain in piles. Haritaki powder is made into paste with equal amount of jaggery and is taken orally before food to reduce pain, itching, and size of pile mass in hemorrhoids (S.S.Ci. 6/13). Haritaki fried in ghrita and mixed with jaggery and Pippali is advisable in piles (C.S.Ci. 14/138).
4. **Grahani roga** (sprue): Haritaki stem bark powder with Takra alleviates grahani associated with ama and rakta (B.S.grahani/168).
5. **Yakrita pleehodara** (enlargement of liver and spleen): Haritaki, Rohitaka kwath mixed with Yavakshara and Pippali should be taken in the morning for alleviating yakritapleehodara, udarroga, and gulma (S.G. 2/2/121).
6. **Raktapitta** (hemorrhage): Haritaki powder impregnated seven times with Vasa swarasa control raktapitta (C.D. 9/27).
7. **Prameha** (diabetes): Phalatrikadi kwath is used as a anupana in diabetes or regular consumption of Haritaki powder in a dose of 3 g with honey helps in controlling blood sugar level in diabetes (A.S.Ci. 14/5).
8. **Kushta** (skin disease): Regularly intake of Haritaki and Nimba powder alleviates kushta within a month (VM. 51/58).
9. **Shotha** (edema): Haritaki powder should be taken with gomutra to alleviate edema of kaphaj origin (C.S.Ci. 12/21) (A.H.Ci. 17/2).
10. **Rasayana** (rejuvenation): Regular intake of Haritaki powder fried in ghrita, followed by intake of ghrita for a month prevents aging, impart youthfulness, and strength (A.H.U. 39/148).
11. **Bradhna** (inguinal hernia): Haritaki paste fried in Eranda taila mixed with Pippali and saindhava should be used in inguinal hernia (B.S.bradhna ci/3).
12. **Aamvata** (rheumatoid arthritis): One should take Haritaki regularly with Eranda taila in Aamvata, gradharsi, and vriddhi roga (VM. 25/11) (BP.Ci. 26/51).

Officinal Part Used

Fruits

Dose

Powder: 3 to 6 g

Formulation

Triphala churna, Abhayarishta, Pathyadi vati, Pathyadi kvatha, Vyaghriharitaki, Chitrakaharitaki, Agastiharitaki, Dantiharitaki, Pathyadi churna, Abhayadi guggulu, Abhayamalakiya rasayana.

Toxicity/Adverse Effects

Due to its ruksha properties, it should not be consumed in excess by weak, malnourished individuals, during fasting, depression, pregnant women, and person who have lost considerable amount of blood.

Substitution and Adulteration

Fruits of *Terminalia citrina* Roxb. ex Flem., in East India and *Terminalia pallida* in Southern India are used in the name of Haritaki (Sharma et al 2005).

Points to Ponder

- Haritaki exhibit numerous pleiotropic actions like antiaging, antioxidant, antidiabetic, renoprotective, hepatoprotective, cardioprotective, antianaphylactic, immune modulatory, and adaptogenic.
- For diseases prevention and maintenance of healthy state, seasonal rasayana regimen Ritu haritaki should be followed.

Suggested Readings

Bag A, Bhattacharyya SK, Chattopadhyay RR. The development of *Terminalia chebula* Retz. (Combretaceae) in clinical research. Asian Pac J Trop Biomed 2013;3(3):244–252

Bag A, Bhattacharyya SK, Chattopadhyay RR. The development of Terminalia chebula Retz. (Combretaceae) in clinical research. Asian Pac J Trop Biomed 2013;3(3):244–252

Evans W. Trease and Evan's Pharmacology. 14th ed. Philadelphia: W.B. Saunders; 1996:493

Gogte VM. Ayurvedic Pharmacology and Therapeutic Uses of Medicinal Plants: Dravyaguna vigyan. New Delhi: Chaukha

Mahadev GV. Ayurvedic Pharmacology and Therapeutic Uses of Medicinal Plants (Dravyagunavignyan). Mumbai: Bharatiya Vidya Bhavan; 2000:515–516

Mammen D, Bapat S, Sane R. An investigation to variation in constituents in the fruits of *Terminalia chebula* Retz. at different maturity stages. Int J Pharma Bio Sci 2012;3(1):416–419

Sharma PC, Yelne MB, Dennis TJ. Database on Medicinal Plants used in Ayurveda, Vol. 3. New Delhi: CCRAS Department of Indian Systems of Medicine and Homeopathy (I. S. M. & H.), Ministry of Health and Family Welfare, Government of India; 2005:282–292.

The Ayurvedic Pharmacopeia of India, Part I, Vol. 1. New Delhi: Department of AYUSH, Ministry of Health and Family Welfare, Government of India; 1989:63

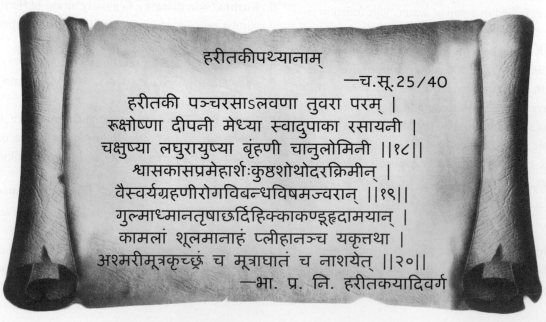

हरीतकीपथ्यानाम्
—च.सू. 25/40
हरीतकी पञ्चरसाऽलवणा तुवरा परम् ।
रूक्षोष्णा दीपनी मेध्या स्वादुपाका रसायनी ।
चक्षुष्या लघुरायुष्या बृंहणी चानुलोमिनी ॥१८॥
श्वासकासप्रमेहार्शःकुष्ठशोथोदरक्रिमीन् ।
वैस्वर्यग्रहणीरोगविबन्धविषमज्वरान् ॥१९॥
गुल्माध्मानतृषाछर्दिहिक्काकण्डूहृदामयान् ।
कामलां शूलमानाहं प्लीहानञ्च यकृत्तथा ।
अश्मरीमूत्रकृच्छ्रं च मूत्राघातं च नाशयेत् ॥२०॥
—भा. प्र. नि. हरीतकयादिवर्ग

40. Hingu *[Ferula asafoetida Linn.]*

Family:	*Apiaceae (Umbelliferae)*
Hindi name:	*Hing*
English name:	*Asafoetida, Devil's dung, Stinking gum*

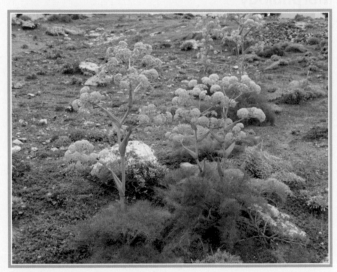

Plant of *Ferula asafoetida* Linn.

> *The organosulfides are primarily responsible for the strong odor and flavor of Hingu. In order to reduce its pungency and strong sulfurous odor it is advised to heat it in oil or ghee before use.*

Introduction

Hingu is an oleo-gum-resin obtained from the rhizome and root of the *Ferula asafoetida* plant. The Latin name "ferula" means *carrier* or *vehicle*. Asa is a Latinized form of Persian word "aza" meaning a resin, and the word "foetida" means a bad stinking smell which refers to its strong sulfurous odor.

In the middle ages, a small piece of Hingu was tied around the neck and arms to keep one safe from seasonal, bacterial, and viral illnesses such as cough, cold, and fever. In Persia, the herb is so highly esteemed as a condiment that it is popularly known as Food of the God (Kareparamban et al 2012). In Jamaican customary, it is traditionally applied to anterior fontanelle of babies because it is believed to protect them from evil spirits and demons. In the African American hoodoo tradition, Hingu is used in magic spells, as it is believed to have the power both to protect and to curse (Mahendra and Bisht 2012).

For several centuries, Hingu has been in constant use as a tempting spice and trusted medicine in many systems of medicine like Ayurveda, Unani, Siddha, Chinese, Persian, etc. It is a popular household remedy and is used in many prescriptions in traditional healing (Mahendra and Bisht 2012). In Charaka Samhita, it is described in Aharyogivarga (C.S.S. 27/299) and bhedniyayavagu (C.S.S. 2/29). In the treatment of santarpanjanya rog, it is mentioned as a content of vyoshadisattu and kusthadi churna (C.S.S. 23/1, 20). It is also described as sangyaprabodhan dravya in sanyasa chikitsa (C.S.S. 24/49). Sushrut described Hinguniryas as deepan, pachandravyain shakavarga (S.S.Su. 46/228) and shirovirechak dravya (S.S.Su. 39/6). Ashtang Hridaya mentioned it in oushadivarga as deepan, pachan, rochan, pitta kopakdravya (A.H.Su. 6/152). Hingu is used in preparation of tikshankshar (A.H.Su. 30/21) and as dhupan dravya in vrana chikitsa (A.H.Su. 29/25).

In nutshell, Hingu is used as a digestive aid in food, as a flavoring agent in curries, fried or barbecued meat, dal, pickles, etc. and as a constituent of many spice mixtures. The whole plant is used as a fresh vegetable and as an antidote in opium poisoning.

Vernacular Names

Arabic: Haltit, Tyib
Assamese: Hin
Bengali: Hing
Chinese: Asafoetida, awei
Farsi: Anghuzeh
German: Stinkasant, Teufelsdreck
Greek: Aza
Gujarati: Hing, Vagharni
Kannada: Hing, Ingu
Kashmiri: Eng
Malayalam: Kayam
Marathi: Hing, Hira, Hing
Oriya: Hengu, Hingu
Punjabi: Hing
Spanish: Asafetida
Tamil: Perungayam
Telugu: Inguva
Urdu: Hitleet, Hing

Synonyms

Sahasravedhi: Its strong odor can pierce thousands of substances and remain intact.
Jatuka: Its exudate is similar to Laksha.
Bahlika: The plant is native to Arabian region.
Ramatha: It is a well-known trade commodity.
Atyugra: It is highly odorous.
Bhootnashan: It has antibacterial properties.
Jaran: It increases digestive power.
Jantughna: The plant has antimicrobial action.

Classical Categorization

Charak Samhita: Deepaniya, Shwasahara, Sangyasthapana
Sushrut Samhita: Pippalyadi, Ushakadi, Shirovirechana
Ashtang Hridaya: Ushakadi, Vatsakadi
Dhanvantari Nighantu: Shatpushpadi varga
Madanpal Nighantu: Sunthyadi varga
Kaiyadev Nighantu: Oushadi varga
Raj Nighantu: Pippalayadi varga
Bhavaprakash Nighantu: Haritakyadi varga

Distribution

The plant is native to Iran and Afghanistan. Nowadays it is distributed throughout the Mediterranean region to central Asia. In India, it is cultivated in Kashmir and Punjab.

Morphology

Hingu is a monoecious perennial herb of 2 to 3 m height. The upper part of fully developed herb appears as circular mass of 30 to 40 cm. All parts of the plant have distinctive fetid smell.

- **Stem:** Flowering stems are 10 cm thick and hollow with a number of schizogenous ducts in the cortex region containing the resinous gum.
- **Leaves:** Compound, two to four pinnate, pubescent, segments oblong, entire, obtuse, stem leaves cauline with sheathing petiole.
- **Flowers:** Pale greenish-yellow in large compound umbels (**Fig. 40.1**).
- **Fruits:** Broadly oblong to suborbicular 1 cm × 8 mm, winged, oval, flat, thin reddish-brown, and have milky juice.
- **Root:** Large pulpy, thick carrot-shaped tap root.
- **Exudate:** Initially milky white, highly aromatic, aroma like garlic, hardens and turns brown on exposure to air (**Fig. 40.2**).

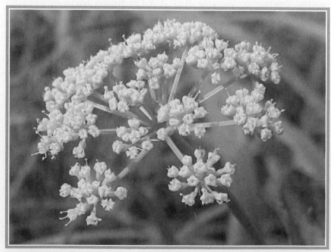

Fig. 40.1 Flowers.

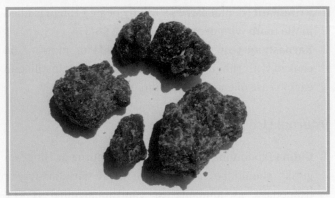

Fig. 40.2 Exudate.

The plant is propagated through seeds and vegetative methods.

Method of Collection of Hingu

Hingu is extracted from the roots of at least 4 to 5 years old plants. Before the flowering starts, the upper part of the root is open and bare; an incision is made at the lowest part of the stem close to the crown of the root. Milky white oleo-gum-resin exudate is obtained from the incised area, which hardens and turns brown on exposure to air. The exudate is collected after some days and fresh incisions are made. The process of collection of oleo-gum-resin and making incision is repeated until root stops exudation, i.e., about 3 months after the first cut (Anonymous 2002).

Phenology

Flowering time: April to June
Fruiting time: April to June

Key Characters for Identification

➤ *A monoecious perennial herb of 2 to 3 m height with distinctive fetid smell.*
➤ *Leaves are pinnate compound, pubescent with oblong segments.*
➤ *Flowers are pale greenish-yellow in large compound umbels.*
➤ *Fruits are small, oblong to suborbicular, thin, flat, reddish-brown.*
➤ *Roots are thick, pulpy, carrot-shaped tap root.*
➤ *Exudate is initially milky white which turns brown on exposure to air and has garlic-like smell.*

Types

Hingu is available in market in three forms which is as under (Anonymous 2002):

- Tear: Purest form, rounded or flattened in shape with gray color
- Mass: Most common form consisting of stuck tears of oleo-gum-resin and forms a mass mixed with fragments of soil, etc.
- Paste: Contains soil and woody matter

Rasapanchaka

Guna	Laghu, Snigdha, Tikshna
Rasa	Katu
Vipak	Katu
Virya	Ushna

Chemical Constituents

Asafoetida contains three main fractions, i.e., resins (40–60%), gum (20–25%), and volatile oil (10–15%). The resin fraction contains ferulic acid, assaresinotannol, assafoetidnol A, B, farnesiferols A, B, C, epiconferidone, colladonin, galbanic acid, coumarins, sesquiterpene coumarins, and other terpenoids. The gum includes glucose, galactose, 1-arabinose, rhamnose, glucuronic acid, polysaccharides and glycoproteins, and the volatile oil contains sulfur-containing compounds (2-butyl 1-propenyl disulfide, 1-(methyl thio) propyl 1-propenyl disulfide and 2-butyl 3-(methyl thio)-2-propenyl disulfide), monoterpenes (α & β-pinene, etc.), valeric acid, free ferulic acid, and traces of vanillin and other volatile terpenoids (Iranshahy and Iranshahi 2011; Kajimoto et al 1989; Duan et al 2002).

Identity, Purity, and Strength

- Foreign matter: Not more than 2 %
- Total ash: Not more than 15%
- Acid-insoluble ash: Not more than 3%
- Alcohol-soluble extractive: Not less than 50%
- Water-soluble extractive: Not less than 50%

(Source: The Ayurvedic Pharmacopeia of India 1989)

Karma (Actions)

Ayurvedic classical texts have attributed deepan (appetizer), pachan (digestive), rochan (relish), artavajanan (emmenagogue), anuloman (laxative), bhedaniya (purgative), hridya (cardio tonic), chakshusya (beneficial for vision), balya (tonics), shoolaghna (antispasmodic), and krimighna (anthelmintic) properties to it.

- Doshakarma: Kapha vatahara and Pitta vardhak
- Dhatukarma: Deepan, Balya
- Malakarma: Anulomana, Sara

Pharmacological Actions

Antispasmodic, analgesic, antimicrobial, antifungal, antiviral, antioxidant, antidiabetic, antiulcer, smooth muscle relaxant, anticancer, anticytotoxicity, antiobesity, anthelmintic, anxiolytic, hepatoprotective, antihemolytic, chemoprotective, nephroprotective, antihypertensive, anti-flatulence, neuroprotective, memory enhancer, digestive enzyme promoter, and antagonistic effects (Amalraj and Gopi 2017; Sultana et al 2015).

Indications

In Ayurvedic classics, Hingu is used in shola (colic), gulma (abdominal lump), udararoga (abdominal disease), aanaha (obstruction/constipation), agnimandhya (loss of appetite), hridyaroga (heart disease), kasa (cough), shwasa (asthma), apasmara (epilepsy), unmada (insanity), krimi (worm infestation), artavaroga (menstrual-related diseases), vibandh (constipation), netraroga (eye disease), pliharoga (spleen disease), arsha (piles), bastishool (bladder pain), krimidanta (dental carries), and karnashool (earache).

In traditional folklore medicine, it is used to treat worm infections, hysteria, convulsions, asthma, bronchitis, ulcers, whooping cough, as well as snake and insect bites.

Therapeutic Uses

External Use

1. **Vishamjwar** (intermittent fever): Snuffing with Hingu mixed with jeernaghrita prevents chaturtha kvisham jwar (VJ. 1/53).

2. **Krimidant** (dental carries): Mildly heated Hingu is filled in the tooth with dental carries (VM. 58/37).
3. **Karnashool** (ear pain): Hingvadi taila or mustard oil cooked with Hingu, Tumburu, and Shunthi is instilled in ears in case of earache and tinnitus (VM. 59/16).

Internal Use

1. **Gulma** (abdominal lump): Hingvadi churna or Hingvadi gutika should be taken before meal with madya or ushnodaka as anupana in vatakaphajgulma (C.S.Ci. 5/79-84).
2. **Udarshoola** (abdominal pain): Decoction of Shunthi, Eranda, and Yava added with Hingu and Pushkarmool gives relief in udarshool. Intake of Eranda, Yava, Hingu, and Suvarchalalavan also gives the same effect (VM. 26/8-9).
3. **Madatyay** (alcoholism): Hingu and Maricha mixed with suvarchallavan should be given with madya and amlakanji till the person regains consciousness (C.S.S. 24/49).
4. **Udavrata** (retention of feces, urine, and flatus): Powder prepared by mixing Hingu, Yavani, Vida lavan, Shunthi, Jeerak, Haritaki, Pushkarmool, and Kushta is used in pleeha, udarroga, ajeerna, and vishuchika (C.S.Ci. 26/22).
5. **Unmada** (insanity): Daily intake of ghrita prepared from Vyastha, Hingu, and Choraka is beneficial in unmada (C.S.Ci. 9/57).
6. **Vatavyadhi** (neuromuscular disease): Hingvadivati one tablet daily in the morning is prescribed in vatavyadhi (S.S.Ci. 5/28).

Officinal Part Used

Gum-resin

Dose

Powder: 125 to 500 mg

Formulations

Hingvadivati, Hingvastak churna, Raja pravartinivati, Hingutriguna taila, Hingukarpura gutika, Ayaskriti, Agnimukha churna, Kumaryasava, Hingvadhya ghrita, Hingvadi gutika.

Toxicity/Adverse Effects

If used within therapeutic doses, it does not show any toxicity or adverse effects. But consumption in large doses may lead to bulging in the mouth, diarrhea, flatulence, nervousness, and headache.

Shodhana

By giving bhavna of padmapatra swaras for 1 yam in sun heat (Shastry 2002).

Substitution and Adulteration

It is adulterated with wheat flour, small stone particles, starch powder, other cheap oleo-gum resins, etc. For its purity testing, mix a small quantity of Hingu in water; the water will turn milky white. In fire, pure Hingu burns completely (Sharma et al 2000).

Points to Ponder

- *Iran and Afghanistan are the largest producers of Hingu.*
- *Besides being a popular culinary spice, Hingu is widely used in treatment of digestive, respiratory, and gynecological disorders aggravated due to vatadosha.*

Suggested Readings

Amalraj A and Gopi S. Biological activities and medicinal properties of Asafoetida: a review. J Trad Complement Med 2017;7(3):347–359

Anonymous. The wealth of India, Vol. IV, 1st ed. New Delhi: CSIR; 2002:20–21

Duan H, Takaishi Y, Tori M. Polysulfide derivatives from Ferula asafoetida. J Nat Prod 2002;65:1667–1669

Iranshahy M, Iranshahi M. Traditional uses, phytochemistry and pharmacology of asafoetida (*Ferula asafoetida* oleo-gum-resin): a review. J Ethnopharmacol 2011;134:1–10

Kajimoto T, Yahiro K, Nohara T. Sesquiterpenoid and disulphide derivatives from *Ferula asafoetida*. Phytochemistry 1989;28: 1761–1763

Kareparamban JA, Nikam PH, Jadhav AP and Kadam VJ, *Ferula foetida* "*Hing*": a review. Res J Pharm Biol Chem Sci 2012;3(2):775–786.

Mahendra P and Bisht S. *Ferula asafoetida*: traditional uses and pharmacological activity. Pharmacogn Rev 2012;6(12):141–146

Sharma PC, Yelne MB, Dennis TJ. Database on medicinal plants used in Ayurveda, Vol. 1. New Delhi: CCRAS; 2000:217

Shastry L, ed. Yogaratnakara, with Vidyotini Hindi commentary, 7th ed. Varanasi: Chaukhamba Sanskrit Sansthan; 2002:171

Sultana A, Asma K, Khaleequr R, and Shafeequr R. Oleo-gum-resin of *Ferula asafoetida*: a traditional culinary spice with versatile pharmacological activities. Res J Recent Sci 2015;4:16–22

The Ayurvedic Pharmacopeia of India. Part I, Vol. 1. New Delhi: Department of AYUSH, Ministry of Health and Family Welfare, Government of India; 1989:65

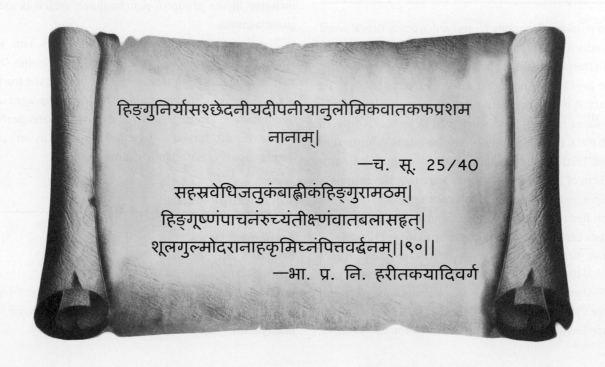

हिङ्गुनिर्यासश्छेदनीयदीपनीयानुलोमिकवातकफप्रशमनानाम्।
—च. सू. 25/40
सहस्रवेधिजतुकंबाह्लीकंहिङ्गुरामठम्।
हिङ्गूष्णंपाचनंरुच्यंतीक्ष्णंवातबलासहृत्।
शूलगुल्मोदरानाहकृमिघ्नंपित्तवर्धनम्॥९०॥
—भा. प्र. नि. हरीतक्यादिवर्ग

41. Jambu *[Syzygium cumini (L) Skeels]*

Synonym:	*Eugenia jambolana Lamk*
Family:	*Myrtaceae*
Hindi name:	*Jamun, Jaman*
English name:	*Jaman, Jambolan, Black plum*

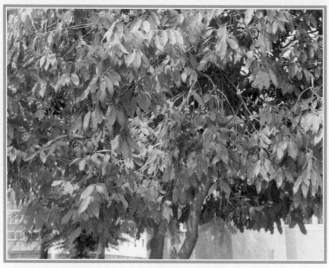

Plant of *Syzygium cumini* (L) Skeels.

Jambu is popularly known as the Fruit of God as it is believed that Lord Rama survived on Jamun fruits for years during his exile from Ayodhya.

Introduction

The genus name *Syzygium* is derived from a Greek word *syzygos* which means yoked together, referring to the paired leaves in the plant (Janick and Paull 2008).

Since ages Jambu has been a sacred tree to Hindus and Buddhists. It is customary to plant at least one Jambu tree in Lord Rama temples as it is believed to be his favorite. In Mahabharata, the body color of Sri Krishna is compared to this fruit. Lord Megha is said to have descended on earth in the form of Jambu tree. Puranas state that the cosmos is split into seven concentric island continents in the center of which lies the Jambudvipa. Its leaves are used in many auspicious ceremonies and decorating marriage pandals.

Charak has mentioned it as best vatajanaka dravya (C.S.Su. 25/40 & 27/140), and included it in Phalasava (C.S.Su. 25/2). Sushrut has included it in phalvarga as grahi and excessive vata aggravating fruit (S.S.Su. 46/166). Vagabhatt has described it as guru, visthambhi, sangrahi, vatavardhak,

and akanthya dravya (A.H.Su. 6/127). Its tender leaves are included in the group of panchpallava, which is used for gandhakarma.

The ripe fruits are used for making juices, jam, jellies, wines, squashes, etc. The seeds are used in tisanes (herbal tea) for diabetics (Helmstadter 2008). Besides the fruits, the plant is used as timber, fodder, fuel, making agricultural equipment, in tanning leather and making soaps, perfumes, etc. Leaves are served as food for silkworm in sericulture. Young shoots are used for cleaning teeth.

Vernacular Names

Assamese: Jam
Bengali: Jaam, Kalajam
Burma: Thabyebyu
Gujarati: Jambu, Jambuda
Kannada: Merale, Jamneralae, Jambu, Neralamara
Malayalam: Njaval, Naval

Marathi: Jambhool
Oriya: Jamukoli, Jamu, Jam
Punjabi: Jammu
Tamil: Naaval, NavvalSambu, Mahamaram, Nagal
Telugu: Nesedu, Neredu
Urdu: Jamun, Jaman, Phalenda

Synonyms

Phalendra: Its fruits are considered best among all fruits.
Mahaphala: The plant bears large fruits.
Surbhipatra: Its leaves are aromatic.
Mahajambu: The plant bears big-sized fruits.
Nilaphala: Fully ripe fruit is bluish-purple in color.
Nilanjanachhada: The young leaves have bluish tinge.
Maharasa: The fruit is profusely juicy in nature.
Mahaskandha: The tree has a big trunk.
Meghamodini: The plant bears fruits in rainy season.

Classical Categorization

Charak Samhita: Mutra-sangrahaniya, Purisha-virajaniya, Chhardi-nigrahaniya
Sushrut Samhita: Nyagrodhadi
Ashtang Hridaya: Nyagrodhadi
Dhanvantari Nighantu: Amraadi phalvarga
Madanpal Nighantu: Phal varga
Kaiyadev Nighantu: Oushadivarga
Raj Nighantu: Amraadivarga
Bhavaprakash Nighantu: Amradiphalvarga

Distribution

The plant is native to India, Indonesia, Malaysia, Pakistan, and Afghanistan. In India, it is commonly found in plains, forest, and hilly regions up to 1,800 m. It is planted in Bihar, Odisha, upper Gangetic plains, West Bengal, Konkan, and in southern states along the river banks.

Morphology

It is a fast growing, large or medium-sized evergreen tree reaching up to a height of 15 to 30 m and can live for more than 100 years.

- **Bark:** Light gray to ash colored, 0.5 to 2.5 cm thick, external surface more or less rough or rugged, internal surface rough, fibrous, and reddish-brown (**Fig. 41.1**).
- **Leaves:** Simple, opposite, variable in sizes 8–14 × 4–7 cm, petiolate, elliptic, ovate-oblong, acute-acuminate apex, smooth, glabrous surface (**Fig.41.2**).
- **Flowers:** Greenish-white in trichotomies panicle, sweet scented, sessile (**Fig. 41.3**).
- **Fruits:** Ovoid or globose berries, pink initially and turning black purple when fully mature, smooth, fleshy, crowned with a truncate calyx cap (**Fig. 41.4**).
- **Seed:** Single seeded, oval or round, smooth, brownish-black, enclosed in a cream colored, coriaceous covering. The plant is propagated by seeds (**Fig. 41.5**).

Phenology

Flowering Time: March to April
Fruiting Time: May to July

> ### Key Characters for Identification
>
> ➤ *A fast growing, medium-sized, evergreen tree of 15 to 30 m.*
> ➤ *Leaves: Simple, ovate-elliptical, opposite, smooth and in variable sizes.*
> ➤ *Flowers: Sweet scented in greenish-white panicles.*
> ➤ *Fruits: Smooth, fleshy, ovoid berries, single seeded, purple–black colored.*

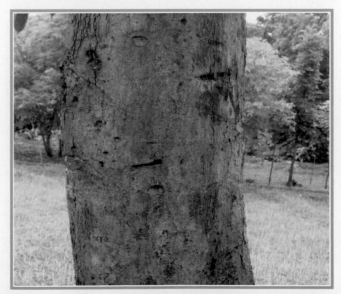

Fig. 41.1 Bark.

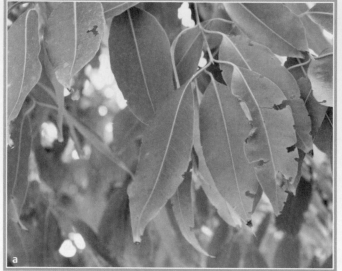

Fig. 41.2 **(a)** Leaves. **(b)** Tender leaves.

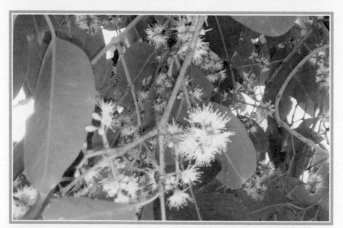

Fig. 41.3 Flowers.

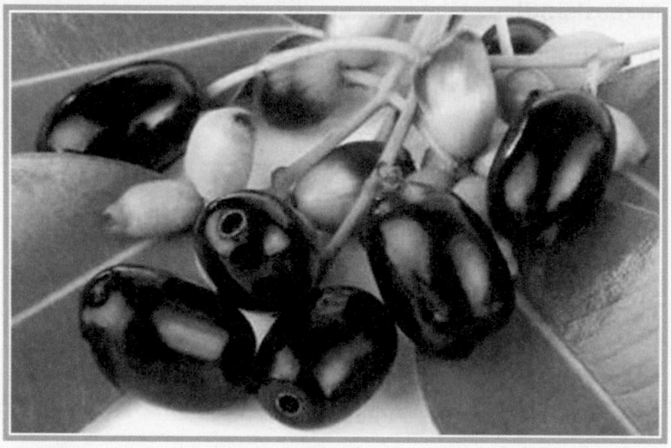

Fig. 41.4 Fruits.

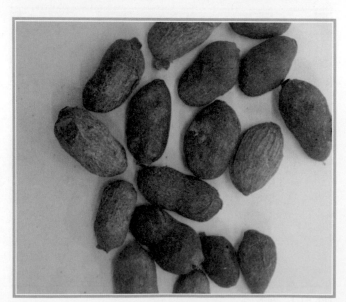

Fig. 41.5 Seeds.

Types

- Bhavaprakash: Two types: Raj jambu, Kshudrajambu
- Kaiyadev and Dhanvantari: Three types: Mahajambu, Kshudrajambu, Kakjambu
- Raj Nighantu: Three types: Mahajambu, Kakjambu, Bhumijambu

Rasapanchaka

Guna	Guru, Ruksha,
Rasa	Kashaya, Madhura, Amla
Vipak	Katu
Virya	Sheeta

Chemical Constituents

The plant is reported to be rich in compounds like anthocyanins, glucoside, ellagic acid, isoquercetin, kaempferol, and myrecetin. The seeds are reported to have jambosine (alkaloid), jamboline or antimelin (glycoside), flavonoids, phenolic compound, protein, calcium, etc. The leaves have acylated flavonol glycoside, quercetin, myrcetin, triterpenoids, esterase, galloyl carboxylase, tannins (Mortan 1987). The stem bark is rich in betulinic acid, friedelin, epifriedelinol, β-sitosterol, eugenin, quercetin, kaempferol, gallic acid, ellagic acid, gallo and ellagic-tannins. The flowers are rich in kaempferol, quercetin, myricetin, isoquercetin, oleanolic acid, eugenol-triterpenoid A &B (Nair and Subramaniam 1962). The fruits are rich in raffinose, glucose, fructose, citric acid, anthocyanins, gallic acid, malic acid, delphinidin-3-gentiobioside, petunidin-3-gentiobioside, cyanidin diglucoside, malvidin, and minerals like calcium, potassium, iron, vitamins A, B, C. The essential oil extracted from different parts of the plant contains β, α pinene, camphene, limonene, myrcene, cis and trans ocimene, terpinene, terpinolene, bornyl acetate, α copaene, β caryophyllene, α-Humulene, cadinene (Vijayanand et al 2001).

Identity, Purity, and Strength (Stem bark)

For Stem Bark

- Foreign matter: Not more than 2%
- Total ash: Not more than 11%
- Acid-insoluble ash: Not more than 1%
- Alcohol-soluble extractive: Not less than 9%
- Water-soluble extractive: Not less than 11%

For Seeds

- Foreign matter: Not more than 1%
- Total ash: Not more than 5%
- Acid-insoluble ash: Not more than 1%
- Alcohol-soluble extractive: Not less than 6%
- Water-soluble extractive: Not less than 15%

(Source: The Ayurvedic Pharmacopeia of India 1999)

Karma (Actions)

Ayurvedic classics described it as sangrahi (astringent), vatala (cause flatulence), vistambhi (constipative), rochan (relish), deepan (appetizer), pachan (digestive), mutrasangrahaniya (urinary astringent), stambhaka (inhibitory action), kanthya (beneficial for throat), lekha (scraping), krimighna (anthelmintic), dahaprasasmana (cooling effect), chardinigrahan (antiemetic), yakrituttejaka (hepatic stimulant), balya (tonic), hridya (cardiotonic), and viryavardhaka (spermatopoetic).

- Doshakarma: Kapha-pitta hara
- Dhatukarma: Rochan, hridya
- Malakarma: Visthambhi

Pharmacological Actions

Different parts of the plant are reported to have antihyperglycemic, antioxidant, antimicrobial, antibacterial, anti-inflammatory, antifungal, antidiarrheal, antifertility, anorexigenic, cardioprotective, gastroprotective, antiulcerogenic, radioprotective, anti-HIV, antileishmanial activity (Sagrawat et al 2006).

Indications

Ayurvedic classics attribute its use in atisaar (diarrhea), pravahika (dysentery), raktasrava (hemorrhage), prameha (diabetes), raktapitta (bleeding disorders), chardi (vomiting), vibandha (constipation), adhyaman (flatulence), kantharoga (throat infections), shwasa (asthma), kasa (cough), daha (burning sensation), jwara (fever), yoniroga (vaginal diseases), pradar (excessive discharge per vagina), shrama (excessive fatigue), shosha (emaciation), krimi (worm infestation), twakroga (skin diseases), hridyaroga (heart diseases), updansha (soft chancre).

Traditional healers throughout the country have been using its seeds for generations as an effective therapy for controlling blood sugar (Ratasimamanga 1998). Tribals in Tamil Nadu use seed extracts to treat cough, cold, fever, skin diseases, throat infections, intestine, and genitourinary ulcers (Chandrasekaran and Venkatesalu 2004). In Unani medicines, it is used as liver tonic, blood purifier, strengthening agent for tooth, gums, and as antifungal lotion in ringworm infections of head (Sagrawat et al 2006).

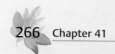

Therapeutic Uses

External Use

1. **Vyanga** (freckles): Paste prepared with tender leaves of Jambu, Amra, Haridra, Daruharidra, and nav guda mixed with mastu when applied on face removes freckles (A.H.U. 32/22).
2. **Vranaropana** (wound healing): Dusting the wounds with powdered bark of Arjuna, Udumbar, Ashvattha, Lodhra, Katphala, and Jambu enhances the healing process (C.S.Ci. 25/113).
3. **Kukunaka** (ophthalmia neonatorum): Washing the eyes with decoction of Jambu, Amra, Amalaki, and Ashmantaka is recommended in kukunaka (S.S.U. 19/13).
4. **Krimikarna** (maggots in ear): Instilling lukewarm juice of Jambupatra and pakwa phal expels out maggot from ears (G.N. 3/2/66).

Internal Use

1. **Atisaar** (diarrhea): Powder of seed kernel of Jambu, Amra, Bilwa, Kapitha, Shunti should be taken with liquid gruel in atisaar (C.S.Ci. 8/127).
2. **Raktaatisaar** (diarrhea associated with blood): Juice extracted from the leaves of Jambu, Amra, Amalaki should be taken with ajadugdh and madhu to control diarrhea associated with blood (CD. 3/68).
3. **Raktapitta** (hemorrhage): Intake of cold infusion of Jambu, Amra, and Arjuna is beneficial in controlling raktapitta (S.S.U. 45/23).
4. **Grahani** (Sprue): Juice extracted from Jambutwak mixed with an equal quantity of ajadugdha is beneficial for children affected with grahani (CD. 64/46).
5. **Chardi** (vomiting): Cooled decoction of tender leaves of Jambu and Amra mixed with honey is used to control vomiting (C.S.Ci. 20/30). Cooled decoction of tender leaves of Amra, Jambu, Ushira, Vatashung, and avroha with honey is also used in chardi (A.H.Ci. 6/14-15).
6. **Agnimandhya** (loss of appetite): Consumption of Jambuswarasa or Jambu prepared in vinegar improves digestion (S.B. 4/267-71).

Officinal Parts Used

Fruit, seed, bark, leaves

Dose

Powder: 3 to 6 g
Decoction: 50 to 100 mL
Juice: 10 to 20 mL

Formulations

Pancha-pallav yoga, Pathyadyachurna, Amradikwath, Karanjadighrita, Jambavaditaila, Pushyanugchurna, Jambuphalasava.

Toxicity/Adverse Effect

No adverse reactions or toxicity have been noted.

Substitution and Adulteration

None

Points to Ponder

- *Owing to its immense nutritional values, Jambu fruit is considered as a great nutraceutical food supplement.*
- *Therapeutically, it is widely used in the treatment of diabetes, diarrhea, sore throat, liver ailments, and bleeding disorders.*

Suggested Readings

Chandrasekaran M, Venkatesalu V. Antibacterial and antifungal activity of Syzygium jambolanum seeds. J Ethnopharmacol 2004;91: 105–108

Helmstadter. Syzygiumcumini (L.) Skeels (Myrtaceae) against diabetes: 125 years of research. Pharmazie 2008;62:91–101.

Janick J, Paull RE. The Encyclopedia of Fruit & Nuts. Wallingford: CABI; 2008:954

Morton J. Fruits of Warm Climates. Miami: Julia F. Morton Publication; 1987:375–378

Morton JF. Jamaica cherry. In: Fruits of Warm Climates. Miami, FL: Julia F. Morton; 1987:65–69

Nair RAG, Subramaniam SS. Chemical examination of the flowers of Eugenia jambolana. J Sci Ind Res 1962;21(B):457–458

Ratasimamanga U. Native plants for our global village. TWAS Newsl 1998;10:13–15

Sagrawat H, Mann AS, Kharya MD. Pharmacological potential of Eugenia jambolana: a review. Pharmacognosy 2006;2:96–104

Shukla R. Jambu (Syzygiumcumini): a fruit of gods. Ayurpharm: Int J Ayurveda Allied Sci 2013;2(4):86–91

The Ayurvedic Pharmacopeia of India. Part I, Vol. 2. New Delhi: Department of AYUSH, Ministry of Health and Family Welfare, Government of India; 1999:58–60

Vijayanand P, Rao LJ, Narasimham P. Volatile flavor components of Jamun fruits (Syzygiumcumini(L.). Flavour Fragrance Journal 2001;16:47–49

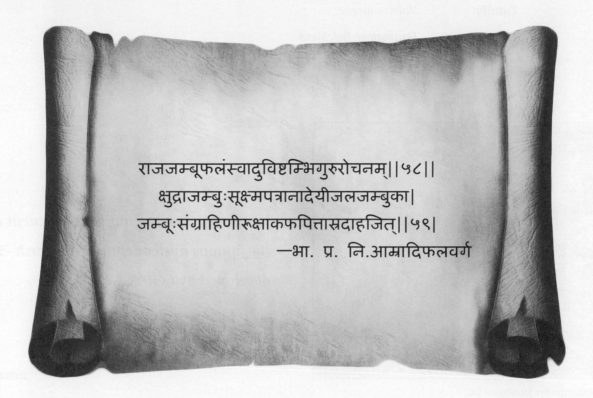

राजजम्बूफलंस्वादुविष्टम्भिगुरुरोचनम्||५८||
क्षुद्राजम्बुःसूक्ष्मपत्रानादेयीजलजम्बुका|
जम्बूःसंग्राहिणीरूक्षाकफपित्तास्रदाहजित्||५९|
—भा. प्र. नि.आम्रादिफलवर्ग

42. Jatamamsi *[Nardostachys jatamamsi DC]*

Family: *Valerianaceae*

Hindi name: *Jatamamsi, Balchhad*

English name: *Spikenard, Indian Nard, Nardus root, Jatamamsi, Musk root*

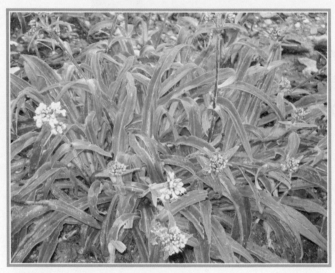

Plant of *Nardostachys jatamamsi* DC.

Jatamansi root is a major constituent of the famous antiepileptic drug Ayush–56 developed by CCRAS, New Delhi.

Introduction

Jatamamsi is a well-known herb used in traditional system of medicines since ages for the treatment of mental ailments. The herb is known by the name of Jatamansi because its roots resemble the matted hairs of Himalayan sages. The plant has found a reputed place in ancient Greek, Roman, Egyptian, and Arabian texts. It is included in the group of 11 drugs used as incense in the holy temple of Jerusalem. Priests used the herb in religious rituals and for embalming. Hippocrates used it in sweetened and spiced wine drinks. The European used the herb for seasoning food (Andrew 2000). It is also used for making perfumes, aromatic medicated oils, and as a sedative soothing drink. Since ancient times, Jatamamsi oil is a demanded article of luxury and a valuable medicinal agent.

In Samhitas and Nighantus, it is mentioned in the name of Mamsi and Jatila. Charak used its rhizome as a content in prayogik dhumnetra (C.S.Su. /21) and its fumigation in treating diseases like kushta, kasa, hikka, shwasa, shotha, chardi, etc. Sushrut used it as an ingredient of sadhyuvrana ropana taila (S.S.Ci. 2/75) and in the treatment of dushi visha, mudhagrabha, kasa, vrana. Due to overexploitation and large-scale destruction of natural habitat, it is rated as a critically endangered species by International Union for Conservation of Nature (IUCN) (Nayar and Sastry 1988).

Vernacular Names

Assamese: Jatamansi, Jatamangshi
Bengali: Jatamamsi
Gujarati: Baalchad, Kalichad
Kannada: Bhootajata, Ganagila maste
Kashmiri: Bhutijata
Malayalam: Manchi, Jatamanchi
Marathi: Jatamansi
Oriya: Jatamansi
Punjabi: Billilotan, Balchhar, Chharguddi

Tamil: Jatamanji
Telugu: Jatamams
Urdu: Sumbul-ut-teeb

Synonyms

Bhutajata: The hairy rhizome is used to dispel evil organisms.
Jatamansi: The rhizome is covered profusely with hairs.
Jatila: The rhizome bears abundant root hairs.
Mamsi: It is an efficacious drug in mental disorders.
Mata: Being sedative in action, it helps in inducing sound sleep like a mother.
Nalda: The rhizome is highly aromatic.
Sulomasa: The rhizome is beautifully covered by blackish-gray hair.
Tapaswini: The hairy rhizome looks like the matted hairs of sages.

Classical Categorization

Charak Samhita: Sanjnasthapana, Kandughna, Shukrajanana
Sushrut Samhita: Eladi
Ashtang Hridaya: Anjanadi, Eladi
Dhanvantari Nighantu: Chandanadi varga
Madanpal Nighantu: Karpuradi varga
Kaiyadev Nighantu: Oushadi varga
Raj Nighantu: Chandanadi varga
Bhavaprakash Nighantu: Karpuradi varga

Distribution

The plant is native to the Alpine and sub-Alpine regions of India, Pakistan, Nepal, Bhutan, Tibet, and China. It usually grows between 3,300 and 5,000 m above sea level in the regions of Jammu and Kashmir, Himachal Pradesh, Uttarakhand, Assam, and Sikkim.

Morphology

An erect, perennial herb about 10 to 60 cm height, with stout, long, and woody root stocks, densely covered with fibrous or lamellar remains of old sheaths.

- **Leaves:** Simple, glabrous, basal one elongated, spatulate, 10–25 cm × 2–3 cm narrowed into a petiole. Cauline leaves is opposite, oblong, sessile about 8 cm long, five-nerved at base (**Fig. 42.1**).
- **Flowers:** Rose or pale pink colored, appears in terminal corymbose cymes (**Fig. 42.2**).
- **Fruits:** Small, hairy, and crowned by persistent calyx teeth.
- **Root:** Deeply seated, dark gray rhizomes are crowned with reddish-brown tufted fibers, aromatic, highly agreeable odor, size ranges from 2.5 to 7.5 cm. Shape is elongated and cylindrical (**Fig. 42.3**). The plant is propagated by vegetative methods like rhizome cuttings.

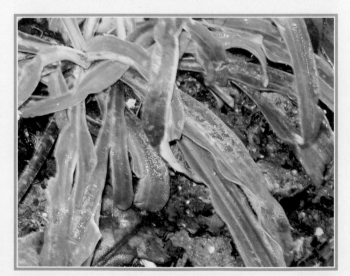

Fig. 42.1 Leaves.

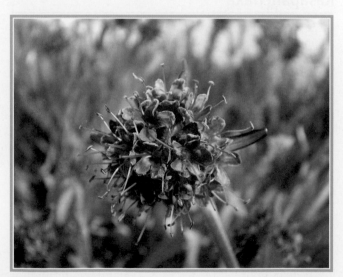

Fig. 42.2 Flowers.

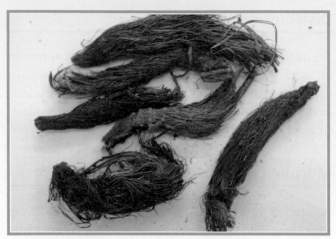

Fig. 42.3 Rhizomes.

Phenology

Flowering Time: April to June

Fruiting Time: May to June

Key Characters for Identification

➤ *An erect, perennial herb about 10 to 60 cm height with hairy rootstock.*

➤ *Leaves are simple, long, narrow, spatulate, and glabrous.*

➤ *Flowers are rose or pale pink in terminal cymes.*

➤ *Fruits are small, hairy with persistent calyx.*

➤ *Rhizomes are cylindrical, aromatic, dark gray, crowned with reddish-brown tufted fibers.*

Rasapanchaka

Guna	Laghu, Ruksha,
Rasa	Tikta, Kashaya, Madhura
Vipak	Katu
Virya	Sheeta
Prabhav	Bhutaghna

Chemical Constituents

The main active constituents reported from the roots are sesquiterpenes (volatile component), coumarin, alkaloids,

lignans, and neolignanes (Chatterji and Prakashi 1997). Jatamansone or valeranone is the principal sesquiterpene, and others are α-patcho-ulense, jatamansic acid, nardin, nardal, nardol, valerenal, angelicin, β-eudesmol, β-atchoulense, β-sitosterol, calarene, jatamansin, jatamansinol, valeranal, valeranone, nardostachnol, nordostachnol, and jatamansic acid (Rastogi and Mehrotra 2001). Other nonvolatile components include jatamansin (coumarine), actidine (alkaloid), propionate, cyclohexanol ester, essential oil, resin, and sugar (Chatterjee et al 2000).

Identity, Purity, and Strength

- Foreign matter: Not more than 5%
- Total ash: Not more than 9%
- Acid-insoluble ash: Not more than 5%
- Alcohol-soluble extractive: Not less than 2%
- Water-soluble extractive: Not less than 5%
- Volatile oil: Not less than 0.1%

(Source: The Ayurvedic Pharmacopeia of India 1999)

Karma (Actions)

Traditional Ayurveda texts attribute medhya (brain tonic), rasayan (rejuvenative), pachan (digestive), balya (provide physical strength), kantiprada (complexion promoter), nidrajanana (promotes sleep) manas-roga gana (alleviates mental diseases), kasa-shwasa hara (cure cough and asthma), keshya (hair tonic), dahaprasamana (alleviates burning sensation), vranaropaka (wound healing), and kusthaghna (alleviates skin diseases) properties to it.

- Doshakarma: Tridoshashamaka
- Dhatukarma: Rasayan, Medhya, Balya
- Malakarma: Malashodhak

Pharmacological Actions

Its rhizomes are reported to show marked tranquilizing activity, antioxidant, antipyretics, antibacterial, antiasthmatic, antifungal, hepatoprotective, antihypertensive, antidepressants, antidiabetic, anticancerous, anticonvulsant, neuroprotective, cognition and memory improvement, hypolipidemic, cardioprotective, and nootropic activities (Muthuraman and Nithya 2016; Ahmad et al 2013).

Indications

Ayurvedic classics used it in the treatment of unmada (insanity), apasmara (epilepsy), bhootbadha (evil spirits), anidra (insomnia), visha (poisoning), visarp (erysipelas), daha (burning sensation), kushta (skin diseases), vrana (wounds), kasa (cough), shwasa (asthma), vatavyadhi (neuromuscular disease), hridya roga (heart diseases), palitya (graying of hair), chardi (vomiting), etc.

Its essential oil is used to maintain a balance in emotional, spiritual, and physical energies. It is applied locally in anxiety, stress, fear, hysteria, emotional breakdown, nervousness, irritability, vertigo, seizures as a tranquillizing, relaxant, nervine tonic, soothing, antianxiety medication.

Therapeutic Uses

External Use

1. **Kushta** (skin disease): Local application of paste prepared with Jatamamsi, Marich, lavan, Haridra, Tagar, Snuhi, grahadhoom, mutra, pitta, and Palash kshar destroys kushta (C.S.Ci. 7/87).
2. **Hikka and shwasa** (hic-cough and bronchial asthma): Dhumavarti of Jatamamsi is useful in hikka and shwasa (C.S.Ci. 17/78).
3. **Kasa** (cough): Inhaling smoke of Manashila, Madhuk, Jatamamsi, Musta, and Ingudi followed by lukewarm milk and jaggery gives relief in kasa (C.S.Ci. 18/69) (S.S.U. 52/22).
4. **Vatarakta** (gout): Application of Madhuka, Ashvatha twak, Jatamamsi, Vira, Udumbar, and Durva paste after raktasravana in vatarakta gives relief in redness, pain, and burning sensation (C.S.Ci. 29/131). It is also an ingredient of madhuparnyadi taila and mahapadmaka taila used in treating vatarakta (C.S.Ci. 29/92,112).
5. **Sadhyovrana** (accidental wounds): Applying oil prepared with Talish, Padmaka, Jatamamsi, Harenu, Agaru, Chandana, Haridra, Daruharidra, Padma beej, Ushira, and Madhuka accelerates healing of wounds (S.S.Ci. 2/75-76).
6. **Keshvardhana** (hair growth): Powdered Mamsi, Kushta, Kala tila, Sariva, and Nilotpala are pounded with milk and then mixed with madhu. The paste is applied in root hairs to promote hair growth (A.H.U. 24/41).
7. **Kumarasayana** (rejuvenation for children): Intake of ghrita cooked with Siddharthak, Vacha, Jatamamsi, Payasa, Apamarga, Shatavari, Sariva, Brahmi, Pippali, Haridra, Kushta, and Saindhav promotes health, strength, and intellect in children (S.S.Sa. 10/45).

Internal Use

1. **Unmada** (insanity): Intake of mahapaisachika ghrita is useful in unmada and apasmara (C.S.Ci. 9/45-48).
2. **Chhardi** (vomiting): Kalka of Chandana, Chavya, Jatamamsi Draksha, Balaka, and gaireka should be taken with cold water to control vomiting (C.S.Ci. 20/33).
3. **Vatavyadhi** (neuromuscular disease): It is an important ingredient of Balataila used in vata-vyadhi (C.S.Ci. 28/153).

Officinal Part Used

Root/Rhizome

Dose

Powder: 2 to 4 g

Formulations

Mamsyadi kwath, Rakshoghna ghrita, Sarvosoudhi Snana, Lavangadya churna.

Toxicity/Adverse Effect

Jatamamsi oil is reported to be nontoxic, nonirritating, and nonsensitizing.

Substitution and Adulteration

Jatamamsi is substituted and adulterated with *Selenium vaginatum* Clarke, *Valeriana officinalis*, *Valeriana jatamamsi*, *Cymbopogon schoenanthus* Spreng., *Nymphoides macrospermum* L., and other species of Nardostachys like *N. chinensis*, *N. grandiflora* (Sagar 2014; Bell 2004).

The roots of *Cymbopogon schoenanthus* Spreng and *Nymphoides macrospermum* L. are used as substitutes to Nardus rhizome (root). Rhizome of *Selinum vaginatum* Clarke and *Selinum tenuifolium* Wall. ex Clarke are used as an adulterant.

Points to Ponder

- *Jatamamsi is a reputed drug in Ayurveda which has been used in treating psychological disorders for centuries.*
- *It is a critically endangered herb which requires immediate sustainable conservation strategies.*
- *It is well known for its medhya, rasayan, vrana ropana, keshya, kantivardhak, balya, nidrajanan properties.*

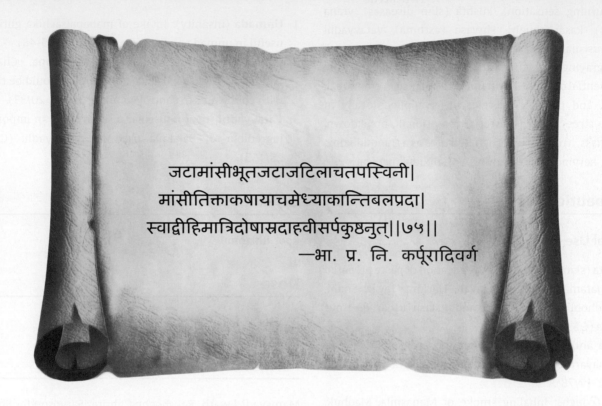

जटामांसीभूतजटाजटिलाचतपस्विनी।
मांसीतिक्ताकषायाचमेध्याकान्तिबलप्रदा।
स्वाद्वीहिमात्रिदोषास्रदाहवीसर्पकुष्ठनुत्।।७५।।
—भा. प्र. नि. कर्पूरादिवर्ग

43. Jatiphala [*Myristica fragrans* Houtt]

Family: *Myristicaceae*

Hindi Name: *Jaiphala*

English Name: *Nutmeg, True nutmeg, False aril, Mace tree, Fragrant nut tree*

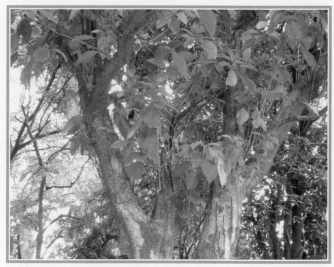

Tree of *Myristica fragrans* Houtt.

Myristica fragrans is a dioceious plant. However, the plants are identified as male and female after they bloom (about 6–7 years).

Introduction

The name Jatiphala is a combination of two words "Jati" and "phala." The word "Jati" literally means aroma and phala is fruit, referring to the aromatic nature of the fruit. The seed is popularly known as jayaphal and the fleshy red covering on the seed, i.e., mace is known as Javitri or Jatikosha.

Since ages both Jayaphala and Javitri are used as ingredients of garam masala in Indian homes. It is customary to use Jayaphala seed rubbed in water or seed paste for gastric troubles, diarrhea, vomiting, and stomachache in infants. The Arabians introduced Jatiphala as a trade commodity and spread it in Europe, China, and India. The Europeans used it as condiment, fumigant, and a hot food to counteract the effects of cold. Butter derived from its seeds is used in tobacco, perfumery, and toothpaste (Rosengarten 1969).

In traditional folklore medicine, Jayaphal and Javitri are used as stimulant, carminative, emmenagogue, and abortifacient drug (Nadkarni 1988). Classical texts such as Charak, Sushrut, and Ashtang described it as a refreshing and purifying drug for oral cavity (C.S.Su./77) (S.S.Su. 46/203). Keeping small pieces of Jayaphal pacifies throat infections, cleanses oral cavity, teeth, tongue, strengthens tooth and jaws, and removes foul odor of mouth (S.S.Ci. 24/21-23). In Ashtang Hridya, Jayaphal is included in the contents of Khadiradi gutika (A.H.U. 22/93), whereas in Gadanigrah, Jatiphaladi churna is indicated in kasa. Sharangdhar used jatiphala as deepana pachana, grahi, and shukrastambhaka dravya.

Besides medicinal importance, Jayaphal and Javitri are used as spices, preservative, flavoring agent in food, perfumes, in manufacture of synthetic camphor, pine oil, and as component of herbal tea, soft drinks, milk, etc. (Van Gils and Cox 1994).

Vernacular Names

Arabic: Jiansiban, Jouzbawwa
Bengali: Jaiphala, Jaitri, Jayapatri, Jotri, Japatri
Cambodia: Bochkak
Chinese: TouK'ou, JouTouK'ou
German: Muskatnuss, Muskatnussbaum
Greek: Kaaryonaromatikon, Moscharion
Gujarati: Jaiphala, Jayfar, Javantari
Italian: Moscatero, Nocemoscata
Kannada: Jadikai, Jaykai, Jaidikai, Jaji, Jajipatri
Kashmiri: Jafal
Malayalam: Jatika, Jatikosha, Jatipatri, Surabhi
Marathi: Jaiphal, Jayapatri
Oriya: Jaiphal
Punjabi: Jaiphal, Jauntari
Russian: Muskatnoetrava
Tamil: Sathikkai, Jathikkai, Jadhikai, Jadhikkai Adiphalam, Sivigaram, Kosham
Telugu: Jajikaya, Jaji, Jati, Jajipatri, Lavangamu
Urdu: Jauzbuwa, Jaiphal

Synonyms

Jatikosha: The aromatic fruit has a netted aril over the seed inside it.
Jatiphala: The fruit is aromatic in nature.
Kosha: The seed is enclosed inside the aril.
Malatiphala: The fruit bears aroma.

Classical Categorization

Charak Samhita: not mentioned
Sushrut Samhita: not mentioned
Ashtang Hridaya: not mentioned
Dhanvantari Nighantu: Chandanadi varga
Madanpal Nighantu: Karpuradi varga
Kaiyadev Nighantu: Oushadi varga
Raj Nighantu: Chandanadi varga
Bhavaprakash Nighantu: Karpuradi varga

Distribution

It is indigenous to the Moluccas and Banda Island in the South Pacific and is seldom found truly wild. It is now cultivated in tropical regions, especially in Indonesia, Grenada in West Indies, and Sri Lanka. In India, it is cultivated in high rainfall zone of Western Ghats including Kerala, Karnataka, and Tamil Nadu up to the 700 to 800 m elevation. Nilgiri, Salem, Tirunelveli, Ramanathapuram, Coimbatore, Kanyakumari, and Madurai districts of Tamil Nadu are famous for its cultivation.

Morphology

An aromatic evergreen tree of 5 to 15 m height with grayish-black, lenticellate bark outside and red inside.

- **Leaves:** Simple, alternate, petiolate, entire margin, lamina oblong to lanceolate, about 5–15 cm × 2–7 cm, acuminate apex, upper surface shiny, dull beneath (**Fig. 43.1**).
- **Flower:** Dioecious, occasionally both male and female flowers found on same tree. Female flowers arise in groups of one to three, while male flowers in groups of one to ten. Flowers are pale yellow, fragrant, in umbellate cymes, waxy, fleshy, and bell shaped. Male flowers are 5 to 7 mm, and female flowers are up to 1 cm.
- **Fruits:** Fleshy, globose or pyriform, drooping, yellow, smooth, 6 to 9 cm long with a longitudinal ridge (**Fig. 43.2**). On maturity, it splits into two halves revealing a purplish-brown shiny seed (nutmeg) surrounded by a red aril (mace) (**Fig. 43.2**).
- **Seed** (nutmeg): Ovoid, 2 to 3 cm long, firm, fleshy, white, transverse red-brown veins, and covered by red aril (**Fig. 43.3a, b**). The plant is propagated by seeds and vegetative methods.

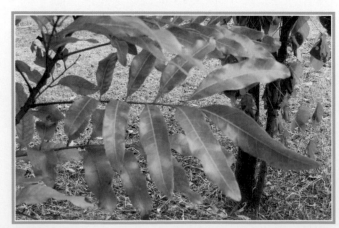

Fig. 43.1 Leaves.

Phenology

Flowering Time: November to March
Fruiting Time: March to May

Key Characters for Identification

➤ A medium-sized, evergreen, aromatic tree with gray bark.
➤ Leaves: Simple, alternate, oblong-lanceolate, shiny above dull beneath.
➤ Flowers: Dioecious, pale yellow, fragrant, in umbellate cymes, bell shaped.
➤ Fruits: Fleshy, globose, smooth, yellow-colored, splits into two halves on maturity, enclosing an ovoid seed covered by a red aril (mace).

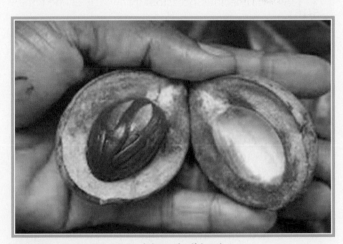

Fig. 43.2 Fruits.Fig. 43.3 **(a)** Seeds. **(b)** Aril.

Rasapanchaka

Guna	Laghu, Tikshna
Rasa	Tikta, Katu
Vipak	Katu
Virya	Ushna

Chemical Constituents

Fruits of Jatiphala contain derivatives of alkyl benzene (myristicin, elemicin, safrole, etc.), terpenes, myristic acid, essential oil, sabinene, α-thujene, α-pinene, β-pinene, limonene, γ-terpinene, terpinolene, terpinene-4-0l, methyl eugenol, trimyristin, formic acid, phytosterol, furfural, geraniol, geranyl-acetate, iron, calcium, magnesium, sodium, phosphorus, manganese, zinc, riboflavin, thiamin, fat, protein, and fibers. Its oil chiefly consists of terpenes, miristic oil, trimistin, glycerides, stearic, lauric, linoleic, and palmitic acids (Kirtikar and Basu 1984; Qiu et al 2004; Yang et al 2008).

Identity, Purity, and Strength

For Seed

- Foreign matter: Not more than 1%
- Total ash: Not more than 3%
- Acid-insoluble ash: Not more than 0.5%

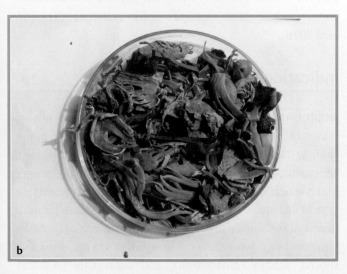

Fig. 43.2 Fruits.Fig. 43.3 **(a)** Seeds. **(b)** Aril.

- Alcohol-soluble extractive: Not less than 11%
- Water-soluble extractive: Not less than 7%
- Ether-soluble extractive: Not less than 25%
- Volatile oil: Not less than 5%

(Source: The Ayurvedic Pharmacopeia of India 1999)

Karma (Actions)

Ayurvedic classics describe it as deepan (appetizer), pachana (digestive), grahi (fecal astringent), rochan (relish), swarya (beneficial for voice), sugandhi (aromatic), madaka (narcotic), vrishya (aphrodisiac), hridya (cardio tonic), yakritut tejaka (hepatic stimulant), krimighna (anthelmintic), kushthaghna (antipruritus), jwarghna (antipyretics), varnya (complexion promoter), akshepahara (anticonvulsant), durgandhnashaka (fragrance/remove foul smell), vedanasthapaka (anodynes), vataanulomaka (carminative), and shothahara (reduce swelling).

- Doshakarma: Kaphavatahara
- Dhatukarma: Deepan, vrishya, jwaraghna
- Malakarma: Vataanulomaka, maladurgandhyanashak

Pharmacological Actions

The kernel and mace is reported to have carminative, deodorant, stimulant, aphrodisiac, antidiarrheal, anthelminthic, hypolipidemic, hypocholesterolemic effect, antidepressant, antidiabetic, cytotoxicity, memory-enhancing activity, antioxidant, hepatoprotective, pesticidal activity, antibacterial, antifungal, anticonvulsant, anti-inflammatory, smooth muscle relaxant, analgesic, expectorant, diuretics, emmenagogue, and antispasmodic activities (Tripathi et al 2016).

Indications

Jatiphal and Javitri are used in the treatment of atisaar (diarrhea), shwasa (asthma), kasa (cough), peenasa (common cold), krimi (worms), kushta (skin disease), grahani (sprue), agnimandhya (loss of appetite), ajeerna (indigestion), mukhavairasya (tastelessness of mouth) shukrameha (a type of diabetes), chardi (vomiting), vrana (wounds), anidra (insomnia), shool (pain), akshepa (convulsions), rajorodha (amenorrhea), jwar (fever), hridyaroga (heart diseases), shosha, kshaya (emaciation), and vatavyadhi (diseases originated due to aggravated vata). The oil is applied externally in mild ringworm infections, cracked feet, skin diseases, rheumatism, paralysis, and sprains.

As per folklore medicine, Sugali tribe of Chittoor and Cuddapah applies its oil on the umbilical cord to prevent infections. People of Nandurbar tribes of Maharashtra use its seed kwath for preventing hiccough and vomiting (Tayade and Patil 2010).

Therapeutic Uses

External Use

1. **Atisaar** (diarrhea): Jatiphala paste prepared with water is applied on the navel region to check atisaar (B.R.atisaar ci./30).
2. **Vyanga** (freckles): Local application of paste of Jatiphala or its aril (Jatipatri) removes freckles (B.P.Ci. 61/42) (R.M. 5/16).
3. **Vipadika** (cracked feet): Paste of Jatiphala is applied locally to cure cracked feet (B.S. kusta ci./118).

Internal Use

1. **Atisaar** (diarrhea): Jatiphala and Shunthi pounded with cold water are given to check diarrhea (S.B. 4/141). Oral intake of Jatiphala, Lavang, Jeeraka, and tankana powder mixed with madhu and sharkara controls all types of diarrhea (B.R.atisaar ci./30).
2. **Visuchika** (cholera): In case of thirst and mild nausea, water boiled with Lavanga or Jatiphala should be given (C.D. 6/91).

Officinal Parts Used

Seed, oil, mace

Dose

Power: 0.5 to 1 g
Oil: 1 to 3 drops

Formulations

Jatiphaladi churna, Jatiphaladi vati, Garbhachintamani rasa, Mahagandhaka vati, Ahiphenasava, Kasturibhairava rasa, Khadiradi gutika.

Toxicity/Adverse Effects

Intake of nutmeg in large doses may cause intoxication symptoms like profuse sweating, flushed face, tachycardia, delirium, altered state of mind, euphoria, dry throat, etc. within 6 hours of ingestion. Myristicin, the chief active constituent, in large doses can cause fatty degeneration of liver (Anonymous 1995; Beyer et al 2006; Hallström and Thuvander 1997).

Substitution and Adulteration

Fruits of *Myristica malabarica* Lamk. and *M. dactyloides* Gaertn. are used as adulterant to Jatiphala (Sharma et al 2002).

Points to Ponder

- *The kernel and aril of Jatiphala are highly demanded drugs domestically as well as internationally as spices, medicine, and nutritional supplements.*
- *It is a drug of choice for diarrhea, flatulence, stomach ache, and rheumatism.*

Suggested Readings

Anonymous. The Wealth of India: Raw Materials, Vol. 6(L-M). New Delhi: Publications and Information Directorate, CSIR;1995: 474–490

Beyer J, Ehlers D, Maurer HH. Abuse of nutmeg (*Myristica fragrans* Houtt.): studies on the metabolism and the toxicologic detection of its ingredients elemicin, myristicin, and safrole in rat and human urine using gas chromatography/mass spectrometry. Ther Drug Monit 2006;28(4):568–575

Hallström H, Thuvander A. Toxicological evaluation of myristicin. Nat Toxins 1997;5(5):186–192

Kirtikar KR, Basu BD. Indian Medicinal Plants, Vol. III. 2nd ed. Deharadun; 1984:2141.

Nadkarni KM. *Myristica fragrans*. In: Indian Materia Medica. 3rd ed. Mumbai: Bombay Popular Prakashan; 1988:830–840

Qiu Q, Zhang G, Sun X, Liu X. Study on chemical constituents of the essential oil from *Myristica fragrans* Houtt. by supercritical fluid extraction and steam distillation. Zhong Yao Cai 2004;27(11): 823–826

Rosengarten F Jr. The Book of Spices. 1st ed. Livingston Publishing Company; 1969:489.

Sharma PC, Yeine MB, Dennis TJ. Database on Medicinal Plants Used in Ayurveda, Vol. 4. New Delhi: Central Council for Research in Ayurveda and Siddha, Department of I. S. M. & H., Ministry of Health and Welfare, Government of India; 2002:216–217

Tayade SK, Patil DA. Ethnomedicinal applications of spices and condiments in Nandurbar District (Maharashtra). J Ecobiotechnol 2010;2/8:08–10

Tripathi N, Kumar V, Acharya S. Myristica fragrans: a comprehensive review. Int J Pharm Sci 2016;8(2):27–30

Van Gils C, Cox PA. Ethnobotany of nutmeg in the spice islands. J Ethnopharmacol 1994;42(2):117–124

Yang XW, Huang X, Ahmat M. New neolignan from seed of *Myristica fragrans*. Zhongguo Zhongyao Zazhi 2008;33(4):397–402

Nagja T, Vimal K, Sanjeev A. Myristica fragrans: a comprehensive review. Int J Pharm Pharm Sci 2016;8(2):27–30

The Ayurvedic Pharmacopeia of India. Part I, Vol. 1 New Delhi: Department of AYUSH, Ministry of Health and Family Welfare, Government of India; 1999:70

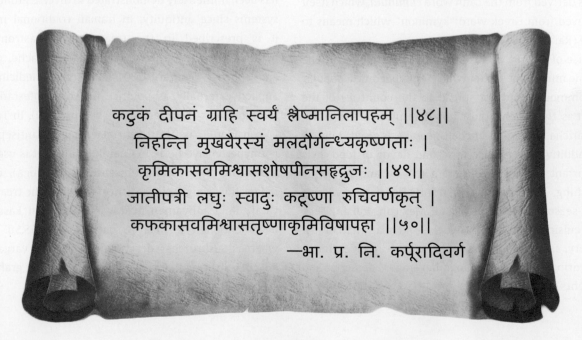

कटुकं दीपनं ग्राहि स्वर्यं श्लेष्मानिलापहम् ||४८||
निहन्ति मुखवैरस्यं मलदौर्गन्ध्यकृष्णताः |
कृमिकासवमिश्रासशोषपीनसहृद्रुजः ||४९||
जातीपत्री लघुः स्वादुः कटूष्णा रुचिवर्णकृत् |
कफकासवमिश्रासतृष्णाकृमिविषापहा ||५०||
—भा. प्र. नि. कर्पूरादिवर्ग

44. Jeeraka *[Cuminum cyminum Linn.]*

Family:	*Apiaceae (Umbelliferae)*
Hindi name:	*Jira, Safed jira*
English name:	*Cumin seed*

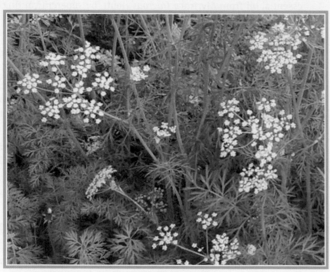

Plant of *Cuminum cyminum* Linn.

Khorasan region of Iran is the largest producer and exporter of Jeeraka in the world.

Introduction

Cumin is derived from the Latin word *cuminum*, which itself was derived from Greek word "kyminon" which means to enhance (Rai et al 2012).

The use of Jeeraka as a culinary spice started in Europe during the middle ages. After which it has become a popular trade commodity and got spread to the countries of the world. It is the second most popular spice in the world after Maricha. In Indian kitchen, Jeeraka is used daily as a food additive to enhance taste and flavor of food. It is an important ingredient of garam masala and Jal zeera, a refreshing, appetizer Indian drink. Jeeraka powder is used as seasoning spice in Indian, Mexican, Italian, Thai, Spanish cuisines. Cumin oil is widely used in aromatherapy, perfumery, as a seasoning in soups, sausage, pickles, meat, and flavoring agent in alcoholic beverages, desserts, and condiments (Farrell 1985).

Jeeraka is not only a popular spice, but has diverse medicinal applications too. The medicinal use of Jeeraka has been immensely demonstrated in diverse ethnomedical systems since antiquity. In Iranian traditional medicine, it is prescribed in the treatment of gastrointestinal, gynecological, respiratory disorders, toothache, diarrhea, and epilepsy (Zargary 2001). In Arabic medicines, it is applied externally as poultice in worm infestations and scorpion bites (Leporatti and Ghedira 2009). In Tunisia, it is considered as abortive, galactagogue, antiseptic, and antihypertensive herb. In Charak Samhita, it is used in the treatment of abdominal diseases (udar roga), diarrhea, indigestion, cough, piles. Sushrut used it in the treatment of vataj gulma, adhyaman, madatyay, mutraghat, kasa. Charak has mentioned jeeraka in harit varga (C.S.Su. 27/172) whereas Sushrut has described it in shaka varga (S.S.Su. 46/221). Sharangdhar quotes it in examples of grahi dravya (Sh.S.P. 4/11).

Vernacular Names

Assamese: Jira

Arabic: kammun, kemouyn

Malaysia: jintan puteh

Sinhalese: cheeregum, jeera

Tamil: Sheeragam, Chirakam, Jeerakam

Bengali: Jira, Sadajira

French: Cumin

German: Kreuzkümmel, Romische Kümmel

Italian: Cumino

Gujarati: Jirautmi, Jirn, Jiraugi, Jeeru, Jirun

Kannada: Jirage, Bilejirege

Kashmiri: Safed Zoor

Malayalam: Jeerakam

Marathi: Pandhare jire

Oriya: Dhalajeera, Dalajira, Jira

Punjabi: Safed Jira, Chitta Jira

Spanish: Comino

Telugu: Jilakarra, Tella Jilakarra

Urdu: Zirah, Zirasafed

Synonyms

Jarana: The fruit has digestive, carminative properties.

Ajaji: It stimulates digestive fire.

Kana: The fruit looks like grains.

Deerghajeeraka: This variety is longer in comparison to other varieties.

Auttarapatham: The plant is abundantly cultivated in northern region.

Deepak: It stimulates digestive fire.

Deerghakam: The fruit is quiet long.

Peetabham: The fruit is yellowish in color.

Medhyam: It is brain tonic in action.

Ruchyam: It improves taste in food.

Classical Categorization

Charak Samhita: Shoolaprasamanam

Sushrut Samhita: Pippalyadi

Ashtang Hridaya: Pippalyadi

Dhanvantari Nighantu: Shatpushpadi varga

Madanpal Nighantu: Sunthyadi varga

Kaiyadev Nighantu: Oushadi varga

Raj Nighantu: Pippalyadi varga

Bhavaprakash Nighantu: Haritakyadi varga

Distribution

The plant is a native of Egypt but now it has been extensively cultivated in the Middle East, India, China, Iraq, Libya, Turkey, and other Mediterranean countries. In India, Gujarat, Rajasthan, Maharashtra, Punjab, and Uttar Pradesh are the major cumin-producing states.

Morphology

Annual delicate herbaceous plant 15 to 50 cm high, somewhat angular and tends to drop under its own weight. The plant has deep-seated long, white roots.

- **Leaves:** Five to ten cm long, tri- to multipinnate, thread-like leaflets, bluish-green in color, glabrous, and lamina finely pinnatifid with oblong-linear tips (**Fig. 44.1**).
- **Flower:** Flowers are in umbels radiating in groups of three to five, petals are white or pink. Bracts are long and simple, style is short and turned outward at the end (**Fig. 44.2**).

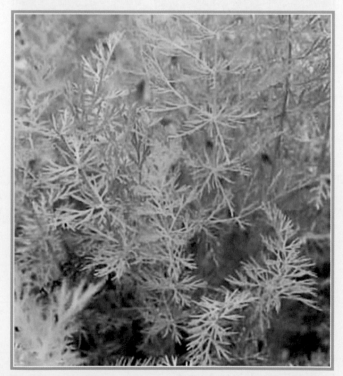

Fig. 44.1 Leaves.

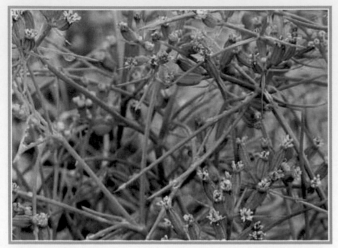

Fig. 44.2 Flower.

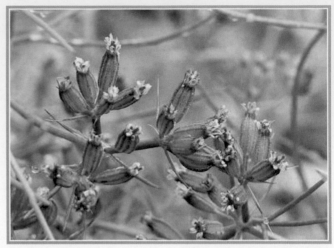

Fig. 44.3 Fruit.

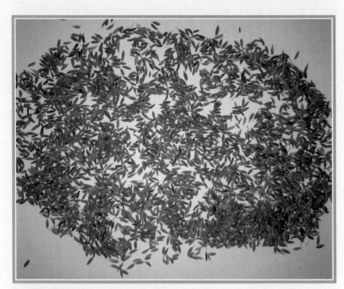

Fig. 44.4 Seeds.

- **Fruit:** A schizocarp often separated into mericarp, brownish-gray with light-colored ridges, ellipsoidal, elongated, 4 to 6 mm long × 2 mm wide, tapering at both ends containing single seed. Mericarps with five longitudinal hairy primary ridges from base to apex alternating with four secondary ridges that are flatter (**Fig. 44.3**). The plant is propagated by seeds (**Fig. 44.4**).

Phenology

Flowering Time: May to June
Fruiting Time: July to August

Key Characters for Identification

➤ An annual, weak, aromatic herb of 15 to 50 cm height.
➤ Leaves are bluish-green, thread-like, pinnate compound.
➤ Flowers are in white or pink umbels, in a group of three to five.
➤ Fruits are -aromatic schizocarp, brownish-gray with ridges on surface, tapering at both ends, separated into mericarp.

Types

Bhavaprakash and Kaiyadev Nighantu classified it into three types, namely, Sweta Jeeraka (*Cuminum cyminum* Linn.), Krishna Jeeraka (*Carum carvi* Linn.), and Kalajaji (*Nigella sativa* Linn.).

Dhanvantari Nighantu: three types—Shukla Jeeraka, Krishna Jeeraka, Brihatpali (vanyajir).

Raj Nighantu: four types—Gour ajaji, Shyah Jeeraka, Prithvika, Brihatpali.

Rasapanchaka

Guna	Laghu, Ruksha
Rasa	Katu
Vipaka	Katu
Virya	Ushna

Chemical Constituents

The fruit contains alkaloid, anthraquinone, coumarin, flavonoid, glycoside, dietary fibers, protein, resin, saponin, tannin, steroid, 3 to 4% volatile oil, and 10% fixed oil. Cuminaldehyde, γ-terpinene, o-cymene, limonene, β-pinene, α-pinene, eugenol, tetradecane γ-terpinene, β-ocimene, p-mentha-2-en-ol, α-terpinyl acetate, α-terpinolene, and myrcene cuminoside A and B are the major constituents of cumin oil (Takayanagi et al 2003; Chaudhary et al 2014). The roots, stems, leaves, and flowers are rich in tannins and phenolic compounds like p-coumaric acid, quercetin, rosmarinic acid, trans-2-dihydrocinnamic acids, resorcinol, and vanillic acid (Bettaieb et al 2010). The fruit is also rich in carbohydrate, fats, vitamin A, B, C, K, α-carotenoid, β-carotene, calcium, iron, sodium, zinc, palmitic, oleic, linoleic acid, and omega 6 fatty acids (Parthasarathy 2008).

Identity, Purity, and Strength

For Fruit

- Foreign matter: Not more than 2%
- Total ash: Not more than 8%
- Acid-insoluble ash: Not more than 1%
- Alcohol-soluble extractive: Not less than 7%
- Water-soluble extractive: Not less than15%

(Source: The Ayurvedic Pharmacopeia of India 1989)

Karma (Actions)

In Ayurveda classics, Jeeraka is described as deepan (appetizer), pachan (digestive), rochan (relish), grahi (astringent), medhya (intellect promoter), jwaraghna (antipyretics), vrishya (aphrodisiac), balya (physical strength promoter), chakshusya (beneficial for vision), garbhasayavishudhakaraka (uterine cleansing), vishaghna (antidotes), krimighna (anthelmintic) dravya. .

- Doshakarma: Kapha vatahara
- Dhatukarma: Deepan, srotoshodhan
- Malakarma: Vataanulomana

Pharmacological Actions

Jeeraka and its oil is reported to possess antimicrobial, anti-inflammatory, analgesic, hepatoprotective, antiflatulent, insecticidal, antiestrogenic, antidiabetic, bronchodilator, antioxidant, blood platelet aggregation, anticancer, anti-infertility, contraceptive, neuroprotective, antistress, antifungal, hypocholesterolemic, antiepileptic activities (Al-Snafi, 2016).

Indications

Jeeraka is widely prescribed in the treatment of gulma (abdominal lump), adhmana (distension), aruchi (loss of interest/ageusia), atisara (diarrhea), grahani (sprue), kushta (skin disease), krimi (worm infestation), visha (poisoning), jwara (fever), chardi (vomiting), agnimandhya (loss of appetite), arsha (piles), mutravrodha (retension of urine), ashmari (calculus), kasa (cough), pratishyay (common cold), shotha (swelling), vrana (wound), sarpa dansha (snake bite), vrishchik dansha (scorpion sting) rajoavrodh (amenorrhea), and netraroga (eye diseases).

Therapeutic Uses

External Use

Vrishchik dansha (scorpion sting): Lukewarm paste of Jeeraka mixed with ghrita and saindhav is applied locally to get relief in pain of scorpion sting (C.D. 65/23).

Internal Use

1. **Vishamjwara** (irregular fevers or malaria): Jeeraka paste with jaggery should be taken in vishamjwara. It also improves appetite and destroys diseases caused by vata (A.S.Ci. 2/93) (V.M. 1/228).
2. **Chardi** (vomiting): Leha prepared with Jeeraka, Sauvarchal lavan, sharkara, Maricha, and madhu is used to check vomiting (V.M. 15/18).
3. **Amlapitta** (acidity): Intake of ghrita processed with paste of Jeeraka and Dhanyaka gives relief in amlapitta, aruchi, mandagni, and vaman (C.D. 52/51).

Official Part Used

Fruit

Dose

Powder: 3 to 6 g

Formulations

Jeerakadi modaka, Jeerakadya churna, Jeerakadyarista, Jeerakadyataila, Hingwastak churna, Dhatri rasayana, Yograj guggul.

Toxicity/Adverse Effect

Not reported on proper administration of designated therapeutic dose.

Substitution and Adulteration

Adulterated with oil extracted samples of Jeeraka.

Points to Ponder

- *Jeeraka is a popular daily utility culinary spice with great neutraceutical value.*
- *Jeeraka is a renowned drug for gastrointestinal diseases like gulma, grahni, atisaar, agnimandhya, udar shool, vibandha, arsha, aruchi, chardi.*

Suggested Readings

Al-Snafi AE. The pharmacological activities of *Cuminum cyminum*: a review. IOSR J Pharm 2016;6(6):46–65

Bettaieb I, Bourgou S, Wannes WA, Hamrouni I, Limam F, Marzouk B. Essential oils, phenolics, and antioxidant activities of different parts of cumin (*Cuminum cyminum* L.). J Agric Food Chem 2010;58(19):10410–10418

Chaudhary N, Husain SS, Ali M. Chemical composition and antimicrobial activity of volatile oil of the seed of *Cuminum cyminum* L. World J Pharm Pharm Sci 2014;3(7):1428–1441

Farrell KT. Spices, Condiments and Seasonings. Westport, CT: The AVI Publishing Co., Inc.; 1985:98–100.

Leporatti ML, Ghedira K. Comparative analysis of medicinal plants used in traditional medicine in Italy and Tunisia. J Ethnobiol Ethnomed 2009;5:31–39

Parthasarathy VA, Chempakam B, Zachariah TJ. Chemistry of Spices. Oxfordshire and Cambridge, MA: CAB International; 2008: 211–226.

Rai N, Yadav S, Verma AK, Tiwari L, Sharma RK. A monographic profile on quality specifications for a herbal drug and spice of commerce: *Cuminum cyminum* L. Int J Adv Herbal Sci Technol 2012;1(1):1–12

Takayanagi T, Ishikawa T, Kitajima J. Sesquiterpene lactone glucosides and alkyl glycosides from the fruit of cumin. Phytochemistry 2003;63(4):479–484

The Ayurvedic Pharmacopeia of India, Part I, Vol. 1. New Delhi: Department of AYUSH, Ministry of Health and Family Welfare, Government of India; 1989:143

Zargary A. Medicinal Plants. 5th ed. Tehran: Tehran University Publications; 2001:35

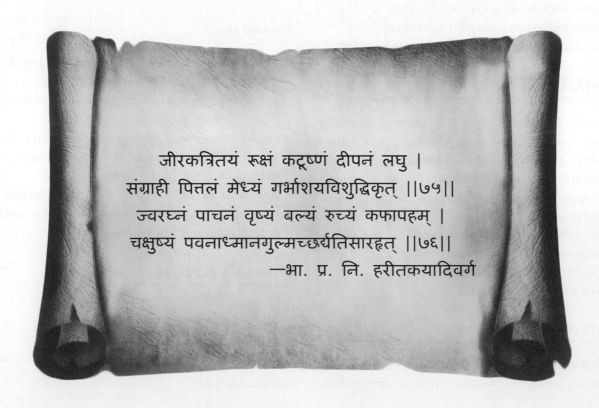

जीरकत्रितयं रूक्षं कटूष्णं दीपनं लघु |
संग्राही पित्तलं मेध्यं गर्भाशयविशुद्धिकृत् ||७५||
ज्वरघ्नं पाचनं वृष्यं बल्यं रुच्यं कफापहम् |
चक्षुष्यं पवनाध्मानगुल्मच्छर्द्यतिसारहृत् ||७६||
—भा. प्र. नि. हरीतक्यादिवर्ग

45. Jyotishmati [Celatrus paniculatus Willd.]

Family:	*Celastraceae*
Hindi name:	*Malkangini*
English name:	*Climbing staff tree, Black oil plant*

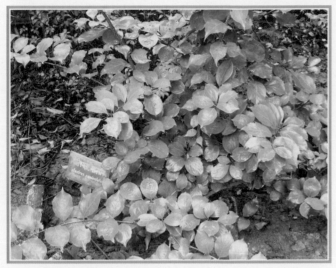

Plant of *Celatrus paniculatus* Willd.

Jyotishmati is popularly known as the Intellect tree as it miraculously improves cognitive function, learning, memory, and mental acuity.

Introduction

Jyotishmati is named after its ability to enhance cognitive function and natural luminosity (jyoti) of the mind (mati). Since time immemorial, it has been used to treat brain-related diseases and enhance learning and memory.

The plant has a long history of usage as medicine. In Unani and Siddha medical system, Jyotishmati is used for treating facial paralysis, backache, gout, paraplegia, fatigue, and neurasthenia (Singh et al 2010). Thai practitioners used it for fever, diarrhea, and dysentery (Premuan-sappakun-ya 1964). In Chinese traditional medicine, Jyotishmati oil is used as a natural insecticide and for treatment of arthritis, swellings, chill, fever, pain, and infections (Chen and Liang 1999). In Charak Samhita, Jyotishmati is mentioned in shirovirechan (C.S.Su. 2/5) and moolini dravya (C.S.Su. 1/79). Sushrut has described the properties of Jyotishmati taila in taila varga. Its oil is considered as laghu, katu rasa, katu vipaki, ushna virya, mriduvirechaka in action,

and is used in the treatment of krimi, kushta, prameha, shiroroga (S.S.Su. 45/115). Oil is also used for purification and healing of wounds (S.S.Ci. 8/51). Dalhana described it as kakamardanika whereas Vagabhatta mentioned it in dravya for tikshan dhumapana (A.H.Su. 21/17).

Ruthless and indiscriminate use of Jyotishmati seed and oil has led to its inclusion under highly vulnerable/ endangered plant species in Eastern and Western Ghats. It is also reported to be critically endangered in Uttar Pradesh and Uttrakhand (Pattanaik et al 2009; Rajasekharan and Ganeshan 2002).

Vernacular Names

Assamese: Kapalphotla
Gujarati: Malkangani
Kannada: Doddaganugae, Gangunge beeja, Gangunge humpu, Kangondiballi
Malayalam: Ceruppunnari, Uzhinja, pololuvam

Marathi: Malkangoni, Kanguni
Oriya: Malkanguni, Korsana
Punjabi: Malkangoni
Tamil: Valuluvai
Telugu: Malkangani, Peddamaveru
Urdu: Malkangani
Bengali: Kijri

Synonyms

Agnibha: The plant is similar to fire in action.
Durjaraa: The seeds do not digest easily.
Jyotishska: Improves digestive fire and is ushna virya in nature.
Kakandi: Shape of the fruit resembles crow's eggs.
Kanguni: The seeds look like millet grains.
Katabhi: The seeds are katu/pungent in rasa.
Lata: It is a climber.
Medhya: It promotes intellect.
Paravatapadi: Its roots resemble the pigeon's foot.
Peetataila: The extracted oil is yellow colored.
Pinyaa: It is a famous trade commodity.
Sukshmaphala: The plant bears small fruits.
Suvarnalatika: The climber has yellow flowers that resemble the color of gold.
Vega: It is a fast growing plant.

Classical Categorization

Charak: Shirovirechanopaga
Sushrut: Adhobhagahara, Shirovirechana, Arkadi
Ashtang Hridaya: Arkadi
Dhanvantari Nighantu: Guduchyadi varga
Madanpal Nighantu: Abhyaadi varga
Kaiyadev Nighantu: Oushadi varga
Raj Nighantu: Guduchyadi varga
Bhavaprakash Nighantu: Haritakyadi varga

Distribution

The plant is native to Indian subcontinent and is found throughout India up to an elevation of 1,800 m, including the Himalayas, Eastern Ghats, Western Ghats, and other high-altitude regions.

It is also known to grow wildly in Australia, China, Taiwan, Cambodia, Indonesia, Malaysia, Myanmar, Nepal, Sri Lanka, Thailand, Vietnam, etc.

Morphology

It is a woody climbing or scrambling shrub with terete branches. Young branches are pendulous.

- **Stem:** Rough, pale, reddish-brown exfoliating bark covered with densely small elongated white lenticels. Stem up to 6 m in length and 10 cm in diameter (**Fig. 45.1**).
- **Leaves:** Simple, alternate, broad, oval to obovate or elliptic in shape, leathery and smooth. Short petiole, apex acute, acuminate, base-cuneate, obtuse or rounded, margin toothed (**Fig. 45.2**).
- **Flowers:** Unisexual yellowish-green, borne in terminal drooping panicles. Male flowers: minute, pale green, calyx lobes suborbicular toothed, petals oblong or obovate-oblong entire, disk copular. Female flowers have sepals, petals, and disc similar to those of male flowers (**Fig. 45.3**).
- **Fruits:** Capsule, depressed, globose, three-valved, three-celled, bright yellow in color, 1 to 1.3 cm in diameter, three to six seeds per capsule (**Fig. 45.4**).
- **Seeds:** Grow in side capsule, ellipsoid or ovoid, yellowish to reddish-brown, enclosed in orange–red fleshy aril (**Fig. 45.5**). The plant is propagated by seeds.

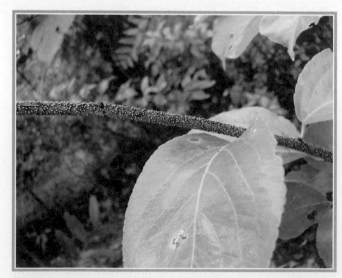
Fig. 45.1 Stem.

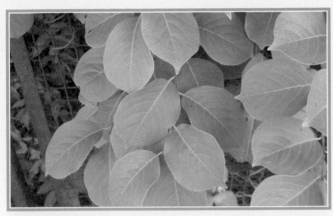

Fig. 45.2 Leaves.

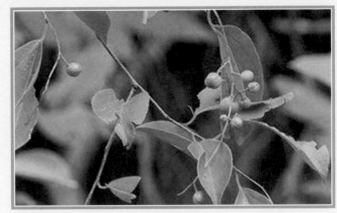

Fig. 45.4 Fruits.

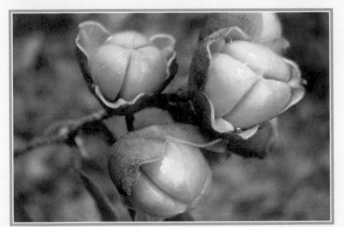

Fig. 45.3 Flowers.

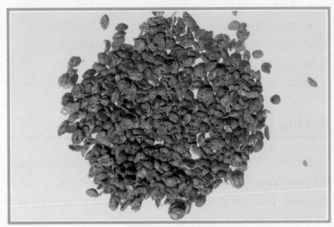

Fig. 45.5 Seeds.

Phenology

Flowering Time: March to June

Fruiting Time: June to September

Key Characters for Identification

➤ *A woody climber or shrub with young drooping branches.*

➤ *Stem is rough, reddish-brown, exfoliating, marked with white lenticels.*

➤ *Leaves are alternate, oval to obovate, dentate, acuminate apex, leathery.*

➤ *Flowers are unisexual, yellowish-green, in terminal drooping panicles.*

➤ *Fruits are yellow capsule, globose, three-valved, three-celled.*

➤ *Seeds are 3-6 per capsule, ovoid yellow to reddish-brown.*

Types

None

Rasapanchaka

Guna	Tikshna
Rasa	Katu, Tikta
Vipak	Katu
Virya	Ushna (Atyushna)

Chemical Constituents

The seeds mainly contain alkaloid (celastrine, wifornine, paniculatine A and B), sesquiterpene alkaloids (celapanin, celapanigin, celapagin), sesquiterpene esters/polyol ester (malkanguniol, malkangunin, celapanin, celapanigine, agrofuran), quinone methide/phenolid tri terpenoids (celastrol, pristimerin, zeylasterol, zeylasterone), carbolic acids (acetic acids, benzoic acid), fatty acids (oleic, linoleic, palmitic, stearic, crude lignoceric acids), crystalline substances (tetracosanol, sterol). Leaves are rich in saponin content whereas the bark and root have β-sitosterol, pistimerin, zeylasteral, terpenes (Gamlath et al 1990; Warsi 1940).

Identity, Purity, and Strength (Seed)

- Foreign matter: Not more than 2%
- Total ash: Not more than 6%
- Acid-insoluble ash: Not more than 1.5%
- Alcohol-soluble extractive: Not less than 20%
- Water-soluble extractive: Not less than 09%
- Oil content: Not less than 45%

(Source: The Ayurvedic Pharmacopeia of India 1999)

Karma (Actions)

Ayurvedic classics described Jyotishmati seeds and taila as deepan (appetizer), pachan (digestive), medhya (intellect promoter), shirovirechana, vamak (induce vomiting), sara (laxative), vatahara (pacify vata dosha), vedanasthapana (anodynes), uttejaka (stimulant), nadibalya (neurotonics), vatanulomana (carminative), hridyauttejaka (cardiac stimulants), shothahara (reduce swelling), mutral (diuretics), artavajanana (emmenogogue), vajikarana (aphrodisiac), kushthaghna (antipruritus), swedajanana (diaphoretics), jwaraghna (antipyretics)..

- Doshakarma: Kaphavatahara
- Dhatukarma: Medhya, deepana
- Malakarma: Vataanulomana, swedajanan

Pharmacological Actions

In vivo and in vitro studies on Jyotishmati showed antihistaminic, sedative, anticonvulsant, antiprotozoal, antiviral, antipyretic, antiulcerogenic, antiemetic, antibacterial, antimalarial, emmenagogue, hypotensive, stimulant, central muscle relaxant, antiarthritic, wound healing, hypolipidemic, antiatherosclerotic, spasmolytic, tranquillizer, analgesic, anti-inflammatory, antifertility (antispermatogenic), and memory enhancer activities (Gatinode et al 1957; Bhanumathy et al 2010).

Indications

Jyotishmati seeds and oil are used in the treatment of unmada (insanity), apasmara (epilepsy), vrana (wounds), agnimandhya (loss of appetite), udarroga (abdominal disorders), shiroroga (cephalagia), bhootbadha (evil spirits), vibandha (constipation), gulma (abdominal tumor), visarp (erysipelas), pandu (anemia), pakshaghata (paralysis), ardita (facial paralysis), sandhivata (arthritis), gridhrasi (sciatica), katishoola (backache), vatavikara (neuromuscular diseases), mastishkaroga (brain disorders), nadidaurbalya (neuropathy), hridyamandata (cardiac debility), shotha (inflammations), kasa (cough), shwasa (asthma), mutrakrichchhta (dysuria), kashtartava (dysmenorrhea), klaibya (infertility), kushta (skin diseases), kandu (pruritus), and jwar (fever).

Tribals of Bastar region in Chhattisgarh use Jyotishmati beej in a gradual increasing dose of 1 to 100 seeds daily in treating weak memory. Traditional healers throughout the length and breadth of the country use Jyotishmati taila to improve memory, intellect, retention, and recalling power, to alleviate mental fatigue, stress, and minor joint pains (Nadkarni and Nadkharni 1976). Seed oil mixed with lavang, jayaphal, javitri, etc. is used to treat beri-beri (vit-B1 deficiency disease) and anxiety neurosis (Kirtikar and Basu 1935).

Therapeutic Uses

External Use

1. **Sidhma** (a type of dermatosis): Local application of Jyotishmati taila processed with Apamarga kshara jal decanted for seven times cures sidhma (A.H.Ci. 19/75).
2. **Tandra** (drowsiness): Taking nasya of Jyotishmati taila and Pindaraka root removes drowsiness in fever (B.S. jwar ci./490).
3. **Vranashodhana** (cleansing of wounds): Decoction of Jyotishmati is used for washing wounds (S.S.Ci.8/39).

Internal Use

1. **Udara roga** (abdominal disease): Oil extracted from the fruit of Jyotishmati mixed with Svarjik kshara and Hingu should be taken with milk (S.S.Ci. 14/10) (B.S. udarrog ci.56).

2. **Artavaavrodha** (amenorrhea): Intake of Japa flower, kanji, and fried leaves of Jyotishmati induces menstruation (C.D. 62/25).

Officinal Parts Used

Seed, seed oil, leaves, bark

Dose

Seed powder: 1 to 2 g
Oil: 5 to 10 drops

Formulations

Jyotishmati taila, Vishyandana taila, Smritisagara rasa, Laghuvishagarbha taila, Chitrakadi taila, Mahapaishachika ghrita.

Toxicity/Adverse Effects

If seeds are taken in more than the recommended dose, it may cause diarrhea and vomiting (Sharma et al 2002).

Substitution and Adulteration

Lavang taila is used as substitute to Jyotishmati taila (Sharma et al 2002).

Points to Ponder

- *Drug of choice for neurodegenerative diseases, memory loss, dementia, neuropathy, cephalalgia, and beri beri.*
- *Jyotishmati is a potent medhya, shirovirechan, vamak, vatahara, and swedajanan dravya.*

Suggested Readings

Bhanumathy M, Chandrasekar S.B., Chandur Uma, Somasundaram T. Phyto pharmacology of *Celastrus paniculatus*: an overview. Int J Pharm Sci Drug Res 2010;2(3):176–181

Chen PD, Liang JY. The progress of studies on constituents and activities of genus *Celastrus*. Strait Pharm J 1999;11:3

Gamlath CB, Gunatilaka AAL, Tezuka Y, Kikuchi T, Balasubramaniam S. Quinone-methide, phenolic and related triterpenoids of plants of Celastraceae: further evidence for the structure of celastranhydride. Phytochemistry 1990;29:3189–3192

Gatinode BB, Raiker KP, Shroff FN, Patel JR. Pharmacological studies with malkanguni: an indigenous tranquilizing drug (preliminary report). Curr Pract 1957;1:619–621

Kirtikar KR, Basu BD. Indian Medicinal Plants, Vol. II. 2nd ed. Allahabad, India: Lalit Mohan Basu; 1935:1492.

Nadkarni KM, Nadkharni AK. The Indian Materia Medica. Bombay: Popular Prakashan, Bombay; 1976:810.

Pattanaik C, Reddy CS, Reddy KN. Ethnobotanical survey of threatened plants in Eastern Ghats, India. Our Nat 2009;7:122–128

Premuan-sappakun-ya Thai. Part I. Old Style Doctor Association. Bangkok: Am-Phon-Pittaya; 1964:25.

Rajasekharan PE, Ganeshan S. Conservation of medicinal plants biodiversity: an Indian perspective. Curr Res Med Aromat Plants 2002;24:132–147

Sharma PC, Yeine MB, Dennis TJ. Database on Medicinal Plants used in Ayurveda, Vol. 2. New Delhi; Department of I. S. M. & H., Central Council for Research in Ayurveda and Siddha, Ministry of Health and Welfare, Government of India; 2002:216–217.

Singh H, Krishna G, Baske PK. Plants used in the treatment of joint diseases (rheumatism, arthritis, gout, lumbago) in Mayurbhunj district of Odisha, India. Report Botanical Survey of India 2010; 2:22–26

The Ayurvedic Pharmacopeia of India, Part I, Vol. 2. New Delhi: Department of AYUSH, Ministry of Health and Family Welfare, Government of India; 1999:66

Warsi SA. The chemical examination of *Celastrus paniculatus*. Curr Sci 1940;9:134–135

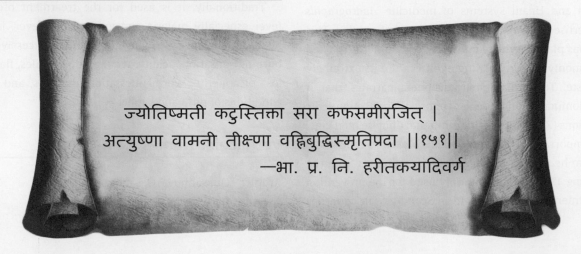

ज्योतिष्मती कटुस्तिक्ता सरा कफसमीरजित् ।
अत्युष्णा वामनी तीक्ष्णा वह्निबुद्धिस्मृतिप्रदा ॥१५१॥
—भा. प्र. नि. हरीतकयादिवर्ग

46. Kalmegh *[Andrographis paniculata (Burm.f.) Wall.ex Nees]*

Family:	*Acanthaceae*
Hindi name:	*Chirayata, Kirayat, Kalpanath, Mahatita, Kalmegh*
English name:	*Green chiretta, Creat, King of Bitters*

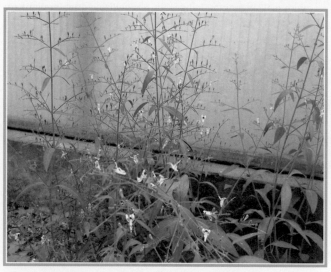

Plant of *Andrographis paniculata* (Burm.f.) Wall.ex Nees.

Andrographis was selected by the Ministry of Public Health as one of the medicinal plants to be included in "The national list of essential drugs A.D. 1999" in Thailand.

—Pholphana et al 2004

Introduction

Andrographis paniculata is a well-known plant in Bengal by the name "kalmegh." Kalamegha means "dark cloud." It is also known as Bhui-neem, meaning "neem of the ground." It is the main herb of the domestic remedy known as "Alui" which is given to infants from ancient times, in both Ayurveda and Unani systems of medicine. *Andrographis* was advertised in England as a substitute of quinine. This herbaceous plant is widely cultivated in Southern Asia and it is commonly known as "King of bitters" for its extremely bitter taste. The Indian pharmacopoeia narrates that it is a predominant constituent of more than 26 Ayurvedic formulations (Zhang 2004). In traditional Chinese medicine, it is an important "cold property" herb used to relieve the body from heat, as in fevers and to dispel toxins from the body (Dang 1978). It is commonly used for the prevention and treatment of common cold in Scandinavian countries

(Cacres et al 1997). In Malaysia, *A. paniculata* is traditionally known as "hempedubumi" (bile of the earth).

The plant is sometimes sold under the name of "Chireta" in the market. The plant, however, is not the actual Chireta but "Kalmegh" of Ayurveda, though it possesses antimalarial properties. The ethnomedical uses of the plant is comparable with *Swertia chirayita* in south-eastern India.

Traditionally, it is used for the treatment of chronic fever especially malaria and intermittent fever, jaundice, hepatitis, hepato-splenomegaly, anemia, excessive thirst, burning sensation, acidity, wound, ulcers, piles, flatulence, loss of appetite, worm infestation, diabetes, and vitiated conditions of pitta and kapha.

Vernacular Names

Arabic: Quasabhuva, Qasabuzzarirah
Assamese: Chiorta, Kalmegh

Azerbaijani: Acılar Şahı, Acılar Xanı (khanı)

Bengali: Kalmegh, Mahatita

Burmese: Se-ga-gyi

Chinese: Chuan Xin Lian

French: Chirette verte, Roidesamers

Gujarati: Kariyatu, Kiryata, Olikiryat, Kiryato

Indonesian: Sambiroto, Sambiloto

Japanese: Senshinren

Kannada: Nelaberu, Nela-bivinagida

Konkani: Vhadlem Kiratyem

Lao: La-Sa-Bee

Malay: Hempedu Bumi, Sambiloto

Malayalam: Nelavepu, Kiriyattu

Manipuri: Vubati

Marathi: Oli-kiryata, Kalpa

Mizo: Hnakhapui

Oriya: Bhuinimba

Punjabi: Chooraita

Persian: Nain-e Havandi

Philippines: Aluy, Lekha, and Sinta

Russian: Andrografis

Scandinavian: Green Chiratta

Sinhalese: Hın Kohomba or Heen Kohomba, Nin-bin-kohomba

Spanish: Andrografis

Tamil: Nilavembu, Shirat-kuchchi

Telugu: Nilavembu

Thai: Fa-Talai-Jorn, Fah-talai-jon (jone)

Turkish: Acılar Kralı, Acı Pas¸a, Acı Bey

Urdu: Kalmegh, Kariyat, Mahatita

Vietnamese: Xuy^en T^am Li^en

Synonyms

Bhunimba: It is the Neem of the ground (smaller than Neem) and has bitter taste like Neem.

Kalmegh: It is compared to dark cloud.

Classical Categorization

Categorization is not mentioned in Brihatrayee and famous Nighantus.

Distribution

A. paniculata is native to Taiwan, Mainland China, and India. It is also commonly found in the tropical and subtropical Asia, Southeast Asia, and some other countries including Cambodia, Caribbean islands, Indonesia, Laos, Malaysia, Myanmar, Sri Lanka, Thailand, and Vietnam. This plant is also found in different phytogeographical and edaphic zones of China, America, West Indies, and Christmas Island (Niranjan et al 2010; Wu et al 1996; Benoy et al 2012).

It is found throughout India, specifically in Maharashtra, Karnataka, Uttar Pradesh, Tamil Nadu, Andhra Pradesh, and Madhya Pradesh. It is cultivated to some extent in Assam and West Bengal (Kokate et al 2006).

Morphology

It is an annual, herbaceous plant erecting to a height of 30 to 110 cm in moist shady places.

- **Stem:** Acutely quadrangular, much branched, easily broken due to its fragile texture (**Fig. 46.1**).
- **Leaves:** Simple, opposite, lanceolate, glabrous, 2 to 12 cm long, 1 to 3 cm wide with acute entire margin or slightly undulated, and upper leaves often bractiform with short petiole, acute at both ends, upper surface dark green, lower surface whitish-green (**Fig. 46.2**).
- **Flowers:** Inflorescence of the plant is characterized as patent, terminal, and axillary in panicle, 10 to 30 mm long with small bract and short pedicel. The flowers possess calyx with five sepals which are small and

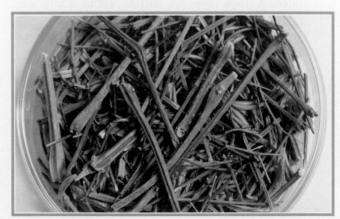

Fig. 46.1 Dry rectangular stem.

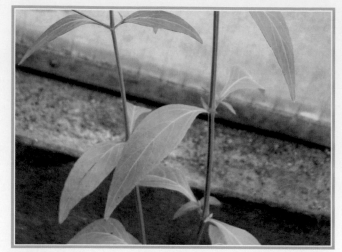

Fig. 46.2 Leaves.

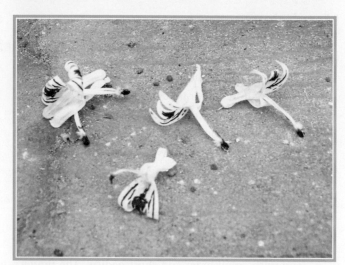

Fig. 46.3 Flowers.

linear. Corolla tubes are narrow, about 6 mm long, bilabiate, upper lip oblong, white with a yellowish top, whereas the lower tips are broadly cuneate, three-lobed, white with violet markings; stamens two, inserted in the throat and far exerted; anther basally bearded. Superior ovary, two-celled; style far exerted (**Fig. 46.3**).

- **Fruit:** Capsule of the plant is erect, linear-oblong, 1 to 2 cm long and 2 to 5 mm wide, compressed, longitudinally furrowed on broad faces, acute at both ends, thinly glandular-hairy (**Fig. 46.4**).
- **Seeds:** Very small, numerous, subquadrate, and yellowish-brown in color (Niranjan et al 2010; Zhang 2004).

It is normally grown from seeds in its native areas. Moist shady places, forests, and wastelands are preferable

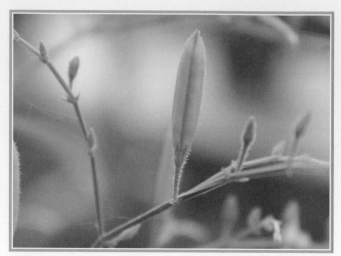

Fig 46.4 Fruit.

for their well development. In India, it is cultivated during rainy phase of summer season (Kharif) crop.

Phenology

Flowering Time: August to November
Fruiting Time: October to January

Key Characters for Identification

➤ *It is an annual 1 m heighted herbaceous plant with acutely quadrangular stem.*
➤ **Leaves:** *Simple, opposite, lanceolate, glabrous, 2 to 12 cm long, 1 to 3 cm wide, acute at both ends, highly bitter.*
➤ **Flowers:** *Inflorescence in terminal and axillary panicle, 10 to 30 mm long with small bract and short pedicel, white flower with violet marking.*
➤ **Fruits:** *Linear-oblong capsule, 1 to 2 cm long and 2 to 5 mm wide, acute at both ends, thinly glandular-hairy.*
➤ **Seeds:** *Very small, numerous, subquadrate, and yellowish-brown in color.*

Rasapanchaka

Guna	Laghu, Ruksha
Rasa	Tikta
Vipaka	Katu
Virya	Ushna

Chemical Constituents

The primary active constituent of *A. paniculata* is the andrographolide (Chen and Liang 1982). It is colorless, bitter, crystalline substance and is known as diterpene lactone.

The other major chemical constituents present in *A. paniculata* are andrographin, panicolin, andrographolide, diterpene, glucoside-neoandrographolide, andrographidines, neo-andrographolide, chlorogenic, myristic acid, homoandrographolide, andrographiside andropanoside, α- and β-sitosterol, apigenin, etc.

Identity, Purity, and Strength

- Foreign matter: Not more than 2%
- Total ash: Not more than 15%
- Acid-insoluble ash: Not more than 3%
- Alcohol-soluble extractive: Not less than 8%
- Alcohol (60%) soluble extractive: Not less than 24%
- Water-soluble extractive: Not less than 20%

(Source: Sharma et al 2001)

Karma (Actions)

This plant is described as a deepana (increases digestive fire), yakrituttejaka (hepatoprotective, liver stimulant), pittasaraka (cholagogue), rechana (purgative), kushtaghna, (antidermatosis), krimighna (anthelmintic), rakta shodhaka (blood purifier), swedajanana (diaphoretic), jwaraghna (antipyretic), vishamajwarahara (subside intermittent fever), and shothhara (anti-inflammatory/reducing swelling) in Ayurveda.

- Doshakarma: Kaphapittashamaka
- Dhatukarma: Rakta shodhaka (blood purifier)
- Malakarma: Rechana (purgative), swedajanana

Pharmacological Actions

The plant has pharmacological actions like hepatoprotective, abortifacient, antiperiodic, antipyretic, analgesic, anti-inflammatory antibacterial, antithrombotic, antiviral, cancerolytic, cardioprotective, choleretic, antivenom, depurative, digestive, expectorant, hypoglycemic, immune enhancement, laxative, sedative, thrombolytic, vermicidal (Mishra 2007), anti-HIV, antioxidant, hypotensive, cholinergic, antimicrobial (Sharma et al 2001), antiulcer, microfilaricidal, antidiarrheal, and antiallergic (Gupta and Tandon 2004).

Indications

It is indicated in kaphapittavikar (diseases of kapha and pitta), agnimandya (loss of appetite), yakritvridhi (hepatomegaly), vibandha (constipation), krimi (worm infestation), raktavikar, shotha (edema), charmaroga (skin disease), jeernajwara (chronic fever), vishamjwara (intermittent fever), jwarottaradaubalya (weakness after recovering fever).

Contraindications

In vivo studies in mice and rabbits suggested that *A. paniculata* may have abortifacient activity (Hancke 1997; Panossian et al 1999). It may not be used during pregnancy or lactation in higher doses.

Therapeutic Uses

Internal Use

1. **Jeernajwara** (chronic fever): Regular consumption of decoction prepared from whole parts of Kalmegh twice daily prevents the occurrence of all types of fever.
2. **Kamala** (jaundice): Decoction prepared from 1 g Kalmegh powder, 2 g Bhumiamalaki, and 2 g Mulethi powder is an effective remedy in jaundice, hepatitis, hepatomegaly, and anemia.
3. **Ajeerna** (indigestion): Three grams of Kalmegh powder with equal quantity of jaggery is given twice per day in indigestion, flatulence, and chronic constipation.
4. **Charmaroga** (skin diseases): Soak 3 g of Kalmegh powder and 3 g of Amla powder in a glass of water at night. Filter and drink it next morning to get rid of all types of skin diseases.
5. **Asrikdara** (menorrhagia): Fresh leaf juice is given to prevent excessive bleeding during menstruation.

Officinal Parts Used

Aerial parts of the plant, whole plant, and roots are most commonly used. Traditionally, the plant was used as an infusion, decoction, or powder, either alone or in combination with other medicinal plants. Commercial preparations have standardized the extracts of the whole plant in modern times and also in many controlled clinical trials.

Dose

Powder: 1 to 3 g
Juice: 5 to 10 mL
Decoction: 20 to 40 mL
Liquid extract: 0.5 to 1 mL (Sharma et al 2001)

Formulations

Tiktaka ghrita, Bhunimbadi kwath, Panchtikta kasaya, Devdarvayadi kwath churna, Pathyadi kwath churna, Nimbadi kwath churna, Aragvadhadi kwath churna.

Toxicity/Adverse Effects

The plant is safe at its therapeutic dose and is neither associated with any serious toxicity nor any side effects. However when it is administered at higher dose it may cause gastric discomfort, vomiting, and loss of appetite. These side effects occur due to the bitter taste of andrographilide. Injection of the crude drug extract (extract of stem and leaves) may lead to anaphylactic shock (Zhang 2004). Male reproductive toxicity (Akbarsha and Murugaian 2000) and cytotoxicity (Nanduri et al 2004) of *A. paniculata* have also been reported.

The LD-50 of the alcohol extract, obtained by cold maceration, is 1.8 g/kg (Rana and Avadhoot 1991). The LD-50 of andrographolide (yield 0.78% w/w from whole plant) in male mice through intraperitoneal route is 11.46 g/kg (Handa and Sharma 1990).

Substitution and Adulteration

A. paniculata (Burm.f.) Wall.ex Nees is used as a substitute of Kiratatikta (*S. chirayita* Buch-Ham). *A. echinoides* (Linn.)

Nees is used as an adulterant and substitute for kalmegh (*A. paniculata* (Burm.f.) Wall.ex Nees) (Sharma et al 2001).

> ### Points to Ponder
>
> - *A. paniculata (Burm.f.) Wall.ex Nees is used as substitute of Kiratatikta (S. chirayita Buch-Ham).*
> - *It is commonly known as "King of bitters" for its extremely bitter taste.*
> - *It is used in agnimandya (loss of appetite), yakritvridhi (hepatomegaly), vibandha (constipation), krimi (worm infestation), raktavikar, shotha (edema), charmaroga (skin disease), jeernajwara (chronic fever), vishamjwara.*

Suggested Readings

Akbarsha MA, Murugaian P. Aspects of the male reproductive toxicity/male antifertility property of andrographolide in albino rats: effect on the testis and the cauda epididymidal spermatozoa. Phytother Res 2000;14(6):432–435

ang WL. Preliminary studies on the pharmacology of the andrographis product dihydroandrographolide sodium succinate. Newsletter Chin Herb Med 1978;8:26–28

Benoy GK, Animesh DK, Aninda M, Priyanka DK, Sandip H. An overview on *Andrographis paniculata* (burm. F.) Nees. Int J Res Ayurveda Pharm 2012;3(6):752–760

Caceres DD, Hancke JL, Burgos RA, Wikman GK. Prevention of common colds with Andrographis paniculata dried extract: a pilot double blind trial. Phytomedicine. 1997;4:101–104

Chen W, Liang X. Deoxyandrographolide 19-β-D-glucoside from the leaves of *Andrographis paniculata*. Planta Med 1982;15:245–246

Cáceres DD, Hancke JL, Burgos RA, Wikman GK. Prevention of common colds with *Andrographis paniculata* dried extract: a pilot double blind trial. Phytomedicine 1997;4(2):101–104

Gupta AK, Tandon N. Reviews on Indian Medicinal Plants. Vol. 2. New Delhi: Alli-Ard, ICMR; 2004:283–298

Hancke J. Reproductive toxicity study of *Andrographis paniculata* extract by oral administration of pregnant Sprague-Dawley rats. Cato. de Chile: Santiago, Pontifica Univer; 1997

Handa SS, Sharma A. Hepatoprotective activity of andrographolide from *Andrographis paniculata* against carbon tetrachloride. Indian J Med Res 1990;92:276–283

Jarukamjorn K, Nemoto N. Pharmacological aspects of *Andrographis paniculata* on health and its major diterpenoid constituent andrographolide. J Health Sci 2008;54(4):370–381

Kokate CK, Puroht AP, Gokhale, SB. Pharmacognosy. Pune, India: Nirali Publication; 2006, (34), 251–252

Manual for Cultivation, Production and Utilization of Herbal Medicines in Primary Healthcare. Nonthaburi: Department of Medical Sciences, Ministry of Public Health; 1990

Medicinal plants in VietNam. Manila, World Health Organization. WHO Regional Publications; 1990. Western Pacific Series, No. 3

Mishra SK, Sangwan NS, Sangwan RS. *Andrographis paniculata* (Kalmegh): a review. Pharmacogn Rev 2007;1(2):283–298

Mishra SK, Sangwan NS, Sangwan RS. Andrographis paniculate (Kalmegh): a review. Pharmacognosy review 2007;1:283–298

Nanduri S, Nyavanandi VK, Thunuguntla SS, et al. Synthesis and structure-activity relationships of andrographolide analogues as novel cytotoxic agents. Bioorg Med Chem Lett 2004;14(18):4711–4717

Niranjan A, Tewari SK, Lehri A. Biological activities of Kalmegh (*Andrographis paniculata* Nees) and its active principles: a review. Indian J Nat Prod Resour 2010;1(2):125–135

Panossian A, Kochikian A, Gabrielian E, et al. Effect of *Andrographis paniculata* extract on progesterone in blood plasma of pregnant rats. Phytomedicine 1999;6(3):157–161

Pharmacopoeia of the People's Republic of China. Vol. 1 (English ed.). Beijing: Chemical Industry Press; 1997

Pholphana N, Rangkadilok N, Thongnest S, Ruchirawat S, Ruchirawat M, Satayavivad J. Determination and variation of three active diterpenoids in *Andrographis paniculata* (Burm.f.) Nees. Phytochem Anal 2004;15(6):365–371

Rana AC, Avadhoot Y. Hepatoprotective effects of *Andrographis paniculata* against carbon tetrachloride-induced liver damage. Arch Pharm Res 1991;14(1):93–95

Sharma M, Sharma R. Identification, purification and quantification of andrographolide from *Andrographis paniculata* (burm. F.) Nees by HPTLC at different stages of life cycle of crop. J Curr Chem Pharm Sci 2013;3(1):23–32

Sharma PC, Yelne MB, Dennis TJ. Database on Medicinal Plants used in Ayurveda, Vol. 4. New Delhi: C.C.R.A.S, Department of I.S.M. & H., Ministry of Health and Family Welfare, Government of India; 2001:34–60

Sher H, Elyemeni M, Hussain K and Sher H. Ethnobotanical and economic observations of some plant resources from the northern parts of Pakistan. Ethnobot Res App 2011;9:27–41

Standard of ASEAN Herbal Medicine. Vol. 1. Jakarta: ASEAN Countries. 1993

Thai Herbal Pharmacopoeia. Vol. 1. Bangkok: Prachachon Co.; 1995

Valdiani A, Kadir MA, Tan SG, Talei D, Abdullah MP, Nikzad S. Nain-e Havandi *Andrographis paniculata* present yesterday, absent today: a plenary review on underutilized herb of Iran's pharmaceutical plants. Mol Biol Rep 2012;39(5):5409–5424

Wu Z, Raven PH, Hong DY, Garden MB. Flora of China: Cucurbitaceae through Valerianaceae with Annonaceae and Berberidaceae. Beijing, China: Science Press; 1996

Zhang X. World Health Organization. WHO Monographs on Selected Medicinal Plants. Vol. 2. Geneva: AITPBS Publications and Distributors; 2004:12–34

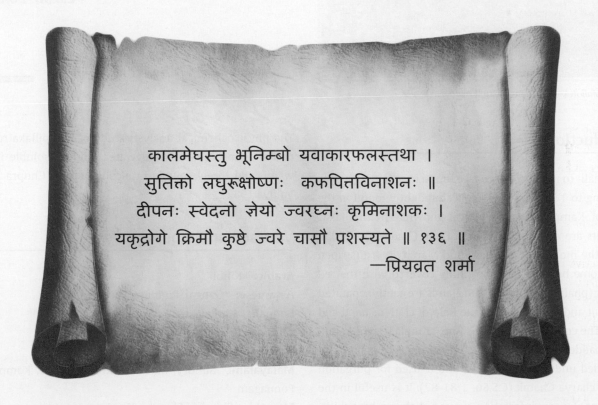

कालमेघस्तु भूनिम्बो यवाकारफलस्तथा ।
सुतिक्तो लघुरूक्षोष्णः कफपित्तविनाशनः ॥
दीपनः स्वेदनो ज्ञेयो ज्वरघ्नः कृमिनाशकः ।
यकृद्रोगे क्रिमौ कुष्ठे ज्वरे चासौ प्रशस्यते ॥ १३६ ॥
—प्रियव्रत शर्मा

47. Kampillaka [*Mallotus philipinensis* Muell Arg.]

Family: *Euphorbiaceae*

Hindi name: *Kabila, Sindur, Rohini, Kambhal*

English name: *Kamala Tree, Monkey-face Tree*

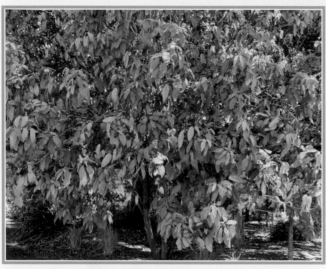

Plant of *Mallotus philipinensis* Muell Arg.

Kampillak processed with buttermilk (Takrasidhha kampillaka) is virudhhakarak (incompatible)

—C.S.Su. 26/84

Introduction

It is a small- to medium-sized tree found in outer Himalayas ascending to 1,500 m. The tree is abundantly found in the region of Kampilla, that's why it is known as Kampillaka.. The fruits are collected in Vasanta ritu (Nadakarni 2005). During the months of February and March, its fruits ripen and become brick-red in color, fully covered with the red covering (phalaraja); the hair and glands are gently separated from fruit and collected with the help of cloth or hand and stored. The collected material is fine, granular powder, dull red or madder red in color, which floats on water. This plant is included under phalinidravya and is used for purgation as per Acharya Charak (C.S.Su. 1/81-87). It is useful in the treatment of worm infestation, wound, diabetes, bronchitis, abdominal diseases, and spleen enlargement.

Even though it is a herbal drug, because of its usefulness in mercurial preparations, it has been included under sadhranarasas in Rasashastra (Vaghabhattacharya 2003).

The physicochemical analysis study of Kampillaka reveals that it is insoluble in cold water, slightly soluble in hot water, and freely soluble in alcohol, ether (Chopra 1994; Vaidya 1982).

Vernacular Names

Arabic: Kinbil

Assamese: Gangai, Puddum, Lochan

Bengali: Kamala, Kamalagundi

Gujarati: Kapilo

Kannada: Kampillaka, Kunkumadamara

Malayalam: Sundry, Manawa, Kuramatakku, Kampipala, Ponnagam

Marathi: Shindur, Shendri, Kapila

Oriya: Bosonto-gundi, Kumala, Sundragundi, Kamalagundi

Persian: Kanbela

Punjabi: Kumila, Kamal, Kambal, Kamela

Santhal: Rora

Tamil: Kapli, Kungumam, Kurangumanjanatti, Kamala, Manjanai, Kunkumam, Kamala

Telugu: Kunkuma, Chendra-sinduri, Kapila, Vassuntagunda, Sundari, Vasanta, Kumkumamu

Urdu: Kamila

Synonyms

Kampillak: It is a tree mostly found in the region of Kampilla.

Karkasha: Fruits of this plant are rough to touch due to hairs.

Raktanga: Fruits are covered with red powder.

Raktachurnaka: Fruits are covered with red powder.

Patodaka: It is useful for dyeing of cloth.

Ranjanaka: Powder of fruit is commonly used for dyeing of cloth.

Raktashamana: It pacifies rakta vikar and is used as blood purifier.

Vranashodhana: It is useful in wound cleansing.

Rechana: It has purgative action with removal of krimi.

Rochanaka: It has appetizer properties.

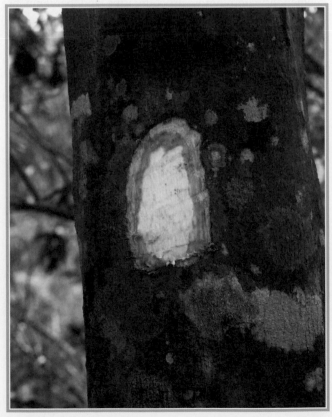

Fig. 47.1 Bark.

Classification

Charak Samhita: Phalini dravya

Sushrut Samhita: Shyamadi gana

Dhanwantari Nighantu: Chandanadi varga

Madanpal Nighantu: Abhayadi

Kaiyadev Nighantu: Aushadhi varga

Raj Nighantu: Suvarnadi varga

Bhavaparakash: Haritakyadi varga

Distribution

It is widely distributed in tropical and subtropical regions of outer Himalayas up to 1,500 m in India. It is also found in China, Myanmar, Sri Lanka, Thailand, and throughout Malaysia to Australia (Warier 1995; Hooker 1890).

Morphology

It is a small- to medium-sized tree, up to 25 m tall and a trunk diameter of 40 cm with many branches.

- **Bark:** The gray bark is smooth, or with occasional wrinkles or corky bumps. Small branches are grayish-brown in color, with rusty covered small hairs toward the end. Leaf scars are evident (**Fig. 47.1**).
- **Leaves:** Simple, alternate, more or less leathery, ovate-lanceolate, 8–20 × 3–9 cm, cuneate to round with two glands at base. Leaves are mostly acute or acuminate at apex, three-nerved at base, glabrous above, pubescent and with many red glands beneath, veins raised and evident under the leaf. Petiole size is 1 to 4 cm long, and is puberulous and reddish-brown in color (**Fig. 47.2**).

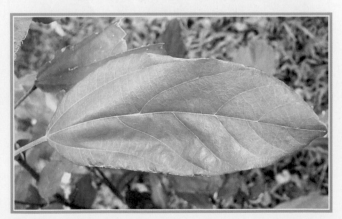

Fig. 47.2 Leaf.

- **Flowers:** Small, dioecious, male flowers in terminal and axillary position, 2 to 10 cm long, solitary or fascicled paniculate spikes; each flower is with numerous stamens, small; female flowers have spikes or slender racemes; each flower with a stellate hairy, three-celled ovary with three papillose stigmas. Ovary is covered with red glands (**Fig. 47.3**).
- **Fruits:** Globose, three-lobed capsule, 8 to 12 mm in diameter, covered with bright red powder and minute hairs which can be easily removed. There is one small black globular seed in each of the three parts of the capsule (**Fig. 47.4**).
- **Seeds:** Subglobose, black, 3 to 4 mm across (**Fig. 47.5**). Fresh seed is advised for germination (Orwa et al 2009; Zafar 1994).

Phenology

Flowering time: March to April
Fruiting time: July to August

Key Characters for Identification

➤ Its powder is soft and crimson colored.
➤ The pure Kampillaka floats on the water and impurities like sand, mud, brick powder, etc., settles down at the bottom.
➤ It may produce yellow line on white paper when rubbed with wet fingertip.
➤ It produces sparking when put on fire (Sharma 2001).

Chemical Constituents

Rottlerin and isorottlerin are obtained from capsule hairs and glands. Red compound and yellow compound are also obtained from kamala.

Seeds contain cardenolides-corotoxigenin L-rhamnoside and coroglaucigenin, L-rhamnoside. Fatty oil is obtained from seeds.

Phenolic compounds: Isocoumarins and bergenin are isolated from the heart wood, the bark, and the leaves of *M. philippinensis*.

Chalcone derivatives: Mallotophilippens C, D, and E are found from the fruit.

The stem bark contains kamaladiol-3-acetate and friedelin. Nitrogen and ash found in leaves.

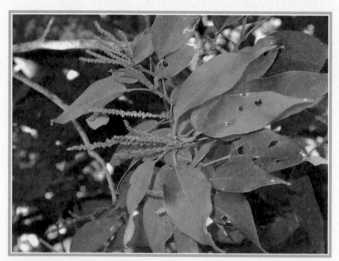

Fig. 47.3 Flower.

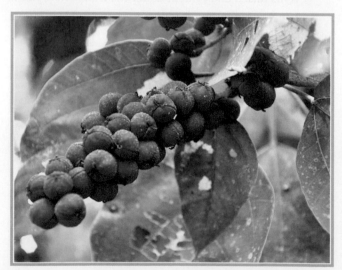

Fig. 47.4 Fruits.

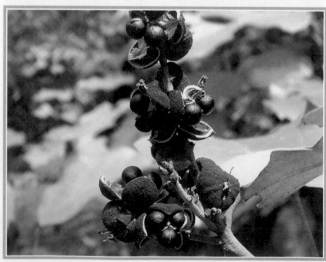

Fig. 47.5 Black seeds.

Identity, Purity, and Strength

- Foreign matter: Not more than 2%
- Total ash: Not more than 6%
- Acid-insoluble ash: Not more than 4%
- Alcohol-soluble extractive: Not less than 50%
- Water-soluble extractive: Not less than 1.0%

(Source: The Ayurvedic Pharmacopeia of India 2003)

Rasapanchaka

Guna	Laghu, Ruksha, Tikshna
Rasa	Katu
Vipak	Katu
Virya	Ushna

Karma (Actions)

Rechana (purgative), krimighna (anthelmintic), deepan (increases appetite), garbha nirodhaka (contraceptive), kustaghna (antidermatosis), raktashodaka (blood purifier), vrana ropana (wound healing).

Leaves are bitter, cooling, and appetizer. All parts of plant like glands and hairs from the capsules or fruits are used as heating, purgative, anthelmintic, vulnerary, detergent, maturant, carminative, and alexiteric agent.

- Doshakarma: Kapha pittahara
- Dhatukarma: Raktashodaka
- Malakarma: Rechana

Pharmacological Actions

The plant has antibacterial, antifungal, antifertility, anti-filarial, anti-inflammatory, immunoregulatory, anti-oxidant, antiradical, protein inhibition implicated in cancer processes, hepatoprotective in vitro cytotoxicity against human cancer cell, anticestodal, veterinary applications, purgative, anthelmintic, antituberculosis, antiallergic, anti-leukemic, antiproliferative, anti-HIV activity, antitumor, wound healing, mesenchymal stem cell (MSC) proliferation, coloring agent–dye, hypoglycemic, and hemostatic actions.

Indications

It is mainly used in krimi (worms), gulma (abdominal lumps), udararoga (abdominal diseases), vrana (wound), prameha (diabetes), anaha (tympanitis), ashmari (urinary calculus), visha (poison), raktapitta (bleeding disorders).

It is useful in the treatment of bronchitis, abdominal diseases, and spleen enlargement, if taken with milk or curd (yoghurt). It can be quite useful for expelling tape-worms (Usmanghani et al 1997). It is also used as an oral contraceptive. The powder and other parts of this plant are used externally for healing of ulcers and wound. It is used to treat parasitic infections of the skin like scabies, ringworm, and herpes.

Therapeutic Uses

External Use

Vrana (wound): The oil prepared from Kampillaka or cooked with Durva juice is used externally for wound healing (C.S.Ci. 25/93).

Internal Use

1. **Gulma** (abdominal lumps): (a) Kampillaka mixed with honey is taken orally to induce purgation and cures Pittaja Gulma (V.M. 30/14). (b) The powder of kampillaka is given with sugar and honey to facilitate bowel and cures Raktaja Gulma (BP.Ci. 32:49).
2. **Krimi** (worms): Half tola of Kampillaka powder is given with jaggery which expels all types of worms from the bowel without any doubt (B.P.Ci 7/22).
3. **Prameha** (diabetes): To treat the kapha-pittaja Prameha, powder of Kampillaka Saptaparna, Shala, Bibhitaka, Rohitaka, Kutaja, and flower of Kapittha is given with honey or paste in the dose of 1 tola with the juice of Amalaki (C.S.Ci. 6/35-36).

Officinal Part Used

Phala raja (dry powder of glands and hairs of fruits)

Dose

Powder: 500 mg to 1 g (The Ayurvedic Pharmacopeia of India 2003)

Formulations

Krimighatini Gutika, Kampillaka churna, Kampillkadi churna, Patoladhi churna, Shaladi yoga, Kampillakadi gutika, Krumignadivarti, Triphaladyaghrita, Dhanvantaraghrita, Kampillakadighrita, Kampillaka taila, Mahavajraka taila.

Substitution and adulteration

It is commonly adulterated with the dye of *Bixa orellana* Linn., ferric oxide, brick powder, fruit powder of *Ficus benghalensis*, flower powder of *Carthamus tinctorius*, ferruginous sand, hairs of fruits of *Flemingia macrophylla*, etc. (Zafar and Yadav 1993; Ahmad and Hashmi 1995; Sharma et al 2002).

Toxicity/Adverse Effects

Hazards and/or side effects are not known for proper therapeutic dosages. Large doses may cause colic, cramping, diarrhea, GI distress, and nausea. It may cause mild nausea, occasional vomiting, and loose motion.

Seeds of *Mallotus philippinensis* ethereal extract have adverse effects on various parameters of female rats. Even the extract reduces serum levels of gonadotropins in treated animals at high dose of 100 mg/kg body weight. Reduced weights of ovary and uterus, follicular development, and increased atretic follicular in the ovary are due to subnormal levels of steroid hormones. Thus, pregnancy is very difficult in female rats treated with kamala seed extract (Thakur et al 2005).

The approximate lethal dose of rottlerin in rat was 750 mg/kg. The plant extract was found lethal to trematodes; alcoholic extract being most effective in vitro and in vivo. Death of worms commenced 60 and 90 min after addition of alcoholic extract (1:100 concentration) and aqueous extract (1:25 concentration), respectively. This herb may cause nausea or gripping before purging. No other information about the safety of this herb is available (Zafar et al 1993).

Purification of Kampillaka

Kampillaka is subjected thrice to bhavana with juices of matulunga (*Citrus medica* Linn.) and adraka (ginger) (Mookerjee 2004). Kampillaka is also purified by swedan (boiling) with haritakikashaya (decoction of *Terminalia chebula*) or kanji (gruel) by means of dolayantra (Neelakanta 2007).

> **Points to Ponder**
>
> - *Phalaraja: Brick red powder collected from mature fruit of M. philippinensis is used for medicinal purpose.*
> - *Kampillak comes under sadharana rasa in Rasashastra.*
> - *It is mainly indicated in krimi, guma, vrana, and prameha.*

Suggested Readings

Ahmad F, Hashmi S. Adulteration in commercial Kamila (*Mallotus philippinensis* Muell.): an anthelmintic drug of repute. Hamdard Med 1995;38:62–67

Chopra RN. Indigenous Drugs of India. Calcutta: Academic Publishers; 1994:359

Hooker JD. *Mallotus philippinensis* muell. in the flora of British India, Vol. V. Authority of the Secretary of State for India in Council; 1890:443

Mookerjee B. Rasajalanidhi. Ch. 3. Varanasi: Chaukhamba Orientalia; 2004:212

Nadakarni KM. Indian Materia Medica. Mumbai: Popular Prakashana Pvt. Ltd; 2005:762

Neelakanta KB. Basavarajeeyam. Hindi translation by V. Rangacharya, 25th chapter/181. Hyderabad: Bharateeya Ayurvijnana Itihas Sansthan; 2007:886

Orwa C, Mutua A, Kindt R. Agroforestree Database: A Tree Reference and Selection guide. Version4.0; 2009

Sharma PC, Yelne MB, Denris TJ. Kampillaka: *Mallotus philippinensis.* In: Database of Medicinal Plants Used in Ayurveda. New Delhi: CCRAS; 2002:104

Thakur SC, Thakur SS, Chaube SK, Singh SP. An etheral extract of Kamala (*Mallotus philippinensis* (Moll.Arg) Lam.) seed induce adverse effects on reproductive parameters of female rats. Reprod Toxicol 2005;20(1):149–156

The Ayurvedic Pharmacopoea of India, Part 1, Vol. 1. New Delhi: Department of AYUSH, Ministry of Health and Family Welfare, Government of India; 2003:55

Tryambaknath S. Rasamitra (Practical Rasashastra). Varanasi: Chaukhamba Sanskrit Series; 2001:96

Usmanghani K, Saeed A, Alam MT. Indusynic Medicine. Karachi. Research Institute of Indusyunic Medicine; 1997:285–287

Vaghabhattacharya. Rasaratna Samuchchaya. Ch. 3/126-127. Varanasi: Chaukhamba Orientalia; 2003:37

Vaidya B. Some Controversial Drugs in Indian Medicine. Ch. 6. Varanasi: Chowkambha Orientalia; 1982:185

Warier PK. *Mallotus philippinensis* muell. Arg, in Indian Medicinal Plants, Vol. III. Madras, India: Orient Longman Ltd; 1995:375.

Zafar R, Yadav K. Pharmacognostical and phytochemical investigations on the leaves of *Mallotus philippinensis* Muell. Arg. Hamdard Med 1993;36(3):41–45

Zafar R. Medicinal Plants of India. 1st ed. 1994 (P.NO.89-104)

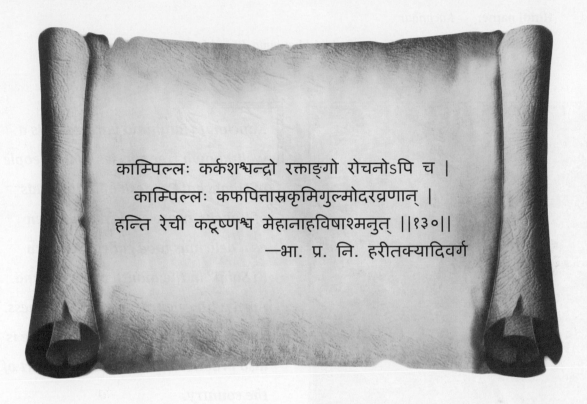

कार्म्पिल्लः कर्कशश्चन्द्रो रक्ताङ्गो रोचनोऽपि च |
कार्म्पिल्लः कफपित्तास्रकृमिगुल्मोदरव्रणान् |
हन्ति रेची कटूष्णश्च मेहानाहविषाश्मनुत् ||१३०||
—भा. प्र. नि. हरीतक्यादिवर्ग

48. Kanchanara [*Bauhinia variegata* Linn.]

Family:	*Fabaceae*
Hindi name:	*Kachnaar*
English name:	*Mountain Ebony, Buddhist bauhinia, Camel foot tree, Poor man's orchid*

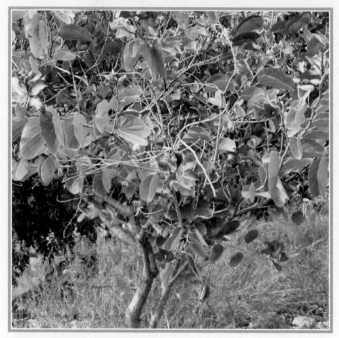

Plant of *Bauhinia variegata* Linn.

> *Kanchnar (Bauhinia variegata) is a well-known tree species to the people of Himachal Pradesh of India. Buds of Kanchnar are cooked and eaten as a delicious food called "Karalen Ki Sabji" in the month of March and April with celebration and happiness. Eating Kanchnar buds as vegetable is also practiced in Northeastern part of the country.*
>
> *—Nariyal and Sharma (2017)*

Introduction

Different species of Bauhinia are known and used as Kanchnar in Indian system of medicine. Kanchnar is not described in Brihattrayi. Kovidara and Karbudara are mentioned in Samhitas which are now known as Kanchnar. Both these plants (Kovidar and Karbudar) are mentioned in vamanopaga mahakasaya of Charak Samhita (C.S.Su. 4/13) and Urdhwabhagahar gana of Sushrut Samhita (S.S.Su. 39/3). Acharya Chakrapani interpreted Karbudar as Sweta kanchan at above context of Charak Samhita and as Kanchnar in the context of enema recipes for parikarta (sawing pain; C.S.Si. 10/34-35). Acharya Dalhan clarified that Kovidar is one variety of Kanchnar (S.S.Su. 46/181). From these references it becomes clear that Kovidar and

Karbudar are two different varieties of Kanchnar. But it becomes confusing or controversial when Dhanwantari Nighantu and Raj Nighantu mentioned that Kanchnar and Kovidar are synonymous to each other. Bhavaprakash Nighantu has mentioned two types of Kanchnar (i.e., Kanchnar and Kovidar) and different Sanskrit names have been given to them. Kanchnar bears red-colored flowers.

Watt (1972) has described *Bauhinia variegata* Linn. as Rakta Kanchnar and *B. racemosa* Linn. as Shveta Kanchnar. Besides *B. variegata* Linn., *B. purpurea* Linn., *B. tomentosa* are also mentioned under Peeta Kanchnar in the Hindi commentary of Bhavaprakash Nighantu (Chunekar and Pandey 1982). Professor Priyavrat Sharma (1978) has described *B. variegata* Linn. as Kanchnar in his book Dravyaguna Vijnanam. *B. variegata* Linn. has been considered as Kanchnar by many modern scientists and *B. purpurea* Linn. has been regarded as Kovidara (Raghunathan and Mitra 1999).

Charak has mentioned that both Kovidara and Karbudara flowers are Grahi and Raktapitta shamaka (C.S.Su. 27/104). Sushruta has mentioned that Kovidara flower is sweet (madhura rasa) in taste and can improve metabolism (vipaka) and can cure bleeding disorders (Raktapitta shamaka) (S.S.Su. 46/ 281) while Karbudara is sweet (madhura rasa) in taste and can improve metabolism (vipaka) and cure vatapittashamaka (S.S.Su. 45/120).

Bauhinia is a large genus under which about 250 species are present. *B. variegata* is also known as Butterfly tree as its leaves are in the shape of "butterfly," which is common to many Bauhinia species. The genus was named after Bauhin brothers, Swiss-French botanists. The leaves share the double-leaf configuration of a heart, or more popularly, that of a butterfly.

Vernacular Names

Assamese: Kancan, Kanchan

Bengali: Kanchana, Rakta Kanchana

Burmese: Bwaycheng, Bwechin

Canarese: Arisinantige, Ayata, Bilikanjivala, Irkubalitu, Kanjivala, Karalabhogi, Kempukanjivala, Kempumandara, Mandara, Ulipe

French: Arbe de saint Thomas, Bauhinie panachee

Gujarati: Champakati, Kanchnar, Kachnar

Kannada: Keyumandar, Kanchavala

Kashmiri: Kalad

Malayalam: Chuvanna Mandharam

Marathi: Kanchana, Raktakancana

Oriya: Kachana, Kaniara

Punjabi: Kanchnar

Tamil: Sigappu mandarai, Sihappu mantarai

Telugu: Deva Kanchanam, Kanjanamu, Mandara, Mandari

Urdu: Kachnal

Synonyms

Kanchanar: This plant bears golden yellow-colored flowers.

Kovidar: It germinates by forcefully piercing through the soil.

Kuddala: It germinates by forcefully piercing through the soil.

Kundali: Its flower resembles the shape of kundali and protects from diseases.

Charmarika: It has smooth and beautiful bark.

Gandaari: Kanchnara is an effective drug for Gandamala.

Shonpushpak: It has copper- or red-colored flower.

Tamrapuspa: It has copper- or red-colored flower.

Ashfotaka: It bears dehiscent fruits or pods.

Swalpkeshari: The stamens of this plant are very few.

Yugapatraka: The leaves of Kanchnara are bifid or cleft in nature.

Yugmapatrak: The leaves of Kanchnara are bifid or cleft in nature.

Classical Categorization

Charak Samhita: Vamanopaga

Sushruta Samhita: Urdhva bhaagahara

Dhanwantari Nighantu: Guduchyadi varga

Madanpal Nighantu: Abhayadi varga

Kaiyadev Nighantu: Aushadhi varga

Raj Nighantu: Karviradi varga

Bhavaprakash Nighantu: Guduchyadi varga

Distribution

B. variegata was planted in garden, park, and roadsides as ornamental plant in many warm temperate and subtropical regions. It was native to Southeast Asia and grows in tropical and subtropical climate (Hocking 1993; Sinha and Verma 2012).

In India, it is distributed in sub-Himalaya and outer Himalaya of the Punjab and Sikkim states. It is also found in Burma and China and tropical countries, including Africa and South America (Anonymous 1995; Filho 2009).

Morphology

It is a medium-sized deciduous tree reaching up to 15 m in height.

- **Bark:** Grayish-brown with several vertical cracks. Sometimes with silvery patches, rough, compact, exfoliating in woody strips and scales (**Fig. 48.1**).

- **Leaves:** Simple, alternate, 6 to 15 cm across, bifid, cleft one-fourth to one-third way down, broadly ovate, cordate at the base, entire margin, apex obtuse, pubescent beneath when young, subcoriaceous, 10 to 12 nerved, petiole 2 to 4 cm long (**Fig. 48.2**).
- **Flowers:** Bisexual, large, fragrant, white or pink, uppermost petal darker and variegated, usually appears before the leaves or appear on leafless branches in short axillary or terminal racemes. Calyx 2 to 2.7 cm long, pubescent, and toothed at apex while petals are 4 to 5 cm long, ovate-obovate, the uppermost darker with purple veins. The light green, fairly hairy calyx forms a pointed five-angled bud and splits open on one side, remaining attached; petals five, slightly unequal, wavy margined, and narrowed to the base; five curved stamens; very slender, stalked, curved pistil, with narrow, green, one-celled ovary, style and dot-like stigma (**Fig. 48.3**).
- **Fruits:** Flat, hard, glabrous, self-dehiscent pods of 15 to 30 cm long and 2 to 4 cm width, unripe fruit is green in color and it becomes reddish-brown after ripening (**Fig. 48.4a, b**).
- **Seeds:** Each pod contains 10 to 15 seeds. Seeds are flat, round, and brown in color (**Fig. 48.5**).

It is propagated through seeds, stump planting, and stem cutting (Rawat and Bhatt 2002).

Phenology

Flowering time: February to April

Fruiting time: May to June

Key Characters for Identification

➤ *A medium-sized deciduous tree 15 m tall with gray brown bark.*

➤ *Leaves: Simple, alternate, bifid, broadly ovate, cordate at the base, entire margin, obtuse apex.*

➤ *Flower: Bisexual, white or pink, uppermost petal darker and variegated appears in leafless branches in short axillary or terminal racemes.*

➤ *Fruit: Flat, hard, glabrous, self-dehiscent brown pods of 15 to 30 cm long and 2 to 4 cm width.*

➤ *Seeds: Flat, round, and brown.*

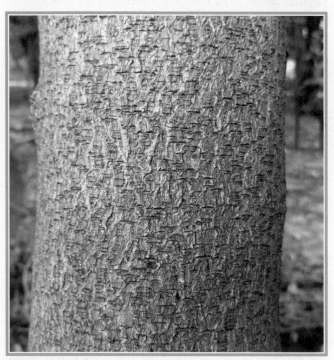

Fig. 48.1 Bark.

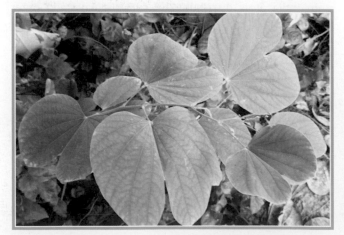

Fig. 48.2 Leaves.

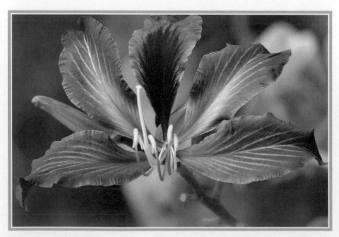

Fig. 48.3 Flower.

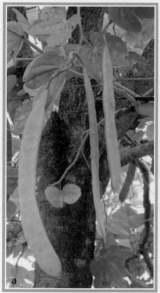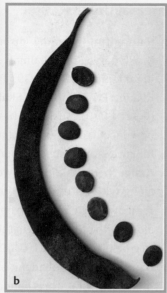

Fig. 48.4 **(a)** Young fruit. **(b)** Mature fruit with seeds.

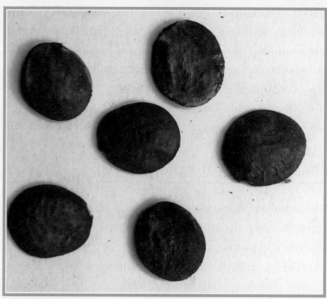

Fig. 48.5 Seeds.

Types

Two types of Kanchnar have been described in Bhavaprakash Nighantu: Kanchnar and Kovidar. In Nighantu Ratnakar, three types of Kanchnar have been described according to the color of the flower, viz. yellow, red, and white varieties of Kanchnar. All varieties have similar properties.

Rasapanchaka

Rasa	Kasaya
Guna	Laghu, Ruksha
Virya	Sheeta
Vipaka	Katu
Prabhava	Gandamalanashana

Chemical Constituents

The main constituents of *B. variegata* are as follows:

- Root: Flavonol glycosides 5,7,3',4 tetrahydroxy-3-methoxy-7-o-α-L-rhamnopyranosyl (1→3)–o-β-d-galactopyranoside, new flavonone (2S)-5, 7-dimethoxy-3,4 methylenedioxy flavonone and new dihydrodibenzoxepin, 5,6b dihydro-1,7-dihydro-1,7-dihydroxy-3,4-dimethoxy-2methyldibenz (b,f) oxepin

- Stem bark: Quercitroside, Kaempferol-3-glucoside, lupeol and beta-sitosterol isoquercitroside, rutoside, myricetol glycoside, and kaempferol glycosides
- Flowers: Quercitroside, isoquercitroside rutoside, taxifoline rhamnoside, kaempferol-3-glucoside, myricetol glycoside
- Leaves: Lupeol, alkaloids, fat, glycoside, phenolics, lignin, saponins, terpenoids, β-sitosterol, tannins, kaempferol-3-glucoside, rutin, quercetin, apigenin, apigenin-7o-glucoside amides, carbohydrates, protein, vitamin C, calcium, and phosphorus
- Seeds: Protein, fatty oil containing oleic acid, linoleic acid, palmitic acid, and stearic acid (Singh et al 2016).

Identity, Purity, and Safety

- Foreign matter: Not more than 2%
- Total ash: Not more than 11%
- Acid-insoluble ash: Not more than 0.2%
- Alcohol-soluble extractive: Not less than 2%
- Water-soluble extractive: Not less than 6%

(Source: The Ayurvedic Pharmacopeia of India 1989)

Karma (Actions)

This plant possesses properties such as sangrahi (astringent), vranaropana (wound healing), kusthaghna (antileprotic), krimighna (anthelmintic), deepan (appetizer), mutrasangrahaniya (urinary astringent), shothahara (swelling reducing), vamanakarak (causes vomiting), raktastambhak (hemostatic), kasahara (antitussive) as per various classical texts and Nighantus of Ayurveda.

- Doshakarma: Kapha pittashamaka
- Dhatukarma: Raktastambhak
- Malakarma: Sangrahi, mutrasangrahaniya

Pharmacological Actions

The reported pharmacological actions of *B. variegata* are anti-inflammatory, antioxidant, antidiabetic, antimicrobial, antitumor/cytotoxic, antiarthritic, antiobesity, anthelmintic, insecticidal, antihyperlipidemic, immunomodulatory, proteinase inhibitor, hepatoprotective, and antiasthmatic, nephroprotective, antiulcer, antigoitrogenic, wound healing (Singh et al 2016), hemagglutinating (Wassel et al 1989), hematinic (Dhonde et al 2007), and anticarcinogenic (Pandey and Agrawal 2009).

Indications

As per Ayurveda, it is used in krimi (worm infestation), kushta (leprosy), charmaroga (skin diseases), gudabhramsha (prolapse rectum), gandamala (scrofula), apaci (cervical lymphadenitis), galaganda (goiter), vrana (wound), raktapitta (bleeding disorders), raktapradara (dysfunctional uterine bleeding), kshaya (consumption), kasa (cough), mutrakuchhra (dysuria), atisara (diarrhea), pravahika (dysentery), lasikagranthi vridhi (lymphadenitis), prameha (diabetes), and medoroga (obesity).

Plant is also useful in the treatment of edema, ulcers, eye diseases, piles, hemorrhoids, and it is an antidote to snake bite (Asima and Satyesh 1992; Khare 2007). Flowers of Kanchnar are used in raktapitta and arsha.

Therapeutic Uses

External Use

Mukha vrana (mouth ulcer): Use Kanchnar bark decoction as a mouthwash as well as gargle with it frequently in mouth ulcers, pyorrhea, and bad breath.

Internal Use

1. **Raktapitta** (bleeding disorders): Flowers of Kovidar, Kaashmarya, and Shalmali should be used as vegetable in raktapitta (C.S.Ci. 4/39). Powder of flowers of Kovidar, Khadir, Priyangu, and Shalmali is given in raktapitta (C.S.Ci. 4/70). Sushruta has also suggested the use of powder of Madhuka, Shobhanjan, Kovidara, and Priyangu for curing bleeding disorders (raktapitta; Su.S.U. 45/19).

2. **Arsha** (hemorrhoids): Powder of root bark of Kovidara along with butter milk with suitable diet is also a good remedy to cure hemorrhoids (A.H.Ci. 8/31). Kovidara along with other drugs in the form of Khad yusha is given to cure bleeding piles (C.S.Ci. 14/202).

3. **Gandamala** (lymphadenitis): The fresh bark of Kanchnar mixed with Shunthi is pounded with sour gruel and given in Gandmala (V.M. 41/19). According to Sharangdhar, one should regularly take bark of Kanchnar stem and Shunthi to cure Gandamala (lymphadenitis; Sha.S. 2/2/124 & BP.Ci. 44/37).

4. **Parikartika** (sawing pain): Acharya Charak has also mentioned about the use of Karbudara and other drugs like Aadhki, Kadam, and Vidula in the form of Vasti to cure Parikartika (C.S.Si.10/34).

5. **Masurika** (pox): Decoction prepared with bark of *B. variegata* should be given with Swarna makshik bhasma (B.P.Chi. 60/49).

6. **Sarpa visha** (snake bite): Sushrut advised to administer Kovidara along with Shirish, Arka, and Katbhi in case of snake bite (Su.S.Ka. 5/17).

7. **Hyperthyroidism:** Daily intake of 40 mL bark decoction of Kanchnar twice a day helps in reducing the elevated levels of thyroid hormone and regulates its functioning. Kanchnar guggulu two tablets twice a day can also be used.

Officinal Parts Used

Stem bark, root, flower, flower buds, gum, leaf, and fruits.

Dose

Bark powder: 3 to 6 g
Decoction: 40 to 80 mL

Flower juice: 10 to 20 mL (Chunekar and Pandey 1982; Sharma 1978).

Formulations

Kanchnar Guggulu, Kanchan gutika, Gandamala kundan rasa, Gulkand Kanchnar and Kanchanaradi Kwatha. Ushirasava, Chandanasava, Vidangarishta, Kanchnar drava, Kanchnar Varuna Kwatha (Anonymous 1978, 2000; Singh 2002).

Toxicity/Adverse Effects

Aqueous and ethanolic extracts of stem and root of *B. variegata* Linn. given to rats did not show any mortality or noticeable behavioral changes in the trial subjects. These extracts were found to be safe up to 2,000 mg/kg body weight (Rajani and Ashok 2009).

Substitution and Adulteration

Different species of *Bauhinia* viz. *B. purpura* Linn., *B. malabarica* Linn., *B. racemose* Linn., *B. tomentosa* Linn. resemble morphologically as well as medicinally with *B. variegate* Linn. Bark of these plants is sold in the market under the name of Kanchnar (Garg 1992; Prasad and Prakash 1972).

Points to Ponder

- *Bauhinia variegata Linn. is considered as Rakta Kanchnar, B. racemosa Linn. as Shveta Kanchnar, and B. purpurea Linn. as Kovidara.*
- *Kovidar and Karbudar terms are used for Kanchnar in Samhita.*
- *Kanchnar is used in raktapitta, arsha, galaganda, gandamala, kushta, krimi, apaci, etc.*

Suggested Readings

Anonymous. The Ayurvedic Formulary of India, Part I. 1st ed. New Delhi: Department of I.S.M. and H., Ministry of Health and Family Welfare, Government of India; 1978.

Anonymous. The Ayurvedic Formulary of India, Part II. 1Ist English ed. New Delhi: Department of I.S.M. and H., Ministry of Health and Family Welfare, Government of India; 2000

Anonymous. The Wealth of India: Raw Materials, Vol. IV. New Delhi: Publication and Information Directorate, CSIR; 1995

Asima C, Satyesh CP. In the Treatise of Indian Medicinal Plants, Vol. 2. New Delhi: Publication and Information Directorate CSIR; 1992: 24-26

Chunekar KC, Pandey GS. Bhavaprakash Nighantu of Bhavamishra. Hindi Translation & Commentary. 6th ed. Varanasi: Chaukhambha Bharati Academy; 1982:337-339

Dhonde SM, Siraskar BD, Kulkarni AV, Kulkarni AS, Bingi SS. Haematinic activity of ethanolic extract of stem bark of *Bauhnia variegata* Linn. Int J Green Pharmacy 2007;1(3-4):28–33

Filho CV. Chemical composition and biological potential of plants from the genus *Bauhinia*. Phytother Res 2009;23(10):1347–1354

Garg S. Substitute and Adulterant Plants. New Delhi: Periodical Experts Book Agency; 1992:29-30

Hocking D. Trees for Dry Lands. New Delhi: Oxford & IBH Publishing Co.; 1993

Khare CP. *Bauhinia variegata* Indian Medicinal Plants: An Illustrated Dictionary. Springer; 2007:86-87

Nariyal V, Sharma P. Kanchnar (*Bauhinia variegata*) as a medicinal herb: a systematic review. Int J Adv Res (Indore) 2017;5(9):587–591

Pandey S, Agrawal RC. Effects of *Bauhinia variegata* bark extract on DMBA induced mouse skin carcinogenesis: a preliminary study. Glob J Pharmacol 2009;3(3):158–162

Prasad S, Prakash A. Pharmacognostical Study of *Bauhinia variegate*. Ind J Pharm 1972;34(6):170

Raghunathan K, Mitra R. Pharmacognosy of Indigenous Drugs, Vol. I. New Delhi: CCRAS; 1999:466

Rajani GP, Ashok P. In vitro antioxidant and antihyperlipidemic activities of *Bauhinia variegata* Linn. Ind J Pharmacol 2009; 41(5):227–232

Sharma PV. Dravyaguna Vijnana, Vol. II. Varanasi: Chaukhambha Sanskrit Bharati Academy; 1978:234-235

Singh KL, Singh DK, Singh VK. Multidimensional uses of medicinal plant Kachnar (*Bauhinia variegata* Linn.). Am J Phytomed Clin Therap 2016;4(02):58-72

Singh RR, Kumar BV. Natures Pharmacopeia: Medicinal Plant Diversity in Doon Valley. Dehradun; 2002

Singh RS. Vanaushadhi Nirdeshika. 3rd ed. Uttar Pradesh Hindi Sansthana; 2002:62

Sinha K, Verma AK. Evaluation of antimicrobial and anticancer activities of methanol extract of in vivo and in vitro grown *Bauhinia variegata* L. Int Res J Biol Sci 2012;1(6):26–30

Suresh TRCC, Sanghamitra D. Gagandeep K, Kumar GR. Kanchnara (*Bauhinia variegata* Linn.): a critical review. Int J Ayurv Pharma Res 2015;3(7):39–46

The Ayurvedic Pharmacopoea of India, Part 1, Vol.1. New Delhi: Department of AYUSH, Ministry of Health and Family Welfare, Government of India; 2003:56-57

Wassel GM, Wahab SMA, Ammar SA. Seed proteins of selected *Bauhinia* species & their haemagglutinating effect. Herba Hungarica 1989;23(12):123–125

Watt G. Dictionary of Economic Products of India, Vol. I. Delhi: Periodical Experts; 1972:425-426

काञ्चनारः काञ्चनको गण्डारिः शोणपुष्पकः |

कोविदारश्चमरिकः कुद्दालो युगपत्रकः |

कुण्डली ताम्रपुष्पश्चाश्मन्तकः स्वल्पकेशरी ||८८||

काञ्चनारो हिमो ग्राही तुवरः श्रेष्मपित्तनुत् |

कृमिकुष्ठगुदभ्रंशगण्डमालाव्रणापहः ||८९||

कोविदारोऽपि तद्वत्स्यात्तयोः पुष्पं लघु स्मृतम् |

रूक्षं संग्राहि पित्तास्रप्रदरक्षयकासनुत् ||९०||

—भा. प्र. नि गुडूच्यादिवर्ग

49. Kantakari [*Solanum xanthocarpum* Schrad & Wendl.*]

Family:	*Solanaceae*
Hindi:	*Bhatkataiya, Chhotikateri Kateli, Bhui Ringani*
English:	*Yellow-berried night-shade, Febrifuge plant*

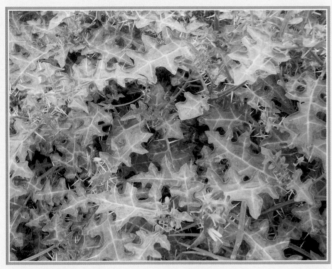

Plant of *Solanum xanthocarpum* Schrad & Wendl.

Brihati, Kantakari, and Agnidamana are collectively known as kantakatraya.

Introduction

Solanum xanthocarpum Schrad & Wendl. (Syn: *Solanum surattense* Burmi) of Solanaceae family is a prickly herb having immense importance in traditional systems of medicine. This plant is covered with plenty of thorns that is why it is called Kantakari. It is one of the key ingredients of famous formulations like dashamoola, laghu panchmool, and panchtikta. Kantakari is a prime drug for kasa (cough) as per Vagabhatta. This plant is mainly known for its shwasahara, kasahara, jwarahara properties in different dosage forms.

Brihati and Kantakari are collectively known as Brihati dwaya. Vaidya Bapalal ji added agnidamana (Vallibrihati: *Solanum trilobatum*) to Brihati dwaya and opinionated Kantakatraya. Bhavaprakash mentioned Kankakari with white flower has garbhakar action. Fruits of both Kantakari dwaya have Shukrarechan properties.

Vernacular Names

Assamese: Katvaedana, Kantakar
Bengali: Kantakari
Gujarati: Bhoringani
Kannada: Nelagulla, Kiragulla
Malayalam: Kantakari Chunda
Marathi: Bhauringani, Kataringani
Orissa: Bhejibaigana, Ankarati, Chakada Bhaji
Punjabi: Kandiari
Tamil: Kandangatri, Kandan Katri, Kandanghathiri
Telugu: Nelamulaka, Pinnamulaka, Mulaka, Chinnamulaka, Vakudu

Synonyms

Kantakari: This herb is covered with lots of thorn.
Kantakarika: It is a thorny plant.

Kantakini: The plant is full of thorns.

Dushsparsha: It is very difficult to touch due to presence of thorns.

Dhavani: It is a straggling herb.

Vyaghri: This plant is useful in the diseases of nose and promotes voice.

Kantalika: It is a very prickly herb.

Kshudra: It is a small herb in comparison to Brihati. It also enhances digestive fire and that is why it is called kshudra.

Kasaghnou: It cures cough.

Nidigdhika: The plant grows very fast and removes mucous coating from the respiratory tract.

Kuli: Fruits are found in cluster.

Kshudraphala: It has small fruits.

Chitraphala: It bears small variegated fruit.

Dravani: It liquefies the shlesma (cough) and acts as expectorant.

Rastrika: It is a common plant available everywhere.

Classification

Charak Samhita: Kasahara, Sothahara, Hikkanigrahana, Kanthya, Angamardaprasamana, Sheetaprasamana

Sushrut Samhita: Brihatyadi, Laghupanchamoola, Varunadi

Ashtanga Sangraha: Vidarigandhadi, Varunadi, Kanthya, Hikkanigrahana, Kasahara, Sheetaprashamana, Angamardaprashamana, Shotahara

Ashtanga Hridaya: Vidarigandhadi Varunadi Laghupanchamoola

Dhanwantari Nighantu: Guduchyadi varga

Madanpal Nighantu: Abhayadi varga

Kaiyadev Nighantu: Aushadhi varga

Raj Nighantu: Shatahwadi varga

Bhavaprakash: Guduchyadi varga

Distribution

It is a distributed in Australia, Ceylon, India, Malaysia, Polynesia, and Southeast Asia (Parmar et al 2010; Parmar et al 2017). It is commonly found throughout India, ascending to 2,200 m on the Himalaya as wild growing plants along the roadsides and dry waste lands (Sharma et al 2001; Anonymous 1998).

Morphology

It is prickly, diffused, bright-green perennial herb, about 1.2 m tall usually with woody base.

- **Stem:** Profusely branched, somewhat zigzag, young stems are clothed with dense satellite and tomentose hairs, spines are compressed, straight, yellow, glabrous, and shining, often exceeding 1.3 cm (**Fig. 49.1**).

- **Leaves:** Ovate-elliptic, sinuate or subpinnatified, usually five to ten in number, 2.5 to 6 cm in length, hairy on both sides, long, sharp, yellow spines on mid ribs and veins, unequal base, petiole 1.3 to 2.5 cm long (**Fig. 49.2**).

- **Flowers:** Bluish-pink in extra-axillary racemes, calyx-persistent, calyx lobes 5, free, obovate, densely hairy, and prickly. Corolla broadly ovate-triangular, lobes 5, acute, tube short, globule lobes are 10 to 12 mm long, linear-lanceolate. Filaments are 2 mm long, glabrous,

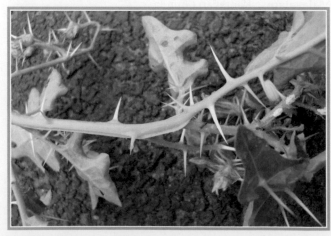

Fig. 49.1 Stem.

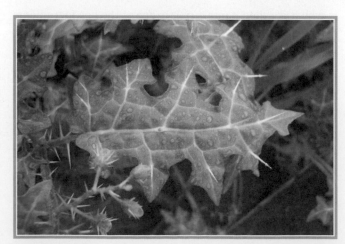

Fig. 49.2 Leaf.

anthers 8 mm long. Ovary is ovoid and glabrous (**Fig. 49.3**).

- **Fruits:** Berries are globose with persistent calyx; young fruits are greenish with white stripes. It turns yellow when mature (**Fig. 49.4a, b**).
- **Seeds:** Numerous, circular, flat, and smooth, 1 to 2 mm in diameter (Singh and Singh 2010; Kirtikar and Basu 2005). It can be propagated by seeds or vegetative method by stem cuttings.

Phenology

Flowering time: January to June
Fruiting time: January to June

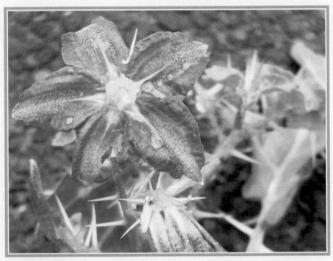

Fig. 49.3   Flower.

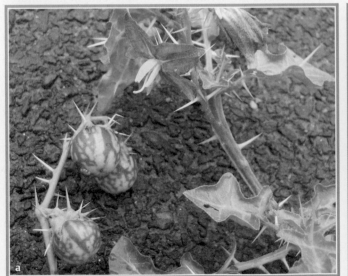

Fig. 49.4   **(a)** Young green fruits. **(b)** Mature fruit.

Key Characters for Identification

➤ *It is prickly, diffused, bright-green, perennial herb, about 1.2 m tall.*
➤ *Stem: Zigzag, clothed with dense satellite and tomentose hairs.*
➤ *Leaves: Ovate-elliptic, sinuate or subpinnatified, hairy on both sides with long, sharp, yellow spines.*
➤ *Fruits: Berries are globose with persistent calyx, greenish with white stripes in young fruit, yellow when mature.*

Chemical Constituents

S. xanthocarpum plant contains alkaloids, sterols, saponins, flavonoids, and their glycosides. In addition to this, carbohydrates, fatty acids, amino acids, etc. are also present.

The chemical constituents reported to be present in Kantakari are carpesterol, gluco alkaloid solanocarpine, solanine-S, solasodine, solasonine, solamargine, cyclo-artanol, stigmasterol, campesterol, cholesterol, sitosteryl-glucoside, stigmasteryl glucoside, solasurine, galactoside of sitosterol, methyl ester of 3,4-dihydroxycinnamic acid and 3,4-dihydroxycinnamic acid (caffeic acid), isochlorogenic, neochlorogenic, chlorogenic acids (fruit); flavonal glycoside, quercetin-3-0-D-glucopyranosyl-0-D-mannopyranoside, apigenin, sitosterol (flower); solanocarpine and amino acids (seeds); coumarins, scopolin, scopoletin, esculin, and esculetin (leaves, roots, and fruits); carpesterol, tomatidenol,

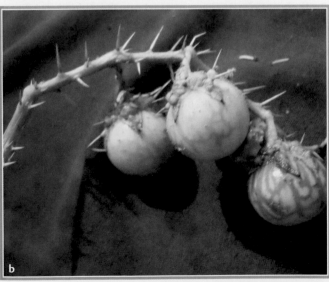

norcarpesterol, and solasonine (plant; Jayakumar and Murugan 2016; Khanam and Sultana 2012; The Ayurvedic Pharmacopeia of India 2001).

Identity, Purity, and Strength

- Foreign matter: Not more than 2%
- Total ash: Not more than 9%
- Acid-insoluble ash: Not more than 3%
- Alcohol-soluble extractive: Not less than 6%
- Water-soluble extractive: Not less than 16%

(Source: The Ayurvedic Pharmacopeia of India 2001)

Rasapanchaka

Guna	Laghu, Ruksha, Ushna
Rasa	Tikta, Katu
Vipaka	Katu
Virya	Ushna

Karma (Actions)

The main actions of Kantakari are deepana (appetizer), pachana (digestive), sothahara (reduce swelling), kasaghna (relieves cough), hikkanigrahana (reduce hic-cough), shwasahara (antiasthmatic), vedanasthapana (pain reliever), swedajanana (increases sweating), jwaraghna (antipyretic), rechana (purgative), bhedana (drastic purgative), krimighna (anthelmintic), amahara, raktashodhaka (blood purifier), mootrala (diuretics), garbhashayasankochaka (uterine contraction), vajikarana (aphrodisiac).

- Doshakarma: Kaphavatashamak
- Dhatukarma: Sukrarechan (BPN)
- Malakarma: Rechana, mootrala

Pharmacological Actions

The recent studies on various medicinal properties of *S. xanthocarpum* is reported as antifertility, hypoglycemic, antifilarial, anticancer, antiasthmatic, anti-inflammatory, hepatoprotective, antitussive, antipyretic, antihistaminic, antihyperlipidemic, apoptosis-inducing activity, mosquito larvicidal, antianaphylactic, and antiandrogenic activities (Reddy and Reddy 2014).

Indications

It is mainly indicated in kasa (cough), shwasa (asthma), jwara (fever), pinasa (rhinitis), parswapeeda (pain in lateral sides), krimi (worm infestation), hridaya roga (heart disease), hikka (hic-cough), vatakaphaja vikara, krimidanta (dental carries), dantashoola (toothache), karnaroga (ear diseases), apatantraka (hysteria), apasmara (epilepsy), angamarda (bodyache), sandhivata (osteoarthritis), agnimandya (loss of appetite), udavarta (flatulence), vibandha (constipation), arsha (piles), raktavikara (diseses related to blood), shotha (swelling), swarabheda (hoarseness of voice), ashmari (urinary calculus), pooyameha (a type of diabetes), mootrakrichchhara (dysuria), rajorodha (amenorrhea), kashtaprasava (dysmenorrhea), klaibya (impotency), charmaroga (skin disease), netrabhishyanda (conjunctivitis).

The whole plant is used traditionally for curing various ailments. Decoction of the plant is used in gonorrhea; paste of leaves is applied to relieve pain; seeds act as expectorant in cough and asthma; roots are expectorant and diuretic, useful in the treatment of catarrhal fever, coughs, asthma, and chest pain. Charaka and Sushruta used the extract of entire plant and fruits in internal prescription for bronchial asthma, tympanitis, misperistalsis, piles, and dysuria, and for rejuvenation. Kantkari Ghrita of Charaka is specific for cough and asthma. Linctuses prepared from the stamens of flowers is prescribed for chronic cough in children (Bangasena).

The plant is useful in fever, cough, asthma, costiveness and pain in chest (Nadkarni 2009). The stem, flowers, and fruits are prescribed for treating burning sensation in the feet accompanied by vesicular eruptions and watery eruption (Pingale 2013). Juices of the berries are useful in sore throat, asthma, chronic bronchitis, and also for cardiac stimulation (Govindan et al 2004).

The hot aqueous extract of dried fruits is used for treating cough, fever, and heart diseases (Joy et al 2001). Juice of fruit of *S. xanthocarpum* is used in sore throats and rheumatism.

It was reported in a clinical trial that oral administration of dry powder of *S. xanthocarpum* at a dose of 300 mg thrice daily for 3 days was found to be very effective in controlling mild-to-moderate bronchial asthma and the bioactivity is equivalent to that of administration of 200 mg of deriphylline (Govindan et al 1999).

Therapeutic Uses

External Use

Yuvanpidika (acne): The fruit paste is applied externally to the affected area for treating pimples and swellings (Gupta and Dutt 1938).

Internal Use

1. **Kasa** (cough): (a) Kantakari is the best medicine for kasa (A.H.U. 40-56). The juice prepared from the whole plant of Kantakari by putapak vidhi is given with Pippali powder to treat kasa, shwasa, and kaphaja vyadhi (Sh.S. 2.1.35). (b) Decoction prepared from Kantakari, Guduchi, and Shunthi is given with Pippali powder to cure kasa, shwasa, and pinasa (Sh.S. 2.2.48). (c) The soup prepared with black gram and Kantakari is taken with Amalaki juice to cure all types of cough (C.S.Ci. 18/184). Kantakari ghrita is given in kasa (C.S.Ci. 18/35,125-128).
2. **Shwasa** (asthma): The mixture of 6 g of Kantakari (Amalaki pramana) and 3 g of Hingu (1/2 of Kantakari) is licked with honey to cure shwasa within 3 days (S.S.U. 51/55).
3. **Apasmara** (epilepsy): The fruit juice of Kantakari is given as nasya to cure the attack of epilepsy and restore the consciousness quickly (S.B. 4/456).
4. **Mutraghata** (retention of urine): Juice of Kantakari is given with honey to get relief from mutraghata (AS.Ci. 13.5, AH.Ci. 11/11, GN. 2.28.29).
5. **Chronic cough in children:** Avaleha (linctus) prepared from flower of Kantakari is given to get relief from chronic cough in children (Bangasen, Balaroga, 59, Bh.P.Ci. 71/161).
6. **Pinasa** (chronic coryza): Vyaghritailam (Sh.S. 2.9.180) is used in pinasa.
7. **Ashmari** (urinary calculus): Roots of Gokshur, Ikshuraka, Eranda, Brihati, and Kantakari are pounded with milk and taken with sweet curd for a week to break the calculus (C.S.Ci. 26/22).

Officinal Parts Used

Root and whole plant

Dose

Decoction: 50 to 100 mL

Formulations

Dashamooladi kwath, Kantakaryadi kwath, Laghupanchamool kwath, Guduchyadi kwath, Sudarsana Choorna, Brahma rasayana, Chyavanprash avaleha, Kantakari avaleha, Vyaghri haritaki, Kantakari ghrita. Panchtikta ghrita, Vyaghri ghrita, Vyaghri taila, Dashmoolarista.

Toxicity

Studies on rats have shown that the hot water extract of the drug could be toxic at 200 mg/kg dose. But no clinical data has reported any toxicity on humans (Anonymous 2002).

> **Points to Ponder**
>
> - *Brihati and Kantakari are known as Brihatidwaya.*
> - *Kantakari is also a member of panchtikta.*
> - *Kantakari is considered as best to cure kasa (A.H.U. 40/56).*
> - *It is mainly indicated in kasa, shwasa, pinasa, parswapida, hikka, etc.*

Suggested Readings

Anonymous. Indian Herbal Pharmacopoeia, Vol. 1. Jammu Tawi: Indian Drug Manufacturers' Association Regional Research Laboratory; 1998:139-146.

Anonymous. Indian Herbal Pharmacopoeia. Revised ed. Mumbai: IDMA; 2002.

Govindan S, Viswanathan S, Vijayasekaran V, Alagappan R. A pilot study on the clinical efficacy of *Solanum xanthocarpum* and *Solanum trilobatum* in bronchial asthma. J Ethnopharmacol 1999;66(2):205–210

Govindan S, Viswanathan S, Vijayasekaran V, Alagappan R. Further studies on the clinical efficacy of *Solanum trilobatum* in bronchial asthma. Phytother Res 2004;18:805–809

Gupta MP, Dutt S. Chemical examination of the seeds of *Solanum xanthocarpum*. II. Constituents. J Indian Chem Soc 1938;15:95–100

Jayakumar K, Murugan K. Solanum alkaloids and their pharmaceutical roles: a review. J Anal Pharm Res 2016;3(6):00075

Joy PP, Thomas J, Mathew S, Skaria BP. Medicinal Plants Tropical Horticulture, Vol. 2, Bose TK, Kabir J, Das P, Joy PP, editors. Calcutta: Naya Prakash; 2001:449-632.

Khanam S, Sultana R. Isolation of β-sitosterol and stigmasterol as active immunomodulatory constituent from the fruits of *Solanum xanthocarpum* (Solanaceae). IJPSR 2012;3(4):1057–1060

Kirtikar KR, Basu BD. Indian Medicinal Plants, Vol. III. International Book Distributors; 2005:1759-1761.

Nadkarni KM. Indian Materia Medica, Vol. I. 3rd ed. Mumbai: Popular Publication; 2009:1156-1158

Parmar KM, Itankar PR, Joshi A, Prasad SK. Anti-psoriatic potential of *Solanum xanthocarpum* stem in Imiquimod-induced psoriatic mice model. J Ethnopharmacol 2017;198:158–166

Parmar S, Gangwal A, Sheth N. *Solanum xanthocarpum* (Yellow Berried Night Shade): a review. Der Pharmacia Lett 2010;2(4):373–383

Pingale SS. Evaluation of acute toxicity for *Solanum xanthocarpum* fruits. BioMedRx 2013;1(3):330–332

Reddy NM, Rajasekhar Reddy N. *Solanum xanthocarpum*: chemical constituents and medicinal properties: a review. Scholars Acad J Pharm 2014;3(2):146–149 (SAJP)

Sharma PC, Yelne MB, Dennis TJ. Database on Medicinal Plants used in Ayurveda, Vol. 4. New Delhi: CCRAS, Department of I.S.M. & H., Ministry of Health and Family Welfare, Government of India; 2001: 269-287.

Singh OM, Singh TP. Phytochemistry of *Solanum xanthocarpum*: an amazing traditional healer. J Sci Ind Res (India) 2010;69:732–740

Tekuri SK, Pasupuleti SK, Konidala KK, Amuru SR, Bassaiahgari P, Pabbaraju N. Phytochemical and pharmacological activities of *Solanum surattense* Burm. f.: a review. J Appl Pharm Sci 2019;9(03): 126–136

The Ayurvedic Pharmacopoeia of India, Part I, Vol. I, 1st ed. New Delhi: Department of I.S.M. & H., Ministry of Health and Family Welfare, Government of India; 2001:59-60

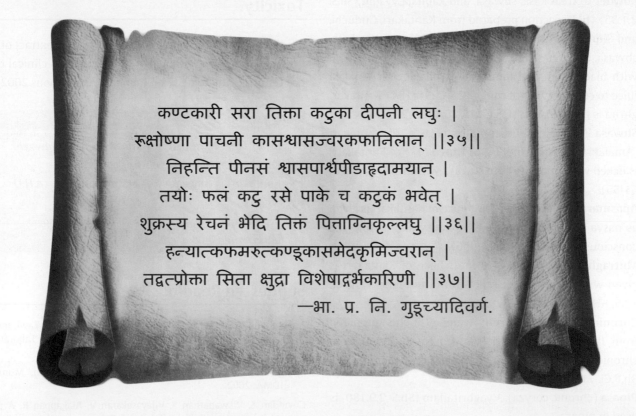

कण्टकारी सरा तिक्ता कटुका दीपनी लघुः |
रूक्षोष्णा पाचनी कासश्वासज्वरकफानिलान् ||३५||
निहन्ति पीनसं श्वासपार्श्वपीडाहृदामयान् |
तयोः फलं कटु रसे पाके च कटुकं भवेत् |
शुक्रस्य रेचनं भेदि तिक्तं पित्ताग्निकृल्लघु ||३६||
हन्यात्कफमरुत्कण्डूकासमेदकृमिज्वरान् |
तद्वत्प्रोक्ता सिता क्षुद्रा विशेषाद्गर्भकारिणी ||३७||
—भा. प्र. नि. गुडूच्यादिवर्ग.

50. Kapikachchhu [*Mucuna prurita* Hook.]

Family: *Fabaceae*

Hindi name: *Kevanch, Kaunch*

English name: *Cowhage, Cowitch*

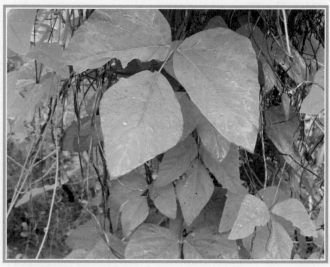

Plant of *Mucuna prurita* Hook.

It significantly increases the sexual desire, penile rigidity, erection, and duration of ejaculation with orgasm.

Introduction

Kapi means monkey and kachhu means itching. It causes severe pruritus or itching to monkey when they sit on this plant. It also causes itching to human when it touches their skin.

Kapikachu (*Mucuna pruriens* Bek. or *M. prurita* of Fabaceae family) is a famous vrishya (aphrodisiac) drug mentioned in Ayurvedic texts right from Charaka and Sushruta Samhita period. It is an established herbal drug used for the management of male infertility, nervous disorders, and also as an aphrodisiac. It has been shown that its seeds have potential of substantial medicinal importance. Traditionally, this plant is used in Parkinson disease. In current research, it is found that *M. pruriens* has been shown to have anti-Parkinson and neuroprotective effects, which may be related to its antioxidant activity.

M. pruriens is a tropical legume and is commonly known as velvet bean or cowitch or cowhage or Alkushi. It is one of the most popular medicinal plants of India and is a constituent of more than 200 indigenous drug formulations. It is widespread and is found in the plains of India (Sastry and Kavathekar 1990). The demand for *Mucuna* in Indian as well as international drug markets has increased many fold only after the discovery of the presence of L-3,4dihydroxy phenyl alanine (L-DOPA), an anti-Parkinson disease drug, in the *Mucuna* seeds (Farooqi et al 1999).

It showed good improvement in seminal parameters like sperm count, volume of semen, pH of semen, and motility of sperms (Jadhao 2013).

Vernacular Names

Assamese: Bandar Kekowa
Bengali: Alkusa, Alkushi
Chinese: Ci mao li dou
French: Pois mascate
Gujarati: Kivanch

Himachal (Kangri): Gajelbeliyan

Jamaica, Barbados: Cowitch

Kannada: Nasugunni

Konkani: Khavalyavali, Majram

Malayalam: Nayikuruma, Shoriyanam

Marathi: Kuhili

Myanmar: Khway Hlay Ya

Nepal: Kauchho/Kauso

Nigeria (Bini language): Iyekpe

Oriya: Baidanka

Punjabi: Kawanchi, Gugli, Kavanch

Sinhala: Wandhuru mae

Tamil: Punaikkali, Poonaikkate

Telugu: Dulagondi, Pilliadagu

Thai: Mah mui

Synonyms

Adhyanda: Seeds of this plant resemble testicles.

Ajada: Seeds are potent aphrodisiac.

Atmagupta: The plant protects itself naturally, as the hair on its fruit causes itching.

Duhsparsha: It is difficult to handle because it causes severe itching.

Kachura: It causes itching.

Kandura: Hair present on its fruit produces intense itching.

Kapikachhu: Hair of the fruit of this plant produces intense itching like monkey.

Kapiromaphala: Legumes are covered with stiff hair like that of monkey.

Languli: Legumes are shaped like a monkey's tail.

Markati: Legumes are covered with stiff hair like that of monkey. It is a potent aphrodisiac drug.

Pravrushayani: The plants grow in rainy season.

Shukashimbi: Legumes are covered with stiff hair.

Vanashukari: It grows wildly.

Vrishya: It has aphrodisiac property.

Vrusabhi: Seeds are potent aphrodisiac.

Vrusyabeeja: Seeds are potent aphrodisiac.

Vyanga: Fruits of the plant are curved.

Classification

Charak Samhita: Balya, Purishvirajaneeya, Vamanopaga

Sushrut Samhita: Vidarigandhadi, Vatasamshamana, Kakolyadi

Ashtanga Sangraha: Vidaryadi, Durvadi gana

Ashtanga Hridaya: Vidaryadi gana

Dhanwantari Nighantu: Guduchyadi varga

Madanpal Nighantu: Abhayadi varga

Kaiyadev Nighantu: Aushadhi varga

Raj Nighantu: Guduchyadi varga

Bhavaprakash: Guduchyadi varga

Sodhala Nighantu: Guduchyadi varga, Lakshmanadi varga

Distribution

It grows naturally right from lower Himalayan range to entire tropical plains of India (Muralia and Pathak 2013). It is cultivated in Uttar Pradesh, Madhya Pradesh, and Andaman and Nicobar Islands of India. It is also found in tropical regions, especially Africa, West Indies, tropical America, the Pacific Islands, and the United States.

Morphology

It is an annual, herbaceous creeper that can reach 15 m in length. Young plants are almost covered with fuzzy hairs while older ones are completely free of hairs (Sahaji 2011).

- **Leaves:** The leaves are trifoliate, alternate or spiraled, gray-silky beneath. Leaflets are membranous, broadly ovate, elliptic or rhomboid ovate, unequal at the base; terminal leaflets are smaller, lateral, very unequal sized; petioles are long and silky, 6.3 to 11.3 cm (**Fig. 50.1**).

- **Flowers:** Flowers are dark purple, white or lavender in color, 6 to 30 in numbers, pealike but larger, with distinctive curved petals, and occur in drooping racemes (**Fig. 50.2**).

- **Fruits:** Longitudinal pods are curved, four to six seeded and about 4 to 13 cm long and 1 to 2 cm wide, sigma shaped, densely clothed with persistent pale brown or gray bristles that cause a severe itch if they come in contact with skin. The husk is very hairy and carries up to seven seeds. The chemical compounds responsible for the itch is a protein, mucunain. Young fruit is green and it turns to brown when it matures (**Fig. 50.3a, b**; Agharkar 1991) and serotonin (Kumar et al 2009).

- **Seeds:** The seeds are flattened, uniform, ellipsoid, shiny black, 1 to 1.9 cm long, 0.8 to 1.3 cm wide,

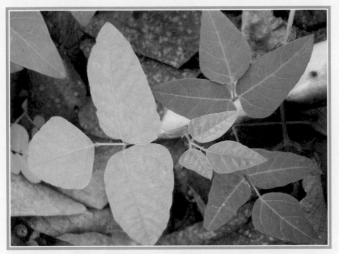

Fig. 50.1 Trifoliate leaf.

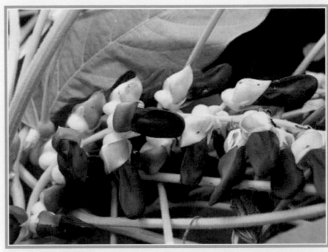

Fig. 50.2 Flower.

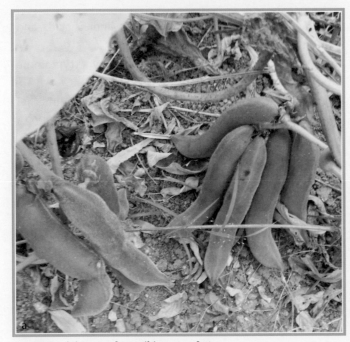

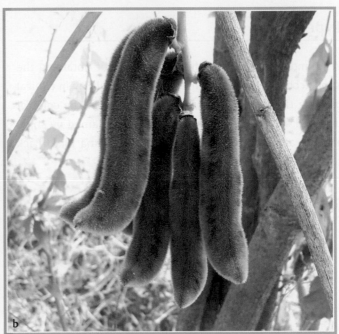

Fig. 50.3 **(a)** Young fruits. **(b)** Mature fruits.

and 4 to 6.5 mm thick. Hilum is prominent white to pale yellow (**Fig. 50.4a, b**).

This plant can be propagated through seeds.

Phenology

Flowering time: August to September

Fruiting time: September to February

Key Characters for Identification

➤ It is an annual, herbaceous creeper.
➤ Leaves: Trifoliate, alternate, gray-silky beneath, broadly ovate or elliptic, terminal leaflets are smaller.
➤ Flowers: Plenty lavender, white- or purple-colored flowers.
➤ Fruits: Sigma shaped 4 to 13 cm long and 1 to 2 cm wide longitudinal pods, covered with pale brown hairs which cause itching.
➤ Seeds: Ellipsoid, shiny black seed.

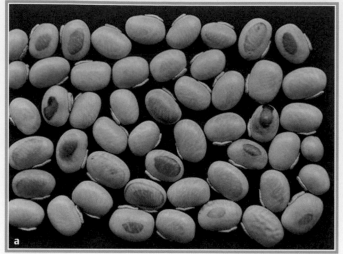
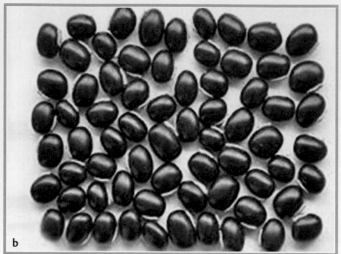

Fig. 50.4   (a) White seeds. **(b)** Black seeds.

Types

Wild and cultivated are the two sources of obtaining the Kapikacchu. The former variety has better utility in clinical practice than cultivated variety. According to the color of the seed, two types of Kapikachhu are explained by some authors as Sveta bija (white seed) and Krisna bija (black seed) (Gupta and Samgraha 2002).

Rasapanchaka

Rasa	Madhura, Tikta
Guna	Guru, Snigdha
Vipak	Madhura
Virya	Ushna

Chemical Constituents

Mucuna is a rich source of protein, carbohydrate, lipid, fiber, minerals, and amino acids. Other phytoconstituents are:
- **Seeds:** It contains high concentrations of L-Dopa (about 3.1–6.1%) with trace amounts of 5-hydroxy tryptamine (serotonin), nicotine, dimethyl tryptamine (DMT), bufotenine, 5-MeO-DMT, and beta-carboline. Other constituents are mucunine, mucunadine, mucunanidine, prurieninine, pruriendine, tryptamine, steroids flavonoids. L-Dopa is present in the seeds as well as in the stem, leaves, and roots.

- **Seed oil:** Stearic, palmitic, myristic, linoleic acids, and sterol.
- **Hair:** Amines such as 5-hydroxy tryptamine (serotonin), mucuanain.
- **Leaf:** It contains about 0.5% L-DOPA, 0.006% dimethyl tryptamine, and 0.0025% 5-MeO-DMT (Erowid 2002).

Identity, Purity, and Strength

- Foreign matter: Not more than 1%
- Total ash: Not more than 5%
- Acid-insoluble ash: Not more than 1%
- Alcohol-soluble extractive: Not less than 3%
- Water-soluble extractive: Not less than 23%
- Fixed oil: Not less than 3%

(Source: The Ayurvedic Pharmacopoeia of India 2001)

Karma (Actions)

It is highly vrusya (aphrodisiac), bruhmana karaka (increases body mass), and balya (strength promoting), vatahara (pacify vata), stanya janana (galactogogue), raktadoshanashak (pacifyies rakta dosha).

The seeds are astringent, laxative, anthelmintic, aphrodisiac, and tonic. They are useful in gonorrhea, sterility, vitiated conditions of vata, and general debility (Anonymous 2002).
- Doshakarma: Vata pittahara, Kapha hara
- Bhavaprakash: Seed is vatahara
- Dhatukarma: Vrishya, Brimhana, Balya
- Malakarma: Mutrala

Pharmacological Actions

The actions include antivenom, hypoglycemic, aphrodisiac, antimicrobial, anti-Parkinson activity, antidepressant, anti-inflammatory, antitumor, antidiabetic, antiprotozoal, anthelmintic, hypotensive, spasmodic, hypocholesterolemic, antifungal, nervine tonic antioxidant, neuroprotective effects (Sharma et al 2000). Seed diet produces hypoglycemic effect in normal rats (Anonymous 2006).

Indications

It is indicated in vata vyadhi (neuromuscular diseases), kampavata (tremor), vajikara (aphrodisiac), atisara (diarrhea), yoni roga (gynecological diseases), vandhyata (infertility), rakta pitta (bleeding disorders), dushtavrana (wound), klaivya (impotency), daurbalya (weakness).

The main use of this herb is to treat the symptomatic effects in Parkinson disease. The seeds are traditionally used as nervine tonic, emmenagogue, astringent, aphrodisiac, spermatorrhea, depressive neurosis, urinary troubles, leucorrhea, and paralysis. The hairs of the pods are vermifuge, mild vesicant, and treated for round worm infections and diseases of liver and gallbladder. The root is used in vaginal laxity.

The chief benefits of Kapikachhu are improved sleep (promotes deep sleep), reduced body fat, decreased cellulite, decreased wrinkles, improved skin texture and appearance, increased bone density, reversal of osteoporosis, increased lean muscle mass, improved mood and sense of well-being, enhanced libido and sexual performance, increased energy levels, improved cholesterol profile, regeneration of organs (heart, kidney, liver, lungs), and dramatically strengthening of immune system.

Therapeutic Uses

External Use

Sandhi shool (rheumatic pain): Bark powder mixed with dry ginger is used for rubbing over painful rheumatic joints (Nadkarni 1982).

Internal Use

1. **Vrishya** (used as aphrodisiac): (a) Wheat flour and seed powder of Kapikachchhu is cooked with milk and then it is taken with ghee followed by intake of milk (S.S.Ci. 26/30). (b) One tablet of Vanari gutika with milk is taken twice daily for aphrodisiac action (B.P.Ci. 72/71-75). (c) Powder of Kapikachhu and Ikshuraka and sugar is taken with warm milk to increase semen (S.S.Ci. 26/33).

2. **Krimi** (worm infestation): The fruit hairs of Kapikachchhu are kept within the pulp of jaggery and swallowed twice or thrice daily after anointing the lips and mouth with ghee. It cures worms, gastroenteritis, and hematemesis (S.B. 4/280).

3. **Vata Vyadhi** (neuromuscular diseases): Intake of decoction of Kapikachchhu for 1 month helps to regain the strength of arms (CD 22/27).

Officinal Parts Used

Seed, root, hair of fruit

Dose

Seed powder: 3 to 6 g
Decoction (root): 50 to 100 mL
Hair: 125 mg

Formulations

Vanari gutika, Mushalyadi pachana, Bramha rasayana, Vrisya pupalika, Maha paisachika Ghrita, Swadamstradi Ghrita, Tryusanadya Ghrita, Vrishya yoga pupalika, Kapikachu churna, Nagabala ghrita, Amrita taila, Maha mayura Ghrita, Svayam Gupta Churna Yoga, Agastya Rasayana, Vidaryadi Ghrita, Svayan guptadi churna, Rati modaka, Kameswara modaka, Madana kamadeva rasa, Mahakameswara modaka, Gokshuradi yoga.

Toxicity/Adverse Effects

The toxic principle in *Mucuna* seed is held to be L-Dopa, 3-(3,4 dihydroxyphenyl alanine), a compound chiefly used in treating the symptoms of Parkinson disease. In addition to gastrointestinal disturbances like nausea, vomiting, and anorexia, the most serious effects are reported to be aggression, paranoid delusions, hallucinations, delirium, severe depression, with or without suicidal behavior, and unmasking of dementia. Psychotic reactions are more likely in patients with postencephalitic Parkinsonism or a history of mental disorders (Reynolds 1989).

The hair of the cowhage bean pod is a strong irritant and can cause severe itching, burning, and swelling if it is taken by mouth or applied to the skin.

Substitution and Adulteration

M. utilis Wall., *M. cochinchinensis* (Lour.) (white seed), and *M. cochinchinensis* (Lour.) (black seed) are sold as Kapikachhu in the markets of North India and Southern parts of the country, respectively (Garg 1992; Lucas 2013).

Points to Ponder

- *Kapikachhu is considered as one of the best aphrodisiacs and nervine tonic.*
- *Its seed contains high concentrations of L-Dopa and is used for the treatment of Parkinson disease.*
- *It increases sperm count as well as sperm motility.*

Suggested Readings

Agharkar SP. Medicinal Plants of Bombay Presidency. Jodhpur, India: Scientific Publication; 1991:1–2

Anonymous. Indian Medicinal Plants: A Compendium of 500 Species. Orient LongMan Publisher; 2002:68-72

Anonymous. The Ayurvedic Pharmacopoeia of India, Part-I, Vol. III, 1st ed. New Delhi: Department of I.S.M. & H., Ministry of Health and Family Welfare, Government of India; 2001:23-24

Anonymous. The Wealth of India: 1st Supplement Series, Vol. 4. New Delhi: NISCAIR Publishing; 2006:166–167

Erowid. *Mucuna pruriens*. Created 2002-APR-22. International Legume Database and Information Service. Genus *Mucuna*. Version 10.01; 2002

Farooqi AA, Khan MM, Sundhara MA. Production Technology of Medicinal and Aromatic Crops. Bangalore: Natural Remedies Pvt. Ltd; 1999:26–28

Garg S. Substitute and Adulterant Plants. New Delhi: Periodical Expert Book Agency; 1992:82

Gupta KA, Samgraha A. With Hindi Commentary. Vol. 1 & 2. Varanasi: Krishnadas Academy; 2002:136

Jadhao SR. Physiological study of Shukravaha Srotas and clinical study of kapikacchu churna in klaibya with special Ref. to oligozoospermia. Thesis. PG Department of Sharir kriya, NIA Jaipur; 2013:141-145

Kumar A, Rajput G, Dhatwalia VK, Srivastav G. Phytocontent screening of *Mucuna* seeds and exploit in opposition to pathogenic microbes. J Biol Environ Sci 2009;3(9):71–76

Lucas DS. Dravyagun Vijnana Study of Dravya: Materia Medica, Vol. 2. Varanasi: Choukhambha Bharati Academy; 2013:123-126.

Muralia S, Pathak AK. Database of Medicinal Plant Used in Ayurveda: Medicinal and Aromatic Plants' Cultivation and Uses. Raj Publishers Distributors; 2003:185-187.

Nadkarni AK. The Indian Materia Medica, Vol. I. India: Popular Prakashan Private Limited; 1982:817–820

Reynolds JEFM. The Extra Pharmacopeia. London: Pharmaceutical Press; 1989:1015-1020

Sahaji PS. Acute oral toxicity of *Mucuna pruriens* in albino mice. Int Res J Pharm 2011;2(5):162–163

Sastry CST, Kavathekar YY. Plants for Reclamation of Wastelands. New Delhi: Publications and Information Directorate; 1990:317–318

Sharma PC, Yelne MB, Dennis TJ. Database Medicinal Plants Used in Ayurveda, Vol. 1. New Delhi: CCRAS;2000

Yadav MK, Upadhyay P, Purohit S. Pandey BL, Shah H. Phytochemistry and pharmacological activity of *Mucuna pruriens*: a review. Int J Green Pharm 2017;11(2):69–73

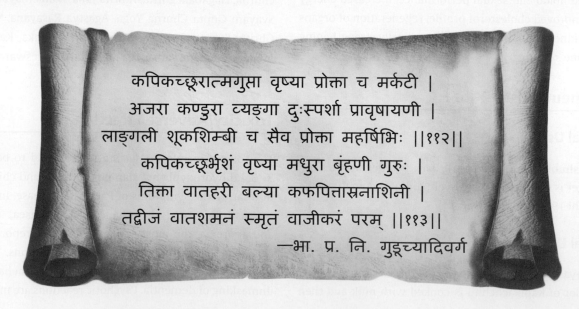

कपिकच्छूरात्मगुप्ता वृष्या प्रोक्ता च मर्कटी |
अजरा कण्डुरा व्यङ्गा दुःस्पर्शा प्रावृषायणी |
लाङ्गली शूकशिम्बी च सैव प्रोक्ता महर्षिभिः ||११२||
कपिकच्छूर्भृशं वृष्या मधुरा बृंहणी गुरुः |
तिक्ता वातहरी बल्या कफपित्तास्रनाशिनी |
तद्बीजं वातशमनं स्मृतं वाजीकरं परम् ||११३||
—भा. प्र. नि. गुड्च्यादिवर्ग

51. Karkatashringi [*Pistacia integerrima stewart* ex brandis]

Family: *Anacardiaceae*

Hindi: *Kakdashingi, Kakarsingi, Kakra, Kakkatasimgi,,Kangar Masna, Sumak, Tungu, Tanbari, Shne, Karkarshingi*

English name: *Pistacia gall, Crab's claw*

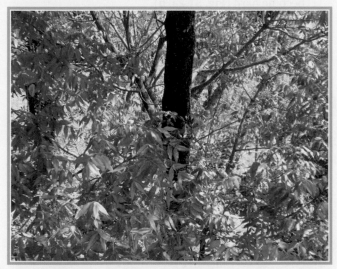

Plant of *Pistacia integerrima stewart* ex brandis.

The galls of Pistacia integerrima is exported to many countries from various parts of Pakistan like Dir valley, Swat valley, etc. to various local and international markets.

Introduction

Karkatashringi (*Pistacia integerrima*) is a multibranched, single-stemmed, deciduous shedding tree belonging to the family of Anacardiaceae. It is found in North-West Himalaya including the Siwalik ranges/Rohilkhand from Indus to Kumaon between 500 and 2,500 m altitudes (Anonymous 2005). Typical types of worms make horn-shaped galls on the branches and leaves (Jindal et al 2012). These galls are pale greenish-brown or pinkish, elongated, horn-shaped, hollow, twisted, curved, or straight. When young, they are coriaceous, but later become hard. This gall is caused by the insect *Dasia aedifactor* (Homoptera). Plant produces resin against insect. They make these galls by sucking juice from the leaves and these galls are called Karkatashringi (Jindal et al 2012).

The galls are considered store houses of secondary metabolites, and hence they have importance in Indian traditional medicine system (Chopra et al 1982).

Vernacular Names

Assamese: Kakiasrngi

Bengali: Kakra, Kakrashingi, Kandashringi

Gujarati: Kakadasingi, Kakra, Kakarshingi

Kannad: Kakada shrungi, Karkataka shrungi, Dushtapuchattu

Kashmiri: Kakkar, Kamaladina, Drak, Gurga, Kakrasingi

Malayalam: Karkata shringi, Karkktakasingi

Marathi: Karkadasringi, Kakra, Kakarsingi, Kakadshingi

Oriya: Kakadashrungi, Kakadashringi

Punjabi: Kakar, Kakarshingi, Drek, Gurgu, Kakkeran, Kakkrangehe, Kakala, Kakrain, Kangar, Khakkar, Masna, Sarawan, Shne, Tanbari, Tungu, Sumak, Kakarsingi

Tamil: Karkata shrungi, Kakkatashingi

Telugu: Kakar Singi, Karkataka shrungi, Kakarasimga

Urdu: Kakrasinghi, Kakra

Synonyms

Karkashringi: The gall resembles the leg of crab/it kills the krimi (jiva).

Shringi: It cures many diseases.

Kuliravishanika: The gall resembles the claws of young crab.

Ajashringi: It looks like horn of a goat.

Chakra: Sometimes it is round in shape.

Karkatakhya: The gall has crab-like appearance.

Ghosha: It is bell shaped.

Mahaghosha: It is bell shaped.

Vakra: The useful part, gall is curved.

Samhitokta Classification

Charak Samhita: Kasahara, Hikkanigrahana

Sushrut Samhita: Kakolyadi, Padmakadi

Dhanwantari Nighantu: Guduchyadi varga

Madanpal Nighantu: Abhayadi varga

Kaiyadev Nighantu: Aushadhi varga.

Raj Nighantu: Pippalyadi varga

Bhavprakash Nighantu: Haritakyadi

Distribution

It is found in North-West Himalaya including the Siwalik ranges/Rohitkhand from Indus to Kumaon between 800 and 1,900 m altitudes. It is native to Asia and is widely distributed in East Afghanistan, Pakistan, India, Japan, China. It is cultivated in Punjab, India (Pant and Samant 2010).

Morphology

It is a deciduous multibranched tree, having dark gray to blackish bark trees which grow up to 18 m.

- **Leaves:** Leaves are 20 to 25 cm in length, with or without terminal leaflet; leaflets are four to five pairs, lanceolate, coriaceous, pari or imparipinnate and base oblique, dark and green color which turns bright red in autumn. The terminal leaflet is much smaller than the lateral ones or is even reduced to a micro size. Leaves are very often affected by insect-forming conical galls (**Fig. 51.1**).

- **Flower**: Flowers are small, reddish in color, and are arranged in panicles.
- It is unisexual, dioecious, male panicles are short and compact in comparison to female. Inflorescence is red.
- **Fruits:** Globular with a bony endocarp, apiculate, 5 to 6 mm in diameter, purplish or blue at maturity.
- **Gall:** Characteristic galls are produced on the leafy branches. Galls are pale greenish-brown or pinkish, elongated, horn-shaped, hollow, twisted, curved, or straight. When young they are coriaceous, but later become hard (**Fig. 51.2a, b**).
- **Bark**: Dark gray or blackish (Sher et al 2011; Padulosi et al 2002).

It can be propagated by seeds and by vegetative method.

Phenology

Flowering time: March to May

Fruiting time: June to October

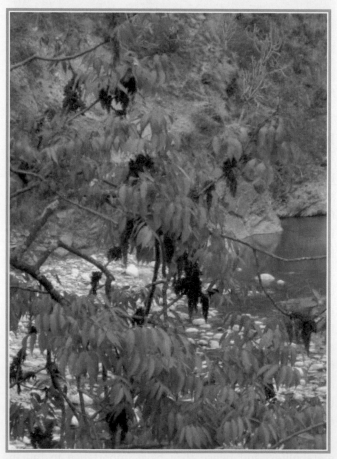

Fig. 51.1 Leaves.

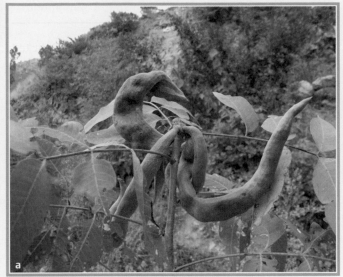 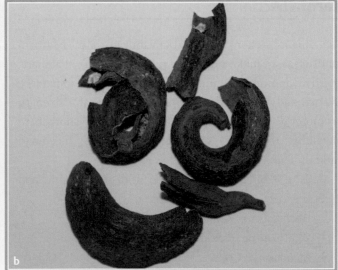

Fig. 51.2 **(a)** Fresh gall. **(b)** Dry gall.

Rasapanchaka

Guna	Guru, rukshya
Rasa	Kasaya, tikta
Vipaka	Katu
Virya	Ushna

Chemical Constituents

Generally, *P. integerrima* contains different phytochemicals including alkaloids, flavonoids, tannins, saponins, sterols, and essential oils.

- **Gall:** Chiefly, it contains resin, two isomeric triterpenic acids (pistacienoic acids A and B), tannins, a triterpene alcohol (tirucallol), beta-sitosterol, tetracyclic triterpenes, pistacigerrimones A, B, C
- **Seed:** Alpha-piene, beta-piene, camphene, DL-limonene, 1:8-cinol, alpha-terpineol, beta-terpineol, aromadendrin, lactonic stearoptene, caprylic acid, alpha-d-pinene, alpha and beta-phallandrene, amino acids, dihydromalyalic acid, protein
- **Seed oil:** Hydrocarbons, sterols, triterpenoids
- **Leaves, bark:** Tannins

(Source: Jindal et al 2012; Joshi and Mishra 2009; Prajapati et al 2006; Uddin et al 2011)

Majorly, gall contains resins, pistacienoic acid, tetracyclic triterpenes, camphene, luteolin, pistancin, pistacinin, amino acids, dihydromavalic acids, sterols, and tannins (Warrier et al 1995).

Identity, Purity, and Strength

- Foreign matter: Not more than 2%
- Total ash: Not more than 7%
- Acid-insoluble ash: Not more than 0.2%
- Alcohol-soluble extractive: Not less than 30%
- Water-soluble extractive: Not less than 30%

(Source: The Ayurvedic Pharmacopeia of India 2001)

Karma (Actions)

The main actions of Karkatashringi are kasahara (antitussive), hikka-nighrana (anti-hiccough), vatahara, vrushya (aphrodisiac), grahi (absorbent), dipana (appetizer), jwaraghna (antipyretics), balya (physical strength promoter), kaphanissaraka (expectorant), shothahara (swelling reducing), raktarodhaka (checks bleeding), vatanulomana (carminative).

Galls of *P. integerrima* are bitter in taste, aromatic, and used as expectorant as well as tonic.

- Doshakarma: Kaphavatashamak
- Dhatukarma: Raktarodhaka, balya
- Malakarma: Grahi

Pharmacological Actions

Galls of *P. integerrima* were reported to have significant analgesic, anti-inflammatory, antimicrobial, antioxidant, antispasmodic, carminative, antiamoebic, antigastrointestinal motility effect and anthelmintic properties. It has been reported to have depressant, antinociceptive, and hyperuricemic effect disorder (Ansari and Ali 1996; Ahmad et al 2010; Ansari et al 1993). Galls of *P. integerrima* were also known to lower uric acid content in mice in a dose-dependent manner (Ahmad et al 2006).

Indications

It is mainly used in kasa (cough), shwasa (asthma), arti (pain), kshaya (consumption), chhardi (vomiting), trishna (thirst), aruchi (anorexia), urdwavata, kaphavata (diseases of kaphavata), atisara (diarrhea), raktapitta (bleeding disorder), and jwara (fever).

These galls are useful in dysentery, ulcers, bronchitis, fever, irritability of stomach, leprosy, psoriasis, skin diseases, vitiated conditions of tridosha, dyspepsia, inflammation, pharyngitis, leucorrhea, and general debility. It is also very effective in children at the time of teething. In Pakistan, the galls of *Pistacia chinensis* var. are used for the treatment of hepatitis and liver. Roasted galls are taken with honey for cough, asthma, and diarrhea in northern areas of Pakistan (Abbasi et al 2010).

Therapeutics Uses

1. **Kasa** (cough): Powder of Karkatashringi should be licked with oil in vatik kasa (C.S.Ci. 18/50). Its powder mixed with ghee, sugar, and honey is taken, followed by intake of milk (A.S.Ci. 4/32).
2. **Shwasa and hikka** (asthma and hic-cough): (a) Powder of Karkatashringi and seed of radish mixed with honey and ghee is given to children to treat asthma (B.S balaroga 62). (b) Yavagu (gruel) prepared with Karkatashringi is beneficial in hiccough and asthma (C.S.Ci-17/101).
3. **Vajikarana** (aphrodisiac): Paste of Karkatashringi mixed with milk is given to improve the libido. During this period, the patient is advised to take the diet mixed with sugar, ghee, and milk (A.S.U 50/44).
4. **Chhardi** (vomiting): Powder of Karkatashringi and Musta is given with honey to check vomiting (C.S.Ci. 20/38).

Officinal Part Used

Gall

Dose

Gall powder: 1 to 3 g, but it can be given in the dose of 3 to 6 g (The Ayurvedic Pharmacopeia of India 2001).

Formulations

Balachatubhadrachoorna, Chyavanprashaavaleha, Dasamoolarista, Shrungadi choorna, karkatadi choorna, khadiradi gutika, shivagutika, chaturbhadra choorna, kameswar modak, Brihat talisadi churna, Devadarvayadi kwath churna, shatavaryadi ghrit, Kanta karyavaleha .

Toxicity/Adverse Effects

No acute toxicity was reported in oral administration of extracts (Ahmad et al 2010).

Essential oil of gall has a depressant action on the central nervous system of guinea pigs and white rats when given in sublethal doses. The animals become deeply unconscious in about an hour. Lethal dose (m.l.d. 0.1 mL/100 g body wt.) causes deep narcosis leading to death within a few hours.

The oil has a slight irritant action on the skin and mucous membrane (Anonymous 2005).

Substitution and Adulteration

Galls found in the plants like *Rhus succedanea* Linn., *Garuga pinnata* Roxb., *Terminalia chebula* Retz. are also available in the name of Karkatashringi in the market (Anonymous 2005).

Points to Ponder

- *Horn-shaped gall on the branches and leaves of P. integerrima by a certain type of insect is called Karkatashringi.*
- *It is found in North-West Himalaya between 800 and 1,900 m altitudes.*
- *It is mainly used for kasa, shwasa, hikka, atisara, jwara, liver diseases, etc.*

Suggested Readings

18. Sher H, Elyemeni M, Hussain K, Sher H. Ethnobotanical and economic observations of some plant resources from the northern parts of Pakistan. Ethnobot Res App 2011;9:27–41

Abbasi AM, Khan MA, Ahmad M, Zafar M. Herbal medicines used to cure various ailments by inhabitants of Abbottabad district, North West Frontier, Pakistan. Ind J Trad Know 2010;9:175–183

Ahmad NS, Farman M, Najmi MH, Mian KB, Hasan A. Activity of polyphenolic plant extracts as scavengers of free radicals and inhibitors of xanthine oxidase. J Basic Appl Sci 2006;2:1–6

Ahmad S, Ali M, Ansari SH, Ahmed F. Phytoconstituents from the galls of *Pistacia integerrima* Stewart. J Saudi Chem Soc 2010;14(4): 409–412

Anonymous. The database on medicinal plants used in Ayurveda. New Delhi: Central Council for Research in Ayurveda and Siddha, Government of India; 2005:169

Ansari SH, Ali M, Qadry JS. Essential oils of *Pistacia integerrima* galls and their effect on the central nervous system. Int J Pharmacogn 1993;31(2):89–95

Ansari SH, Ali M. Analgesic and antiinflammatory activity of tetracyclic triterpenoids isolated from *Pistacia integerrima* galls. Fitoterapia (Milano) 1996;67:103–105

Chopra RN, Chopra IC, Handa KL, Kapoor LD . Indigenous Drugs of India. 2nd ed. Delhi: Academic Publishers; 1982:377–379

Jindal A, Vashist H, Gupta A, Jalhan S. Physicochemical and phytochemical evaluation of *Pistacia integerrima* stew ex brand. J Global Pharma Technol 2012;4(7):24–27.

Joshi UP, Mishra SH. In vitro anti-oxidant activity of galls of *Pistacia integerrima*. Pharmacol Online 2009;2:763–768

Padulosi S, Hodgkin T, Williams J, Haq N. Managing plant genetic diversity. Wallingford: IPGRI/CABI Publishing; 2002:323–338

Pant S, Samant SS. Ethnobotanical observations in the Mornaula reserve forest of Kumoun, West Himalaya, India. Ethnobot Leafl 2010;14:193

Prajapati ND, Purohit SS, Sharma AK, Kumar T. A Handbook of Medicinal Plants, 3rd ed. Jodhpur: Agrobios Hindustan Printing Press; 2006

Sharma PV. Dravyaguna-Vijnana, Vol. II. Varanasi: Chaukhambha Bharti; 1981:132–137

The Ayurvedic Pharmacopeia of India. Part 1, Vol. 1. New Delhi: Department of ISM&H, Ministry of Health and Family Welfare, Government of India; 2001:66

The wealth of India: A dictionary of Indian raw materials and industrial products, Vol. VIII. New Delhi: Publication and Information Directorate, CSIR; 1998:120

Uddin G, Rauf A, et al. Phytochemical screening of *Pistacia cccchinensis* var. integerrima. Middle-East J Sci Res 2011;7(5):707–711

Warrier PK, Nambiar VPK, Ramankutty C. Indian Medicinal Plants: A Compendium of 500 Species, Vol. 4; 1995:304

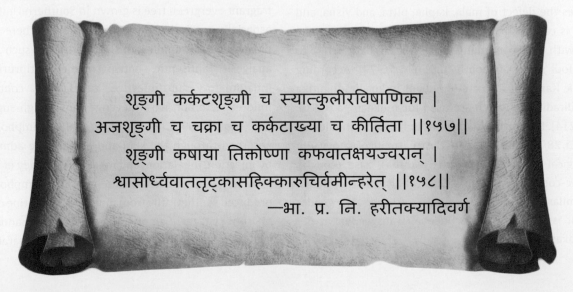

शृङ्गी कर्कटशृङ्गी च स्यात्कुलीरविषाणिका ।
अजशृङ्गी च चक्रा च कर्कटाख्या च कीर्तिता ॥१५७॥
शृङ्गी कषाया तिक्तोष्णा कफवातक्षयज्वरान् ।
श्वासोर्ध्ववाततृट्कासहिक्कारुचिर्वमीन्हरेत् ॥१५८॥
—भा. प्र. नि. हरीतक्यादिवर्ग

52. Karpura [*Cinnamomum camphora* (Linn.) Nees & Eberm]

Family: *Lauraceae*

Hindi name: *Karpura*

English name: *Camphor tree , Camphor laurel, Japanese camphor*

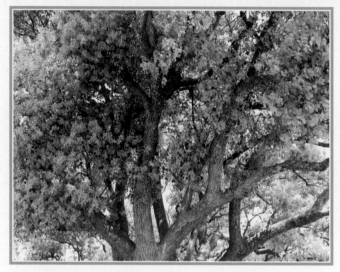

Plant of *Cinnamonum camphora* (Linn.) Nees & Eberm.

> *Camphor is obtained through steam distillation, purification, and sublimation of wood, twigs, and bark of Cinnamonum camphora (Linn.).*
>
> —*Paolo 2009*

Introduction

Karpur is not described in any gana of Brihattrayee of Ayurveda, but it is mentioned in different vargas of various Nighantus. The plant of Karpur has aromatic exude that eliminates the defect of mala, kapha, pitta, and visha, and hence it is called Karpur. Acharya Charak advised to take Karpur with other aromatic drugs in tambul (betel) to remove foul smell of mouth (C.S.Su. 5/76-77). According to Charak, Karpur is also an ingredient in khadiradi gutika and khadiradi taila which are used for mukharoga (C.S.Ci. 26/206-214). Karpur is also present in balataila (medicated oil) (C.S.Ci. 28/148-156) used for the treatment of vatavyadhi (neurological disorder), shwasa (asthma), kasa (cough), hikka (hic-cough), etc. Acharya Sushrut also has mentioned about similar types of uses for mouth refreshers. The gender of Karpur is pumsi (male) or kleeba (transgender) as per Bhavaprakash Nighantu.

Camphor (*Cinnamomum camphora*) is a white, crystalline substance with a strong odor and pungent taste, derived from the wood of camphor laurel (*C. camphora*) and other related trees of Laurel family. Camphor tree is native to China, India, Mongolia, Japan, and Taiwan, and a variety of this fragrant evergreen tree is grown in Southern United States, especially in Florida (Frizzo et al 2000). There are many pharmaceutical applications for camphor, such as topical analgesic, antiseptic, antispasmodic, antipruritic, anti-inflammatory, anti-infective, rubefacient, contraceptive, mild expectorant, nasal decongestant, cough suppressant, etc. (Paolo 2009; Chelliah Abiya 2008). Camphor is easily absorbed through the skin and can also be administrated by injection, inhalation, and ingestion (Sydney et al 1978).

A large proportion of the world's camphor is now produced synthetically from pinene, a turpentine derivative, or from coal tar. Camphor is used in the manufacture of celluloid, in disinfectants, and chemical preparations, and has a wide range of medicinal uses. Safrole, produced from the residual oil after camphor extraction, is used in soap and perfume manufacture. *C. camphora* has been used medicinally for thousands of years to fight toothache, clear up urinary tract infections, and soothe stomach irritation. It has a broad range of historical uses in different cultures, including the treatment of diarrhea, arthritis, and various menstrual disorders. *C. camphora* is used for religious purposes also.

Vernacular Names

Bengali: Karpur
Chinese: Xiang-zhang, Zhang-shu
Creole: Kafm, bom zangle
Dutch: Kamferboom
French: Camphrier, camphre, baume anglais, Arbre a camphre
German: Kampferßaum
Gujarati: Karpur
Italian: Canfora, confora
Japanese: kkusu-no-ki, kuso-no ki, hon-sho
Kannada: Pache karpoora
Marathi: Karpur
Nepali: Kapur
Portuguese: Alcanforeira
Sanskrit: Karpura
Spanish: Alcanfor, alcanforero, alcanfor delJapón
Swahili: Mkafuri maita
Swedish: Kamfertraed
Tamil: Karpooram, Pachai Karpooram
Telugu: Karpooram Chettu

Synonyms

Chandrasanjya: It has properties like those of the moon.
Chandra: Its color is bright white like the moon.
Ghanasara: Its exudate is solid in form.
Himabaaluka: It is cool to touch and found in powder form.
Himanaama: It is white in color and has a cooling effect.
Karpura: The plant has aromatic exude which eliminates the defect of mala, kapha, pitta, and visha.
Shishir: It is cool to touch and has a cooling effect.
Shitabhra: Its extract resembles white clouds.

Shitalarajah: It is cool to touch and found in powder form.
Sphatika: Its extract is found in sphatik (blocks) form.

Classification

Dhanwantari Nighantu: Chandanadi varga
Madanpal Nighantu: Karpuradi varga
Kaiyadev Nighantu: Aushadhi varga
Raj Nighantu: Chandanadi varga
Bhavaprakash Nighantu: Karpuradi varga

Distribution

This plant is distributed across Taiwan, Japan, and China. Now-a-days, it is grown in many tropical and subtropical forests of India, Sri Lanka, South Africa, United States, etc. In India, it is found in Tamil Nadu, Kerala, and Karnataka (Frizzo et al 2000).

Morphology

It is a medium-sized evergreen tree about 15 to 25 m tall. The bark is rough on the outside and smoother inside. All parts of the tree have peculiar fragrance of camphor.

- **Trunk:** Bark is thick and grooved (**Fig. 52.1**).
- **Leaves:** Shiny leaves, 5 to 12.5 cm long and 2.5 to 5 cm broad, yellowish-green in color with a leathery texture. Its leaves resemble the leaves of Tejpatra

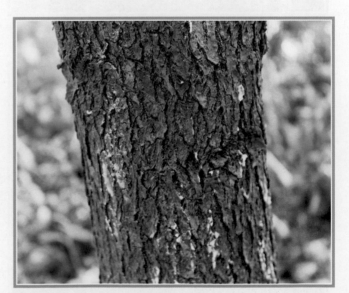

Fig. 52.1 Trunk.

also known as Indian bay leaves. Simple, alternate, coriaceous, long petiolate, glabrous on upper side, three-nerved at the base, ovate or oblong, or elliptic-ovate, at both ends attenuate-acute (**Fig. 52.2**).

- **Flowers:** Flowers are small, yellowish-white in color, and occur in clusters in axillary panicles (**Fig. 52.3**).
- **Fruits:** Fruits are dark green in color resembling peas (globose berry), dark green when unripe, and black when mature (**Fig. 52.4**).
- **Seeds:** Seeds are small and have peculiar fragrance of Karpura.

It is propagated through seeds.

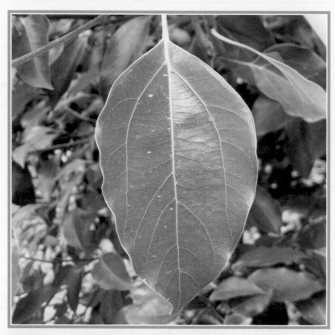

Fig. 52.2 Leaves.

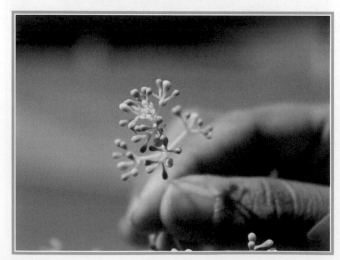

Fig. 52.3 Flower.

Phenology

Flowering time: There are different cultivation seasons for this plant according to their regions. In India and China, flowers flourish in April to May and in Vietnam, it occurs in April to May.

Fruiting time: In India and China, fruiting starts during September to November, and in Vietnam, it starts in November to January.

Key Characters for Identification

➤ It is a medium-sized evergreen tree about 15 to 25 m tall.
➤ Leaves: Simple, alternate, coriaceous, 5 to 12.5 cm long and 2.5 to 5 cm broad, long petiolate, glabrous on upper side, three-nerved at the base, ovate or oblong, or elliptic-ovate.
➤ Flowers: Small, yellowish-white in color, and occur in clusters in axillary panicles.
➤ Fruits: Globose berry, dark green when unripe, and black when mature.

Types

As per Bhavaprakash Nighantu, it is of two types: (a) Pakwa and (b) Apakwa. Apakwa is considered better than the pakwa variety.

Kaiyadeva explained three varieties: Ishaavaasa, Hima sanjnaka, and Potashraya. Ishaavaasa is bright white, Hima is pandura varna (pale white color), and Potashraya is white

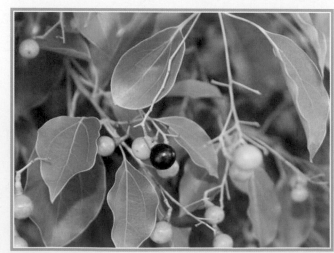

Fig. 52.4 Fruit.

in color. Ishaavaasa is more potent in comparison to the other two. According to him, camphor that has no eyes and has the appearance of sphatika (alum) is considered as best.

Later, he explained that there are two types based on their processing: Pakva and Apakva. Pakva is of two types: Sadala and Nirdala. Apakva is of three types: Ishaavaasa, Hima sanjnaka, and Potashraya. Apakva is better than the Pakva variety (K.N. Aushadhi varga/1280-1286).

Raj Nighantu explained around 14 types of Karpura on the basis of rasa, guna, and glow. As per the origin, Karpura is of three types: Shira, Madhya, and Tala. These are produced in upper, middle, and lower parts, respectively (R.N. Chandanadi varga/62-66).

Chunekarji explained four varieties of camphor, viz.

- Bhimseni or Baras Karpura (*C. camphora*)
- Chini or Japani Karpura (*C. camphora*)
- Patri or Nagi Karpura: *Blumea balsamifera, B. lacera, B. densiflora*, etc.
- Krutima Karpura: Synthetic variety camphor

Rasapanchaka

Guna	Laghu
Rasa	Katu, Tikta, Madhura
Vipak	Katu
Virya	Sheeta

Chemical Constituents

The major phytoconstituents are eugenol, isoeugenol, cineol, linalool, limonene, safrole, α-pinene, β-pinene, β-myrecene, α-humulene, p-cymene, nerolidol, cinnamaldehyde, cinnamate, cinnamic acids, and numerous essential oils, caryophyllene, limonene, carvacrol, azulene, etc. (Frizzo et al 2000; Chelliah Abiya 2008).

Major oil constituents of *C. camphora* are camphor, linalool, borneol, camphene, dipentene, terpineol, safrole, and cineole (Chelliah Abiya 2008).

Karma (Actions)

The main actions of Karpur are lekhana (scraping property), vishahara (antitoxic), chakshushya (improves vision, good

for eyes), madakaraka (produces intoxication), yogavahi (acts as a catalyst), dahahara (being a coolant, it relieves burning sensation), vrushya (acts as aphrodisiac in lower dose but higher doses decrease sexual performance), medhya (improves intelligence), kruminashana (relieves intestinal worm infestation), daurgandha nashana (removes foul smell).

- Doshakarma: Kapha pittahara
- Dhatukarma: Vrusya, lekhana, medoghna
- Malakarma: Mutral (diuretic)

Pharmacological Actions

The antitussive, nasal decongestant, and expectorant actions of camphor and of its derivatives were the first ones to be systematically investigated (Inoue and Takeuchi, 1969). Other actions are cardiac stimulant, emollient, diaphoretic, thermogenic, antiseptic, anodyne, antioxidant, antispasmodic, anti-inflammatory, strong decongestant, fungicide, aphrodisiac, narcotic, antiarthritic, anesthetic and nervous pacifier, antitussive, nasal decongestant and expectorant, anthelmintic, antibacterial, increases sperm motility and sperm viability, attenuates and enhances sexual behavior properties (Rao and HuaGan 2014).

Indications

It is used in daha (burning sensation), trishna (thirst), asyavairasya (tastelessness), medoroga (obesity), daurgandhya (foul smell), mukhashosa (dryness of mouth), kushta (leprosy), kandu (itching), vrana (wound), netra roga (eye diseases).

Camphor is today mostly used in the form of inhalants and camphorated oil, a preparation of 19% or 20% camphor in a carrier oil, for the home treatment of colds (Theis and Koren 1995) and as a major active ingredient of liniments and balms used as topical analgesics (Xu et al 2005). Camphor is readily absorbed from all the sites of administration, after inhalation, ingestion, or dermal exposure (Baselt and Cravey 1990). Peak plasma levels were reached by 3 hours postingestion when 200 mg camphor was taken alone, and 1 hour postingestion when it was ingested with a solvent (Tween 80; Koppel et al 1988). In case of dermal application, the volume of the absorption is relatively low in comparison with the speed of the process.

The antitussive, nasal decongestant, and expectorant actions of camphor and of its derivatives were one of the first ones to be systematically investigated (Inoue and Takeuchi 1969).

It is used against a wide spectrum of diseases like bronchitis, colds, congestion, diarrhea, dysentery, edema, flu, gas, metabolic and heart strengthening, hiccups, indigestion, liver problems, menorrhagia, melancholy, muscle tension, nausea, and vomiting. It assists uterine contractions during labor and menstrual pain from low metabolic function. In Unani medicine, it is used as a cephalic tonic and cardiac stimulant and for the treatment of coughs. Flowers are used in the European tradition as a blood purifier. *C. camphor* may find its way to a diabetic's daily diet. It contains a chemical called methoxy hydroxy chalcone polymer, which can reduce the blood glucose level.

The concentration of 3 to 11% has been approved by the FDA for topical use as a pain reliever and anesthetic (Paolo 2009).

Contraindications

Camphor is distributed throughout the whole body and can permeate the placenta. Hence, it must be avoided during pregnancy and lactation (Sweetman 2005).

Therapeutic Uses

External Use

Shirashool (headache): It is used locally to treat headaches and pain.

Internal Use

1. **Shwasa** (asthma): Vati prepared from Karpur and jaggery is given to get relief from asthma quickly (S.B.-4/386).
2. **Netra roga** (eye diseases): Fine powder of Karpur and latex of Vata are mixed and used as anjana (coryllium) to treat Shukragata roga of eye (corneal opacity) (V.M-61/97, BS.Netra.175).
3. **Sadya vrana** (traumatic wound): Fresh wound caused by any accident or trauma is filled with Karpur and ghee and covered by bandage to prevent infection and pus and accelerate healing of the wound (C.D.-44/55).

4. **Kustaja vrana** (leprotic wound): Karpur taila is used locally as pichu to heal the leprotic wound rapidly (VM-16/15).
5. **Trishna** (thirst): Camphor powder is kept in mouth in order to check thirst (KS.Vishesh kalpa).
6. **Mutraghata** (retention of urine): (a) Camphor powder is introduced into the urethra to treat retention of urine (C.D. 33/13). (b) Camphor powder treated with goat's urine or sheep's urine is introduced into the urethra to get relief from retention of urine (B.P.Ci-36/32).

Officinal Parts Used

Niryasa (exudates) and oil

Dose

Powder: 125 to 375 mg

Formulations

Karpura rasa, Karpuradi Vati, Karpurasava, Hingukarpuradi Vati, Arkakarpur.

Toxicity/Adverse Effects

Camphor occurs in nature in its dextrorotatory form (D-camphor), while the laevorotatory form (L-camphor) exists only as a synthetic form. These two forms produce different profiles of toxicity. D-camphor, L-camphor, and their racemic mixture were tested for toxicity in mice. The natural form was nontoxic at 100 mg/kg body weight while the synthetic form induced different kinds of toxic and behavioral effects such as body jerks and hunched posture; the racemic mixture showed similar effects to the L-form (Chatterjie and Alexander 1986).

Camphor intoxication has been reported in humans and especially children but mostly because of accidental ingestion or exceeding the recommended dose (Paolo 2009).

More than 100,000 cases of ingestion exposures to camphor-containing products were registered between 1990 and 2003 (Manoguerra et al 2006), causing a range of symptoms that comprise convulsion, lethargy, ataxia, severe nausea, vomiting, and coma (Koppel et al 1988; Manoguerra et al 2006).

Points to Ponder

- *Camphor is obtained from Cinnamomum camphora.*
- *It is mainly used for obesity, foul smell, dryness of mouth, leprosy, itching, wound, and eye diseases.*
- *It must be avoided during pregnancy and lactation.*
- *The gender of Karpur is pumsi (male) or kleeba (transgender).*

Suggested Reading

Baselt RC, Cravey RH. Disposition of Toxic Drugs and Chemicals and Drugs. 3rd ed. Year Book Medical Publishers Inc.; 1990

Chatterjie N, Alexander GJ. Anticonvulsant properties of spirohydantoins derived from optical isomers of camphor. Neurochem Res 1986;11(12):1669–1676

Chelliah Abiya D. Biological activity prediction of an ethno medicinal plant *Cinnamomum camphora* through bioinformatics. Ethnobotan Leafl 2008;12:18190

Frizzo CD, Santos AC, Paroul N, et al. Essential oils of Camphor tree (*Cinnamomum camphora* Nees & Eberm) cultivated in Southern Brazil. Braz Arch Biol Technol 2000;43(3), 1–4

Inoue Y, Takeuchi S. Expectorant-like action of camphor derivatives. Nippon Ika Daigaku Zasshi 1969;36(4):351–354

Kirtikar KR, Basu BD. Indian Medicinal Plants, Vol. 9. 2nd ed. Varanasi: Oriental Enterprises; 1972.

Koppel C, Martens F, Schirop Th, Ibe K. Hemoperfusion in acute camphor poisoning. Intensive Care Med 1988;14:431–433.

Köppel C, Martens F, Schirop T, Ibe K. Hemoperfusion in acute camphor poisoning. Intensive Care Med 1988;14(4):431–433

Manoguerra AS, Erdman AR, Wax PM, et al; American Association of Poison Control Centers. Camphor poisoning: an evidence-based practice guideline for out-of-hospital management. Clin Toxicol (Phila) 2006;44(4):357–370

Paolo Z. Camphor: risks and benefits of a widely used natural product. J Appl Sci Environ Manag 2009;13(2):69–74

Rao PV, HuaGan S. Cinnamon: A Multifaceted Medicinal Plant. Hindawi Publishing Corporation Evidence-Based Complementary and Alternative Medicine Volume; 2014, Article ID 642942, 12 pages.

Sweetman SC, ed. Martindale: The Complete Drug Reference. 34th ed. London: The Pharmaceutical Press; 2005

Sydney S, Cohen SN, John F, et al. Camphor: who needs it? Am Acad Pediatr 1978;62(3):40406

Theis JG, Koren G. Camphorated oil: still endangering the lives of Canadian children. CMAJ 1995;152(11):1821–1824

Xu H, Blair NT, Clapham DE. Camphor activates and strongly desensitizes the transient receptor potential vanilloid subtype 1 channel in a vanilloid-independent mechanism. J Neurosci 2005;25(39):8924–8937

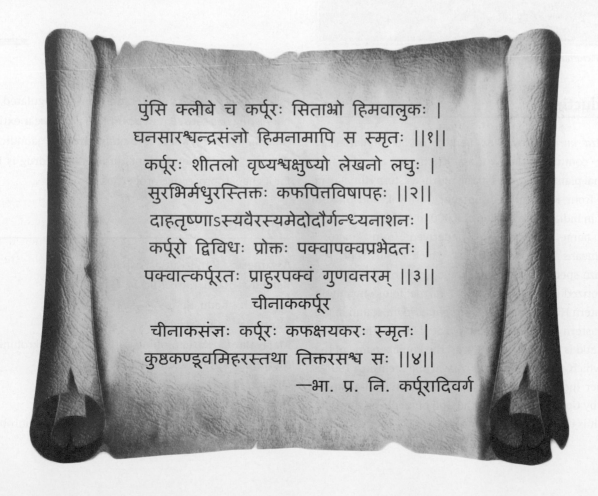

पुंसि क्लीबे च कर्पूरः सिताभो हिमवालुकः |
घनसारश्चन्द्रसंज्ञो हिमनामापि स स्मृतः ||१||
कर्पूरः शीतलो वृष्यश्चक्षुष्यो लेखनो लघुः |
सुरभिर्मधुरस्तिक्तः कफपित्तविषापहः ||२||
दाहतृष्णाऽस्यवैरस्यमेदोदौर्गन्ध्यनाशनः |
कर्पूरो द्विविधः प्रोक्तः पक्वापक्वप्रभेदतः |
पक्वात्कर्पूरतः प्राहुरपक्वं गुणवत्तरम् ||३||
चीनाककर्पूर
चीनाकसंज्ञः कर्पूरः कफक्षयकरः स्मृतः |
कुष्ठकण्डूवमिहरस्तथा तिक्तरसश्च सः ||४||

—भा. प्र. नि. कर्पूरादिवर्ग

53. Katuki *[Picrorhiza kurroa Royle ex Benth.]*

Family: *Scrophulariaceae*

Hindi name: *Katuka, Kuru, Kutki*

English name: *Picrorhiza, Hellebore*

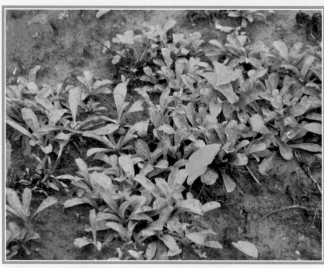

Plant of *Picrorhiza kurroa* Royle ex Benth.

> *Rhizomes of this plant are generally used in the Tibetan and Chinese traditional medicine to treat various ailments like liver disease, fever, asthma, jaundice.*
>
> —Chin et al (2006) and Bantawa et al (2011)

Introduction

Picrorhiza kurroa Royle ex Benth. (of Scrophulariaceae family), commonly known as "Kutki," is a high-value medicinal plant that grows in the north-western Himalayan region, from Kashmir to Kumaon, Garhwal, and Sikkim regions in India at an altitude of 3,000 to 4,500 m.

The name "Picrorhiza" is derived from "picros," which means bitter, and "rhiza," which means root. The Picrorhiza species belongs to the genus *Picrorhiza* and are characterized into two species: *P. kurroa*, found mainly in dry western Himalayas, and *P. scrophulariflora*, found in the moist eastern Himalayas (Bantawa et al 2011). The specific name kutki is derived from "Karu," the Punjabi name of the plant, which also means bitter (Aswal and Mehrotra 1994).

As per Indian mythology, the drug "Katuki" is administered by God Dhanwantari (the God of medicine) himself. Hence, it is called Dhanwantary-grastya (Elizabeth 2002).

The plant is self-regenerating but unregulated, over-harvesting has caused it to be threatened to near extinction (Chauhan 1999). Kutki is mainly used in jaundice, bile disorders, and other ailments of liver. This drug is known for its hepatoprotective properties.

Vernacular Names

Assamese: Katki, Kutki, Kash Kour

Bengali: Katki, Kuru, Kutkr

Gujarati: Kadu, Katu

Kannada: Katvkarohini

Malayalam: Katukurohini, Katurohini, Kadukrohini

Marathi: Kutaki, Kutuki, Katikulki

Oriya: Katuki

Punjabi: Nilkant, Kamalphul, Kaur

Tamil: Katukurohini, Kadugu-rohini, Katugurhorohmi

Telugu: Katuka-rogoni, Katuka-rani, katukarohini, Kati
Urdu: Rutakisqfed, Kutafdsiyah

Synonyms

Amaghni: It reduces ama.
Arista: It safeguards against diseases.
Ashoka: It relieves pain and cures diseases.
Ashokarohini: It is a regenerative drug. It cures many diseases by strengthening liver and purifying blood.
Chakrangi: It has circular marking on the surface.
Kandaruha: It regenerates or propagates by stem cutting.
Katambhara: It has pitta virechaka (choleretic) action.
Katuka: It has pitta virechaka (choleretic) action.
Katurohini: It is a regenerative drug. It cures many diseases by strengthening liver and purifying blood.
Katvi: It is (aswadu) unpalatable.
Krushnabheda: On braking of rhizome, blackish portion is seen in the middle of it. It is purgative in nature.
Matsyapitta: It is bitter in taste like bile of a fish.
Matsyashakala: It bears covering like scale of fish.
Rohini: It is a regenerative drug. It cures many diseases by strengthening liver and purifying blood.
Shakuladani: It is bitter in taste like bile of a fish.
Tikta: It is bitter in taste.

Classical Categorization

Charak Samhita: Bhedaniya, Lekhaniya, Stanya shodhan
Sushruta Samhita: Patoladi, Pippalyadi, Mustadi
Dhanwantari Nighantu: Guduchyadi varga
Madanpal Nighantu: Abhayadi varga
Kaiyadev Nighantu: Aushadhi varga
Raj Nighantu: Pippalyadi varga
Bhavaprakash: Haritakyadi varga

Distribution

It is a high-altitude plant, found in alpine Himalayan region from Kashmir to Sikkim at an elevation of 2,500 to 4,500 m. The plant grows in mountainous places and bare hill sides as well as on the ledges of rocks. It is also found in Pakistan, Tibet, west of China, and north Burma (Anonymous 1999; Coventry 1927; Anonymous 2007).

Chamba, Kangra, Mandi, Shimla, Kinnaur, Lahaul, and Spiti districts are the important habitat in Himachal Pradesh of India for this plant (Uniyal et al 2006).

Morphology

It is a small herb with creeping rhizome, is bitter in taste, and grows in rock crevices and moist, sandy soil. It is 6 to 10 inch tall.

- **Leaves:** Leaves are basal, alternate, acuminate, serrate, stalked, winged, oblanceolate, or narrowly spathulate; each leaf is 2 to 6 cm long and 0.5 to 1.2 cm wide, usually 10 to 20 per rosette; serrate in upper half; surfaces glabrous or sparingly short-glandular-hairy, and leaves turn black on drying (**Fig. 53.1**).
- **Flower:** Flowers are white or pale purple and borne on a tall spike. Calyx is generally five in number; corolla has four lobes, 9 to 10 mm long and bilabiate; stamens are slightly di-dynamous almost equaling corolla, stamens 4, inserted on corolla tube, stigma capitate (**Fig. 53.2**).
- **Fruits:** Fruits are ovoid and swollen capsules, tapered at top, dehiscing into four valves and 6 to 10 mm long.
- **Seeds:** Seeds are numerous and ellipsoid; seed coat is very thick and transparent.
- **Rhizome:** Subcylindrical, straight, or slightly curved, 2.5 to 12.0 cm long and 0.3 to 1.0 cm thick, externally grayish-brown, surface rough due to longitudinal wrinkles, circular scars of roots and bud scales, sometimes roots attached, tip ends in a growing bud surrounded by a tufted crown of leaves (**Fig. 53.3**).

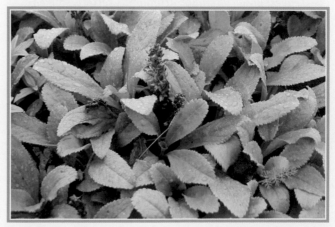

Fig. 53.1 Leaves.

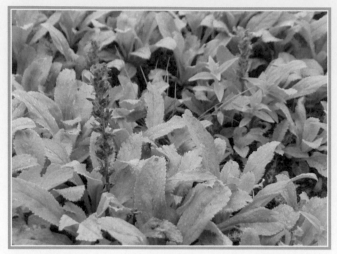

Fig. 53.2 Flower.

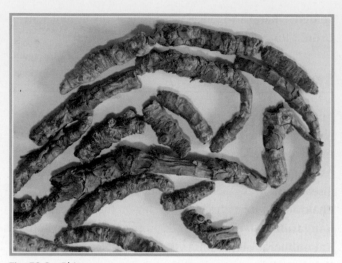

Fig. 53.3 Rhizome.

- **Root:** Thin, cylindrical, 5 to 10 cm long and 0.5 to 1.0 mm in diameter, straight or slightly curved with a few longitudinal wrinkles and dotted scars, mostly attached with rhizomes, dusty-gray; fracture short, inner surface black with whitish xylem (Anonymous 2007, 2008; Kirtikar and Basu 1999).

It is propagated by rhizomes.

Phenology

Flowering time: June to August
Fruiting time: September to November

Key Characters for Identification

➤ *It is a small, hairy, perennial herb, 15 to 25 cm tall.*
➤ *Leaves: Basal, alternate, acuminate, serrate, stalked, winged, oblanceolate, or narrowly spathulate; each leaf is 2 to 6 cm long and 0.5 to 1.2 cm wide.*
➤ *Flowers: White or pale purple color, and borne on a tall spike; calyx is generally five in number; corolla has four lobes, and bilabiate, stamens 4, stigma capitate.*
➤ *Fruits: Ovoid and swollen capsules, tapered at top, dehiscing into four valves and 6 to 10 mm long.*
➤ *Rhizome: Long, externally grayish-brown with longitudinal wrinkles and bitter in taste.*
➤ *Root stacks: Irregularly curved and thick as the little fingers.*

Rasapanchaka

Guna	Ruksha, Laghu
Rasa	Tikta
Vipak	Katu
Virya	Sheeta

Chemical Constituents

The active constituents are obtained from the root and rhizomes. The principal active constituent is known as "kutkin" and it is a mixture of kutkoside and picroside I, II, and III (bitter glycosides). Other identified active constituents are apocynin, drosin, and nine cucurbitacin glycosides (Weinges et al 1972; Stuppner and Wagner 1989; Singh and Rastogi 1972).

Apocynin is a catechol that has been shown to inhibit neutrophil oxidative burst in addition to being a powerful anti-inflammatory agent (Simons et al 1990) while the cucurbitacins have been shown to be highly cytotoxic and possess antitumor effects (Stuppner and Wagner 1989).

Nonbitter substance: kurrin, D-mannitol, vanillic acid, alcohol, kutkiol, sterol kutkisterol, kutkoside, minecoside, picrorhizin (Kumar et al 2013).

Identity, Purity, and Strength

- Foreign matter: Not more than 2%
- Total ash: Not more than 7%
- Acid-insoluble ash: Not more than 1%
- Alcohol-soluble extractive: Not less than 10%
- Water-soluble extractive: Not less than 20%

(Source: The Ayurvedic Pharmacopoeia of India 1999)

Karma (Actions)

The main actions of Katuki are bhedana (purgative), deepan (appetizer), pachana (digestive), hrudya (cardiotonic), krimighna (anthelmintic), jwaraghana (antipyretics), sthanya shodhan (purification of milk), and raktadosha shamak (pacify blood abnormalities).

- Doshakarma: Kaphapittahara
- Dhatukarma: Sthanya shodhan, raktadosha shamak
- Malakarma: Bhedana

Pharmacological Actions

It is most valued for its hepatoprotective effect, but it also shows anti-inflammatory, antioxidant, choleretic, and immunomodulatory actions. Other pharmacological actions are antipyretic, smooth muscle relaxant, antispasmodic, antiviral, antibacterial, cholagogue, hypocholesterolemic, antioxidant, free radical scavenger, antimicrobial, antihepatotoxic, antiasthmatic, digestive, antidiabetic, antiarthritic, hypolipemic effects. (Shetty et al 2010; Singh et al 1993; Sultan et al 2017).

Indications

It is mainly used in kamala (jaundice), prameha (diabetes), shwasa (asthma), kasa (cough), raktaja vikara (blood disorders like jaundice, anemia), daha (burning sensation), kaphaja vikara (diseases of kapha), arochaka (anorexia), visham jwara (intermittent fever), pittajwar (fever caused by pitta), visha (poisoning), hridroga (cardiac diseases), kushta (skin disease), and krimi (worm infestation).

Kutki is mainly known for its hepatoprotective properties. It is effective in jaundice, bile disorders, and other ailments of liver (Lee et al 2006).

The dried roots and rhizomes are used as hepatoprotective, immunomodulatory agent particularly for liver disorders and jaundice, fever, dysentery, and diarrhea (Anonymous 2007; Vaidya et al 1996). It is also useful in epilepsy, cough, swollen piles, leucoderma, and ascites (Rasool et al 2016).

P. kurroa rhizome powder was shown to be hepatoprotective in a double-blind clinical trial in patients with viral hepatitis (Vaidya et al 1996). An Ayurvedic formulation (Arogyavardhini Vati containing 50% *P. kurroa*) was also found effective in a double-blind trial in viral hepatitis.

Intervention with standardized plant extracts of *P. kurroa* regressed several features of nonalcoholic fatty liver diseases like lipid content of the liver tissue, morphological regression of fatty infiltration, hypolipidemic activity, and reduction of cholestasis (Shetty et al 2010).

Therapeutic Uses

1. **Kushta** (skin disease): Ativisha, Chandana, Katuki, and Usheera are given for the treatment of kushta (C.S.Ci-7/132).
2. **Hridroga** (heart disease): Yastimadhu and Katuki is given in kalka form (as paste) with sugar water (C.S.Ci-26/91).
3. **Pandu** (anemia): 10 g of Katuki and juice of Dronapuspi with sugar is applied as anjana (collyrium) and is snuffed with Devadali juice in the treatment of pandu (S.B-4/282).
4. **Jwara** (fever): Fine powder of Katuki mixed with sugar is used in pittaja jwara (fever caused by pitta) (A.S.Ci-1/76 & G.N.2.1.238). 10 g of Katuki mixed with sugar is given with warm water to cure kaphapittaja jwara (fever caused by kapha and pitta) (VM.1.128).
5. **Amlapitta** (hyperacidity): Katuki mixed with sugar is given to get relief from hyperacidity (VM.53/14).
6. **Sthanya shodhan** (purification of breast milk): Decoction of Katuki is given for the purification of breast milk (C.S.Ci.30/261-162).
7. **Hikka** (hic-cough): Gairik (Red-ochre) and Katuki are mixed and given in the treatment of hic-cough (S.S.U-50/27-28).

Officinal Part Used

Dried rhizomes

Dose

Powder: 500 mg to 1 g
For purgation: 3 to 6 g

Formulations

Arogyavardhini gutika, Tiktakadi kwath, Tiktaka ghrita, Katukadya taila, Sarvajvarahara lauha, Mahatikataka ghrita

Toxicity/Adverse Effects

Picrorhiza is not readily soluble in water while it is soluble in ethanol. The bitter taste of the drug makes tinctures unpalatable; it is therefore usually administered as a standardized (4% kutkin) encapsulated powder extract. Typical adult dosage is 400 to 1,500 mg/day. Sometimes, it is recommended in the dose of 3.5 g/day for fevers. No adverse effects of Picrorhiza root have been reported in India. The LD50 of kutkin is greater than 2,600 mg/kg in rats with no data available for humans (Annual Report 1989-1990).

Substitution and Adulteration

The rhizomes of Katuka are commonly adulterated with the stems and roots of the same plant. *Gentiana kurroa* Royle, *G. decumbens* Linn. f., *G. tenella* Fries, *Helleborus niger* Linn. are used as substitutes for Katuka (Raghunathan and Mitra 1982).

Roots of *P. scrophulariiflora* Pennell, *Actaea spicata*, *Cimicifuga foetida*, *Coptis teeta*, *Coscinium fenestratum*, *Swertia chirata* are sold in the drug market under the names Kutaki or Karu (Anonymous 2007).

Roots of *Lagotis glauca* Gaertn. are sometimes advertently collected and found mixed with the material obtained from Kashmir and Kullu regions (Sarin 1996).

Points to Ponder

- *Picrorhiza rhizome or "Indian gentian" is obtained from Picrorhiza kurroa.*
- *It is used in India to treat liver ailments, blood disorders, prameha, and kushta (skin diseases), etc.*
- *Swertia chirata (Kirata tikta) is sold in the market under the name Kutaki.*

Suggested Readings

Annual Report. India: Regional Research Laboratory, Council for Scientific and Industrial Research; 1989-1990

Anonymous. Agro Techniques of Some Selected Medicinal Plants, Vol. I. New Delhi: National Medicinal Plants Board, Department of AYUSH, Ministry of Health and Family Welfare, Government of India; 2008.

Anonymous. Convention on International Trade in Endangered Species of Wild Fauna and Flora. Fourteenth meeting of the Conference of the Parties, The Hague (Netherlands), CoP 14 Prop. 27;2007:1-14.

Anonymous. Pharmacopoeia of the People's Republic of China. Beijing: Chemical Industry Press; 2005.

Anonymous. The Ayurvedic Pharmacopoeia of India, Part I, Vol. 2. New Delhi: Department of AYUSH, Ministry of Health and Family Welfare, Government of India; 2007:91-93.

Aswal BS, Mehrotra BN. Taxonomic Notes on Picrorhiza and Neopicrorhiza; 1994:484-485

Bantawa P, Ghosh SK, Bhandari P, Singh B, Mondal T, Ghosh PD. Micropropagation of an elite line of *Picrorhiza scrophulariiflora*, Pennell: an endangered high valued medicinal plant of the Indo China Himalayan region. Med Aromat Plant Sci Biotechnol 2011;4(1):1-7

Chauhan NS. Medicinal and Aromatic Plants of Himachal Pradesh. New Delhi: Indus Publishing Company; 1999:306.

Chin YW, Balunas MJ, Chai HB, Kinghorn AD. Drug discovery from natural sources. AAPS J 2006;8(2):E239-E253

Coventry BO. Wild Flowers of Kashmir, Vol. 2. 1984, Dehradun: Bishen Singh Mahendra Pal Singh; 1927:89-90, pl. XLV.

Elizabeth WM. Major Herbs of Ayurveda. The Dabur Research foundation and Dabur Ayurvet Limited; 2002:220-222

Kirtikar KK, Basu BD. Indian Medicinal Plants. 2nd ed. International Book Distributors; 1999:1824-1826.

Kumar N, Kumar T, Sharma SK. Phytopharmacological review on genus *Picrorhiza*. Int J Universal Pharm Bio Sci 2013;2(4):334-347

Lee HS, Yoo CB, Ku SK. Hypolipemic effect of water extracts of *Picrorhiza kurroa* in high fat diet treated mouse. Fitoterapia 2006;77(7-8):579-584

Raghunathan K, Mitra R. Pharmacognosy of Indigenous Drugs, Vol. 1. New Delhi: Central Council for Research in Ayurveda and Siddha; 1982.

Rasool S, Khan MH, Hamid S, Sultan P, Qazi PH, Butt T. An overview and economical importance of few selected endangered medicinal plants grown in Jammu and Kashmir region of India. Ann Phytomed 2016;5(2):27-37

Sarin YK. Illustrated Manual of Herbal Drugs Used in Ayurveda. New Delhi: Indian Council of Scientific and Industrial Research; 1996:54

Shetty SN, Mengi S, Vaidya R, Vaidya AD. A study of standardized extracts of *Picrorhiza kurroa* Royle ex Benth in experimental nonalcoholic fatty liver disease. J Ayurveda Integr Med 2010; 1(3):203-210

Simons JM, Hart BA, Ip Vai Ching TR, Van Dijk H, Labadie RP. Metabolic activation of natural phenols into selective oxidative burst agonists byactivated human neutrophils. Free Radical Bio and Med 1990;8:251-258

Singh B, Rastogi RP. Chemical examination of *Picrorhiza kurroa* Benth. Part VI. Reinvestigation of kutkin. Indian J Chem 1972; 10:29–31

Singh GB, Bani S, Singh S, et al. Anti-inflammatory activity of the iridoids Kutkin, Picroside-1 and Kutkoside from *Picrorhiza kurroa*. Phytother Res 1993;7:402–407

Stuppner H, Wagner H. New cucurbitacin glycosides from *Picrorhiza kurroa*. Planta Med 1989;55(6):559–563

Sultan P, Rasool S, Hassan QP. *Picrorhiza kurroa* Royle ex Benth: a plant of diverse pharmacological potential. Ann Phytomed 2017; 6(1):63–67

Uniyal SK, Singh KN, Jamwal P, Lal B. Traditional use of medicinal plants among the tribal communities of Chhota Bhangal, Western Himalaya. J Ethnobiol Ethnomed 2006;2:14

Vaidya AB, Antarkar DS, Doshi JC, et al. *Picrorhiza kurroa* (Kutaki) Royle ex Benth as a hepatoprotective agent: experimental & clinical studies. J Postgrad Med 1996;42(4):105–108

Weinges K, Kloss P, Henkels WD. Natural products from medicinal plants. XVII. Picroside-II, a new 6-vanilloyl-catapol from *Picrorhiza kurroa* Royle and Benth. Justus Liebigs Ann Chem 1972;759: 173–182

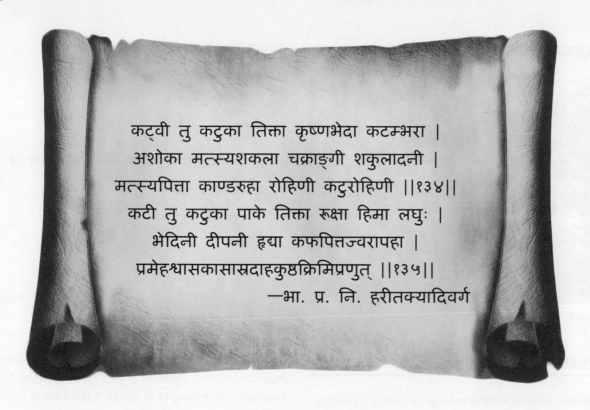

कट्वी तु कटुका तिक्ता कृष्णभेदा कटम्भरा ।
अशोका मत्स्यशकला चक्राङ्गी शकुलादनी ।
मत्स्यपित्ता काण्डरुहा रोहिणी कटुरोहिणी ॥१३४॥
कटी तु कटुका पाके तिक्ता रूक्षा हिमा लघुः ।
भेदिनी दीपनी हृद्या कफपित्तज्वरापहा ।
प्रमेहश्वासकासास्रदाहकुष्ठक्रिमिप्रणुत् ॥१३५॥
—भा. प्र. नि. हरीतक्यादिवर्ग

54. Khadir [*Acacia catechu* (Linn.f.) Willd.]

Family:	*Fabaceae*
Hindi name:	*Khair, Khaira*
English name:	*Cutch tree, Black catechu*

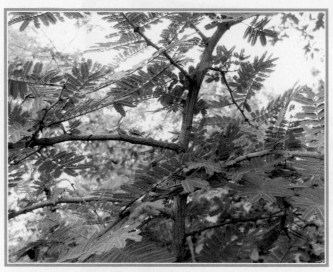

Plant of *Acacia catechu* (Linn.f.) Willd.

Khadir is praised as "Filler of Wound" in Atharva Veda.

Introduction

Khadir (*Acacia catechu* Willd.) belongs to family "Fabaceae" and its subfamily is "Mimosoideae." It is also known as black catechu. The generic name "acacia" comes from the Greek word "akis," meaning a point or a barb. The species name comes from "cutch," a tanning extract isolated from its heartwood. It alleviates the diseases and stabilizes the body and provides strength to the teeth that is why it is called Khadir.

Khadir is considered as best drug for kushta or skin disease as per Ayurveda (C.S.Su. 25/40). The plant is useful internally as well as externally. It is mainly used in skin disorders, itching problems, diseases of teeth, diseases of mouth and throat, cough, obesity, and worms.

A. catechu is a multipurpose tree species. The heartwood of the tree is mainly used for extracting katha and cutch (decoction obtained after filtration), which are sold in the market. Katha is commonly used in Ayurvedic preparations.

Besides this, it serves as one of the major components in masticatory, i.e., chewing of betel leaf (pan) in India and Pakistan (Sangthong et al 2012). It is useful in dental, oral, throat infections and as an astringent for reducing oozing from chronic ulcers and wounds. It dries up the mucous secretions and regains the taste sensation (Sani et al 2012).

Heartwood extract of Khadir is also used as a preservative for fishing nets, dyeing, and leather tanning and as a viscosity regulator for oil drilling (Roy et al 2011). Wood of Khadira is used as firewood and in furniture manufacturing also.

Vernacular Names

Assamese: Kharira, Khara, Khayar
Bengali: Khera, Khayera
Gujarati: Khair, Kathe, Kher
Kannada: Kaggali, Kaggalinara, Kachinamara, Koggigida
Kashmiri: Kath
Malayalam: Karingali

Marathi: Khaira, Khair
Oriya: Khaira
Punjabi: Khair
Tamil: Karungali, Karungkali
Telugu: Chandra, Kaviri
Urdu: Chanbe Kaath

Synonyms

Bahusara: The heartwood is strong and firm.
Bahushalya: The plant bears many thorns.
Balapatra: Leaves or leaflets are very small.
Dantadhavana: Twigs of this plant are used as tooth brush for teeth cleaning.
Galaroganut: It is useful in throat diseases.
Gayatri: It gives protection to the voice or throat of singers.
Jihwashalya: The spine is curved.
Kantaki: It is a wild, thorny tree.
Kanthi: It is beneficial for the throat.
Khadir: It alleviates the diseases and stabilizes the body. It also provides strength to the teeth.
Kustaghni: It is considered as a specific drug for the treatment of kushta (leprosy).
Kustari: It is used in the treatment of kushta.
Medoghna: It cures obesity.
Raktasara: The heartwood is red colored.
Saradruma: The heartwood is strong and firm.
Vakrakanta: It has hooked spines.
Yajngiya: Wood is regarded as holy and used in sacrifices.

Classical Categorization

Charak Samhita: Kustaghna, Udardaprasamana, Mutrasangrahaniya
Sushruta Samhita: Salasaradi
Dhanvantari Nighantu: Guduchyadi varga
Madanpal Nighantu: Vatadi varga
Kaiyedev Nighantu: Aushadhi varga
Raj Nighantu: Shalmalyadi varga
Bhavaprakash Nighantu: Vatadi varga

Distribution

It is common in the sub-Himalayan tract and outer Himalayas ascending from 900 to 1,200 m from Jammu to Assam. It is found widely in Jammu, Punjab, Himachal Pradesh, Uttar Pradesh, Madhya Pradesh, Bihar, Andhra Pradesh, and Odisha (Anonymous 1985).

This plant is native to India, Myanmar, Nepal, Pakistan, and Thailand but now-a-days it is also cultivated in Indonesia, Kenya, and Mozambique.

Morphology

It is a small- to moderate-sized deciduous tree, 9 to 12 m in height.

- **Bark:** The bark is dark gray and rough with short hooked spines. The branches are thin and spike-like because tiny thorns grow around the exterior (**Fig. 54.1**).
- **Leaves:** Bipinnate compound leaves, 30 to 40 pairs of leaflets, main rachis pubescent with a large gland near the middle of rachis; leaflets are very small (**Fig. 54.2**).
- **Flowers:** White to pale yellow, sessile, found in 5 to 10 cm peduncle axillary spikes. Pentamerous with a campanulate calyx, 11.5 mm long, and a corolla 2.5 to 3 mm long; stamens are numerous and far exerted from the corolla, with white or yellowish-white filaments (**Fig. 54.3**).
- **Fruits:** 5 to 12 cm long flat brown pods, shiny and with a triangular peak at the apex and narrowed at base (**Fig. 54.4**).

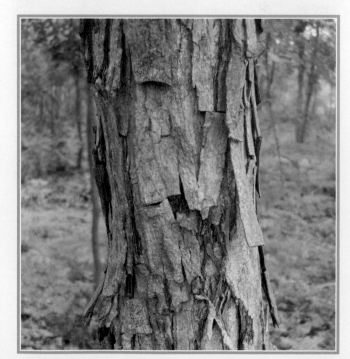

Fig. 54.1 Bark.

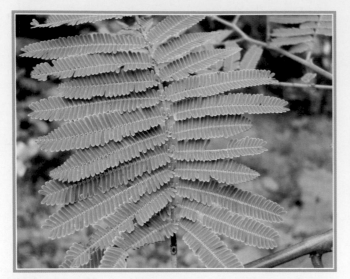

Fig. 54.2 Leaves.

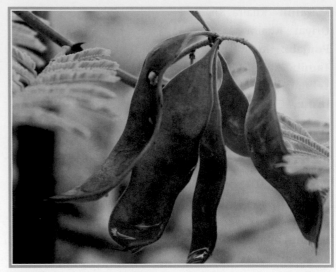

Fig. 54.4 Fruits.

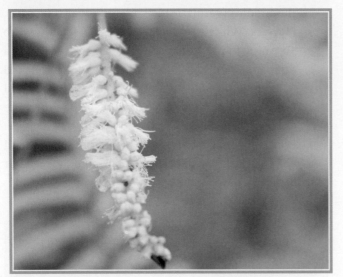

Fig. 54.3 Flowers.

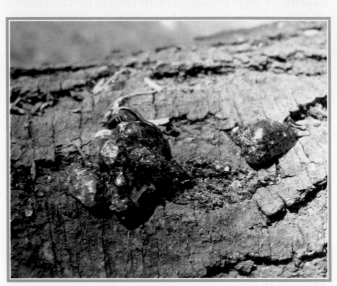

Fig. 54.5 Gum.

- **Seeds:** 3 to 10 seeds per pod, broadly ovoid.
- The gummy extract of the wood is called katha or cutch (**Fig. 54.5**). The sap wood of this plant is large and yellowish-white and heart wood is small and red in color (Saini et al 2008; Guleria et al 2011).

It can be propagated through its seeds.

Phenology

Flowering time: August to October
Fruiting time: November to February

Key Characters for Identification

➤ It is a small- to moderate-sized deciduous tree, 9 to 12 m tall.
➤ The bark is dark gray and rough with short hooked spines.
➤ Leaves: Bipinnate, 30 to 40 pairs of leaflets, leaflets are very small.
➤ Inflorescence: Axillary pedunculate spike.
➤ Flowers: Scented flowers, creamy white.
➤ Fruits: 5 to 12 cm long flat brown pods, shiny and with a triangular peak at the apex, and narrowed at base, 3 to 10 seeded.
➤ Heart wood: Small and red in color.

Types

Dhanwantari Nighantu described two types of Khadir: Khadir and Somavalka (also known as Kadar). As per Bhavaprakash Nighantu, it is of three types: Khadir (*A. catechu*), Shweta khadir/Kadara (*Acacia suma* kurg), and Irimeda/Vit khadir (*Acacia farnaciana* Willd.). Five types of Khadir are mentioned in Raj Nighantu: Khadir, Somavalka, Tamrakantaka/Rakta Khadir, Vit Khadir, and Irimeda.

In India, there are three varieties of *A. catechu*, namely, catechu, catechuoides, and Sundra catechu (*Acacia sundra*). These are commercially used to obtain katha (a concentrated filtered extract) in North India. *A. catechu* is widely distributed in Jammu, Punjab, Himachal Pradesh, Uttar Pradesh, Madhya Pradesh, Bihar, Andhra Pradesh, and Odisha. *A. catechuoides* is found in terrain region of Sikkim, Assam, and West Bengal, whereas *A. sundra*, generally known as Lal Khair (red catechu), is found in Deccan, Gujarat, Rajasthan, and southern Maharashtra (Anonymous 1985).

Rasapanchaka

Guna	Laghu, Ruksha
Rasa	Tikta, Kasaya
Vipak	Katu
Virya	Sheeta
Prabhav	Kustaghna

Chemical Constituents

Major chemical constituents of *A. catechu* are catechin, epicatechin, epicatechin gallate, procatechinic acid, tannins, alkaloids, quercetin and kaempferol, and porifera sterol glucosides. (+)-Afzelechin gum is also present in minor quantity.

- Heartwood: Flavanoids: Catechin, (-)epicatechin, epigallocatechin, epicatechin gallate, epigallocatechin gallate, rocatechin, phloroglucinol, procatechuic acid, catecutannin acid, quercetin, quercitrin
- Leaves: Alkaloids, kaempferol, dihydrokaempferol, taxifolin, (+)-afzelchin gum
- Bark: Glycosides: Poriferasterol, poriferasterol acylglucosides
- Tannin: Gallic acids, phlebotannin

- Sugar: D-galactose, d-rhamnose, I- arabinose (Lakshmi et al 2011; Singh and Lal 2006).

Identity, Purity, and Strength

- Foreign matter: Not more than 2%
- Total ash: Not more than 2%
- Acid-insoluble ash: Not more than 1.2%
- Alcohol-soluble extractive: Not less than 1%
- Water-soluble extractive: Not less than 3%

(Source: The Ayurvedic Pharmacopoeia of India 1989)

Karma (Actions)

The main actions of Khadir are kustaghna (antileprotic), kandughna (antipruritic), kasaghna (anticough), medoghna (antiobesity), krimighna (anthelmintic), pachan (digestive), ruchivardhaka (appetizer), stambhana (astringent), shoni-tasthapana (hemostatics), mutrasangrahana (urinary astringent), vrana ropaka (wound healing), raktashodhaka (useful as blood purifier), kaphapittahara (alleviates kapha and pitta dosha), and dantya (beneficial for teeth) (Sharma et al 2000).

- Doshakarma: Kaphapittashamak
- Dhatukarma: Medoghna
- Malakarma: Mutrasangrahana

Pharmacological Actions

Catechin which is found in Khadir is biologically highly active and it is used as a hemostatic. Another important constituent is taxifolin and it has antibacterial, antifungal, antiviral, anti-inflammatory, and antioxidant activities. Other important pharmacological properties of *A. catechu* are wound healing, anticancer, antimicrobial, antidiarrheal, antimicrobial, hypoglycemic, immunomodulatory, antipyretic, antisecretory, antidiabetic, hepatoprotective, antimycotic, and antiulcer (Lakshmi et al 2011). It possesses anthelmintic, antidysenteric, and antipyretic and hypotensive properties (Sham 1984).

Indications

It is mainly used in kushta (leprosy), krimi (worm infestation), kandu (itching), prameha (diabetes), jwara (fever), vrana (wound), aruchi (anorexia), sthaulya (obesity), switra (leucoderma), shotha (swelling), raktapitta (hemorrhagic disease), pandu (anemia), kaphaja vikara (diseases of kapha), kasa (cough), arsha (piles), bhagandara (fistula-in-ano), atisara (diarrhea), kaphaja kasa (cough caused by kapha), twakaroga (skin diseases), jeernajwara (chronic fever), etc.

The bark, wood extracts, fruits, gum, and flowering tops of *A. catechu* are used for medicinal purpose. The plant is used both internally and externally. It is also used in melancholia, conjunctivitis, hemoptysis, chest pain, asthma, colicky pain, gravel, bronchitis, etc. (Joshi 2000).

Khadir is one of the most potent drugs used for various skin diseases. Khadirarista is a famous preparation used for that purpose. Decoction prepared from this plant is extremely beneficial in vaginal diseases, leucorrhea, menorrhagia, etc. Khadira and Yastimadhu helps in healing the wounds and ulcers in vaginal and anal mucosa. Decoction prepared with bark of Khadir and Triphala is given with ghee and Vidanga powder in anal fistula. The decoction of Khadira and Amalaki is used with Bakuchi powder in skin infections caused due to kapha dosha (Lakshmi et al 2011).

A. catechu is used in treating skin disorders, itching problems, diseases of teeth, diseases of mouth and throat, cough, obesity, worms, diabetes, fever, vitiligo, swelling, wound, bleeding disorders, anemia, eruptive boils, filaria, and is also used as rasayana (longevity enhancer).

Contraindication

The use of *A. catechu* is contraindicated in pregnant or breast-feeding women and patients undergoing immuno-suppressive therapy.

Therapeutic Uses

External Use

1. **Gum bleeding:** It is used externally as a powder to check bleeding from gums.
2. **Twak roga** (skin diseases): The bath of its decoction is an effective panacea for various skin affections. The paste is used externally in skin eruption, boils, ulcer, and wounds.
3. **Swar bheda** (sore throat): The popular preparation Khadiradi gutika is beneficial for chewing in sore throat,

hoarseness of voice, and tonsillitis due to vitiation of kapha doshas. The decoction is an effective gargle in sore throat, cough, and hoarseness of voice.

Internal Use

1. **Kushta** (leprosy): The decoction of Khadira is used as drink, to sprinkle, in tub-bath, etc. (S.S.Ci.9/5). Khadira is the best drug for all types of kushta (C.S.Su. 25/40). Khadira and Bijaka remove all types of kushta (S.S.Ci-6/19). Heartwood of Khadir is used in all types of kushta (A.H.U. 40/50).
2. **Sweta kushta** (vitiligo): Whatever remedies are prescribed for kushta are also applicable for sweta kushta. Out of these decoctions, Khadira is the best medicine for using both externally and internally in vitiligo (C.S.Ci-7/166).
3. **Twak roga** (skin diseases): Decoction of Khadira is used as kalka (paste), lepa (ointment), bath, food, and drink in all types of skin diseases (VM-51/74).
4. **Prameha** (shanaimeha and madhumeha): Khadira kasaya and Khadira Kramuka kasaya are used in shanaimeha and madhumeha, respectively (S.S.Ci- 11/6-9).
5. **Vranashodhan** (wound cleaning): Decoction of Triphala, Khadir, Daruharidra, Nyagrodhadi, Bala, Kush, and Nimba leaves is used for cleaning of wounds (C.S.Ci-25/84).
6. **Danta roga** (diseases of teeth): Decoction of Khadira, Yavani, or root of Neem relieves dental disease (Harita Samhita 3/46.14).
7. **Mukha roga** (diseases of oral cavity): Khadiradi gutika and taila are given for diseases of mouth (C.S.Ci.26/199-207).
8. **Shlipada** (filaria): Paste of heart wood of Khadir, Bijaka, and Sala mixed with honey is taken with cow's urine in morning to cure filariasis (GN.4.2.42).

Officinal Parts Used

Bark, wood extracts, fruits, gum, and flowering tops of *A. catechu.*

Dose

Bark powder: 1 to 3 g
Decoction: 50 to 100 mL
Khadirsara: 0.5 to 1 g

Formulations

Khadiradi vati, Khadirastaka, Khadirarista, Khadiradi kwath, Nagabala rasayana, Brahma rasayana, Indrokta rasayana, Chandandi taila, Madhwasava, Kanakabindu arishta, Khadira ghrita, Maha khadira ghrita, Khadiradi gutika taila, Erimedadi Taila, Lavangadi vati, Kanakabindu arishta, Samvardhana ghrita, etc.

Points to Ponder

- *Khadir is considered as best drug for kushta (skin disease; C.S.Su. 25/40).*
- *As per Bhavaprakash Nighantu, it is of three types: Khadir (Acacia catechu), Shweta khadir/Kadara (Acacia suma kurg.), and Irimeda/Vit khadir (Acacia farnesiana Willd.).*
- *Khadir is mainly used in skin disorders, itching problems, diseases of teeth, diseases of mouth and throat, cough, obesity, worms, diabetes, fever, vitiligo, swelling, wound, bleeding disorders, anemia, eruptive boils, filariasis.*

Suggested Readings

13. Singh KN, Lal B. Notes on traditional uses of khair (*Acacia catechu* Willd.) by inhabitants of Shivalik range in Western Himalaya. Ethnobotan Leafl 2006;10:109–112.

Anonymous. The Wealth of India: Raw Materials, Vol. I-A (Rev.). New Delhi: CSIR;1985:24-30.

Catechu Natural Medicine and Comprehensive Database, hptt://naturaldatabase.therapeuticresearch.com

Guleria S, Tiku A, Singh G, Vyas D, Bhardwaj A. Antioxidant activity and protective effect against plasmid DNA strand scission of leaf, bark, and heartwood extracts from *Acacia catechu*. J Food Sci 2011;76(7):C959–C964

Joshi SH. Medicinal Plant. New Delhi: Oxford and IBH Pub Co Pvt Ltd;2000:271

Lakshmi T, Geetha RV, Anitha R. In vitro evaluation of antibacterial activity of heartwood extract of *Acacia catechu* willd. Int J Pharm Bio Sci 2011; 2(2):188

Roy A, Geetha RV, Lakshmi T. In vitro evaluation of anti mycotic activity of heartwood extract of *Acacia catechu* Willd. J Pharm Res 2011;4(7):1–2

Saini ML, et al. Comparative pharmacognostical and antimicrobial studies of *Acacia* species (Mimosaceae). J Med Plants Res 2008; 2(12):378–386

Sangthong S, Pintathong P, Chaiwut P. Comparison of microwave-assisted methods on extraction of cosmetic bioactivities from *Areca catechu* L. In: Proceeding of International Conference; 2012: 271–274.

Sani IM, Iqbal S, Chan KW, Ismail M. Effect of acid and base catalyzed hydrolysis on the yield of phenolics and antioxidant activity of extracts from germinated brown rice (GBR). Molecules 2012; 17:7584–7594

Sham JS. Hypotensive effect of *Acacia catechu*. Planta Med 1984;50(2): 177–180

Sharma PC, Yelne MB, Denni TJ. Database on Medicinal Plants Used in Ayurveda, Vol. 1. New Delhi: Central Council For Research in Ayurveda and Siddha, Department of ISM & H, Ministry of Health & Family Welfare, Government of India;2000:216–224.

The Ayurvedic Pharmacopoeia of India, Part I, Vol. 1. New Delhi: Department of AYUSH, Ministry of Health & Family Welfare, Government of India; 1989:70

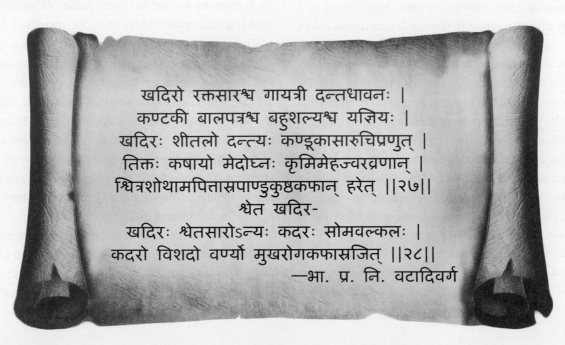

खदिरो रक्तसारश्च गायत्री दन्तधावनः |
कण्टकी बालपत्रश्च बहुशल्यश्च यज्ञियः |
खदिरः शीतलो दन्त्यः कण्डूकासारुचिप्रणुत् |
तिक्तः कषायो मेदोघ्नः कृमिमेहज्वरव्रणान् |
श्वित्रशोथामपित्तास्रपाण्डुकुष्ठकफान् हरेत् ||२७||
श्वेत खदिर-
खदिरः श्वेतसारोऽन्यः कदरः सोमवल्कलः |
कदरो विशदो वर्ण्यो मुखरोगकफास्रजित् ||२८||
—भा. प्र. नि. वटादिवर्ग

55. Kiratatikta [*Swertia chirayita* (Roxb. ex Fleming) H. Karst.]

Family:	*Gentianaceae*
Hindi name:	*Chirayata*
English name:	*Chireta*

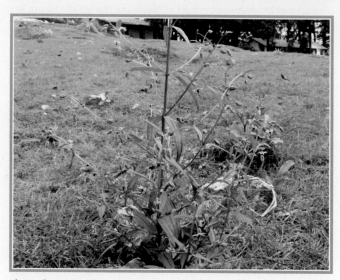

Plant of *Swertia chirayita* (Roxb. ex Fleming) H. Karst.

> *S. chirayita was first described by Roxburgh under the name of Gentiana chirata in 1814.*
>
> —*Scartezzini and Speroni (2000)*

Introduction

Swertia chirayita (Syn: *Swertia chirata*, Buch.-Ham) is a medicinal plant belonging to the family Gentianaceae. It is an important medicinal plant aboriginal to clement Himalayas in India, Nepal, and Bhutan. In India, 40 species of *Swertia* are recorded (Clarke 1885; Kirtikar and Basu 1984), of which *S. chirayita* is considered the most important for its medicinal properties. Its medicinal usage is declared in American and British pharmacopoeias, Indian Pharmaceutical codex (Joshi and Dhawan 2005) and in different conventional systems of medicines like Ayurvedic, Unani, and Siddha. In India, it is known as Chirayata. It is found in high altitude areas of Himalayas, particularly in kirata region (north east) and is bitter in taste; hence it is called Kiratatikta.

The plant is used as a bitter tonic in treatment of fever, liver disorders, and for curing various skin diseases. *S. chirayita* has an established domestic (Indian) and international market, which is increasing at a rate of 10% annually. The increasing national and international demand for *S. chirayita* has led to unscrupulous collection from the wild and adulteration of supplies. The increasing high usage of *S. chirayita*, mostly the underground tissues, as well as the illegal overharvesting combined with habitat destruction resulted in a drastic reduction of its populations and has brought this plant to the verge of extinction. According to the International Union of Conservation of Nature (IUCN) criteria, *S. chirayita* conservation status has been categorized as "critically endangered" (Joshi and Dhawan 2005). *S. chirayita* is among the 32 most highly prioritized medicinal plants of India as identified by The National Medicinal Plant Board, Government of India.

The current speed of extinction through human interferences is estimated to be approximately 100 to 1,000 times faster than the natural speed of extinction (Chapin et al 2000). Due to its excessive overexploitation from the natural habitat, narrow geographic occurrence (Bhat et al 2013), and unresolved inherent problems of seed viability and seed germination (Badola and Pal 2002; Joshi and Dhawan 2005), alternative approaches for propagation and conservation are urgently required to avoid the possible extinction of this important species. Good conservation practices and sustainable supply of raw drug is very much essential to conserve this critically endangered medicinal plant.

This will require innovative tools that utilize biotechnological interventions, including micropropagation under a controlled environment, cryopreservation, and bioreactors, for the conservation as well as for raising commercial production (Kumar and Van Staden 2015).

Vernacular Names

Arabic: Qasabuzzarirah
Bengali: Chireta
Burma: Sekhagi
Deccan: Charayatah
Gujarati: Chirayata
Kannada: Nilavebu
Malayalam: Nilaveppu
Marathi: Chirayita
Nepal: Cherata
Punjabi: Charaita
Persian: Nenilawandi, Qasabuzzarirah
Tamil: Nilavembu, Shirattakuchi
Telugu: Nilavembu
Urdu: Chiarayata

Synonyms

Anaryatikta: It is found in kirata region (north east) and has bitter taste.
Bhunimba: It is a small herb having bitter taste like Nimba.
Haima: It grows on high altitudes of Himalaya.
Kairata: It is found in kirata region (north east) and has bitter taste.
Kandatikta: Its stem is bitter.
Katutiktaka: It has katu tikta (pungent and bitter) taste.
Kirata: It is found in kirata region (north east) and has bitter taste.

Kiratatiktaka: It is found in high altitude areas of Himalaya, particularly in kirata region (north east) and it is bitter in taste.
Ramasenaka: It is found in kirata region (north east) and has bitter taste.

Classical Categorization

Charak Samhita: Stanya Shodhana, Trishna Nigrahana
Sushruta Samhita: Aragwadhadi
Dhanwantari Nighantu: Guduchyadi varga
Madanpal Nighantu: Abhayadi varga
Kaiyadev Nighantu: Aushadhi varga
Raj Nighantu: Prabhadradi varga
Bhavaprakash: Haritakyadi varga

Distribution

It is a critically endangered medicinal herb indigenous to the mountainous districts of northern India growing at high altitude in the subtemperate region of Himalayas in between 1,200 and 3,000 m from Kashmir to Bhutan and in Khasi hills in Meghalaya at 1,200 to 1,500 m (Joshi and Dhawan 2005; Anonymous 2007; Kirtikar and Basu 1984; Clarke 1885). It can be grown in subtemperate regions between 1,500 and 2,100 m altitudes (Bentley and Trimen 1880).

Morphology

It is an annual or biannual erect herb of 0.5 to 1.5 m height.

- **Stem:** Two to three feet long, middle portion is cylindrical while upper portion is quadrangular, orange brown or purplish in color (**Fig. 55.1**).
- **Leaves:** Simple, opposite, sessile, lanceolate, apex is acuminate whereas base is cordate, five to seven nerved, and 4 cm long (**Fig. 55.2**).
- **Flowers:** Small numerous, tetramerous, large leafy panicles, greenish-yellow color and tinged with purple or white hairs. The calyx is gamophyllous with four lobes, corolla-lobes four twisted and superimposed, united at the base where they have pairs of nectaries on each lobe covered with long hairs. Four stamens, opposite the corolla lobe, at the base of the corolla.

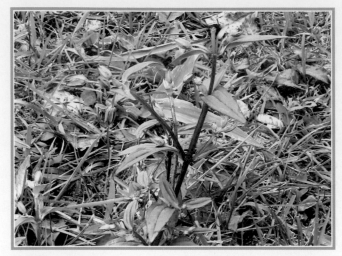

Fig. 55.1 Stem.

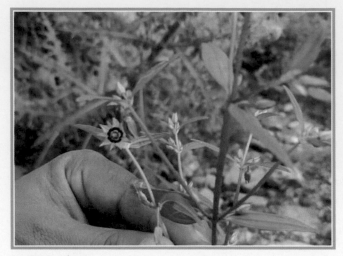

Fig. 55.3 Flowers.

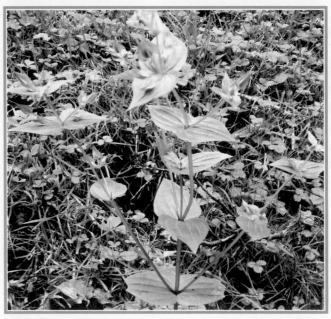

Fig. 55.2 Leaves.

Phenology

Flowering time: July to September
Fruiting time: September to November

Key Characters for Identification
➤ It is an annual or biannual erect herb of 0.5 to 1.5 m height.
➤ Stem: Orange brown or purplish in color.
➤ Leaves: Simple, opposite, sessile, lanceolate, apex is acuminate, cordate base.
➤ Flowers: Small numerous, tetramerous, large leafy panicles, greenish-yellow color.
➤ Fruits: Egg-shaped capsule, two-valved with dark brownish numerous seeds, dehiscent.
➤ Root: Small, light brown, twisted, and tapering root.

Ovary unilocular with ovules laminal placentation parietal, two stigmas (**Fig. 55.3**).

- **Fruits:** Egg-shaped capsule, two-valved with a transparent yellowish pericarp, dehiscent.
- **Seeds:** Numerous, very small, dark brownish color.
- **Root:** The roots are generally small, 5 to 10 cm in length, light brown, somewhat twisted, and gradually tapering (Scartezzini and Speroni 2000; Chandra et al 2012; Joshi and Dhawan 2005; Bentley and Trimen 1880).

Seeds should be sown in nursery and seedlings transplanted later in the field (Anonymous 1992).

Rasapanchaka

Guna	Laghu, Ruksha
Rasa	Tikta
Vipak	Katu
Virya	Sheeta

Chemical Constituents

The major phytoconstituents are amarogentin (chirantin), swertiamarin, amaroswerin, gentianin, swerchirin, xanthones, mangiferin, lignan, triterpenoids, pentacyclic triterpenoids, gentiocrucine, lupeol, swertanone, terxerol, β-amyrine, β-sitosterol, sweroside, amaroswerin, and gentiopicrin (Kumar et al 2015).

Identity, Purity, and Strength

- Foreign matter: Not more than 2%
- Total ash: Not more than 6%
- Acid-insoluble ash: Not more than 1%
- Alcohol-soluble extractive: Not less than 10%
- Water-soluble extractive: Not less than 10%

(Source: The Ayurvedic Pharmacopeia of India 1989)

Karma (Actions)

The main actions of Kiratatikta are sara (laxative), jwaraghna (antipyretics), sthanyashodhan (galactopurifier), kushtaghna (antileprotic), deepan (appetizer), pachan (digestive), raktadoshahara (blood purifier), vranashodhana (wound cleansing), trishnanashak (antithirst).

- Doshakarma: Kapha pittahara
- Dhatukarma: Raktadoshahara
- Malakarma: Sara (Virechana)

Pharmacological Actions

The main pharmacological actions of Kiratatikta are antibacterial, antifungal, antiviral, antioxidant, anti-inflammatory, hypoglycemic, antidiabetic, antimalarial, hepatoprotective, antileishmanial, anticarcinogenic, anthelmintic, antipyretic, antidiarrheal, anti-HIV, CNS depressant, mutagenicity, antileprosy, anticholinergic, antihepatitis-B virus, dyslipidemia, gastroprotective, wound healing, anesthetics, antihistaminic, anticonvulsant, hypotensive, antipsychotic, diuretic, chemopreventive (Aleem and Kabir 2018).

Indications

It is used in sannipatika jwara, shwasa (asthma), kasha (cough), shotha (swelling), trishna (thirst), daha (burning sensation), kushta (skin diseases), prameha (diabetes), jwara (fever), vrana (wound), krimi (worm infestation), raktaja vikara (blood diseases), etc.

It is used to cure ulcers, gastrointestinal diseases, skin diseases, cough, hiccup, liver and kidney diseases, neurological disorders, and urogenital tract disorders. It is also used to purify breast milk and for laxative and carminative purpose (Garg 1965; Sharma 1986).

The wide range of medicinal uses include the treatment of chronic fever, malaria, anemia, bronchial asthma, hepatotoxic disorders, liver disorders, hepatitis, gastritis, constipation, dyspepsia, skin diseases, worms, epilepsy, ulcers, scanty urine, hypertension, melancholia, and certain types of mental disorders, secretion of bile, blood purification, and diabetes (Karan et al 1999; Banerjee et al 2000; Rai et al 2000; Saha et al 2004; Chen et al 2011).

Therapeutic Uses

External Use

1. **Vrana** (wound): Decoction of Kiratatikta is used for cleansing of wound (Sharma 1986).
2. **Vispotaka** (eruptive boils): Bhunimbadi Kashaya is used in vispotaka (G.N/2.40.66).

Internal Use

1. **Jwar** (fever): Hot infusion of Kiratatikta is given with leaves of Dhanyaka to alleviate fever quickly (S.B. 4/32).
2. **Sthanya shodhana** (purification of breast milk): Decoction of Kiratatikta is administered to purify breast milk (C.S.Ci. 30/261-262).
3. **Chhardi** (vomiting): Paste of Kiratatikta is given along with honey and sugar to get relief from nausea and vomiting (H.S. 3.51.6).
4. **Shotha** (edema): Paste of Kiratatikta and Shunthi is taken to cure tridoshajanya chronic edema (C.S.Ci. 12/42).
5. **Sarvanga Shotha** (whole body edema/anasarca): Intake of paste of Kiratatikta and Shunthi followed by Punarnava kwatha removes generalized edema (V.M. 39/17).
6. **Raktapitta** (intrinsic hemorrhage): Kiratatikta, Kramuka, Musta, etc. are separately mixed with sandal and administered in raktapitta (C.S.Ci. 4/79).

Officinal Part Use

Panchanga (whole plant)

The whole plant is used in traditional remedies but the root is mentioned to be the most bioactive part (Kirtikar and Basu 1984).

Dose

Powder: 1 to 3 g
Decoction: 50 to 100 mL

Formulations

Important formulations of Kiratatikta are Sudarshana churna, Kiratadi kwatha, Bhunimbadi kwatha, Chandanasava, Lodhrasava, Chandraprabhavati, Sarvajwara lauha.

Proprietary medicines such as ayush-64, diabecon, mensturyl syrup, and melicon V ointment 2–4 contain Chirata extracts in different amounts for its antipyretic, hypoglycemic, antifungal, and antibacterial properties.

Toxicity/Adverse Effects

So far, no serious side effects or toxicity of *S. chirayita* have been reported, but further toxicological studies are still needed to confirm the safety of *S. chirayita* in humans. Efforts are required for further studies, especially evaluating its biological activities in vivo and toxicological and mutagenic properties in order to better validate the safety of these different plant-derived compounds (Kumar and Van Staden 2015).

Substitution and Adulteration

Many species of *Swertia* of Gentianaceae family are used as substitution of Kiratatikta which are mentioned as under:

- *S. purpurascens* Wall
- *S. decussata* Nimmo Gah
- *S. chinensis* Franchet
- *S. paniculata* Wall
- *S. parennis* Linn
- *S. corymbosa* Wight
- *S. affinis* Clerke
- *Enicostemma littorale* Blume
- *S. lawii* Burkill

- *Exacum bicolor* Roxb.
- *Erythraea roxburghii* G. Don.
- *Exacum tetragonum* Roxb

(Source: Aleem and Kabir 2018; Joshi and Dhawan 2005; Kumar et al 2017).

Adulterants

Following drugs are adulterated in the name of Chirayata.

- *S. angustifolia* Buch (Fam: Gentianaceae)
- *S. alata* Royle ex D.Don (Fam: Gentianaceae)
- *Andrographis paniculata* Nees (Fam: Acanthacea)
- *Rubia cordifolia* Linn. (Fam: Rubiaceae)

The true chirata can be distinguished from other substitutes and adulterants by its intense bitterness, brownish-purple stem (dark color), continuous yellowish pith, and petals with double nectaries (Verma and Kumar 2001).

Points to Ponder

- *Bhunimba is the synonym used for both Kiratatikta and Kalmegh.*
- *Kiratatikta is a critically endangered medicinal herb.*
- *It is used for fever, skin disease, cough, asthma, diabetes, etc.*

Suggested Readings

Aleem A and Kabir H. Review on *Swertia chirata* as traditional uses to its phytochemistry and pharmacological activity. J Drug Deliv Ther. 2018;8(5-s):73–78

Anonymous. The Unani Pharmacopoeia of India, CCRUM, Vol. 2. New Delhi: Department of AYUSH, Ministry of Health & Family Welfare, Government of India, Seema Offset Press, 1992:117–125

Anonymous. The Unani Pharmacopoeia of India. New Delhi: Rakmo Press, CCRUM, Department of AYUSH, Ministry of Health and Family Welfare, Government of India; 2007.

Badola HK, Pal M. Endangered medicinal plants in Himachal Pradesh. Curr Sci 2002;83(7):797–798

Banerjee S, Sur TP, Das PC, and Sikdar S. Assessment of the anti-inflammatory effects of *Swertia chirata* in acute and chronic experimental models in male albino rats. Indian J. Pharmacol. 2000;32:21–24

Bentley R and Trimen H, eds. Medicinal plants. London: J and A Churchill, 1880:183

Bhat AJ, Kumar M, Negi AK, Todaria NP. Informants' consensus on ethnomedicinal plants in Kedarnath Wildlife Sanctuary of Indian Himalayas. J Med Plants Res 2013;7:148–154

Chandra S, Kumar V, Bandopadhyay R, and Sharma MM. SEM and elemental studies of *Swertia chirayita*: a critically endangered medicinal herb of temperate Himalayas. Curr Trends Biotechnol Pharm. 2012;6:381–388

Chapin FS III, Zavaleta ES, Eviner VT, et al. Consequences of changing biodiversity. Nature 2000;405:234–242

Chen Y, Huang B, He J, Han L, Zhan Y, and Wang Y. In vitro and in vivo antioxidant effects of the ethanolic extract of *Swertia chirayita*. J. Ethnopharmacol. 2011;136:309–315

Clarke CB. The flora of British India, JD Hooker, ed., Vol. IV. London: L. Reeve and Co. 1885:124

Garg DS. Dhanvantri-Banaushdhi Vishesh Ank, Vol. 3. Aligarh: Dhanvantri Karyalaya; 1965:94

Joshi P and Dhawan V. *Swertia chirayita*–an overview. Curr Sci, 2005: 635–640

Karan M, Vasisht K, and Handa SS. Morphological and chromatographic comparison of certain Indian species of Swertia. J Med Aromat Plant Sci. 1999;19:995–963

Kirtikar KR and Basu BD, eds. Indian Medicinal Plants, Vol. III. Dehradun: Dehradun Publishers;1984:1664–1666

Kumar N, Chaubey S, Yadav C, Singh R. Review on *Swertia chirata* Buch.-Ham. Ex Wall: a bitter herb W.S.R. to its phytochemistry and biological activity. Int Ayurv Med J. 2017;5(9):3414–3419

Kumar V & Van Staden J. A review of *Swertia chirayita* (Gentianaceae) as a traditional medicinal plant. PMC, 2015;6:PMC4709473.

Kumar V and Van Staden J. A review of *Swertia chirayita* (Gentianaceae) as a traditional medicinal plant, PMC,V.6. 2015: PMC4709473

Rai LK, Prasad P, and Sharma E. Conservation threats to some medicinal plants of the Sikkim Himalaya. Biol Cons. 2000;93:27–33

Saha P, Mandal S, Das A, Das PC and Das S. Evaluation of the anti-carcinogenic activity of *Swertia chirata* Buch. Ham: an Indian medicinal plant, on DMBA-induced mouse skin carcinogenesis model. Phytother Res: Int J Pharmacol Toxicol Eval Nat Prod Deriv. 2004;18(5):373–378

Scartezzini P and Speroni E. Review on some plants of Indian traditional medicine with antioxidant activity. J Ethnopharmacol. 2000;71:23–42

Sharma PV. Dravyaguna-vijnana, Vol. 2. Varanasi: Chaukhambha Bharti Academy, 1986

The Ayurvedic Pharmacopoeia of India, Part I, Vol. 1. New Delhi: Ministry of Health & Family Welfare, Department of Ayush, Government of India, 1989:71

Verma NK and Kumar A. Isozyme polymorphism and genetic diversity among Swertia species-endangered medicinal plants of Himalayas. Indian J Plant Gen Res. 2001;14:74–77

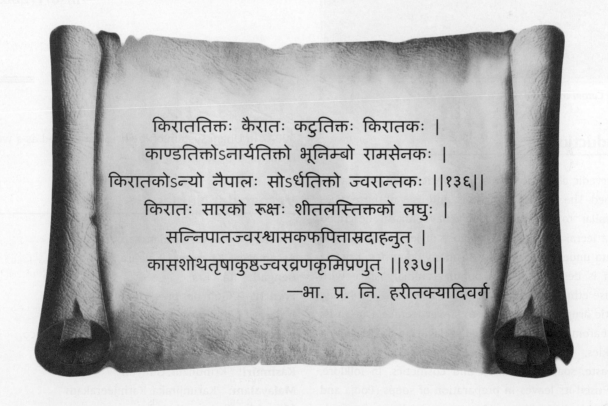

किराततिक्तः कैरातः कटुतिक्तः किरातकः |
काण्डतिक्तोऽनार्यतिक्तो भूनिम्बो रामसेनकः |
किरातकोऽन्यो नैपालः सोऽर्धतिक्तो ज्वरान्तकः ||१३६||
किरातः सारको रूक्षः शीतलस्तिक्तको लघुः |
सन्निपातज्वरश्वासकफपित्तास्रदाहनुत् |
कासशोथतृषाकुष्ठज्वरव्रणकृमिप्रणुत् ||१३७||
—भा. प्र. नि. हरीतक्यादिवर्ग

56. Krishna Jeeraka *[Carum carvi Linn.]*

Family: *Apiaceae (Umbeliferae)*

Hindi: *Kalajeera, vilayati jeera*

English: *Black caraway*

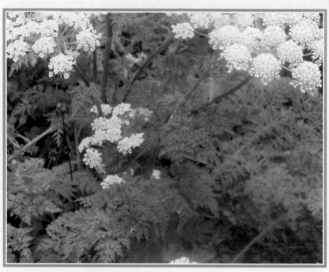

Plant of *Carum carvi* Linn.

Arabian physicians used to import kala jeera from Kerman city of the Iran that is why it is also known as Zeera Kermani.

–Ansari (2009)

Introduction

In Ayurvedic classics, mainly four varieties of Jeeraka are described. The properties, actions, and uses of these types are similar to a great extent. Bhavaprakash described Krishna Jeeraka under the category of Jeeraka tritya and Sushruta under Jeeraka dvay. In many countries, Krishna Jeeraka is designated as a popular culinary spice with immense ethnomedicinal use. Krishna Jeeraka is a highly aromatic drug in comparison to shwet Jeeraka. Due to its distinct aroma, its seeds are used as flavoring and seasoning of pickles, soups, sauce, meat, beverages, mouthwash, toothpaste, soaps, perfumes, and cosmetics. In folklore, people used its leaves in preparation of soups (Pooja and Singh 2014). In traditional Moroccan medicine, its seeds are used to treat diabetes and hypertension (Tahraoui et al 2007). It is also used to treat pneumonia and eczema in Russia and Indonesia, respectively (Sadowska and Obidoska 2004). In Unani system of medicine, it is used as a weight-reducing drug in obesity.

Vernacular Names

Arabic: Carawya, Kardiah, karoya

Assamese: Krisnjeera, Kalajira, Kaljira

Bengali: Kala jira

French: Cumin des pres, Cumin romain

Gujarati: Shahjirun, Shahjiru

Italian: Caro, Comino dei prati, Cumino Tedesco

Kannada: Kari jeerige, Shahajeerige

Kashmiri: Krihunzur, Gunyun

Malayalam: Karunjiraka, Karinjeerakam

Marathi: Shahira, Shahajire

Oriya: Kalajira

Persian: Karbya, Jirah rumi

Punjabi: Zira Siyah, Kalajira

Russian: Timon
Tamil: Karamjiragam, Shimai shambu, Kekku-virai
Telugu: Nalla Jeelakarra, Shimai sapu
Urdu: Zira Siyah, Kala Zira

Synonyms

Kashmirajeeraka: It is abundantly cultivated in Kashmir.
Jarana: It stimulates digestive fire.
Karavi: It is a potent carminative drug.
Sugandhi: The fruit is highly aromatic in nature.
Udagarashodhan: It purifies belching.
Kali: The fruit is black in color.
Bahugandha: The fruit exhibits multiple odors.
Ruchya: It improves taste of food.

Classical Categorization

Charaka Samhita: not mentioned
Sushruta Samhita: not mentioned
Ashtang Hridaya: not mentioned
Dhanvantari Nighantu: Shatpushpadi varga
Madanpal Nighantu: Sunthyadi varga
Kaiyadev Nighantu: Oushadi varga
Raj Nighantu: Pippalyadi varga
Bhavaprakash Nighantu: Haritakyadi varga

Distribution

The plant is extensively cultivated in Europe, Asia, and Africa. However in India it occurs wildly in a limited area of Western Himalaya, Jammu & Kashmir, Chakrata hill of Uttarakhand, and Chamba of Himachal Pradesh. It is also cultivated in the hills of North India and South India (Anonymous 1992).

Morphology

It is an erect, glabrous, biennial herb of 1.5 to 2 feet in height, with fleshy, fusiform tap root. Stem is erect, angular, grooved, filled with latex, branched from the ground up, smooth, hollow, and 30 to 60 cm in height.

- **Leaves:** Soft-fern-like leaves with thread-like division, bi or tripinnate, narrowly triangular to linear oblong, basal one forming into rosette, cauline leaves alternate, both are glabrous (**Fig. 56.1**).

- **Flower:** The main stem and the side branches terminate in a compound flowering umbel of 8 to 16 umbel rays; epicalyx and calyx are almost nonexistent; flowers are small, white, pink, or red colored (**Fig. 56.2**).

- **Fruit:** It is a schizocarp which is glabrous, oblong, and ellipsoid, consists of two mericarps, 3 to 6 mm long, sickle-shaped, brown colored with five angular ribs. The plant is propagated by seeds (**Fig. 56.3**).

Phenology

Flowering time: May to August
Fruiting time: May to August

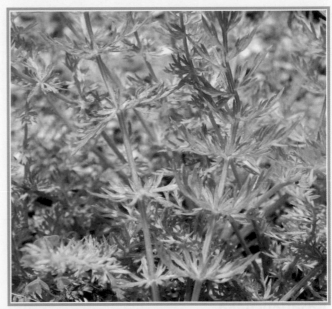

Fig. 56.1 Leaves.

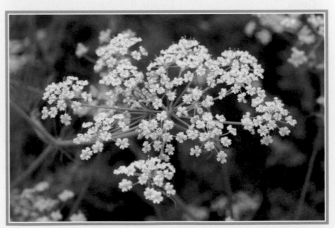

Fig. 56.2 Flowers.

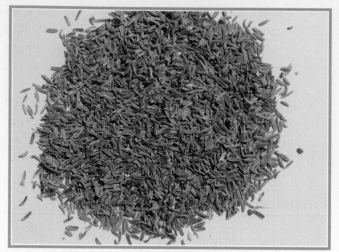

Fig. 56.3 Seeds.

> **Key Characters for Identification**
>
> ➤ *An erect, glabrous, biennial herb of 1.5 to 2 feet.*
> ➤ *Leaves are soft-fern-like bi or tripinnate, triangular to oblong.*
> ➤ *Flowers are white, pink, or red, in a compound umbel of 8 to 16 rays.*
> ➤ *Fruits are brown schizocarp, sickle-shaped, 3 to 6 mm long with angular ribs.*

Types

It is one of the types of Jeeraka as described in Bhavaprakash, Kaiyadev, and Raj Nighantu.

Rasapanchaka

Guna	Laghu, Ruksha
Rasa	Katu
Vipaka	Katu
Virya	Ushna

Chemical Constituents

Krishna Jeeraka seeds contain 1 to 9% essential oils, volatile oil, protein, dietary fibers, total lipids, carbohydrates, vitamins, minerals, fatty acids glucosides, galactosides, psoralens, sterol, umbelliferon, scopoletin, and herniarin. The major phytoconstituents of essential oil are carvone, carvacrol, carvenone, limonene, α-pinene, β-pinene, cis-carveol, β-myrcene, monoterpene hydrocarbon, sesquiterpenes, aldehydes, ketones, camphene, γ-terpinene, β-ocimene, p-cymene, caryophyllene, α-terpineol, germacrene A & D (Sedlakova et al 2003; Anonymous 1992; Wichtmann and Stahl-Biskup 1987).

Identity, Purity, and Strength

For Seeds:

- Foreign matter: Not more than 2%
- Total ash: Not more than 9%
- Acid-insoluble ash: Not more than 1.5%
- Alcohol-soluble extractive: Not less than 2%
- Water-soluble extractive: Not less than 12%
- Volatile oil: Not less than 3.5%

(Source: The Ayurvedic Pharmacopeia of India 1989)

Karma (Actions)

In Ayurvedic classics, Krishna Jeeraka is described as rochak (relish), deepan (appetizer), pachan (digestive), param grahi (highly absorbent), durgandhnashan (removes foul smell), chakshusya (eye tonic), hridya (cardiotonic), jwaraghna (antipyretic), garbhasayashodhan (uterine purificator), vataanulomana (laxative), shothghna (anti-inflammatory), stanyajanan (galactogouge), sugandhi (aromatic) dravya.

- Doshakarma: Kaphavatahara
- Dhatukarma: Rochan, hridya
- Malakarma: Vataanulomana

Pharmacological Actions

The plant is reported to exhibit antimicrobial, antifungal, antibacterial, anticancer, antioxidant, analgesic, antispasmodic, antiobesity, emmenagogue, hypolipidemic, antidiabetic, bronchodilator, diuretics, antistress, nootropic, hepatoprotective, nephroprotective, and aphrodisiac activities (Khan et al 2016).

Indications

Krishna Jeeraka is an effective remedy for mukhadurgandh (halitosis), aruchi (distaste), ajeerna (indigestion), agnimandhya (dyspepsia), udarshool (abdominal pain), adhyaman (flatulence), chardi (vomiting), hrillasa (horripilation), grahni (sprue), atisaar (diarrhea), gulma (abdominal lump), arsha (piles), krimi (worm infestation), shotha (inflammation), hridyaroga (cardiac diseases), prasuti vikara (diseases after puerperium), and jeernajwar (chronic fever).

Seeds of Krishna Jeeraka are also used in spasmodic gastrointestinal pain, morning sickness, headache, enhancing lactation, menstrual cramps, stomatitis, hoarseness of voice, eczema, leukoderma, malaria, lumbar pain, rheumatism, eye ailments, and genitourinary diseases (Khare 2004). In uterine pain and inflammations, decoction is used as sitz bath (Lubhaya 2004). Water prepared with Krishna Jeeraka is used to treat gastric trouble in children (Ali 1993). In epistaxis, inhalation of its powder with vinegar gives relief (Baitar 2003).

Therapeutic Uses

External Use

Vyanga (freckles): Paste of Jeerak dvay, Krishna tila, and Sharsap prepared with milk is applied on face to get relief in vyanga and lanchan (A.H.U. 32/18).

Internal Use

1. **Vishmajwara** (malaria): Intake of Krishna Jeeraka along with guda and a bit of maricha powder checks malarial fever (B.P.Ci. 1/755).
2. **Aruchi** (anorexia): Krishna Jeeraka, Jeerak, Draksha, Vrikshamla, Dadima, and Suvarchal lavan mixed with madhu guda cure all types of aruchi (C.S.Ci. 26/212).

Officinal Parts Used

Seed and seed oil

Dose

Powder: 1 to 3 g

Formulations

Saraswata churna, Laghulayi churna, Madhusnuhi rasayan, Jeerakadi modaka, Jirakadyaristha, Ashtangavleha, Gaganadi lauha.

Toxicity/Adverse Effects

Long-term use of Krishna Jeeraka may cause yellow color hyperpigmentation of skin and can affect lung and intestine (Ghani 2011). It is not suitable for Pitta dominant prakriti individuals (Baitar 2003).

Substitution and Adulteration

Fruits of *Carum gracile* Lindle, *Carum villosum* Haines, *Bunium persicum* (Boiss.), *B. cylindricum* Drude, *Bupleurum lanceolatum* Wall.ex.DC, *Apium graveolens* L., *Borreria articularis* L.f., *Bupleurum falcatum* L., and *Aegopodium podograria* are often used as substitutes or adulterants of Krishna jeeraka (Sharma et al 2002).

> **Points to Ponder**
>
> - *In Ayurvedic classics, Krishna Jeeraka is described as a type of Jeeraka. Its properties, actions, and usage are very much similar to Jeeraka (Cuminum cyminum L.)*
> - *Krishna Jeeraka is recommended to use in indigestion, flatulence, diarrhea, halitosis, chronic purulent wounds, and chronic fever.*

Suggested Readings

Ali SS. Unani Advia Mufaradah. 6th ed. New Delhi: Taraqqui Urdu Buero; 1993:178-179

Anonymous. The Wealth of India: A Dictionary of Indian Raw Materials and Industrial Product, Vol. 3 (Ca-Ci). New Delhi: Publication & Information Directorate, CSIR; 1992:313–316

Ansari MU. Munafe-ul-Mufredat. New Delhi: Ayejaz Publishing House; 2009:366-367

Baitar I. Al-Jame le Mufradat al Advia wal Aghzia (Urdu translation), Vol. IV. New Delhi: CCRUM; 2003:198-200

Ghani N. Khazainul Advia. New Delhi: Idara Kitab al Shifa;2011:775

Khare CP. Encyclopedia of Indian Medicinal Plants. New York: Verley; 2004:130-132

Lubhaya R. Goswami Bayanul Advia, Vol. 1. Delhi: Goswami Pharmacy; 2004:305-306

Mohiyuddin KR, Wasim A, Minhaj A, Azhar H. Phytochemical and pharmacological properties of *Carum carvi* L. Eur J Pharm Med Res 2016;3(6):231–236

Mohiyuddin KR, Wasim A, Minhaj A, Azhar H. Phytochemical and pharmacological properties of Carum carvi L. Eur J Pharm Med Res 2016;3(6):231–236

Pooja A, Singh DK. A review on the pharmacological aspects of *Carum carvi*. J Biol Earth Sci 2014;4(1):M1–M13

Sadowska A, Obidoska G. Caraway. In: Nemeth E, ed. The Genus *Carum*. USA: CRC Press; 2004:11

Sedlakova J, Kocourkova B, Lojkova L, Kuban V. Determination of essential oil content in caraway (*Carum carvi* L.) species by means of supercritical fluid extraction. Plant Soil Environ 2003;49(6):277–282

Sharma PC, Yeine MB, Dennis TJ. Database on Medicinal Plants Used in Ayurveda, Vol 6. New Delhi: Central Council for Research in Ayurveda and Siddha, Department of I.S.M. and H., Ministry of Health and Welfare, Government of India; 2002:86–90

Tahraoui A, El-Hilaly J, Israili ZH, Lyoussi B. Ethnopharmacological survey of plants used in the traditional treatment of hypertension and diabetes in south-eastern Morocco (Errachidia province). J Ethnopharmacol 2007;110(1):105–117

The Ayurvedic Pharmacopeia of India, Part I, Vol. 1. New Delhi: Department of AYUSH, Ministry of Health and Family Welfare, Government of India; 1989:102

Wichtmann EM, Stahl-Biskup E. Composition of the essential oils from caraway herb and root. Flavour Fragrance J 1987;2(2):83–89

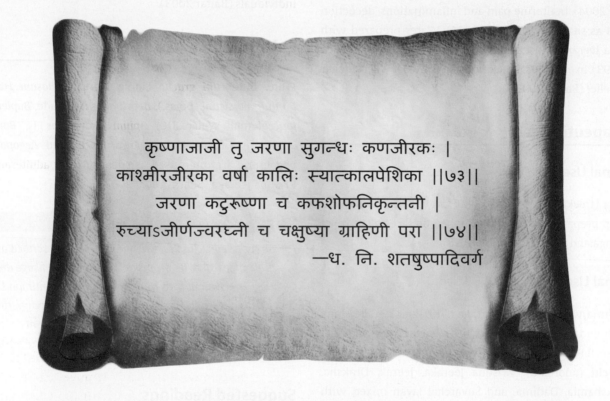

कृष्णाजाजी तु जरणा सुगन्धः कणजीरकः ।
काश्मीरजीरका वर्षा कालिः स्यात्कालपेशिका ॥७३॥
जरणा कटुरूष्णा च कफशोफनिकृन्तनी ।
रुच्याऽजीर्णज्वरघ्नी च चक्षुष्या ग्राहिणी परा ॥७४॥
—ध. नि. शतपुष्पादिवर्ग

57. Kumari [*Aloe barbadensis* Mill. Syn. *Aloe vera* (Linn.) Burm.f.]

Family: *Liliaceae*

Hindi name: *Ghikunwar, Ghikumari*

English name: Indian aloe, Curacao aloe, Barbados aloe, Jaffarabad aloe

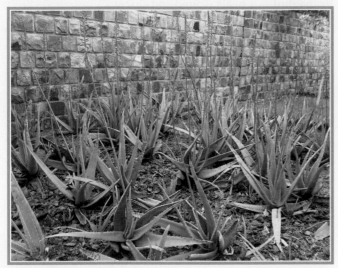
Plant of *Aloe vera* (Linn.) Burm.f.

> *The Egyptians called Aloe "The plant of immortality."*

Introduction

The name *Aloe vera* derives from the Arabic word "Alloeh" meaning shining bitter substance, while *Vera* in Latin means true. Two thousand years ago, the Greek scientists regarded *Aloe vera* as the universal panacea. Today, the *Aloe vera* plant is used for various purposes in dermatology (Itrat and Zarnigar 2013).

In Ayurveda, Aloe is known as Kumari or "young girl," because aloe is believed to bring back youthfulness, energy, and femininity. Aloe is used as a tonic for the female reproductive system. There is no direct description of Kumari in Brihattrayee. In the context of Madhur skanda drugs of Charak Samhita, Acharya Chakrapani listed Kumari for the drug Kshudrasaha (C.S.Vi.8/139,Chakrapani). First time, the plant Kumari is mentioned in Dhanwantari Nighantu (10th century AD) in Amradi varga (D.N. Amradi/147-148).

The earliest recorded human use of *Aloe vera* comes from the Ebers Papyrus; an Egyptian medical record, which is from the 16th century BC. Ancient Egyptians considered *Aloe vera* as the plant of immortality (as per the literature published in the *Indian Journal of Dermatology*). Egyptian queens, Nefertiti and Cleopatra used the leaves of this plant as part of their regular beauty regimes. Alexander the Great and Christopher Columbus also used it to treat the wounds of their soldiers. The first reference to *Aloe vera* in English was a translation by John Goodyew in AD 1655 of Dioscorides' Medical treatise *De Materia Medica* (Davis 1997). *Aloe vera* was in use as a laxative since the 1800s, in the United States. By the mid-1930s, a turning point occurred when it was successfully used to treat chronic and severe radiation dermatitis (Davis 1997). There are also recorded evidences that the plant has been in use for many centuries in countries like China, Japan, India, Greece, Egypt, Mexico, and Japan (Marshall 1990).

It is commonly called aloe, burn plant, lily of the desert, and elephant's gall. It is a cactus-like plant with green, dagger-shaped leaves that are fleshy, tapering, spiny, marginated, and filled with a clear viscous gel (Cheesbrough 2000; Joseph and Raj 2010; Manvitha and Bidya 2014).

Vernacular Names

Arabic: Sibr
Assamese: Musabhar, Machambar
Bengali: Ghritakumari, Kanya
Chinese: Lu Hui
Cuba: Sabilla
Dutch: Aloe
French: Aloes
German: Aloe
Greek: Aloi
Gujarati: Kumarpathu, Kunawar, Eliyo
Haiti: Laloi
Italian: Aloe
Japanese: Rokai
Kannada: Kathaligida, Lolesara, Kumari, Karilola
Kashmiri: Musabbar
Korian: Nohwa
Malayalam: Kattuvala, Kattarvala
Marathi: Korphad
Oriya: Kumari, Mushaboro
Persian: Sibr
Punjabi: Elwa, Musabbar
Russian: Aloe, Aloi, Sabur
Tamil: Kattalai, Sirukattalai, Bhottu katrazhae
Telugu: Kalabanda
Thai: Wan hang Jo
Urdu: Musabbar, Ailiva, Siber, Ailwa
Vietnam: Lohoi

Synonyms

Amaraa: This plant does not destroy easily.
Ambudhisrava: It gives watery jelly-like secretion on cutting its leaves.
Bahupatra: It bears many leaves.
Deerghapatrika: It has long leaves.
Ghritakumarika: It contains ghee-like jelly substance in its leaves.
Gruhakanya: This plant is treated as daughter of every house because of its sweet qualities.
Kantakapravruta: It has thorns on its leaves.

Kanya: It is well known for its rasayan properties.
Kumari: It requires very little water to grow and provides cooling effects. Due to rasayan properties it provides strength and nourishment.
Saha: It sustains even hot weather.
Sthuladala: Its leaves are very thick.
Sukantaka: It has thorny leaves.
Taruni: Young girls use this plant for multiple purposes.
Vipulasarva: Its leaves give rise to excessive secretion on cutting.
Vranaghni: It heals wound and abscess.

Classical Categorization

Dhanwantari Nighantu: Amradi varga
Madanpal Nighantu: Abhayadi varga
Kaiyadev Nighantu: Aushadhi varga
Raj Nighantu: Parpatadi varga
Bhavaprakash Nighantu: Guduchyadi varga

Distribution

It is native to southern and eastern Africa along the upper Nile in the Sudan. Later on, it is introduced into North Africa and many other countries across the globe. Countries like India, South Africa, the United States of America, Venezuela Aruba, Bonaire, Haiti, etc. cultivate this plant for commercial purposes (African Pharmacopoeia 1985; Yeh et al 2003). The Aloe grown in desert of Southern California is considered as the finest quality. The plant can resist temperatures up to 104 F and can also withstand below freezing temperatures until root is not damaged.

In India, it is found in Rajasthan, Andhra Pradesh, Gujarat, Maharashtra, Uttarakhand, Himachal Pradesh, and Tamil Nadu.

Morphology

It is a dwarf, succulent, perennial herb with short stem and shallow root system.

- **Leaves**: Radical, 30 to 60 cm long, 10 cm broad, and 1.8 cm thick, fleshy, in rosettes, sessile, often crowded with horny prickles on margins, surface pale green with irregular white blotches, narrowed from base to apex, convex below. Leaves are filled with a

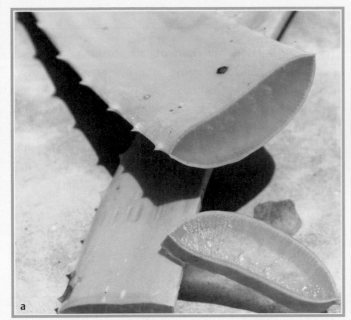

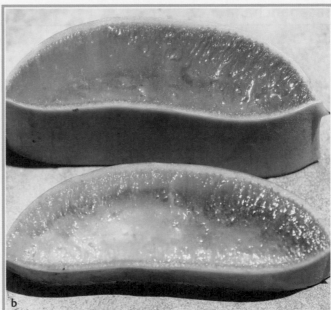

Fig. 57.1 **(a)** Leaves. **(b)** Slimy jelly.

translucent slimy juice. It becomes blackish-brown on drying, shiny, and brittle (**Fig. 57.1a, b**).

- **Flowers**: Bright yellowish-orange tubular flowers in terminal racemes about 2.5 cm long, peduncle spongy, green, simple or few branched, up to 40 cm long. Stamens are frequently projected beyond the perianth tube (**Fig. 57.2**).
- **Fruit**: Capsular, 1.5 x 1.0 cm, cylindrical or ellipsoid-oblong. Fruits contain many seeds (Yeh et al 2003).

It is propagated by suckers.

Phenology

Flowering time: September to December
Fruiting time: December to February

Key Characters for Identification

➤ *A dwarf, succulent, perennial herb.*
➤ *Leaves: Radical, 30 to 60 cm long, 10 cm broad, and 1.8 cm thick, fleshy, in rosettes, sessile, crowded, prickles on margins, surface pale green with irregular white blotches. Leaves are filled with a translucent slimy juice.*
➤ *Flowers: Yellow-orange in terminal racemes.*
➤ *Fruit: Capsular, 1.5 × 1.0 cm, cylindrical or ellipsoid-oblong.*

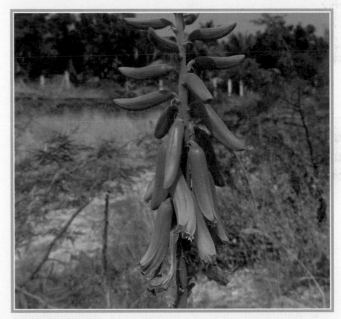

Fig. 57.2   Flowers.

Types

There are several species under the genus *Aloe*, including *Aloe vera*, *Aloe barbadensis*, *Aloe ferox*, *Aloe chinensis*, *Aloe indica*, and *Aloe perryi*. Among these, *Aloe vera* Linn. syn. *Aloe barbadensis* Miller is accepted unanimously as the correct botanical source of Aloe (Chandegara and Varshney 2013).

Rasapanchaka

	Leaves	Dried juice
Guna	Guru, Snigdha, Pichchhila	Laghu, Ruksha, Teekshna
Rasa	Tikta, Madhura	Tikta, Madhura
Vipaka	Katu	Katu
Virya	Sheeta	Ushna

Chemical Constituents

The *Aloe vera* leaf gel contains about 98% water (Pandey and Singh 2016). *Aloe vera* contains 200 potentially active constituents; vitamins, enzymes, minerals, sugars, lignin, saponins, salicylic acids, and amino acids, which are responsible for the multifunctional activity of Aloe (Gautam and Awasthi 2007; Sharrif and Verma 2011; Sahu et al 2013). The details are as under:

- Vitamins: It contains Vitamins A (beta-carotene), C, E, B12, folic acid, and choline.
- Enzymes: It contains eight enzymes: aliiase, alkaline phosphatase, amylase, bradykinase, carboxypeptidase, catalase, cellulase, lipase, and peroxidase. Bradykinase helps to reduce excessive inflammation when applied to the skin topically, while others help in the breakdown of sugars and fats.
- Minerals: It provides calcium, chromium, copper, selenium, magnesium, manganese, potassium, sodium, and zinc.
- Sugars: It provides monosaccharides (glucose and fructose) and polysaccharides (glucomannans/polymannose).
- Anthraquinones: It provides 12 anthraquinones, which are phenolic compounds traditionally known as laxatives. It provides Aloe emodin, aloetic acid, alovin, anthracene.
- Fatty acids: It provides four plant steroids; cholesterol, campesterol, β-sisosterol, and lupeol.
- Amino acids: It provides 20 of the 22 required amino acids and 7 of the 8 essential ones.
- Hormones: Auxins and gibberellins (Shelton 1991; Atherton 1998; de Rodríguez et al 2005; Vogler and Ernst 1999; Coats 1979).

Karma (Actions)

The main actions of Kumari are brimhan (increase body mass), balya (improve physical strength), vrisya (aphrodisiac), vatashamak (pacify vata), vishaghna (antidote), dahashamak (subsides burning sensation), chakshushya (beneficial for eyes), rasayan (rejuvenation), bhedan (purgative), jwaraghna (antipyretics), kusthaghna (antidermatosis), twachya (complexion promoter), vranashodhan and ropan (wound cleansing and healing).

- Doshakarma: Kaphapittashamaka
- Dhatukarma: Brimhan, balya, vrisya, twachya
- Malakarma: Bhedan

Pharmacological Actions

Aloe vera gel have bitter, cooling, anti-inflammatory, anthelmintic, liver stimulant, analgesic, purgative, digestive, carminative, depurative, diuretic, stomachic, aphrodisiac, antibacterial, rejuvenator, and tonic properties, antidiabetic, antitumor, anticancer, antibacterial, antiviral, antifungal, moisturizing actions, wound-healing effects, antiaging agent, laxative effects, antiseptic, cosmetic and skin protection, immunomodulatory effects, radio protective, and antimutagenic effects (Anonymous 2003; Lanka 2018; Sharma et al 2014; Sahu et al 2013; Pareek et al 2013).

Indications

Aloe vera is a miraculous herb that includes a self-healing house. Since time immemorial, it has been used in traditional system in day-to-day practice. Its juice is used in dyspepsia, anartava (amenorrhea), kastartava (dysmenorrhea), dagdha (burns), shoola (colic), yakrit and pleeha vridhi (liver and spleen enlargement), kushta (leprosy), twacharoga (skin diseases), constipation (vibandha), krimi (worm infestation), carbuncles, painful inflammations (shotha), granthi (cyst), vrana (wound), visphota (chronic ulcers), catarrhal and purulent eye infections, gulma (abdominal lump), raktapitta (bleeding disorders), kaphajwara (fever caused by kapha), shwasa (asthma), and (ajeerna) indigestion. It is an incredible herb for skin. It is an ingredient of many soaps, facial masks, toners, face wash, and scrubs.

The plant is useful in everyday life as it soothes a variety of skin ailments such as mild cuts, antidote for insect stings, bruises, poison ivy, and eczema along with skin moisturizing and antiaging, maintains health of digestive tract, blood and lymphatic circulation, and functioning of kidney, liver, and gall bladder, and hence, makes it a boon to human.

Contraindications

Aloe should not be given or prescribed to patients with inflammatory intestinal diseases, such as appendicitis, Crohn disease, ulcerative colitis, irritable bowel syndrome, or diverticulitis, or to children less than 10 years of age. Aloe should not be used during pregnancy or lactation except under medical supervision after evaluating benefits and risks. Aloe is also contraindicated in patients with cramps, colic, hemorrhoids, nephritis, or any undiagnosed abdominal symptoms such as pain, nausea, or vomiting (Gilma et al 1990; Bisset 1994). Aloe is also contraindicated in patients with intestinal obstruction or stenosis, atony, severe dehydration with electrolyte depletion or chronic constipation (WHO Monograph 1999).

Therapeutic Uses

External Use

1. **Guhya charmakila** (penile wart): Wrapping of green leaf of *Aloe vera* cures the wart (RM. 24/1 and BP.Ci. 52/5).
2. **Inflammation in penis**: Jeerak pounded with juice of *Aloe vera* is applied as paste locally on abscess. It reduces the inflammation and pacifies burning sensation (R.R.S. 25/18).
3. **Vrana** (abscess): Unripe, ripening, or ripe abscess should be covered with the steamed leaves devoid of pulp. Decoction of Kumari, Tila, and sour gruel ripens the abscess (V.M. 16/101-102).
4. **Sthanavyatha** (mastitis): Root of *Aloe vera* is mixed with Haridra and applied as paste on breast to relieve pain (GN. 6.8.23).
5. **Dagdha** (burn): Regular application of *Aloe vera* gel on the affected area gives tremendous relief in itching and burning sensation caused by radiotherapy, sun exposure, chemical burn, and fire burn.
6. **Cosmetic use**: Daily application of *Aloe vera* gel on the face improves complexion, reduces dark spot and acne, hydrate, rejuvenate, moisturize, and tone up the skin.

Its regular use prevents the skin from sun tanning and imparts a glowing effect.

7. **Hair fall**: Massage the Juice of *Aloe vera* mixed with coconut milk and wheat germ oil on scalp before shampooing hair. If used continuously, it helps in regrowth of hair. *Aloe vera* also helps in the reduction of dandruff.

Internal Use

1. **Phleehavridhi** (spleen enlargement): The juice of Kumari is taken with Haridra powder to treat splenomegaly and apache (scrofula) (Sh.S.2.1.15).
2. **Apasmara** (epilepsy): Ghee cooked with juice of *Aloe vera* and decoction of Madhuka is given with sugar in epilepsy and palpitation of heart (SB. 4.453).
3. **Mutrakrichha** (dysuria): Juice of Kumari or decoction of laghupanchmool is given in dysuria during fever (V.M.7/10).
4. **Kamala** (jaundice): Kumari juice is taken as snuff to remove jaundice (BP.Ci. 8/44).
5. **Gulma** (abdominal lump): 5 g of pulp of Kumari mixed with cow's ghee, fine powder of Trikatu, Haritaki, and salt should be taken in gulma (BP.Ci. 32/44).
6. **Rajarodha** (amenorrhea): Kumarika vati or rajapravartani vati is given in amenorrhea (BR.P.1182-83).

Official Parts Used

Leaf, leaf-juice, dried juice of leaf

Dose

Leaf juice: 10 to 20 mL
Dried juice: 100 to 300 mg

Formulations

Kumaryasava, Rajapravartani vati, Pradarantaka rasa.

Toxicity/Adverse Effects

- Topical: It may cause redness, burning and stinging sensation, and rare generalized dermatitis in sensitive individuals. Allergic reactions are mostly due to anthraquinones, such as aloin and barbaloin. It is best to apply it to a small area first to test for possible allergic reaction.

- Oral: Abdominal spasms and pain may occur after even a single dose, and overdose can lead to colicky abdominal spasms and pain, as well as the formation of thin, watery stools. Chronic abuse of anthraquinone stimulant laxatives can lead to hepatitis (Beuers et al 1991) and electrolyte disturbances (hypokalemia, hypocalcemia), disturbs cardiac rhythm in heart patients, and can cause metabolic acidosis, malabsorption, weight loss, albuminuria, and hematuria (Müller-Lissner 1993; Godding 1976). Prolong use of anthraquinone laxatives causes melanotic pigmentation of the colonic mucosa (pseudomelanosis coli). After discontinuation of the drug, pigmentation is reversible within 4 to 12 months and it is clinically harmless (Müller-Lissner 1993). Prolonged use has been reported to increase the risk of colorectal cancer (Chinnusamy et al 2009; Salazar et al 2010; Sundarkar 2011; Kareman 2013; Akev 2015; Ahmad et al 2016).

- Larger doses lead to accumulation of blood in pelvic region and reflux stimulation of uterine muscles and may bring about abortion or premature birth in late pregnancy. Toxic doses may cause kidney damage (Sharma et al 2001).

Substitution and Adulteration

Acacia catechu Willd. (black catechu), iron pieces, and stones are mixed for the adulteration of *Aloe vera* (Sharma et al 2001).

Points to Ponder

- *Aloe barbadensis Miller is accepted unanimously as the correct botanical source of Aloe.*
- *Its juice is used in dyspepsia, amenorrhea, dysmenorrhea, burns, colic pain, liver and spleen enlargement, skin diseases, and constipation.*
- *Aloe should not be used during pregnancy or lactation.*

Suggested Readings

African Pharmacopoeia, Vol. 1. Lagos: Organization of African Unity, Scientific, Technical & Research Commission;1985

Ahmad M, Khan MP, Mukhtar A, Zafar M, Sultana S, Jahan S. Ethnopharmacological survey on medicinal plants used in herbal drinks among the traditional communities of Pakistan. J Ethnopharmacol 2016;184:154–186

Akev N, Can A, Sutlupınar N, et al. Twenty years of research on *Aloe vera*. Istanbul Ecz. Fak. Derg. J. Fac. Pharm. Istanbul 2015;45(2):191–215

Anonymous. The Wealth of India, Vol. 1. New Delhi: NISCAIR; 2003: 191-193

Anonymous. Unani Pharmacopeia of India, Part 1, Vol. 1. New Delhi: Department of AYUSH;2007:82-83

Atherton P. *Aloe vera* revisited. Br J Phytother 1998;4:176–183

Beuers U, Spengler U, Pape GR. Hepatitis after chronic abuse of senna. Lancet 1991;337(8737):372–373

Bisset NG. Sennae folium: Max Wichtl's Herbal Drugs & Phytopharmaceuticals. Boca Raton, FL: CRC Press;1994

Chandegara VK, Varshney AK. *Aloe vera* L. Processing and products: a review. Int J Med Aromat Plants 2013;3(4):492–506

Cheesbrough M. Medical Laboratory Manual for Tropical Countries. Oxford: Butterworth;2000:260

Chinnusamy K, Nandagopal T, Nagaraj K, Sridharanet S. *Aloe vera* induced oral mucositis: a case report. Internet J Pediatr Neonatol 2009;9(2)

Coats BC. The Silent Healer: A Modern Study of *Aloe vera*. Garland, TX;1979

Davis RH. *Aloe vera*: A Scientific Approach. New York: Vantage Press Inc.; 1997:290-306

de Rodríguez DJ, Hernández-Castillo D, Rodríguez- García R, Angulo-Sanchez JL. Antifungal activity in vitro of *Aloe vera* pulp and liquid fraction against plant pathogenic fungi. Ind Crops Prod 2005;21(1):81–87

Gautam S, Awasthi P. Nutrient composition and physiochemical characteristics of *Aloe vera* (*Aloe barbadensis*) powder. J Food Sci Technol 2007;44:224-225

Gilman AG, Nies AS, Rall TW. Goodman and Gilman's the Pharmacological Basis of Therapeutics. 8th ed. New York: McGraw Hill; 1990

Godding EW. Therapeutics of laxative agents with special reference to the anthraquinones. Pharmacology 1976; 14(1, Suppl 1) 78–101

Itrat M, Zarnigar K. *Aloe vera*: a review of its clinical effectiveness. Int Res J Pharm 2013;4:75–79

Joseph B, Raj SJ. Pharmacognostic and phytochemical properties of *Aloe vera* linn: an overview. Int J Pharm Sci Rev Res 2010;4(2):106–110

Kareman ES. A self-controlled single blinded clinical trial to evaluate oral lichen planus after topical treatment with *Aloe vera*. J GHR 2013;2(4):503–507

Lanka S. A review on *aloe vera*-the wonder medicinal plant. J Drug Deliv Ther 2018;8(5-s):94–99

Manvitha K, Bidya B. *Aloe vera*: a wonder plant its history, cultivation and medicinal uses. J Pharmacogn Phytochem 2014;2(5):85–88

Marshall JM. *Aloe vera* gel: what is the evidence? Pharm J 1990;24: 360–362

Müller-Lissner SA. Adverse effects of laxatives: fact and fiction. Pharmacology 1993;47(Suppl 1):138–145

Nadkarni KM. Indian Plants and Drugs. New Delhi: Shishti Book Distributors;2004:28-29

Pandey A, Singh S. *Aloe vera*: a systematic review of its industrial and ethno-medicinal efficacy. Int J Pharm Res Allied Sci 2016;5:21–33

Pareek S, Nagaraj A, Sharma P, Naidu S, Yousuf A. *Aloe-vera:* a herb with medicinal properties. IJOCR 2013;1(1):47–50

Sahu PK, Giri DD, Singh R, et al. Therapeutic and medicinal uses of *Aloe vera*: a review. Pharmacol Pharm 2013;4:599–610

Sahu PK, Giri DD, Singh R, et al. Therapeutic and medicinal uses of *Aloe vera*: a review. Pharmacol Pharm 2013;4:599–610

Salazar-Sánchez N, López-Jornet P, Camacho-Alonso F, Sánchez-Siles M. Efficacy of topical *Aloe vera* in patients with oral lichen planus: a randomized double-blind study. J Oral Pathol Med 2010;39(10):735–740

Sharma P, Kharkwal AC, Kharkwal H, Abdin MZ, Varma A. A review on pharmacological properties of *Aloe vera*. Int J Pharm Sci Rev Res 2014; 29(2):31-37

Sharma PC, Yelne MB, Dennis TJ. Database on Medicinal Plants used in Ayurveda, Vol. 1. New Delhi: CCRAS, Department of ISM & H, Ministry of Health and Family Welfare, Government of India; 2001:225-243

Sharrif MM, Verma SK. *Aloe vera* their chemicals composition and applications: a review. Int J Biol Med Res 2011;2:466–471

Shelton RM. *Aloe vera*: its chemical and therapeutic properties. Int J Dermatol 1991;30(10):679–683

Sundarkar P. Use of *Aloe Vera* in dentistry. J Indian Acad Oral Med Radiol 2011;23(3):S389–S391

Vogler BK, Ernst E. *Aloe vera*: a systematic review of its clinical effectiveness. Br J Gen Pract 1999;49(447):823–828

WHO Monograph on Selected Medicinal Plants, Vol. 1. Geneva: WHO; 1999:33-40

Yeh GY, Eisenberg DM, Kaptchuk TJ, Phillips RS. Systematic review of herbs and dietary supplements for glycemic control in diabetes. Diabetes Care 2003;26(4):1277–1294

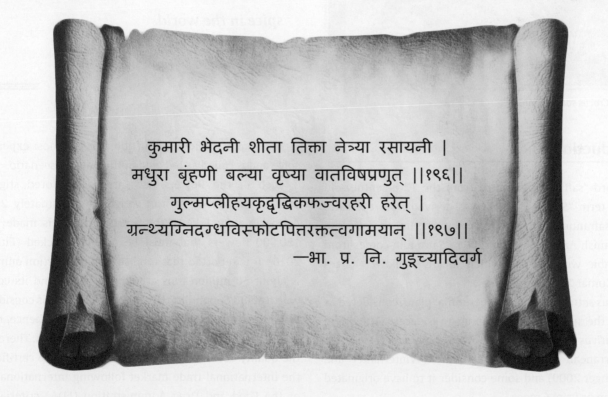

कुमारी भेदनी शीता तिक्ता नेत्र्या रसायनी |
मधुरा बृंहणी बल्या वृष्या वातविषप्रणुत् ||१९६||
गुल्मप्लीहयकृद्वृद्धिकफज्वरहरी हरेत् |
ग्रन्थ्यग्निदग्धविस्फोटपित्तरक्त्वगामयान् ||१९७||
—भा. प्र. नि. गुडूच्यादिवर्ग

58. Kumkum–Kesara [*Crocus sativus* Linn.]

Family:	*Iridaceae*
English name:	*Saffron, Crocus*
Hindi name:	*Kesar, Zaffran*

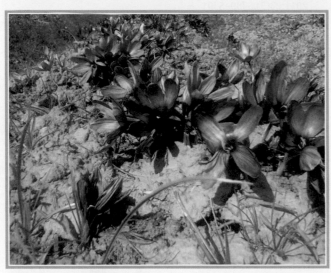

Plant of *Crocus sativus* Linn.

> *The world's annual saffron production is estimated around 300 tons per year (Iran produces 76% of total) and is considered to be the most expensive spice in the world.*

Introduction

The word "saffron" originated from the 12th-century-old French term "Safran," which was derived from the Latin word "safranum." It is also related to the Italian Zafferano and Spanish Azafran (Harper 2001). Safranum comes from the Arabic word "asfar" which means "yellow" (Katzer 2001; Kumar 2006).

Crocus sativus L. is a small perennial plant, considered as king of the spice world. It belongs to Iridaceae. The origin of *C. sativus* is not clearly known; some suggest eastern Mediterranean as its endemic place (Winterhalter and Straubinger 2000) and some consider it to have originated from Iran or from Greece.

The genus *Crocus* consists of about 90 species and some are being cultivated for flower. The flowering time in case of *C. sativus* is autumn. The traditional methods of saffron cultivation and flower harvesting are very tedious and labor extensive, and it leads to increased cost of saffron. Due to its high demand and low production, it is the most expensive spice and is called as red gold in the present scenario.

Each of the flowers has three red-colored stigmas, and one stigma of saffron weighs approximately 2 mg. Approximately 1 kg of this valuable spice is made from 150,000 flowers that must be carefully picked (Pitsikas 2016). It is reported that total saffron production annually is about 50 million tons around the globe and its cost is worth about $50 million (Negbi 2003). Saffron is considered to be the most expensive spice in the world; hence, there are efforts for its artificial production or defraud. Therefore, the quality conservation of saffron needs to be certified in the international trade market following international ISO or the Food and Drug Administration (FDA) criteria and standards.

Collection of saffron flowers and isolation of stigmas are not easy. It is started just after the appearance of the first flower in the field because the flowers remain only for 3 to 4 days. If the flowers remain under warm weather and sunlight or wind, then the quality of color and odor will change and decrease. The appropriate season for collection is related to the first watering time. At the flowering stage, the flowers are handpicked and allowed to dry under shade. This is a traditional method but is considered poor because it produces less saffron, leading to its high economic value. In India, cultivation of *C. sativus* is restricted to Jammu and Kashmir only. The saffron produced in Jammu and Kashmir is world famous for its quality. To enhance the potential capabilities to cultivate saffron to get the maximum yield, various biotechnological approaches (considered as most feasible techniques) were employed. In India, many institutions such as Indian Agricultural Research Institute (ICAR), Department of Biotechnology (DBT), and Council of Scientific and Industrial Research (CSIR) are involved in developing methods to enhance the production of saffron at both in vitro and in vivo levels. The biotechnological tools lead to the establishment of protocol for mass multiplication of disease-free clones and also provide the insights via rDNA technology to get the transgenic lines.

The flowers of *C. sativus* contain three key components known as crocin, picrocrocin, and safaranal (Shahnawaz et al 2017). These three components are reported to be responsible for the color, taste, and aroma of the saffron, respectively. *C. sativus* possesses a number of medicinally important activities such as antigenototoxic and cytotoxic effects, antioxidants, and antidepressants. It also improves memory and learning skills, and increases blood flow in retina and choroid.

Besides the medicinal importance, saffron is being used as a spice (regarded as all-time king of spice world) (Ferrence and Bendersky 2004), as a dye (Basker and Negbi 1983), as perfume (Tarantilis et al 1995), and in food industry.

Vernacular Names

Arab: Zafrah, zipharana
Persian: Zafrah, zipharana
Bengali: Jafran
Marathi: kecara
Gujarati: Keshar
Telugu: Kunkuma-purva, kunkumma-purru
Tamil: Kunkumappu
Malayalam: Kunkumappu
Konkan: Kunkuma-kesara

French: Safran
German: Safran (Nadkarni 2000)

Synonyms

Agnishikham: It looks like fire flame.
Balkhim: It is found in Balhika region.
Ghusrunam: It is a popular cosmetic substance.
Kaashmiraka: It grows in Kashmir.
Kashmiram: It grows in Kashmir.
Kumkum: It is used in shiraroga, vrana, etc.
Kusumbha: It looks like a Safflower.
Kusumodbhavam: It is obtained from flowers of the plant.
Pishunam: It emits intense odor.
Pitakam: It is yellow in color.
Raktam: It is red in color.
Sankocham: It is a popular cosmetic substance.
Shonitabhidhm: It is red in color.
Trivram: It emits intense odor.
Varam: It is a popular cosmetic substance.
Varnyam: It is a popular cosmetic substance to enhance complexion.

Classical Categorization

Charak Samhita: Shonitasthapana
Sushruta Samhita: Eladi
Dhanwantari Nighantu: Chandanadi varga
Madanpal Nighantu: Karpooradi varga
Kaiyadev Nighantu: Aushadhi varga
Raj Nighantu: Chandanadi varga
Bhavaprakash Nighantu: Karpuradi Varga

Distribution

The *C. sativus* believed that Kumkum is originated from Greece, Asia minor, and Persia, spreading eastwards to Kashmir and China (Mathew 1999). It is reported to have been cultivated above 1,600 m elevation in Greece, India, Iran, Afghanistan, Azerbaijan, China, Egypt, France, Iraq, Israel, Italy, Japan, Pakistan, Morocco, Spain, Switzerland, Turkey, United Arab Emirates since ancient times (Vinning 2005; Singla and Bhat 2011). The state of Jammu and Kashmir is the place where saffron is predominately cultivated in India. In fact, Kashmir is considered one of the three prominent cultivating places of saffron all over the world.

Morphology

It is a kind of grass, that is a small perennial herb, with purple- or lilac-colored flowers, 15 to 30 cm high.

- **Leaves:** Gray-green leaves have hairy margins and grow to about 1 or 1-1/2 feet long. Leaves are radical, linear, dark green above, pale green below, enclosed in a membranous sheath, sometimes remaining fresh nearly the whole winter (**Fig. 58.1**).
- **Flowers:** The corm produces a funnel-shaped, reddish-purple (sometimes lilac or white) flower. The flowers are hermaphrodite (has both male and female organs) and are pollinated by bees, butterflies. It is sessile, scented, appearing with leaves in autumn; petals are narrow elliptical, fused below into the corolla tube. The flower has three brick red–colored stigmas (25–30 mm long), which droop over the petals. These stigmas are collected as saffron. There are also three yellow stamens, which lack the active compounds and are not collected. The stigma is attached to a style (orange color), which has little of the active components and is only included with the lower grades of saffron. Each bulb produces from one to seven flowers (**Fig. 58.2**).
- **Fruits:** Loculicidal capsules.

It is propagated by vegetative method. The underground parts of the plant, corms or bulbs, can be used to produce new plant as this plant has no seed propagation.

Key Characters for Identification

➤ *Color: Stigma is dark red to reddish-brown; style is yellowish-brown to yellowish-orange.*
➤ *Odor: Strong, characteristic, and aromatic.*
➤ *Taste: Characteristic and bitter.*
➤ *Size: Stigmas are 25 mm long, and styles are about 10 mm long.*
➤ *Shape: Stigma is trifid and styles are cylindrical (Kokate et al 2006).*

Phenology

Flowering time: Autumn (October to December)
Fruiting time: December

Types

According to Bhavaprakash, Kesara is of three types as per its habitat.

- Kashmiraja: It is found in Kashmir. It is small, red in color and smells like a lotus (Padma Gandhi). It is considered as the best variety.

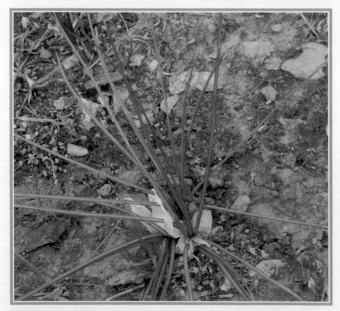

Fig. 58.1 Leaves.

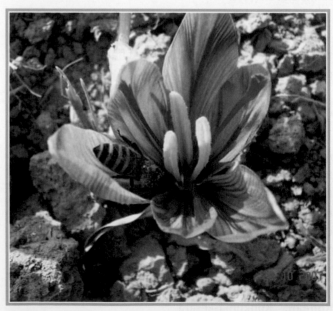

Fig. 58.2 Flowers.

- Balhika: It is found in Balhika region. It is also small, pandur varna (pale yellow color) and smells like a Ketaki plant. Its quality is medium.
- Parasik: Ishat pandur (light pale yellow), smells like honey, and is long. It is considered as worse variety.

Rasapanchaka

Guna	Snigdha
Rasa	Katu, Tikta
Vipak	Katu
Virya	Ushna

Chemical Constituents

Three key components in saffron are crocin, picrocrocin, and safranal (expressed mostly in stigma) (Shahnawaz et al 2017). The red color of the stigma is due to crocin. Picrocrocin is responsible for the bitter taste and safranal is responsible for odor and aroma and is used as flavoring agent.

Saffron has intensive fragrance with slightly bitter taste and produces a bright yellow-orange solution when soaked in warm water (Anjum et al 2015). Its stigma was shown to contain carbohydrates, minerals, mucilage, vitamins B1 and B2, and pigments. Crocin, crocetin, carotene, lycopene, and gigantic (Bhat and Broker 1953), anthocyanin, alpha-carotene, beta-carotene, and zeaxanthin are the oil-soluble pigments that can be found in the stigma (Nørbæk and Kondo 1998).

Identity, Purity, and Strength

Identification

When sulfuric acid is sprinkled on it, the stigmas turn blue immediately, gradually changing to purple and finally purplish-red.

Stamens of safflower and florets of marigold should be absent; should be free from artificially dyed corn silk or fibers.

Absence of fixed oil or glycerin: When pressed between clear filter paper, the paper does not display translucent oily spots.

Foreign organic matter: Not more than 2 %. Styles not more than 10%.

Loss on drying: Loses not more than 14% of its weight, when dried at 100°C.

Ash: Not more than 7.5%

Acid-insoluble ash: Not more than 1%

(Source: The Ayurvedic Pharmacopeia of India 2004)

Karma (Actions)

Varnya (complexion promoter), blood purifiers, chhardinashak (antiemetic), jantunashak (kills worm), twakdoshahara (alleviate skin problems), vranahara (heals wound), vishaghna (antidote), rochana (enhance taste).

- Doshakarma: Tridoshahara
- Dhatukarma: Raktashodhak
- Malakarma: Rechana

Pharmacological Actions

Pharmacological properties like anodyne, emmenagogue, diuretic, anticancer, laxative, anticonvulsant, antidepressant, relaxant, antioxidant, antitussive, antihyperlipidemic, antibacterial, antiseptics, antifungal, and antiflatulent are reported.

Anti-Alzheimer activities are found in Kesara. It is reported that it has antitumoral and anticarcinogenic activities and its cytotoxic and antimutagenic effects have also been reported. It is also used as a tonic and promoter of defenses in Ayurvedic medicine, for some disorders in the central nervous system in Chinese medicine, and for homeopathic preparations (Abdullaev 2002).

Xuan et al (1999) reported that crocin analogs isolated from saffron significantly increased the blood flow in the retina and choroid as well as facilitated retinal function recovery and it could be used to treat ischemic retinopathy and/or age-related macular degeneration.

Ahmad (2005) revealed that crocetin, which is an important ingredient of saffron, may be helpful in preventing parkinsonism. Salomi et al (1991) reported that crocin and dimethyl-crocetin isolated from saffron are nonmutagenic.

Indications

Bhavaprakash advised to use Kesara in headache, vomiting, wound, acne, and worm infestation. It is used as cardiotonic and nervine tonic. Traditionally, it is used as aphrodisiac, antispasmodic, and expectorant, and in treating ailments of stomach.

It is mainly used in chhardi (vomiting), kasa (kasa), vrana (wound), vyanga (freckles), shira roga (diseases of head), drustiroga (eye diseases), kantha roga (throat problem), sidhma (one type of skin disease), mutrashotha (inflammatory diseases of urinary system), udavartta (flatulence), mutraghata (urinary obstruction), suryavartta (headache), ardhava bhedaka (a type of headache; The Ayurvedic Pharmacopeia of India 2004).

It has also been used for the treatment of ocular and cutaneous conditions (Xuan et al 1999); lowering blood pressure (Soeda et al 2001); for wounds, fractures, and joint pain; to prevent plague and other epidemics; to cure anemia, migraines, and insomnia; in promoting and regulating menstrual periods (Akhondzadeh et al 2004, 2007); as a cardiotonic (Bathaie and Mousavi 2010); and in the treatment of sores and respiratory disorders (Xi et al 2007; Xiang et al 2006).

Saffron and its constituents are able to increase the uterine motility tone (Chang et al 1964) by acting as an emmenagogue agent and, at higher dose, by producing metrorrhagia and even abortion. Paradoxically, it has also been reported that saffron has a uterine sedative property which is useful in dysmenorrhea and the menstrual syndrome (Leclere 1983). These effects at the uterine level have dictated its use in folk medicine, but at least one death has been attributed to the ingestion of 1.5 g (Basker and Negbi 1983).

In the present scenario, saffron water extract (carotenoid) has proven to have medicinal potential to treat cancer, and cerebrovascular and cardiovascular complications (Rios et al 1996; Nair et al 1991; Abdullaev 1993).

It is also reported to have various other activities in different parts of the world. For example, in the Middle East, it is used as antispasmodic, aphrodisiac, carminative, cognition enhancer, emmenagogue, and thymoleptic, and in traditional Chinese system of medicine, saffron is used to treat amenorrhea, high-risk deliveries, menorrhagia, and postpartum lochiostasis (Rios et al 1996).

Besides its medicinal uses, it is also used as spice, dye, perfume, and food.

Contraindications

It is contraindicated in pregnancy (Khare 2004). The Complete German Commission E Monographs have not approved this plant for use in cramps or asthma (Blumenthal 1998).

Therapeutics Uses

External Use

Sheet (cold): Kumkum, Aguru, Nakha Kasturi, Ela, Devadaru, Saileya, Musta, Rasna, Vacha, and Kushta drugs are used in combination or separately as single drug and applied externally as lepa (paste) to pacify cold (A.S.Ci-2/87).

Internal Use

1. **Vatavyadhi** (neuromuscular disease): Kumkum, Agaru, Tamala patra, Kushta, Ela, Tagara should be taken to get relief from Vatavyadhi (S.S.Ci. 4/24-25).
2. **Shirashool** (headache): Ghee processed with Kumkum and sugar is given as nasya in headache caused by rakta and pittaja (A.H. 4-24/7).
3. **Mutraghata** (suppression of urine): One karsha (about 1 2 g) of Kumkum should be put in honey water for overnight. Then in the next morning it is taken orally which renders immediate relief (S.S.Ci-58/31).

Officinal Part Used

Dried stigma

Dose

Powder: 0.5 to 1 g

Formulations

Kumkumadi ghrita, Kumkumadya taila, Kumkumadi lepa, Karpuradyarka, Balarka Rasa, Yakuti, Mahanarayana taila, Pusyanuga churna.

Toxicity

Saffron is nontoxic in animal studies (LD50: 20.7 g/kg) and noncytotoxic in in vitro studies. The corms are toxic to young animals. In respect to LD50 values and maximum nonfatal doses, the stigma extracts were more toxic than the petals' extract and have been reported as 1.6 g/kg, i.p., and 3.38 g/kg, i.p., in mice. According to a toxicity classification, stigma and petal extracts are "relatively toxic" and "low toxic," respectively. Treatment with the *C. sativus* extract also significantly prolonged the life span of cisplatin-treated mice almost threefold (Nair et al 1991).

Toxicity studies showed that the hematological and the biochemical parameters were within normal range with saffron extract (Nair et al 1991).

Substitution and Adulteration

Beet, pomegranate fibers, and red-dyed silk fibers are occasionally mixed to decrease the cost of original saffron. The yellow stamens of saffron have been mixed with the saffron stigma or powder to increase the product mass. Sometimes flowers of other plants like *Carthamus tinctorius*, or safflower, *Calendula officinalis*, or marigold, arnica, and tinted grasses are intentionally added to the genuine stigmas. Turmeric powder, paprika, and other substances of similar color are also mixed with saffron powder (Kafi 2002; Hagh-Nazari and Keifi 2007).

Kusumbha puspa is substituted for Kumkum as per Bhavaprakash.

Points to Ponder

- It is regarded as all-time king of spices and is also called "red gold" in the present scenario.
- Kusumbha puspa is substituted for Kumkum as per Bhavaprakash.
- Brick red–colored stigmas are collected as saffron.
- It is used in headache, vomiting, wound, acne, and worm.

Suggested Readings

Abdullaev Fl. Biological effects of saffron. Biofactors 1993;4(2):83–86

Abdullaev Fl. Cancer chemopreventive and tumoricidal properties of saffron (*Crocus sativus* L.). Exp Biol Med (Maywood) 2002;227(1):20–25

Abdullaev JF, Caballero-Ortega H, Riverón-Negrete L, et al. In vitro evaluation of the chemopreventive potential of saffron. Rev Invest Clin 2002;54(5):430–436

Ahmad AS. Biological properties and medicinal use of saffron. Pharmacol Biochem Behav 2005;81:805–813

Akhondzadeh BA, Moshiri E, Noorbala AA, Jamshidi AH, Abbasi SH, Akhondzadeh S. Comparison of petal of *Crocus sativus* L. and fluoxetine in the treatment of depressed outpatients: a pilot double-blind randomized trial. Prog Neuropsychopharmacol Biol Psychiatr 2007;31(2):439–442

Akhondzadeh S, Fallah-Pour H, Afkham K, Jamshidi AH, Khalighi-Cigaroudi F. Comparison of *Crocus sativus* L. and imipramine in the treatment of mild to moderate depression: a pilot double-blind randomized trial [ISRCTN45683816]. BMC Complement Altern Med 2004;4:12

Anjum N, Pal A, Tripathi YC. Phytochemistry and pharmacology of saffron: the most precious natural source of colour, flavour and medicine. SMU Med J 2015;2:335–347

Basker D, Negbi M. Uses of saffron. Econ Bot 1983;37:228–236

Bathaie SZ, Mousavi SZ. New applications and mechanisms of action of saffron and its important ingredients. Crit Rev Food Sci Nutr 2010;50:761–786

Bhat JV, Broker R. Riboflavine and thiamine contents of saffron, *Crocus sativus* Linn. Nature 1953;172(4377):544

Blumenthal M. The Complete German Commission E Monographs. Boston: American Botanical Council; 1998

Chang VC, Lin YL, Lee MJ, Show SJ, Wang CJ. Inhibitory effect of crocetin on benzopyrene genotoxicity and neoplastic transformation in C3H1OT1=2 cells. Anticancer Res 1996; 765:3603–3608.

Ferrence SC, Bendersky G. Therapy with saffron and the goddess at Thera. Perspect Biol Med 2004;47(2):199–226

Hagh-Nazari S, Keifi N. Saffron and various fraud manners in its production and trades. Acta Hortic 2007; (739):411–416 (ISHS)

Harper D. Saffron. Online Etymology Dictionary;2001. <http:// www.etymoline.com/index.php?search=saffron&search mode=none

Kafi M. Saffron: Production Technology and Manufacture. Mashhad: Ferdowsi University Publication;2002

Katzer G. Saffron (*Crocus sativus* L.). Gernot Katzer's Spice;2001

Khare CP. Encyclopedia of Indian Medicinal Plants. Germany: Springer; 2004:166

Kirtikar and Basu. Indian Medicinal Plants. 2nd ed. Vol. 4. 1993:2463

Kokate CK, Purohit AP, Gokhale SB. Pharmacognosy. Pune: Nirali Prakashan; 2006; 390

Kumar V. The Secret Benefits of Spices and Condiments. Sterling;2006: 103

Mathew B. Botany, Taxonomy and Cytology of *C. sativus* L. and Its Allies. In: M. Negbi, ed. Saffron. Amsterdam: Hardwood Academic Publishers; 1999

Nadkarni KM. Indian Materia Medica, Vol. 1. Bombay: Popular Prakashan; 2000:390-391

Nair SC, Pannikar B, Panikkar KR. Antitumour activity of saffron (*Crocus sativus*). Cancer Lett 1991;57(2):109–114

Negbi M. Saffron: *Crocus sativus* L. CRC Press; 2003

Nørbæk R, Kondo T. Anthocyanins from flowers of *Crocus* (Iridaceae). Phytochemistry 1998;47:1–4

Pitsikas N. Constituents of saffron (*Crocus sativus* L.) as potential candidates for the treatment of anxiety disorders and schizophrenia. Molecules 2016;21(3):303

Rios JL, Recio MC, Ginger RM, Manz S. An update review of saffron and its active constituents. Phytother Res 1996;10:189–193

Salomi MJ, Nair SC, Panikkar KR. Cytotoxicity and nonmutagenicity of *Nigella sativa* and saffron (*Crocus sativus*) in vitro. Proc Ker Sci Congr 1991; 5:244

Salomi MJ, Nair SC, Panikkar KR. Inhibitory effects of *Nigella sativa* and saffron (*Crocus sativus*) on chemical carcinogenesis in mice. Nutr Cancer 1991;16(1):67–72

Shahnawaz M, Sangale MK, Qazi HA, et al. An attempt of in vivo cultivation of *Crocus sativus* L. in Western Maharashtra, India. Int J Adv Res (Indore) 2017;5:1403–1407

Singla RK, Bhat VG. Crocin: an overview. Indo Global J Pharmac Sci 2011;1:281–286

Soeda S, Ochiai T, Paopong L, Tanaka H, Shoyama Y, Shimeno H. Crocin suppresses tumor necrosis factor-alpha-induced cell death of neuronally differentiated PC-12 cells. Life Sci 2001;69:2887–2898

Tarantilis PA, Morjani H, Polissiou M, Manfait M. Inhibition of growth and induction of differentiation of promyelocytic leukemia (HL-60) by carotenoids from *Crocus sativus* L. Anticancer Res 1994;14(5A):1913–1918

The Ayurvedic Pharmacopoea of India, Part 1, Vol. 4. New Delhi: Govt. of India, Ministry of Health and Family Welfare, Department of AYUSH; 2004:52-54

Vinning G. Saffron: issues in international marketing. Paper deposited on SNV MAP. August 2005

Wang CJ, Shiah HS, Lin JK. Modulatory effect of crocetin on aflatoxin B1

Winterhalter P, Straubinger M. Saffron—renewed interest in an ancient spice. Food Rev Int 2000;16:39–59

Xiang M, Qian ZY, Zhou CH, Liu J, Li WN. Crocetin inhibits leukocyte adherence to vascular endothelial cells induced by AGEs. J Ethnopharmacol 2006;107:25–31

Xi L, Qian Z, Du P, Fu J. Pharmacokinetic properties of crocin (crocetin digentiobiose ester) following oral administration in rats. Phytomedicine 2007;14(9):633–636

Xuan B, Zhou YH, Li N, Min ZD, Chiou GC. Effects of crocin analogs on ocular blood flow and retinal function. J Ocul Pharmacol Ther 1999;15(2):143–152

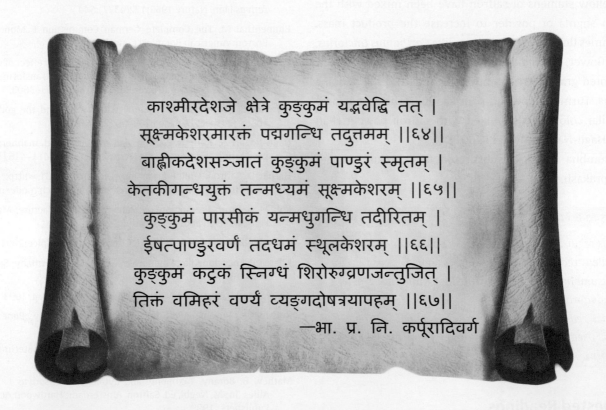

काश्मीरदेशजे क्षेत्रे कुङ्कुमं यद्भवेद्धि तत् |
सूक्ष्मकेशरमारक्तं पद्मगन्धि तदुत्तमम् ||६४||
बाह्लीकदेशसञ्जातं कुङ्कुमं पाण्डुरं स्मृतम् |
केतकीगन्धयुक्तं तन्मध्यमं सूक्ष्मकेशरम् ||६५||
कुङ्कुमं पारसीकं यन्मधुगन्धि तदीरितम् |
ईषत्पाण्डुरवर्णं तदधमं स्थूलकेशरम् ||६६||
कुङ्कुमं कटुकं स्निग्धं शिरोरुग्व्रणजन्तुजित् |
तिक्तं वमिहरं वर्ण्यं व्यङ्गदोषत्रयापहम् ||६७||
—भा. प्र. नि. कर्पूरादिवर्ग

59. Kupilu *[Strychnus nux-vomica Linn.]*

Family:	*Loganiaceae (Syn: Strychnaceae)*
Hindi name:	*Kuchala*
English name:	*Nuxvomica, Strychnine tree, Poison nut-tree*

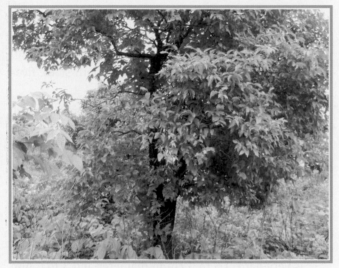

Plant of *Strychnus nuxvomica* Linn.

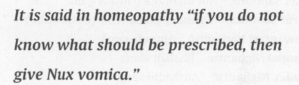

It is said in homeopathy "if you do not know what should be prescribed, then give Nux vomica."

Introduction

Strychnos nux-vomica (Kupilu) is derived from a Greek word "Strychnos," which means poisonous, and "nuxvomica," which means having vomiting effects (Suresh et al 2014). Kupilu is a poisonous drug of vegetable origin, included in upavisha varga. Literature claims that though it is a poisonous drug, it can be used for therapeutic purposes after its purification. Crude drug Kuchala is used in the treatment of anemia, lumbago, asthma, bronchitis, constipation, diabetes, malarial fever, skin disease, paralysis, muscle weakness, and appetite loss (Gruenwald 2000). Seeds of *S. nux-vomica* are used as nervine tonic, alexiteric, aphrodisiac, anthelmintic, digestive, purgative, and stimulant. Detoxified Kuchala seeds are used as an important ingredient in various Ayurvedic medicines like agnitundi vati, navjeevan rasa, and vishatinduka vati (Lavekar 2008).

According to the Pharmacopoeia of the People's Republic of China, *nux-vomica* is bitter in flavor and warm in nature, and is attributive to the liver and spleen meridians. It has been shown to remove obstruction in the channels, relieve pain, and subdue swelling. However, due to its severe toxicity, *nux-vomica* should be processed before oral usage, should not be taken over a long time period of time, and its dosage should be strictly controlled. Furthermore, it is contraindicated in pregnant women.

Vernacular Names

Arabian: Ajaraki, Habbul Gurav
Bengali: Kunchila
Gujarati: Jherkuchala, Zerkochala
Malayalam: Kaajjeel
Marathi: Kajara
Parsi: Kuchula, Phuloosemaahi
Tamil: Yettikottai
Telugu: Mushini Ginjalu, Mushti Vittulu

Synonyms

Tinduka: Its fruits resemble Tindu.
Jalada: It grows in watery place.
Deerghapatraka: It has long leaves.
Kupilu: It is an inferior variety of pilu.
Kakatinduka: This is considered as Tinduk for crow.
Vishatindu: It is the poisonous variety of Tinduk.
Garadruma: It is a poisonous plant.
Other synonyms are Kakapiluka, Kakendu, Markatatinduka, Karaskara, Kulaka, and Vishamusti.

Classical Categorization

Charak Samhita: Not mentioned in any gana
Sushrut Samhita: Surasadi, phala visha (beeja visha)
Dhanwantari Nighantu: Amradi varga
Madanpal Nighantu: Phaladi varga
Kaiyadev Nighantu: Aushadhi varga
Raj Nighantu: Amradi varga
Bhavaprakash Nighantu: Amradiphala varga
Rasatarangini: Sthavara Vanaspatik vish Upavisha

Distribution

Nux-vomica is native to tropical and subtropical regions of South East Asia and Australia (Pawar 2017). In India, it is commonly observed in moist deciduous and semi-evergreen forests of West Bengal, Bihar, Maharashtra, Odisha, Central and South India up to an altitude of 500 m (Pulliah and Rani 2011).

Morphology

- **Habit:** It is a shrub or small tree that is 5 to 25 m in height with irregular branches and ash-colored bark. The young shoots are deep green color with a shiny coat.
- **Leaves:** Simple, oppositely decussate arrangement and are papery; leaf blade is suborbicular, broadly elliptic or ovate, 5 to 18 cm in length and 4 to 13 cm in width, short stalked, smooth on both sides, five-nerved from base (**Fig. 59.1**).
- **Flower:** Its five-merous flower is funnel shaped, greenish-white in color. They bloom in the cold season and have a foul smell (**Fig. 59.2**).
- **Fruit:** Indehiscent brownish-yellow globular berries. Its size is like small oranges, 4 to 6 cm in diameter, and contains a gelatinous pulp in which one to five seeds are embedded (**Fig. 59.3**).
- **Seeds:** Flattened disc/discoid shaped, dried ripe seed is very hard, 1.5 to 3 cm in diameter and 3 to 6 mm in thickness, much compressed, covered with hair radiating from center, has no odor but tastes very bitter (**Fig. 59.4**).

It is propagated by seed and vegetative methods.

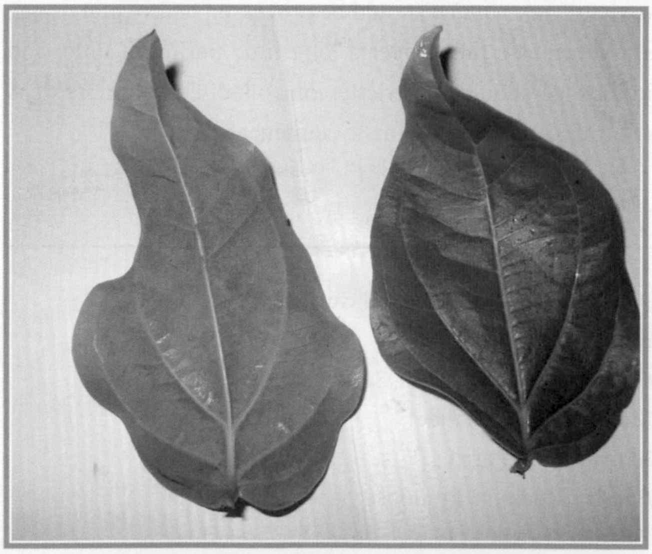

Fig. 59.1 Leaves.

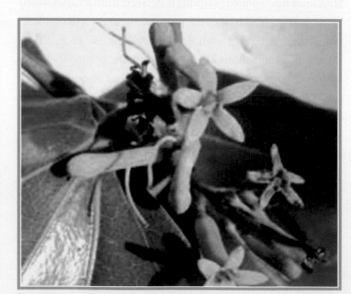

Fig. 59.2 Flower.

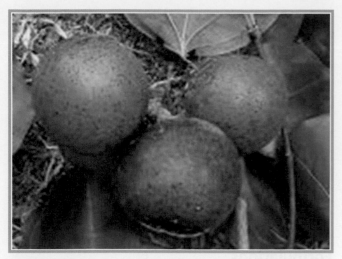

Fig. 59.3 Fruits.

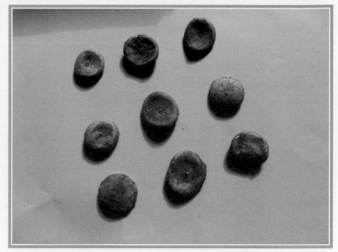

Fig. 59.4 Seeds.

Phenology

Flowering time: November to February

Fruiting time: March to May

Key Characters for Identification

➤ Shrub or small tree, 5 to 25 m tall with irregular branches and ash-colored bark.

➤ Leaves: Simple, oppositely decussate, elliptic or ovate, short stalked, smooth, five-nerved from base.

➤ Flower: Funnel-shaped, greenish-white colored flower.

➤ Fruit: Indehiscent brownish-yellow globular berries, which is like small oranges in size. It contains a gelatinous pulp in which one to five seeds are embedded.

➤ Seeds: Flattened disc/discoid shaped, dried ripe seed is very hard, 1.5 to 3 cm in diameter and 3 to 6 mm in thickness.

Chemical Constituents

Many chemical compounds, including alkaloids, iridoid glycosides, flavonoid glycosides, triterpenoids, steroids, and organic acids, have been isolated and identified from *S. nux-vomica*. Of these, the alkaloids are the principal chemical component.

Strychnine and brucine are considered to be the major bioactive and principal toxic compounds among these

alkaloids. The dried seeds of *S. nux-vomica* contain 2.6 to 3% total alkaloids, out of which 1.25 to 1.5% is strychnine, 1.7% is brucine, and the rest are vomicine and igasurine (Nadkarni 1954).

Other minor alkaloids are iso-strychnine, iso-brucine β-colubrine, icajine, 16-hydroxy α-colubrine, brucine N-oxide, novacine, iso-brucine-N-oxide, iso-strychnine-N-oxide, 4-N-hydroxymethyl strychnidin 17 acetic acid, 10,11-dimethoxy-4-N-hydroxymethyl strychnine 17 acetic acid, pseudostrychnine, pseudobrucine.

They also contain vomicine, colubrine, logamine, logamine glycosides, and fatty substances.

Identity, Purity, and Strength

- Total ash: 4.23 ± 0.25 % w/w
- Acid-insoluble ash: 3.06 ± 0.05% w/w
- Water-soluble ash: 0.93 ± 0.05% w/w
- Loss on drying: 7.83 ± 0.28% w/w
- Swelling index: 53.33 ± 11.54% v/v

(Source: Bhati et al 2012)

Karma (Actions)

The important actions of Kupilu are vedanasthapana (analgesic), shothahara (anti-inflammatory), deepan (appetizer), pachan (digestive), grahi (absorbent), nadibalya (nerve stimulant), kasahara (antitussive), kustaghna (antidermatosis), kandughna (antipruritus), madakaraka (intoxication), vajikarana (aphrodisiac).

- Doshakarma: Kaphapittahara and Vatakara
- Dhatukarma: Vajikaran
- Malakarma: Grahi

Pharmacological Actions

Actions include analgesic, anti-inflammatory, anti-convulsant, antitumor effect, antiamnesic, antidiarrheal, antidysenteric, antispasmodic, febrifuge, stimulant, aphrodisiac and tonic, immunomodulatory effects on the nervous system, antisnake venom activity, hepatoprotective, antipyretic, etc. (Katiyar et al 2010; Deng et al 2006; Kwon et al 2009).

Indications

It is used in kushta (skin disease), amavata (rheumatoid arthritis), sandhivata (osteoarthritis), krimi (worm infestation), shwasa (asthma), kasa (cough), gulma (abdominal lump), aruchi (anorexia), visuchika (cholera), arsha (piles), kapha roga (diseases of kapha), vrana (wound), dhwajabhangha (erectile dysfunctions), kampa (tremor), badhirya (deafness), ardita (facial paralysis), pakshaghata (hemiplegia), andria (insomnia), raktavikara (diseases of rakta), vatarakta (gout), vishamajwara (intermittent fever).

Contraindications

It is contraindicated in pregnancy, during breast-feeding, and in contact dermatitis.

Therapeutic Uses

1. **Jwara** (fever): Purified Kupilu with equal quantity of Maricha powder is mixed with the decoction of Indrayava to make pills. It eliminates constipation and vatika jwara (fever) (S.B. 4/101).
2. **Visuchika** (cholera): Kupilu, Hingu, and Navasadara are fried in fire separately and then mixed and rubbed with water to make vati (pills). It cures visuchika (S.B. 4/277)

3. **Agnimandya** (loss of appetite): Kupilu, Hingu, and Navasadara are rubbed with lemon juice and made into pills and taken orally to increase appetite (S.B. 4/256).

Officinal Part Used

Seeds

Dose

60 to 25 mg

Formulations

Navajeevan rasa, Agnitundi vati, Laxmivilas rasa, Vishamusti, Krimi mudgar rasa, Kupilu Hinwadi vati, Vishatindukadi lepa, Vatagajankush, Kupilubeejadi kwath, Vishatinduk taila, Maha Vishagarbha taila.

Toxicity/Adverse Effects

Toxicity features are reported if drug is administered in high dose and unpurified form. In Chinese Pharmacopoeia it is classified as a highly toxic medicine (Committee for the Pharmacopoeia of China 2015). Strychnine and brucine the most abundant alkaloids of *nux-vomica* are highly toxic to humans and animals (Patocka 2015). Both compounds are neurotoxic and competitive antagonist of the glycine receptors in the central nervous system of vertebrate. Lethal doses of strychnine induce convulsions of the central nervous system and death through respiratory or spinal paralysis or cardiac arrest. The common cause of death is respiratory failure (Chen et al 2012). The lethal dose of strychnine was found to be 30 to 120 mg for an adult individual and 15 mg for a child (Patocka 2015). Brucine is poisonous but its toxic effects are only one-eighth of that of strychnine. Lethal concentration causes life-threatening complications like rhabdomyolysis and acute renal failure. The lethal dose of brucine for an adult individual is 1,000 mg (Maji and Banerji 2017). Excess dose of *nux-vomica* causes convulsions and tetanus-like symptoms. Symptoms include chest discomfort, contractions of all limb muscles, carp pedal spasm, muscle pain, numbness, hyperventilation, confusion, nystagmus (rapid movement of the eyes), knee-jerks, tiredness, and seizures (Pawar 2017). Complications consist of hyperthermia, renal failure, and rhabdomyolysis.

Treatment

If jaws are not closed, then stomach pump is used at once. Stomach is washed in dilute solution of potassium permanganate. Suspension of animal charcoal is given to absorb any free strychnine and then removed from the body. If the strychnine is not removed, then death is must. Inject large dose of potassium bromide and chloral hydrate per rectum. Artificial respiration, oxygen, and supportive therapy may be given. Antidote may be used.

Purification of Kupilu

Various methods are mentioned in classical Ayurvedic texts for the purification of Kupilu. Processing/detoxification of *nux-vomica* seeds is very essential before its therapeutic use. Use of different factors like cow's urine, milk, ghee (purified butter), kanji (sour gruel), castor oil, ginger juice, sand, vinegar, etc. for processing is described lucidly in different pharmacopoeias. Every purification process directs toward reducing the levels of alkaloids and has some therapeutic rationale.

Shodhan (purification) in cow's milk: Seeds are boiled in cow's milk for 3 hours by Dolayantra method. Then its outer covering is removed and the seeds dried in sunlight. When dried properly, it is pulverized. According to Ras Tarangini, it is the method of attaining uttam shuddhi.

Shodhan in cow's urine: Seeds are soaked in cow's urine for 7 days. Fresh cow's urine is used each day. After 7 days they are cleaned with warm water. The outer covering is removed, and the seeds are dried in sunlight followed by pulverization.

Shodhana in cow's urine and cow's milk: Seeds are soaked in cow's urine for 7 days, then seeds are cleaned with warm water, then boiled in cow's milk for 3 hours by Dolayantra method. Then the outer covering is removed and then seeds are dried in sunlight properly and then pulverized (siddhayoga sangraha).

Shodhana is also done in cow's ghee, kanji, cow's dung, cow's ghee, cow's urine, and cow's milk.

Points to Ponder

- *Paribhadra (Erythrina variegata) is used as antidote of Kupilu.*
- *Before use, the seeds of Kupilu must be detoxified properly with cow's milk, urine, or ghee.*
- *It is not safe to use in pregnant women and lactating mothers. Avoid it in children.*
- *As per the Drugs and Cosmetics Act, the medicines containing nux-vomica should be taken only under strict medical supervision.*

Suggested Readings

Ambikadatta S, Commentary SH. Rasratnasammucchaya. 8th ed. Varanasi: Chaukhamba Amarbharati Prakashan; 1988:170

Ambikadatta S, ed. Sushrutsamhita-klp.3/3. Varanasi: Chukhambha Sanskrit Sansthan; 2000:16

Anonymous. The Wealth of India, Vol. 10. New Delhi: National Institute of Science Communication, Council of Scientific & Industrial Research; 1998;:62

Bhati R, Singh A, Saharan VA, Ram V, Bhandari A. *Strychnos nux-vomica* seeds: pharmacognostical standardization, extraction, and antidiabetic activity. J Ayurveda Integr Med 2012;3(2):80–84

Cai BC, Wu H, Yang XW, Hattori M, Namba T. Analysis of spectral data for 13CNMR of sixteen Strychnos alkaloids. Yao Xue Xue Bao 1994;29:44–48

Chen J, Wang X, Qu YG, et al. Analgesic and anti-inflammatory activity and pharmacokinetics of alkaloids from seeds of *Strychnos nux-vomica* after transdermal administration: effect of changes in alkaloid composition. J Ethnopharmacol 2012;139(1):181–188

Deng XK, Yin W, Li WD, et al. The anti-tumor effects of alkaloids from the seeds of *Strychnos nux-vomica* on HepG2 cells and its possible mechanism. J Ethnopharmacol 2006;106(2):179–186

Gruenwald J. PDR for Herbal Medicines. 2nd ed. Montvale: Thomson Healthcare; 2000:548

Katiyar C, Kumar A, Bhattacharya SK, Singh RS. Ayurvedic processed seeds of nux-vomica: neuropharmacological and chemical evaluation. Fitoterapia 2010;81(3):190–195

Kirtikar KR, Basu BD. Indian Medicinal Plants, Vol. 3. 2nd ed. Dehra Dun: Bishen Singh Mahendra Pal Singh; 2003:1646

Kwon SH, Kim HC, Lee SY, Jang CG. Loganin improves learning and memory impairments induced by scopolamine in mice. Eur J Pharmacol 2009;619(1-3):44–49

Lavekar GS. Database on Medicinal Plants Used in Ayurveda and Siddha, Vol. 5. New Delhi: CCRAS; 2008:139

Liu XK, Li W. Chemical constituents of Maqianzi (*Strychno nux-vomica*). Zhong Cao Yao 1998;29:435–438

Maji AK, Banerji P. *Strychnos nux-vomica*: a poisonous plant with various aspects of therapeutic significance. J Basic Clin Pharm 2017;8:S087–S103

Nadkarni KM. Indian Materia Medica, Vol. 2. 3rd ed. Mumbai: Popular Prakashan; 1954:1179

Nighantu B. Commentary by Dr. Krishnachandra Chunekar. Edited by Dr. Pandey. Varanasi: Chaukhamba Bharti Academy; 2006:568

Patocka J, ed. Handbook of Toxicology of Chemical Warfare Agents. Academic Press; 2015:215

Pawar RP. Isolation and characterization of alkaloids of nux-vomica by instrumental technique. J Med Chem Drug Discov 2017;2(3):5461

Pulliah T, Rani SS. Flora of Eastern Ghats, Vol. 4. New Delhi: Regency Publication; 2011:135–139

Sharma DN. Rasratna Sammuchaya. 2nd ed. New Delhi: Motilal Banarasidas Publication; 1996:15684

Sharma PV. Dravyaguna-Vigyana, Vol. 2. Varanasi: Chukhambha Bharti Academy; 2005:85

Sharma SN, Shastri KN. Rasatarangini. 11th ed. New Delhi: Motilal Banarasidas Publication; 2000:676-689

Shastry JLN. Dravyaguna Vijnana, Vol. 2. 3rd ed. Varanasi: Chukhambha Orientalia; 2008:353

Shastry PK. Rasatarangini. 11th ed. New Delhi: Motilal Banarasidas Publication; 1979:675

Suresh NP, Pullaiah T, Varalakshmi D. Textbook of Pharmacognosy, Vol. II. 1st ed. New Delhi: Ikon Books and CBS Publishers; 2014:244

Trease GE, Evans WC. Trease and Evans' Pharmacognosy. 15th ed. Philadelphia: W.B. Saunders Company Ltd.; 2000:378

Warrier PK, Nambiar VP, Ramankutty C. Indian Medicinal Plants: A Compendium of 500 Species, Vol. 5. Hyderabad: Orient Longman; 1996:202

Yang XW, Yan ZK, Cai BC. Studies on the chemical constituents of alkaloids in seeds of *Strychnos nux-vomica* L. Zhongguo Zhongyao Zazhi 1993;18(12):739–740, 763–764

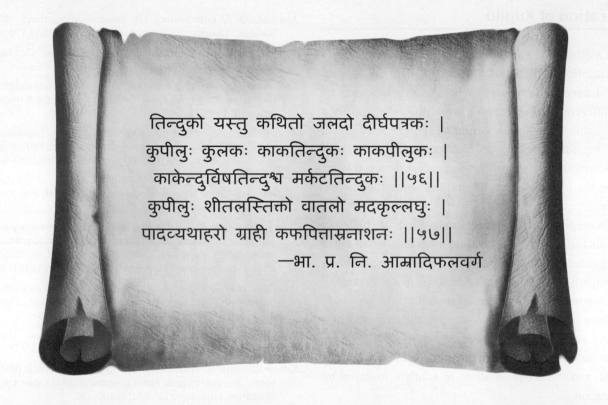

तिन्दुको यस्तु कथितो जलदो दीर्घपत्रकः |
कुपीलुः कुलकः काकतिन्दुकः काकपीलुकः |
काकेन्दुर्विषतिन्दुश्च मर्कटतिन्दुकः ||५६||
कुपीलुः शीतलस्तिक्तो वातलो मदकृल्लघुः |
पादव्यथाहरो ग्राही कफपित्तास्रनाशनः ||५७||
—भा. प्र. नि. आम्रादिफलवर्ग

60. Kushta [*Saussurea lappa* C.B. Clarke]

Synonyms:	*Saussurea costus (Fale) Lipschitz*
Family:	*Asteraceae*
Hindi name:	*Kooth*
English name:	*Costus root*

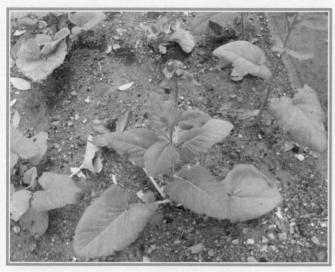

Plant of *Saussurea lappa* C.B. Clarke

> *The water-based recipes of meda (fat), payah (milk), rakta (blood), and Kushta are used in the evening and morning for irrigation of Punnaga, Nagakeshar, and Bakula plants during their flowering season to notably improve the fragrance of the treated plants.*
>
> —*Vrikshaayurveda/250*

Introduction

Saussurea lappa C.B. Clarke (Family: Asteraceae) commonly known as Qust-e-shireen is a long, erect herb found mostly in northern mountainous regions of Pakistan and India (Gupta and Ghatak 1967). This plant is endemic to the valley of Kashmir and is distributed between 2,400 and 3,000 m above the sea level. This species is used to prepare ritual scents and various medicines, and is also used as a tonic, carminative, and stimulant, as well as a good remedy for the treatment of asthmatic spasms, chronic skin diseases, rheumatism, cough, cholera, scabious itching, and incurable sores (Singh 1935; Chang and Kim 2008).

S. *lappa* has been declared critically endangered (Butola and Samant 2010; Anonymous, 1973; Nayar and Shastry 1987, 1988, 1990) and has been included in Appendix I of the Convention on International Trade in Endangered Species (CITES) of Wild Fauna and Flora to promote its conservation. In light of the fact that this plant is an economically viable MAP (Medicinal and Aromatic Plants) for cultivation in temperate zones, the National Medicinal Plants Board of the Government of India has given priority to the development of agro-technology for the cultivation of this crop. In vitro propagation techniques for this endangered species are in place (Arora and Bhojwani 1989; Guo et al. 2007) because the annual trade volume of *S. lappa* is estimated between 300 and 400 metric tons (Sinha 2011). It is currently under cultivation in areas of Himachal Pradesh and Uttarakhand (Kuniyal et al. 2005).

Being an endangered species, it has been prioritized among the species of high conservation concern (Khoshoo 1993; Badola and Pal 2002; Ved et al. 2003). Its trade is strictly prohibited under Foreign Trade Development Act, 1992.

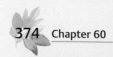

Vernacular Names

Arabi: Kuste
Assamese: Kud, Kur
Bengali: Kudo, Kood
Chinese: Mu Xiang
Farsi: Kust-E-Talkh
French: Costus elegant
German: Practige kostwurz
Gujarati: Kudu, Upaleta
Kannada: Changal Kustha, Koshta
Kashmiri: Kuth
Malayalam: Kottam, Seyuddi
Marathi: Upleta, Kustha
Oriya: Kudha
Punjabi: Kuth
Tamil: Goshtam, Kosbtham, Kottam
Telugu: Changalva Koshtu, Kustham
Urdu: Minal, Qust

Synonyms

Kushta: The drug is useful in leprosy/skin diseases.
Rogahwaya: It cures all types of diseases.
Vapya: It grows in cold and marshy places.
Paribhavya: The drug is considered a safeguard from diseases.
Utpala: It grows in watery place like utpala or lotus plant.
Pakala: It protects from diseases.
Ruk: It can be used freely without any doubts.
Kashmiraja: The natural habitat of the plants is Kashmir.

Classical Categorization

Charak Samhita: Lekhaniya, Shukrashodhan, Asthapanopag
Sushruta Samhita: Eladi
Dhanwantari Nighantu: Chandanadi varga
Madanpal Nighantu: Abhayadi varga
Kaiyadev Nighantu: Aushadhi varga
Raj Nighantu: Chandanadi varga
Bhavaprakash Nighantu: Haritakyadi varga

Distribution

It is native to the Himalayan region and is distributed in Alpine and sub-Alpine regions of Himalaya between 2,500 and 3,000 m altitude. Its natural population is reported from the higher elevations of Jammu and Kashmir and Himachal Pradesh. It is now cultivated in Kashmir, Himachal Pradesh, and in some parts of Uttarakhand. Population status/Cause for Rare Endangered and Threatened (RET): It is critically endangered due to indiscriminate collection (for its roots) and destruction of habitat. Its commercial cultivation was taken up during 1920s and 1930s in Kashmir, Lahul, and Garhwal in its natural habitat. It is also cultivated in Leh.

Morphology

It is an erect, perennial, robust herb.

- **Stem:** Simple 1 to 2 m high, fibrous with radical leaves.
- **Leaves:** Basal leaves are scaberulous above, glabrate beneath, margins irregularly toothed. These are very large, 50 cm to 115 cm, with long petiole. Petiole is 60 to 90 cm long, lobately winged, whereas cauline leaves are semi-amplexicaul, 15 to 30 cm long, sessile, or with shorter petiole. Leaves are almost clasping the stem (**Fig. 60.1a, b**).
- **Flower:** Bluish-purple to almost black, stalkless head, hard, rounded, often two to five clustered together in axillary or terminal. Involucral bracts many, ovate lanceolate, purple, long, and pointed. Receptacle bristles, very long, corolla-tubular, blue-purple or almost black, anthers tails fimbriate (**Fig. 60.2**).
- **Fruits:** Achenes are curved, compressed, and 8 mm long.
- **Root:** Roots are stout, inverted cone-shaped, up to 60 cm long, grayish to dull brownish, with characteristic penetrating odor (**Fig. 60.3**).

It is propagated through seeds.

Phenology

Flowering time: June to August
Fruiting time: August to September

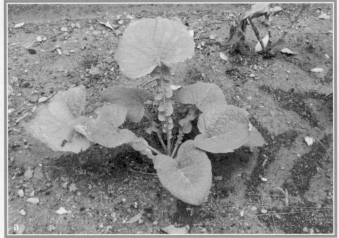

Fig. 60.1 **(a, b)** Leaves.

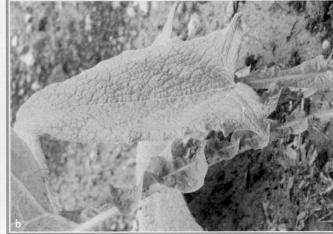

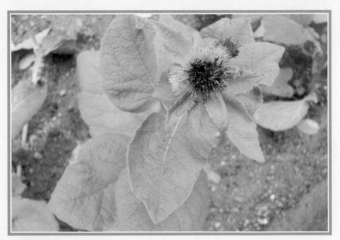

Fig. 60.2 Flower.

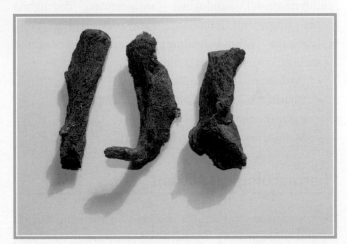

Fig. 60.3 Root.

Key Characters for Identification

➤ *It is 1 to 2 m tall, with a thick fibrous stem.*
➤ *Leaves are radical with long lobately winged stalks.*
➤ *Flowers are dark purple or black in color.*
➤ *Roots are stout, carrot-like, 60 cm long, possessing a characteristic penetrating odor.*

Rasapanchaka

Guna	Laghu
Rasa	Katu, Tikta, Madhura
Vipak	Katu
Virya	Ushna

Chemical Constituents

Plant contains phytoconstituents such as resins, alkaloids, steroids, and flavonoids. Costunolide is one of the major bioactive constituents of *S. lappa* root. Other constituents are costunolide, dihydrocostunolide, 12-methoxydihydrocostunolide, dihydro costus lactone, α-hydroxydehydrocostus lactone, β-hydroxydehydro-costus lactone, betulinic acid, 1 saussure amines a-c, α-cyclocostunolide, saussureal, and has also three anthraquinones compound: β-sitosterol, palmitic acid, and linoleic acid.

The costus oil, a pale yellow or brownish viscous emollient, is obtained from the roots either by steam distillation or through extraction with solvents. The oil contains resinoids, essential oils, inulin, saussurine, and other alkaloids (Kuniyal et al. 2005).

Identity, Purity, and Strength

- Foreign matter: Not more than 2%
- Total ash: Not more than 4%
- Acid-insoluble ash: Not more than 1%
- Alcohol-soluble extractive: Not less than 12%
- Water-soluble extractive: Not less than 20%

(Source: The Ayurvedic Pharmacopeia of India 1989)

Karma (Actions)

The main actions of Kushta are shukrala (spermopoietic), kashahara (antitussive), shwasahara (antiasthmatic), jwaraghna (antipyretics), vishaghna (antidote), kushaghna (antidermatosis), kandughna (antipruritus), dadrughna (cures ringworm infection), rasayana (rejuvenation), vranaropaka (wound healing), vranashodhaka (wound cleansing), krishakaraka (fat reducing).

- Doshakarma: Vata kaphahara
- Dhatukarma: Shukrashodhan, Vajikaran, Raktashodhaka
- Malakarma: Mutrala, Swedajanana

Pharmacological Actions

The pharmacological actions reported for the plant Kushta are anti-inflammatory, antibacterial , anticancer, cytotoxic, antispasmodic, hepatoprotective, immunomodulator, antiepileptic, hypolipidemic, hypoglycemic, antiparasitic, antimicrobial, antidiarrheal central nervous system depressant, anticonvulsant, antiulcerogenic, angiogenesis, etc.

Indications

It is used in gout (vatarakta), visarpa (erysipelas), shwasa (bronchial asthma), kasa (cough), throat infection, kushta (skin disease), convulsion, jwara (fever), krimi (worm infestation), hikka (hic-cough), visha (poisoning), kandu (itching), etc.

Therapeutic Uses

1. **Gulma** (abdominal lump): Sarjikshara, Kushta, and Saindhava are mixed together and given with warm water (S.S.U-42/46, V.M.30/10).

2. **Arunsika** (head boils): Kushta is roasted in an earthen pan then powdered and mixed with oil. Its external application reduces itching, discharge, pain, burning sensation (A.H.U. 24/23).

3. **Medhya** (intellect promoter): Suvarna bhasma, Kushta, and Vacha are mixed together with honey and ghrita and this preparation is taken as leha (linctus) to promote physical strength and intellect in children (S.S.Sha. 10/68-70).

4. **As Rasayana** (rejuvenation): Kushta is used as rasayana (A.S.U. 49/218).

5. **Unmada** (insanity) and **apasmara** (epilepsy): Old ghee processed with Brahmi juice, Vacha, Kushta, and Shankhapuspi eliminates insanity, epilepsy, and sinful act (C.S.Ci. 10/25).

6. **Sarpa visha** (Snake poisoning): 100 g of Tagar and Kushta are mixed with 200 mL honey and ghee and are given in snake poisoning.

7. **Rheumatism:** The dried rootstock is mixed with mustard oil, and the paste obtained is applied locally to treat rheumatism (Siddique et al 2002).

Officinal Part Used

Root

Dose

Powder: 500 mg to 1 g

Formulations

Kushtadi taila, Kushtadi churna, Dashamularista, Sarivadyasava, Kumaryasava, Narayana taila.

Toxicity/Adverse Effects

Large doses of the extract of *S. lappa* cause giddiness, headache, and drowsiness. Inhalation of smoke of powdered root of this plant produces marked CNS depression (Sharma et al 2000).

Substitution and Adulteration

The root of *Saussurea hypoleuca* Spreng. is used as substitute and adulterant to genuine costus root. Following plants are used as adulterant to *S. lappa*:

- *Inula royleana* DC.
- *Inula racemosa* Hook.f.
- *Inula grandiflora* Willd.
- *Euphorbia thomsoniana* Boiss.
- *Salvia lanata* Roxb.
- *Salvia ligularia*
- *Aconitum heterophyllum*
- *Senecio jaquemontianus* (Decne) Benth. ex Hook.f.
- *Costus speciosus*
- *Arctium lappa* Linn.
- *Kyllinga triceps* (Nivisha)

Elecampane (*Inula helenium* Linn.) root oil available in most parts of the world is common adulterant to costus root oil (Sharma et al 2000).

Points to Ponder

- *Saussurea lappa C.B. Clarke is a critically endangered medicinal plant.*
- *Kushta is used as a substitute plant for Puskarmoola, Langali, and Sthouneya.*
- *Kushta is mainly used in kasa, shwasa, hikka, kushta, and for shukrashodhan.*

Suggested Readings

Anonymous. Convention on International Trade in Endangered Species of Wild Fauna and Flora. Signed at Washington, DC on March 3, 1973 and amended at Bonn, Germany on 22 June 1979; 1973

Arora R, Bhojwani SS. In vitro propagation and low temperature storage of *Saussurea lappa* C.B. Clarke: an endangered, medicinal plant. Plant Cell Rep 1989;8(1):44–47

Badola HK, Pal M. Endangered medicinal plants in Himachal Pradesh. Curr Sci 2002;83(7):797–798

Butola JS, Samant SS. *Saussurea* species in Indian Himalayan region: diversity, distribution and indigenous uses. Int J Plant Biol 2010;1(e9):43–51

Chadha YR. The Wealth of India, Vol. IX: Rh-So. New Delhi: CSIR; 1972:196

Chang K, Kim G. Comparison of volatile aroma component of *Saussurea lappa* C.B. Clarke root oil. Prev Nutr Food Sci 2008;13:128–133

Chopra RN, Nayer SL, Chopra IC. Glossary of Indian Medicinal Plants. National Institute of Science Communication; 1996:141

Guo B, Gao M, Liu CZ. In vitro propagation of an endangered medicinal plant *Saussurea involucrata* Kar. et Kir. Plant Cell Rep 2007;26(3):261–265

Gupta OP, Ghatak BJ. Pharmacological investigations on *Saussurea lappa* (Clarke). Indian J Med Res 1967;55(10):1078–1083

Khoshoo TN. Himalayan biodiversity conservation: an overview. In: Dhar U, ed. Himalayan Biodiversity: Conservation Strategies. Nainital: Himavikas Publication, Gyan Prakash; 1993:5-38

Kuniyal CP, Rawat YS, Oinam SS, Kuniyal JC, Vishvakarma SCR. Kuth (*Saussurea lappa*) cultivation in the cold desert environment of the Lahaul valley, northwestern Himalaya, India: arising threats and need to revive socio-economic values. Biodivers Conserv 2005;14:1035–1045

Nadkarni KM. Indian Materia Medica. 2nd ed. Bombay: Popular Book Depot; 1954:76-78

Nayar MP, Shastry ARK. Red Data Book of Indian Plants, Vol. I, II, & III. Calcutta: Botanical Survey of India; 1987, 1988, 1990:187

Samant SS, Dhar U, Palni LMS. Medicinal Plants of Indian Himalaya: Diversity, Distribution, Potential Values, Vol. 13. Nainital: Himavikas Publication; 1998:43-47

Sharma PC, Yelne MB, Denni TJ. Database on Medicinal Plants Used in Ayurveda, Vol. 7. New Delhi: Central Council for Research in Ayurveda and Siddha, Dept. of ISM & H, Min. of Health & Family Welfare, Govt. of India; 2000:244–264

Sharma PV. Classical Uses of Medicinal Plants. Varanasi: Chaukhambha Visvabharati; 1996:109

Sharma PV. Dravyaguna-Vijnana, Vol. II. Varanasi: Chaukhambha Bharati Academy; 1981:572

Siddique MAA, Wafai BA, Mir RA, Sheikh SA. Conservation of Kuth (*Saussurea costus*)—a threatened medicinal plant of Kashmir Himalaya. In: Samant SS, Dhar U, Palni LMS, eds. Himalayan Medicinal Plants: Potential and Prospects. Nainital: Gyanodaya Prakashan; 2002:197–204

Singh BS. The ecology and culture of Kuth (*Saussurea lappa*, Clarke). Indian For 1935;2:80–89

Sinha S. A review of the status of *S. costus* (Falc.) Lipsch. In: India and the Impact of Its Listing in CITES, Appendix I: A Study by TRAFFIC India (Draft Report); 2011:1–19

Stainton A. Flowers of the Himalaya: A Supplement. Delhi: Oxford University Press; 1988:81-84

The Ayurvedic Pharmacopoeia of India. Part I, Vol. 1. New Delhi: Department of AYUSH, Ministry of Health & Family Welfare, Government of India; 1989:76

Ved DK, Kinhal GA, Ravikumar K, et al. CAMP Report: Conservation Assessment and Management Prioritisation for the Medicinal Plants of Jammu & Kashmir, Himachal Pradesh & Uttaranchal. Workshop, Shimla, Himachal Pradesh. FRLHT, Bangalore, India; 2003

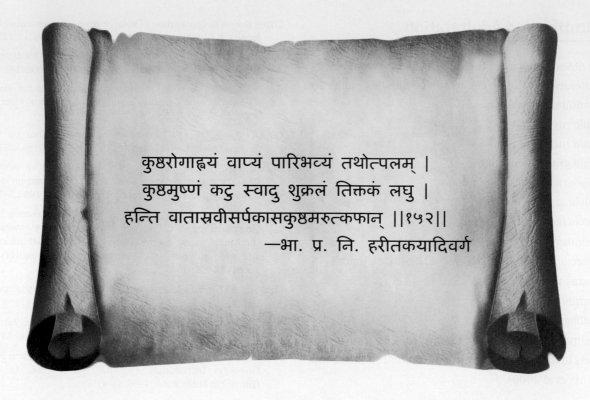

कुष्ठरोगाह्वयं वाप्यं पारिभव्यं तथोत्पलम् ।
कुष्ठमुष्णं कटु स्वादु शुक्रलं तिक्तकं लघु ।
हन्ति वातास्रवीसर्पकासकुष्ठमरुत्कफान् ॥१५२॥
—भा. प्र. नि. हरीतकयादिवर्ग

61. Kutaja *[Holarrhena antidysenterica (L) Wall ex A. DC]*

Family: *Apocynaceae*

Hindi name: *Kurchi, Kuda, Kudaiya, Kuraiya*

English name: *Kurchi bark tree, Conessi bark tree, Tellicherry bark tree*

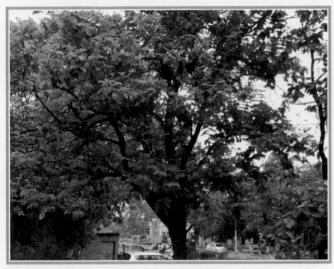

Plant of *Holarrhena antidysenterica* (L) Wall ex A. DC.

During the festival of "Nabanna" (new crops), people of Odisha state of India offer leaves of this plant along with rice to the goddess.

Introduction

Holarrhena antidysenterica is a very significant herbal drug in Ayurvedic and Unani and other Indian system of medicines. Its seed and bark have been used in British Materia Medica also for a long time. This meticulous herb was used to treat a variety of infectious diseases especially in diarrhea, dysentery, skin diseases. It is also reported that it is efficacious against *Staphylococcus aureus*, *Entamoeba histolytica*, and *Escherichia coli*. Acharya Charak mentioned this plant elaborately in a separate chapter in (5th chapter) Kalpasthan of Charak Samhita. This plant is used for vamana karma (to induce emesis). A total of 18 medicinal preparations of Kutaja are described in that chapter by Acharya Charak for vamana karma. Vagabhatta considered this plant as best drug for the treatment of raktarsha (bleeding piles).

Vernacular Names

Assamese: Dudhkuri

Bengali: Karachi, Kurachi

Gujarati: Kudo, Kuda, Kadachhal

Kannada: Korachi, Kodasige, Halagattigida, Halagatti Mara

Kashmiri: Kogad

Malayalam: Kodagapala, Kutakappala

Marathi: Kuda, Pandhra Kuda

Oriya: Kurei, Keruan

Punjabi: Kenara, Kurasukk, Kura

Tamil: Veppalai, Kudasapalai

Telugu: Kodisepala, Kodaga, Palakodisa

Urdu: Tukhm-e-Kurchi, Indarjao Talkh, Kurchi

Synonyms

Girimallika: Plant grows wildly in hilly area with sweet-scented flowers like Jasmine.

Indra: It refers to synonyms of Lord Indra.

Kalinga: It grows wildly in hilly areas, especially in Kalinga region (Odisha state).

Kauto: It grows wildly in hilly areas.

Kootaja: It grows wildly in hilly areas.

Kutaja: It grows wildly in hilly areas.

Mahagandha: The plants bear sweet-scented jasmine-like flowers.

Mallikapuspa: The plants have jasmine-like flowers.

Panduradruma: The bark of this plant is pale.

Pravrushenya: Flowers of Kutaja bloom in early rainy season.

Sangrahi: It has grahi action and is used in diarrhea and dysentery.

Shakra: It is a potent drug.

Shakrashakhi: It has gregarious branches.

Varatikta: It is considered as potent bitter drug.

Vatsaka: It grows wildly in hilly areas of Vatsak Pradesh.

Yavaphala: Fruits of Kutaja have barley-shaped seeds.

Classical Categorization

Charak Samhita: Arshoghna, Kandughna, Stanyashodhana, Astapanopaga

Sushrut Samhita: Aragvadhadi, Pippalyadi, Haridradi, Lakshadi

Dhanwantari Nighantu: Shatapuspadi varga

Madanpal Nighantu: Abhayadi varga

Kaiyadev Nighantu: Aushadhi varga.

Raj Nighantu: Prabhadradi varga

Bhavaprakash Nighantu: Guduchyadi varga.

Distribution

This plant is found throughout the country, especially in Odisha, and deciduous forests of tropical Himalaya up to 900 to 1,200 m altitude. It is also found in subtropical and tropical regions of Asia and Africa.

Morphology

It is a small tree of 2 to 10 m in height with milky latex.

- **Stem bark:** The stem bark is grayish-brown and rough. The stem is white and soft (**Fig. 61.1**).
- **Leaves:** Simple, opposite, sessile, elliptic, or ovate; it is oblong in shape, entire margin, smooth, shortly petiolate, lamina 10–20 cm × 6–10 cm; its base is obtuse, often round or acute; its nerves are in 10 to 14 pairs (**Fig. 61.2**).
- **Flower:** White, small, and arranged in a cluster in terminal corymbose cyme, jasmine-like smell, petals are salver shaped and overlap on right side. The calyx lobe is 2.5 to 3 mm long, oblong-lanceolate, acute, and ciliate. Corolla puberulous outside; tube 8 to 13 mm long, slightly inflated near the base over the stamens, mouth not closed with ring of hair; throat hair inside;

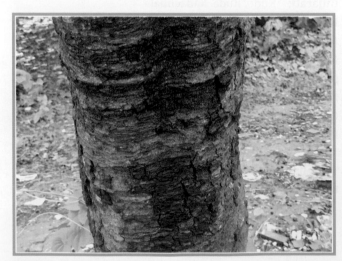

Fig. 61.1 Stem bark.

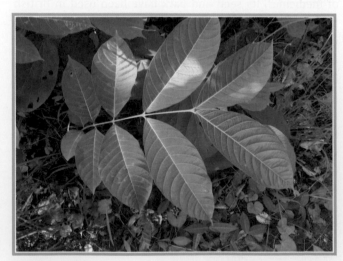

Fig. 61.2 Leaves.

lobes about equaling the tube, oblong, round at the apex, and more or less pubescent (**Fig. 61.3**).

- **Fruits:** Found in pair, elongate, curved, cylindrical, free long follicles, 15–35 cm long × 0.5–0.8 cm diameter, parallel, terete, coriaceous, and obscurely lone lose, usually with dotted white spots (**Fig. 61.4a, b**).
- **Seeds:** Many flat seeds with brown hairs are found in dried fruit, bitter in taste; 8 mm long or more, linear oblong, 25 to 30 seeds found in a follicle (**Fig. 61.5**; Anonymous 1992; Shah et al 1985; Akhtar et al 2010).

Phenology

Flowering time: June to September
Fruiting time: October to February

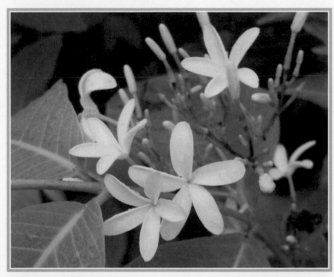

Fig. 61.3 Flowers.

Key Characters for Identification

➤ *Small tree of 2 to 10 m in height with milky latex.*
➤ *The stem bark is grayish-brown and rough. The stem is white and soft.*
➤ *Leaves: Simple, large, opposite, oval-shaped, papery, and smooth or hairy.*
➤ *Flowers: White, small, and arranged in a cluster which looks like flattened top.*
➤ *Fruits: Long follicles, which look like two slender pencils arising from a node. The follicles have white warty spots on the surface. Dried fruits break open releasing numerous flat seeds with brown hairs.*

Types

As per Acharya Charak, Kutaja is of two types:

- Pumkutaja (male Kutaja): Big fruits, white flower, smooth leaves
- Strikutaja (female Kutaja): Shyama (blackish) and Aruna (reddish) flower, puspaphal vrinta anu (very small stalk of flower and fruits).

Rasapanchaka

Guna	Laghu, Ruksha
Rasa	Tikta, Kasaya
Vipak	Katu
Virya	Sheeta

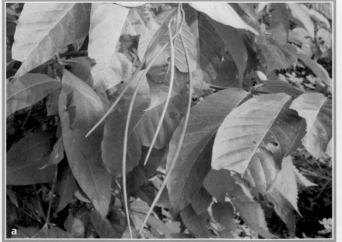

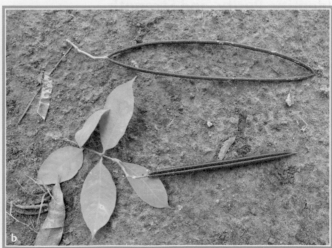

Fig. 61.4 **(a)** Fruits of male Kutaja. **(b)** Fruits of female Kutaja.

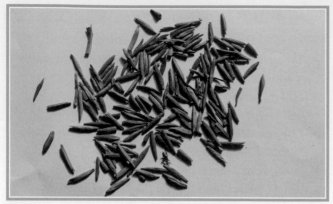

Fig. 61.5 Seeds.

Chemical Constituents

Near about 30 alkaloids have been isolated from the plant, mostly from the bark of Kutaja. The bark contains 2% of alkaloids, namely, conessine, conkurchine, kurchine, holarrhemine, holarrhenine, kurchicine, and conkurchinine. Holacetin, conkurchin, regholarrhenine-A, B, C, D, E, and F, pubescine, norholadiene, kurchinin, kurchinidine, etc. (Shah and Trivedi 1981).

Presence of alkaloids, anthraquinones, coumarins, flavonoids, saponins, sterols, tannins, and terpenes in *H. antidysenterica* are reported (Akinyemi et al 2005).

Various parts of *H. antidysenterica* contain alkaloids, steroidal alkaloid, fats, tannin, and resin. Various alkaloids are reported, such as 3-aminoconanines, 20-aminoconanines, 3-aminopregnans, 20-diaminopregnanes from both seeds and bark.

Seed: Antidysentericine. Seeds are known as Indrayava.

Identity, Purity, and Strength

- Water-soluble extractive: Not less than 10%
- Foreign matter: Not more than 2%
- Total ash: Not more than 7%
- Acid-insoluble ash: Not more than 1%
- Alcohol-soluble extractive: Not less than 18%

(Source: The Ayurvedic Pharmacopeia of India 1989)

Karma (Actions)

The important actions of Kutaja are deepan (appetizer), pachan (digestive), sangrahi (astringent), upashoshana (absorptive), raktapittahara (reduce bleeding), hrudrogahara (prevent cardiac disease), kusthaghna (antidermatosis).

As per Kaiyadev Nighantu, the flower of Kutaja has sheeta virya, tikta and kasaya rasa, laghu guna, and deepan actions while its fruit has katu and tikta rasa, anushna Virya and deepan, pachan and grahi action.

- Doshakarma: Kaphapittashamak; fruit is tridoshashamak; flower is vatakarak and kaphapitta shamak
- Dhatukarma: Raktapittashamak
- Malakarma: Sthambhana, sangrahi

Pharmacological Actions

The pharmacological actions reported are antispasmodic, astringent, anthelmintic, stomachic, febrifuge, diuretic, antibacterial, amoebicidal, antidiabetic, antidiarrheal, anti-inflammatory, and analgesic, antioxidant, antiurolithic, antihemorrhoidal, anthelmintic, antimicrobial, antimalarial, antihyperglycemic and antihyperlipidemic, cytotoxic, antiplasmodial, antimutagenic, immunomodulatory, protection of DNA from radiation, anthelmintic, CNS depressant, inhibition of acetylcholinesterase, analgesic, antipsoriatic. It inhibits growth of various microbes against vaginitis (Hagers 1976; Khare 2007). The fruit extracts have potent anticancer properties (Dhar et al 1968).

Indications

Root and bark is used in pravahika (amoebic dysentery), atisara (diarrhea), shoola (colic dyspepsia), arsha (piles), kushta (skin disease), raktapitta (hemorrhagic diseases), visarpa (erysipelas), trishna (thirst), krimi (worm infestation).

Flowers are used in raktapitta ((hemorrhagic diseases), kushta, atisara, and krimi, and fruits are used in kushta (skin diseases), jwara (fever), visarpa (erysipelas), shoola, guda kila and vatarakta (gout).

The stem bark is found effective against various infections, antidontalgic, febrifuge, antidropsical, diuretic, in piles, colic, dyspepsia, chest affections, and as a tonic in diseases of the skin and spleen properties (Chopra et al 1982).

Seeds are astringent, febrifuge, antidysenteric, anthelmintic, carminative, and used in diarrhea. The leaves are used in chronic bronchitis, and locally for boils and ulcers (Chopra et al 1982; Wealth of India 1959). The seeds are effective in jaundice (Sharma et al 1979).

Therapeutic Uses

External Use

1. **Kushta** (skin disease): External application of paste of Kutaja, Lodhra, Dhataki, Karanja, and Jati is used to cure kushta and other skin diseases (C.S.Ci. 7/95-99). Decoction of Kutaja cures all types of skin diseases (AH. Chi. 19/36).
2. **Vrana** (wound): Decoction prepared with Kutaja, Arka, and Karaveer is used to heal the wound by cleaning (C.S.Ci. 25/87).

Internal Use

1. **Atisara** (diarrhea): Kutaja is the best drug for diarrhea (AH.U. 40/49). Decoction of Shyonak and bark of Kutaja cures all types of diarrhea (Sha.Sa. 2.1.12). Seeds and barks of Kutaja are pounded with honey and Ativisha, and the paste is taken with rice water. It checks diarrhea caused due to pittaja (C.SCi. 19/51).
2. **Raktarsha** (bleeding piles): Kutajadi Rasakriya is used (C.S.Ci. 14/185). Decoction of Shunthi and Kutaja checks mucus and blood.
3. **Shukrasmari** (vesical calculus): Kutaja bark powder is given with curd along with wholesome diet to expel gravels through urethra (Bh.P.Ci. 37/49).
4. **Prameha** (diabetes): Paste of flower of Kutaja, Kapittha, Rohitaka, Bibhitaka, and Saptaparna is useful in prameha (S.S.Ci. 11/8).
5. **Jwara** (fever): Decoction of Indrayava and Katuki in rice water or Yastimadhu cures fever that occurs due to pitta (H.S. 3.2.66).

Officinal Parts Used

Bark, seed, flowers, leaves

Dose

Powder: 3 to 6 g
Decoction: 50 to 100 mL

Formulations

Kutajaghana vati, Kutajarista, Kutajavaleha, Kutajasura, Mahamanjishtadi kashayam, Stanyashodhana kashaya, and Patoladi choornam.

Toxicity/Adverse Effects

Sheikh et al (2016) and Pathak et al (2015) studied the acute oral toxicity and found that all types of extracts (aqueous, ethanolic, hydroalcoholic, etc.) of *H. antidysenterica* seeds are safe up to 2,000 mg/kg body weight (BW) in rats.

Hegde and Jaisal (2014) reported that the ethanolic extract of *H. antidysenterica* leaves is safe up to 2,000 mg/kg single oral dose in rats. It is reported that the ethanolic extract is safe up to 3,000 mg/kg BW (Keshri 2012; Kumar and Yadav 2015).

Ethanolic extract of seed prevents streptozotocin-induced BW loss and hyperglycemia when administered for 28 consecutive days (Kumar and Yadav 2015).

Subchronic toxicity of ethanolic extract of *H. antidysenterica* complexes with polyvinylpyrrolidone at the dose of 270 and 530 mg/kg BW/day (which is 10 and 20 times less than the dosage used for humans), causing hepatotoxicity in rats when given for three consecutive months. Hence, it is suggested that overdoses and prolonged use should be avoided so as to prevent hepatotoxic effects (Permpipat et al 2012).

Substitution and Adulteration

The bark of *H. antidysenterica* is often adulterated with the bark of *Wrightia tomentosa*, *W. tinctoria*, and sometimes with *W. zeylanica*.

> ### Points to Ponder
>
> - *Kutaja is best drug for shlemapittarakta sangrahika (kapha, rakta, and pitta shangrahana) and upashoshna (absorption) (C.S.Su. 25/40).*
> - *Astanga hridaya considered that this is best plant for raktarsha (bleeding piles).*
> - *Sharangadhar placed Kutaja in Sthambana dravya.*
> - *Seed of Kutaja is known as Indrajava.*

Suggested Readings

Akhtar P, Ali M, Sharma MP, Farooqi H, Mir SR, Khan HN. Development of quality standards of *Holarrhena antidysenterica* (Linn.). bark. Recent Res Sci Technol 2010;3:73–80

Akinyemi KO, Oladapo O, Okwara CE, Ibe CC, Fasure KA. Screening of crude extracts of six medicinal plants used in South-West Nigerian unorthodox medicine for anti-methicillin resistant *Staphylococcus aureus* activity. BMC Complement Altern Med 2005;5:6–11

Anonymous. Dictionary of Indian Medicinal Plants. Lucknow: CIMAP; 1992

Chopra RN, Chopra IC, Handa KL, Kapur ID. Chopra's Indigenous Drugs of India. New Delhi: Academic Press; 1982:342

Dhar ML, Dhar MM, Dhawan BN, Mehrotra BN, Ray C. Screening of Indian plants for biological activity: I. Indian J Exp Biol 1968;6(4): 232–247

Hagers. Handbuch der Pharmazeutischen Praxis. New York, NYS: Springer-Verlag; 1976:92–95

Hegde K, Jaisal KK. Anti-diabetic potential of ethanolic extract of *Holarrhena antidysenterica* Linn Leaves. Int J Pharm Sci Res 2014;5:429–435

Keshri UP. Antidiabetic efficacy of ethanolic extract of *Holarrhena antidysenterica* seeds in streptozotocin–induced diabetic rats and its influence on certain biochemical parameters. J Drug Deliv Ther 2012;2:159–162

Khare CP. Indian Medicinal Plants: An Illustrated Dictionary. New York: Springer Science plus Business Media, LLC; 2007

Kumar S, Yadav A. Comparative study of hypoglycaemic effect of *Holarrhena Antidysenterica* seeds and glibenclamide in experimentally induced diabetes mellitus in albino rats. Biomed Pharmacol J 2015;8:477–483

Pathak VK, Maiti A, Gupta SS, Shukla I, Rao CV. Effect of the standardized extract of *Holarrhena antidysenterica* seeds against Streptozotocin-induced diabetes in rats. Int J Pharma Res Rev. 2015;4:1–6

Permpipat U, Chavalittumrong P, Attawish A, Chuntapet P. Toxicity study of *Holarrhena antidysenterica* Wall. Bark. Bull Dep Med Sci. 2012;40:145–157

Shah NC, Gupt G, Bhattacharya N. Bharat Bhaishajya Ratnakar. New Delhi: B. Jains Publishers; 1985

Shah RR, Trivedi KN. Indian J Chem Section B: Org Chem 1981; 20B:210

Sharma RK, Dhyani SK, Sanker V. Some useful and medicinal plants of the district Dehradun and Shivalik. Pharm 1979;34:169

Sheikh Y, Manral MS, Kathait V, Prasar B, Kumar R, Sahu RK. Computation of *in vivo* antidiabetic activity of *Holarrhena antidysenterica* seeds extracts in Streptozotocin-induced diabetic rats. Iran J Pharm Ther. 2016;14:22–27

The Ayurvedic Pharmacopoeia of India, Part I, Vol. 1. New Delhi: Department of AYUSH, Ministry of Health & Family Welfare, Government of India; 1989:78

Wealth of India: Raw Materials, Vol. V, H-K. New Delhi: CSIR; 1959

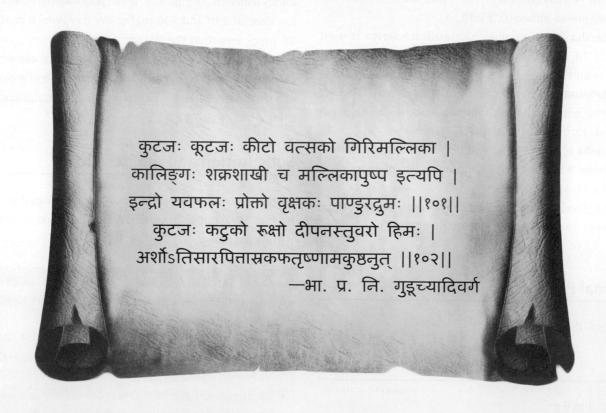

कुटजः कूटजः कीटो वत्सको गिरिमल्लिका |
कालिङ्गः शक्रशाखी च मल्लिकापुष्प इत्यपि |
इन्द्रो यवफलः प्रोक्तो वृक्षकः पाण्डुरद्रुमः ||१०१||
कुटजः कटुको रूक्षो दीपनस्तुवरो हिमः |
अर्शोऽतिसारपित्तास्रकफतृष्णामकुछनुत् ||१०२||
—भा. प्र. नि. गुडूच्यादिवर्ग

62. Lavanga [*Syzygium aromaticum* Linn.]

Synonyms:	*Eugenia caryophyllus Linn., Merit perry*
Family:	*Myrtaceae*
Hindi name:	*Lavang*
English name:	*Clove tree, Clove of commerce*

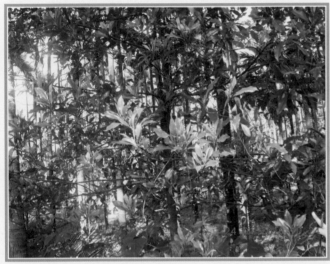

Plant of *Syzygium aromaticum* Linn.

> *The oldest clove tree aged between 350 and 450 years is in Ternate island of Indonesia. The island is the largest producer of clove in the world.*
>
> —*Worall (2012)*

Introduction

The word "clove" is derived from a French word "clou" and English word "clout" meaning a nail, which signifies the similarity of the floral bud to a broad-headed nail.

Lavanga have been used historically as a valuable spice in Mexican, Indian, Italian, and Persian cuisine. The first instance of Lavanga's use as a mouth freshener was cited in Chinese history. The use of clove as a spice started in Europe around 4th century AD, and Arabians started its commercial trading. During the 17th and 18th centuries, the Dutch had monopoly over the clove trade, which was taken over by the French till 19th century. In India, the British East India company introduced clove in 1800 AD. It became a popular trade commodity with pricing equivalent to gold. Clove mixed with tobacco is used to prepare a type of cigarette (kretek) in Indonesia. These cigarettes were smoked throughout Europe, Asia, and United states as a sedative agent (Parle and Khanna 2011).

Lavanga is a valuable spice, great preservative, flavoring agent, and a versatile medicinal plant. Since centuries, it has been used as a painkiller medicine in dental emergencies like toothache, sore gums, and caries. Clove oil is applied on affected areas in rheumatism, muscular cramps, and arthritis. Classical Ayurveda text also supports its multifaceted medicinal uses. Charaka, Sushrut, and Ashtang recommend to retain it in mouth for purification of tongue, oral cavity, reducing foul smell, strengthen gums and teeth, and to pacify diseases of throat (C.S.Su. 5/77) (S.S.Su. 46/202,491) (A.H.U. 22/93). It is used in the treatment of mukharoga, arsha, aruchi, trishna, vrana, and vatavyadhi (C.S.Su. 26/209) (C.S.Su. 28/153).

Lavanga is an important ingredient in preparing homemade garam masala, pickles, masala tea, and biryani. It is added as a flavoring agent in food products like meats, sausages, confectionery, candies, and sauces. Clove oil is used as a germicidal, anesthetic agent in mouthwashes. Oil is also used as a clearing agent in histological slide preparation and in aromatherapy (Khatri et al 2014).

Vernacular Names

Arabic: Kabshqarunfil
Bengali: Lavang
Chinese: Ding Xiang
Dutch: Kruidnagel
French: Giroflier
Gujarati: Lavang, Laving
Indonesian: Cengke, Cengkeh
Kannada: Lavanga, Kirambu
Kashmiri: Rung
Malayalam: Karampu, Karayarnpoovu, Grampu
Marathi: Lavang
Oriya: Labanga
Persian: Mikhak
Punjabi: Laung, Long
Spanish: Clavo de olor
Tamil: Kirambu, Lavangam, Ilavankam, Grambu
Telugu: Lavangamu, Kaaravallu
Urdu: Qarnful, Laung

Synonyms

Devakusum: It is considered as the flower of God and is used for worshipping them.
Divyaganda: The floral bud has divine aroma.
Grahanihara: It is a potent remedy for grahani diseases.
Shriprasunaka: The plant is believed to be originated by goddess Laksmi.
Shrisanja: The plant is denoted by the synonyms of goddess Laksmi.
Varija: Thrives/ borne in water-prone areas.
Chandanpushpaka: Its flowers are aromatic like that of chandan.

Classical Categorization

Charaka Samhita: not mentioned in dashemani
Sushruta Samhita: not mentioned in gana
Ashtang Hridaya: not mentioned in gana
Dhanvantari Nighantu: Chandanadi varga
Madanpal Nighantu: Karpuradi varga
Kaiyadev Nighantu: Oushadi varga
Raj Nighantu: Chandanadi varga
Bhavaprakash Nighantu: Karpuradi varga

Distribution

The plant is indigenous to the Moluccas, known as spice islands of Indonesia. Nowadays it is cultivated abundantly in Indonesia, India, West Indies, Tanzania, Malaysia, Sri Lanka, Brazil, and Madagascar. In India, it mainly grows in Karnataka, Tamil Nadu, and Kerala.

Morphology

It is an aromatic, evergreen, medium-sized tree of about 8 to 10 m in height with semierect, gray, dense branches.

- **Leaves:** Simple, opposite, oblong to elliptic, petiolate, glabrous with many oil glands on lower surface (**Fig. 62.1**).
- **Flowers:** Small, crimson color, borne at terminal ends of branches in cymose inflorescence, each peduncle has three to four stalked flowers. Floral buds are greenish-yellow, glossy initially and turns bright red on maturity. Buds are 1 to 2 cm long, divided into elongated stem and a bulbous globose ovary surrounded by four fleshy sepals (**Fig. 62.2**).

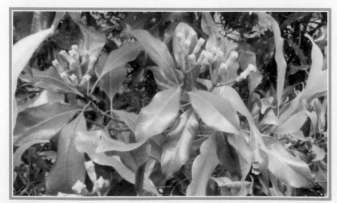

Fig. 62.1 Leaves.

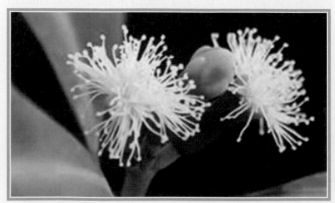

Fig. 62.2 Flower.

The tree starts blooming after 7 years of age. The commercialized part, i.e., floral buds are collected in the maturation phase before flowering.

- **Fruit:** Olive-shaped, single-seeded, fleshy, dark pink drupe crowned by the calyx lobes, popularly referred to as " mother of clove" (**Fig. 62.3a, b**). Most of the parts are aromatic (leaves, flower, and bark). The plant is propagated by seeds.

Phenology

Flowering time: May to June
Fruiting time: August to December

Key Characters for Identification

➤ *An aromatic, evergreen, medium-sized tree of 8 to 10 m.*
➤ *Leaves are simple, opposite, oblong to elliptic with numerous oil glands.*
➤ *Flowers are small, crimson, borne at terminal ends. Floral buds 1 to 2 cm, yellow green and turns bright red on maturity. Divided into elongated stem and globose head with four sepals.*
➤ *Fruits are olive shaped, one-seeded, fleshy berries.*

Types

None.

Rasapanchaka

Guna	Laghu, Snigdha
Rasa	Katu, Tikta
Vipak	Katu
Virya	Sheeta

Chemical Constituents

The floral buds contain 15 to 20% essential oil, carbohydrate, protein, fibers, vitamins, minerals, tannins, alkaloids, terpenoids, glycosides, ketones, and aldehydes. The essential oil is chiefly composed of eugenol 70 to 85%, eugenyl acetate 15%, and α- and β-caryophyllene (12–15%; Jimoh et al 2017). Other compounds of essential oils are vanillin, pyrogallol tannin, gallo tannic acid, eugenin, kaempferol, rhamnetin, eugenitin, oleanolic acid, methyl amyl ketone, methyl salicylate, syringic acid, caffeic acid, eugenitin, isorhamnetin, quercetin, phenyl acetic acid, methyl and dimethyl furfural (Nassar et al 2007).

Identity, Purity, and Strength

- Foreign matter: Not more than 2 %
- Total ash: Not more than 7%
- Acid-insoluble ash: Not more than 1%
- Alcohol-soluble extractive: Not less than 3%

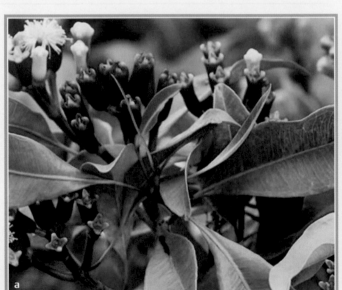
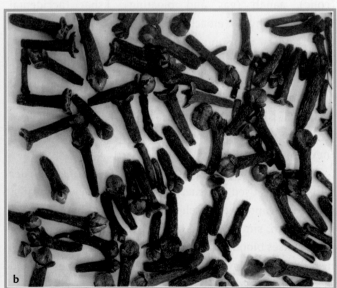

Fig. 62.3 (a, b) Fruit.

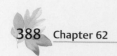

- Water-soluble extractive: Not less than 9%
- Volatile oil: Not less than 15%

(Source: The Ayurvedic Pharmacopeia of India 1989)

Karma (Actions)

It is reported to possess deepan (appetizer), pachan (digestive), rochan (relish), chakshusya (beneficial for vision), vrishya (aphrodisiac), vishaghna (antidote), hridya (cardiotonic), mangalya (beneficial), vedanahara (analgesic), shothhara (reduces swelling), vranaropana (wound healing), stambhan (faecal astringent), durgandhnashan (removes foul smell) properties.

- Doshakarma: Kaphapittahara
- Dhatukarma: Chakshusya, vrishya
- Malakarma: Stambhaka

Pharmacological Actions

Clove and clove oil is reported to possess antimicrobial, analgesic, antioxidant, anticancer, anthelmintic, anti-inflammatory, antithrombotic, cardioprotective, anti-bacterial, antifungal, anesthetic, insecticidal, and chemoprotective activities against liver and bone marrow toxicity (Khatri et al 2014; Kaur and Kaushal 2019).

Indications

Classical texts advise it to be used in treatment of shool (colic), aanah (gas and bloating), kshat (accidental wounds), kshyay (emaciation), raktavikara (diseases of blood), visha (poisoning), trishna (thirst), kasa (cough), shwasa (asthma), hikka (hic-cough), chardi (vomiting), atisaar (diarrhea), amlapitta (hyperacidity), adhyaman (constipation), vrana (wounds), peenasa (rhinitis), shiroroga (headache), mukharoga (diseases of oral cavity), dantshool (toothache), raktapitta (bleeding disorders), and vatavyadhi (neuromuscular diseases).

In traditional folklore medicine, paste of Lavanga powder with honey is used for acne. Clove oil mixed in warm water, inhaled as vapors, gives relief in respiratory conditions like cold, cough, sinusitis, and bronchitis. Application of clove oil increases blood circulation; hence, it is used in frost bite. In some areas, clove oil is used as mosquito repellant and insecticidal drug.

Therapeutic Uses

External Use

1. **Vatajshool** (pain): Lavanga paste pounded in warm water should be applied externally on the affected area (Vd.m.12/6).
2. **Dantshool** (tooth ache): Local application of Lavanga taila reduces pain and inflammation in carious tooth.

Internal Use

1. **Vishuchika** (cholera): Drinking cold infusion of Lavanga is useful in reducing thirst and nausea in cholera (VM. 6/62).
2. **Kasa** (cough): Lavanga and saindhav lavan is chewed thoroughly to ease down cough, throat irritation, and hoarseness of voice. Lavanga taila with madhu is also an effective remedy for recurring cough.
3. **Chardi** (vomiting): Intake of Lavanga powder with madhu helps in preventing emesis.
4. **Mukhvaishadya** (mouth freshener): One should keep Jatiphal, Ela, Lavanga, Kapura, Puga, Tambula, Kankola, Latakasturi in mouth for cleansing oral cavity, improving taste, and refreshing mouth (C.S.Su. 5/77).
5. **Ajeerna** (indigestion): Intake of Lavang satva extracted by soaking Lavanga and Chikkika rasa in patala yantra gives relief in ajeerna and udarshool (S.B. 44/266).

Officinal Parts Used

Flower buds and oil

Dose

Dried flower bud (powder): 500 mg to 2 g (The Ayurvedic Pharmacopeia of India 1989)
Oil: 1 to 3 drops

Formulations

Lavanga divati, Lavangadi churna, Avipatikar churna, Lavang chatusama.

Toxicity/Adverse Effects

Clove oil is a slight irritant and unpleasant in taste. If it is ingested in large dose, it may cause gastric irritation, vomiting, and skin irritation. It should be avoided during pregnancy (Jirovetz and Buchbauer 2006).

Substitution and Adulteration

In the standardized authentic sample of Lavanga, the essential oil content should not be less than 15 to 20 %. Sub-standard, exhausted (oil extracted samples), over-ripe buds, immature buds, clove stalks, mother cloves are mixed with genuine Lavang sample.

Points to Ponder

- *Lavanga has marked antibacterial, analgesic, and antioxidant properties.*
- *Lavanga is an effective drug used in the treatment of mukharoga, kasa, shwasa, chardi, aruchi, shool, and vatavyadhi.*

Suggested Readings

Jimoh SO, Arowolo LA, Alabi KA. Phytochemical screening and antimicrobial evaluation of *Syzygium aromaticum* extract and essential oil. Int J Curr Microbiol Appl Sci 2017;6:4557–4567

Jirovetz L, Buchbauer G, Stoilova I, Stoyanova A, Krastanov A, Schmidt E. Chemical composition and antioxidant properties of clove leaf essential oil. J Agric Food Chem 2006;54(17):6303–6307

Kaur K, Kaushal S. Phytochemistry and pharmacological aspects of *Syzygium aromaticum*: a review. J Pharmacogn Phytochem 2019;8(1):398–406

Khatri M, Mittal M, Gupta N, Parashar P, Mehra V. Phytochemical evaluation and pharmacological activity of *Syzygium aromaticum*: a comprehensive review. Int J Pharm Pharm Sci 2014;6(8):67–72

Nassar IM, Gaara HA, El-Ghorab HA, et al. Chemical constituents of clove (*Syzygium aromaticum*, Fam. Myrtaceae) and their antioxidant activity. Rev Latinoam Quím 2007;35(3):35–38

Parle M, Khanna D. Clove: a champion spice. Int J Res Ayurv Pharm 2011;2(1):47–54

The Ayurvedic Pharmacopeia of India. Part I, Vol. 1. New Delhi: Department of AYUSH, Ministry of Health and Family Welfare, Government of India; 1989:111

Worrall S. The world's oldest clove tree. BBC News Magazine. Retrieved June 23, 2012

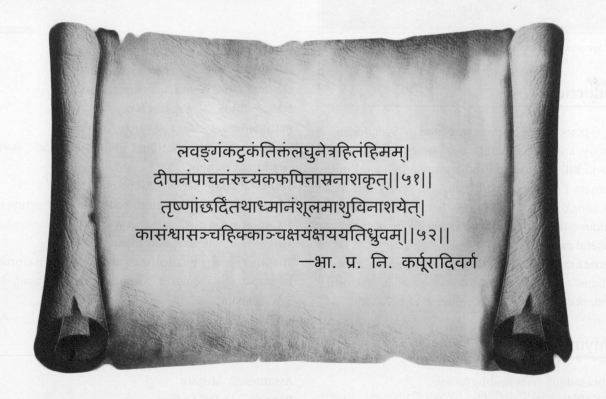

लवङ्गंकटुकंतिक्तंलघुनेत्रहितंहिमम्।
दीपनंपाचनंरुच्यंकफपित्तास्रनाशकृत्।।५१।।
तृष्णांछर्दितथाध्मानंशूलमाशुविनाशयेत्।
कासंश्वासञ्चहिक्काञ्चक्षयंक्षययतिध्रुवम्।।५२।।
—भा. प्र. नि. कर्पूरादिवर्ग

63. Lodhra [*Symplocos racemosa* Roxb.]

Synonyms: *Symplocos beddomei C.B. Clarke*

Family: *Symplocaceae*

Hindi name: *Lodh*

English name: *Chunga, Symplocos bark*

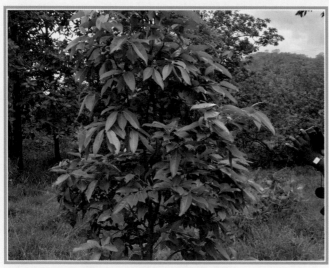

Plant of *Symplocos racemosa* Roxb.

In Europe, it was formerly looked upon as a cinchona bark and had been known at various times as "Ecorce de lautour," "China nova" and "China paraquatan."

—Watt (1972)

Introduction

Herbal plant *Symplocos racemosa* (Symplocaceae) commonly known as Lodhra is a small evergreen tree located in hilly region and most commonly found in the Poorvothara Pradesh of India mainly in planes and lower hills of Bengal, Assam, and Burma. *S. racemosa* Roxb. is an indigenous plant having ample medicinal application. Its main useful part is bark.

In Sanskrit, this tree was known as Lodhra meaning "propitious" and "Tilaka" because it was used in making the Tilaka mark on the forehead (De Silva et al 1979).

Synonyms

Akshaprasadan: It is healthy for eye.

Akshibheshaja: It is useful in eye diseases.

Bhillataru: It is well known to tribal people as Bhilla.

Galab: The bark is used in dyeing industry.

Lodhra: That which causes malavarodha.

Mahalodhra: Size of leaf is big.

Pattikalodhra: It is one variety of Lodhra.

Rodhra: It has healing properties and stambana (astringent) action.

Sthulavalkala: Bark of this plant is thick.

Tilwak: The name given to Lodhra but the action differs according to Charaka.

Tirit: That which relieves diseases.

The other synonyms are Brihatpaksha, Chillak, Hastirodhrak, Jeernapatra, Kandakilak, Kramuka, Lakshaprasad, Pattila, Savara, Shambaro, etc.

Vernacular Names

Assamese: Mugam

Bengali: Lodha, Lodhra

Gujarati: Lodhaz

Kannada: Lodhra

Kashmiri: Kath

Malayalam: Pachotti

Marathi: Lodha, Lodhra

Punjabi: Lodhar

Tamil: Vellilathi, Vellilothram

Telugu: Lodhuga

Urdu: Lodh, Lodhpathani

Classical Categorization

Charaka Samhita: Shonita sthapana, Sandhaniya, Purisha sangrahaniya

Sushruta Samhita: Lodhradi, Nyagrodhadi

Ashtanga Hridaya:

Dhanwantari Nighantu: Chandanadi varga

Madanpal Nighantu: Abhayadi varga

Kaiyadev Nighantu: Aushadhadi varga

Raj Nighantu: Pippaladi varga

Bhavaprakash Nighantu: Haritakyadi varga

Distribution

It is found abundantly in the plains and lower hills throughout north and east India, ascending in the Himalayas up to an elevation of 1,400 m, southwards it extends up to Chhota Nagpur. It is very commonly found in the lower hills of Bengal, Assam, and Burma (The Wealth of India 1976). It is also found in Bangladesh, Myanmar, China, Thailand, Vietnam, and Nepal.

Morphology

It is an evergreen, small tree or shrub, 6 to 8.5 m tall. Stem is shown in **Fig. 63.1**.

- **Leaves**: Simple, alternate, elliptic or oblong, 8-15 × 3-5 cm, base rounded, acute or acuminate apex, dentate margin-saw-like teeth. Papery, hairless, 8 to 10 pairs of nerves **(Fig. 63.2)**.
- **Flowers:** Shortly stalked, bisexual in axillary racemes, whitish-pink and fragrant. The flowers are very small with 1.4 cm diameter and appear mostly white which turn yellow, fragrant in auxiliary, simple or compound racemes. Pedicels as long as calyx tube and stamens are about 100 in number.
- **Fruit:** Drupes, ellipsoid to ovoid 1.5 × 0.5 cm, hairless, dark blue when ripe, turning yellow when dry.
- **Seed:** One to two, oblong.
- **Bark:** Small of varying sizes and thickness, outer surface buff to brownish, longitudinally wrinkled and bearing horizontal lenticels, inner surface brownish, rough and scanty fracture, short and granular, taste acrid and bitter **(Fig. 63.3;** The Wealth of India 1976).

Phenology

It is propagated by seeds and stem cutting.

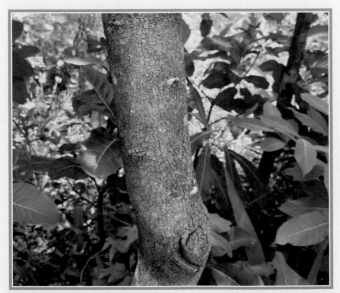

Fig. 63.1 Stem.

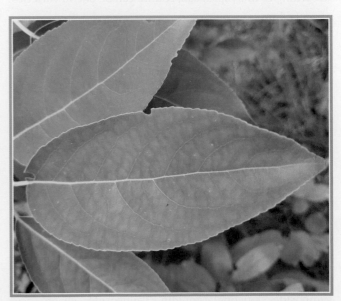

Fig. 63.2 Leaves.

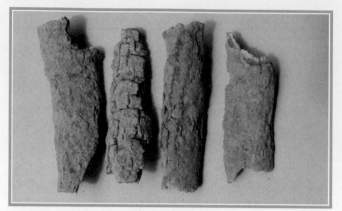

Fig. 63.3 Bark.

Key Characters for Identification

➤ *Evergreen small tree or shrub, 6 to 8.5 m tall*

➤ *Leaves: Simple, alternate, elliptic or oblong, 8-15 × 3-5 cm, base rounded, acute or acuminate apex, dentate margin*

➤ *Flowers: Shortly stalked, bisexual in axillary racemes, whitish-pink turns to yellow, fragrant. Pedicels as long as calyx tube and stamens are about 100 in number.*

➤ *Fruit: Dark blue drupes, ellipsoid to ovoid, 1.5 × 0.5 cm*

➤ *Bark: Small of varying sizes and thickness, outer surface buff to brownish, inner surface brownish and rough.*

Types

According to Bhavaprakash, Lodhra can be of two varieties:
- Lodhra
- Paittika Lodhra

Rasapanchaka

Guna	Laghu, Ruksha
Rasa	Kasaya
Vipak	Katu
Virya	Sheeta

Chemical Constituents

Bark contains flavanol glucosides like symplocoside, symposide, leucopelargonidin 3-glucoside, ellagic acid, flavonol glycoside like rhamnetin 3-digalactoside, triterpenoids like 19 α-hydroxyarjunolic acid-3, 28-O-bis-β-glucopyranosides, 19 α-hydroxyasiatic acid-3, 28-O-bis-β-glucopyranosides, betulin, oleanolic acid, oxalic acids, loturidine, Loturine phytosterol, sugar, β-sitosterol, and α-amyrin (Badoni et al 2010; Nagore et al 2012; Gopal et al 2013).

Identity, Purity, and Strength

- Foreign matter: Not more than Nil%
- Total ash: Not more than 12%
- Acid-insoluble ash: Not more than 1%
- Alcohol-soluble extractive: Not less than 9 %
- Water-soluble extractive: Not less than 15%

(Source: The Ayurvedic Pharmacopeia of India 1986)

Karma (Actions)

Shothaghna (anti-inflammatory), chakshusya (beneficial for vision), grahi (absorbent), rochana (relish), vishaghna (antidote).

- Doshakarma: Kaphapittahara
- Dhatukarma: Raktastambhana
- Malakarma: Grahi

Pharmacological Actions

It has analgesic, anthelmintic, antiacne effect, antiangiogenic and antibacterial, anticancer, anti-inflammatory, antioxidant, and hepatoprotective properties (Wakchaure et al 2010; Raval et al 2009; Kumar et al 2007; Rao et al 2011; Devmurari 2010).

Indications

It is used in atisara (diarrhea), jwaratisara (diarrhea with fever), raktapitta (hemorrhage), shopha (inflammation), shotha (swelling), asrikdara (menorrhagia), trishna (thirst), visha (poisoning).

It is used in eye diseases, acne and pimple, leucorrhea, wound, skin disorders, ascites, hoarseness of voice, fever, menstrual disorders, hemorrhage, diarrhea, dysentery, elephantiasis, liver disease, bowel complaints, ulcer, bleeding gums (Kirtikar and Basu 1999). Lodhra is considered as a drug of choice for gynecological disorders. It has been used to treat the menorrhagia, leucorrhea, and menstrual disorders. It is also used in abortions, miscarriages, and vaginal ulcers.

It is used as emmenagogue and aphrodisiac, and it is a potent remedy for inflammation and clearing uterus in Unani system of medicine. It is used in raktapittam, athisaram, and pradaram as per Siddha (Nadkarni 1954).

Contraindications

None

Therapeutic Uses

External Use

1. **Yuvan pidika** (acne and pimple): Paste of Lodhra and Sphatik should be applied locally (A.S.Sha-37/5).
2. **Eye disease**: Sariba, Lodhra fried in ghee should be applied on lid as paste in the disease of whole eye (C.S.Ci. 26/233).
3. **Kushta** (skin disease): Rubbing and applying powder paste of Lodhra, Dhataki, Indravaya, Karanja, and Jati is useful in skin diseases (C.S.Ci. 7/95).
4. **Vrana** (wound): Power of Dhataki and Lodhra promotes wound healing (C.S.Ci. 25/67-68).
5. **Hemorrhage**: External application of powder of Lodhra, Madhuk, Priyangu, Patanga, Gairik, Sarjarasa, Rasanjan, Shalmalipuspa etc.

Internal Use

1. **Sweta pradara** (leucorrhea): Paste of Lodhra is taken with the decoction of Nyagrodha bark (C.S.Ci. 30/118).
2. **Pravahika** (dysentery): Lodhra with curd is useful in dysentery (BP.Chi-2/120).
3. **Raktapitta** (intrinsic hemorrhage): Lodhra is beneficial for checking hemorrhage (C.S.Ci. 4/73-77).
4. **Diseases of women:** Lodhrasava is a popular formulation for women's diseases (AH.Ci. 12/24-28).

Officinal Part Used

Bark

Dose

Powder: 3 to 5 g
Decoction: 20 to 30 g

Formulations

Brihat Gangadhar churna, Chandanasava, Dashmoolarista, Kumaryasava, Lodhradi kwath, Lodhrasava, Pusyanuga churna, Rodhrasava, Rodhrasava.

Toxicity/Adverse Effects

Not reported yet.

Substitution and Adulteration

Following species are used as substitutes and adulterants of Lodhra:

- *Symplocos crataegoides*
- *Symplocos spicata*

Points to Ponder

- *Lodhra is used effectively in women diseases like rakta pradar, sweta pradar, etc.*
- *It has grahi properties; hence, it is used in raktapitta and other bleeding disorders.*

Suggested Readings

Badoni R, Semwal DK, Kothiyal SK, Rawat U. Chemical constituents and biological applications of the genus Symplocos. J Asian Nat Prod Res 2010;12(12):1069–1080

Bhusnar HU, Nagore DH, Nipanik SU. Phytopharmacological profile of *Symplocos racemosa*: a review. Pharmacologia 2014;76:83

De Silva LB, De Silva ULL, Mahendran M. The chemical constituents of *Symplocos racemosa* Roxb. J Natl Sci Counc Sri Lanka 1979;7:1–3

Devmurari VP. Phytochemical screening study and antibacterial evaluation of *Symplocos racemosa* Roxb. Arch Appl Sci Res 2010;2:354–359

Kirtikar KR, Basu BD. Indian Medicinal Plants. 2nd ed. Dehradun, India: Popular Publications; 1999:878–879

Krishna CG, Divya M, Ramya K, Sheba Dolly R, Phani Kumar K. Pharmacological evaluation of *Symplocos Racemosa* bark extracts on experimentally induced ulceritis in rat model. Elixir Pharmacy 2013;55:12964–12966

Kumar GS, Jayaveera KN, Kumar CKA, et al. Antimicrobial effects of Indian medicinal plants against acne-inducing bacteria. Trop J Pharm Res 2007;6:717–723

Lucas DS, Dravyaguna-Vijnana- Study of Dravya-Materia Medica, Chaukhamba Visvabharati: Varanasi, Reprint: 2013:251

Nadkarni. Indian Materia Medica. 3rd ed. Bombay: Popular Book Depot; 1954:87, 1186

Nagore DH, Kuber VV, Patil PS, Deshmukh TA. Development and Validation of RP-HPLC method for quantification of Loturine from Polyherbal formulation containing *Symplocos racemosa* (Roxb). Int J Pharm Pharm Sci Res 2012;2:79–83

Rao R, Bhavya B, Pavani K, Swapna A, Prasoona CH. Anthelmintic activity of *Symplocos racemosa*. Int J Pharma Bio Sci 2011;1:198–230

Raval BP, Patel JD, Patel BA, Ganure AL. Potent *in vitro* anticancer activity of *Symplocos racemosa* bark. Rom J Biol Plant Biol 2009;54: 135–140

Raval BP, Suthar MP, Patel RK. Potent *in vitro* anti-tumor activity of *Symplocos racemosa* against leukemia and cervical cancer. Electron J Biol 2009;5:89–91

Sharma PV. Classical Uses of Medicinal Plants. 1st ed. Varanasi: Chaukhamba Vishvabharati; 2004:331

The Ayurvedic Pharmacopoeia of India. Part I, Vol. I. 1st ed. New Delhi: Department of Health, Ministry of Health and Family Welfare, Government of India; 1986:112

The Wealth of India. A Dictionary of Indian Raw Materials and Industrial Products: Raw materials. New Delhi: National Institute of Science Communication and Information Resources; 1976:10, 90

Wakchaure D, Jain D, Singhai AK, Somani R. Hepatoprotective activity of Symplocos racemosa bark on carbon tetrachloride-induced hepatic damage in rats. J Ayurveda Integr Med 2011;2(3):137–143

Watt G. Dictionary of the Economic Products of India. New Delhi, India: Periodical Expert Book Agency; 1972

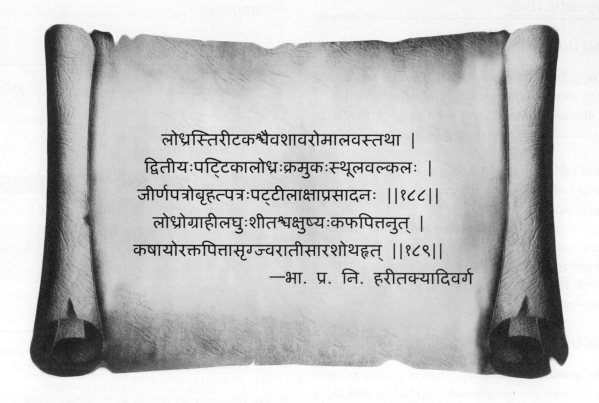

लोध्रस्तिरीटकश्चैवशावरोमालवस्तथा |
द्वितीयःपट्टिकालोध्रःक्रमुकःस्थूलवल्कलः |
जीर्णपत्रोबृहत्पत्रःपट्टीलाक्षाप्रसादनः ||१८८||
लोध्रोग्राहीलघुःशीतश्चक्षुष्यःकफपित्तनुत् |
कषायोरक्तपित्तासृग्ज्वरातीसारशोथहृत् ||१८९||
—भा. प्र. नि. हरीतक्यादिवर्ग

64. Madanphala *[Randia dumetorum (Retz.) Lam.]*

Synonym: *Catunaregam spinosa (Thumb.) Tirveng.*

Family: *Rubiaceae*

Hindi name: *Mainphala, Madan*

English name: *Emetic nut*

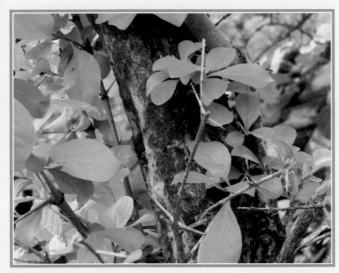

Plant of *Randia dumetorum* (Retz.) Lam.

> *Inside the fruit the seeds are arranged in peculiar manner of four rows and are popularly known as Madanphala pippali. The unripe green fruit is known as Madanphala shalatu.*

Introduction

Madanaphala derived its Latin name *"Randia"* in the memory of famous botanist Sir Issac Rand and *dumetorum* means thorny bushes which corresponds to the presence of many spines or thorns in the plant (Gogte 2000).

Since time immemorial, Madanphala is a popular remedy in traditional medicines for inducing vamana (a biopurification method to detoxify aggravated kapha and pitta dosha via oral route). It is also considered as drug of choice in vamana (therapeutic emesis), asthapan basti (decoction enema), and anuvasana basti (oil enema) (C.S.Su. 25/40). Charaka Samhita, Ashtang Hridaya, and Ashtang Sangraha consider it as vamnopayogi or vamanopaga dravya, and in Sushrut Samhita, it is categorized under urdhvabhaghara dravya. Charaka and Sushrut considered Madanphala as the best drug for inducing emesis (C.S.Ka. 1/13; S.S.Su.43/3) and included it in phalini dravya (C.S.Su.1/84). Its importance can be judged with the fact that

Charaka has devoted a complete chapter Madanphala kalpa in Kalpa sthana describing 133 formulations of Madanphala alone to induce emesis (C.S.Ka. 1/14-26). Sushrut has described 31 emetic formulations of Madanphala (S.S.Su. 43/4,6).

Madanphala is not only a renowned drug of shodhan chikitsa (detoxification therapy) but have marked efficacy in shaman chikitsa (palliative treatment).

It is administered internally or applied externally in the form of paste in painful infections, inflammatory diseases, rheumatism, cold, cough, fever, abscesses, and ulcers. The aqueous extract of the root bark is a potent insecticide and insect repellent (Dastur 1962).

Vernacular Names

Arabic: Jauzulaki, Jijul kai
Assamese: Maen, Behmona
Bengali: Mainaphal, Mayanaphal

Gujarati: Mindhal, Mindhol, Mindhar

Kannada: Mangarikai, Karigidda, Maggrekai, Kari, MaggareKayi

Kashmiri: Madanfal

Malayalam: Malankara, Malamkarakka

Marathi: Ghela, Peralu, Mindhal, Wagatta, Gelphal

Oriya: Maena, Madana, Palova

Punjabi: Mindhal, Rara, Manphal

Tamil: Marukkarai

Telugu: Mranga Kaya, Monga Kaya

Urdu: Mainphal, Jauz-ul-Qai

Synonyms

Chardana: The fruit is used to induce chardi (vomiting).

Karahata: The sharp spines cause injury to hands.

Madana: On ingestion the fruit produces hallucination, horripilation, and malaise.

Maruvaka: The plant grows well in marupradesh, i.e., dry region.

Pindeetaka: Inside the fruit, seeds are arranged in pile mass.

Pindi: The fruit is globose shaped.

Ratha: The fruit is indicated in many disorders.

Shalyaka: The branches bear sharp thorns.

Vishapushpaka: Flowers contain some toxic constituents.

Classical Categorization

Charaka Samhita: Asthapanopaga, Anuvasanopaga, Phalini and Vamana Dravya.

Sushrut Samhita: Aragvadhadi, Muskakadi, Urdhabhagahara

Ashtang Hridaya: Araghvadhadi

Dhanvantari Nighantu: Guduchyadi varga

Madanpal Nighantu: Abhyadi varga

Kaiyadev Nighantu: Oushadi varga

Raj Nighantu: Shalmalyadi varga

Bhavaprakash Nighantu: Haritakyadi varga

Distribution

It is found throughout India in deciduous forests up to an altitude of 1,400 m. It is common in Gujarat, Maharashtra, Tamil Nadu, Rajasthan, Bengal, Bihar, Orissa, Madhya Pradesh, and South India.

Morphology

It is a deciduous, thorny, rigid shrub or tree, reaching up to 9 m height. Bark is rough, dark brown or gray, scaly, studded with strong straight spines.

- **Leaves:** Simple, axillary, usually fascicled on the suppressed branches, 3 to 6 cm long and 2 to 3 cm width, obovate, wrinkled, shining, more or less pubescent above and on the nerves beneath, obtuse apex, tapering into the petiole at the base (**Fig. 64.1**).
- **Flowers**: White colored first, turning yellow when it fades, fragrant, solitary or two to three together at the ends of short leafy branchlets (**Fig. 64.2**).
- **Fruits:** Berries 2 to 3 cm long and 2.5 cm broad, ovoid or subglobose, pale green when unripe and yellow on

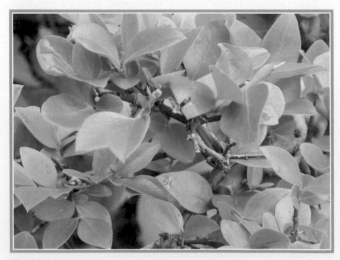

Fig. 64.1 Leaves.

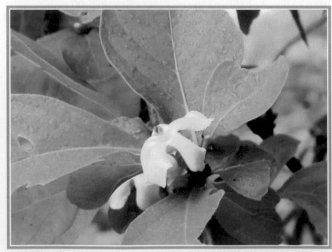

Fig. 64.2 Flower.

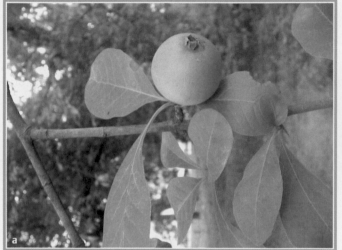
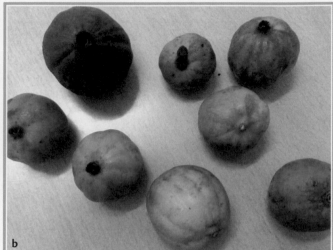
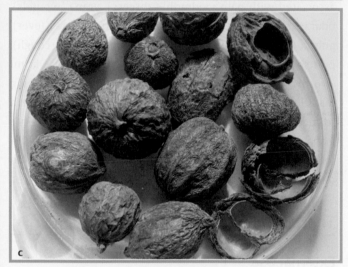

Fig. 64.3   (a) Fruit. (b) Unripe fruits. (c) Dry fruits.

maturity, smooth surface, fleshy, and longitudinally ribbed. Dried fruits are tough but brittle, split up in two masses of closely adherent seeds are seen in two loculi (**Fig. 64.3a–c**). Seeds are numerous, flattened, ovoid to oblong, and light brown in color (Kirtikar and Basu 1991). The plant is propagated by seeds and root suckers.

- **Collection time:** Between vasanta and greeshma in pushya, ashvini, or mrigashira nakshatra (C.S.Ka. 1/13).

Phenology

Flowering time: May to June

Fruiting time: August to December

Key Characters for Identification

➤ A thorny, deciduous shrub or tree of about 9 m height.

➤ Leaves: axillary, fascicled on the suppressed branches, obovate, lustrous.

➤ Flowers are fragrant, white colored, solitary, or in group of two to three.

➤ Fruits are ovoid or subglobose berries, fleshy, pale green, which turns yellow on maturity.

Types

Raj Nighantu has described its two types:

- Varah (mahapinditaka): Big, round, black-colored fruit
- Snigdha pinditaka: Bulky round fruit

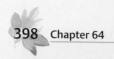

Rasapanchaka

Guna	Laghu, Ruksha
Rasa	Madhura, Tikta (B.P. & K.D); Katu, Tikta (D.N. & Raj); Tikta (M.P.)
Vipaka	Katu
Virya	Ushna
Prabhava	Vamaka

Chemical Constituents

Fully mature fruit contains glycosides, saponins (dumeto-ronins A to F), randianin, randioside A, randia acid, mollisidial triterpenoid, glycosides, leucocyanidin, and mannitol. Seeds are rich in fat (1.5%), protein (14.2%), mucilage, resin, organic acid (1.4%), and volatile oil. The bark contains scopoletin, mannitol, randialic acid, and coumarin glycosides. The root bark has triterpenes and leaves have iridoid glycoside (Patel et al 2011; Agarwal et al 1999).

Identity, Purity, and Strength

- Foreign matter: Not more than 2%
- Total ash: Not more than 6%
- Acid-insoluble ash: Not more than 0.25%
- Alcohol-soluble extractive: Not less than 19%
- Water-soluble extractive: Not less than 16%

(Source: The Ayurvedic Pharmacopeia of India 1989)

Karma (Actions)

Madanphala fruit is reported to have vamaka (emetic), shothahara (anti-inflammatory), vedanasthapana (anodyne), vranashodhana (purifies wounds), nadishamaka (nervine depressant), vatanulomana (carminative), krimighna (anthelminthic), grahi (absorbent), raktashodhaka (blood purifier), kaphanisaraka (expectorant), artava janana (emmenogogue), swedajanan (diaphoretic), kushtaghna (antidermatosis), jwaraghna (antipyretic), lekhana (scrapping), and vishaghna (antidote to poison) actions.

- Doshakarma: Kaphavatashamaka, Kaphapittashamshodhaka
- Dhatukarma: Lekhan, srotoshodhana
- Malakarma: Vamak, vataanulomana, swedajanan

Pharmacological Actions

A scrutiny of literature revealed some notable pharmacological activities of the plant as antibacterial, anti-inflammatory, antiallergic, analgesic, immunomodulatory, antileishmanial, anthelmintic, and anticancer (Ghosh et al 1983; Todkari 2015).

Indications

Ayurveda classics advocated the use of Madanphala in vatavyadhi (neuromuscular diseases), amavata (arthritis), shotha (inflammation), vedanayuktavikara (diseases associated with pain), vidradhi (abscess), vrana (wounds), udarashool (stomachache), kaphapradhana jwara (fever), gulma (abdominal lump), shwasa (asthma), kasa (cough), pratishyaya (common cold), vibandh (constipation), krimi (worms), pravahika (dysentery), raktavikara (bleeding disorders), kashtartava (dysmenorrhea), kashtaprasava (difficult labor), kushta (skin diseases), medoroga (obesity), vishavikara (poisonous affection) (Sharma et al 2001). In folklore medicine, the fruit pulp is used in worm infestation and for inducing abortion (Agarwal et al 1999).

Therapeutical Uses

External Use

1. **Parsvshool** (pain in flanks): Madanphala paste mixed with kanji is applied on navel region to subside pain in flanks (B.S.shool/11).
2. **Garbhsang** (difficult labor): Fumigation of vaginal region with Pinditak is advised in garbhasang (S.S.Sa. 10/11).
3. **Vranaprakshalan** (washing abscess and wounds): Decoction prepared by mixing Madanphala, Triphala, Patol, Nirgundi, and Arka is used for washing the area in chronic abscess, wounds, and ulcers.
4. **Visha** (poisonous bite): Poultice prepared by mixing Madanphala churna with Sarpagandha and Ishwarimool churna in water is applied in snake bite and scorpion sting.

Internal Use

1. **Vaman** (inducing emesis): Soak 3 g Madanphala seed powder in 50 mL water for an hour. Grind it and add

honey and saindhav lavan to it. Drink empty stomach, it will induce emesis and give relief from aggravated Kapha and Pitta conditions. Mixture of Madanphala seed powder, saindhav lavan, and Pippali churna with lukewarm water is also used for inducing emesis (C.S.Ka. 1/13-14) (A.H.Ka. 1.1).

2. **Jwar** (fever): Madanphala, Pippali, Kutaja, Madhuka with lukewarm water is given for inducing emesis in fever (C.S.Ci. 3/228).

3. **Tamakswasa** (asthma): Intake of 1 tsf powdered Madanphala, Arkamula twaka, and Madhuka in equal amount daily helps in expelling phlegm and gives relief in asthma.

4. **Abdominal pain:** Make paste of the fruit with vinegar and apply around the naval region to get relief in severe abdominal pain and distention.

5. **Atisaar** (diarrhea): Taking 20 to 40 mL root decoction twice daily gives relief in diarrhea and dysentery (Chopra et al 1956).

Officinal Parts Used

Fruit and bark

Dose

Fruit powder: 3 to 6 g for emesis
Therapeutic dose: 1 to 2 g

Formulations

Madanadi lepa, Saindhavadi taila, Araghvadadi kasaya, Arimedadi taila, Vardhmana Madanphala kalpa, Tilvaka ghrita, Bilvadi taila.

Toxicity/Adverse Effects

Not reported

Substitution and Adulteration

The fruit is a valuable emetic drug and is used as substitute for ipecacuanha (*Cephaelis ipecacuanha* (Brot.) A.Rich.) (Sharma et al 2001).

> *Points to Ponder*
>
> - *Madanphala is the best emetic drug among all the dravyas.*
> - *It is a renowned drug used in the treatment of shotha, vidradhi, vrana, jwara, kushta, gulma, udarshool, shwasa, kasa, and raktavikara.*

Suggested Readings

Agrawal SS, Singh VK. Immunomodulators-A review of studies on Indian medicinal plants and synthetic peptides, Part- 1, Medicinal plants, Proc. Indian Natl Sci Acad. 1999;65:179–204

Agrawal SS, Singh VK. Immunomodulators: a review of studies on Indian medicinal plants and synthetic peptides. Part I: Medicinal plants. Proc Indian Natl Sci Acad 1999;65:179–204

Chopra RN, Nayar SL, Chopra IC. In Glossary of Indian Medicinal plants. New Delhi, India: Council of Scientific and Industrial Research; 1956:209

Dastur JF. In Medicinal Plants of India and Pakistan. Bombay. D. B. Taraporevala Son's & Co. Pvt. Ltd; 1962:140

Ghosh D, Thejomoorthy P. Veluchamy. Anti-inflammatory and analgesic activities of oleanolic acid 3-/3- Glucoside (RDG-1) from *Randiadumetorum*(Rubiaceae). Indian J Pharmacol 1983;4:31–34

Gogte VM. Ayurvedic Pharmacology and Therapeutic Uses of medicinal Plants(Dravyagunavignyan) Part II, medicinal plants, Plant no.(87), 1st Edition. Bhartiya Vidya Bhavan; 2000:454

Kirtikar KR, Basu BD. Indian Medicinal Plants. Panni office. Bahadurganj, Allahabad: Bhuwaneswari Ashrama; 1991:648–652

Patel Ritesh G, Pathak Nimish L, Rathod Jaimik D, Patel LD, Bhatt Nayna M. Phytopharmacological properties of Randiadumetorum as a Potential Medicinal Tree An overview. J Appl Pharm Sci 2011;1(10):24–26

Sharma PC, Yelne MB, Dennis TJ. Database on Medicinal Plants Used in Ayurveda, Vol.2. New Delhi: CCRAS; 2001:380–356

Todkari DP. Madanaphala (*Randia dumetorum* lam.): A phyto-pharmacological review. Int J Ayurvedic Med 2015;6(2):74–82

The Ayurvedic Pharmacopeia of India. Part 1, Vol. 1. New Delhi: Department of AYUSH, Ministry of Health and Family Welfare, Government of India; 1989:114

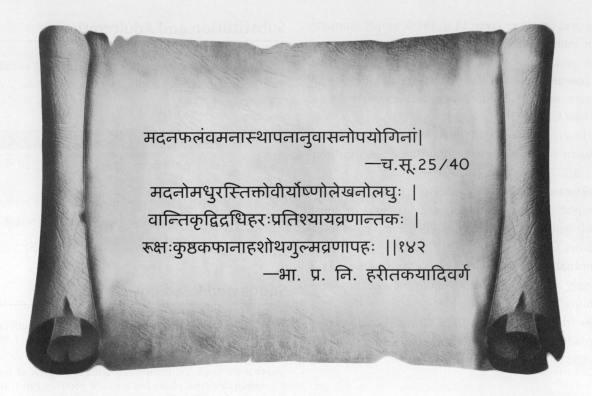

मदनफलंवमनास्थापनानुवासनोपयोगिनां|

—च.सू. 25/40

मदनोमधुरस्तिक्तोवीर्योष्णोलेखनोलघुः |

वान्तिकृद्विद्रधिहरःप्रतिश्यायव्रणान्तकः |

रूक्षःकुष्ठकफानाहशोथगुल्मव्रणापहः ||१४२

—भा. प्र. नि. हरीतकयादिवर्ग

65. Mandukparni *[Centella asiatica Linn. Urban.]*

Synonym:	*Hydrocotyle asiatica Linn.*
Family:	*Apiaceae*
Hindi name:	*Bengsang*
English name:	*Indian Pennywort, waternavel, waterpennywort*

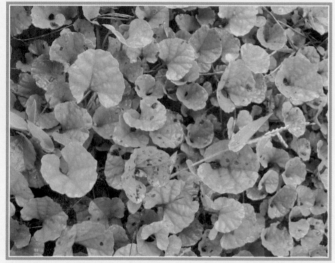

Plant of *Centella asiatica* Linn. Urban.

> *Popularly known as "brain food" for its memory enhancer, nervine tonic, and revitalizing effect on the nerves and brain cells. It is also known as "snow plant" due to its cooling properties.*
>
> —*Nalini et al (1992) and Emboden (1985)*

Introduction

The Latin name "centella" is derived from Latin word "centum" which means hundred referred to the profuse, branched prostate nature of the plant.

Mandukparni is used as a medicinal drug since the period of Atharva Veda. In Agnipurana, its powder is used to get rid of vali and palitya. There is a long history of its use as a memory enhancer drug in different systems of medicines. It is officially enlisted in Chinese, European, and British Herbal Pharmacopeias. In Chinese traditional medicines, it is used in the treatment of diarrhea, dysentery, scabies, tuberculosis, jaundice, measles, difficult urination, epistaxis, and as an endocrine tonic and adaptogen. They called it as "miracle of elixir" and believe that drinking its infusion daily enhances longevity and virility (Leyel 1970). In Malaysian traditional medicine, Centella tea is recommended in hypertension, diarrhea, and urinary tract infections. In Madagascar and

Brazil, the herb is traditionally used for treating leprosy, tuberculosis, elephantiasis, and obesity (Leonard 1998). In Ayurveda, Mandukparni is described in the category of Medhya rasayana (psychotropic) drugs (C.S.Ci. 1/3/30). Charaka has recommended use of Mandukparni swarasa for medhavardhan and considered it as ayushya, bala, agni, swaravardhani, and aamayanashini (pacify diseased state). Charaka and Sushrut mentioned it in shaka varga (C.S.Su. 27/96) (S.S.Su. 46/264) and considered it as hitakari shaka for medha.

In Nighantu period, there is controversy on the identity of Mandukparni because two popular intellect-promoting drugs, *Centella asiatica* and *Bacopa monnieri*, are used by the same name of Brahmi in different parts of India. Bhavaprakash, Madanpal, Kaiyadev, and Raj Nighantus have described Brahmi and Mandukparni together as Brahmi and assigned similar properties to them. Dhanvantari and some other Nighantus described it under the name of suvarchala which further increases the controversy. However, the controversy has been resolved and it is concluded that Brahmi is *Bacopa monnieri* and Mandukparni is *C. asiatica* (Anonymous 1992).

Economically, the plant is used in preparing cosmetic products, hair oils, perfumes, and lotions. In Tamil Nadu and Uttarakhand, leaves are eaten as vegetables to enhance memory power. However, due to its high demand, unrestricted exploitation, limited cultivation, and marked depletion in wild, the species has been listed as threatened and endangered species by the International Union for Conservation of Nature and Natural Resources (IUCN) (Pandey et al 1993; Singh 1989).

Vernacular Names

Assamese: Manimuni
Bengali: Jholkhuri, Thalkuri, Thankuni
Bihari: Chokiora
Chinese: Fo-ti-tieng
Gujarati: Khodabrahmi, Khadbhrammi, Barmi, Moti Brahmi
Kannada: Ondelaga, Brahmi soppu
Malayalam: Kodangal, Kodagam, Kutakm, Kutannal, Muthal, Muttil
Marathi: Karivana, Karinga
Nepali: Ghodtapre
Oriya: Thalkudi
Punjabi: Brahmi
Sinhalese: Hingotukola
Tamil: Vallarai, Babassa
Telugu: Vauari, Bekaparnamu, Bokkudu, Saraswataku, Mandukbrahmmi
Urdu: Brahmi

Synonyms

Bheki: It is denoted by the synonyms of a frog.
Divya: It has many divine properties.
Mahoushadi: It is considered as best among medicinal drugs.
Mandukparnika: The leaf surface is compared with body surface of a frog.

Twastri: The herb is praised by Lord Brahma, i.e., intellect promoting.

Classical Categorization

Charaka Samhita: Vyasthapana, Tiktaskanda
Sushruta Samhita: Tikta varga
Dhanvantari Nighantu: Karviradi varga
Madanpal Nighantu: Abhyadi varga
Kaiyadev Nighantu: Oushadi varga
Raj Nighantu: Parpatadi varga
Bhavaprakash Nighantu: Guduchyadi varga

Distribution

It is widely distributed in the warmer regions of the world including Asia, Africa, Australia, and America. It grows throughout India in wet moist places, along the banks of rivers, canal, shaded areas, open gardens, and near water source.

Morphology

It is a slender, creeping, perennial, stoloniferous, faintly aromatic herb. Stem is long prostrate, stoloniferous, filiform often red in color, with rooting nodes and long internodes.

- Leaves are simple with elongated petioles and sheathing leaf base, orbicular or reniform, 2 to 5 cm long, 3 to 7 cm width, crenate-dentate margin, with five to seven furrowed veins (**Fig. 65.1**).
- Flowers are white-pink, axillary, almost sessile, with three to six flowers in fascicled umbels (**Fig. 65.2**).
- Fruits are laterally compressed, oblong, globular in shape, with two curved round mericarps and seven to nine ridges (**Fig. 65.3a, b**).
- Roots: are stock vertical stout, 3 to 4 inches long.

The plant is propagated by stolon and seeds.

Phenology

Flowering time: April to June
Fruiting time: May to October

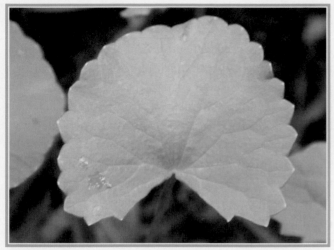

Fig. 65.1 Leaf.

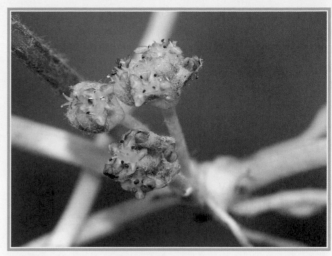

Fig. 65.2 Flowers.

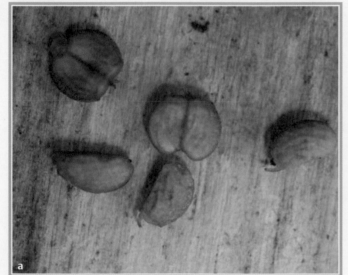

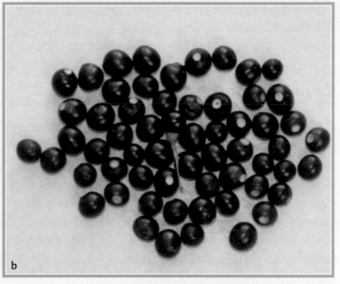

Fig. 65.3 (a, b) Fruits.

Key Characters for Identification

➤ *A perennial creeping stoloniferous herb with rooting at the nodes.*
➤ *Leaves are simple, orbicular or reniform, with crenate-dentate margin.*
➤ *Flowers: white pink, axillary, three to six in fascicled umbels.*
➤ *Fruits: Laterally compressed, oblong and globular in shape.*

Types

None

Rasapanchaka

Guna	Laghu, Sara
Rasa	Tikta, Kashaya, Madhura
Vipaka	Madhura
Virya	Sheeta

Chemical Constituents

The plant is reported to have triterpenoid (thankuniside, isothankunic acid, centellose, asiatic acid, centellic acid, centoic acid and madecassic acids, brahmoside, brahminoside, brahmic acid), alkaloids (hydrocotylin), glycoside (asiaticoside A & B, madecassoside, and centelloside), flavonoids (3-glucosylquercetin, 3-glucosylkaempferol), fatty acids (palmitic, stearic, lignoceric, oleic, linoleic, linolenic acid), and volatile oil. The plant also has resins, tannins, amino acids, minerals, and vitamin B, C, G (Singh and Rastogi 1969; Chopra et al 1956).

Identity, Purity, and Strength (Whole Plant)

- Foreign matter: Not more than 2 %
- Total ash: Not more than 17%
- Acid-insoluble ash: Not more than 5%
- Alcohol-soluble extractive: Not less than 9%
- Water-soluble extractive: Not less than 20%
(Source: The Ayurvedic Pharmacopeia of India 2004)

Karma (Actions)

In Ayurveda classics, Mandukparni is designated as medhya (intellect promoting), rasayana (rejuvenator), ayushya (enhancing life expectancy), swarya (good for voice), smritipada (improves memory), hridya (cardiotonic), vishaghna (antidote to poison), deepan (appetizer), balya (strength promoting), varnya (improves complexion), mutral (diuretic), vyasthapana (antiageing), stanyajanana (galactogogue), stanyashodhana (purifies breast milk), and vranaropaka (wound healing) dravya.

- Doshakarma: Tridoshashamaka
- Dhatukarma: Rasayana, Balya
- Malakarma: Mutral

Pharmacological Actions

The whole plant is reported to have neuroprotective, radioprotective, cardioprotective, anxiolytic, anticonvulsant, antidepressant, antioxidant, memory enhancer, antileprotic, antitubercular, diuretic, febrifuge, adaptogen, immunomodulator, sedative, antiviral, analgesic, wound healing, antifertility, antispasmodic, anticancerous, hepatoprotective, and antiulcer properties (Arora et al 2002; Shakir et al 2007).

Indications

Mandukparni is used in the treatment of unmada (insanity), apasmara (epilepsy), kushta (skin diseases), kandu (pruritus), pandu (anemia), prameha (diabetes), hridadaurbalya (cardiac debility), swarabheda (tonsillitis), gandamala (goiter), shleepada (filariasis), daurbalya (general debility), raktavikara (diseases of aggravated rakta), kasa (cough), shwasa (asthma), shotha (inflammation), aruchi (distaste), visha (poisoning), vrana (wounds/ulcers), and jwara (fever).

It is widely prescribed in epilepsy, schizophrenia, cognitive dysfunction, diseases of skin, nerve, and blood, and acts as a tonic for accelerating nervous activity, and improving youth, longevity, and memory. In other traditional systems, it has been used in the management of cholera, measles, jaundice, leucorrhea, hematemesis, hepatitis, urethritis, toothache, syphilis, smallpox, neuralgia, rheumatism, and venous insufficiency. Poultices are applied locally in sprains, contusions, fractures, and furunculosis (Anonymous 1999).

Therapeutical Uses

External Use

Pitika (boils): Local application of Mandukparni juice or paste subsides boils (G.N. 4/1/119).

Internal Use

1. **Medhya** (intellect promoting): Daily intake of Mandukparni swaras, Madhuka powder, Guduchi swaras, and Sankhpushpikalka with milk is an outstanding intellect-promoting rasayana (C.S.Ci. 1/3/30).
2. **Swarabheda** (hoarseness of voice): Mandukparni, Bilva root, Kushta, Sankhpushpi are mixed with madhu and are taken orally to get relief in swarbheda (B.P.Ci. 1/659).
3. **Unmada** (Insanity): Mandukparni leaves' juice mixed with equal quantity of Dhatura and somavalli is used daily to get relief in epilepsy and insanity (B.S.unmada/22). Medicated ghee prepared with Mandukparni juice is also useful in treating hysteria, insanity, and epilepsy.
4. **Kasa and Shosha** (cough and emaciation): Mandukparni, Yashtimadhu, and Shunthi with milk is used daily as

vardhmana rasayan in kasa and shosha as Nagbala (A.H.Ci. 3/119).

5. **Kamala** (jaundice): Persons suffering from jaundice should take juice of Mandukparni, mixed with madhu, haridra, amalaki, and milk daily in the morning (Vd.M. 10/2).

6. **Peenas** (coryza): Drinking decoction prepared with Mandukparni, Marich, and Kulattha gives relief in chronic coryza (Vd.M. 16/69).

7. **Mutradaha** (burning micturition): 1/4 teaspoon of Mandukparni and Bhumyamalaki leaves' paste with buttermilk or dahi should be used daily to get relief in mutradaha (burning micturition) and raktamutrata (hematuria).

Officinal Part Used

Whole plant

Dose

Juice: 10 to 20 mL
Powder: 3 to 6 g

Formulations

Sarasvatarishta, Brahma rasayana, Brahmipanaka, Brahmi taila, Saraswata ghrita.

Toxicity/Adverse Effects

Literature survey doesn't show any toxicological data. However, asiaticosides are reported as possible skin carcinogens in rodents after repeated topical application (Laerum and Iverson 1972). It may cause allergic contact dermatitis, headache, and may aggravate pruritus on local application (Danese et al 1994).

Substitution and Adulteration

Brahmi and Mandukparni are often substituted for each other in the market under the name of Brahmi (Sharma et al 2000), and plants with similar looking leaves like *Merremia emarginata* Hallier f., *Hydrocotyle javanica* Thunb, *Hydrocotyle rotundifolia* Roxb., and *Malva rotundifolia* Linn. (Bagchi and Puri 1989).

Points to Ponder

- *Mandukparni is a potent medhya rasayan (psychotropic drug).*
- *Besides being sold in the market in the same name, Brahmi and Mandukparni are two different intellect-promoting drugs.*
- *It is the drug of choice for epilepsy, cognitive dysfunction, skin diseases, bleeding disorders, and venous insufficiency.*

Suggested Readings

Anonymous. The Wealth of India: A Dictionary of Indian Raw Materials and Industrial Products – Raw Materials Series, Vol. 3, (Publications and Information Directorate, CSIR, New Delhi), Rev Ser, (Ca–Ci), 1992:428–430

Anonymous. WHO Monographs on Selected Medicinal Plants. Geneva: World Health Organization; 1999:77–85

Arora D, Kumar M, Dubey SD. *Centella asiatica*- A review of its medicinal uses and pharmacological effects. J Nat Rem 2002;2(2):143–149

Bagchi GD, Puri HS. Centella asiatica II; Herba hung. 28, 1989:127–34

Chopra RN, Nayar SL, Chopra IC. Glossary of Indian Medicinal Plants. New Delhi: Council for Scientific and Industrial Research; 1956:58

Danese P, Carnevali C, Bertazzoni MG. Contact dermatitis. 31; 1994:201

Emboden WA. The ethnopharmacology of *Centella asiatica* (L.) Urban (Apiaceae). J Ethnobiol 1985;5(2):101–107

Laerum OD, Iverson OH. Reticuloses and epidermal tumors in hairless mice after topical skin applications of cantharidin and asiaticoside. Cancer Res 1972;32:1463–1469

Leonard BD. Medicine at Your Feet: Healing Plants of the Hawaiian Kingdom *Centella asiatica* (Pohekula); 1998

Leyel CF. Elixirs of Life. New York, NY: Samuel Weiser, Inc.; 1970

Nalini K, Aroor AR, Karanth KS, Rao A. Effect of *Centella asiatica* fresh leaf aqueous extract on learning and memory and biogenic amine turnover in albino rats. Fitoterapia 1992;63:232–237

Pandey NK, Tewari KC, Tewari RN, Joshi GC, Pande VN, Pandey G. Medicinal plants of Kumaon Himalaya, strategies for conservation. In: U Dhar (ed.), Himalaya Biodiversity Conservation Strategies, Vol. 3. Nanital: Himavikas Publication; 1993:293–302

Shakir JS, Qudsia N, Mehboobus S. *Centella asiatica* Linn. Urban. A review. Nat Prod Radiance 2007;6(2):158–170

Sharma PC, Yelne MB, Dennis TJ. Database of Medicinal Plants Used in Ayurveda, Vol. 1. New Delhi: Central Council of Research in Ayurveda and Siddha; 2000:264–270

Singh B, Rastogi RP. A reinvestigation of the triterpenes of *Centellaasiatica* III. Phytochemistry 1969;8:917–921

Singh HG. Himalayan herbs and drugs, importance and extinction threat. J. Sci Res. Plants Med 1989;10:47–52

The Ayurvedic Pharmacopeia of India. Part I, Vol. 4. New Delhi: Government of India, Ministry of Health and Family Welfare, Department of AYUSH; 2004:71

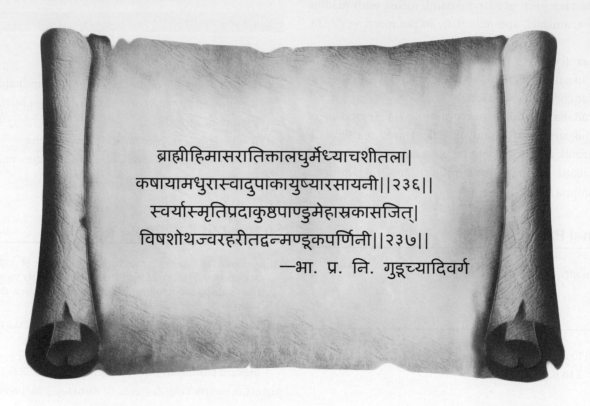

ब्राह्मीहिमासरातिक्तालघुर्मेध्याचशीतला।
कषायामधुरास्वादुपाकायुष्यारसायनी।।२३६।।
स्वर्यास्मृतिप्रदाकुष्ठपाण्डुमेहास्रकासजित्।
विषशोथज्वरहरीतद्वन्मण्डूकपर्णिनी।।२३७।।
—भा. प्र. नि. गुडूच्यादिवर्ग

66. Manjishtha [*Rubia cordifolia* Linn.]

Family: *Rubiaceae*

Hindi name: *Manjith*

English name: *Indian Madder, Dyer's madder*

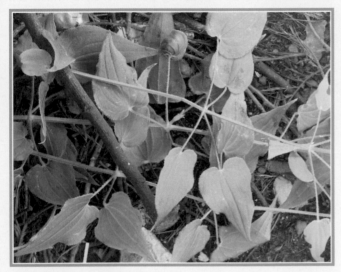

Plant of *Rubia cordifolia* Linn.

Although Manjishtha is recorded to be widespread in India, in some areas it has been regionally assessed as threatened.

Introduction

The Latin name *Rubia cordifolia* is derived from two words "Rubia" (meaning red) and "cordifolia" meaning cordate-shaped leaves of the plant. The plant yields plenty of red-orange coloring pigments which are used for dyeing fabrics.

Manjishtha is an age old ethnic medicinal plant used to cure diverse form of skin ailments. Since ages it is used by women folk as a home remedy for acne, blemishes, imparting natural glow, and complexion enhancing drug. Ancient treatises like Charaka and Sushrut also validate the age-old claims of being the best blood purifier drug. Charaka mentioned Manjishtha in varnyamahakashaya. Bhavaprakash included it as a major ingredient in Laghu, Madhya, Brihat Manjistadikwath (B.P.Kustharogadhikara/ 99-106). Sharangdhar, Chakraduta, and Vrindamadhav also

mention about the uses of Manjishtha in treatment of acne, skin diseases, and bleeding disorders. Acharya Charaka has suggested its use in eczematous dermatitis and pliharoga whereas Sushrut used it in raktarsha, and karnapalichikitsa. Sushrut used ropakghrita prepared with Manjishtha Chandan, Murva, and Lodhra in agnidagdh chikitsa (S.S.Su. 12/26). Manjishtha has also been enlisted in Chinese Pharmacopeia for the treatment of circulatory disorders, uterine disorders, bleeding disorders, and joint disorders. Unani practitioners used it in menstrual disorders, urinary obstructions, detoxification, paralysis, edema, and skin diseases (Patil et al 2009).

Apart from its medicinal value, it is used as natural food colorants, hair dyes, face packs, creams, soaps, cosmetics, dyeing clothes, and in veterinary medicines (Jha 1992). The interest in the isolation of natural dyes and coloring matters is increasing due to its applications in food, drugs, and other human consumptions (Wang et al 1992).

Vernacular Names

Assamese: Phuvva
Bengali: Manjistha, Manjith
Greek: Albisam
Gujarati: Manjitha
Kannada: Manjustha, chitravalli
Kashmiri: Dandu
Malayalam: Manjatti, Manchatti
Marathi: Manjihtha
Persian: Runas, Rudak
Punjabi: Kuparphali, Majit, Khuri
Tamil: Manjitte, ceevalli
Telugu: Manjishtha, Manderti
Urdu: Majeeth

Synonyms

Aruna: The stem is reddish-black in color.
Bhandi: The plant has spreading nature.
Kala: Its dried roots are black colored.
Kalmeshika: It competes with the increasing age, i.e., has antiaging effect.
Lata: Morphologically, the plant is a climber.
Mandukparni: The shape of its leaves resembles the shape of Mandukparni leaves.
Raktaangi: The plant parts, i.e., root, stem are red in color.
Raktayashtika: Its stem is red-colored.
Rasayani: The plant is immune modulator in action.
Samanga: It helps in restoring the normal complexion of entire body.
Vastraranjani: The dye extracted from its roots is used for dyeing clothes.
Viksha: It spreads extensively over the ground.
Yojanvalli: The climber can spread to an area of one yojan.

Classical Categorization

Charaka Samhita: Varnya, Vishaghna, Jwaraghna
Sushrut Samhita: Priyangvadi, Pittasansamana
Ashtang Hridaya: Priyangvadi
Dhanvantari Nighantu: Guduchyadi varga
Madanpal Nighantu: Abhyadi varga
Kaiyadev Nighantu: Oushadi varga
Raj Nighantu: Pippalyadi varga
Bhavaprakash Nighantu: Haritakyadi varga

Distribution

The plant is a native of North East Asia extending from Japan to Africa. It is found throughout India in hilly regions up to an altitude of 3,000 ft from North East Himalayas to Southern peninsula.

Morphology

It is a climbing or scrambling perennial herb which can spread up to 1.5 to 2 m.

- **Stem:** Slender, rectangular, divaricately branched, and prickly hispid (**Fig. 66.1**).
- **Leaves:** Rough, evergreen, arranged in whorl of four per node, oval to cordate shape, 4 to 8 cm long, 2 to 3 cm width; lower leaves are larger than upper, long petiole, having five to seven main nerves (**Fig. 66.2**).
- **Flowers:** Small, greenish-white to red in terminal panicled glabrous dichasial cyme, pentapetalous, sweet scented (**Fig. 66.3**).
- **Fruits:** Round berries of 4 to 6 mm diameter, smooth, shiny, fleshy, green in fresh state, on maturity turns red to black (**Fig. 66.4**).
- **Root:** Long, cylindrical, smooth, about 1 m long and 12 mm thick, bright red or brownish-red in color.

Phenology

Flowering time: June to August
Fruiting time: September to December

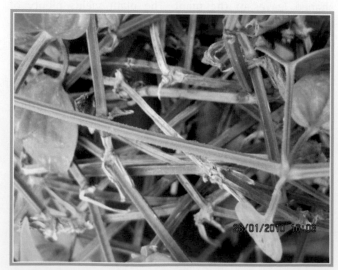

Fig. 66.1 Stem.

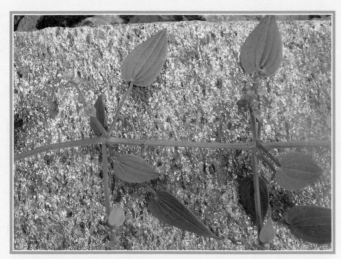

Fig. 66.2 Leaves.

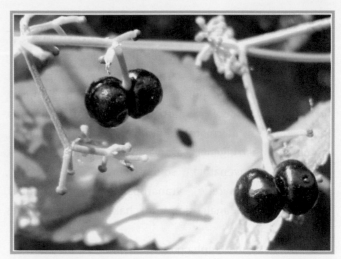

Fig. 66.4 Fruit.

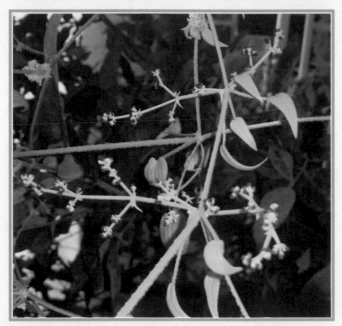

Fig. 66.3 Flowers.

Key Characters for Identification

➤ *A climbing or scrambling perennial herb of about 2 m.*

➤ *Leaves are rough, arranged in whorl of four per node, oval to cordate, two larger, two smaller, long petiole.*

➤ *Flowers are greenish-white in terminal panicled dichasial cyme.*

➤ *Fruits are globose berries, smooth fleshy, unripe green, red on maturity.*

➤ *Roots are long, cylindrical, smooth, red to reddish-brown.*

Rasapanchaka

Guna	Guru, Ruksha
Rasa	Tikta, Kashaya, Madhur
Vipaka	Katu
Virya	Ushna

Chemical Constituents

Different classes of bioactive compounds such as anthraquinones and their glycosides, naphthoquinones, terpenes, hexapeptides, carboxylic acids, iridoids, and saccharides are reported from various parts of Manjishtha. Its root mainly contains purpurin, munjistin (coloring agent), xanthin (yellow) xanthopurpurin, pseudopurpurin, alizarin (orange red), mollugin, garancin, rubimallin, rubicoumaric acid, rubifolic acid, and β-sitosterol naphthohydroquinone, di-β-D-glucoside, daucosterol (Wang et al 1992; Singh et al 2004).

Identity, Purity, and Strength

- Foreign matter: Not more than 2%
- Total ash: Not more than 12%
- Acid-insoluble ash: Not more than 0.5%
- Alcohol-soluble extractive: Not less than 3%
- Water-soluble extractive: Not less than 17%

(Source: The Ayurvedic Pharmacopeia of India 2001)

Karma (Actions)

Ayurvedic classics described Manjishtha as swarya (soothing to throat), vranakrita or varnya (improves complexion), raktshodhaka (blood purifier), krimighna (anthelmintic), vishaghni (antidote), shothghna (anti-inflammatory), kushtaghna (antidermatosis), pramehaghna (antidiabetic), stambhan (astringent), artavajanana (emmenogogue), rasayana (rejuvenator), sonitasthapana (hemostatic), jwaraghna (antipyretic), vranaropaka (wound healing), vedanasthapana (analgesic), and chakshushya (improves vision).

- Doshakarma: Kapha pittashamaka
- Dhatukarma: Rasayana, Raktashodhak
- Malakarma: Virechan

Pharmacological Actions

Several in vivo and in vitro researches proved that Manjishtha root and stem possess astringent, thermogenic, febrifuge, anthelmintic, galactopurifier, antidysenteric, antioxidant, immunomodulator, rejuvenator, antiacne, antiarthritic, anticancer, antitumor, antileukemic, antistress, expectorant, wound healing, antimicrobial, anti-inflammatory, analgesic, nootropic, diuretic, hepatoprotective, neuroprotective, and radioprotective properties (Meena et al 2010; Siddiqui et al 2012).

Indications

Manjishtha is traditionally used in the treatment of visha (poisoning), shotha (inflammations), yoniroga (menstrual disorder), akshiroga (eye disease), karnaroga (ear diseases), raktaatisaar (bleeding diarrhea), visarpa (erysipelas), raktavikara (bleeding disorders), prameha (diabetes), vrana (wounds), kushta (skin disease), sarpavisha (snake bite), arsha (hemorrhoids), bhagna (fracture), vyanga (freckles/blemishes), etc. In other systems of medicines, its root, stem decoction, paste, and juice are widely used for the treatment of edema, eczema, leprosy, leucoderma, chronic ulcers, ringworm, hematuria, hematemesis, fever, menstrual disorders, uterine bleeding, internal external hemorrhage, constipation, stomachache, dysentery, headache, rheumatism, jaundice, pleurisy, bronchitis, cough, urinary disorders, lithiasis, and scorpion sting.

Therapeutic Uses

External Use

1. **Visarpa** (erysipelas): Local application of paste of Manjishtha, Lodhra, and Chandana is advised.
2. **Vyang** (freckles): In vyang, Manjishtha powder pounded and mixed with madhu should be applied on face (A.S.U. 37/24).

Internal Use

1. **Kushta** (skin diseases): Manjishtha root powder mixed with honey is applied externally on blemishes, burn, to remove pimples, freckles, acne, leucoderma, dark spots, discoloration, and to enhance luster and glow of skin. Dried crushed orange peel, Chandan, Haridra, and Manjishtha makes an excellent face pack. Manjisthadi kwath is used internally for same period for better results (S.G. 2/2/38,39).
2. **Garbhasyashodhan** (uterine purification): Decoction of Manjishtha with Ishwarimool and Pippalimool should be given to mother after delivery to purify uterus.
3. **Prameha** (diabetes): One should use decoction of Manjishtha and Chandana daily in Manjisthmeha (S.S.Ci. 11/9).
4. **Raktaarsha** (bleeding piles): Ghee cooked with the decoction of Manjishtha and Shigru is useful in bleeding piles (S.S.Ci. 6/9).
5. **Sarpvisha** (snake poisoning): Intake of ghrita mixed with Manjishtha, grahadhoom, and madhu helps in reducing the toxic effect due to snake poisoning (A.H.U. 36/59).
6. **Asthibhagna** (fracture): Decoction or paste for local application of Manjishtha, Arjuna, Yashtimadhu, and Sugandhbala promotes bone healing in fractures. Local application of Manjishtha and Yashtimadhu mixed with Kanji reduces pain and swelling due to fracture or dislocation (VM. 46/3).

Officinal Parts Used

Root and stem

Dose

Powder: 1 to 3 g
Decoction: 20 to 40 mL

Formulations

Manjisthadi kwath, Mahamanjisthadi kwath, Kumkumadi taila, Chandanasava, Jatyadi ghrita.

Toxicity/Adverse Effects

Manjishtha when administered on prolonged medication in large doses may cause headache, and hematuria that may affect lungs (Siddiqui et al 2012).

Substitution and Adulteration

In crude drug market, stem pieces of Manjishtha are sold as Manjishtha roots. However *R. cordifolia* itself is used as an adulterant of *Swertia chirata* Roxb.ex. flem. (Lavekar et al 2008).

> ### Points to Ponder
>
> - *Manjishtha is a potent drug for skin diseases such as erysipelas, leucoderma, acne, blemishes, discoloration, pimples, freckles, pigmentations.*
> - *Manjishtha is reputed worldwide as an efficient blood purifier, hemostatic, galactopurifier, antiseptic, febrifuge, rejuvenator, and tonic.*

Suggested Readings

Jha MK. The Folk Veterinary System of Bihar: A Research Survey. Gujarat, India: NDDB, Anand; 1992

Lavekar GS, Padhi MM, Joseph GVR, et al. Database on Medicinal Plants Used in Ayurveda. Vol. 5, New Delhi: CCRAS; 2008:176

Meena AK, Pal B, Panda P, Sannd R, Rao MM. A review on Rubia cordifolia: Its phyto constituents and therapeutic uses. Drug Invention Today 2010;2(5):244–246

Patil R, Mohan M, Kasture V, Kasture S. Rubia cordifolia: a review. Orient Pharm Exp Med 2009;9(1):1–13

Siddiqui A, Jamal A, Tajuddin, Amin KMY, Bhat JU. A Review of important medicinal plant Majeeth (*Rubia cordifolia* Linn.) Phytochemical and Pharmacological studies. Int J Universal Pharm Life Sci 2012;2(2):126–142

Singh R. Geetanjali, Chauhan SM. 9, 10-Anthraquinones and other biologically active compounds from the genus *Rubia*. J. Chem. Biodivers. 2004;1:1241–1264

The Ayurvedic Pharmacopeia of India. Part I, Vol. 3 New Delhi: Department of AYUSH, Ministry of Health and Family Welfare, Government of India; 2001:113

Wang SX, Hua HM, Wu LJ, Li X, Zhu TR. Studies on anthraquinones from the roots of *Rubia cordifolia* L. Yao Xue Xue Bao 1992;27(10):743–747

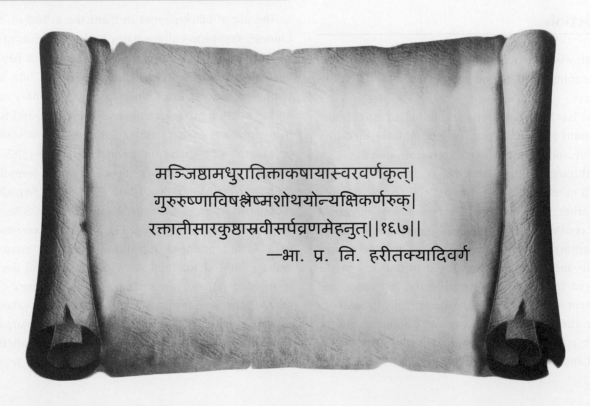

मञ्जिष्ठामधुरातिक्ताकषायास्वरवर्णकृत्।
गुरुरुष्णाविषश्लेष्मशोथयोन्यक्षिकर्णरुक्।
रक्तातीसारकुष्ठास्रवीसर्पव्रणमेहनुत्।।१६७।।
—भा. प्र. नि. हरीतक्यादिवर्ग

67. Maricha [*Piper nigrum* Linn.*]

Family: *Piperaceae*

Hindi name: *Kali Mirch*

English name: *Black pepper*

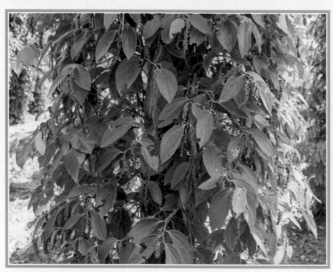

Plant of *Piper nigrum* Linn.

> *Bioperine is a standardized extract from the fruits of Piper nigrum L. It contains 95% piperine and is effective as a food additive in humans and animals. It is also termed as natural thermonutrient and bioavailability enhancer.*
>
> —*Majeed et al (1999)*

Introduction

The English word "pepper" is derived from the Latin word "piper" meaning spirit or energy which is indicative of its hot potency.

Maricha has been used for years in Indian kitchen as a food seasoning spice. It is a popular food additive, medicine, preservative, and biocontrol agent and is considered as "King of spice" throughout the world. The trade of black pepper along with other spices has changed the course of world history. Earlier, the country having monopoly in pepper trade was considered as economically sound and powerful. In 2nd century BC, pepper trade was first dominated by Chinese and was later introduced in Sumatra at the beginning of 15th century. After this, the cultivation and production of Maricha increased exponentially in Southern Asia. Later, the European and American colonization in the area made pepper a precious valuable trade commodity (Aggarwal and Kunnumakkara 2009).

The use of black pepper in medicine in Indian, Syrian, Chinese, European culture dates back thousands of years. The Syrian book of medicine prescribes black pepper in liver diseases, indigestion, gangrene, insect bite, cough, toothache, abscess, etc. Chinese used it in urinary calculus and as a folk remedy in epilepsy, insect bite, and tumors. In Ayurveda text Sharandhara Samhita, it is described as an example of lekhana and pramarthidravyas (Sh.S. 1/4/9, 23). It is an important ingredient of famous formulations such as trikatu and shadushna (B.P.S. 1/62,74). Charaka mentioned Maricha in kusthahar pradeha (C.S.Su. 3/12), ahaaryogi varga (C.S.Su. 26/298), and in the treatment of kasa, kushta, prameha, rajyakshma, unmada, kshatsheen, arsha, grahni, chardi, and yonivyapada. Sushrut described it in sanshodhan, sansamandravya, shakavarga (S.S.Su. 46/224) and used it in the treatment of arsha, vatavyadhi, ashmari, kushta, kshudroga, sopha, apatanaka, sarpavisha, and anuvasanabasti. Black pepper and its other varieties are widely used for culinary purposes, flavoring and seasoning of food, meat, essence, and in preparation of garam masala, masala tea, cookies, sweets, bakery products, etc. (Mathew 1984).

Vernacular Names

Bengali: Golmorich, Kalamorich, Morich
Dutch: Peper
French: Poivre
German: Pfeffer
Gujarati: Kalimori
Kannada: Karimonaru, Menaru
Konkani: Miriyakonu
Malayalam: Kurumulaku
Marathi: Kalamiri
Punjabi: Galmirich, Kalimirch
Tamil: Milagu
Telugu: Miriyalu, Marichamu
Urdu: FilfilSiyah, Kalimirich

Synonyms

Dharampatan: It is a famous export commodity which enhances foreign trade.
Katukam: The fruit is katu in rasa and vipaka.
Krishan: The dried fruit is black colored.
Tikshanam: The fruit is sharp and piercing in nature.
Ushna: The fruit is hot in property and potency.
Vellaj: Morphologically, the plant is a climber.
Vritaphalam: The fruit is round in shape.
Yavneshtha: It is liked by the people of yavan (Europeans).

Classical Categorization

Charaka Samhita: Deepaniya, Shoolprasasmana, Krimighna, Sirovirechana
Sushrut Samhita: Pippalayadi, Trikatu
Ashtang Hridaya: Vatsakadi varga
Dhanvantari Nighantu: Shatpushpadi varga
Madanpal Nighantu: Sunthyadi varga
Kaiyadev Nighantu: Oushadi varga
Raj Nighantu: Pippalyadi varga
Bhavaprakash Nighantu: Haritakyadi varga

Distribution

It is mainly cultivated in the Southern states of Andhra Pradesh, Kerala, Karnataka, Konkon, and Tamil Nadu. It is found wild and is also cultivated in Assam, Darjeeling, Sylhet, Saharanpur, and Dehradun.

Morphology

It is a woody, perennial, shade loving, glabrous, climbing vine that climbs around trees, poles, or any other support reaching up to 4 m, rooting from the nodes.

- **Leaves:** Simple, alternate, cordate shape, glabrous, 5 to 10 cm length and 3 to 6 cm width, with three to seven prominent veins (**Fig. 67.1**).
- **Flowers:** Minute in spikes, usually dioecious, length of spike is variable (**Fig. 67.2**).
- **Fruits:** They occur in pendulous bunches, ovoid or globose, 3 to 4 mm in diameter, one-seeded berry,

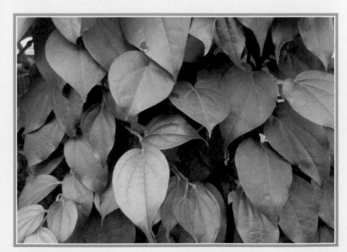

Fig. 67.1 Leaves.

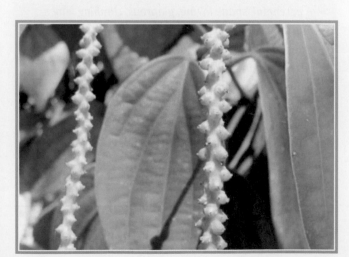

Fig. 67.2 Flower.

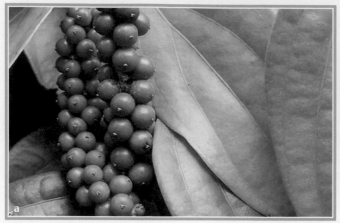
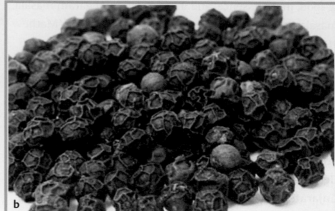

Fig. 67.3 **(a)** Fruits. **(b)** Dried fruits.

fleshy and smooth, green unripe fruit (known as a peppercorn), which turns orangish red on maturity (**Fig. 67.3a**). Dried fruits are externally black, pungent, have rugae surface, and are internally white in color (**Fig. 67.3b**). Dried Maricha fruits are soaked in water overnight, outer cover is removed & dried. Then it is known as Shweta Maricha. The plants bear fruits from fourth or fifth year and continue to bear fruits up to 7 years.

The plant is propagated by vegetative methods.

Phenology

Flowering time: June to November
Fruiting time: February to April

Key Characters for Identification

➤ A perennial, shade loving, glabrous, climbing vine reaching up to 4 m and rooting at nodes.
➤ Leaves are simple, glabrous, cordate shape, three to seven prominent veins.
➤ Flowers are minute in spikes and dioecious.
➤ Fruits are ovoid or globose, fleshy, smooth berries, occur in pendulous bunches. Unripe are green whereas fully mature are red and dried black.

Types

Raj Nighantu has described two types of Maricha:
• Maricha
• Shwet Maricha

On the basis of trade, three types of Maricha are available in the market:
• Black pepper
• White pepper
• Green Pepper

Rasapanchaka

Rasapanchaka	Aadra Maricha	Shushk Maricha
Guna	Guru, Kinchidtikshna	Laghu, Ruksha, Tikshna
Rasa	Katu	Katu
Vipaka	Madhura	Katu
Virya	Na atiushna	Ushna
Doshaghanta	Kapha vatahara	Kapha vatahara Pittakar

Chemical Constituents

Maricha fruits are reported to have diverse group of compounds like phenols, flavonoids, alkaloids, amides, steroids, lignans, neolignans, terpenes, and chalcones. Among these alkaloids, piperine and its isomers isopiperine, chavicine, isochavicine are the principal ones. The other compounds are piperamide, piperamine, piperettine, piper-acide, piperolein, sarmentine, sarmentosine retrofracta-mide A, brachyamide B, N-formylpiperidine, guineensine, isobutyl-eicosadienamide, tricholein, trichostachine, and isobutyl-octadienamide (Parmar et al 1997).

Identity, Purity, and Strength

- Foreign matter: Not more than 2%
- Total ash: Not more than 5%
- Acid-insoluble ash: Not more than 0.5%
- Alcohol-soluble extractive: Not less than 6%
- Water-soluble extractive: Not less than 6%

(Source: The Ayurvedic Pharmacopeia of India 2001)

Karma (Actions)

Ayurveda classics attributed deepan (carminative), pachana (digestive), ruchya (relish), pramarthi (expels out cough), lekhana (scrapping), utejaka (stimulant), vataanulomaka (expels out vata), swedajanan (diaphoretic), jwaraghna (antipyretic), mutral (diuretic), chedana (expectorant), krimighna (anthelmintic), kusthaghna (antidermatosis), medohara (antiobesity), shoolaghna (analgesic), avrishya (non aphrodisiac), and artavajanan (emmenogogue) properties to Shushka Maricha. Aadra Maricha: Guru, kinchit ushna, madhura vipaki, katu, don't aggravate pitta, kaphanisaraka (expectorant), and are slightly teekshan in properties (K.D.N.oushadivarga/1162).

Shwet Maricha is described as vishaghna, bhootnashan, avrishya, and rasayana (R.N. pippalyadivarga/38).

- Doshakarma: Kapha vatahara and Pittavardhaka
- Dhatukarma: Lekhan, chedana
- Malakarma: Vataanuloman, mutral, swedajanan

Pharmacological Actions

Maricha fruit is also reported to exhibit antimicrobial, antioxidant, analgesic, anti-inflammatory, antispasmodic, anticancer, antitumor, antihypertensive, antiplatelets, antidiarrheal, digestive, bioavailability enhancer, insecticidal, larvicidal, expectorant, immunomodulator, hepatoprotective, antiasthmatics, and antipyretic properties (Damanhouri and Ahmad 2014).

Indications

It is used for the treatment of kasa (cough), shwasa (asthma), pratishyay (common cold), agnimandhya (decrease digestive fire), ajeerna (indigestion), udarshool (abdominal pain), adhyaman (flatulence), krimi (worm infestation), hridyaroga (heart diseases), shivitra (leucoderma), kilasa (a type of skin disease), dantashool (toothache), dantakrimi (tooth caries), Jwar (fever), rajorodha (amenorrhea), mutrakricchta (dysuria).

Therapeutic Uses

External Use

1. **Yuvanpidika** (pimples): To get rid of pimples in puberty one should apply daily Maricha powder mixed with ox bile or water (S.G. 3/11/11).
2. **Dantashool** (toothache): Decoction of Maricha is used as gargles to relieve toothache.
3. **Marichadi taila:** It is used for external application in skin diseases, rheumatoid arthritis, osteoarthritis, and paralysis.

Internal Use

1. **Grahaniroga** (sprue): Intake of Marichadi churna (B.S.ajeerna/91) alone or March churna with Chitrak and Suvarchala with takraas anupana gives relief in grahani, udarshool, pleeha, mandagni, gulma, and arsha (S.G.2/6/53).
2. **Kasa** (cough): Daily intake of Maricha powder mixed with mishri, ghrita, and madhu in the form of leha is an effective remedy in cough (S.S.U. 52/18).
3. **Shwasa, Hikka** (asthma, hic-cough): In hikka and shwasa, Maricha powder mixed with Bharangi and Yavakshara is used with warm water (A.S.Ci. 6/34).
4. **Pratishyay, peenasa** (common cold, coryza): Maricha powder mixed with guda along with the diet of dahi and sour food cures newly formed coryza (VM. 60/21).
5. **Sthoulya** (obesity): In obesity one should take 1 betel leaf with 10 grains of Maricha followed by intake of cold water for 2 months daily (Vd.M. 12/31).
6. **Pama** (eczema): Maricha powder should be taken orally with fresh go-ghrita to alleviate eczema, scabies (Vd.M. 11/49).

Officinal Part Used

Fruit

Dose

Powder: 0.5 to 1 g

Formulations

Trikatu churna, Marichyadi gutika, Marichyadi taila.

Toxicity/Adverse Effects

Administration of Maricha or its formulations for prolonged duration may cause burning sensation, hyperacidity, nausea, fever, and headache.

Substitution and Adulteration

Maricha fruits are often adulterated with dried papaya seeds.

Points to Ponder

- *Piperine is the main active alkaloid in Maricha. It increases the bioavailability of drugs and nutrients.*
- *Shushka Maricha is pitta aggravating, katu vipaki whereas Aadra Maricha is madhura vipaki and not so pitta aggravating in properties.*

Suggested Readings

Aggarwal BB, Kunnumakkara AB. Molecular Targets and Therapeutic Uses of Spices: Modern Uses for Ancient medicines. Singapore: World Scientific Publishing Pvt. Ltd; 2009:25–28

Damanhouri ZA, Ahmad A. A Review on Therapeutic Potential of Piper nigrum L. (Black Pepper): The King of Spices. Med Aromat Plants 2014;3(3):1–6

Majeed M, Badmaev V, Rajendran R. BioPerine Nature's Own Thermonutrient and Natural Bioavailability Enhancer. Piscataway, NJ: Nutriscience Publishers Inc.; 1999

Mathew AG. Pepper. J Plant Crops 1984;12:94–97

Parmar VS, Jain SC, Bisht KS, et al. Phytochemistry of the genus *Piper*. Phytochemistry 1997;46:597–673

The Ayurvedic Pharmacopeia of India. Part I, Vol. 3. New Delhi: Government of India, Ministry of Health and Family Welfare, Department of AYUSH; 2001:116

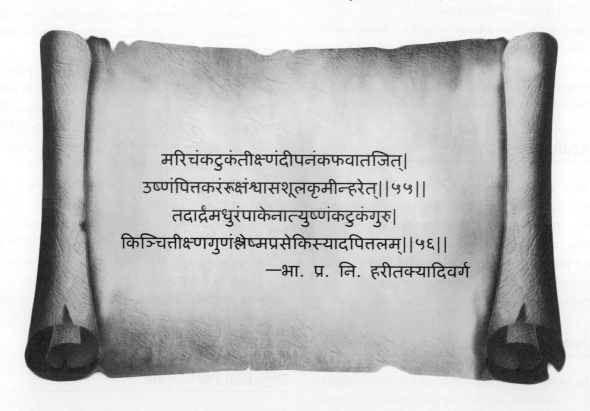

मरिचंकटुकंतीक्ष्णंदीपनंकफवातजित्।
उष्णंपित्तकरंरूक्षंश्वासशूलकृमीन्हरेत्।।५५।।
तदार्द्रंमधुरंपाकेनात्युष्णंकटुकंगुरु।
किञ्चित्तीक्ष्णगुणंश्लेष्मप्रसेकिस्यादपित्तलम्।।५६।।
—भा. प्र. नि. हरीतक्यादिवर्ग

68. Musta *[Cyperus rotundus Linn.]*

Family: *Cyperaceae*

Hindi name: *Motha*

English name: *Nut grass, purple nut grass, sedge*

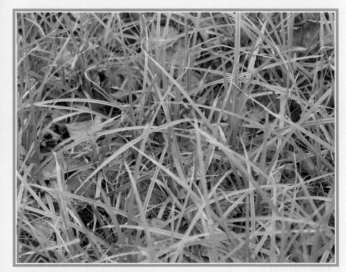

Plant of *Cyperus rotundus* Linn.

> *The herb grows abundantly in potato fields and is difficult to dug out from the soil; thus, it becomes a great nuisance for potato cultivators.*

Introduction

The Sanskrit word "Musta" is derived from the verse *musta sanghate iti* which means the one who grows in cluster of tubers. The word *Cyperus* is derived from Greek *kuperos* and *rotundus* is a Latin word which means round, highlighting the shape of the tuber.

Musta is a perfect example of medicinal weed with innumerable qualities and a long history of folklore use. The plant is praised in Ayurvedic, Siddha, Unani, Homeopathic, Naturopathic, Chinese, and American traditional systems of medicine. In Ayurveda, Charaka attributes sangrahi deepaniya pachaniya properties to it (C.S.Su. 25/40). Ashtang described it as the best drug for jwara along with Parpata (A.H.Su.) which attributes apasmarhara property to it. Acharya Charaka considered it as an important drug in the management of madatyaya and vangasena in apasmara. Shodhala used it for external application in vrana. It is also one of the ingredients of trikarshika, chaturbhadra, and sarvaoushadi gana. Bhavaprakash considered the Musta which grows in anoopdesha as best. Its oil is used in making perfumes and as essence in food and cosmetics.

Vernacular Names

Bengali: Mutha, Musta

Burmese: Vomonniu

Chinese: Suo cao, Xiang fu zi

German: Knolliges Zypergras

Gujarati: Moth, Nagarmothaya

Kannada: Konnari Gadde

Malayalam: Muthanga, Kari Mustan

Marathi: Moth, Nagarmoth, Motha, Bimbal

Punjabi: Mutha, Motha

Tamil: Korai, Korai-Kizhangu

Telugu: Tungamustalu

Urdu: Sad Kufi

Synonyms

Gangeyi: It grows naturally near the banks of river Ganga.

Granthila: The tuber is nodular in shape.

Krodeshtha: The tuber is eaten by pigs in abundance.

Kuruvinda: It grows naturally in Kuru Pradesh.

Mustaka: It grows in clusters, i.e., has gregarious nature.

Rajkasheruka: The tuber is similar in appearance to kaseru fruit.

Sugandhi: The tuber is aromatic in nature.

Varidanamakam: It is known by the other synonyms of water or clouds.

Classical Categorization

Charaka Samhita: Lekhaniya, Trishna nigrahana, Triptighna, Stanyashodhana, Kandughna

Sushruta Samhita: Mustadi, Vachadi

Ashtang Hridaya: Mustadi, Vachadi

Dhanvantari Nighantu: Guduchyadi varga

Madanpal Nighantu: Abhyadi varga

Kaiyadev Nighantu: Oushadi varga

Raj Nighantu: Pippalyadi varga

Bhavaprakash Nighantu: Karpuradi varga

Distribution

Musta grows naturally in tropical, subtropical, and temperate regions of the world. Throughout India, it occurs as a weed in wastelands, fields up to an altitude of 1,500 ft.

Morphology

It is a perennial glabrous grass of about 20 to 30 cm height with slender stolon and triquetrous aerial stem.

- Leaves are radical, dark green, numerous, narrowly linear, flat, sheathed, one nerved (**Fig. 68.1**).
- Flower inflorescence consists of four to six brown purple spikes radiating from a long, slender, triangular stalk; spikelets are purplish green, in compound umbels (**Fig. 68.2**).
- Fruit is gray-black-colored trigonus nut, single-seeded.
- Rhizome is tuberous; tuber is of conical shape with wiry, slender root, 1 to 3 cm long, aromatic, external surface reddish-brown, rough, and internally white in color (**Fig. 68.3**). The plant is propagated by vegetative method from tuber.

Phenology

Flowering time: Throughout the year
Fruiting time: Throughout the year

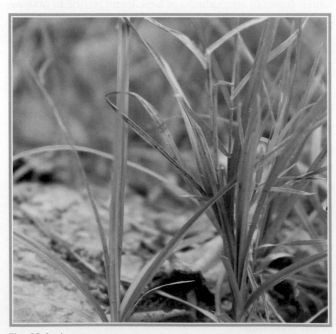

Fig. 68.1 Leaves.

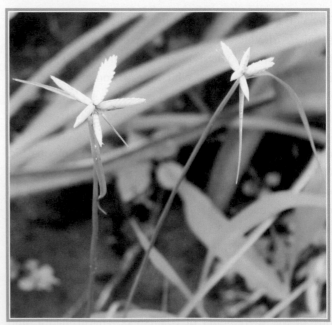

Fig. 68.2 Flowers.

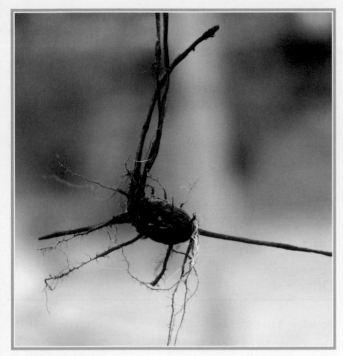

Fig. 68.3 Tuber.

Key Characters for Identification

➤ *A perennial glabrous grass of 20 to 30 cm height.*
➤ *Leaves are narrowly linear, dark green, flat, and sheathed.*
➤ *Inflorescence of four to six brown-purple spikes radiating from a slender stalk.*
➤ *Fruits are trigonus nut, gray-black-colored.*
➤ *Rhizome is tuberous; tubers are conical, aromatic, rough, black-brown externally and white internally.*

Types

Bhavamishra has described three types of Musta:

- Bhadra Musta: *C. rotundus* L.
- Nagar Musta: *Cyperus scariosus*—Best among the three
- Kaivart/Jal Musta: *Cyperus esculentus*

Rasapanchaka

Guna	Laghu, Ruksha
Rasa	Katu, Tikta, Kashaya
Vipaka	Katu
Virya	Sheeta

Chemical Constituents

The tuber contains essential oil, flavonoids, terpenoids, sesquiterpenes, fats, sugar, gum, carbohydrates, albumins, and fibers. The essential oil has cyperene I & II, cyperol, isocyperol, cineol, α-cyperone, α-pinene, cyperenone, kobusone, mustakone, cyperotundone, α- & β-selinene and β-sitosterol cyproterone, cypera-2,4-diene, α-copaene, cyperene, aselinene, rotundene, valencene, gurjunene, trans-calamenene, g-calacorene, epi-a-selinene, and α-muurolene (Rai et al 2010; Joulain and Konig 1998).

Identity, Purity, and Strength

For Rhizome

- Foreign matter: Not more than 2%
- Total ash: Not more than 8%
- Acid-insoluble ash: Not more than 4%
- Alcohol-soluble extractive: Not less than 5%
- Water-soluble extractive: Not less than 11%
- Volatile oil: Not less than 1%

(Source: The Ayurvedic Pharmacopeia of India 2001)

Karma (Actions)

Musta possesses grahi (absorbent), deepana (appetizer), pachana (digestive), krimighna (antimicrobial), swedajanan (diaphoretic), shothahara (anti-inflammatory), triptighna (antisaturative), vishaghna (antidote to poison), medohara (antiobesity), trishnanigrahana (thirst restraining), stanya-shodhan (galactopurificator), jwaraghna (antipyretic). Its oil is bactericidal and fungicidal.

- Doshakarma: Kapha pittashamak
- Dhatukarma: Medohara, Grahi
- Malakarma: Swedajanan

Pharmacological Actions

Its rhizome is reported to have anti-inflammatory, diaphoretic, antidiarrheal, antitussive, insecticidal, antibacterial, antioxidant, anticancer, antipyretic, analgesic, antispasmodic, anticonvulsant, antiulcer, antiallergic, antimalarial, neuroprotective, hypolipidemic, antiplatelet, wound healing, antidiabetic, hepatoprotective, emmenagogue, vermifuge, and tonic properties (Das et al 2015; Sivapalan 2013).

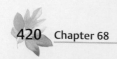

Indications

Ayurvedic texts advocated to use Musta in trishna (thirst), jwara (fever), jantu (microbial infections), aruchi (distaste), krimi (worm infestation), visha (poisoning), agnimandya (loss of appetite), ajeerna (indigestion), kasa (cough), mutrakricchta (dysuria), vaman (vomiting), sutikaroga (diseases after puerperium), atisaar (diarrhea), aamvata (arthritis).

In folklore and traditional practices, Musta is used in dysmenorrheal, menstrual irregularities, abdominal complaints, skin diseases, malaria, insect bite, wounds, boils, blisters, and in deficient lactation (Oliver-Bever 1986).

Therapeutic Uses

External Use

1. **Vrana** (wounds): Fresh rhizome made into paste and mixed with ghrita is applied locally on wounds and ulcers (CD. 6/91).
2. **Stanyavridhi** (galactogogue): For inducing lactation, Musta powder mixed with water is applied on the breast.

Internal Use

1. **Jwara** (fever): Water mixed with Musta, Parpata, Ushira, Chandana, Sugandhbala, and Shunthi powder is boiled till it reduces to half. Then it is kept aside and cooled. This water is known as Shadangpaniya. It should be given regularly to the person suffering from fever and thirst (C.S.Ci. 3/145).
2. **Atisaar** (diarrhea): Intake of decoction of Musta alone mixed with honey gives relief in diarrhea (S.S.U. 40/72). To control diarrhea associated with mucous and blood, one should take Mustaka ksheerpaka with madhu daily (S.S.U. 40/47). In aamatisar, Musta and Shunthi powder mixed with madhu is given (C.S.Ci. 19/22).
3. **Madatyaya** (alcoholism): Consumption of water boiled with Musta helps in reducing the effect of excessive alcohol intake (C.S.Ci. 24/167).
4. **Kasa** (cough): Kasa caused by vitiated kapha and pitta is relieved by taking sharkaradi formulation with Musta and Maricha (C.S.Ci. 20/38).

5. **Vatarakta** (gout): Vatarakta associated with kapha is cured by taking decoction of Musta, Amalaki, and Haridra (B.P.Ci. 29/78).
6. **Granthi-visarp** (erysipelas): Using Sattu prepared with Musta, Bhallataka, and madhu in diet is efficacious in granthi-visarp (C.S.Ci. 21/130).
7. **Hallimaka** (a form of jaundice): Musta powder and loha bhasm should be taken with Khadira kwath in hallimaka (B.P.Ci. 8/45).

Officinal Part Used

Tuber

Dose

Powder: 3 to 6 g
Decoction: 50 to 100 mL

Formulations

Mustakadi churna, Mustakadi leha, Mustakarishta, Gangadhar churna.

Toxicity/Adverse Effects

Not reported

Substitution and Adulteration

Mixed with other similar looking rhizomes.

Points to Ponder

- *Musta which grows around a water source or water prone area is considered as best quality.*
- *Musta is a popular traditional herb widely used as digestive, analgesic, antispasmodic, antimalarial, antidiarrheal, antibacterial.*

Suggested Readings

Das B, Pal DK, Haldar A. A review on *Cyperus rotundus* as a tremendous source of pharmacologically active herbal medicine. Int J Green Pharm 2015;9(4):198–203

Joulain D, Konig WA. The Atlas of Spectral Data of Sesquiterpene Hydrocarbons. Hamburg: EB-Verlag; 1998

Oliver-Bever B. Medicinal Plants in Tropical West Africa. Cambridge: Cambridge University Press; 1986:200

Rai PK, Kumar R, Malhotra Y, Sharma D, Karthiyagini T. Standardization and preliminary phytochemical investigation on *Cyperus rotundus* Linn. rhizome. Int J Res Ayurveda Pharm 2010;1:536–542

Sivapalan R. Medicinal uses and pharmacological activities of *Cyperus rotundus* Linn.: a review. Int J Scient Res Publications 2013;3(5):1–8

The Ayurvedic Pharmacopeia of India. Part I, Vol. 3. New Delhi: Department of AYUSH, Ministry of Health and Family Welfare, Government of India; 2001:131

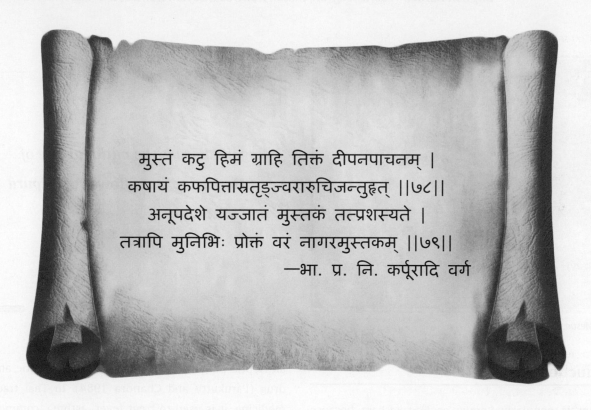

मुस्तं कटु हिमं ग्राहि तिक्तं दीपनपाचनम् |
कषायं कफपित्तास्रतृड्ज्वरारुचिजन्तुहृत् ||७८||
अनूपदेशे यज्जातं मुस्तकं तत्प्रशस्यते |
तत्रापि मुनिभिः प्रोक्तं वरं नागरमुस्तकम् ||७९||
—भा. प्र. नि. कर्पूरादि वर्ग

69. Nagakeshara *[Mesua ferrea Linn.]*

Family: *Clusiaceae*

Hindi name: *Nagkesar*

English name: *Cobra's saffron, Indian Ironwood, Ceylon Ironwood*

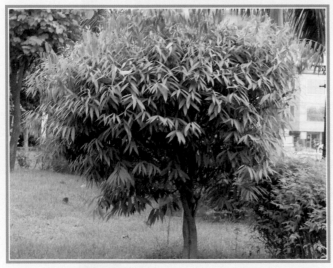

Plant of *Mesua ferrea* Linn.

Nagakeshara is the national tree of Sri Lanka and state flower of Tripura and Mizoram.

Introduction

The plant is popularly known as Nagakeshara because snakes are attracted toward the saffron-like aroma of the flowers. It is believed that snakes reside near the plant.

Since time immemorial, Nagakeshara is being extensively used in folklore, therapeutics, and commercial industry. It is a beautiful evergreen tree cultivated widely for its timber, fragrant flowers, and foliage. It is not included in any of the dashemani gana but Charaka used it in the treatment of arsha, visarpa, and vataroga. Sushrut considered it as a vishaghna dravya and used in hikka and water purification. Bangsena considered Nagakeshara as best rakt sangrahak (hemostatic) drug. It is also a famous ingredient in many Siddha formulations like elathi churna, inji churna, kanthaga rasayanam, parangipattai rasayanam, narathai legium, karisalai legium, and thalisathi vadagam (Anonymous 1992). The tribals of Assam used it as an antiseptic, purgative, blood purifier, anthelmintic, and tonic drug (Parukutty and Chandra 1984). In Thai traditional medicine, it is used to treat fever, asthma, common cold, and as antipyretic, carminative, expectorant, cardiotonic, and diuretic drug (Foundation of Resuscitate and Encourage Thai Traditional Medicine 2005). The plant is commercially popular in the market because of its oil which is known as kesar oil, extracted from the seeds. In north Canada, the oil is used in rheumatism and itching (Kritikar and Basu 1981).

Apart from medicinal uses, its seed oil is being used commercially in polymer industry (Dutta and Karak 2005), painting, as firewood, dye, cosmetic, substitute for gasoline (Konwer and Baruah 1984), and leaf extract in preparation of silver nanoparticles (Konwarh et al 2010). The seeds are burnt like candles, the wood is used for making golf club heads, and flowers and stamens are used to stuff pillows for bridal bed (Sahni 1998).

Vernacular Names

Arabic: Narae Kaisar
Assamese: Negeshvar, Nahar
Bengali: Nageshvara, Nagesar
Burmese: Gungen, Kenga
German: Nagassamen
Gujarati: Nagkesara, Sachunagkeshara, Nagchampa, Pilunagkesar
Italian: Croco di cobra
Kannada: Nagsampige, Nagakesari
Malayalam: Nangaa, Nauga, Peri, Veluthapala, Nagppu, Nagappovu
Marathi: Nagkesara
Oriya: Nageswar
Punjabi: Nageswar
Russia: Mezuia zheleznaia
Singapore: Sembawang
Tamil: Naugu, Naugaliral, Nagachampakam, Sirunagappu
Telugu: Nagachampakamu
Urdu: Narmushk, Nagkesar

Synonyms

Ahipushpa: The flowers are liked by snakes.
Champey: The flower is golden colored.
Kanak: The flower has golden stamen.
Kanchaaha: It is denoted by the other synonyms of gold.
Kanchan: The color of the stamen is golden yellow.
Kesar: The useful part of the plant is stamen.
Nagpushpa: The flower is characterized by its hooded petals.
Tung: It is a synonym of snake.

Classical Categorization

Charaka Samhita: Not mentioned
Sushruta Samhita: Eladi, Vachadi, Anjanadi, Priyangvadi
Ashtang Hridaya: Eladi, Vachadi, Anjanadi, Priyangvadi
Dhanvantari Nighantu: Shatpushpadi varga
Madanpal Nighantu: Karpuradi varga
Kaiyadev Nighantu: Oushadi varga
Raj Nighantu: Pippalyadi varga
Bhavaprakash Nighantu: Karpuradi varga

Distribution

The plant is native to tropical countries like India, Sri Lanka, Burma, Bangladesh, China, Russia, etc. In India, it is widely distributed in evergreen forests up to an altitude of 1,500 m. It is mostly distributed in the states of Assam, Karnataka, West Bengal, Maharashtra, Tamil Nadu, and Kerala, and is cultivated in the gardens of North India for decoration.

Morphology

It is a medium- to large-sized, glabrous, evergreen tree with beautiful foliage that can attain a height of 18 to 30 m.

Bark is reddish-brown to gray, smooth, and peels off in thin flakes; its wood is extremely hard (**Fig. 69.1**).

Leaves are simple, opposite, leathery, lanceolate, 6-15 cm long by 2-4 cm wide; immature leaves are coppery red covered in a waxy bloom below, acute-acuminate apex, nerves inconspicuous (**Fig. 69.2a, b**).

Flowers are sweet, scented, up to 7.5 cm in diameter, solitary or paired, axillary or terminal, white colored with numerous golden yellow stamens; stamen is shorter than the length of the petals and style is twice as long as the stamens (**Fig. 69.3**).

Fruits are ovoid shape, with a conical point, 2.5 to 5 cm long. It is green when unripe, and becomes brown on drying, with woody pericarp that contains 1-4 pyriform, smooth, shiny, brown seeds (**Fig. 69.4**).

The plant is propagated by seeds.

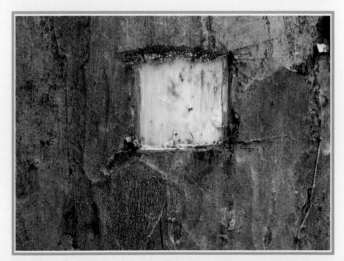

Fig. 69.1 Bark.

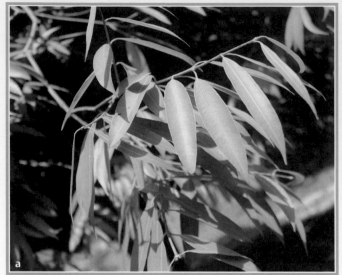

Fig. 69.2 **(a)** Leaves. **(b)** Tender leaves.

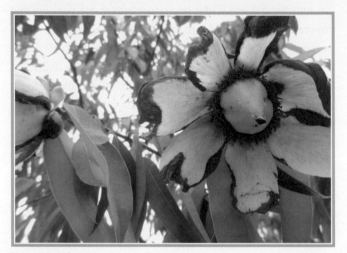

Fig. 69.3 Flowers.

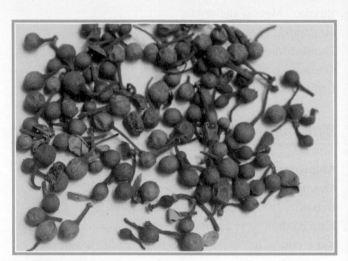

Fig. 69.4 Fruits.

Phenology

Flowering time: January to April
Fruiting time: April to October

Key Characters for Identification

➤ Medium- to large-sized, evergreen tree with brown-gray bark.
➤ Leaves are opposite, leathery, lanceolate, immature coppery red.
➤ Flowers are scented, axillary, or terminal, white colored with numerous golden yellow stamens.
➤ Fruits are of oval shape, with a conical point containing 1-4 pyriform seeds.

Rasapanchaka

Guna	Laghu, Ruksha
Rasa	Kashaya, Tikta
Vipaka	Katu
Virya	Ushna

Chemical Constituents

Phytochemical studies revealed that the plant is rich in phenyl coumarins, xanthones, and triterpenoids. Other constituents are mesuaferrol, leuco anthocyanidin, mesuone, and euxanthone.

Stamens have α- and β-amyrin, β-sitosterol, biflavonoids-mesuaferrones A and B, mesuanic acid, mesuaferrol, manneisin 1,5-dihydroxyxanthone, euxanthone 7-methyl ether, and β-sitosterol.

Stem bark and heartwood have 4-alkylcoumarins ferruols A and B, triterpenoid guttiferol, mesuaxanthones A and B, ferraxanthone, hydroxyxanthone, methoxyxanthone, anthocyanidin β-sitosterol, and meauxanthone A and meauxanthone B.

The kernels contain about 75% of oil which is rich in fatty acids like linoleic, oleic, stearic, and arachidic acids.

Seed oil contains phenylcoumarins like mesuol, mesuagin, mammeisin, mammeigin, and mesuone (Sahu et al 2014; Chow and Quon 1968).

Identity, Purity, and Strength

- Foreign matter: Not more than 2%
- Total ash: Not more than 6%
- Acid-insoluble ash: Not more than 3%
- Alcohol-soluble extractive: Not less than 15%
- Water-soluble extractive: Not less than 12%

(Source: The Ayurvedic Pharmacopeia of India 1999)

Karma (Actions)

Ayurveda classics have attributed deepan (carminative), aamachana (digestive), grahi (absorbent), raktasangrahi (haemostatic), durgandhanashana (removes foul odour), swedapanayana (checks excessive sweat), vishaghna (antidote), shothhara (antiinflammatory), trishnanigrahana (antithirst), chardinigrahana (antiemetic), krimighna (anthelmintic), kandughna (antipruritis), kusthaghna (antidermatosis), mutrajanan (diuretic), vedanasthapana (analgesic), jwaraghna (antipyretic), and balya (tonic) alya (tonic) properties to it.

- Doshakarma: Kaphapittahara
- Dhatukarma: Raktasangrahi, Pachan
- Malakarma: Mutral, swedapanayana

Pharmacological Actions

The scientific screening of this plant also reported its antioxidant, hepatoprotective, antiasthmatic, antiallergic, CNS depressant, anticonvulsant, analgesic, anti-inflammatory, antimicrobial, antiseptic, blood purifier, anthelmintic, cardiotonic, diuretic, expectorant, antipyretic, purgative, antispasmodic, antineoplastic, antivenom, and immunostimulant activities (Chahar et al 2013).

Indications

Pungkesar (stamen) is used in the treatment of jwara (fever), kandu (itching), trishna (thirst), atisweda (excessive sweat), raktapitta (bleeding disorders), chardi (vomiting), hrullas (nausea), agnimandya (loss of appetite), ajirna (indigestion), dourgandhya (foul smell), kushta (skin diseases), krimi (worm infestation), visarpa (erysipelas), visha (poison), vrana (wounds), raktapradara (uterine bleeding), mutraghata (dysuria), raktarsha (bleeding piles), pravahika (dysentery), and sandhivata (arthritis).

Leaves and flowers are antidotes for snake bite and scorpion sting. Oil is used for cutaneous infection, sores, scabies, wounds, and rheumatism. Kernels are used to poultice wounds and in skin eruptions. The decoction or infusion of bark and roots is useful in gastritis, bronchitis, uterine bleeding, leucorrhea, bleeding diarrhea, excessive sweat, chronic cough, and burning micturition.

Therapeutic Uses

External Use

1. **Visha** (poisoning): Local application of Nagakeshara leaves or flower paste is used as antidotes for snake bite and scorpion sting.
2. **Daha** (burning sensation): Nagakeshara powder mixed with Shatadhauta ghrita is applied on palm and sole to reduce burning sensation of palm and sole.

Internal Use

1. **Rakta atisaar** (bleeding diarrhea): Nagakeshara powder with rice water is an excellent remedy to prevent bleeding associated in diarrhea (B.S.atisaar Ci./119) .
2. **Rakta arsha** (bleeding piles): Daily intake of Nagakeshara powder with butter and sharkara checks bleeding in hemorrhoids. Local application of Shatadhauta ghrita mixed with Nagakeshara powder is also beneficial (C.S.Ci. 14/210).

3. **Pradar** (leucorrhea/menorrhagia): Intake of Nagakeshara powder along with buttermilk for 3 days cures both types of pradara (B.S.striroga Ci./34).

4. **Atisweda** (excessive sweat): If excessive sweat production occurs in a person, then application of Nagakeshara flower paste locally or oral intake of its powder is used to check its production.

5. **Hikka** (hic-cough): In hikka one should take Nagakeshara churna mixed with madhu sharkara along with madhuka and ikshu rasa (S.S.U. 50/23).

6. **Garbhasthapana** (for conception): Intake of Nagakeshara and Puga churna helps in garbhasthapana (B.S.striroga Ci./145).

Officinal Part Used

Stamen

Dose

Powder: 1 to 3 g

Formulations

Eladi churna, Pushyanug churna, Dashmoolarista, Suparipaka, Drakshaasava, Brahmi vati, Pradarnashaka churna.

Toxicity/Adverse Effects

Hematological, biochemical, and acute toxicity studies on different extracts of Nagakeshara do not report any toxicity or adverse effect (Udayabhanu et al 2014).

Substitution and Adulteration

Punnaga (*Calophyllum inophyllum* Linn.), Tamala (*Cinnamomum wightii* Meissn.), and Jatiphala (*Myristica fragrans* Houtt.) are used as substitutes for Nagakeshara. In herbal drug markets of Gujarat and Bombay, unripe buds of Surpunnaga (*Ochrocarpus longifolius* Benth. & Hook. f.) are sold in the name of ratan Nagakeshara. Unripe fruits of Tamala (*Cinnamomum tamala* Nees & Eberm.) or *C. wightii* are sold as kala Nagakeshara. In South Indian markets, fruits of *Dillenia pentagyna* Roxb. is known as Malabar

Nagakeshara and Nattu Nagakeshara resembles *C. wightii*. Buds of *Mammea suriga* Kost. and *Calophyllum inophyllum* Linn. are its reported adulterants (Sharma et al 2000; Prakash et al 2013).

> **Points to Ponder**
>
> - *Nagakeshara is an excellent medicine for jwar, atisweda, chardi, raktapitta, pradar, kushta, and dourgandhya.*
> - *It is a natural herbal substitute for gasoline and diesel, has great industrial application as polymer, dyeing agent, and is used for preparation of silver nanoparticles.*

Suggested Readings

Anonymous. The Siddha Formulary of India, Part I. New Delhi: Ministry of Health and Family Welfare, Government of India; 1992

Chahar MK, Sanjaya KDS, Geetha L, Lokesh T, Manohara KP. *Mesua ferrea* L: a review of the medical evidence for its phytochemistry and pharmacological actions. Afr J Pharm Pharmacol 2013;7(6): 211–219

Chow YL, Quon HH. Chemical constituents of the heartwood of *Mesua ferrea*. Phytochemistry 1968;7:1871

Dutta S, Karak N. Synthesis, characterization of poly (urethane amide) resins from Nahar seed oil for surface coating applications. Prog Org Coat 2005;53:147–152

Foundation of Resuscitate and Encourage Thai Traditional Medicine. Thai Pharmaceutical Book. Bangkok: Pikanate Printing Center Co-operation; 2005

Konwarh R, Kalita D, Mahanta C, Mandal M, Karak N. Magnetically recyclable, antimicrobial, and catalytically enhanced polymer-assisted "green" nanosystem-immobilized Aspergillus niger amylo-glucosidase. Appl Microbiol Biotechnol 2010;87(6):1983–1992

Konwer D, Baruah K. Refining of the crude oil obtained from *Mesua ferrea* L. seeds. Chem Ind 1984;413–414

Kritikar KR, Basu BD. Indian Medicinal Plants. Vol. 1. 2nd ed. Dehradun: International Book Distributors; 1981:274

Parukutty B, Chandra GS. Studies on the medicinal uses of plants by the Boro tribals of Assam-II. J Econ Taxon Bot 1984;5:599–604

Prakash O, Jyoti AK, Pavan K, Niranjan KM. Adulteration and substitution in Indian medicinal plants: an overview. J Med Plant Stud. 2013;1(4):127–132

Sahni KC. The Book of Indian Trees. Mumbai: Bombay Natural History Society; 1998

Sahu AN, Hemalatha S, Sairam K. Phyto-pharmacological review of *Mesua ferrea* Linn. International Journal of Phytopharmacology 2014;5(1):6–14

Sharma PC, Yelne MB, Dennis TJ. Database on Medicinal Plants used in Ayurveda, Vol. 1. New Delhi: CCRAS Department of Indian Systems of Medicine and Homeopathy (ISM&H), Ministry of Health and Family Welfare, Government of India; 2000:283

The Ayurvedic Pharmacopeia of India. Part I, Vol. 2. New Delhi: Department of AYUSH, Ministry of Health and Family Welfare, Government of India; 1999:126

Udayabhanu J, Kaminidevi S, Thangavelu T. A study on acute toxicity of methanolic extract of *Mesua ferrea* L. in Swiss albino mice. Asian J Pharm Clin Res 2014;7:66–68

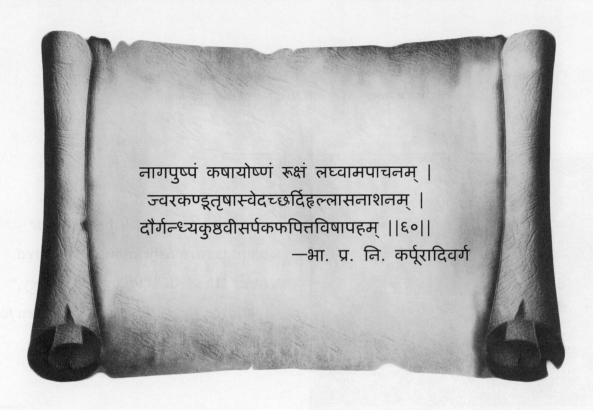

नागपुष्पं कषायोष्णं रूक्षं लघ्वामपाचनम् |
ज्वरकण्डूतृषास्वेदच्छर्दिहृल्लासनाशनम् |
दौर्गन्ध्यकुष्ठवीसर्पकफपित्तविषापहम् ||६०||
—भा. प्र. नि. कर्पूरादिवर्ग

70. Nimba *[Azadirachta indica A. Juss.]*

Family:	*Meliaceae*
Hindi name:	*Neem*
English name:	*Margosa Tree, Neem Tree, Indian lilac*

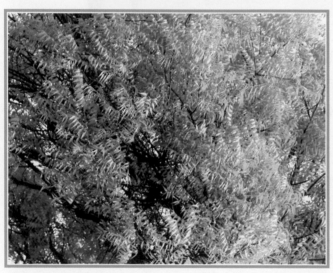

Plant of *Azadirachta indica* A. Juss.

Owing to its versatile benefits, the plant is variously known as "Sacred tree," "Heal All," "Village Pharmacy," "Nature's Drugstore," and "Panacea for all diseases."

Introduction

The Latin name *Azadirachta indica* is derived from the Farsi word *azad darakht* which means the "free or noble tree of India," suggesting its multiple use and easy availability in India.

The history of Nimba use in social, cultural, spiritual, nutrition, medicine, and pharmaceutical application dates back over 5,000 years. It is an age-old belief to plant Nimba tree in the house so as to ward off evil spirits and to ensure passage to heaven. During celebrations and wedding ceremony, people used to decorate their homes and main entrance with Nimba leaves and flowers. In Tamil Nadu, it is an old tradition to decorate the Goddess Mariamman statue with garlands of Nimba flowers. In Maharashtra during Gudi padva, it is customary to drink Nimba juice or eat Nimba paste on that day with some food to avoid negative side-effects of the season or change of seasons. Hindus used to worship Nimba tree to protect their children from chickenpox because it is believed that Sithala mata, the Goddess of chickenpox, lives in the tree. Newly born babies are laid upon the Nimba leaves to provide them with the protective aura. Before burying, Muslims used to give bath to the dead body with Nimba water.

All parts of the tree have medicinal properties and are used to prepare different medical preparations. Nimba tea is taken to reduce headache and fever. Traditionally, Nimba twigs are used as toothbrush to clean teeth. People used to apply Nimba taila to hair to kill head lice (Biswas et al 2009). Charaka has recommended consuming its tender leaves as a prophylactic measure for disease prevention. Charaka advocated using Nimba decoction, paste, ghrita in skin diseases, vrana, arsha, shotha, luta visha, netraroga, etc. Sushrut recommended the use of Nimba leaves smoke for fumigation and nimbi taila as shodhan dravya (C.S.Su. 45/115). In many parts of India and Myanmar, its tender shoots and flowers are eaten as a vegetable.

Apart from the medicinal uses, Nimba cake is used as manure or fertilizer, Nimba gum as a food additive, leaves as an insecticidal agent, bark in tanning, dyeing, wood in preparing furniture, seed pulp for industrial fermentations, and oil in cosmetics (for preparing herbal soaps, shampoo, oil, creams, balms, mouthwash).

Vernacular Names

Arabic: Neeb

Assamese: Mahanim

Bengali: Nim, Nimgacha

Burmese: Tamar

Gujarati: Kadvo Limbdo

Kannada: Bevu, Kahibevu, Nimba, Oilevevu

Konkani: Beva-rooku

Malayalam: Veppu, Aruveppu

Marathi: Balantanimba, Kadunimb, Limba

Oriya: Nimba

Persian: Azad dirakht

Punjabi: Nim, Nimba, Bakam

Tamil: Veppai, Vembu, Vempu, Veppam

Telugu: Vemu, Vepa, Yapachettu

Thai: Sadao

Urdu: Neem

Synonyms

Arishta: It is used to eradicate a number of diseases.

Hinguniryasa: Like hingu, on excision, the plant exudates a gum.

Krimighna: It has anthelmintic action.

Pichumarda: It destroys skin diseases.

Puyari: The plant is a potent drug for purulent wounds.

Sutiktak: The plant is best among tikta dravyas.

Tiktak: The plant is tikta rasa dominant.

Vartvach: Stem bark is the best among all the parts used.

Classical Categorization

Charak Samhita: Kandughna, Tikta skanda

Sushrut Samhita: Araghvadi, Guduchyadi, Lakshadi

Ashtang Hridaya: Araghvadi, Guduchyadi, Lakshadi

Dhanvantari Nighantu: Guduchyadi varga

Madanpal Nighantu: Abhyadi varga

Kaiyadev Nighantu: Oushadi varga

Raj Nighantu: Prabhadradi varga

Bhavaprakash Nighantu: Guduchyadi varga

Distribution

It is found almost everywhere in India.

Morphology

It is a large, highly branched, evergreen tree of 40 to 50 ft height.

- **Leaves:** Compound, imparipinnate, alternate, 20 to 35 cm long, leaflets 7 to 13 in number, leaflets subopposite, falcate-lanceolate shape, oblique at base, bluntly serrate, up to 7 x 3 cm, glabrous, green above, pale beneath (**Fig. 70.1a, b**).

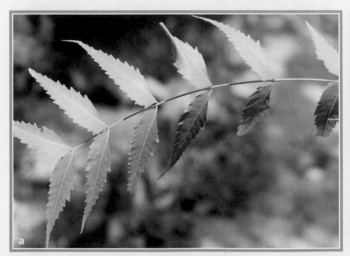
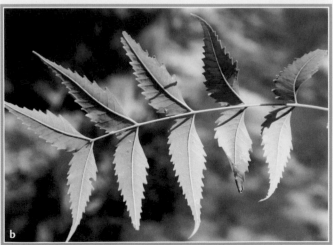

Fig. 70.1   (a) Leaves, **(b)** ventral surface of leaves.

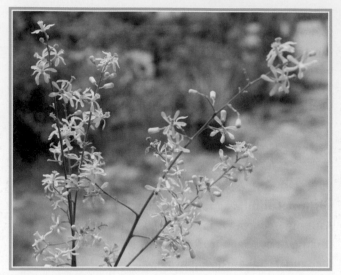

Fig. 70.2 Flowers.

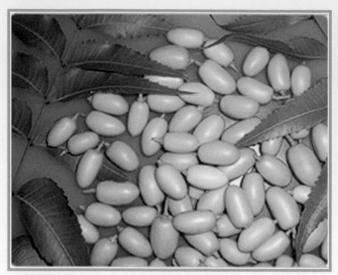

Fig. 70.3 Fruits.

- **Flowers:** White or greenish yellow, small, many, in long, slender, axillary panicles (**Fig. 70.2**).
- **Fruit:** Drupes, when fresh, green in color, turning yellow on ripening, oblong or ovoid shape, single seeded. Seeds are dirty brown, 1 cm in length, 4 to 5 mm in width, taste bitter, characteristic odor (**Fig. 70.3**).
- **Bark:** Channeled, tough, fibrous, brownish-black with a rough scaly surface. Internally, yellowish, laminated, and coarsely fibrous (**Fig. 70.4**).

The methods of propagation are seeds, stem cutting, and root suckers.

Phenology

Flowering time: March to April
Fruiting time: June to July

Key Characters for Identification
➤ A branched, evergreen tree of 40 to 50 ft height.
➤ Leaves are compound, imparipinnate, falcate-lanceolate shape, leaflets 7 to 13 in number, oblique at the base.
➤ Flowers are white or greenish yellow in long axillary panicles.
➤ Fruits are oblong or ovoid drupe, green when unripe, yellow when ripe, and black when dry.
➤ Bark is channeled, fibrous, brownish black, rough surface.

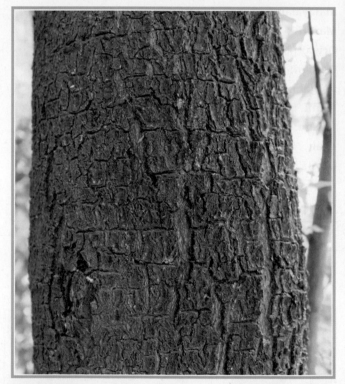

Fig. 70.4 Bark.

Rasapanchaka

Rasa	Tikta, Kashaya
Guna	Laghu
Vipaka	Katu
Virya	Sheet

Chemical Constituents

The most important active constituent of Nimba is azadirachtin, and the others are nimbin, nimbidin, nimbidol, sodium nimbinate, gedunin, salannin, nimbolinin, azadiractol, azadiractone, nimbidine, nimbol, nimbidiol, nimocin, nimbocetin, nimolimone, margosin, quercetin, ß-sitosterol, polyphenolic flavonoids, benzyl alcohol, and high amount of tocopherol, arachidic acid, linoleic, margosic, and palmitic acids. Leaves contain nimbin, nimbanene, 6-desacetylnimbinene, nimbandiol, nimbolide, ascorbic acid, n-hexacosanol, amino acid, and nimbiol (Hossain et al 2013; Ghimeray et al 2009).

Identity, Purity, and Strength

- Foreign matter: Not more than 2%
- Total ash: Not more than 7%
- Acid-insoluble ash: Not more than 1.5%
- Alcohol-soluble extractive: Not less than 6%
- Water-soluble extractive: Not less than 5%

(Source: The Ayurvedic Pharmacopeia of India 1999)

Karma (Actions)

Various Ayurveda texts assign krimighna (anthelmintic), kandughna (antipruritis), kusthaghna (antidermatosis), jantughna (antibacterial), vranashodhaka (wound purifier), vranaropana (wound healing), grahi (absorbent), ahridaya (noncardiotonic), raktashodhaka (blood purifier), putihara (removes foul smell), dahaprasasmana (refrigerant), pachana (digestive), jwaraghna (antipyretic), vedanastha-pana (analgesic), uttejaka (stimulant), and shothahara (anti-inflammatory) properties to Nimba.

- Nimba patra: netrya, vishaghna, krimighna, vranashodhan
- Nimba pushp: chakshusya, vishaghna, krimighna
- Nimba phal: bhedana, krimighna, kushthaghna
- Nimba taila: pratidushaka (antiseptic), jantughna (antibacterial)
- Beej majja: krimighna, kushthaghna
- Doshakarma: Kapha pittashamaka
- Dhatukarma: Katu paushtika (bitter tonic), grahi
- Malakarma: Sarak, putihara

Pharmacological Actions

Several experimental and biological studies on bark, leaves, fruits, flowers, oil of Nimba revealed that it exhibits antibacterial, antiviral, antifungal, insecticidal, antipyretic, antiseptic, liver stimulant, anthelmintic, analgesic, anti-inflammatory, antitubercular, blood purifier, expectorant, antifertility, hypoglycemic, hypolipidemic, antiulcer, diuretic, antimalarial, anticancer, hepatoprotective, immunomodulatory, CNS depressant, and antineoplastic activities (Gupta and Tandon 2004).

Indications

Ayurveda classics advocated the use of Nimba in kandu (pruritus), kushta (skin diseases), krimi (intestinal worms), vidradhi (abscess), granthi (tumors), vrana (wounds), apachi (tubercular glands), nadivrana (sinus), kasa (cough), shwasa (asthma), jwara (fever), netraroga (eye diseases), raktapitta (bleeding disorders), hridyadaha (heartburn), aruchi (distaste), gulma (abdominal tumor), arsha (piles), meha (diabetes), kshat (injury), kshaya (emaciation), mada (hallucination), daha (burning sensation), shrama (fatigue), raktavikara (diseases of aggravated raktadosha), palitya (graying of hair), abhishyandi (obstructed channels), phiranga (syphilis), sutikaroga (puerperal diseases), and jeerna and visham jwara (intermittent and malarial fevers). Its flowers have pittashamaka property and therefore are specially used in aruchi. Nimba taila is applied locally in chronic skin diseases, leucoderma, eczema, syphilitic sores, ulcer, ringworm, scabies, and leprosy (Sharma et al 2000).

Therapeutic Uses

External Use

1. **Twak roga** (skin diseases): Local application of Dhatura, Nimba, Tambula patra swarasa is recommended in skin diseases like pama, dadru, vicharchika, kandu, raksha (Sh.S. 3/11/52-53).
2. **Shotha** (edema): Tub bath in the decoction of Nimba, Ankola, Eranda, Tarkari, Kutaja, Karanja, and Kadali leaves is beneficial in all types of inflammatory diseases (K.S./344).

3. **Padminikantaka** (acne): An ointment of Nimba Aragvadha paste is useful in padminikantaka (A.H.U. 37/6).

4. **Palitya** (graying of hairs): Regular application of Neem oil in the scalp or taken as nasya (snuff) for a month with mild diet is useful in preventing premature graying of hairs (A.H.U. 24/34) (SG. 2/9/152).

5. **Dantaroga** (tooth diseases): Decoction of Nimbamool is used as mouthwash in diseases of teeth and gums (Ha.S. 3/46/14).

6. **Vranashodhan** (for wound washing): Decoction of Nimba leaves is used for washing the wounds (C.S.Ci. 25/84).

7. **Netraroga** (eye diseases): Powdered Nimba patra and Lodhra is kept in a cotton pouch and dipped in water. The tincture is instilled in the eyes to reduce netra shotha, kandu, and shool (B.S.netra ci./117).

Internal Use

1. **Krimi** (worm infestation): Consuming leaf juice of Dhatura or Nimba mixed with madhu daily expels out worms from the intestine (B.P.Ci./7/24).

2. **Kushta** (skin diseases): Decoction of Nimba, Patola is an efficacious remedy in all types of kushta (C.S.Ci. 7/97-99). If the affected part becomes purulent and is eaten by maggots, decoction of Nimba, Vidanga mixed with gomutra should be used for snana (bathing), pana (oral intake), and pralepa (local application) (C.S.Ci. 7/157). In case of maggots, regular intake of decoction prepared from Nimba, Arka, Alarka, and Saptaparna is recommended (S.S.Ci. 9/52).

3. **Sheetpitta** (urticaria): Regular oral intake of Nimba leaves and Amalaki (Fruit) mixed with ghrita prevent urticaria and other skin diseases (CD. 51/9). Decoction of its leaves is also used for bathing purpose and for washing chronic wounds.

4. **Meha** (diabetes): Daily intake of decoction prepared with patra, mool, phal, pushpa, twak of Nimba, Aragvadh, Saptaparna, Murva, Kutaj, Soma, and Palasha helps in controlling all types of diabetes (S.S.Ci. 11/8).

5. **Raktapitta** (intrinsic hemorrhage): Tender leaves of Patola, Nimba, Vetagra, Plaksh, and Vetasa should be consumed as vegetable in raktapitta (B.P.Ci. 9/18).

6. **Vatarakta** (gout): Drinking the decoction of Patola and Nimba leaves pacifies vatarakta (B.S.3/23/ 7-8).

7. **Amalpitta** (acidity): Churna prepared by adding 1 part Panchnimba, 2 parts Vridhdaru, and 10 parts sattu (parched grains) mixed with madhu sharkara should be taken with cold water in amalpitta (VM. 53/19).

8. **Kamala** (jaundice): Decoction of Triphala or Guduchi or Darvi or Nimba with madhu should be taken in the morning (C.S.Ci. 16/63).

9. **Stanyashodhan** (galacto-depurant): Yusha prepared with Nimba, Vetagra, Patola, Vartaka, and Amalaki mixed with trikatu and saindhava is used to purify breast milk (C.S.Ci. 30/259).

10. **Visha pratishedh** (antidote to poison): Nimba beej should be taken with ushna jal to neutralize poison (Ha.S. 3/56/11).

Officinal Parts Used

Bark, oil, leaves, flower

Dose

Bark powder: 1 to 2 g
Leaves juice: 10 to 20 mL
Oil: 5 to 10 drops

Formulations

Nimba taila, Nimbarishta, Nimbadi churna, Nimbharidrakhand, Panchtikta ghrita, Mahamarichyadi taila, Panchnimba churna, Mahagandhaka vati.

Toxicity/Adverse Effects

Not reported

Substitution and Adulteration

The leaves of Aralu (*Ailanthus excelsa*) and Mahanimba (*Melia azadirachta*) are used as the substitute and adulterant of Nimba.

Points to Ponder

■ *Nimba is the cheapest, versatile, multifarious tree with immense therapeutic potentials.It is a renowned drug for skin diseases, wound healing, abscess, tumors, and blood-borne diseases.*

Suggested Readings

Biswas K, Chattopadhyay I, Banerjee RK, Bandyopadhyay U. Biological activities and medicinal properties of Neem (*Azadirachta indica*). Curr Sci 2002;82(11):1336–1345

Ghimeray AK, Jin CW, Ghimire BK, Cho DH. Antioxidant activity and quantitative estimation of azadirachtin and nimbin in *Azadirachta indica* A. Juss grown in foothills of Nepal. Afr J Biotechnol 2009;8(13):3084–3091

Gupta AK, Tandon N. Reviews on Indian Medicinal Plants, Vol. 3(Are - Azi). New Delhi: Indian Council of Medical Research; 2004: 320–395

Hossain MA, Al-Toubi WAS, Weli AM, Al-Riyami QA, Al-Sabahi JN. Identification and characterization of chemical compounds in different crude extracts from leaves of Omani neem. Journal of Taibah University for Science 2013;7(4):181–188

Sharma PC, Yelne MB, Dennis TJ. Database on Medicinal Plants used in Ayurveda, Vol. 1. New Delhi: CCRAS Department of Indian Systems of Medicine and Homeopathy (ISM&H), Ministry of Health and Family Welfare, Government of India; 2000:289–293

The Ayurvedic Pharmacopeia of India. Part I, Vol. 2. New Delhi: Department of AYUSH, Ministry of Health and Family Welfare, Government of India; 1999:134

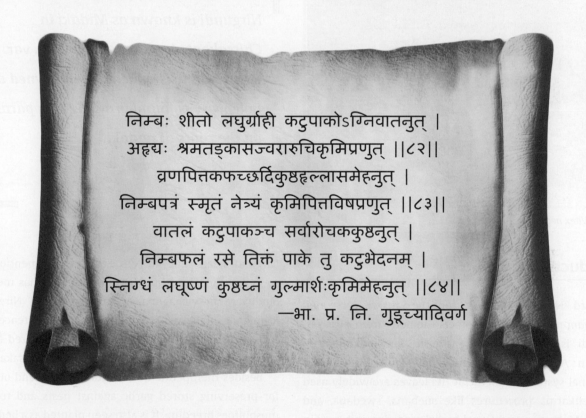

निम्बः शीतो लघुर्ग्राही कटुपाकोऽग्निवातनुत् ।
अह्रद्यः श्रमतड्कासज्वरारुचिकृमिप्रणुत् ॥८२॥
व्रणपित्तकफच्छर्दिकुष्ठहल्लासमेहनुत् ।
निम्बपत्रं स्मृतं नेत्र्यं कृमिपित्तविषप्रणुत् ॥८३॥
वातलं कटुपाकञ्च सर्वारोचककुष्ठनुत् ।
निम्बफलं रसे तिक्तं पाके तु कटुभेदनम् ।
स्निग्धं लघूष्णं कुष्ठघ्नं गुल्मार्शःकृमिमेहनुत् ॥८४॥
—भा. प्र. नि. गुड्च्यादिवर्ग

71. Nirgundi *[Vitex negundo Linn.]*

Family:	Verbenaceae
Hindi name:	Samhalu
English name:	Five-leaved chaste

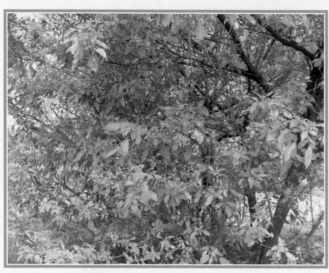

Plant of *Vitex negundo* Linn.

> *Nirgundi is known as Midaki in Chitrakoot. A. parasitica A. Rich. var. Chitrakutensis which is a renowned drug in leprosy is found growing as a parasite on the roots of midaki.*

Introduction

The word "Nirgundi" derived from the Sanskrit verse *gudi rakshayam* means which protects the body from diseases. Nirgundi is a well-known analgesic, anti-inflammatory plant in Ayurveda, Unani, Siddha, Chinese, European traditional systems of medicine. Its leaves are widely used in panchkarma procedures like snehana, swedana, and basti. In Malaysian traditional herbal medicine, it is used in gynecological disorders, for regulating the menstrual cycle, for increasing lactation, fibrocystic breast disease, and postpartum remedies (Wan Hassan 2010). In Sri Lanka, it is used in dentistry and joint disorders whereas in Bangladesh it is potent remedy for malaria and catarrhal fever. In Indian folklore medicine, Nirgundi is a popular drug for malaria and snake bite.

In classical Ayurvedic texts, two plants are available in the name of Nirgundi, i.e., *Sinduvara* and *Nirgundi*. Sinduvara is described as the variety of *Vitex* having white flowers and Nirgundi bears blue flowers. Sushrut also mentioned sita pushpi and neel pushpi Nirgundi. Charaka has mentioned Sinduvara in vishaghna mahakashaya and Nirgundi in krimighna mahakashaya indicating the existence of two types of Nirgundi. Ashtang Sangraha considered Nirgundi as a krimighna drug similar to undrukarni (musakarni).

Besides therapeutic use, Nirgundi leaves and oil is used for preserving stored garlic against pests and to control mosquitoes breeding. It is also seen planted as a hedge plant along the roadsides.

Vernacular Names

Assamese: Aslak, Pasutia, Aggla chitta
Bengali: Nirgundi, Nishinda
Gujarati: Nagoda
Kannada: Lakkigida, Nekkigida, Nekka
Konkani: Lingad
Malayalam: Indranee, Nirgundi, Karunocci

Marathi: Nirgundi, Nisind
Oriya: Beyguna, Begundia, Indrani
Punjabi: Sambhalu, Banna
Tamil: Karunochchi, Nocchi
Telugu: Nallavavilli, Vavili
Urdu: Poast-e-sambhalu, Panjangusht

Synonyms

Indranika: It is a highly efficacious drug.
Sheetsah: The plant is resistant to cold, i.e., is hot in potency.
Shephali: The plant bears beautiful flowers.
Sinduvara: The plant checks the accumulation of fluid in the body.
Sugandhika: The leaves and flowers are aromatic in nature.
Suvaha: It facilitates the displusion of mala and dosha.

Classical Categorization

Charaka Samhita: Vishaghna, Krimighna
Sushruta Samhita: Surasadi
Ashtang Hridaya: Surasadi
Dhanvantari Nighantu: Karviradi varga
Madanpal Nighantu: Abhyadi varga
Kaiyadev Nighantu: Oushadi varga
Raj Nighantu: Shatvahadi varga
Bhavaprakash Nighantu: Guduchyadi varga

Distribution

Nirgundi is globally distributed from tropical to temperate regions of the world. Native to Indo-Malaysia and cultivated in Europe, Asia, America, and West Indies. It is found throughout India, ascending to 1,500 m in waste lands, on roadside, river banks, streams, or in moist places near deciduous forests.

Morphology

It is an aromatic, large shrub or small tree, of about 3 m height, with dense, whitish, tomentose, quadrangular branches.

- **Stem bark:** Thin, corky, yellowish-gray, occurs in channeled pieces, rough, with lenticels, and transversely cracked (**Fig. 71.1**).
- **Leaves:** Opposite long petiole, digitately compound, leaflets 3 to 5, lanceolate, unequal, terminal leaflet bigger than lateral leaflets, serrate margin, acute to acuminate apex, upper surface dark green, lower surface silvery white, tomentose (**Fig. 71.2**).
- **Flowers:** Blue-purple, crowded in short cymes, forming erect, narrow, tapering, terminal, or axillary panicles (**Fig. 71.3**).
- **Fruits:** Globose or ovoid, drupe, 2 to 3 mm across, black when ripe. Seeds 2 to 4, in bony endocarp. Seeds are known as Renuka beej.
- **Root:** Woody, fairly thick, 8 to 10 cm in diameter, external surface brownish and rough.

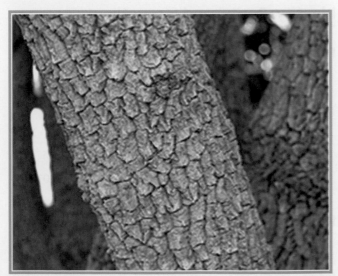

Fig. 71.1   Bark.

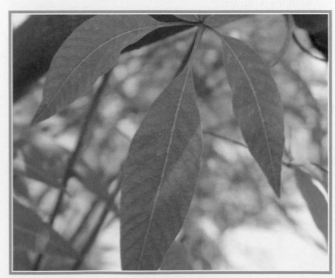

Fig. 71.2   Leaves.

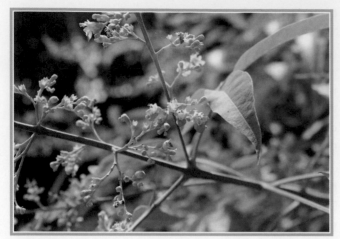

Fig. 71.3 Flowers.

The plant is propagated by seeds, shoot cutting, and root suckers.

Phenology

Flowering time: June to August
Fruiting time: December to January

Key Characters for Identification
➤ *A large shrub or small tree with tomentose, quadrangular branches.*
➤ *Stem bark is thin, corky, yellowish gray.*
➤ *Leaves are opposite, digitately compound, leaflets 3 to 5, lanceolate shape.*
➤ *Flowers are blue-purple and occur in terminal or axillary panicles.*
➤ *Fruits are globose or ovoid drupe with two to four seeds.*
➤ *Roots are brown, woody, thick, 8 to 10 cm in diameter.*

Types

Nighantu	Types	Names
Sushrut	2	Shwet pushpi and Neel pushpi
Dhanvantari	2	Sephalika and Nirgundi
Kaiyadev	3	Nirgundi, Sinduvara, Sephalika
Raj	3	Sinduvara, Nirgundi, and Sephalika

Nighantu	Types	Names
Sodhala	2	Sinduvara (white) and Sephalika (blue)
Bhavaprakash	2	Sinduvara and Nirgundi
Nighantu Ratnakar	2	Kartari and Aranya Nirgundi

Rasapanchaka

Guna	Laghu, Ruksha
Rasa	Katu, Tikta, Kashaya
Vipaka	Katu
Virya	Ushna

Chemical Constituents

Phytochemical studies revealed the presence of essential oil, triterpenes, diterpenes, sesquiterpenes, flavonoids, flavones, iridoid glycosides, lignan, and stilbene derivative in various parts of Nirgundi. The active constituents among them are negundoside, nishindaside, agunoside, mussaenoside, eurotoside, casticin, vitexin, vitricine alkaloid, aucubin, α pinenes, camphene, caryophyllene, vanilic acid trimethoxyflavone, β sitosterol, hentriacontane, artemetin, orientin, and terpinyl acetate (Ladda and Magdum 2012; Suganthi and Dubey 2016).

Identity, Purity, and Strength

For Leaves

- Foreign matter: Not more than 2%
- Total ash: Not more than 8%
- Acid-insoluble ash: Not more than 1%
- Alcohol-soluble extractive: Not less than 10%
- Water-soluble extractive: Not less than 20%

(Source: The Ayurvedic Pharmacopeia of India 2001)

Karma (Actions)

Ayurvedic texts have described it as having keshya (hair tonic), sophahara (anti-inflammatory), chakshushya (eye tonic), vishaghna (antidote to poison), smritiprada (enhances memory power), anulomana (facilitate downward movement of vata), krimighna (antimicrobial), kasahara (expectorant), kandughna (antipruritic), vedanasthapana (analgesic), kushtaghna (antileprotic), jwaraghna (antipyretic), vranashodhana (purifies wound), deepana (appetizer), pachana (digestive) properties.

- Doshakarma: Kaphavatashamaka
- Dhatukarma: Vishaghna, Keshya
- Malakarma: Anulomana, Mutral

Pharmacological Actions

Various in vivo and in vitro studies showed that Nirgundi exhibits analgesic, anti-inflammatory, antispasmodic, antiseptic, anthelmintic, expectorant, carminative, digestive, antifertility, estrogenic, hepatoprotective, antiallergic, CNS depressant, antipyretic, diuretic, depurative, anticonvulsant, antiarthritic, rejuvenating, antipsychotic, and mosquito repellent activities (Sharma et al 2005).

Indications

Nirgundi is used in the treatment of shool (pain), shotha (edema), aamdosha, vatavyadhi (diseases of aggravated vata dosha), kushta (skin diseases), kasa (cough), shwasa (asthma), pratishyay (common cold), aamvata (rheumatoid arthritis), pradara (excessive discharge per vagina), gulma (abdominal tumor), aruchi (distaste), krimi (worm infestation), vrana (wounds), adhyaman (flatulence), pleeha roga (diseases of spleen), medoroga (obesity), jwara (fever), netra roga (eye diseases), karna roga (ear diseases), kshaya (general debility), kshata (accidental injury), mutraghata (dysuria), sutika rog (puerperal diseases), shirashool (headache).

Therapeutic Uses

External Use

1. **Gandmala** (cervical adenitis): Nirgundi taila or root powder pounded with water should be used as nasya in gandmala (VM. 41/24,52; SG. 2/9/195).
2. **Shotha** (inflammation): Fomentation with decoction of Nirgundi, Erand, Arka leaves gives immediate relief in pain and inflammation of any body part.

3. **Putikarna** (fetid ear): Instilling oil prepared with Nirgundi swaras, sindhuj lavan, raj, guda mixed with madhu helps in removing foul smell in ear diseases (B.S.karnarog/89).

Internal Use

1. **Aamvata** (rheumatoid arthritis): Regular intake of 2 g root powder of Nirgundi twice daily with Raasnadi kwath helps in reducing the pain and inflammation due to Arthritis. Oral intake of Nirgundi root powder with oil is beneficial in sandhivata, kativata, and kampavata (RRS. 21/164).
2. **Vatavyadhi** (diseases of aggravated vata): Taking Nirgundi swaras and Eranda taila separately pacifies aggravated vata in katipradesh (Vd.M. 12/8).
3. **Snayuka krimi** (guinea worm): Snayuka krimi are destroyed by taking go ghrita and Nirgundi swaras alternatively for 3 days each (VM. 55/18).
4. **Nadivrana** (sinus): Oil prepared from Nirgundi moola and patra swarasa is beneficial in kushta, nadivrana, vatavyadhi, pama, apachi in the form of pan (oral), abhyanjana (anointment), and puran (filling) (C.S.Ci. 28/134 -135).
5. **Kshayksheen** (consumption): Intake of ghrita prepared with Nirgundi root, flowers, and patra swaras removes the state of consumption (CD. 10/82).
6. **Sutika roga** (puerperal diseases): Daily intake of Nirgundi, Rasona, and Shunthi decoction mixed with pippali churna pacifies all the sutika roga (Y.R./425).
7. **Kasa, shwasa** (cough, asthma): Taking decoction of Nirgundi, Guduchi, Haritaki, and Marich in equal parts mixed with lavan gives relief in kasa and shwasa (Vd.M. 3/11).
8. **Apasmara** (epilepsy): Nirgundi mula churna is beneficial in apasmara (RRS. 21/57).
9. **Angaghata** (paralysis): Decoction prepared with equal quantity of Nirgundi, Raasna, Arka, and Eranda mool churna is given twice daily in hemiplegia, paraplegia, facial palsy, and other Vataj diseases.

Officinal Parts Used

Root, leaves, seed

Dose

Leaf juice: 10 to 20 mL
Root powder: 3 to 6 g
Seed powder: 3 to 6 g

Formulations

Nirgundi ghrita, Nirgundi taila, Nirgundi kalpa.

Toxicity/Adverse Effects

Adverse effects with its use are rare; however, minor gastrointestinal upset, mild skin rash, and itching have been reported in some cases (Rastogi et al 2010).

Substitution and Adulteration

Nirgundi seeds are substituted with Tulasi beej and its root and leaves are adulterated with other species of the same genus such as *Vitex trifolia* Linn.f., *Vitex rotundifolia*, *Vitex agnus castus*.

Points to Ponder

- *Nirgundi is one of the best painkillers and anti-inflammatory medicines in Ayurveda.*
- *The Vitex species with white flower is known as Sinduvara and the one with blue flowers is known as Nirgundi.*

Suggested Readings

Ladda PL, Magdum CS. *Vitex negundo* Linn.: ethnobotany, phytochemistry and pharmacology—a review. Int J Adv Pharm Biol Chem 2012;1(1):115

Rastogi T, Kubde M, Farooqui IA, Khadabadi SS. A review on ethanomedicinal uses and phyto-pharmacology of anti-inflammatory herb *Vitex negundo*. Int J Pharm Sci Res 2010;1(9):23–28

Sharma PC, Yelne MB, Dennis TJ. Database on Medicinal Plants used in Ayurveda. C.C.R.A.S. Department of Indian Systems of Medicine and Homeopathy (ISM&H). Ministry of Health and Family Welfare, Government of India. 2005;3:452–455

Suganthi N, Dubey S. Phytochemical constituents and pharmacological activities of *Vitex negundo* Linn. J Chem Pharm Res 2016;8(2): 800–807

The Ayurvedic Pharmacopeia of India. Part I, Vol. 3. New Delhi: Department of AYUSH, Ministry of Health and Family Welfare, Government of India; 2001:144

Wan Hassan WE. Ulam: Salad Herbs of Malaysia. Masbe Sdn. Bhd. 2010:106–107

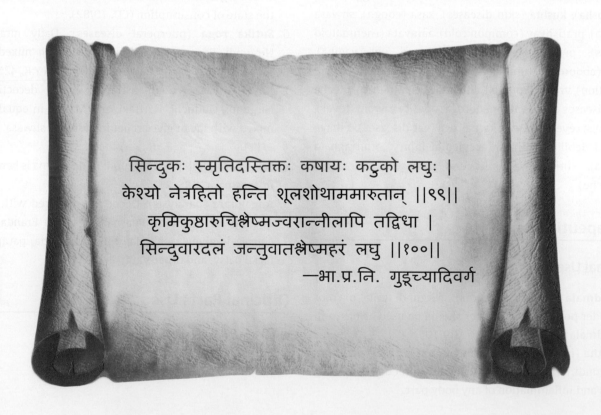

सिन्दुकः स्मृतिदस्तिक्तः कषायः कटुको लघुः |
केश्यो नेत्रहितो हन्ति शूलशोथाममारुतान् ||९९||
कृमिकुष्ठारुचिक्ष्रेष्मज्वरान्नीलापि तद्विधा |
सिन्दुवारदलं जन्तुवातक्ष्रेष्महरं लघु ||१००||
—भा.प्र.नि. गुडूच्यादिवर्ग

72. Palash *[Butea monosperma Lam. Kutze]*

Synonym:	*Butea frondosa Koenig ex Roxb.*
Family:	*Fabaceae*
Hindi name:	*Dhak, Teshu*
English name:	*Bastard peak, Flame of forest*

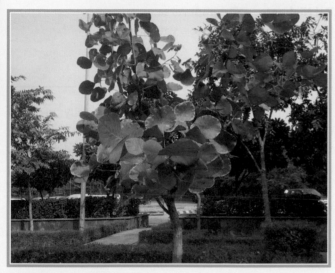

Plant of *Butea monosperma* Lam. Kutze.

In navagraha vatika, Palasha should be planted in South-East direction as it represents the planet Moon (chandra graham/soma). Its roots are used for samidha in ritual ceremonies (yagya) to pacify the negative effect of Chandra graha.

Introduction

The tree attains its Sanskrit name because of its beautiful foliage. The genus *Butea* is named after the Earl of Bute, a patron of botany, and *monosperma* means single seeded.

In Hindu mythology, Palasha is considered an auspicious tree. It is believed that the tree is a form of Agni deva, the God of fire (Murti et al 1940). Its flowers are offered to Goddess Kali as a substitute of blood in sacrifice rituals (Ambasta 1994). Its wood is used in sacrificial ceremonies (yagya) to God. This sacred tree is known as the treasurer of God.

Ancient scriptures described Palasha as a plant with immense medicinal and economical potential. Chakradutta has advised to use its gum for external application. Sharangdhar considered its seeds wormicidal. Sodhala used its root juice in netraroga, flowers in blindness, seeds in worm infestation, and stem as rasayana drug. Sushrut described its shaka as kapha pitta guna and its oil madhura,

kashaya (S.S.Su. 45/121). Charaka used it in basti dravya and as lepa in kushta (C.S.Su. 3/16). The gum obtained from the incision in the stem is used as a hemostatic agent and is known as Bengal kino or Butea kino. In folklore medicine, the gum is used in the treatment of mouth ulcers, sore throat, leucorrhea, diarrhea, and excessive perspiration. Acharya Charaka has advocated using it in treatment of arsha, atisaar, raktapitta, rakta gulma, visha, mukharoga, yoni roga, rajyakshma, and kshatasheen.

Besides medicinal uses, Palasha leaves are used in rural areas for preparation of pattal (leaf plates), donas (cups), wrapping biddi, and as cattle fodder. The flowers yield an orange dye which is used to make natural Holi colors.

Bark fibers are used for making cordage. The gum is added in food dishes and leather industry. The wood pulp is suitable for newsprint manufacturing and production of natural lac because the tree is a good host to the lac insect (Ambasta 1994).

Vernacular Names

Bengali: Palash Gachha, Palas
Bihari: Faras, Paras
Gujarati: Kesudo, Khakharo, Khakhapado
Kannada: Muttug, Muttugamara, Muttala
Kashmiri: Dhak
Konkani: Palash
Malayalam: Plasu, Camata, Plas, Pilacham
Marathi: Palas, Khakara, Khakharo
Oriya: Porasur
Persian: Palah
Punjabi: Palash, Dhak, Tesu, Chichra
Tamil: Purasu, Paras, Camata
Telugu: Moduga, Modugu, Chettu
Urdu: Dhak, Palaspara

Synonyms

Brahmavrisha: It is considered as the sacred tree to worship Lord Brahma.
Kinshuka: The shape of flower resembles the parrot's beak.
Ksharshreshtha: The alkali obtained from the plant is best, i.e., highly efficacious.
Raktapushpaka: The flowers are bright red colored.
Samidvara: Its wood is used for samidha in yagya.
Triparna: The plant bears characteristic trifoliate leaves.
Vatapotha: The plant is renowned drug to pacify vatu diseases.
Yagyiya: The wood of the plant is used in sacrificial ceremonies (*yagya*).

Classical Categorization

Charaka Samhita: not mentioned
Sushrut Samhita: Rodhradi, Nyaygrodhadi, Mushkakadi, Ambashthadi
Ashtang Hridaya: Lodhradi, Nyaygrodhadi, Mushkakadi, Ambashthadi
Dhanvantari Nighantu: Amradi varga
Madanpal Nighantu: Vatadi varga
Kaiyadev Nighantu: Oushadi varga
Raj Nighantu: Karviradi varga
Bhavaprakash Nighantu: Vatadi varga

Distribution

The plant is native to South Asia, especially in Indo-Gangetic plains, Malaysia, Nepal, Indonesia, Laos, Cambodia, Vietnam, Bangladesh, Sri Lanka, Myanmar, and Thailand. It is distributed throughout India in dry deciduous forests of Himalayas, Maharashtra, Kerala, Karnataka, Rajasthan, Gujarat, and Madhya Pradesh.

Morphology

A medium-sized deciduous tree, 30 to 40 ft in height. Trunk is crooked and twisted with irregular branches and rough, gray bark (**Fig. 72.1**).

- **Leaves:** Trifoliate, long petiolate, in which terminal leaflet is big, rhomboidal in shape, lateral leaflets are ovate, coriaceous, thick, leathery in touch, ash green colored, glabrous above, finely silky beneath (**Fig. 72.2**).

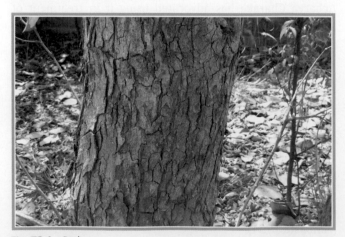

Fig. 72.1 Bark.

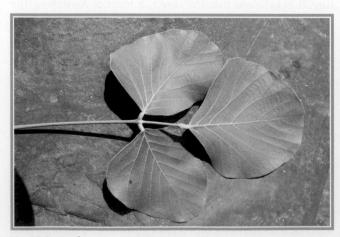

Fig. 72.2 Leaf.

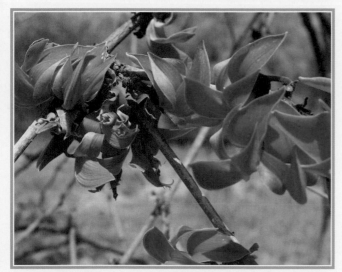

Fig. 72.3   Flower.

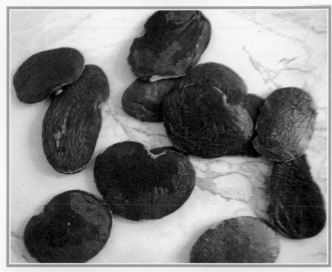

Fig. 72.5   Seeds.

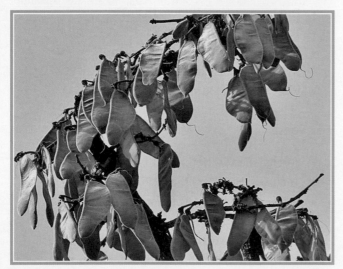

Fig. 72.4   Fruits.

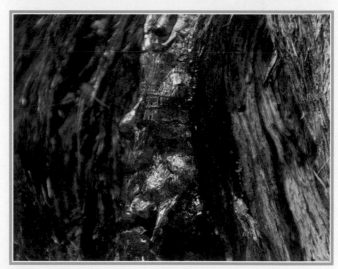

Fig. 72.6   Gum.

- **Flowers:** Bright orange-red, large, in rigid racemes, velvety, borne on leafless branches from January to March. Each flower consists of five petals comprising one standard, two smaller wings and a curved beak-shaped keel (**Fig. 72.3**). It is this keel which gives it the name of parrot tree.

- **Fruit:** Indehiscent, flat thin, silky, stalked tomentose pod, 10 to 13 cm long, pendulous, thickened at the sutures, containing single seed (**Fig. 72.4**). Seeds are flat, kidney shape, wrinkled surface, reddish brown in color (**Fig. 72.5**). The plant is propagated by seeds and root suckers. Gum from the plant is shown in **Fig. 72.6**.

Phenology

Flowering time: February to April
Fruiting time: May to June

Key Characters for Identification

➤ A medium-sized deciduous tree with rough gray bark.
➤ Leaves trifoliate, terminal leaflet rhomboidal and lateral leaflets oval, leathery, silky beneath.
➤ Flowers orange-red, in racemes, velvety, borne on leafless branches.
➤ Fruits flat indehiscent tomentose pod 10 to 13 cm long.
➤ Seeds flat, reddish-brown, kidney shape.

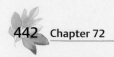

Types

Raj Nighantu has mentioned its four types on the basis of flower color:

- Rakta
- Peeta
- Sita: Best variety
- Neel

Rasapanchaka

	Bark, leaf, seed, gum	Flowers
Rasa	Katu, Tikta, Kashaya	Tikta, Katu, Kashaya
Guna	Laghu, Ruksha	Laghu, Snigdha
Vipaka	Katu	Madhura
Virya	Ushna	Sheeta
Doshaghanta	Kaphavatashamaka	Kaphapittashamaka

Chemical Constituents

The plant is rich in alkaloids, flavonoids, glycosides, phenolic compounds, amino acids, glycosides, resin, saponin, steroids, and fatty acids. Some of the important constituents are as follows:

- **Bark:** It consists of gallic acid, kino-tannic acid, pyrocatechin, allophanic acid, butolic acid, shellolic acid, butrin, butein, butin, alanind, palasitrin, cyanidin, histidine, palasimide, miroestrol, methoxyiso-flavones; cajanin and isoformononetin, buteaspermin A, buteaspermin B and
- buteasperminol, medicarp, cajanin, formononetin, isoformonentin, and cladrin.
- **Flower:** It contains triterpene butrin, isobutrin, coreopsin, sulphurein, isocoreopsin, monospermoside, isomonospermoside, chalcones, aurones, steroids, glycosides, and flavonoids.
- **Seed:** It has palasonin, isomonospermoside, mono-spermoside, allophonic acid, flavone glycoside, fixed oil, and fatty acids.
- **Gum:** It contains tannins, resins, pyrocatechin, and mucilaginous material.

- **Leaves:** Have kino-oil containing oleic, linoleic, lignoceric, and palmitic acid (Tiwari et al 2019; Gupta et al 2012).

Identity, Purity, and Strength

For Stem Bark

- Foreign matter: Not more than 2%
- Total ash: Not more than 12%
- Acid-insoluble ash : Not more than 1.5%
- Alcohol soluble extractive : Not less than 10%
- Water-soluble extractive : Not less than 14%

For Gum

- Foreign matter: Not more than 2%
- Total ash: Not more than 3%
- Acid-insoluble ash: Not more than 1%
- Alcohol soluble extractive: Not less than 69%
- Water-soluble extractive: Not less than 63%

For Seeds

- Foreign matter: Not more than 1%
- Total ash: Not more than 7%
- Acid-insoluble ash: Not more than 0.5%
- Alcohol soluble extractive: Not less than 9%
- Water-soluble extractive: Not less than 25%

(Source: The Ayurvedic Pharmacopeia of India 1999, 2004)

Karma (Actions)

Ayurveda classics attributed deepan (carminative), vrishya (aphrodisiac), sara (laxative), sangrahi (absorbent), sandhaniya (union promoter), krimighna (anthelmintic), stambhaka (hemostatic), sheetal (refrigerant), kusthaghna (antidermatosis), jwaraghna (antipyretic), mutral (diuretic), and rasayana (rejuvinator) properties to it. However, different parts showed different karma which are enlisted as under:

- Pushpa (flowers): Grahi (absorbent), sheetal (coolant), sugandhi (aromatic), raktastambhaka (hemostatic), dahaprasasmana (pacify burning sensation).
- Phal (fruit): Laghu, ushna

- Beeja (seeds): Katu, ushna, snigdha, krimighna (anthelmintic), kusthaghna (antileprotic), vishaghna (antidote to poison)
- Niryasa (gum): Grahi, sandhaniya (union promoting), vrishya (aphrodisiac), balya (tonic), kashaya (astringent)
- Twak (bark): Deepan (carminative), grahi, uttejaka (stimulant), stambhaka (hemostatic), sandhankara
- Pravala: Krimivataharam param
- Doshakarma: Tridoshashamaka
- Dhatukarma: Rasayana
- Malakarma: Stambhaka, Soshaka

Pharmacological Actions

Its reported pharmacological actions are anthelmintic, analgesic, anticonvulsant, antidiabetic, anticancer, anti-inflammatory, antidiarrheal, antiestrogenic, antifertility, antimicrobial, antifungal, antibacterial, antihyperglycemic, antihyperlipidemic antispasmodic, antistress, chemo-preventive, hemagglutinating, hepatoprotective, osteo-protective, free radical scavenging, thyroid inhibitory, antioxidant, and wound-healing activities (Tiwari et al 2019; Sharma and Deshwal 2011).

Indications

The entire plant is widely used in the treatment of diverse ailments like:

- Pushpa (flowers): Daha (burning sensation), mutrakricchta (dysuria), trishna (thirst), vatarakta (gout), kushta (skin diseases), kandu (pruritus), shool (pain), raktapitta (bleeding disorders), jwara (fever), pradara (discharge from vagina)
- Phal (fruit): Meha (diabetes), arsha (piles), krimi (worm infestation), kushta (skin diseases), udar roga (abdominal diseases), gulma (abdominal tumors), pleeha (diseases of spleen)
- Beeja (seeds): Krimi (worm infestation), kushta, visha (poisoning), kandu, and pama and dadru (minor skin ailments)
- Niryasa (gum): Vrana (wounds), dourbalya (debility), raktasrava (hemorrhage)
- Twak (bark): Vrana, bhagnasandhankara (fracture healing), grahni (irritable bowel syndrome [IBS]),

gulma, atisaar (diarrhea), yoni roga (uterine disorders), krimi, shool
- Kshara: Udara shool, udarroga, adhyaman (flatulence), vibandha (constipation)

Therapeutical Uses

External Use

1. **Daha** (burning sensation): In case of burning sensation due to fever apply cold paste prepared by Palasha patra, Badar or Nimba pounded in kanji (B.P.Ci. 1/360).
2. **Vrischika dansha** (scorpion sting): Paste prepared with Palasha beeja impregnated with Arka ksheer is applied locally to subside pain in scorpion bite (A.S.U. 43/70).
3. **Garbhanirodhan** (contraceptive): Finely powdered Palasha beeja mixed with madhu ghrita should be applied in vagina for contraception (G.N. 6/1/60).

Internal Use

1. **Krimi roga** (worm infestation): Regular consumption of Palash Beeja, Kampillaka, and Vidanga powder pounded with Guda with Takra (butter milk) helps in expelling out round worms from intestine. Intake of Palasha beej swarasa or kalka with tandulodaka destroys worms (S.S.U. 54/25).
2. **Rakta pitta** (bleeding disorders): To check intrinsic hemorrhage, Palasha pushpa mixed with double quantity of sugar should be taken with milk (SB. 4/304).
3. **Atisaar** (diarrhea): Drinking Palasha phala decoction mixed with milk followed by warm milk is advised in atisaar (C.S.Ci. 19/60).
4. **Rasayana** (rejuvenator): Intake of Palasha beeja, Vidanga beeja mixed with Amalaki swarasa with madhu ghrita for a month gives antiageing effect (RM. 33/5).
5. **Kasa** (cough): Daily intake of powdered Palasha beeja, Udumbara, and Maricha for 3 days cures cough (VD. 3/16).
6. **Udarshool** (colic): Yusha prepared with Palasha or Dhanyaka mixed with sharkara should be taken (S.S.U. 42/107).

Officinal Parts Used

Seed, bark, fruit, flower, gum, and kshara (alkali)

Dose

Seed powder: 3 to 6 g

Bark decoction: 50 to 100 mL

Gum: 1 to 3 g

Formulations

Palashkshara ghrita, Palashbeejadi churan, Krimikuthara rasa, Mahanarayana taila, Janam ghutti.

Toxicity/Adverse Effects

Not reported in humans. However, mild-to-moderate toxicity in seeds has been reported in mice, earthworm, dogs, and rabbits (Sharma et al 2000).

Substitution and Adulteration

Not reported

Points to Ponder

- *All parts of Palasha possess therapeutic efficacy. The bark, seeds, gum, leaves are hot in potency except flowers which are madhura and sheeta in properties.*
- *Palasha beeja churna is a drug of choice for worm infestation especially for round worm infestation.*

Suggested Readings

Ambasta BP. The Useful Plants of India, Vol. 1. New Delhi: CSIR; 1994:91

Gupta P, et al. Phytochemical and pharmacological review on *Butea monosperma* (Palash). Int J Agron Plant Prod 2012;3(7):255–258

Murti P. Bhaskara, R. and Krishnaswamy, H. Proceedings of the Indian Academy of Sciences, Section A 12A; 1940:472–476

Sharma AK, Deshwal N. An overview: On phytochemical and pharmacological studies of *Butea monosperma*. Int J Pharm Sci Res 2011;3:864–867

Sharma PC, Yelne MB, Dennis TJ. Database on Medicinal Plants used in Ayurveda, Vol. 1. New Delhi: CCRAS Department of Indian Systems of Medicine and Homeopathy (ISM&H), Ministry of Health and Family Welfare, Government of India; 2000:336–338

The Ayurvedic Pharmacopeia of India. Part I, Vol. 2. New Delhi: Department of AYUSH, Ministry of Health and Family Welfare, Government of India; 1999:137

The Ayurvedic Pharmacopeia of India. Part I, Vol. 4. New Delhi: Department of AYUSH, Ministry of Health and Family Welfare, Government of India; 2004:92 & 94

Tiwari P, Jena S, Sahu PK. *Butea monosperma*: phytochemistry and pharmacology. Acta Sci Pharma Sci 2019;3(4):19–26

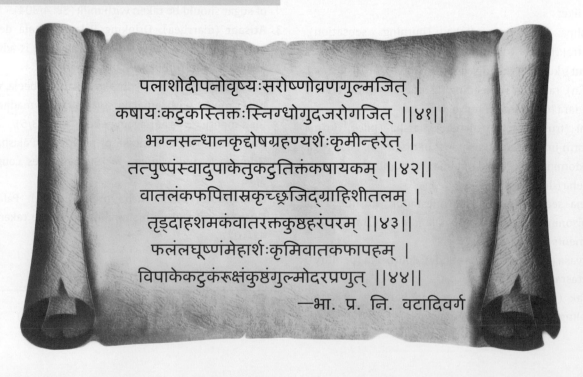

पलाशोदीपनोवृष्यःसरोष्णोव्रणगुल्मजित् |

कषायःकटुकस्तिक्तःस्निग्धोगुदजरोगजित् ||४१||

भग्नसन्धानकृद्दोषग्रहण्यर्शःकृमीन्हरेत् |

तत्पुष्पंस्वादुपाकेतुकटुतिक्तंकषायकम् ||४२||

वातलंकफपित्तास्रकृच्छ्रजिद्ग्राहिशीतलम् |

तृड्दाहशमकंवातरक्तकुष्ठहरंपरम् ||४३||

फलंलघूष्णंमेहार्शःकृमिवातकफापहम् |

विपाकेकटुकंरूक्षंकुष्ठंगुल्मोदरप्रणुत् ||४४||

—भा. प्र. नि. वटादिवर्ग

73. Parpata [*Fumaria indica* Pugsley]

Synonym:	*Fumaria parviflora Lam.*
Family:	*Fumariaceae*
Hindi name:	*Pittapapda, Dhamgajra*
English name:	*Five-leaved fumitory*

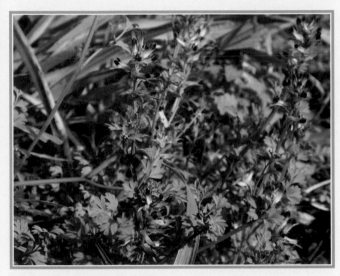

Plant of *Fumaria indica* Pugsley.

Musta Parpata is considered as best drug for Jwara.

Introduction

The Latin name *Fumaria* is derived from the word "fumus terrae" which means smoke of the earth (Orhan et al 2015) or unpleasant smell, and parviflora consists of two words "parvi" (small) and "flora" (flowers) which collectively means that the plant bears small flowers having unpleasant odor.

Parpata is widely used in traditional and folklore systems of medicine as a drug of choice for pitta aggravated jwara. Charaka and Sushrut recommended it for treatment of fever, vomiting, and blood disorders. Chakradutta considered Parpata as the best drug for alleviating pitta jwara. Charaka and Sushrut have described it in shakavarga. In Turkey, it is used against hepatobiliary dysfunction, and in the Unani traditional system, it is prescribed to treat gastrointestinal and respiratory ailments (Jameel et al 2014).

Vernacular Names

Arabian: Bukslat-ul- mulik, Shahtaraja
Assamese: Shahtaraj
Bengali: Vanshulpha, Bansulpha
German: Erdrauch
Gujarati: Pittapapada, Pitpapado, Pittapapado
Kannada: KalluSabbasige, Parpatu, Chaturasigide
Kashmiri: Shahterah
Marathi: Pittapada, Shatara, Pitpapda
Nepalese: Kairuwa
Persian: Shatra, Shahtarah
Punjabi: Shahtara, Pittapapara
Sinhalese: Pathapadaga
Tamil: Tura, Tusa, Thura
Telugu: Parpatakamu, Chatarashi
Urdu: Shahatra

Synonyms

Kavachnamak: The plant protects the users from diseases.

Panshuprayay: It bears all the synonyms of sand or dust because of its cooling effect.

Sukshmapatra: The leaves of the plant are minute in size, i.e., pinnatisect.

Vartikta: It is considered as the best drug among tiktadravya.

Classical Categorization

Charaka Samhita: Trishnanigrahan

Dhanvantari Nighantu: Guduchyadi varga

Madanpal Nighantu: Abhyadi varga

Kaiyadev Nighantu: Oushadi varga

Raj Nighantu: Parpatadi varga

Bhavaprakash Nighantu: Guduchyadi varga

Distribution

The plant is native to Europe, Africa, and Asia especially Middle East. It is found throughout India as weed in rice and wheat fields, wastelands, open areas, etc., from Himalayas to Indo-Gangetic plains down to the Nilgiris.

Morphology

It is a diffuse, erect or procumbent, annual herb of about ½ to 1 ft height. Branches are grooved, glabrous, and pubescent.

- **Leaves:** Alternate, 5 to 10 cm long, two to three times pinnatisect, with linear-acute, mucronate segments, light green color (**Fig. 73.1**).
- **Flowers:** Purple-pink colored, occurs in terminal raceme inflorescence of about 4 to 10 cm long (**Fig. 73.2**).
- **Fruits:** Indehiscent, globose, nutlet of 1 to 2 mm diameter, short stalk, single seeded.

The plant is propagated by its seeds.

Phenology

Flowering time: January to February

Fruiting time: March to April

Key Characters for Identification

- ➤ A diffuse, erect or procumbent, annual herb of about ½ to 1 ft.
- ➤ Leaves are alternate, pinnatisect, with linear-acute, mucronate segments.
- ➤ Flowers are purple-pink, occurs in terminal raceme.
- ➤ Fruits are globose, nutlet, indehiscent, single seeded.

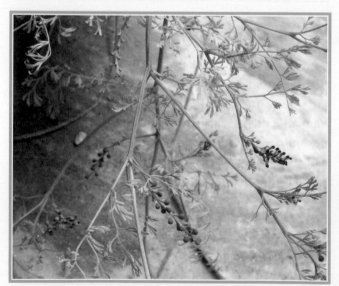

Fig. 73.1 Leaves.

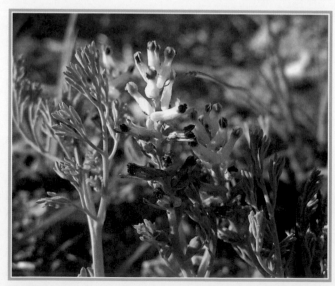

Fig. 73.2 Flowers.

Types

None

Rasapanchaka

Guna	Laghu, Ruksha
Rasa	Tikta
Vipaka	Katu
Virya	Sheeta

Chemical Constituents

Phytochemical analysis of Parpataka revealed the presence of flavonoids, glycosides, tannins, saponins, steroids, triterpenoids, phenols, alkaloids, and anthraquinones. The major constituents among them are protopine, narceimine, tetrahydrocoptisine, narlumidine, methyl fumarate, bicuculine, adlumiceine, coptisine, cryptopine, fumaricine, fumariline, fumaritine, fumarophycine, benzo-phenanthridine, β-sitosterol, stigmasterol, campesterol, tetrahydroxy flavone-3-arabinoside, 3'-4'-dihydroxy flavone and 3,7,4'-trihydroxy flavones, and capric, myristic, lauric, linoleic acids (Popova et al 1982; Hilal et al 1993; Jameel et al 2014).

Identity, Purity, and Strength

- Foreign matter: Not more than 2%
- Total ash: Not more than 30%
- Acid-insoluble ash: Not more than 10%
- Alcohol-soluble extractive: Not less than 7%
- Water-soluble extractive: Not less than 29%

(Source: The Ayurvedic Pharmacopeia of India 2004)

Karma (Actions)

Classical texts attributed sangrahi (absorbent), jwarahara (antipyretic), trishnanigrahan (antithirst), swedjanaka (diaphoretic), krimighna (antimicrobial), mutral (diuretic), raktapittahara (pacifies bleeding disorders), raktashodhaka (blood purifier), raktastambhaka (hemostatic), chardighna

(antiemetic), dahaprashmana (alleviates burning sensation) properties to it.

- Doshakarma: Pittakaphahara
- Dhatukarma: Sangrahi, Trishnanigrahan
- Malakarma: Mutral, Swedajanan

Pharmacological Actions

The plant exhibits antipyretic, anthelmintic, laxative, cholagogue, muscle relaxant, sedative, hepatoprotective, antispasmodic, analgesic, anti-inflammatory, hypotensive, inotropic, antibacterial, antiarrhythmic, and blood purifier properties (Billore et al 2005).

Indications

In traditional systems of medicine, it is used for the treatment of raktapitta (bleeding disorders), bhram (giddiness), murchchha (fainting), trishna (thirst), jwara (fever), daha (burning sensation), mada (hallucination), aruchi (dyspepsia), krimi (worm infestation), pandu (anemia), kamala (jaundice), atisaar (diarrhea), hridyadaha (acidity), vatarakta (gout), kushta (skin diseases), tuberculosis, leprosy, diarrhea, headache, liver disorders, and inflammatory disorders.

Therapeutic Uses

External Use

1. **Vrana** (wounds): Paste of leaves is applied externally on wounds, sore, ulcers, and skin diseases.
2. **Netraabhishyandi** (conjunctivitis): Instillation of Parpata leaves juice in the infected eyes gives relief in conjunctivitis.

Internal Use

1. **Jwara** (fever): Parpatak decoction alone or combined with Guduchi and Amalaki swarasa is used in pittajjwara, daha, sosha, and bhram (A.S.Ci. 1/75) (B.P.Ci. 1/347). Parpata decoction when prepared with Shunthi alleviates all types of fever (R.M. 21/3).
2. **Chardi** (vomiting): Intake of cold decoction of Parpata mixed with madhu is helpful in controlling vomiting (VM. 15/9).

3. **Trishna** (thirst): To reduce thirst, burning sensation, coryza, and fever, Sadangapaniya made up of Musta, Parpata, Chandan, Ushira, Sugandhbala, and Shunthi is used twice daily.

Officinal Part Used

Panchang (whole plant)

Dose

Powder: 3 to 6 g

Formulations

Sadangapaniya, Parpatadikwath, Parpatarishta, Tiktakaghrita, Mahatiktakaghrita, Parpatadighrita.

Toxicity/Adverse Effects

Not reported any

Substitution and Adulteration

In different parts of the country, different plants are used in the name of Parpata. In North India, Punjab, *Fumaria parviflora*, *F. officinalis*, *Oldenlandia corymbosa* L. in Bengal, Maharashtra, *Polycarpaea corymbosa* Lam in Uttar Pradesh, and *Justicia procumbens* in Mumbai, *Rungia repens* Nees in Gujarat, *Mollugo stricta* L. in Madras, Malabar, South India, *Peristrophe bicalyculata* Nees in Mumbai are substituted or adulterated as Parpata (Billore et al 2005).

> **Points to Ponder**
> - *Parpata is the drug of choice for jwara, trishna, chardi, bhrama, mada, daha, and raktapitta.*
> - *Parpata is a controversial drug. In different regions of India, different plants are taken as Parpata.*

Suggested Readings

Billore KV, Yelne MB, Dennis TJ, Chaudhari BG. Database on Medicinal Plants used in Ayurveda, Vol. 7. New Delhi: C.C.R.A.S. Department of Indian Systems of Medicine and Homeopathy (ISM&H), Ministry of Health and Family Welfare, Government of India; 2005: 340–343

Gupta PC, Sharma N, Rao ChV. A review on ethnobotany, phytochemistry and pharmacology of Fumaria indica (Fumitory). Asian Pac J Trop Biomed 2012;2(8):665–669

Hilal SH, Aboutabl EA, Youssef SAH, Shalaby MA, Sokkar NM. Lipoidal matter, flavonoid content, uterine stimulant and gonadal hormone-like activities of Fumaria parviflora Lam growing in Egypt. Plantes Medicinales et Phytotherapie 1993;26:383–396

Jameel M, Ali A, Ali M. New phytoconstituents from the aerial parts of Fumaria parviflora Lam. J Adv Pharm Technol Res 2014;5(2):64–69

Orhan IE, Ozturk N, Sener B. Antiprotozoal assessment and phenolic acid profiling of five Fumaria (fumitory) species. Asian Pac J Trop Med 2015;8(4):283–286

Popova ME, Simánek V, Dolejš L, Smysl B, Preininger V. Alkaloids from Fumaria parviflora and F. kralikii. Planta Med 1982;45(2):120–122

The Ayurvedic Pharmacopeia of India. Part I, Vol. 4. New Delhi: Department of AYUSH, Ministry of Health and Family Welfare, Government of India; 2004:98

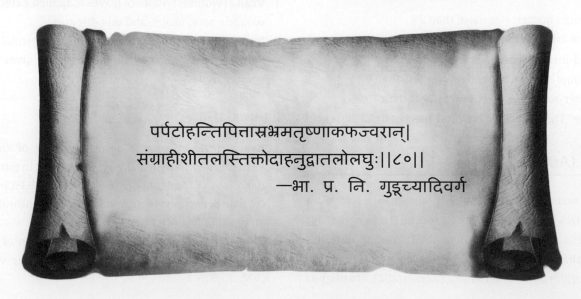

पर्पटोहन्तिपित्तास्रभ्रमतृष्णाकफज्वरान्।
संग्राहीशीतलस्तिक्तोदाहनुद्वातलोलघुः॥८०॥
—भा. प्र. नि. गुड्च्यादिवर्ग

74. Pashanbheda [*Bergenia ciliata* (Haw.) Sternb]

Family:	*Saxifragaceae*
Hindi name:	*Patharchatta, Shilaphod*
English name:	*Velvet leaf, Rock foil*

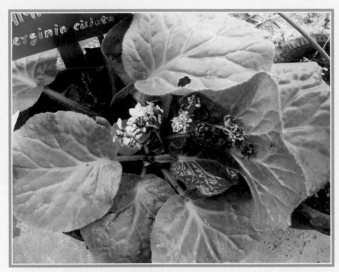

Plant of *Bergenia ciliata* (Haw.) Sternb.

> *Bergenia ciliata and its other species are included in vulnerable species by IUCN.*
>
> *—Ved et al (2003)*

Introduction

The plant derived its name Pashanbheda (Pashan means rock, bheda means piercing) because of its lithotriptic property. The species name *ciliata* refers to the presence of innumerable hair in every plant part.

Pashanbhed is an important diuretic drug used since ages for the treatment of ashmari. Charaka, Sushrut, Ashtang, Chakradutta, Bhavamishra all recommended to use it in ashmari, mutraghata, mutrakricchta chikitsa. It is a promising folklore medicine used in Jammu and Kashmir, Nepal, Bhutan, Tibet, Pakistan, etc. In Sudh-Mahadev region of Himalayas, it is used in vertigo and headache. In Jammu and Kashmir, it is reported to be used in treatment of asthmatic disorders. Root is also used as a tonic, in uterine diseases, fever, pulmonary infection, and in eye diseases (Bhattarai 1991). It has also been used as a poultice, for boils, ulcers, cuts, carbuncle, and wounds in Kashmir; hence, it is known as Zakhmehayat. In Sikkim and West Bengal, the juice of the rhizome is used as an effective remedy for cough and cold.

Leaves and rhizomes are used in veterinary medicine. In local festival called "Phool Sangran" in Uttaranchal, people used to offer its flowers as a good luck charm to their neighbors. The flowers are also cultivated for their aesthetic value.

Vernacular Names

Arabic: Barghienia-mehdiyata
Assamese: Patharkuchi
Bengali: Patharchuri, Himasagara, Patrankur
German: Steinbrech
Gujarati: Pashanbheda, Pakhanbheda
Japanese: Yukinosita
Kannada: Alepgaya, Pahanbhedi, Hittaga, Pasanaberu, Hittulaka
Kashmiri: Pashanbhed

Malayalam: Kallurvanchi, Kallurvanni, Kallorvanchi
Marathi: Pashanbheda
Nepalese: Pakanabadha
Oriya: Pasanbhedi, Pashanabheda
Punjabi: Kachalu, Pashanbhed
Sinhalese: Pahanabeya
Tamil: Sirupilai
Telugu: Kondapindi
Unani: Mukha
Urdu: Pakhanabeda, Zakham-e-hayat

Synonyms

Ashmabheda: The one which has the potency to break stones.
Giribhida: The plant has the capability to emerge from the cracks of mountains.
Bhinnayojini: The plant is originated through the cracks in the mountains.
Ashmaghna: The plant has antilithitic property.
Pashanabhedaka: The plant has the property of breaking calculus in the body.

Classical Categorization

Charaka Samhita: Mutravirechaniya
Sushrut Samhita: Veertarvadi
Ashtang Hridaya: Veertarvadi

Dhanvantari Nighantu: Guduchyadi varga
Madanpal Nighantu: Abhyadi varga
Kaiyadev Nighantu: Oushadi varga
Raj Nighantu: Parpatadi varga
Bhavaprakash Nighantu: Haritakyadi varga

Distribution

The plant is native to Central Asia, from Afghanistan to China. It is found throughout Himalayan region from Kashmir to Bhutan between altitudes of 1,000 and 3,000 m.

Morphology

It is an evergreen perennial herb with stout rootstocks attaining height of 30 cm or more, emerging from the cracks of mountains and lying flat over the surface of mountains.

- **Leaves:** Radicle origin of leaves (i.e., tuft of leaves above and stout rootstocks below). Leaves few, spreading, fleshy, soft, fully studded with minute hairs, glabrous, suborbicular to orbicular in shape, base cordate or round, margin entire to occasionally denticulate at top, ciliate, upper surface is bright green whereas lower surface is brownish red (**Fig. 74.1**).
- **Flowers:** White, pink, or purplish red, pedicellate, in long terminal cymose panicles, sepals pink to red, styles 7 mm long, carpels and styles green or pink (**Fig. 74.2**).

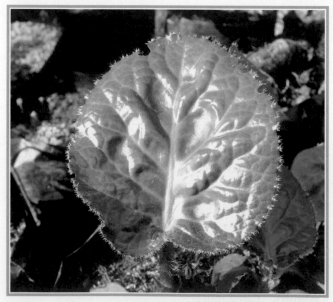

Fig. 74.1 Leaf.

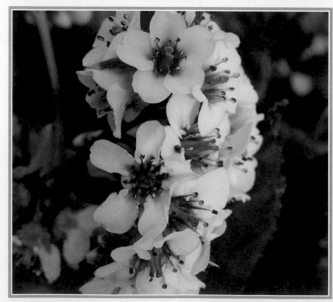

Fig. 74.2 Flowers.

- **Fruit:** Capsules, 13 × 6 mm, round, with numerous albuminous seeds (**Fig. 74.3**).
- **Rootstock:** It is stout, compact, solid, barrel shaped, cylindrical, 1.5 to 3 cm long and 1 to 2 cm in diameter with irregular, longitudinally wrinkled, ridged, furrowed outer surface, covered with brown leaf scars, with characteristic camphoraceous odor (**Fig. 74.4a, b**).

The plant is propagated by seeds and root stocks.

Phenology

Flowering time: February to April
Fruiting time: March to July

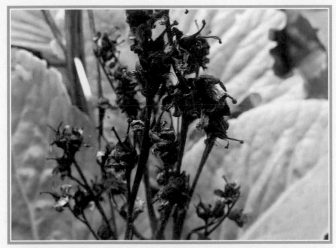

Fig. 74.3 Fruits.

> ### Key Characters for Identification
>
> ➤ An evergreen perennial herb of about 30 cm heightLeaves: Few, spreading, fleshy, fully studded with minute hairs, glabrous, orbicular shape, lower surface reddish brown
> ➤ Flowers: White, pink or purplish red, in terminal cymose paniclesFruits: Round, capsulatedRhizome: Stout, solid, barrel shaped, 1.5 to 3 cm long, wrinkled surface

Types

Raj Nighantu has described its four types:
- Pashanbheda
- Vatapatri
- Shilavalka
- Chatushpatri

Rasapanchaka

Guna	Laghu, Snigdha, Tikshna
Rasa	Kashaya, Tikta
Vipaka	Katu
Virya	Sheeta
Prabhava	Ashmabhedana

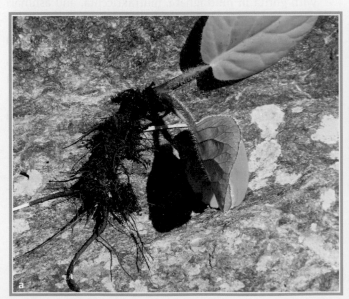

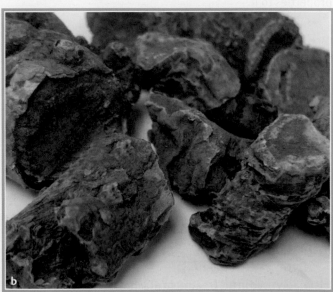

Fig. 74.4 **(a)** Root. **(b)** Dried root.

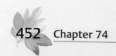

Chemical Constituents

The roots are reported to contain many glycosides, sterols, terpenoids, flavonoids, saponins, starch, minerals, vitamins, mucilage, and ash. The principal compounds among them are bergenin (glycoside), β sitosterol, catechin, afzelechin, lactone, galloyl epicatechin, galloyl catechin, leucocyanidin, gallic acid, methyl gallate, quercetin-3-O-β-D-xylopyranoside, arbutin, p-hydroxybenzoic acid, and protocatechuic acid (Fujii et al 1996; Singh et al 2009).

Identity, Purity, and Strength

For Rhizome

- Foreign matter: Not more than 2%
- Total ash: Not more than 13%
- Acid-insoluble ash: Not more than 0.5%
- Alcohol-soluble extractive: Not less than 9%
- Water-soluble extractive: Not less than 15%

(Source: The Ayurvedic Pharmacopeia of India 1989)

Karma (Actions)

Ayurvedic classics have attributed ashmaribhedana (antilithiatic), mutral (diuretic), bastishodhana (purifies urinary system), shothahara (anti-inflammatory), vranaropana (wound healing), stambhana (astringent), raktapittashamaka (antihemorrhagic), hridya (cardiotonic), jwaraghna (antipyretic), and vishaghna (antitoxin) properties to it.

- Doshakarma: Tridoshashamaka
- Dhatukarma: Bhedana, stambhana
- Malakarma: Mutral

Pharmacological Actions

The plant is reported to have antilithiatic, diuretic, antioxidant, antitussive, antiulcer, antineoplastic, laxative, analgesic, antibacterial, antidiabetic, antiscorbutic, antimalarial, antipyretic, anti-inflammatory, wound-healing, and hemostatic properties (Saini et al 2012).

Indications

It is widely used in the treatment of ashmari (urinary calculus), mutraghata (retention of urine), mutrakricchta (dysuria), mutradaha (burning micturation), mutravikara (urogenital disorders), trishna (thirst), daha (burning sensation), arsha (piles), gulma (abdominal tumors), hridyaroga (heart diseases), yoni roga (uterine disorders), prameha (diabetes), shool (pain), raktapradar (menorrhagia), jwara (fever), raktapitta (bleeding disorders), atisara (diarrhea), pravahika (dysentery), and vrana (wound).

In traditional practices, juice/decoction of its rhizome is used in worm infestation, malaria, postpartum diseases, asthma, boils, spleen enlargement, pulmonary infections, and dysentery.

Therapeutic Uses

External Use

1. **Abhighatajvrana** (traumatic injury): Make a poultice by crushing four to five leaves or root paste of Pashanbheda and apply it on traumatic wounds, boils, cuts, ulcers, burns, and in conjunctivitis.
2. **Raktasrava** (hemorrhage): Leaf juice or paste is applied on the affected area to arrest bleeding.
3. **Karnashool** (earache): Lukewarm leaf juice of Pashanbeda is instilled in earache.

Internal Use

1. **Mutraghata** (retention of urine), **Mutrakricchta** (dysuria): One should take Nala, Pashanbheda, Darbha, Ikshu, Trapusha, Ervarukabeeja boiled in milk added with ghrita in mutraghata, mutrakricchta, and ashmari (S.S.U. 58/47).
2. **Ashmari** (calculus): Decoction prepared with equal quantity of Shunthi, Varuna, Gokshura, Pashanbheda, and Makoya mixed with guda and yavakshar pacifies all types of ashmari (CD. 34/28). Pashanbhedyadhya ghrita is also indicated for vataashmari (CD. 34/8).Pashanbhed churna is indicated in ashmari chikitsa (C.S.Ci. 26/60).

Officinal Parts Used

Rhizome and leaf

Dose

Powder: 3 to 6 g
Decoction: 50 to 100 mL

Formulations

Pashanabhedadikvatha, Pashanabhedadya ghrita, Ashmarihara kashaya, Varunadikvatha, Mootravirechaniya kashaya, Pashanbhedadi churna, Shilodbhidadi taila, Brihadagokshuradya leha, Sarasvata ghrita, Stanyashodhana kashaya.

Toxicity/Adverse Effects

Toxicological studies reveal that Pashanbheda causes acute systematic toxicity which includes edema, erythema, breathing problem, bleeding diarrhea, cardiotoxicity, and CNS depression (Islam et al 2002).

Substitution and Adulteration

Since beginning, Pashanbheda has been considered as a controversial drug. In different parts of the country, different plants were used in the name of Pashanbheda (Sharma et al 2000). These are as follows:

- *Berginialigulata* Engl. in Himalayas and North India
- *Aervalanata* Juss ex Schult. in Rajasthan and Gujarat
- *Kalanchoepinnata* Pers. in Bengal
- *Coleus aromaticus* Benth. in Bengal
- *Ocimumbasillicum* Linn.
- *Homonoiariparia* Lour. in South India
- *Rotula aquatica* Lour. in Mangalore, Mysore
- *Brideliamontana* Willd. in Goa
- *Ammaniabacifera* Linn. in Kerala

Points to Ponder

- *Pashanbheda is a highly controversial drug. Many plants are used in the name of Pashanbheda. However, Bergenia ciliata (Haw.) Sternb. is the accepted botanical source of Pashanbheda.*
- *Pashanbheda is the drug of choice for ashmari, mutraghata, mutrakrichhta, and other urinary tract disorders.*

Suggested Readings

Bhattarai NK. Folk herbal medicines of Makawanpur district, Nepal. Int J Pharmacol 1991;29(4):284–295

Fujii M, Miyaichi Y, Tomimori T. Studies on Nepalese Crude Drugs. XXII: On the Phenolic Constituents of the Rhizome of *Bergenia ciliata* (Haw.) Sternb. Natural Medicines 1996;50(6):404–407

Islam M, Azhar I, Usmanghani K, Gill MA, Ahmad A, Shahabuddin. Bioactivity evaluation of Bergenia ciliata. Pak J Pharm Sci 2002; 15(1):15–33

Saini R, Chauhan R, Sharma S, Dwivedi J. Polypharmacological activities of *Bergenia* species. Int J Pharm Sci Rev Res 2012;13(1):100–110

Sharma PC, Yelne MB, Dennis TJ. Database on Medicinal Plants used in Ayurveda, Vol. 1. New Delhi: CCRAS Department of Indian Systems of Medicine and Homeopathy (ISM&H), Ministry of Health and Family Welfare, Government of India; 2000:348–351

Singh N, Juyal V, Gupta AK, Gahlot MH. Preliminary phytochemical investigation of extract of root of *Bergenia ligulata*. J Pharm Res 2009;2(9):1444–1447

The Ayurvedic Pharmacopeia of India. Part I, Vol. 1 New Delhi: Department of AYUSH, Ministry of Health and Family Welfare, Government of India; 1989:121

Ved DK, Kinhal GA, Ravikumar K, et al. Conservation assessment and management prioritization for the Medicinal plants of Jammu & Kashmir, Himachal Pradesh and Uttaranchal. Bangalore: Foundation for Revitalisation of Local Health Traditions; 2003

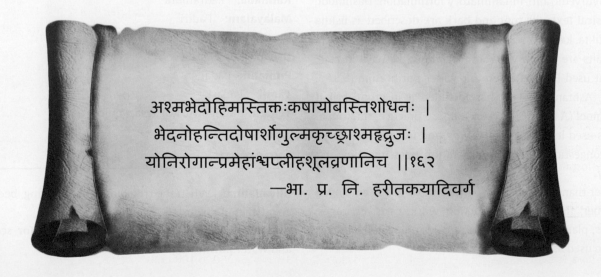

अश्मभेदोहिमस्तिक्तःकषायोबस्तिशोधनः ।
भेदनोहन्तिदोषार्शोगुल्मकृच्छ्राश्महृद्रुजः ।
योनिरोगान्प्रमेहांश्चप्लीहशूलव्रणानिच ।।१६२
—भा. प्र. नि. हरीतकयादिवर्ग

75. Patala *[Stereospermum suaveolens DC]*

Family:	*Bignoniaceae*
Hindi name:	*Patal, Padher*
English name:	*Trumphet flower*

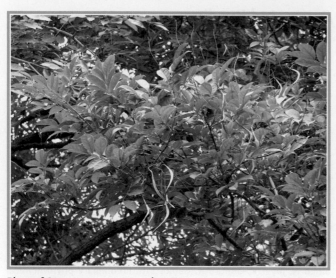

Plant of *Stereospermum suaveolens* DC.

> *Vriksha Ayurveda advocated irrigating Patala tree with water mixed with milk to promote flowering profusely.*
>
> *—Vk.a.14/153*

Introduction

Patala is a traditional plant endowed with immense medicinal properties. Almost all the plant parts are used in managing various ailments. Its root is one of the ingredients of an Ayurvedic anti-inflammatory formulation: Dashmool. In classical texts, its root and bark are described as ushna virya, tikta, kashaya rasa predominant, whereas its flowers and fruits are sheeta virya and madhura, kashaya in rasa. Sushrut used Patala flowers for water purification (S.S.Su. 45/13). Ashtang Hridaya has included it in group brihat panchmool (A.H.Su. 6/167). In folklore practice, traditional healers used its bark, roots, leaves, and flowers in malaria, chest congestion, body ache, eructation, piles, migraine, and obesity.

Other than medicinal properties, the wood is employed in timber, firewood, construction work, carts, carriages, wagons, planks, beams, furniture, and tool making. Leaves are also used as fodder.

Vernacular Names

Assamese: Parul
Bengali: Parul, Parlu
Gujarati: Podal
Kannada: Padramora
Malayalam: Padiri
Marathi: Padal
Oriya: Boro, Patulee
Punjabi: Padal
Tamil: Padari
Telugu: Kaligottu, Kokkesa, Podira

Synonyms

Alivallabha: When the tree blossoms in spring, bee wasp are attracted toward it.
Ambuvasini: Its fragrant flowers are used for scenting and water purification.

Amogha: It is believed to be an unfailing remedy.

Kaachsthali: Leaves have black-colored peduncle.

Kharaschhada: The surface of leaves is rough and leathery.

Krishanvrinta: The petiole of leaves is black colored.

Kuberakshi: Shape of the seeds is like eye ball.

Kumbhipushpi: The shape of the flower resembles a pitcher.

Madhudoot: The plant blossoms in spring.

Phaleruha: The plant is regenerated from its seeds.

Tamrapushpi: The plant bears copper-colored flowers.

Classical Categorization

Charaka Samhita: Shothahara, Triptighna, Virechanopaga

Sushruta Samhita: Aragvadhadi, Brihatpanchmool, Adhobhagahara

Ashtang Hridaya: Aragvadhadi

Dhanvantari Nighantu: Guduchyadi varga

Madanpal Nighantu: Abhyadi varga

Kaiyadev Nighantu: Oushadi varga

Raj Nighantu: Karviradi varga

Bhavaprakash Nighantu: Guduchyadi varga

Distribution

It is found in thick, deciduous forests of Bengal, Bihar, Himalayan Tarai, Kerala, and Tamil Nadu.

Morphology

It is a large, deciduous tree reaching up to a height of 15 to 20 m and 1.8 m in girth. Bark is gray, exfoliating into irregular flakes (**Fig. 75.1**).

- Leaves are compound, imparipinnate, opposite, 30 to 60 cm long, leaflets 3 to 4 pairs, broadly ovate-elliptic-oblong shape, acuminate often serrulate—entire margin (**Fig. 75.2a, b**).

- **Flowers:** Crimson colored, funnel shaped, sweet scented, occurs in inflorescence of large, trichotomous, hairy terminal panicles (**Fig. 75.3**).

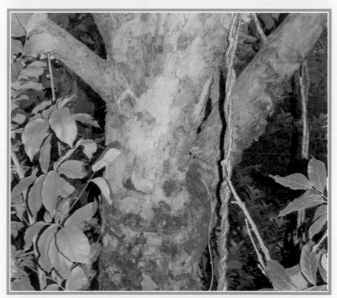

Fig. 75.1 Bark.

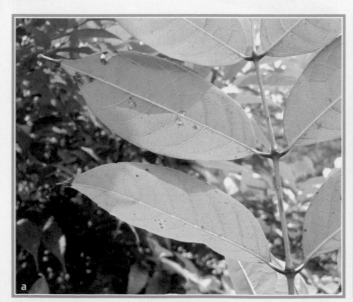
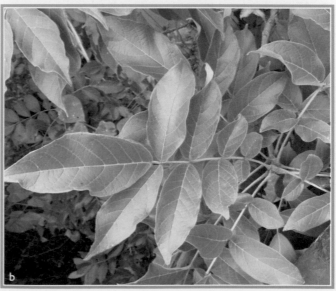

Fig. 75.2 (a) Leaves dorsal surface. (b) Leaves ventral surface.

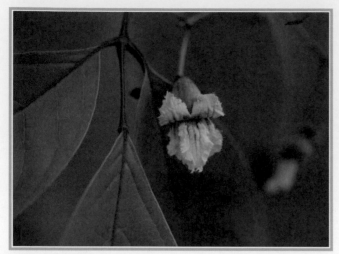

Fig. 75.3 Flower.

- **Fruits:** Elongate, cylindrical pod, four-ribbed, 30 to 40 cm long, rough with lenticels. Seeds are many, 2 to 3 cm long, with papery wings on both sides (**Fig. 75.4**).
- **Roots:** The outer surface of its root is dark brown and pale yellow to cream in color, rough with longitudinal striation, characteristic odor, and bitter taste.

The plant is propagated by its seeds (**Fig. 75.5**).

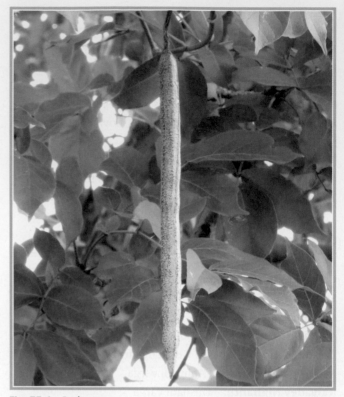

Fig. 75.4 Pod.

Phenology

Flowering time: March to June
Fruiting time: September to February

Key Characters for Identification

➤ *A large deciduous tree of 15 to 20 m height.*
➤ *Leaves are opposite, imparipinnate, leaflets 3 to 4 pairs, ovate to elliptic.*
➤ *Flowers are funnel shaped, scented, crimson colored.*
➤ *Fruits are cylindrical pod, 30 to 40 cm long, rough with lenticels.*

Types

- Bhavaprakash Nighantu: two types—Patala and Ghantapatala
- Raj Nighantu: two types—Patala and Sita Patala
- Kaiyadev and Dhanvantari Nighantu: two types—Patala and Kasta Patala
- Shaligrama Nighantu: three types—Bhumipatala, Kshudra patala, and Vallipatala

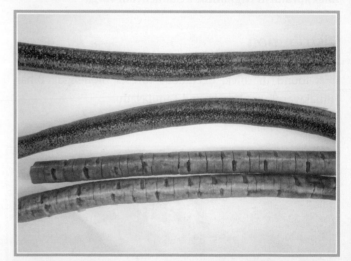

Fig. 75.5 Pod and seeds.

Rasapanchaka

Guna	Laghu, Ruksha
Rasa	Kashaya, Tikta
Vipaka	Katu
Virya	Anushna

Chemical Constituents

The plant is rich in flavonoids, saponins, phenolic compounds, and tannins. Bark has sterekunthal A & B, lapachol (naphthoquinones), dehydro-α-lapachone, sterochenol A & B, apigenin (flavonoid). Roots are rich in p-coumaric acid, triacontanol, cetyl alcohol, oleic, palmitic, stearic acid, lapachol, dehydro-α-lapachone, dehydrotectol, β-sitosterol, sterequinone C, streochenols A and B. Its leaves have scutellarein, 6-hydroxy luteolin, stereolensin, and dinatin (Ghani 2003; Khare 2007).

Identity, Purity, and Strength

For Stem Bark

- Foreign matter: Not more than 2%
- Total ash: Not more than 8%
- Acid-insoluble ash: Not more than 1%
- Alcohol-soluble extractive: Not less than 12.5%
- Water-soluble extractive: Not less than 25%

For Root

- Foreign matter: Not more than 2%
- Total ash: Not more than 8%
- Acid-insoluble ash: Not more than 6%
- Alcohol-soluble extractive: Not less than 10%
- Water-soluble extractive: Not less than 20%

(Source: The Ayurvedic Pharmacopeia of India 2001, 2004)

Karma (Actions)

Ayurvedic texts attributed shothhara (anti-inflammatory), adhobhagahara (pacifies diseases of urogenital system), vishaghna (antitoxin), deepana (carminative), chedana (incision), raktapittashamaka (antihemorrhagic), chardighna (antiemetic), hikkanigrahana (antihic-cough), jwaraghna (jwarghna), vedanasthapana (analgesic), and mutral (diuretic) properties to its root, whereas its flowers have hridya (cardiotonic), sheeta (coolant), kanthya (voice promoter), balya (tonic), poushtika (nutrient), and vajikara (aphrodisiac) properties.

- Doshakarma: Tridoshahara
- Dhatukarma: Shothahara, hridya, balya
- Malakarma: Mutral, vataanulomana

Pharmacological Actions

Scientific studies evidenced that its root and flowers possess anti-inflammatory, analgesic, anticancer, hepatoprotective, antihyperglycemic, antibacterial, antiviral, leishmanicidal, antitubercular, antioxidant, neuroprotective, and wound-healing properties (Chopra et al 1956; Moniruzzaman et al 2018).

Indications

Traditionally, its roots are used in the treatment of shotha (inflammations), adhyamana (flatulence), shwasa (asthma), sanipatika jwara (intermittent fever), vaman (vomiting), shrama (fatigue), shosha (wasting), aruchi (distaste), and trishna (excessive thirst). Flowers are used in hikka (hic-cough), daha (burning sensation), and pitta atisaar (diarrhea of paitika origin). Fruits are given in mutrakrichta (dysuria) and raktapitta (bleeding disorders). Leaves are used in maniacal cases, malarial fever, chronic dyspepsia, otalgia, odontalgia, wounds, and rheumatism. Traditional practitioners in Chhattisgarh used its bark in gout and piles (Kritikar and Basu 1999).

Therapeutic Uses

External Use

1. **Vranabandhana** (for wrapping wounds): Tender leaves of Kadamb, Arjuna, Nimba, Patala, Ashwathva, and Arka are used to cover wounds (C.S.Ci. 25/95).
2. **Adhkapari** (hemicrania): Patala beeja kalka is applied on forehead and temple region in hemicranias.
3. **Dagdhvrana (burn)**: Katu taila processed with decoction and paste of Patala on external application gives relief in pain and discharge in dagdhvrana, reduces burning sensation and blister formation (VM. 45/22).

Internal Use

1. **Hikka** (hic-cough): Flowers and fruit juice are taken with honey to control hiccups (S.S.U. 50/27).
2. **Ashmari and Mutraghata** (calculus and retention of urine): Seven times decanted Kshara of Patala mixed with oil is used in mutravikara (S.S.U. 58/46; VM. 33/4).
3. **Ashmari** (urinary calculus): Kshara of Patala and Karavira should be taken in ashmari (S.S.Ci. 7/22).

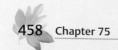

4. **Medovriddhi** (obesity): To reduce weight in obesity decoction of Patala, Chitraka mixed with Hingu, and Shatpushpa should be taken twice daily (B.P.Ci. 39/20).

Officinal Parts Used

Root bark, flowers, leaves, and kshara (alkali)

Dose

Decoction: 50 to 100 mL
Kshara: 1 to 3 g

Formulations

Dashmoolarishta, Brihatpanchmoolkwath, Dhanvantaram taila, Chyavanaprasa, Agastyarasayana.

Toxicity/Adverse Effects

Not reported.

Substitution and Adulteration

The other species of *Stereospermum* like *S. tetragonum* DC, *S. chelonoides* DC are used in place of each other (Billore et al 2004).

> **Points to Ponder**
>
> - *Botanically, two types of Patala are available Patala (Stereospermum suaveolens DC) and Sita or Kasta or Ghanta Patala (Stereospermum chelonoides DC).*
> - *Patala is a renowned drug for shotha, hikka, chardi, ardhavabhedaka, and amlapitta.*

Suggested Readings

Billore KV, Yelne MB, Dennis TJ, Chaudhari BG. Database on Medicinal Plants Used in Ayurveda, Vol. 6. New Delhi: C.C.R.A.S. Department of Indian Systems of Medicine and Homeopathy (ISM&H), Ministry of Health and Family Welfare, Government of India; 2004: 288–291

Chopra RN, Nayar SL, Chopra IC. Glossary of Indian Medicinal Plants. New Delhi: Council of Scientific and Industrial Research; 1956:235

Ghani A. Medicinal Plants of Bangladesh: Chemical Constituents and Uses. 2nd ed. Dhaka: Asiatic Society of Bangladesh; 2003

Khare CP. Indian Medicinal Plants: An Illustrated Dictionary. 1st ed. New York, NY: Springer; 2007:626–627

Kritikar KR, Basu BD. Indian Medicinal Plants, Vol. 2. Dehradun: International Book Distributors; 1999:1848

Moniruzzaman I, Kuddus MR, Haque MR, Chowdhury AMS, Rashid MA. *Stereospermum suaveolens* (Roxb.) DC: shows potential in vivo and in vitro bioactivities. Dhaka Univ J Pharm Sci 2018;17(2):257–263

The Ayurvedic Pharmacopeia of India. Part I, Vol. 3. New Delhi: Department of AYUSH, Ministry of Health and Family Welfare, Government of India; 2001:149

The Ayurvedic Pharmacopeia of India. Part I, Vol. 4. New Delhi: Department of AYUSH, Ministry of Health and Family Welfare, Government of India; 2004:100

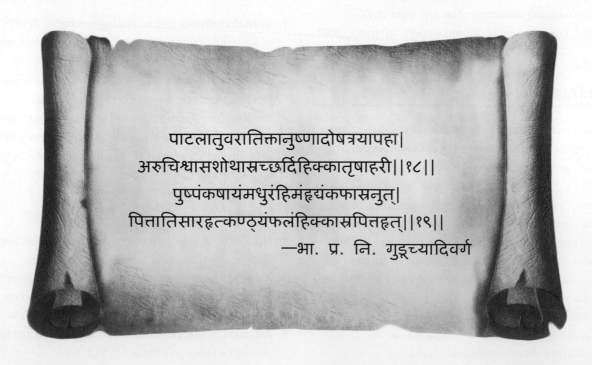

पाटलातुवरातिक्तानुष्णादोषत्रयापहा।
अरुचिश्वासशोथास्रच्छर्दिहिक्कातृषाहरी॥१८॥
पुष्पंकषायंमधुरंहिमंहृद्यंकफास्रनुत्।
पित्तातिसारहृत्कण्ठ्यंफलंहिक्कास्रपित्तहृत्॥१९॥
—भा. प्र. नि. गुडूच्यादिवर्ग

76. Pippali-Pippalimula [*Piper longum* Linn.]

Family:	*Piperaceae*
Hindi name:	*Pippali*
English name:	*Long pepper*

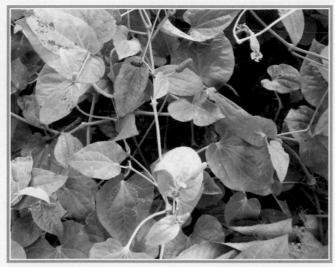

Plant of *Piper longum* Linn.

Pippali is a major ingredient of famous digestive and carminative formulations such as Trikatu, Chaturushna, Panchkola, and Shadaushna.

Introduction

The name Pippali is derived from English word *pepper*. Pippali along with black pepper is a famous trade item since time immemorial. It was used for preparing spice mixture in European cuisine. Hippocrates first described long pepper as a medicament and a spice. It is widely used in seasoning food, preparing spices, and making pickles. It is believed that Pippali originated during the time of *samudra manthan* (churning of ocean). In Brahmanas, Upanishads, and Puranas, Pippali is used as an aphrodisiac drug. Since then it is used as single drug or in combination to treat various ailments related to respiratory and digestive system. Pippali when taken with other drugs increases the bioavailability and absorption of the other active ingredients. Nowadays Pippali is used as a popular bioenhancer drug.

Ashtang considered Pippali as the best remedy for splenomegaly (A.H.U. 40/48). Charaka has included this in shirovirechana, vaman, and santarpaniya dravya (C.S.Su. 2/3,7). It is stated that Pippalimula is the best deepana, pachana, and aanahahshamaka dravya (C.S.Su. 25/40). Pippali is a major ingredient in many yavagus like shoolghna, krimighna, pipasaghna, vataanulomani, and kanthya (C.S.Su. 2/18,23,24,29,31). Charaka has included it in aharayogi varga whereas Sushrut has described it under shaka varga (S.S.Su. 46/223). Acharya Charaka has elucidated yogavahi karma of Pippali; due to this special property it is used in various formulations as a medicine and adjuvant. In C.S.Ci. 26 where virudhavirya dravyas are mentioned, katu rasa dravyas are described as avrishya dravya but Pippali and Shunthi are quoted as exception to it.

Vernacular Names

Arabian: Dra-filfil
Bengali: Pipulmul
Gujarati: Gantoda, Ganthoda, Lindipipal, pipal
Kannada: Modikaddi, Hippali, Tippali, Modi

Malayalam: Kattuthippaliver, Tippaliveru, Lada, Mulagu
Marathi: Pimpli
Oriya: Baihehi, Krykola, Mogodha, Pippoli
Punjabi: Pippali, Maghapipal, Pipal, Filfildaras
Persian: Filfilidray, Pipal, Filfil-i-daras
Sindhi: Tippali
Tamil: Kanda Tippili, Ambinadi Desavaram
Telugu: Modi, Madikatta, Pippallu, pipili, Pippalikatte
Urdu: Filfil Daraz

Synonyms

Chapala: On oral intake, the fruits produce tingling sensation.
Kana: The fruits appear in small berries pattern.
Krishna: The dried fruit is black in color.
Magadhi: It is commonly found in Magadha region.
Shaundi: The fruits are arranged in spike pattern like elephant trunk.
Tikshnatandula: The dried fruit is sharp and pungent in taste.
Upakulya: It easily grows around the water source.
Ushna: The fruit is hot in action and potency.
Vaidehi: It is commonly found in Vaidehi region.

Classical Categorization

Charaka Samhita: Deepaniya, Sheetaprashamana, Shoolprashamana, Kasahara, Hikkanigrahana, Kanthya, Triptighna, Asthapanopaga, Shirovirechanopaga

Sushrut Samhita: Pippalayadi, Amalakyadi, Trikatu, Urdhvabhaghara
Ashtang Hridaya: Pippalayadi
Dhanvantari Nighantu: Shatapushpadi varga
Madanpal Nighantu: Sunthyadi varga
Kaiyadev Nighantu: Oushadi varga
Raj Nighantu: Pippalayadi varga
Bhavaprakash Nighantu: Haritakyadi varga

Distribution

Pippali is native to India–Malaysian region. It is found growing in wild as well as in cultivation in tropical, subtropical rain forests of India, Nepal, Sri Lanka, and adjoining areas. It occurs throughout the hotter parts of India mostly in Assam, West Bengal, Konkan, Kerala, Karnataka, and Andaman and Nicobar.

Morphology

It is a slender, aromatic climber with perennial woody roots. Stems creeping, jointed, erect, subscandent, swollen, and produce roots at the nodes.

- **Leaves:** Simple, axillary, alternate, lower one broadly ovate to cordate, upper one oblong, oval in shape, subacute apex, margin entire, shiny, glabrous, and dark green (**Fig. 76.1**).
- **Flowers:** Yellowish-green, dioecious, which occurs in solitary cylindrical spikes, pedunculate; male flowers are large and slender whereas female flowers are small (**Fig. 76.2**).

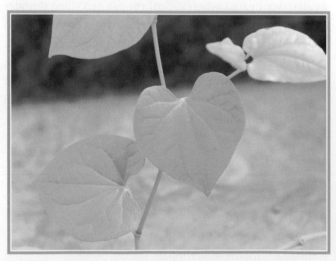

Fig. 76.1 Leaves.

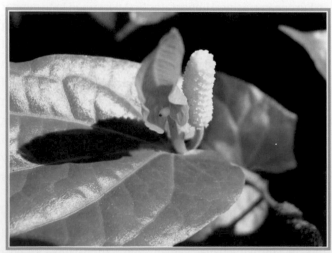

Fig. 76.2 Flower.

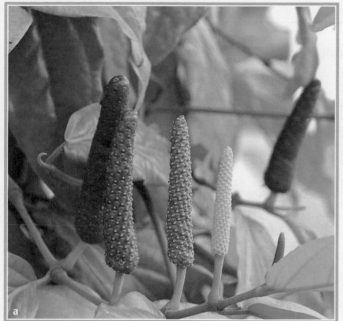

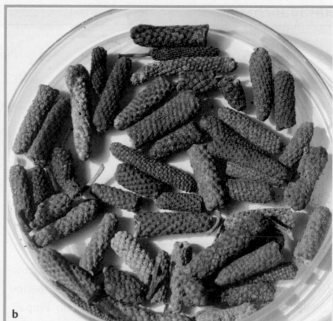

Fig. 76.3 **(a)** Raw fruits. **(b)** Dried fruits.

The plant is propagated by its seeds, root suckers, and air layering method.

Phenology

Flowering time: October to December
Fruiting time: October to December

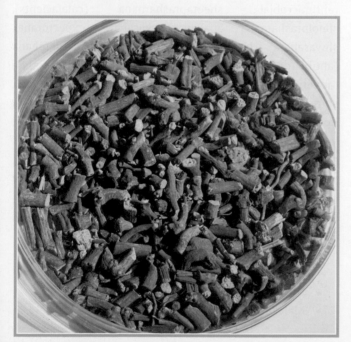

Fig. 76.4 Pippalimula.

- **Fruits:** Oblong berries, small, unripe green which turns to yellowish orange and red when fully ripe and when completely dried, it turns black in color which is completely sunk in solid fleshy spike (**Fig. 76.3a**). Mature and dried spikes form the commercial form of Pippali (**Fig. 76.3b**).
- Roots are slender, brown, and pungent in taste, known as Pippalimula (**Fig. 76.4**).

> ### Key Characters for Identification
>
> ➤ *An aromatic climber with perennial woody roots and creeping stem.*
> ➤ *Leaves alternate, oval to cordate shape, dark green with shiny surface*
> ➤ *Flowers occur in cylindrical spikes, color yellowish green*
> ➤ *Fruits oblong berries, unripe green, mature red-orange and dried black in colorRoots are slender, brown, and pungent*

Types

Raj Nighantu has described four types of Pippali:
- Pippali
- Gaja pippali
- Sanhali pippali
- Vanya pippali

Rasapanchaka

	Pippali (shushka)	Pippali (aadra)	Pippalimula
Guna	Laghu, snigdha, tikshna	Guru, snigdha	Laghu, ruksha
Rasa	Katu	Katu	Katu
Vipaka	Madhura	Madhura	Katu
Virya	Anushna sheeta	Sheeta	Ushna
Doshaghanta	Kapha vatashamaka	Kapha vardhaka	Kapha vatashamaka

Chemical Constituents

Pippali fruit contains alkaloids, amides, volatile oils, saponins, carbohydrates, amygdalin, starch, and protein. Piperine (alkaloid) is the major and active constituent in Pippali. Other constituents are piperlongumine, pipernonaline, pipercide, sesamine, methyl piperine, piperettine, asarinin, pellitorine, piperundecalidine, retrofractamide A, pergumidiene, brachystamide-B, propenal, piperoic acid, β-sitosterol, caryophyllene, sesquiterpenes, and essential oils (Zaveri et al 2010; Rastogi and Malhotra 1993).

Identity, Purity, and Strength

For Mula

- Foreign matter: Not more than 2%
- Total ash: Not more than 5.5%
- Acid-insoluble ash: Not more than 0.2%
- Alcohol-soluble extractive: Not less than 4%
- Water-soluble extractive: Not less than 12%

For Fruit

- Foreign matter: Not more than 2%
- Total ash: Not more than 5.5%
- Acid-insoluble ash: Not more than 0.2%
- Alcohol-soluble extractive: Not less than 4%
- Water-soluble extractive: Not less than 12%

(Source: The Ayurvedic Pharmacopeia of India 1999, 2004)

Karma (Actions)

Ayurvedic classics describe dried Pippali fruit as deepana (appetizer), pachana (digestive), rochan (relish), vrishya (aphrodisiac), rasayana (rejuvenator), rechana (mild laxative), jwaraghna (antipyretic), medhya (brain tonic), hridya (cardiotonic), krimighna (antimicrobial), sheetaprashamana (calefacients), shoolprashamana (analgesic), kasahara (expectorant), shwasahara (bronchial antispasmodic), hikkanigrahana (antihic-cough), kanthya (voice promoter), triptighna (appetizers), asthapanopaga (adjuvant in nonoily enema), shirovirechan (errhines), raktotkleshaka (aggravated rakta dosha), jantughna (antibacterial), vatahara (pacify vata), vatanulomana (laxative), yakriduttejaka (liver stimulant), mutrala (diuretic), kushthaghna (antidermatosis), vishamjwarapratibandhaka (cures irregular fever), balya (tonic), and garbhashayasankochaka (uterine astringent).

- Pippalimula: Deepana, krimighna, rochana, pittakopaka, vatahara, pachana, bhedana
- Doshakarma: Tridoshashamaka, Pittaprakopaka (shushka), Pittashamaka (aadra)
- Dhatukarma: Rasayana, Vrishya
- Malakarma: Rechana, vataanulomana, mutral

Pharmacological Actions

It is reported to exhibit antibacterial, antidiarrheal, antipyretic, analgesic, anti-inflammatory, antioxidant, insecticidal, antimalarial, anticancer, antitumor, CNS stimulant, antitubercular, anthelmintic, antiobesity, hypoglycemic, antispasmodic, neuroprotective, cough suppressor, immunomodulator, hepatoprotective, radioprotective, cardioprotective, anticonvulsant, antiplatelet, antinarcotic, antiulcerogenic, and antiasthmatic activities (Kumar et al., 2011).

Indications

Pippali is advocated to be used in the treatment of shwasa (asthma), kasa (cough), hikka (hic-cough), trishna (thirst), jwara (fever), prameha (diabetes), udarroga (abdominal diseases), gulma (abdominal tumors), shool (colic), adhyamana (flatulence), kushta (skin diseases), arsha (piles), pleeharoga (splenomegaly), katishool (lumbago), shotha (edema), medovriddhi (obesity), vatavyadhi (diseases of aggravated vata), pakshaghata (paralysis), yakritavikara (hepatic disorders), jeernajwara (chronic fever), agnimandhya (anorexia), ajeerna (indigestion), aruchi (dyspepsia), vibandh (constipation), hridyadourbalya (cardiac debility), pandu (anemia), krimiroga (worm infestation), kshaya (wasting), sheetayukta vedana (pain due to cold), amavata (arthritis), sandhivata (osteoarthritis), mutravrodha (urinary retention), mastishka daurbalya (mental debility), raktavikara (bleeding disorders), yakshma (tuberculosis), shukradaurbalya, daurbalya (general debility), rajorodha (amenorrhea), and kashta prasava (difficult labor).

Pippalimula is indicated specifically in vatoudara (a type of abdominal disease), krimiroga (anthelmintic), adhyamana (flatulence), pleeharoga (spleenomegaly), gulma (abdominal tumour), shwasa (asthma), kshaya (emaciation), agnimandhya (loss of appetite), and vatavyadhi (diseases of aggravated vata).

The fruits are used after child birth to check postpartum hemorrhage, as a cholagogue in bile duct and gall bladder obstruction. Unripe fruit is used as an alternative and tonic. A decoction of immature fruits and roots is used in chronic bronchitis, cough, and cold, and is also used in palsy, gout, rheumatism, and lumbago.

Therapeutic Uses

External Use

1. **Shushkakasa** (dry cough): Pippali kept in mouth with malyavacha, yavani, and betel leaf as lozenge prevents dry cough (B.P.Ci. 1/335).

2. **Hikka** (hic-cough): Pippali mixed with sharkara is taken as nasya in hikka (G.N. 2/11/50).

3. **Dantshool** (toothache): Pippali mixed with madhughrita should be kept in mouth in dantashool (VM. 8/17).

Internal Use

1. **Pleehavridhi** (splenomegaly): Pippali powder mixed with lohabhasma should be taken with milk in enlarged spleen (GN. 2/32/49). Consumption of Pippali impregnated with Palashakshara alleviates gulma and pleeha (VM. 37/40).

2. **Vardhman Pippali Rasayana** (rejuvinator): It is a special treatment procedure in which administration of Pippali powder is done in increasing dose for few days then it is decreased and finally withdrawn. It is prescribed in jeernajwara, vatarakta, aruchi, pandu, gulma, pleeha, arsha, udarroga, shotha, kshaya, shosha, garhni, etc. Starting with 1 g powder twice a day on the first day, it is increased by 1 g daily up to a maximum of 5 g on the fifth day, then it is decreased by 1 g daily to a dose of 1 g. Total duration of the treatment is 15 days (C.S.Ci. 1/3/38).

3. **Vishamjwara** (irregular fever): Intake of Pippali, Triphala, dadhi, takra, panchagavya ghrita, and dugdha is recommended in vishamjwara (C.S.Ci. 3/303). Pippali mixed with equal quantity of guda gives relief in jeernajwara and agnimandhya (VM. 1/206).

4. **Kasa** (cough): Intake of 0.5 g of Pippali churna with madhu helps in curing dry cough (B.P.Ci. 12/34). Daily consumption of 1 to 2 tsf Avleha prepared from Draksha and Pippali powder helps in alleviating phlegm, and eases cough and asthma.

5. **Shwasa** (asthma)**:** Powdered Pippali, Amalaki, Shunthi mixed with madhusharkara gives immediate relief in asthma and hic-cough (CD. 12/7).

6. **Arsha** (hemorrhoids): Pippali and Abhya mixed with guda should be taken in arsha (H.S. 3/11/33).

7. **Udarroga** (abdominal diseases): 1,000 Pippali fruits impregnated with snuhidugdha should be gradually consumed in udarroga (S.S.Ci. 14/10) or vardhmana Pippali rasayana should be used.

8. **Gradharsi** (sciatica): Intake of Pippali powder with gomutra and Eranda taila subsides chronic sciatica (B.P.Ci. 24/139).

9. **Garbhanirodh** (contraceptive): Intake of equal amount of Vidangabeeja, tankana, and Pippali churna with milk during the season prevents pregnancy (B.P.Ci. 70/33).

10. **Kshaya and Shosha** (wasting): Intake of linctus prepared with Pippali, Ashvagandha, sharkara with madhughrita is beneficial in kshaya and shosha (CD. 10/14).

11. **Medoroga** (obesity): Pippali churna singly or trikatu along with madhu is administered to treat obesity.

12. **Krimiroga** (worm infestation): Pippalimula should be taken with ajadugdha in worm infestation (S.S.U. 54/32).

13. **Urustambha** (stiffness of thigh): Decoction or paste of Pippali, Pippalimula, and Bhallataka mixed with madhu should be taken daily (G.N. 2/21/22,28).

14. **Stanyavardhana** (galactogogue): Dugdha mixed with Maricha and Pippalimula should be consumed to increase milk production (H.S. 3/53/3).

15. **Nidranasha** (insomnia): Intake of Pippalimula churna with guda is recommended in nidranasha (B.P.Ci. 1/326).

Officinal Parts Used

Fruit and root

Dose

Powder: 0.5 to 1 g

Formulations

Trikatu, Guda Pippali, Pippali khanda, Chausathprahari pippali, Vardhmaan Pippali Rasayana, Sitopaladi churna, Pippalyasava, Ashtangavaleha, Pugakhanda, Vyaghriharitaki avaleha.

Toxicity/Adverse Effects

Since Pippali is ushna, tikshna in properties, it should be avoided in pregnancy and lactation. It is also reported not to use Pippali with barbiturates and phenytoin. However, chronic toxicity studies revealed no untoward effects.

Substitution and Adulteration

The dried fruits of Pippali are often adulterated with other *Piper* species like *Piper peepuloides* Roxb., *Piper retrofractum* Vahl, and *Piper betle* Linn. Pippalimula is adulterated with stem pieces of Pippali and its other allied species (Sharma et al 2001).

Points to Ponder

- *Pippali is used in both dried and wet form. In dried form, it is Pittaprakopaka and in wet form it pacifies pitta (pittashamaka).*
- *Vardhmana Pippali rasayana is the most popular formulation of Pippali.*
- *Pippali is the drug of choice in jeerna jwara, visham jwara, pleehavriddhi, yakritaroga, kasa, shwasa, vatavyadhi, udarroga, and gulma.*

Suggested Readings

Kumar S, Kamboj J, Suman, Sharma S. Overview for various aspects of the health benefits of Piper longum linn. fruit. J Acupunct Meridian Stud 2011;4(2):134–140

Rastogi RP, Malhotra BN. Compendium of Indian Medicinal Plants. Lucknow and New Delhi: NISC, CDRI; 1993:504–857

Sharma PC, Yelne MB, Dennis TJ. Database on Medicinal Plants Used in Ayurveda, Vol. 3. New Delhi: CCRAS Department of Indian Systems of Medicine and Homeopathy (ISM&H), Ministry of Health and Family Welfare, Government of India; 2001:472–476

The Ayurvedic Pharmacopeia of India. Part I, Vol. 2. New Delhi: Department of AYUSH, Ministry of Health and Family Welfare, Government of India; 1999:142

The Ayurvedic Pharmacopeia of India. Part I, Vol. 4. New Delhi: Department of AYUSH, Ministry of Health and Family Welfare, Government of India; 2004:106

Zaveri M, Khandar A, Patel S. Chemistry and pharmacology of *Piper longum* L. Int J Innov Pharmaceut Sci Res 2010;5(1):67–76

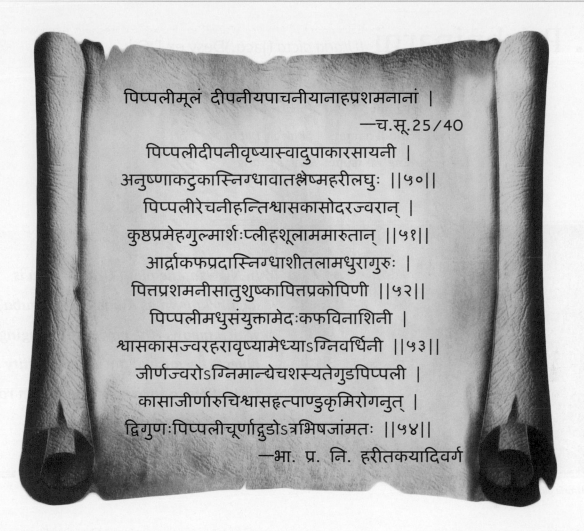

पिप्पलीमूलं दीपनीयपाचनीयानाहप्रशमनानां |

—च.सू. 25/40

पिप्पलीदीपनीवृष्यास्वादुपाकारसायनी |
अनुष्णाकटुकास्निग्धावातश्लेष्महरीलघुः ||५०||

पिप्पलीरेचनीहन्तिश्वासकासोदरज्वरान् |
कुष्ठप्रमेहगुल्मार्शःप्लीहशूलाममारुतान् ||५१||

आर्द्राकफप्रदास्निग्धाशीतलामधुरागुरुः |
पित्तप्रशमनीसातुशुष्कापित्तप्रकोपिणी ||५२||

पिप्पलीमधुसंयुक्तामेदःकफविनाशिनी |
श्वासकासज्वरहरावृष्यामेध्याऽग्निवर्धिनी ||५३||

जीर्णज्वरोऽग्निमान्द्येचशस्यतेगुडपिप्पली |
कासाजीर्णारुचिश्वासहृत्पाण्डुकृमिरोगनुत् |
द्विगुणःपिप्पलीचूर्णाद्रुडोऽत्रभिषजांमतः ||५४||

—भा. प्र. नि. हरीतक्यादिवर्ग

77. Prishniparni [*Uraria picta* (Jacq.)Desv.ex.DC.]

Family: *Fabaceae (Papilionaceae)*

Hindi name: *Pithivan, Dabra*

English name: *Indian Uraria*

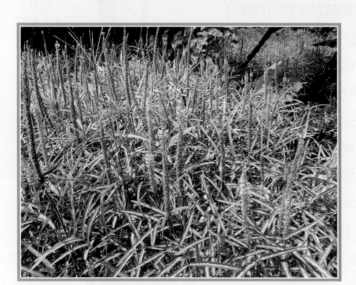

Plant of *Uraria picta* (Jacq.) Desv.ex.DC.

In Nigeria, the plant Uraria picta is locally known as Alupayida (Yoruba) which means "the power of changing object" because of the unique ability of its leaflets to turn inside out when rolled and beaten together.

Introduction

The plant is assigned the name Prishniparni or Prithakparni due to its variegated/blotched pattern found on the surface of leaves. Since ages, it has been widely used as a content of Laghupanchmula and Dashmoola, a famous anti-inflammatory formulation. In classical texts, Prishniparni is described under chatusparni, i.e., Shalaparni, Prishniparni, Mudgaparni, and Mashaparni. Charaka has used it in preparation of pachani, grahi, and atisaar har yavagu (C.S.Su. 2/19-21) and included it in dravyas used for asthapana basti (C.S.Su. 2/11). Charaka considered it as the best deepan, vrishya, sangrahi, and vatahara dravya (C.S.Su. 255/40). Sushrut has recommended using Prishniparni siddha ghrita during fourth month so as to maintain pregnancy smoothly (S.S.Sa. 10/4). Ashtang Hridaya also advocated using it in threatened abortion (A.H.Sa. 2/56).

Prishniparni is a popular medicine in folklore and among traditional practitioners. In folklore, its root decoction is employed for fracture union and heart diseases. In Bihar, the root and fruit are used to treat anal prolapse in children. In Madhya Pradesh, tribal people apply its root paste in snake bite (Parrotta 2001).

Vernacular Names

Bengali: Salpani, Chhalani, Chakule
Gujarati: Pithavan, Selman
Kannada: Murele Honne, Ondele honne, Prushniparni
Malayalam: Orila, Pulatti
Marathi: Pithvan, Prushnipamee, Radbhal
Oriya: Prushnipamee, Shankarjata
Punjabi: Detedarnee
Tamil: Oripai
Telugu: Kolakuponna
Urdu: Shalwan

Synonyms

Chitraparni: The lamina is stripped in different colors.

Dhavani: The plant spreads easily on the ground.

Guha: The plant has deep-seated roots.

Kalashi: It is vrishya (aphrodisiac) in action.

Kroshtuvinna: The inflorescence resembles the tail of jackal or tiger.

Prithakparni: Its leaves' lamina is stripped giving it a distinct appearance.

Sinhapuchchhi: The terminal inflorescence resembles tail of jackal or tiger.

Classical Categorization

Charaka Samhita: Sandhaniya, Angamarda prashasmana, Shothahara

Sushrut Samhita: Vidarigandhadi, Haridradi, Laghupanchamool

Ashtang Hridaya: Haridradi

Dhanvantari Nighantu: Guduchyadi varga

Madanpal Nighantu: Abhyadi varga

Kaiyadev Nighantu: Oushadi varga

Raj Nighantu: Shatvahadi varga

Bhavaprakash Nighantu: Guduchyadi varga

Distribution

It is widely distributed in Australia, Africa, and all parts of Asia. It is usually found in grasslands, waste places, open deciduous forests, and in open plains all over India up to an altitude of 1,800 m.

Morphology

It is an erect, unbranched, annual herb or undershrub, reaching up to 1 m in height.

- **Leaves:** Compound, imparipinnate, 20 to 30 cm long. Leaflets on the upper part of the stem are five to seven in number, 10 to 20 cm long, 2 cm wide, linear, lanceolate, oblong, acute apex, blotched with white irregular-shaped spots throughout the length of the leaves, minutely pubescent beneath, base rounded (**Fig. 77.1**).
- **Flowers:** Pink or purple, in close spicate fascicles along the rachis of cylindrical 15 to 30 cm long racemes, rachis and pedicels downy with hooked hair (**Fig. 77.2**).
- **Fruits:** Pods, pale lead-colored, four to six in number, jointed together, 4 to 5 cm long, smooth, polished with light brown reniform-shaped seeds.
- **Root:** Tap root up to 30 cm long, 1 to 2 cm wide, tough woody externally light yellow to grayish buff in color, internally pale yellow. Fracture fibrous, odor indistinct, taste slightly acrid.

The plant is propagated by its seeds.

Phenology

Flowering time: March to April

Fruiting time: July to December

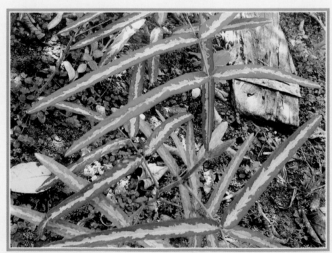

Fig. 77.1 Leaves.

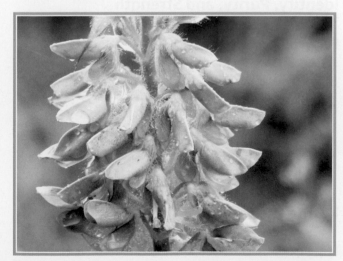

Fig. 77.2 Flowers.

Rasapanchaka

Guna	Laghu, Snigdha
Rasa	Madhura, Tikta
Vipaka	Madhura
Virya	Ushna

Chemical Constituents

Prishniparni roots are reported to be rich in flavonoids, isoflavanones, triterpenes, steroids, stigmasta-4, 22-diene-3-one, β-sitosterol, amino acids, and fatty acids (Rahman et al 2007). 5,7-Dihydroxy-2'-methoxy-3',4'-methylenedioxy isoflavanone and 4',5-dihydroxy-2',3'-dimethoxy-7-(5-hydroxyoxychromen-7yl)-isoflavanone are the active ones.

Identity, Purity, and Strength

For Whole Plant

- Foreign matter: Not more than 2%
- Total ash: Not more than 11%
- Acid-insoluble ash: Not more than 4%
- Alcohol-soluble extractive: Not less than 7%
- Water-soluble extractive: Not less than 8%

(Source: The Ayurvedic Pharmacopeia of India 2004)

Karma (Actions)

Prishniparni is described as sangrahi (absorbent), vrishya (aphrodisiac), sara (laxative), balya (strength promoting), digestive, deepana (carminative), shothahara (anti-inflammatory), shoolaprasasmana (analgesic), jwaraghna (antipyretic), chardighna (antiemetic), vishaghna (antitoxin), kaphanisaraka (expectorant), and mutral (diuretic).

- Doshakarma: Tridoshashamaka
- Dhatukarma: Vrishya, balya
- Malakarma: Sara, mutral

Pharmacological Actions

The root is reported to exhibit anti-inflammatory, antimicrobial, antithrombotic, hepatoprotective, antioxidant, antianxiety, antidepressant, hypolipidemic, and cardioprotective activities (Hem et al 2017).

Indications

The root is widely used in the treatment of daha (burning sensation), jwara (fever), kasa (cough), shwasa (asthma), raktaatisaar (bleeding diarrhea), rakta arsha (bleeding piles), rakta pravahika (dysentery associated with blood), shotha (inflammation), trishna (excessive thirst), vaman (vomiting), vataroga (diseases of aggravated vata), unmada (insanity), vrana (wound), visha (poison). The leaves are antiseptic and are used in gonorrhea. Pods are used in mouth ulcers. Roots and leaves are used for typhoid and tetanus (Chopra et al 1956).

Therapeutic Uses

External Use

1. **Sarpadansha** (snake bite): Fresh juice extracted from Prishniparni panchang is applied on the affected area in snake poison, scorpion sting, and other insect bite.
2. **Vranaropana** (wound healing): Ghrita prepared with Prishniparni, Kapikacchu, Haridra, Malati, sharkara, and drugs of Kakolyadi gana should be used for vranaropana (S.S.Su. 37/25).

Internal Use

1. **Raktaatisaar** (bleeding diarrhea): Peya (liquid gruel) prepared with Prishniparni checks bleeding in diarrhea (C.S.Su. 2/21).

2. **Raktaarsha** (bleeding piles): Lajapeya processed with Bala and Prishniparni controls bleeding in arsha (C.S.Ci. 14/199).

3. **Raktapitta** (hemorrhagic disorders): Yavagu prepared with Masura and Prishniparni added with madhu sharkara checks internal hemorrhage (C.S.Ci. 4/46-48).

4. **Bhagna** (fracture): Intake of Prishniparni mool churna with manshrasa for 3 weeks unites the fracture bone (B.P.Ci. 48/30).

5. **Vatarakta** (gout): Prishniparni cooked in Aja dugdha and mixed with madhu sharkara is beneficial in vatarakta (S.S.Ci. 5/7).

6. **Madatyaya janya trishna** (thirst due to alcoholism): Water processed with Prishniparni should be used as drink in excessive thirst due to alcoholism (C.S.Ci. 24/165).

Officinal Parts Used

Root and leaves

Dose

Root decoction: 50 to 100 mL

Formulations

Prishniparnayadi kwath, Dashmula kwath, Dashmularishta.

Toxicity/Adverse Effects

Not reported.

Substitution and Adulteration

In crude drug market in the name of Prishniparni root (content of dashmula), stem or whole plant is available. Prishniparni is mixed with other similar looking species of genus *uraria* like *Uraria crinite, U. lagopodioides,* and *U. neglecta* (Billore et al 2004).

> **Points to Ponder**
>
> - *Prishniparni is an important constituent of Laghupanchmool and Dashmoola.*
> - *It is a renowned shothahara, asthi sandhaniya, sangrahi, deepana, vrishya, vatahara dravya in Ayurveda.*

Suggested Readings

Billore KV, Yelne MB, Dennis TJ, Chaudhari BG. Database on Medicinal Plants Used in Ayurveda, Vol. 6. New Delhi: CCRAS Department of Indian Systems of Medicine and Homeopathy (ISM&H), Ministry of Health and Family Welfare, Government of India; 2004:314–316

Chopra RN, Nayar SL, Chopra IC. Glossary of Indian Medicinal Plants. New Delhi: CSIR; 1956:250

Hem K, Singh NK, Singh MK. Anti-inflammatory and hepato-protective activities of the roots of *Uraria picta.* Int J Green Pharm 2017;11(1):166–173

Parrotta JA. Healing Plants of Peninsular India, USDA Forest Service, International Institute of Tropical Forestry, Puerto Rico, USA. United Kingdom: CABI Publishing; 2001:393–394, 418–419

Rahman MM, Gibbons S, Gray AI. Isoflavanones from Uraria picta and their antimicrobial activity. Phytochemistry 2007;68(12):1692–1697

The Ayurvedic Pharmacopeia of India. Part I, Vol. 4. New Delhi: Government of India, Ministry of Health and Family Welfare, Department of AYUSH; 2004:115

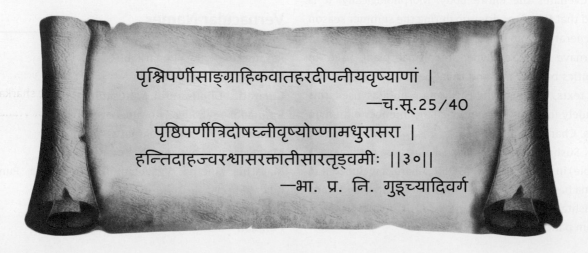

पृश्निपर्णीसाङ्ग्राहिकवातहरदीपनीयवृष्याणां |
—च.सू.25/40
पृष्ठिपर्णीत्रिदोषघ्नीवृष्योष्णामधुरासरा |
हन्तिदाहज्वरश्वासरक्तातीसारतृड्वमीः ||३०||
—भा. प्र. नि. गुड्च्यादिवर्ग

78. Punarnava [Boerhavia diffusa Linn.]

Family:	Nyctaginaceae
Hindi name:	Sathi
English name:	Hogweed, Horse Purslene, Gadapurna

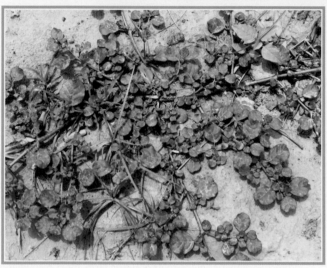

Plant of *Boerhavia diffusa* Linn.

The Genus was named Boerhavia in honor of Hermann Boerhaave, a famous Dutch physician of the 18th century.

Introduction

There are about 40 tropical and subtropical species of *Boerhavia*, out of which 6 are found in India, namely, *B. diffusa*, *B. chinensis*, *B. erecta*, *B. repens*, *B. rependa*, and *B. rubicund*. In Atharva Veda, Punarnava is described as a herb that rejuvenates the entire body. Morphologically, it is observed that the plant dries up during the summer season and regenerates again during the rainy season.

Punarnava is a renowned medicinal plant used in therapeutics by endemic and tribal people since ages. Our ancient texts, Charaka and Sushruta Samhitas used this plant widely for the treatment of a large number of human ailments. Charaka considered it as rasayana and kasahara whereas Sushrut described its shaka as best pathyashaka (vegetable) in shotha (S.S.Su. 46/255). Charaka included it in asthapana basti dravya whereas Sushrut in vata sansamana varga. Ashtanga Hridaya has included it in the group of madhyam panchmool (A.H.Su. 6/169).

The fresh leaves and roots are eaten as vegetables in curries and soups by the tribals. Roots and seeds are added to cereals, pancakes, and other food as nutrient source. Seeds are also served as bird feed. The leaves are given to cattle as fodder so as to increase milk yield (Anonymous 1988).

Vernacular Names

Assamese: Ranga Punarnabha
Bengali: Rakta punarnava
Gujarati: Dholisaturdi, Motosatodo
Kannada: Sanadika, Kommeberu, Komma
Kashmiri: Vanjula Punarnava
Malayalam: Chuvanna Tazhutawa
Marathi: Ghetuli, Vasuchimuli, Satodimula, Punarnava, Khaparkhuti
Oriya: Lalapuiruni, Nalipuruni
Punjabi: ltcit (lal), Khattan

Tamil: Mukurattai (Shihappu)

Telugu: Atikamamidi, Erra galijeru

Synonyms

Deerghapatrika: It bears extra megaphyllous leaves.

Mandalpatrika: The shape of leaves is round.

Rakta: The stem is red colored.

Raktpushpa: The plant bears red-colored flowers.

Shilatika: Therapeutically, it is a useful drug.

Shothaghni: It is a potent anti-inflammatory drug.

Shwetmoola: The plant has white roots.

Varshketu: The plant regenerates every year in rainy season.

Classical Categorization

Charaka Samhita: Vyasthapana, Kasahara, Swedopaga, Anuvasanopaga

Sushrut Samhita: Vidarigandhadi

Ashtang Hridaya: Vidaryadi gana (described as vrischira)

Dhanvantari Nighantu: Guduchyadi varga

Madanpal Nighantu: Abhyadi varga

Kaiyadev Nighantu: Oushadi varga

Raj Nighantu: Parpatadi varga

Bhavaprakash Nighantu: Guduchyadi varga

Distribution

It is found throughout India as weed up to an altitude of 2,000 ft. It grows abundantly in waste places, fields, and marshy places during rainy season.

Morphology

It is a perennial diffuse herb with stout root stock and many procumbent branches.

- **Leaves:** Simple, opposite or subopposite, short petiole, broadly unequal pairs, green above and reddish beneath, ovate or suborbicular shape, acute-obtuse apex, round or subcordate at the base (**Fig. 78.1**).
- **Flowers:** Pink, red, or purple, small, short stalked, in irregular clusters of axillary or terminal corymbs (**Fig. 78.2**).
- **Fruits:** Ovoid or subellipsoid, rounded above, slightly cuneate below, five-ribbed with glandular, viscid hair, easily detachable, single seeded, indehiscent with a thin pericarp.

The stem and root are shown in **Fig. 78.3 and Fig. 78.4**, respectively.

Phenology

Flowering time: May to August

Fruiting time: May to August

Key Characters for Identification

➤ *A perennial diffuse herb with many procumbent branches*

➤ *Leaves: Simple, opposite, unequal pairs, ovate or suborbicular shape*

➤ *Flowers: Small pink or purple, occurs in axillary or terminal corymbsFruits: Ovoid or subellipsoid, five-ribbed, with viscid hairs*

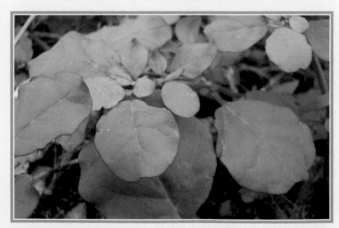

Fig. 78.1 Leaves.

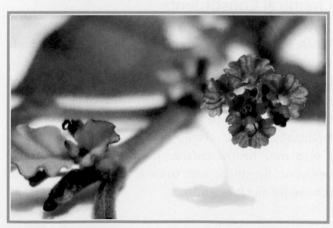

Fig. 78.2 Flowers.

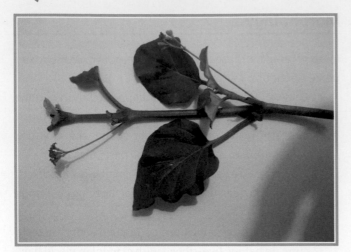

Fig. 78.3 Stem.

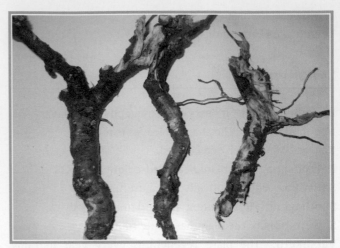

Fig. 78.4 Root.

Types

- Bhavaprakash Nighantu: Two types: Shweta Punarnava and Rakta Punarnava
- Dhanvantari Nighantu: Two types: Punarnava and Krura (punarnava vishesh)
- Raj Nighantu: Three types: Shweta Punarnava, Rakta Punarnava, and Neel Punarnava

Rasapanchaka

Guna	Laghu, Ruksha
Rasa	Katu, Kashaya
Vipaka	Katu
Virya	Sheeta

Chemical Constituents

Whole plant contains a large number of active compounds such as flavonoids, alkaloids, steroids, triterpenoids, lipids, lignins, carbohydrates, proteins, and glycoproteins. Root mainly contains alkaloids punarnavine, punernavoside, boeravinone A-F, boerhavin, boerhaavic acid, hypoxanthine larabinofuranoside, ursolic acid, arachidic acid, α- & β-sitosterol, hentriacontane, β-ecdysone, tetracosanoic, hexacosonoic, stearic acid, palmitic acid, and triacontanol (Chatterjee and Prakash 2013).

Identity, Purity, and Strength

Shothaghna (anti-inflammatory), sara (laxative), deepan (carminative), rochana (improves taste), pandughna (cures anemia), mutravirechana (diuretic), anulomana (facilitate downward movement of vata), hridya (cardiotonic), raktavardhaka (haemopoietic), kasahara (expectorant), vrishya (aphrodisiac), swedadopaga (adjuvant to sudation therapy), netrya (eye tonic), kushtaghna (antidermatosis), jwaraghna (antipyretic), rasayana (rejuvinator), vishaghna (antitoxin).

For Root

- Foreign matter: Not more than 2%
- Total ash: Not more than 10%
- Acid-insoluble ash: Not more than 0.8%
- Alcohol-soluble extractive: Not less than 4%
- Water-soluble extractive: Not less than 10%

(Source: The Ayurvedic Pharmacopeia of India 2001)

Karma (Actions)

Ayurveda classics attributed shothaghna, sara, deepan, rochana, pandughna, mutravirechana (diuretic), anulomana, hridya, raktavardhaka, kasahara, vrishya, swedadopaga, netrya, kushtaghna, jwaraghna, rasayana, vishaghna properties to it.

- Doshakarma: Kapha pittahara
- Dhatukarma: Shothaghna, rasayana
- Malakarma: Mutravirechan, swedopaga

Pharmacological Actions

Previous scientific studies demonstrated that Punarnava possesses immunomodulator, antioxidant, diuretic, hepatoprotective, anti-inflammatory, antibacterial, antinociceptive, hypoglycemic, antiproliferative, antiestrogenic, anticonvulsant, adoptogenic, antimetastatic, antifertility, radioprotective, insecticidal, anthelmintic, chemopreventive, antifibrinolytic activities (Gupta et al 2004).

Indications

Roots are prescribed to be used in treatment of shotha (inflammatory diseases), jaloudar (ascites), aruchi (dyspepsia), udararoga (abdominal diseases), pandu (anemia), jaundice, hepatotoxicity, prameha (diabetes), ashmari (calculus), abhishyanda (conjunctivitis), agnimandya (loss of appetite), vibandha (constipation), hridroga (heart diseases), kasa (cough), shwasa (asthma), urakshata (pulmonary cavitation), raktapradara (menorrhagia), mutrakrichchta (dysuria), madaatyaay (alcoholism), arsha (piles), shool (pain), kushta (skin diseases), jwara (fever), dansha (scorpion sting, snake bite).

Therapeutic Uses

External Use

1. **Abhishyandi** (conjunctivitis): In conjunctivitis, application of root paste of Punarnava with madhu reduces inflammation and redness.
2. **Mudhagarbha** (obstructed labor): Punarnava root lubricated with oil is introduced into vagina to expel out fetus in mudhagarbha (G.N. 6/4/38).

Internal Use

1. **Pandu** (anemia): Daily intake of Punarnava leaf juice or two tablets of Punarnava mandoor (C.S.Ci. 16/93-96) or decoction of Punarnava, Nimba, Patola, Shunthi, Tikta, Amrita, Darvi, and Abhya is useful in pandu (VM. 38/3).
2. **Sarvangshopha** (edema): Daily intake of decoction or paste of Punarnava root mixed with Shunthi paste gives relief in all types of inflammatory disorders (S.S.Ci. 23/12). Or intake of Guggulu with decoction of Punarnava, Devdaru, and Shunthi is beneficial in ascites and edema (VM. 39/8).

3. **Ashmari** (calculus): Daily use of decoction of Punarnava, Gokshur, Varun, and Pashanbheda increases urine output, breaks stones, and expels out gravels.
4. **Antarvidhridhi** (internal abscess): To get rid of internal abscess, decoction of Punarnava and Varuna should be used daily (SG. 2/2/128).
5. **Kamala, Yakritashotha** (jaundice, hepatitis): Punarnava root decoction or powder or Punarnava siddha ghrita helps in expulsion of excessive pitta from the body (cholagogue purgative); thus, it gives relief in hepatitis, jaundice, hepatomegaly, skin disease, and other liver diseases.
6. **Rasayana (rejuvinator)**: To attain rejuvenation of entire body, one should take fresh paste of Punarnava root 20 g with milk for a fortnight, 2 months, 6 months, or a year (A.H.U. 39/155).
7. **Hridyaroga** (heart diseases): In heart diseases associated with pedal edema, breathlessness, and chronic obstructive pulmonary disease (COPD), decoction or Punarnava root powder with Kutki, Chirayata, and Shunthi should be given.
8. **Raktavaman** (hemoptysis): Intake of rakta shali prepared with Punarnava churna, Sharkara, Draksha rasa, dugdh, and ghrita prevents hemoptysis (C.S.Ci. 11/26).

Officinal Parts Used

Root and panchang (whole plant)

Dose

Juice: 5 to 10 mL
Decoction: 50 to 100 mL

Formulations

Punarnavasava, Punarnavashtaka kwath, Punarnava mandoor, Punarnavarishta, Punarnava guggulu, Kumaryasava, Shothaghna lepa.

Toxicity/Adverse Effects

Because of its emetic property, vomiting may be induced if taken in large doses (Sharma et al 2000).

Substitution and Adulteration

Trianthema portulacastrum Linn., i.e., varshabhu roots are often adulterated with Raktapunarnava (Sharma et al 2000).

Points to Ponder

- *In Ayurveda classics, Rakta Punarnava is described under the name of Punarnava and Shweta Punarnava as Vrishchira.*
- *Punarnava is the drug of choice for edema, ascites, dysuria, urinary calculus, anemia, jaundice, and hepatitis.*

Suggested Readings

Anonymous. The Wealth of India: Raw Materials, Vol. 2B. Revised edition. New Delhi: Publications & Information Directorate, CSIR; 1988:174–176

Chatterjee A, Prakash SC. The Treatise on Indian Medicinal Plants, Vol. 1. Revised 1st ed. New Delhi: CSIR, National Institute of Science Communication and Information Resource; 2013:93–94

Gupta AK, Sharma M, Tandon N. Review on Indian Medicinal Plants, Vol 4(Ba-By). New Delhi: ICMR; 2004:285–304

Sharma PC, Yelne MB, Dennis TJ. Database on Medicinal Plants Used in Ayurveda, Vol. 1. New Delhi: CCRAS Department of Indian Systems of Medicine and Homeopathy (ISM&H), Ministry of Health and Family Welfare, Government of India; 2000:360–363

The Ayurvedic Pharmacopeia of India. Part I, Vol. 3. New Delhi: Department of AYUSH, Ministry of Health and Family Welfare, Government of India; 2001:159

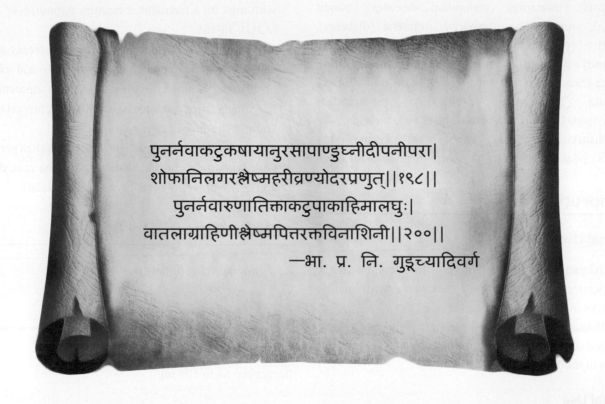

पुनर्नवाकटुकषायानुरसापाण्डुघ्नीदीपनीपरा|
शोफानिलगरश्लेष्महरीव्रण्योदरप्रणुत्||१९८||
पुनर्नवारुणातिक्ताकटुपाकाहिमालघुः|
वातलाग्राहिणीश्लेष्मपित्तरक्तविनाशिनी||२००||
—भा. प्र. नि. गुडूच्यादिवर्ग

79. Pushkarmoola *[Inula racemosa Hook.f.]*

Family:	*Compositae*
Hindi name:	*Pohkarmool*
English name:	*Elicampane root, Orris root*

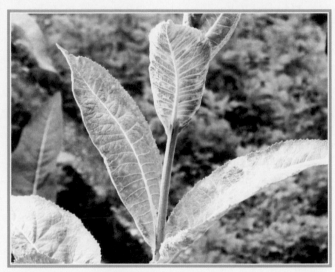

Plant of *Inula racemosa* Hook.f.

Pushkar Guggulu is a popular formulation for ischemic heart disease (IHD), obesity, and hyperlipidemia.

Introduction

The plant is named Pushkarmoola because the fresh root has a strong aromatic odor resembling lotus flower or orris. The plant is first mentioned in Agnipurana as a variety of Kushta (*Saussurea lappa* C.B. Clarke). Since then it is used as a drug of choice kasa, shwasa, hridya shool, and kushta. Charaka has described it as the best drug of hikka, shwasa, and parshvasula (C.S.Su. 255/40). Sushrut and Ashtang have also advocated its use as antiasthmatic, cardiotonic drug.

Other systems of medicines like Unani, Siddha, Tibetan, European, Chinese, and American make free use of Pushkarmool in treating major ailments. The Americans used it for treating tuberculosis and cardiovascular disorders. In Himachal Pradesh, root or leaf paste is applied on swellings and sprains as an antiseptic. Root powder also helps in lowering elevated blood pressure. Roots are also kept with garments to protect them from infestation.

Leaves are used to particulate pollutants chiefly carbon particles (Agarwal 1986).

Due to its indiscriminate overexploitation and destruction of natural habitat, the plant is reported under critically endangered species by IUCN.

Vernacular Names

Assamese: Pohakarmul, Puskar
Bengali: Pushkara, Pushkaramula
Gujarati: Pushkarmula
Kannada: Pushkara Moola
Malayalam: Puskara
Marathi: Pokhar Mool
Oriya: Puskara
Punjabi: Pokhar Mool
Tamil: Pushkarmulam
Telugu: Pushkara Mulamu

Synonyms

Kashmira: The plant grows in high altitude and is native to Kashmir.

Padmapatra: Its leaves resemble lotus leaves

Pouskara: The plant is native to cold regions like the ponds.

Kushta bheda: It is considered a variety of Kushta plant.

Classical Categorization

Charaka Samhita: Shwasahara, Hikkani grahana

Sushrut Samhita: Phala varga

Ashtang Sangraha: Hikkanigrahana

Dhanvantari Nighantu: Guduchyadi varga

Madanpal Nighantu: Abhyadi varga

Kaiyadev Nighantu: Oushadi varga

Raj Nighantu: Pippalayadi varga

Bhavaprakash Nighantu: Haritakyadi varga

Distribution

The plant is abundantly found in India, China, and Europe. In India, it is found in temperate and alpine regions of Western Himalaya at an altitude of 5,000 to 14,000 ft from Kashmir to Kumaon. It is also found in wild among strong alpine vegetation in cold desert of Ladakh (Leh).

Morphology

It is a tall, stout herb of 0.3 to 1.5 m in height. Stem is rough, grooved, and tomentose.

- **Leaves:** Simple, alternate, crenate, leathery, rough above and densely tomentose below, radical or cauline. Upper leaves are lanceolate and stem clasping. Radical leaves are broad and elliptical shaped with long stalk. The cauline leaves are smaller, oblong, and semi-amplexicaule (**Fig. 79.1**).
- **Flowers:** Yellow, very large 3.8 to 5 cm in diameter, many in heads/racemes, born on apical spike-like cluster (**Fig. 79.2**).
- **Fruits:** Reddish, slender, hairless, achene 4 mm long with pappus 8 mm long.
- **Root:** Root stock branched, fresh roots are irregularly fusiform, brownish externally and yellowish white internally. Dry root is dark brown, irregularly wrinkled, camphor-like odor and bitter in taste. The plant is propagated by its seeds and root cuttings (**Fig. 79.3a, b**).

Phenology

Flowering time: July to September

Fruiting time: August to October

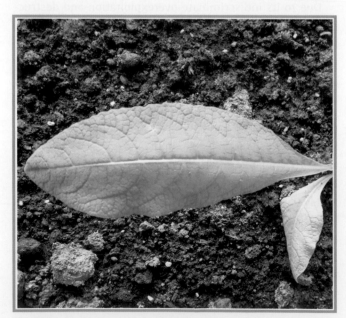

Fig. 79.1 Leaves.

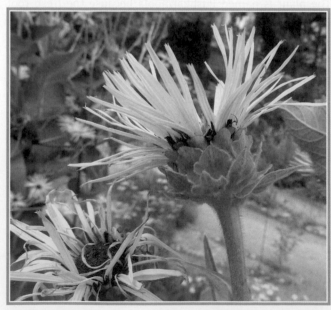

Fig. 79.2 Flowers.

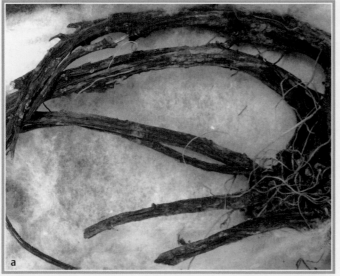

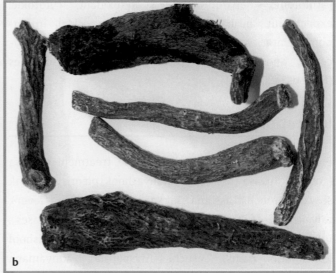

Fig. 79.3 **(a)** Root. **(b)** Dried root.

Key Characters for Identification

➤ *A high altitude tall, stout herb of 0.3 to 1.5 m.*
➤ *Leaves are simple, alternate, crenate, leathery, radical, and cauline*
➤ *Flowers are large, yellow many in heads/racemes. Fruits are reddish, slender hairless achene.*
➤ *Roots are branched, irregularly fusiform, externally brown, internally yellowish white, camphoraceous odor.*

Rasapanchaka

Guna	Laghu, Tikshna
Rasa	Tikta, Katu
Vipaka	Katu
Virya	Ushna

Chemical Constituents

The root has large amounts of sesquiterpene lactones, i.e., alantolactone, isoalantolactone, neo-alantalactone, dihydroisoalanto lactone, inunol, inunolide (germacranolide), dihydroxinunolide, in-unolise, inulin (alkaloid), alantodiene, β-sitosterol, D-mannitol (Bhandari and Rastogi 1983).

Identity, Purity, and Strength

For Root

- Foreign matter: Not more than 2%
- Total ash: Not more than 5%
- Acid-insoluble ash: Not more than 0.6%
- Alcohol-soluble extractive: Not less than 10%
- Water-soluble extractive: Not less than 20%

(Source: The Ayurvedic Pharmacopeia of India 2004)

Karma (Actions)

Ayurvedic classics attributed shothaghna (anti-inflammatory), hikkanigrahan (anti-hic-cough), swashara (anti-asthmatic), jwaraghna (antipyretic), hridya (cardio-protective), jantughna (anti-bacterial), vedanasthapana (analgesic), deepana (appetizer), pachana (digestive), anulomana (antiflatulent), mutrajanan (diuretic), swedajanan (diaphoretic), medohara (antiobesity), vajikara (aphrodisiac), and rasayan (rejuvenator) properties to the plant.

- Doshakarma: Kapha vatahara
- Dhatukarma: Shwasahara, hridya
- Malakarma: Mutral, swedajanan, anulomana

Pharmacological Actions

Pushkarmoola is reported to exhibit bronchodilator, antiallergic, antiasthmatic, anti-inflammatory, analgesic, cardiotonic, hepatoprotective, antioxidant, cytotoxic, expectorant, antibacterial, antifungal, larvicidal, immunomodulator, antimutagenic, adaptogenic, antihyperglycemic, and adrenergic β-receptor blocking activities (Firdous et al 2018).

Indications

Pushkarmoola is administered in the treatment of kasa (cough), shwasa (asthma), parshvashool (pleurisy), tamak shwasa (bronchial asthma), hikka (hic-cough), jwara (fever), rajyakshma (tuberculosis), hridyaroga (heart diseases), medoroga (obesity), shotha (inflammation), sandhishool (rheumatic pains), aruchi (dyspepsia), adhyamana (flatulence), and pandu (anemia).

Therapeutic Uses

External Use

1. **Dantaroga** *(tooth diseases):* *Push*karmoola powder is rubbed on gums and teeth in tooth ache and other diseases of teeth.
2. **Vidradhi** (abscess): Pushkarmoola churna mixed with coconut oil is applied externally in abscess and boils.

Internal Use

1. **Hridaya roga** (heart disease): One to three grams root powder of Pushkarmoola with honey is given in cardiac pain, dyspnea, cough, and hic-cough (VM. 31/12).
2. **Kasa, shwasa** (cough and asthma): Dashmool kwath added with Pushkarmoola churna and madhu should be taken twice daily in kasa, shwasa, hikka parshavashool (VM. 12/18).
3. **Parshavashool** (pleurisy): Pushkarmoola churna is specifically recommended in parshavashool (C.S.Su. 25/40) (A.H.U. 40/56).
4. **Medoroga** (obesity): Pushkarmoola churna with Guggulu is given twice daily in hyperlipidemia, obesity, and cardiac ailments.

Officinal Part Used

Root

Dose

Powder: 1 to 3 g

Formulations

Pushkaradi guggul, Pushkarmulasava, Puskaradi churna, Puskaradi kashaya, Lodhraasava, Kankayana gutika, Kumaryasava.

Toxicity/Adverse Effects

Not reported.

Substitution and Adulteration

The plant Kushta or Eranda moola is used as the substitute of Pushkarmoola (B.P.S. 1/154). Dried roots of *Iris germanica, I. royleana, I. grandiflora, Hedychium spicatum* are intermixed with Pushkarmoola (Lavekar et al 2007).

> **Points to Ponder**
>
> - *Pushkarmoola is a drug of choice for asthma, cough, bronchitis, IHD, tuberculosis, and rheumatic pain.*
> - *Being critically endangered species, roots of Kustha (Saussurea lappa C.B.Clarke) are sold in the market as Pushkarmoola.*

Suggested Readings

Agarwal VS. Economic Plants of India. New Delhi: Deep Printers; 1986:187–188

Bhandari P, Rastogi R. Alloalantolactone: A Sesquiterpene Lactone from Inula-Racemosa, Vol. 22. New Delhi: Council Scientific Industrial Research; 1983:286–287

Firdous Q, Bhat MF, Hussain M. Ethnopharmacology, phytochemistry and biological activity of *Inula racemosa* hook. F: a review. Int J Res Ayurveda Pharm 2018;9(1):95–102

Levekar GS, Chandra K, Dhar BP, et al. Database on Medicinal Plants Used in Ayurveda, Vol. 8. New Delhi: CCRAS Department of Indian Systems of Medicine and Homeopathy (ISM&H), Ministry of Health and Family Welfare, Government of India; 2007:294–300

Sharma S, Sharma RK. Seed physiological aspects of Pushkarmool: a threatened medicinal herb. Curr Sci 2010;99(12):1801–1806

The Ayurvedic Pharmacopeia of India. Part I, Vol. 4. New Delhi: Department of AYUSH, Ministry of Health and Family Welfare, Government of India; 2004:117

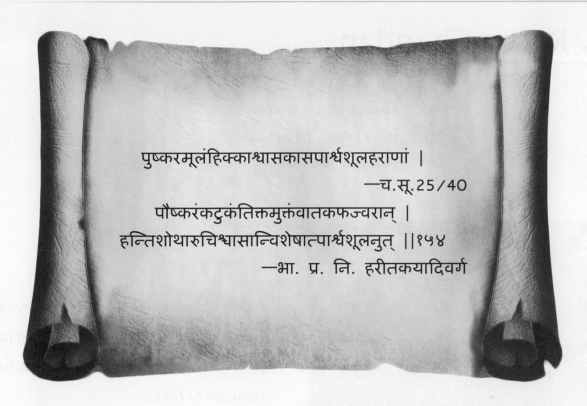

पुष्करमूलंहिक्काश्वासकासपार्श्वशूलहराणां |

—च.सू. 25/40

पौष्करंकटुकंतिक्तमुक्तंवातकफज्वरान् |

हन्तिशोथारुचिश्वासान्विशेषात्पार्श्वशूलनुत् ||१५४

—भा. प्र. नि. हरीतकयादिवर्ग

80. Rakta Chandan [*Pterocarpus santalinus* Linn. F.]

Family: *Fabaceae*

Hindi name: *Lal Chandan*

English name: *Red Sandalwood*

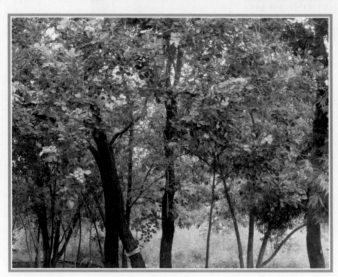

Plant of *Pterocarpus santalinus* Linn. F.

Rakta Chandana is used for kashaya and lepa while Shwet Chandana is used for preparation of churna, leha, asava, and taila (Sh.S. 1/53).

Introduction

The name *Pterocarpus* is derived from a Greek word which means "winged fruit," referring to the unusual shape of the seed pods in the genus. In ancient texts Rakta Chandan is named as Kshudra Chandana which indicated that the properties of both Rakta and Shwet Chandan are almost similar but Rakta Chandan is less potent than Shwet Chandana. In some texts Patrang is used as a substitute drug for Rakt Chandan whereas in Nighantus, Patrang is described under Kuchandana (a type of Chandana).

Rakta Chandan is a well-known drug for diabetes. Vessels made up with its woods have traditionally been used in folklore for drinking water as a treatment of diabetes (Nagaraju and Rao 1989; Latheef et al 2008). Rakta Chandan trees are confined to limited regions of Andhra Pradesh and Karnataka, and because of its ruthless use and illegitimate trade, the species is listed under critically endangered species.

The plant is renowned for its quality timber of exquisite color and is used for making furniture, sculptures, dolls, decorative pieces, and musical instruments. It is also exported to Japan, Malaysia, Sri Lanka, and Germany. The heartwood yields a red color natural dye santalin which is used as a coloring agent in pharmaceutical preparations, foodstuffs, for dyeing wool, cotton, clothes, leathers, as an ingredient of French polish, and for staining other woods. Leaves are used as cattle fodder. In European countries, santalin is used as a coloring agent in medicines.

Vernacular Names

Assam: Sandale, Sandal Ahmar

Bengali: Rakta chandana

French: Santal rouge

Gujarati: Ratanjali, Lalchandan

Kannada: Raktha Chandanam, Agslue, Honne

Malayalam: Rakta Chandanam, Patrangam, Tilaparni

Marathi: Rakta Chandana, Tambada Chandana
Oriya: Raktachandan
Punjabi: Lal Chandan
Spanish: Sándalo rojo
Tamil: Senchandanam, Atti, Semmaram, Sivaffu Chandanam
Telugu: Erra Chandanamu, Agaru gandhamu, Raktachandanam, Rakta ghandhamu
Urdu: Sandal Surkh

Synonyms

Raktang: The parts of plants are red, especially wood.
Kshudra chandan: It is less potent in properties in comparison to Shwet Chandana.
Til parna: Its leaves resemble those of Tila (sesamum) leaves.
Raktasaar: The heartwood is red in appearance.
Praval phal: The fruits are bright red in color like the corals.

Classical Categorization

Charak: Not mentioned
Sushrut: Salasaradi, Patoladi, Sarivadi, Privangadi

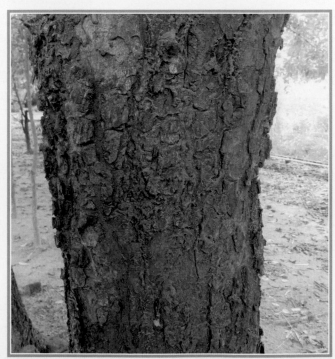

Fig. 80.1 Bark.

Ashtang Hridaya: Guduchyadi, Sarivadi
Dhanvantari Nighantu: Chandanadi varga
Madanpal Nighantu: Karpuradi varga
Kaiyadev Nighantu: Oushadi varga
Raj Nighantu: Chandanadi varga
Bhavaprakash Nighantu: Karpuradi varga

Distribution

Rakta Chandan is widely distributed in the tropical regions of the world, especially in India, Sri Lanka, Taiwan, China, and Nepal. This plant is native to Southern India, especially Chitoor, Cuddapah, Nellore, and Kurnool district of Andhra Pradesh, Tamil Nadu, Kerala, and Karnataka (Anonymous 1969).

Morphology

A glabrous moderate-sized deciduous tree reaching up to a height of 25 to 30 feet.

- **Bark:** Blackish-brown with vertical and horizontal cracks, on injury, copious red sticky thick gum oozes out. Heart wood is dark red or black in color (**Fig. 80.1**).
- **Leaves:** Pinnately compound, imparipinnate, with three to five leaflets, orbicular to ovate shape, 6 to 8 cm length, 5 to 6 cm width, base is round or slightly cordate in shape, emarginated apex, entire margin, glaucous surface (**Fig. 80.2**).

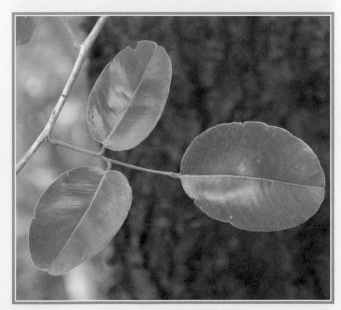

Fig. 80.2 Leaves.

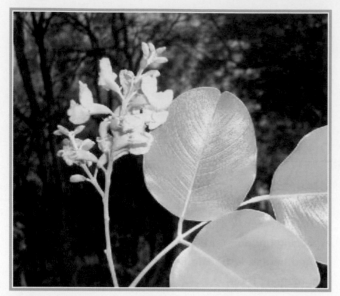

Fig. 80.3 Flower.

- **Flowers:** Yellow, fragrant, about 2 cm long, in short simple axillary and terminal racemes (**Fig. 80.3**).
- **Fruits:** Flat, oblique-orbicular, winged pod with a prominent curved beak. The central hard portion contains the seed (**Fig. 80.4a, b**).
- **Seeds:** One or two per pod, more or less kidney shaped, 1 to 1.5 cm long, smooth, reddish brown. The plant is propagated by seeds and by vegetative methods (**Fig. 80.5**).

Phenology

Flowering time: April to July
Fruiting time: October to January

Key Characters for Identification

➤ *A moderate-sized deciduous tree with reddish brown heartwood*
➤ *Leaves: imparipinnate, three to five leaflets, orbicular to ovate shape*
➤ *Flowers: yellow, fragrant in axillary and terminal racemes*
➤ *Fruits are flat-winged pods, oblique-orbicular, curved beak*
➤ *One or two kidney-shaped seeds, smooth, reddish brown*

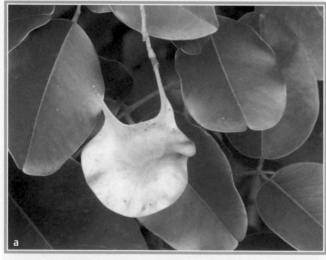

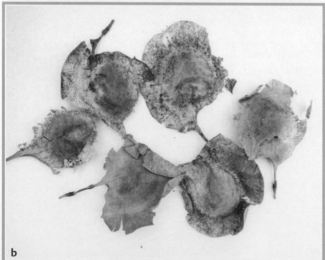

Fig. 80.4 (a) Fruit. (b) Dry sample of fruit.

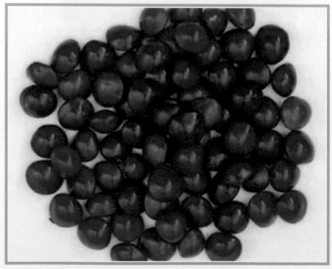

Fig. 80.5 Seeds.

Rasapanchaka

Guna	Guru
Rasa	Madhur, Tikta
Vipaka	Katu
Virya	Sheet

Chemical Constituents

Its heartwood contains various components like carbohydrates, steroids, anthocyanins, saponins, phenols (β-sitosterol; lupeol; epicatechin), triterpenoids, isoflavonoids glycosides, and lignans (savinin, calocedrin). The major bioactive components present in the heartwood are pterocarpol, santalin A & B (red coloring agent), pterocarptriol, pterocarpodilone, lupenediol, santal, ispterocarpolone, pterocarpin, homo pterocarpin, β-eudesmol, cryptomeridiol, pterolinus K and L, and pterostilbenes (Yoganarasimhan 2000; Bulle et al 2016).

Identity, Purity, and Strength

- Foreign matter: Not more than 2%
- Total ash: Not more than 2%
- Acid-insoluble ash: Not more than 0.3%
- Alcohol-soluble extractive: Not less than 3%
- Water-soluble extractive: Not less than 1%

(Source: The Ayurvedic Pharmacopeia of India 2001)

Karma (Actions)

In Ayurvedic classics Rakta Chandan is described as sheet (cooling effect), guru (heavy), netrahitam (beneficial for eye), vrishya (aphrodisiac), vishaghna (antidote), rakshoghna (antibacterial), balya (tonics), chaksushya (beneficial for vision), jantughna (anthelmintics), varnya (complexion promoter), jwaraghna (antipyretics), and raktashodhaka (blood purifier).

- Doshakarma: Kapha pitta shamaka
- Dhatukarma: Balya, varnya, raktashodhaka
- Malakarma: Malashodhana

Pharmacological Actions

In vivo and in vitro research studies showed that the heartwood and bark have exhibited to have coolant, antihyperglycemic (Kameswara et al 2001), antipyretic, antimicrobial, hemostatic, anti-inflammatory, anticancer, antioxidative, neuroprotective, gastroprotective, hepatoprotective (Manjunatha 2006), diaphoretic, anthelmintic, aphrodisiac, and wound-healing properties (Soundararajan et al 2016; Upali Arunakumara et al 2011).

Indications

Traditionally the heartwood is used for the treatment of chardi (vomiting), trishna (thirst), jwara (fever), raktapitta (bleeding disorders), vrana (wounds), visha (poison), kasa (cough), bhranti (gidiness), and bhoot (bacterial infections).

Besides these classical uses, its heartwood is widely used in diabetes (Nagaraju et al 1991), bleeding piles, diarrhea, dysentery, headache, inflammations, skin diseases, bone fracture, leprosy, spider poisoning, scorpion sting, urinary infections, ulcers, general debility, and metal aberrations (Arokiyaraj et al 2008).

Decoction of fruits is used by Kani tribes in chronic dysentery and psoriasis. Heartwood and bark powder taken orally relieves chronic dysentery, worms, hematemesis, vision defects, and hallucination (Chopra et al 1956).

Therapeutic Uses

External Use

1. **Asthibhagna** (fracture): External application of paste of Rakta Chandan, Manjistha, Yasthimadhu, rice flour, and shatdhout ghrita promotes union of fractured bones in bhagna (S.S.Ci. 3/7).
2. **Vyanga** (freckles): Application of paste of Rakta Chandan, Manjistha, Kustha, Lodhra, Priyangu, Vatankura, and Masura on face enhances, tone, luster in Vyanga (A.H.U. 32/17).
3. **Timir** (vision defect): Rakta Chandan pounded with water, madhu, ghrita, and taila is applied daily for a week as anjana (collyrium) which alleviates timir (B.S.netraroga Ci./312).

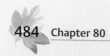

Internal Use

1. **Pittaatisaar** (diarrhea): Decoction or powder of Daruharidra, Duralabha, Bilva, Sugandhbala, and Rakta Chandan checks diarrhea caused by aggravated pitta (S.S.U. 40/63-65).
2. **Prameha** (diabetes): Like Vijaysaar, wooden glasses or vessels made up of its heartwood is used by diabetic patients for drinking water.
3. **Luta visha** (spider poisoning): External application or oral intake of powder of Lodhra, Ushir, Padmak, Mrinaal, Kaleyak, Rakta Chandan, Priyangu pushp, and Dughdhika counteract the effect of all types of spider poisoning (A.H.U. 37/86).

Officinal Part Used

Heartwood

Dose

Powder: 3 to 6 g

Formulations

Chandanadi taila, Chandanasava

Toxicity/Adverse Effect

Not reported yet.

Substitution and Adulteration

Ushira is used as a substitute drug of Rakta Chandan (Bhavmishra 2010).

Points to Ponder

➤ Rakta Chandan is a critically endangered plant and needs large-scale conservation.
➤ Rakta Chandan is chiefly used for the treatment of diabetes, fracture, acne, skin diseases, and poisoning.

Suggested Readings

Anonymous. The Wealth of India: A Dictionary of Indian Raw Material & Industrial Products. Vol. VIII: (Ph-Re). New Delhi: Publication & Information Directorate, CSIR, reprint 2009; 1969:300–306

Arokiyaraj S, Martin S, Perinbam K, Marie Arockianathan P, Beatrice V. Free radical scavenging activity and HPTLC finger print of *Pterocarpus santalinus* L.: an in vitro study. Indian J Sci Technol 2008;1(7):1–3

Bhavmishra: Bhavprakash Nighantu, Commentary by K.C. Chunekar and Edited by G.S. Pandey. Varanasi: Choukhambha Bharati Academy; 2010:960

Bulle S, Reddyvari H, Nallanchakravarthula V, Vaddi DR. Therapeutic potential of *Pterocarpus santalinus* L.: an update. Pharmacogn Rev 2016;10(19):43–49

Chopra RN, Nayar SL, Chopra IC. Glossary of Indian Medicinal Plants. New Delhi: CSIR Publications; 1956:206

Kameswara Rao B, Giri R, Kesavulu MM, Apparao C. Effect of oral administration of bark extracts of *Pterocarpus santalinus* L. on blood glucose level in experimental animals. J Ethnopharmacol 2001;74(1):69–74

Latheef SA, Prasad B, Bavaji M, Subramanyam G. A database on endemic plants at Tirumala hills in India. Bioinformation 2008;2(6): 260–262

Manjunatha BK. Hepatoprotective activity of *Pterocarpus santalinus* L.f.: an endangered plant. Indian J Pharmacol 2006;38(1):25–28

Nagaraju N, Prasad M, Gopalakrishna G, Rao KN. Blood sugar lowering effect of *Pterocarpus santalinus* (red sanders) wood extract in different rat models. Int J Pharmacog 1991;29:141–144

Nagaraju N, Rao KN. Folk-medicine for diabetes from rayalaseema of Andhra Pradesh. Anc Sci Life 1989;9(1):31–35

Soundararajan V, Ravi Kumar G, Murugesan K, Chandrashekar BS. A review on red sanders (*Pterocarpus santalinus* Linn.): phytochemistry and pharmacological importance. World J Pharm Sci 2016;5(6):667–689

The Ayurvedic Pharmacopeia of India. Part I, Vol. 3. New Delhi: Department of AYUSH, Ministry of Health and Family Welfare, Government of India; 2001:157

Upali Arunakumara KKI, Walpola BC, Subasinghe S, Yoon M-H. *Pterocarpus santalinus* Linn. f. (Rath handun): a review of its botany, uses, phytochemistry and pharmacology. J Korean Soc Appl Biol Chem 2011;54(4):495–500

Yoganarasimhan SN. Medicinal Plants of India, Tamil Nadu. Bangalore: Cyber Media; 2000:63

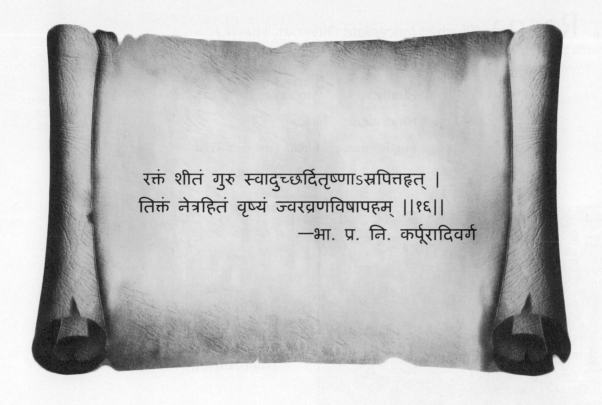

रक्तं शीतं गुरु स्वादुच्छर्दितृष्णाऽस्रपित्तहृत् ।
तिक्तं नेत्रहितं वृष्यं ज्वरव्रणविषापहम् ॥१६॥

—भा. प्र. नि. कर्पूरादिवर्ग

81. Rasna [*Pluchea lanceolata* Oliver et. Hiern.]

Family: *Asteraceae*

Hindi name: *Rasna*

English name: *Indian Camphor weed*

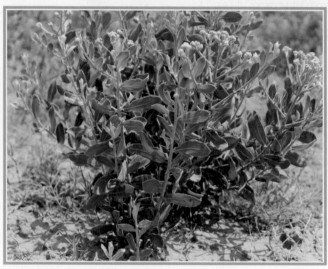

Plant of *Pluchea lanceolata* Oliver et. Hiern.

The genus was named Pluchea in the honor of French naturalist Noël-Antoine Pluche.

Introduction

The plant is assigned the name "Rasna" because of resemblance of its leaves with the tongue. Our tongue is considered as the seat of rasa detection.

Since time immemorial, Rasna has been used in traditional and folklore medicine, to treat various painful afflictions and swelling of the body. Acharya Charak considered Rasna as the best drug for vatavyadhis (C.S.Su. 25/40). Its paste with Agaru is recommended to apply in alleviating cold (C.S.Su. 25/40). Since ancient times, there has been controversy over the correct identity of Rasna. Out of all the drugs, *Pluchea lanceolata* is the most accepted source of Rasna. According to Raj Nighantu, mool and patra Rasna has highest efficacy and trina Rasna has medium potency. Besides being used medicinally, Rasna is also used as fodder for animals.

Vernacular Names

Assamese: Rasnapat
Bengali: Rasna
Kannada: Rasna, Dumme-Rasna
Marathi: Rasna, Rayasana
Punjabi: Reshae
Telugu: Sanna Rashtramu
Urdu: Rauasan, Rasna

Synonyms

Elaparni: The shape of its leaves resembles that of Ela leaves.
Rasna: The shape of leaves is similar to human tongue.
Rasya: It acts on the rasa dhatu.
Shreyashi: The plant is the best drug for vataroga.

Sugandha: The plant emits a pleasant odor.

Surasa: The plant has nourishing property.

Suvaha: It promotes the circulation of rasa dhatu in the srotasa.

Yuktarasa: The plant has fully developed rasa.

Classical Categorization

Charak Samhita: Vyastapana, Anuvasanopaga

Sushrut Samhita: Arkadi, Shlesmsansamana

Ashtang Hridaya: Arkadivarga

Dhanvantari Nighantu: Guduchyadi varga

Madanpal Nighantu: Abhyadi varga

Kaiyadev Nighantu: Oushadi varga

Raj Nighantu: Pippalayadi varga

Bhavaprakash Nighantu: Haritakyadi varga

Distribution

It is found abundantly in tropical and warm temperate regions of India like Punjab, Haryana, Rajasthan, Uttar Pradesh, Delhi, and Madhya Pradesh.

Morphology

It is an erect, undershrub, 30 to 70 cm high. Stem and branches are terete, ashy, and pubescent.

- **Leaves:** Simple, alternate, sessile, very coriaceous, 1 to 3 inch long, 0.5 to 1 inch wide, oblong or lanceolate, obtuse or apiculate apex, ash-green colored, pubescent on both sides (**Fig. 81.1**).
- **Flowers:** Purple in heads of about 5 mm long, forming terminal corymbose panicles, involucre bracts numerous (**Fig. 81.2**).
- **Fruits:** Achene with one seriate pappus hairs, oblong, smooth, distinctly connate base (**Fig. 81.3**). The plant is propagated by its seeds and root stocks (**Fig. 81.4**).

Phenology

Flowering time: April to June

Fruiting time: June to August

Key Characters for Identification
➤ *An erect, undershrub, 30 to 70 cm high with pubescent branches.*
➤ *Leaves: Simple, alternate, sessile, 1 to 3 inch long, lanceolate.*
➤ *Flowers: Purple in heads of about 5 mm long terminal corymbose.*
➤ *Fruits: Achene-type, smooth, oblong with connate base.*

Types

Raj Nighantu has described its three types:

- Mool Rasna: *Alpinia galanga* Willd.
- Patra Rasna: *Pluchea lanceolata* Oliver et. Hiern.
- Trina Rasna: *Vanda roxburghii* R.Br.

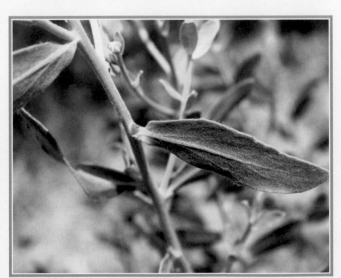

Fig. 81.1 Leaves.

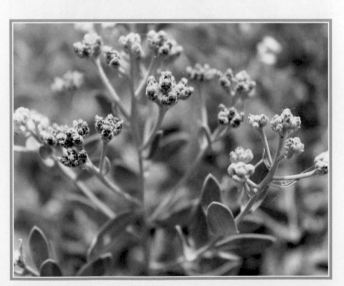

Fig. 81.2 Flowers.

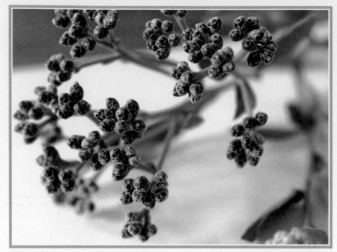

Fig. 81.3 Fruits.

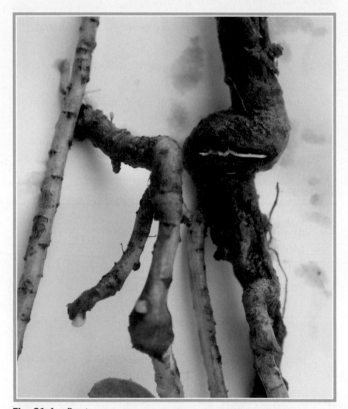

Fig. 81.4 Root.

Rasapanchaka

Guna	Guru
Rasa	Tikta
Vipaka	Katu
Virya	Ushna

Chemical Constituents

The whole plant contains eudesmane-type sesquiter-penoids, quercetin, isorhamnetin, hesperidin (flavonoids), taxifolin (dihydroflavonol), formononetin (isoflavonoid), hexacosanol, quercetin, isorhamnetin, stigmasterol, α- and β-sitosterol, lignan glycosides, and pluchine 7-O-glucoside (Billore et al 2005).

Identity, Purity, and Strength

For Leaves

- Foreign matter: Not more than 2%
- Total ash: Not more than 22%
- Acid-insoluble ash: Not more than 7%
- Alcohol-soluble extractive: Not less than 8%
- Water-soluble extractive: Not less than 23%

(Source: The Ayurvedic Pharmacopeia of India 2001)

Karma (Actions)

Traditionally, the plant is believed to be aampachaka (digestive), shothhara (anti-inflammatory), shoolghna (analgesic), sheetahara (cold alleviating), vishaghna (antidote to poison), jwarahara (antipyretic), raktashodhaka (blood purifier).

- Doshakarma: Vatakaphashamaka
- Dhatukarma: Vedanasthapana, Shothahara
- Malakarma: Vatanulomana, Rechana

Pharmacological Actions

The whole plant is reported to exhibit hepatoprotective, antioxidant, antispasmodic, nervine tonic, diaphoretic, antiarthritic, muscle relaxant, anticancer, laxative, and CNS stimulant properties (Srivastava and Shanker 2012).

Indications

In traditional system of medicines, Rasna is indicated for the treatment of aamvata (rheumatism), sandhivata (osteoarthritis), vatarakta (gout), kampavata (convulsion), visha (poisoning), vishamjwara (intermittent fever), shotha (inflammatory diseases), udarroga (abdominal disorders), hikka (hic-cough), aruchi (dyspepsia), kasa (cough), shwasa (asthma), intestinal and biliary colics, angaghata (paralysis), nadishool (neuritis), katishool (lumbago), mutrakricchta (dysuria), arsha (hemorrhoids), and dustavrana (gangrenous ulcer).

Therapeutic Uses

External Use

1. **Shotha** (inflammatory diseases): Poultice of warm leaves is applied to the inflamed areas.
2. **Vatavyadhi** (neuromuscular diseases): External application of Rasnadi taila gives relief in neuritis, paralysis, backache, palsy, and other vatavyadhis (C.S.Ci. 28/165-170).
3. **Charmadal** (psoriasis): Paste of Rasna, Nakuli, and Gandhnakuli is applied locally in psoriasis (K.S.p. 333).
4. **Arsha** (piles): To give relief in pain and inflammation, fomentation of hemorrhoids with the decoction of Rasna should be done daily.

Internal Use

1. **Aamvata** (rheumatoid arthritis): Taking decoction prepared with Rasna, Guduchi, Eranda, Devdaru, and Shunthi daily gives relief in pain and inflammation in aamvata, sandhivata, katishool, pakshaghata, etc. (VM. 25/6). Rasanasaptakakwath can also be used (VM. 25/7).
2. **Gradharsi** (sciatica): Rasna and Guggulu are mixed together, pounded with ghee and made into pills known as Rasna–Guggulu. It is taken 2 tab twice daily in gridharsi and other vatavyadhis (VM. 22/53) (B.P.Ci. 24/143).
3. **Vatarakta** (gout): Daily intake of decoction made of Rasna, Guduchi, and Aragvadha with Eranda taila is efficacious in vatarakta (VM. 23/6).

Officinal Parts Used

Whole plant, root, leaves

Dose

Decoction: 50 to 100 mL

Formulations

Rasnadi kwath, Rasnasaptaka kwath, Rasnapanchaka kwath, Rasnadi ghrita, Rasnadi taila.

Toxicity/Adverse Effect

Not reported.

Substitution and Adulteration

Rasna is a controversial drug. In different regions of India, different plants are used in the name of Rasna (Vaidya 2005). These are as follows:

- *Pluchea lanceolata* Oliver et. Hiern. in North India, Uttar Pradesh, Gujarat, Punjab
- *Alpinia galanga* Willd. in South India
- *Inula racemosa* Hook.f. in Kashmir, Himachal Pradesh
- *Vanda roxburghii* R.Br. in Bengal, known as Bangiyarasana
- *Saccolabium papillosum* Lindl
- *Viscum album* L. known as Punjabi Rasna
- *Tylophora asthmatica* W.& A.
- *Enicostema littorale* Blume as trina Rasna in Gujarat
- *Aristolochia indica* L. in Bombay, Ceylon
- *Withania coagulans* Dunal. in Sindh, Punjab, Afghanistan, known as Sindhi Rasna

> **Points to Ponder**
>
> - *Rasna is a controversial drug. Many plants are used in the name of Rasna throughout the country but Pluchea lanceolata Oliver et. Hiern. is the authentic accepted source of Rasna.*
> - *Rasna is the drug of choice for vatavyadhis, shotha, shoola, and sheet.*

Suggested Readings

Billore KV, Yelne MB, Dennis TJ, Chaudhari BG. Database on Medicinal Plants Used in Ayurveda, Vol. 7. New Delhi: CCRAS Department of Indian Systems of Medicine and Homeopathy (ISM&H), Ministry of Health and Family Welfare, Government of India;2005:375–378

Srivastava P, Shanker K. *Pluchea lanceolata* (Rasana): chemical and biological potential of rasayana herb used in traditional system of medicine. Fitoterapia 2012;83(8):1371–1385

The Ayurvedic Pharmacopeia of India. Part I, Vol. 3. New Delhi: Department of AYUSH, Ministry of Health and Family Welfare, Government of India; 2001:164

Vaidya B. Some Controversial Drugs in Indian Medicine. 2nd ed. Varanasi: Chaukhambha Orientalia; 2005:31–40

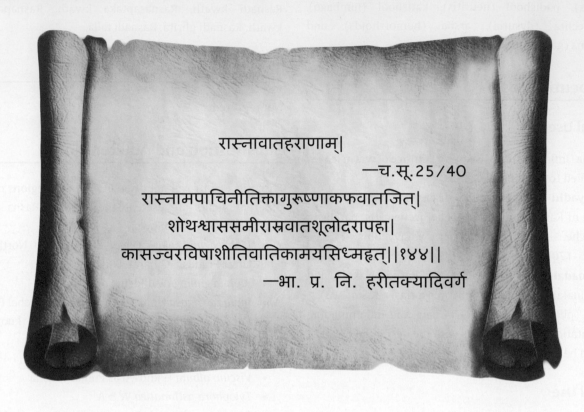

रास्नावातहराणाम्।

—च.सू.25/40

रास्नामपाचिनीतिक्तागुरूष्णाकफवातजित्।

शोथश्वाससमीरास्रवातशूलोदरापहा।

कासज्वरविषाशीतिवातिकामयसिध्महृत्।।१४४।।

—भा. प्र. नि. हरीतक्यादिवर्ग

82. Rasona (Lasuna) *[Allium sativum Linn.]*

Family: *Alliaceae (Liliaceae)*

Hindi name: *Lahsun*

English name: *Garlic, Poorman treacle*

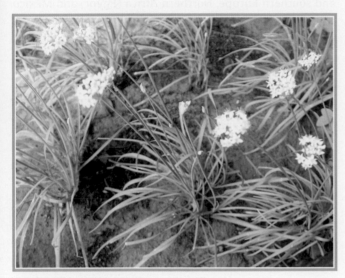

Plant of *Allium sativum* Linn.

> According to the US Food and Drug Administration survey of 900 people, garlic stands as the second most utilized supplement (behind Echinacea), with almost 17% of the population using a garlic supplement.
>
> —Timbo et al (2006)

Introduction

Allium sativum Linn. of Alliaceae family is a cultivated plant distributed in temperate region. According to mythology, when Garuda snatched Amrutha from Lord Indra, a drop of it fell on the earth from which Lasona came into existence. The odor is very peculiarly pungent and disagreeable; taste is acrid and gives warmth to the tongue. It is devoid of only one rasa, i.e., Amla, so it is named "Rasona."

It is not included in any gana of Brihatrayee. But it is extensively mentioned for vatarogachikista and as rasayana. The term "Lasuna" is more used than "Rasona." Vagabhatta considered Lasuna as the best among the vataharadravya. He also emphasized the role of Lasuna rasayana in the treatment of all types of vataavarana except the avarana of rakta and pitta. Kashyap Samhita and Harita Samhita have separate chapters entitled "Lasuna kalpa," which narrate detailed information about Lasuna. Lasuna should be consumed in the winter season (hemanta and shishir ritu);

however, it can also be consumed in spring (vasant ritu) by the kapha predominant person and in rainy season (varsha ritu) by vata predominant person (A.H.U. 39/113-114). Different types of rasa or properties are present in different parts of this plant as per Kashyap and Bhavaprakash.

Originally from Central Asia, garlic is one of the earliest of cultivated plants. The Ebers Codex, and Egyptian medical papyrus dating to about 1550 BCE mentions garlic as an effective remedy for a variety of ailments. Early men of medicine such as Hippocrates, Pliny, and Aristotle espoused a number of therapeutic uses for this botanical plant (Murray 2005). Most of the garlic eaten today comes from China, South Korea, India, Spain, and the United States.

Vernacular Names

Arabic: Saun Taum
Assamese: Maharu
Bengali: Lasuna, Rosun

Chinese: Syun tauh
German: Knoblauch, Lauch
Greek: Allidion, Skorodon
Gujarati: Lasan, Lassun
Italian: Aglio
Kannada: Bulluci
Malayalam: Vellulli, Nelluthulli
Marathi: Lasun
Oriya: Lasun, rasoona
Punjab: Lasan
Tamil: Vellaipoondu
Telugu: Vellulli, Tellapya, Tellagadda
Urdu: Lahsan, Seer

Synonyms

Arista: No evil eyes would affect an individual by using it.
Bhutaghna: It destroys evil organisms.
Lasuna: It is quickly absorbed in body.
Mahakanda: It is a potent drug for all diseases.
Mahaushadha: It is used as one of best medicines.
Mlechchhakanda: It is liked by mlecchas.
Rasona: It is devoid of only one rasa.
Rasonaka: It is devoid of one rasa, i.e., Amla.
Sheetamardaka: It removes cold from body.
Ugragandha: It has prominent pungent smell.
Yavanesta: It is liked by yavana as adjunct food.

Classical Categorization

Not included in any gana of Brihatrayee.
Dhanwantari Nighantu: Karaviradi varga
Madanpal Nighantu: Shakadi varga

Kaiyadev Nighantu: Aushadhadi varga
Raj Nighantu: Pippaladi varga
Bhavaprakash Nighantu: Haritakyadi varga

Distribution

Garlic is cultivated throughout the world. It seems to have originated from Central Asia and then China, the nearest and the Mediterranean region before moving to central and southern Europe, Northern Africa (Egypt) and Mexico. In India, it is mainly cultivated in Punjab, Uttar Pradesh, Madhya Pradesh, Gujarat, Maharashtra, Tamil Nadu, etc.

Morphology

It is a bulbous perennial herb 1 to 2 ft in height.

- **Bulb:** Rounded, composed of about 15 small bulblets known as cloves covered with whitish or pinkish tunic (papery coat) (**Fig. 82.1**).
- **Leaves:** Radical, linear, and flat, 4 to 12 in numbers, green with sheathing base, 20 to 30 cm long (**Fig. 82.2**).
- **Flower:** Borne in a dense, spherical cluster on a spike up to 25 cm long. Individual flower stalks arise from a common point. The young flower head is enclosed in a long beaked pair of bracts which become papery and split to reveal the flower. Flowers are greenish-white or pinkish with six perianth segments (sepals and petals) as shown in **Fig. 82.3**.
- **Fruit:** Globose, three-loculed capsule.
- **Seeds:** Not found in the wild but have been produced under laboratory conditions similar to onion seeds but half in size.

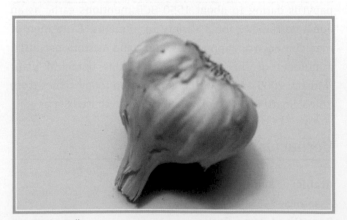

Fig. 82.1 Bulb.

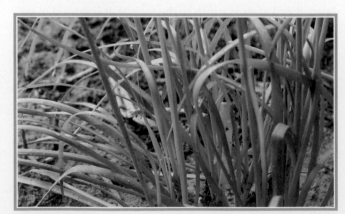

Fig. 82.2 Leaves.

Phenology

Flowering time: January to March

Fruiting time: January to March

Key Characters for Identification

➤ *A bulbous perennial herb 1 to 2 ft in height.*

➤ *Bulb: Rounded, composed of about 15 small bulblets covered with whitish or pinkish papery coat.*

➤ *Leaves: Radical, linear, and flat, 20 to 30 cm long.*

➤ *Flower: Borne in a dense, spherical cluster on a spike up to 25 cm long. Flowers are greenish-white or pinkish with six perianth segments (sepals and petals).*

➤ *Fruit: Globose, three-loculed capsule.*

Rasapanchaka

Guna	Snigdha, Sara, Tikshna, Guru
Rasa	PanchaRasa (Except Amla)
Vipak	Katu
Virya	Ushna

Chemical Constituents

It contains at least 33 sulfur compounds. The most abundant sulfur compound in garlic is alliin (S-allyl cysteine sulfoxide), which is present at 10 and 30 mg/g in fresh and dry garlic, respectively (Lawson 1998). Typical garlic food preparation such as chopping, mincing, and crushing disturbs S-allyl cysteine sulfoxide and exposed it to the allinase enzymes, then quickly converted it to diallyl thiosulfinate, which gives off garlic's characteristic aroma.

- It has several enzymes.
- It has minerals like germanium, calcium, copper, copper, iron, potassium, magnesium, and zinc.
- It has vitamin A, B_1, and C.
- It has amino acids like lysine, histidine, arginine, aspartic acid, etc.

The active constituents of garlic are alliin, allicin, allixin, adenosine, allyl methyl trisulfide, diallyl disulfide, methyl allul trisulfide, 2-Vinyl 1,3-Dithiene, 3-Vinyl 1,3-Dithiene, allyl propyl disulfide, S-allyl cysteine, S-allyl marcaptocysteine.

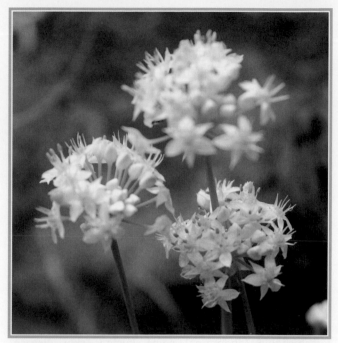

Fig. 82.3 Flowers.

The sulfur compounds contribute to smell as well as taste of garlic.

Identity, Purity, and Strength

- Foreign matter: Not more than 2%
- Total ash: Not more than 4%
- Acid-insoluble ash: Not more than 1%
- Alcohol-soluble extractive: Not less than 2.5%
- Loss on drying: Not less than 60%
- Volatile oil: Not less than 0.1%

Karma (Actions)

Rasona is a very potent drug with properties like balya (increase physical strength), bhagnasandhan (union of fractured bone), brimhana (bulk promoting), deepana (appetizer), hridya (cardiotonic), jantughna (kill worms), kanthya (beneficial for throat), kaphahara (pacify kapha), medhya (intellect promoter), netrya (beneficial for vision), pachan (digestive), rasayana (rejuvenative), varnya (complexion promoter), vrishya (aphrodisiac).

- Doshakarma: Vatakaphahara
- Dhatukarma: Rasayan, brimhana, vrisya
- Malakarma: Vataanulomana

Pharmacological Actions

The various pharmacological actions are antioxidative, antiparasitic, antidiabetic, antibacterial, anticancer, antifungal, antihypertensive, antiprotozoal, antitumor, antiviral, cardioprotective, digestive, diuretic, hepatoprotective, hypocholesterolemic, radioprotective, and wound healing.

Indications

It is used in agnimandya (loss of appetite), ajirna (indigestion), arsha (piles), aruchi (lack of interest in food), bhagna (fracture), gulma (abdominal lump), hridroga (heart disease), jwara (fever), jirnaroga (chronic disease), kukshiroga (abdominal disease), prameha (diabetes), hikka (hic-cough), kasa (cough), krimi (worm infestation), kukshishoola (abdominal pain), kushta (skin disease), shwasa (asthma), sopha (swelling), vatavyadhi (neurological disorder), vibandha (constipation), etc.

It has been used to treat cardiovascular diseases, including atherosclerosis, strokes, hypertension, thrombosis, and hyperlipidemias, as well as has been used in Alzheimer, diabetes, and cancer. It is safe in children.

Contraindications

It is contraindicated for paitika prakriti and garbhini (pregnancy). One should not indulge in doing vyayama (exercise), atapa (sun light exposer), krodha (anger), and should not also take excessive water, milk, and jaggery after use of Lasuna. It is beneficial to take alcohol, meat, and sour drug after the intake of garlic (B.P.N.).

Therapeutic Uses

1. **Vatavyadhi** (neuromuscular diseases)
   (a) Oil cooked with Rasona juice alleviates vata (C.S.Ci. 28/177).
   (b) Rasonakalka (paste) given with til oil is recommended for vatavyadhi (S.G. 2/5/7).
   (c) Rasona should be given with ghee and oil in facial paralysis (arditavata) (B.S.vatavyadhi-103).
   (d) Rasona is the best remedy for vata (A.H.U. 40/52).

2. **Visham Jwar** (malarial fever):
   (a) Rasona mixed with oil should be used before meals (CS.Ci. 30/304).
   (b) Rasona mixed with ghee can be taken every morning (SS.U. 39/213).
3. **Amavata** (rheumatoid arthritis): Rasona should be given with Shunthi and Ingudi in amavata.
4. **Kshaya** (consumption): One should take Lasuna with milk to treat kshaya (S.U. 41/57).
5. **Unmada and Apasmara** (insanity and epilepsy): One should take Lasuna with oil or Shatavari with milk, Brahmi juice, or Kusta or Vacha with honey or Lashunadi ghrita prepared with Lasuna and other drugs to treat insanity and epilepsy.
6. **Gulma** (abdominal lump): Lasunakshira prepared with Dehusked lasuna and milk is given to treat gulma, udarvarta, gidhrasi, hridroga, and shotha (C.S.Ci. 5/94, 95).
7. **Vrana** (wound): Rasona paste is applied to kill organisms present in wound (VM. 44.46).
8. **Stanyajanan** (promotes lactation): Use of Rasona promotes lactation (KS.P. 8).
9. **Visuchika** (cholera): Lasunadi vati is used in visuchika (VJ. 4.13).
10. **Rasayana** (rejuvinator): One pala (50 g) Rasona, two pala (100 g) ghee, and a small amount of honey should be taken with milk keeping the patient on diet of rice with milk. This should be continued for 1 year to achieve good health and longevity (Kashyap Samhita).

Officinal Parts Used

Tuber and oil

Dose

Tuber paste: 3 to 6 g
Oil: 1 to 2 drops

Formulations

Hingutriguna taila, Lasunadi vati, Lasunadya ghrita, Lasunakshirapaka, Rasona Pinda, Rasonastak, Rasonasura, Rasona vati, Vachalasunadi taila.

Toxicity/Adverse Effects

Garlic may also act toxically when overdosed. The main side effect of raw garlic intake is breath odor. Nausea and vomiting are other major side effects. Consumption of garlic also has been reported to be associated with decreased platelet aggregation and bleeding events (Chagan et al 2002). There were several reported allergic reactions to garlic, namely, contact dermatitis, asthma, rhinitis, conjunctivitis, urticaria, anaphylaxis, and angioedema (Gaddoni et al 1994; Rauterberg 1995; Kanerva et al 1996; Armentia and Vega 1997; Roberge et al 1997; Morbidoni et al 2001).

Substitution and Adulteration

Bulb of *Allium ampeloprasm* Linn.

Points to Ponder

- *Five rasas (except amla rasa) are present in Lasuna.*
- *As per Bhavaprakash katu, tikta, kashaya, lavana, and madhur rasas are present in moola, patra, nala, nalagra, and beeja, respectively.*
- *As per Kashyap Samhita, beeja-katu rasa, nala-lavanatikta, patra-kashaya, and vipaka is madhur.*

Suggested Readings

Armentia A, Vega JM. Can inhalation of garlic dust cause asthma? Allergy 1996;51(2):137–138

Chagan L, Ioselovich A, Asherova L, Cheng JW. Use of alternative pharmacotherapy in management of cardiovascular diseases. Am J Manag Care 2002;8(3):270–285, quiz 286–288

Gaddoni G, Selvi M, Resta F, Pasi F. Allergic contact dermatitis to garlic in a cook. Ann Ital Dermatol Clin Sper 1994;48:120–121

Kanerva L, Estlander T, Jolanki R. Occupational allergic contact dermatitis from spices. Contact Dermat 1996;35(3):157–162

Lawson LD. Garlic: a review of its medicinal effects and indicated active compounds. In: Lawson LS, Bauer R, eds. Phytomedicines of Europe: Chemistry and Biological Activity, ACS Symposium Series 691, Am. Chem. Soc. Washington; 1998:176-209

Lucas DS. Dravyaguna-Vijnana: Study of Dravya-Materia Medica. Varanasi: Chaukhamba Visvabharati; 2013:422

Morbidoni L, Arterburn JM, Young V, Mallins D, Mulrow C, Lawrence V. Garlic: its history and adverse effects. J Herb Pharmacother 2001;1:63–83

Murray M, Pizzorno J, eds. Allium sativum (Garlic) in The Textbook of Natural Medicine. 3rd ed. St. Louis, MO: Churchill Livingstone Elsevier; 2006:734

Rauterberg A. Allergic contact dermatitis due to garlic in a cook. Aktuelle Derm 1995;21:317–318

Roberge RJ, Leckey R, Spence R, Krenzelok EJ. Garlic burns of the breast. Am J Emerg Med 1997;15(5):548

Sharma PV. Classical Uses of Medicinal Plants. 1st ed. Varanasi: Chaukhamba Vishvabharati; 2004:321

Sharma PV. Namarupajnanam. 1st ed. Varanasi: Chaukhamba Vishvabharati; 2011:159

The Ayurvedic Pharmacopoeia of India. Part I, Vol. III. 1st ed. New Delhi: Department of Health, Ministry of Health and Family Welfare, Government of India; 1986:108

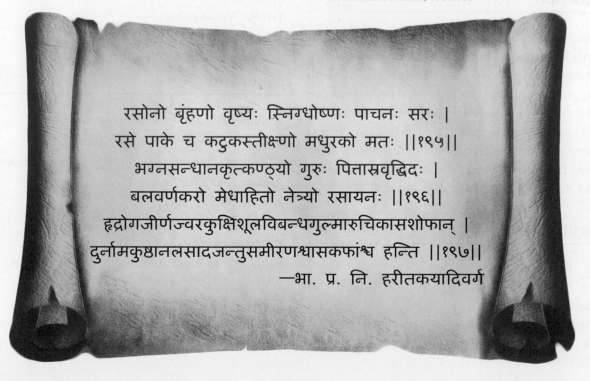

रसोनो बृंहणो वृष्यः स्निग्धोष्णः पाचनः सरः |
रसे पाके च कटुकस्तीक्ष्णो मधुरको मतः ||१९५||
भग्नसन्धानकृत्कण्ठ्यो गुरुः पित्तास्रवृद्धिदः |
बलवर्णकरो मेधाहितो नेत्र्यो रसायनः ||१९६||
हृद्रोगजीर्णज्वरकुक्षिशूलविबन्धगुल्मारुचिकासशोफान् |
दुर्नामकुष्ठानलसादजन्तुसमीरणश्वासकफांश्च हन्ति ||१९७||
—भा. प्र. नि. हरीतक्यादिवर्ग

83. Rohitaka [*Tecomella undulata* G. Don]

Family: *Bignoniaceae*

Hindi name: *Rohida, Roheda*

English name: *Rohida tree*

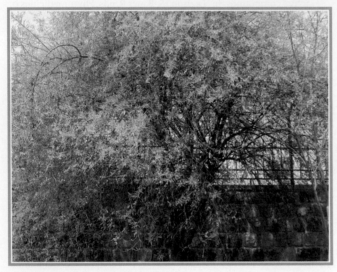

Plant of *Tecomella undulata* G. Don.

It is also known as Desert teak as it is found in arid and semiarid regions of Thar desert. Locally, it is popularly known and traded by the name of Marwar teak or desert teak. The flower of this plant is the state flower of Rajasthan.

Introduction

Tecomella undulata G. Don of Bignoniaceae family is commonly known as desert teak in English and rugtrora in Hindi. The plant Rohitaka is a small shrub or small tree with drooping branches and deciduous or nearly evergreen tree of arid and semiarid regions. It is under threatened condition due to its imprudent harvesting from wild. The plant is very effective to cure leucorrhea, leucoderma, enlargement of spleen, traumatic wounds, hepatitis, piles, anorexia, flatulence, tumors, worm infestations, and syphilis.

Vernacular Names

Bengali: Harinahada, Roda rayana

Gujarati: Rohido

Kannada: Mullumuntala

Malayalam: Chemmaram

Marathi: Rohida

Punjabi: Rohira

Tamil: Malampulvan

Telugu: Rohitaka

Synonyms

Dadimachchhada: It resembles Dadima.

Dadimapuspaka: It resembles Dadima.

Plihaghna: It is very beneficial for spleen disorders.

Raktapuspak: Its flower is red.

Raktavalka: Its bark is red.

Rochana: It has good taste.

Roheetaka: It is a beautiful tree growing wild.

Rohi: It is an efficacious remedy for disorders of liver and spleen.

Rohitaka: It has reddish flowers.

Varatika: It is the best tree among bitter plant categories.

Yakritvairi: It is very beneficial for liver disorders.

Classical Categorization

Charaka Samhita: Not mentioned any gana
Sushrut Samhita: Not mentioned any gana
Dhanwantari Nighantu: Amradi varga
Madanpal Nighantu: Abhayadi varga
Kaiyadev Nighantu: Aushadi varga
Raj Nighantu: Shalmaladi varga
Bhavaprakash Nighantu: Vatadi varga

Distribution

It is a deciduous or nearly evergreen tree of arid and semiarid regions (Chopra et al 1992). This plant originated in India and Arabia (Randhawa and Mukhopadhyay 1986). In India, it is mainly found in western parts of Rajasthan and in Maharashtra, Gujarat, Rajasthan, Punjab, and Haryana. In Rajasthan, it is distributed throughout the districts of Barmer, Jaisalmer, Jodhpur, Pali, Ajmer, Nagaur, Bikaner, Churu, and Sikar (Kritikar and Basu 1993; Nadkarni 2000). In Pakistan, it is found in the regions of Sindh and Baluchistan.

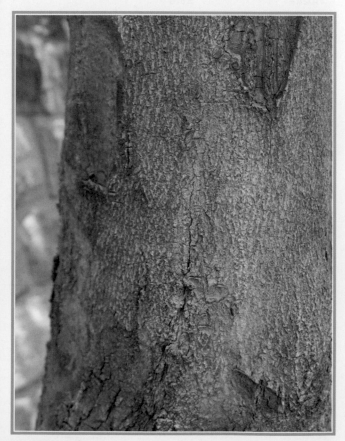

Fig. 83.1   Bark.

Morphology

It is a large shrub or small tree with drooping branches, 2.5 to 5 m in height.

- **Bark:** In young plants, bark is soft and greenish brown, and in trees, it is hard, dark brown, 8 mm thick (**Fig. 83.1**).
- **Leaves:** Grayish-green leaves, simple 5 to 12 cm length by 1 to 3 cm width, narrowly oblong, obtuse and entire with undulating margin (**Fig. 83.2**).
- **Flowers:** Present in corymbose, few flowers racemes, terminating short lateral branches, pedicles 6 to 13 mm long. Flowers are large and beautiful and are found in yellowish-red and orange colors. This flower is the state flower of Rajasthan (**Fig. 83.3a, b**).
- **Calyx:** 9 to 11 mm long, campanulate.
- **Corolla:** 3.5 to 6.5 cm, orange, yellow, campanulate, five subequal lobed, rounded.
- **Stamen:** Exerted, filaments-glabrous.
- **Stigma:** Two laminate, lobes are spatulate-oblong, rounded.
- **Fruit:** Capsule, 20 cm by 1 cm long pod, slightly curved, linear-oblong, acute, smooth (**Fig. 83.4**).
- **Seeds:** 2.5 × 1 cm, winged.

The tree is propagated from seeds and cuttings.

Phenology

Flowering time: April to May
Fruiting time: June to July

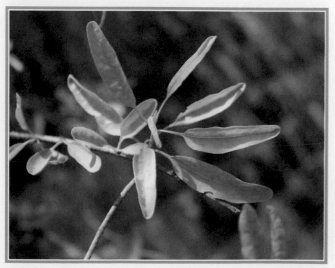

Fig. 83.2   Leaves.

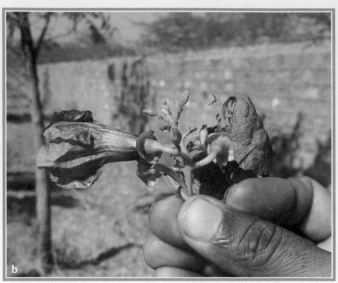

Fig. 83.3 (a, b) Flower.

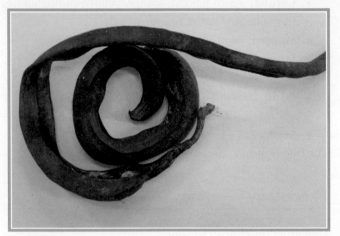

Fig. 83.4 Fruit.

Key Characters for Identification

➤ *Large shrub or small tree with 2.5 to 5 m height.*

➤ *Leaves: Simple, 5 to 12.5 cm × 1 to 3.2 cm, narrowly oblong, obtuse, and entire with undulating margins.*

➤ *Flowers: Large, beautiful, yellow, orange red, and odorless. Pedicles are 6 to 13 mm long.*

➤ *Fruit: Capsule, slightly curved, 15 to 20 cm long pods, 8 mm broad, thin, flattened, and slightly crooked, and seeds are winged, 2 cm long and 8 mm broad.*

➤ *Bark: It is soft and greenish-brown in young plant and hard and dark brown in tree. It is 8 mm and thicker in matured tree.*

Rasapanchaka

Guna	Laghu, Rukhya, Sara
Rasa	Katu, Tikta, Kashaya
Vipaka	Katu
Virya	Sheeta
Prabhav	Pleehaghna

Chemical Constituents

The chemical constituents present are alphanamixin lactone, alphanamixolide, betulinic acid, clutylferulate, crisimaritin, dehydro-α-lapachone, lapachol, oleanic acid, quercetin, radermachol, rohitukin, rutin, stigmasterol, tecomaquinone-1, undulatin, ursolic acid, α-lapachone, β-lapachone, β-sitosterol (Jain et al 2012).

Identity, Purity, and Strength

- Foreign matter: Not more than 2%
- Total ash: Not more than 12%
- Acid-insoluble ash: Not more than 1%
- Alcohol-soluble extractive: Not less than 10%
- Water-soluble extractive: Not less than 15%

(Source: The Ayurvedic Pharmacopeia of India 1986)

Karma (Actions)

It is pungent, astringent, and bitter in taste. Bark is an excellent blood purifier and cholagogue. The drug is capable of following actions: bhedan (purgative), plihaghna (cure diseases of spleen), raktaprasadan (blood purifier), rochan (relish), krimighna (anthelmintic), vranadoshahara (wound healing), etc.

- Doshakarma: Kaphapittahara
- Dhatukarma: Raktaprasadan
- Malakarma: Bhedan

Pharmacological Actions

The various pharmacological actions include analgesic activity, anticancer potential, anti-human immuno-deficiency virus (HIV) potential, anti-inflammatory, antimicrobial, antiobesity, antioxidant, antiproliferative, immunomodulatory, and hepatoprotective activities (Jain et al 2012; Rohilla and Garg 2014).

Indications

It is mainly used in yakrit roga (disease of liver), pliha roga (diseases of spleen), gulma (abdominal lump), udara (abdominal disease), krimi (worm infestation), vrana (wound), raktaja vicar (diseases of blood), and netraroga (eye diseases).

It is used in hepatitis, urinary disorder, splenomegaly, gonorrhea, and leukoderma, and it provides remedy for syphilis and gout. Its bark is also used in treating skin disorder, jaundice, diabetes, cancer, and obesity. Root is used internally for leucorrhea. Bark powder and its decoction are used in enlarged spleen, anemia, intestinal worms, eczema, ascites, piles, anorexia, and tumor.

Therapeutic Uses

1. **Yakritoudar and pleehodar** (hepatomegaly and splenomegaly): Rohitaka stem is kept in the decoction of Haritaki for 7 days and the filtrate is taken to alleviate jaundice, gulma, diabetes, piles, splenomegaly, and other abnormal enlargement and worms (C.S.Ci. 13/81-82; A.H.Ci. 15/91-92). Rohitakghrita is also used for hepatomegaly and splenomegaly (C.S.Ci. 13/85).

2. **Pradar** (leucorrhea): Rohitak root paste is used in pradara (C.S.Ci. 30/116).
3. **Kushta** (skin diseases): Decoction of Khadir, Aragvadha, Arjuna, Rohitaka, Lodhra, Kutaj, Dhava, Nimba, Saptaparna, and Karaveer is used for bath and also used internally for the treatment of kushta (Ch.Chi-7/129).
4. **Prameha** (diabetes): Powder of Kampillak, Saptaparna, Shala, Bibhitaka, Rohitaka, Kutaja, and flowers of Kapittha is taken with honey to treat Kaphapittaja prameha.

Officinal Parts Used

Bark and root

Dose

Powder: 1 to 3 g
Decoction: 50 to 100 mL

Formulations

Rohitak arista, Rohitak ghrita, Rohitakadya choorna, Rohitaka loha, Amlycure, Liv-52, Himoliv.

Substitution and Adulteration

Amoora rohituka W.&A of Meliaceae family is traded as Rohitaka.

Points to Ponder

- *Prabhav of Rohitaka is plihaghna.*
- *Rohitaka is mainly found in dry regions like Rajasthan.*
- *It is mainly used in spleen and liver diseases.*

Suggested Readings

Chopra RN, Nayer SL, Chopra IC. Glossary of Indian Medicinal Plants. New Delhi: National Institute of Science Communication (CSIR); 1992:240

Jain M, Kapadia R, Jadeja RN, Thounaojam MC, Devkar RV, Mishra H. Traditional uses, phytochemistry and pharmacology of *Tecomella undulata*: a review. Asian Pac J Trop Biomed 2012;2:S1918–S1923

Kritikar KR, Basu BD. Indian Medicinal Plants. Dehradun: International Book Distributor; 1993

Lucas DS. Dravyaguna-Vijnana: Study of Dravya-Materia Medica. Varanasi: Chaukhamba Visvabharati; 2013:623

Nadkarni KM. Indian Materia Medica, Vol. 1. Mumbai: Popular Prakashan; 2000:56–57

Randhawa GS, Mukhopadhyay A. Floriculture in India. Mumbai: Allied Publishers; 1986

Rohilla R, Garg M. Phytochemistry and pharmacology of *Tecomella undulata*. Int J Green Pharm 2014;8:1–6

Sharma PV. Classical Uses of Medicinal Plants. 1st ed. Varanasi: Chaukhamba Vishvabharati; 2004:327

Sharma PV. Namarupajnanam. 1st ed. Varanasi: Chaukhamba Vishvabharati; 2011:162

The Ayurvedic Pharmacopoeia of India, Part I, Vol. VI. New Delhi: Department of Health, Ministry of Health and Family Welfare, Government of India; 1986:135

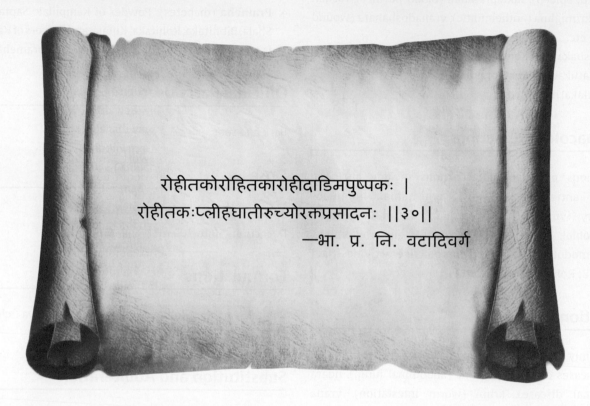

रोहीतकोरोहितकारोहीदाडिमपुष्पकः |
रोहीतकःप्लीहघातीरुच्योरक्तप्रसादनः ||३०||
—भा. प्र. नि. वटादिवर्ग

84. Saireyaka *[Barleria prionitis Linn.]*

Family:	*Acanthaceae*
Hindi name:	*Katsaraiya, Piyabansa, Sahacara, sahachara*
English name:	*Porcupine flower, yellow nail dye plant*

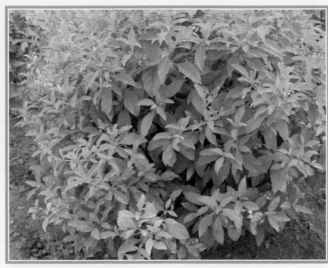

Plant of *Barleria prionitis* Linn.

There are three species of Barleria:
(1) B. prionitis Linn. with yellow flower
(Pitta Saireyaka); (2) B. cristata Linn.
with both red and white flower forms
(Rakta and Sweta Saireyaka); and
(3) B. strigosa with blue flowers (Nila
or Krishna Saireyaka).

Introduction

Barleria prionitis, belonging to Acanthaceae family, is a small spiny shrub, normally familiar as "porcupine flower" with a number of vernacular names. It is an indigenous plant of South Asia and certain regions of Africa. The therapeutical use of its flower, root, stem, leaf, and in certain cases entire plant against numerous disorders including fever, cough, jaundice, and severe pain is recognized by Ayurvedic and other traditional systems.

Acharya Charak has not mentioned Saireyaka in any mahakashaya but he has mentioned about the Krishna Saireyaka (C.S.Ci. 26/266). Sushruta has mentioned Saireyaka dwaya (two varieties of Saireyaka) in viratarvadi gana (S.S.Su. 38/10). Vagabhatta also mentioned two types of Saireyaka in varunadi gana (A.H.Su. 15/21).

Vernacular Names

Assamese: Shinti
Gujarati: Kanta-Saerio, Kantasalio
Kannada: Sahacara
Malayalam: Kirimkurunji, Karim Kurunni
Marathi: Koranta, Koranti, Koreta
Oriya: Dasakeranda
Punjabi: Sahacar
Sanskrit: Kurantaka, Koranda, Kerandaka
Tamil: Sammulli
Telugu: Mulu Gorinta Chettu
Unani: Piyabaasa
Urdu: Pila Bansa, Piya Bansa

Synonyms

Swetapuspa: It has white-colored flower.

Saireyak: It grows in regions fully exposed to the sun such as deserts, naked snowy hill-tops, etc.

Sahachara: This indicates the gregarious habit of occurrence.

Kurantaka: This points toward the presence of piercing structures like thorns in the plant.

Dasi kurantaka: The word "Dasi" may indicate that out of two kurantaka, this may be a smaller than or a close associate of the other.

Rujakara: Thorn of this plant causes pain.

Aartagala: It indicates the oppressed living condition of the plant.

Baana: It indicates the detachment from the parent plants (drop like an arrow) during seedling stage.

Saha and mahasaha: These are also sometimes referred to Saireyak in virtue of their special capacity of toleration and adaptation toward uneasy living conditions and environment.

Classical Categorization

Charak Samhita: Not mentioned in any gana of Charak Samhita

Sushrut Samhita: Varunadi, Aragvadhadi, Veeratarvadi, Kantak panchamoola

Astanga Hridaya: Aragvadhadi, Varunadi

Dhanwantari Nighantu: Guduchyadi varga

Madanpal Nighantu: Abhayadi varga

Kaiyadev Nighantu: Aushadhi varga

Raj Nighantu: Karaviradi varga

Bhavaprakash Nighantu: Puspa varga

Distribution

It is distributed widely throughout Asia including Malaysia, Pakistan, Philippines, Sri Lanka, Bangladesh, Yemen, and tropical Africa. In India, it is commonly found in Assam, Andhra Pradesh, Bihar, Chhattisgarh, Madhya Pradesh, Uttar Pradesh, Tamil Nadu, and West Bengal (Banerjee et al 2012; Vasoya 2012).

Morphology

It is an erect, bushy, perennial shrub 1 to 2 m in height. It possesses two to four sharp, long, axillary spines of 11 mm length.

- **Stem:** Terete, glabrous, much branched with cylindrical, tapering branchlet (**Fig. 84.1**).
- **Leaves:** Simple, opposite, smooth, ovate-elliptic to obovate, acuminate 6-15 cm by 4-6 cm, petiole 0.5 to 3 cm entire margin (**Fig. 84.2**).
- **Flowers:** Sessile, yellow-orange color, equally broad as well as tubular, 3 to 4 cm in length, often solitary in lower axils and spectate in upper axils. Bracts are acute, linear-lanceolate about 1 to 1.5 cm. Corolla is

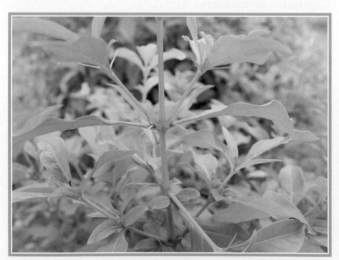

Fig. 84.1 Stem and spine.

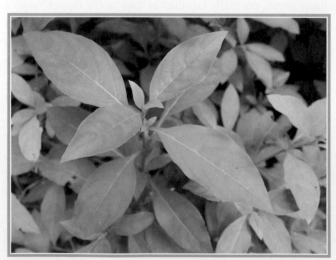

Fig. 84.2 Leaves.

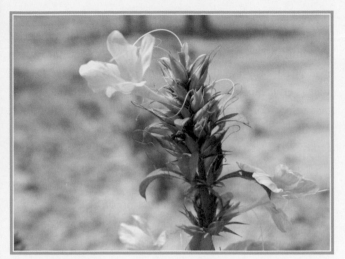

Fig. 84.3 Flowers.

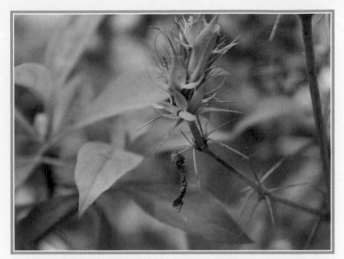

Fig. 84.4 Fruits.

bright golden yellow color. The stamen includes two fertile stamens and two staminoid stamens. The ovary is ovoid and the stigma is long, linear, sticky, and pinkish in color (**Fig. 84.3**).

- **Fruit:** Ovoid and capsular, two-seeded, 1.5-2 cm by 0.6-0.8 cm (**Fig. 84.4**).
- **Seed:** Oval-oblong, flattened, covered with matted hairs, 8 mm by 5 mm (Jain et al 2009; Kala 2005; Kirtikar and Basu 1999; Kaushik and Dhiman 2000; Shendage and Yadav 2010; Dassanayake 1998; Kamble et al 2007).

Phenology

Flowering time: Throughout the year
Fruiting time: Throughout the year

Key Characters for Identification

➤ *It is an erect, thick, thorny undershrub coming up to 1 to 2 m high.*
➤ *Stem: Erect, 1.8 mm thick, terete, hard, glabrous.*
➤ *Leaves: Simple, opposite, smooth, oval-ellipsoid, elliptic whole, variable in scrutinize to 10 cm long and 4 cm wide, petiole short.*
➤ *Flower: Tubular, yellow-orange, 4.0 cm long blooms with distending stalks. Sessile, regularly single in the lower axils, getting to be noticeably spicate above; bracts foliaceous.*
➤ *Fruits: Ovoid and capsular, two-seeded, 1.5-2 cm by 0.6-0.8 cm.*

Types

Bhavaprakash has mentioned four types of Saireyaka as per the color of the flowers with their various synonyms.

- Sweta puspa (*B. cristata* Linn.): This plant has white flowers and other names of this plant is Saireyaka, Swetapuspa Saireyaka, Katu sarika, Sahachara, Bhindi.
- Pitta puspa (*B. prionitis* Linn.): This plant has yellow flower. Other synonyms are Kurantaka.
- Rakta puspa (*B. cristata* Linn.): It has red flower and it is also known as Kurabaka.
- Nila puspa (*B. strigosa* Willd.): The plant has blue flower. Other synonyms are Bana, Baana Dasi, Atargala.

The different species of *Barleria* is the source plant of Saireyaka. These are only classified as per the color of the flowers. The properties and actions of all species are almost similar.

Rasapanchaka

Guna	Laghu
Rasa	Tikta, Madhura
Vipak	Katu
Virya	Ushna

Chemical Constituents

Potassium salt, balarenone, pipataline, lupeol, prioniside-A, B, & C, barlerinoside, verbascosides, shanzhiside, methyl ester, barlerin, acetyl barlerin, 7-methoxydideroside, lupinoside, vanilic acid, p-hydroxybenzoic acids, 6-hydroxyflavanes, β-sitosterol, apigenin 7-0-glucosides, hydroxyl-2,7-dimethyl-3, 6-dimethoxy anthraquinones, 1,3,6,8-tetra methoxy-2, 7-rhamnosyl glucosides (Banerjee et al 2012; Ata et al 2009; Perrin and Amerigo 1996).

Identity, Purity, and Strength

- Foreign matter: Not more than 2%
- Total ash: Not more than 7%
- Acid-insoluble ash: Not more than 1%
- Alcohol-soluble extractive: Not less than 4%
- Water-soluble extractive: Not less than 10%

(Source: The Ayurvedic Pharmacopeia of India 2001)

Karma (Actions)

Kandughna (antipruritus), vishaghna (antidote), kesharanjan (blackening of hairs), keshya (hair tonic), balya (provide physical strength), vrishya (aphrodisiac), kasaghna (antitussive).

- Doshakarma: Kaphavatahara
- Dhatukarma: Vrishya, balya
- Malakarma: Mutral

Pharmacological Actions

The pharmacological actions of *B. prionitis* are anthelminthic, antifertility, antiarthritic, antihypertensive, antibacterial, anticancer, antifungal, anti-inflammatory, antidiabetic, antinociceptive, antioxidant, free radical scavenging, antiviral, CNS depressant, hepatoprotective, gastroprotective, cytotoxic, diuretic, enzyme inhibitory, larvicidal, antidental decay, wound healing (Banerjee et al 2012; Kapoor et al 2014; Naryan and Nikam 2018).

Indications

It is used in kushta (skin disease), vatarakta (gout), kandu (pruritus), vatavyadhi (neuromuscular disease), palitya (premature graying of hairs), shopha (swelling), trishna (thirst), vidaha (burning sensation), visarpa (erysipelas), pandu (anemia), visha (poisoning).

Its leaf is very useful for the treatment of cough, irritation, stiffness of limbs, cold, cataract, enlargement of scrotum, and sciatica (Kumar et al 2011; Sankaranarayanan et al 2010; Singh et al 2012; Mohammed et al 2004). Leaf juice is efficacious as remedy of catarrhal affections, dropsy, gastric problems, pus in ears, whooping cough, glandular swellings, and boils (Mohammed et al 2004; Meena and Yadav 2010). For skin disease and wound, apply crushed leaf on skin (Patil et al 2009; Alam et al 2011). Leaf paste is also very beneficial for curing scabies and toothache (Reddy et al 2010). In case of fever, decoction of leaf extract with honey is given for 7 days (Panda et al 2011). In leucoderma, its ash is applied with butter (Sharma et al 2013).

Therapeutic Uses

External Use

1. **Visarpa** (erysipelas): The paste of Khadira, Saptaparna, Musta, Aragvadha, Dhava, Kurantak, and Devdaru should be applied locally in Khapaja Visarpa (C.S.Ci-21/88).
2. **Vatarakta** (gout): Roots of Sahachar and Jivanti pounded with goat's milk and mixed with ghee should be applied as paste externally (A.H.Ci-22/33).
3. **Graying of hair:** 1 kudava (200 mL) of oil should be cooked with 1 prastha (800 mL) of milk and juice of Bhringaraj, Saireyaka, Tulasi along with 1 pala (50 g) of Yastimadhu and then kept in a stony container or in sheep horn. This oil is used for blackening of hair (A.H.U-24/37-38).

Internal Use

1. **Vatavyadhi** (neuromuscular disease): Oil prepared with the decoction of Sahachar, Devdar, and Shunthi is used in Vatavyadhi.
2. **Mushika visha** (rat poisoning): Root powder of Saireyaka is given with honey and rice water (A.H.U-38/30).

Officinal Parts Used

Root, leaves, whole plant

Dose

Juice: 10 to 20 mL
Decoction: 40 to 80 mL

Formulations

Shahacharadi taila, Nilikadya taila, Astavarga kvatha churna, Rasnarandadi kvatha churna.

Toxicity/Adverse Effects

The toxicity study of alcoholic extract of root and leaves of *B. prionitis* did not show any toxic effect on adult albino rats. No death was reported for the oral administration of extract up to the dose of 2.5 mg/kg body weight for 14 days (Dheer and Bhatnagar 2010). It is also reported that the iridoid glucosides rich aqueous fraction did not produce any sign of abnormalities or any mortality up to the single oral administration of 3,000 mg/kg dose in mice for 15 days of study (Singh et al 2005). However, the intraperitoneal LD_{50} was determined as 2,530 mg/kg dose for aqueous fraction in mice (Singh et al 2005).

> *Points to Ponder*
>
> - *Bhavaprakash has mentioned four types of Saireyaka as per the color of the flowers: sweta, pitta, nila, and rakta puspa Saireyaka.*

Suggested Readings

Alam G, Singh MP, Singh A. Wound healing potential of some medicinal plants. Int J Pharm Sci Rev Res 2011;9(1):136–145

Ata A, Kalhari KA, Samarasekera R. Chemical constituents of *Barleria prionitis* and their enzyme inhibitory and free radical scavenging activities. Phytochem Lett 2009;2(1):37–40

Banerjee D, Maji A, Banerji P. *Barleria prionitis* Linn: a review of its traditional uses, phytochemistry, pharmacology and toxicity. Res J Phytochem 2012;(6):31–41

Dassanayake MD. A Revised Handbook to the Flora of Ceylon, Vol. 12. Boca Raton, FL: CRC Press; 1998: 87

Dheer R, Bhatnagar P. A study of the antidiabetic activity of *Barleria prionitis* Linn. Indian J Pharmacol 2010;42(2):70–73

Jain S, Jain R, Singh R. Ethnobotanical survey of Sariska and Siliserh regions from Alwar district of Rajasthan, India. Ethnobotanic Leafl 2009;1:21

Kala CP. Ethnomedicinal botany of the Apatani in the Eastern Himalayan region of India. J Ethnobiol Ethnomed 2005;1(11):11

Kamble MY, Pal SR, Shendage SM, Dixit GB, Chavan PD, Yadav US, Yadav SR. Promising Indian *Barleria* of ornamental potential. In: Peter KV, ed. Underutilized and Underexploited Horticultural Crops, Vol. 1. New Delhi: New India Publishing Agency; 2007:144

Kapoor A, Shukla S, Kaur R, Kumar R. Preliminary phytochemical screening and antioxidant activity of whole plant of *Barleria prionitis* Linn. Int J Adv Pharma Biol Chem 2014;3(2):410–419

Kaushik P, Dhiman AK. Medicinal Plants and Raw Drugs of India. Dehradun, India: Shiva Offset Press; 2000:412

Kirtikar KR, Basu BD. Indian Medicinal Plants. Dehradun: Bishen Singh Mahendra Pal Singh; 1999:1877–1878

Kumar M, Sheikh MA, Bussmann RW. Ethnomedicinal and ecological status of plants in Garhwal Himalaya, India. J Ethnobiol Ethnomed 2011;7(1):32

Meena K, Yadav B. Some traditional ethnomedicinal plants of southern Rajasthan. Indian J Tradit Knowl 2010;9(3):471–474

Mohammed S, Kasera PK, Shukla JK. Unexploited plants of potential medicinal value from the Indian Thar desert. Nat Prod Radiance 2004;3(2):69–74

Naryan S, Nikam P. A review on pharmacological activities of *Barleria prionitis* linn. World J Pharm Res 2018;7(6):166–180

Panda S, Rout S, Mishra N, Panda T. Phytotherapy and traditional knowledge of tribal communities of Mayurbhanj district, Orissa, India. J Pharmacogn Phytother 2011;3(7):101–113

Patil SB, Naikwade NS, Kondawar MS, Magdum CS, Awale VB. Traditional uses of plants for wound healing in the Sangli district, Maharashtra. Int J Pharm Tech Res 2009;1(3):876–878

Perrin DD, Amerigo WL, eds. Purification of Laboratory Chemicals. 4th ed. New York, NY: Butterworth; 1996

Reddy K, Trimurthulu G, Reddy CS. Medicinal plants used by ethnic people of Medak district, Andhra Pradesh. Indian J Tradit Knowl 2010;9(1):184–190

Sankaranarayanan S, Bama P, Ramachandran J, et al. Ethnobotanical study of medicinal plants used by traditional users in Villupuram district of Tamil Nadu, India. J Med Plants Res 2010;4(12):1089–1101

Sharma P, Shrivastava B, Sharma GN, Jadhav HR. Phytochemical and ethnomedicinal values of *Barleria prionitis* L.: an overview. J Harmo Res Pharm 2013;2(3):190–199

Shendage SM, Yadav SR. Revision of the Genus *Barleria* (Acanthaceae) in India. Rheedea 2010;20:81–130

Singh B, Chandan BK, Prabhakar A, Taneja SC, Singh J, Qazi GN. Chemistry and hepatoprotective activity of an active fraction from *Barleria prionitis* Linn. in experimental animals. Phytother Res 2005;19(5):391–404

Singh B, Kumar D, Singh R. Phytotherapeutics for management and prevention of cataract generation. Phytopharmacology. 2012;3(1):93–110

The Ayurvedic Pharmacopoeia of India, Vol. 3. New Delhi: Ministry of Health & Family Welfare, Department of Ayush, Government of India; 2001:165

Vasoya U. Pharmacognostical and physicochemical studies on the leaves of *Barleria prionitis* (L.). Int J Pharm Sci Res 2012;3(7):2291

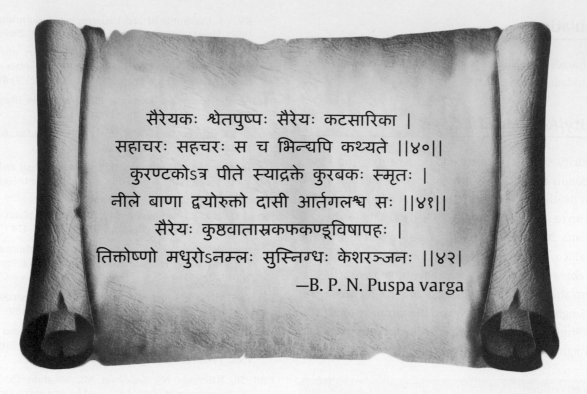

सैरेयकः श्वेतपुष्पः सैरेयः कटसारिका |
सहाचरः सहचरः स च भिन्द्यपि कथ्यते ||४०||
कुरण्टकोऽत्र पीते स्याद्रक्ते कुरबकः स्मृतः |
नीले बाणा द्वयोरुक्तो दासी आर्तगलश्च सः ||४१||
सैरेयः कुष्ठवातास्रकफकण्डूविषापहः |
तिक्तोष्णो मधुरोऽनम्लः सुस्निग्धः केशरञ्जनः ||४२|

—B. P. N. Puspa varga

85. Sarivadvaya [*Hemidesmus indicus* R.Br. *and Cryptolepis buchananii* Roem & Schult]

> *Plant has two varieties, namely, white variety, called "Sweta Sariva," and black variety, "Krishna Sariva." Ayurvedic formulary accepts* Hemidesmus indicus *as white variety, and* Cryptolepis buchananii *Roem. and Schult as black variety.* Ichnocarpus frutescens *is also used as black variety by the people of West Bengal and Kerala.*
>
> —Khare CP (2004)

Introduction

The name "Hemidesmus" is derived from Latin word "Hemidesmos" which means "half bond." It is so named in allusion to subconnate filaments at their base—joint pods and connected stamens. Word "indicus" stands for "of India." *Hemidesmus indicus* belongs to family Asclepiadaceae, which is derived from the word "Askleplos," meaning "God of Medicine" (Gogte 2000). "Anantmul" is a Sanskrit word which means "endless root" (Gupta 2006). It is a white-colored useful twiner spreading extensively that's why it is called Sariva.

H. indicus, commonly known as Anantmool, belongs to the family of Asclepiadaceae. This is a creeper-type plant found in upper Gangetic plain, eastwards to Bengal and Sundarbans and from Central provinces to Travancore and South India. It is a twiner extensively spreading creeper with leaves like serpent's tongue. The useful part is its root which has pleasant aroma like sandal wood. *H. indicus* root is sweet, has cooling effect, and is demulcent. It is very useful as tonic, diuretic, and aphrodisiac. Whole root and root bark are useful in syphilis, leucoderma, hemicrania, rheumatism, and in several liver and kidney disorders.

Vernacular Names

Assamese: Vaga Sariva
Bengali: Anantamul, Shvetashariva
English: Indian Sarasa Parilla
Gujarati: Upalsari, Kabri
Hindi: Anantamul
Kannada: Namada veru, Bili Namadaberu, Anantamool
Kashmiri: Anant mool
Malayalam: Nannari, Nannar, Naruneendi
Marathi: Upalsari, Anantamula
Oriya: Dralashvan Lai Anantamool
Punjabi: Anantmool, Ushbah
Sanskrit: Ananta, Gopasuta, Sariva
Tamil: Ven Nannar
Telugu: Sugandhi Pala, Tella Sugandhi
Urdu: Ushba Hindi

Synonyms

Ananta: It is an extensively spreading creeper.
Aspota: Its fruits are dehiscent.
Chandana: It has sandalwood scent.
Dhavala Sariva: It is a handsome creeper.
Gopa: It protects people from diseases.
Gopakanya: It is reared like a family member.
Gopavalli: It protects people from diseases.
Krushodari: Its stems are thin.
Lata: It is a creeper.
Phanijihwika: Its leaves are like serpent's tongue.
Pratanika: It is a creeper that grows extensively.
Saradi: Its flowers appear in autumn.
Sariva: It is a white useful twiner spreading extensively.
Shyama: It has black color stem (Krishna sariva).

Sugandhimula: Its root is aromatic.

Uttpalasariva: Its aroma is like lotus.

Classification

Charak Samhita: Jwarhara, Dahaprasamana, Stanyasodhana, Kanthya purishasangrahaniya

Sushruta Samhita: Sarivadi, Vidarigandhadi, Vallipanchamoola

Astanga Hridaya: Sarivadi

Dhanwantari Nighantu: Guduchyadi varga

Madanpal Nighantu: Abhayadi varga

Kaiyadev Nighantu: Aushadi varga

Raj Nighantu: Chandanadi varga

Bhavaprakash Nighantu: Guduchyadi varga

Sweta Sariva (*H. indicus* R.Br.)

Family: Asclepiadaceae

English name: Indian sarsaparilla

Hindi name: Anantamool

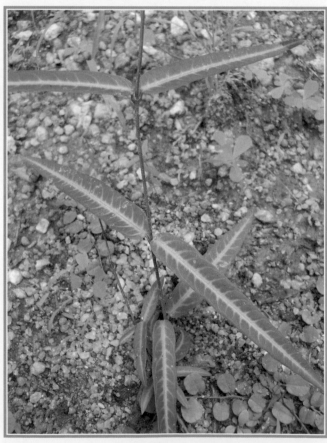

Plant of *Hemidesmus indicus* R.Br.

Distribution

It is found throughout India growing under mesophytic to semi dry condition up to an altitude of 600m .It is also found in Sri Lanka, Pakistan, Iran, and Moluccas. It is generally grows in tropical rainforests and in hot temperate region.

Morphology

It is a slender, laticiferous, perennial, twining, sometimes prostrate, or semierect shrub.

- **Root:** Woody, slender, aromatic, and cylindrical in shape, irregularly bent, 1.5 to 2 cm diameter, externally dark brown, and internally yellowish-brown in color (**Fig. 85.1**).
- **Stems:** Numerous, slender with thickened nodes.
- **Leaves:** Simple, opposites, variable shape, from elliptical oblong to linear lanceolate, 5 to 10 cm long, dark green color (**Fig. 85.2**).

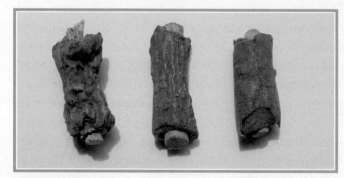

Fig. 85.1 Root.

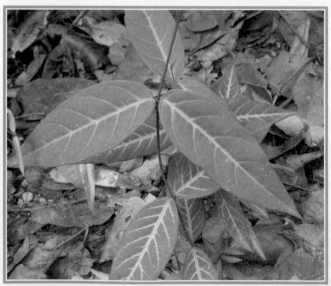

Fig. 85.2 Leaves of Sweta Sariva.

- **Flower:** Greenish-yellow to greenish-purple outside, dull yellow to light purple inside, calyx deeply five-lobed, corolla gamopetalous: about twice to calyx, stamens: 5 in number, inserted near base of corolla with a thick coronal scale.
- Pistil bicarpellary, ovaries free, many ovules with distinct styles.
- **Fruits:** Two straight, slender, narrowly cylindrical, widely divergent follicles, 10-15 cm by 0.5-1 cm.
- **Seeds:** Seeds are many, flat, black, oblong with a long tuft of white silky hairs.

Key Characters for Identification

➤ *It is a slender, laticiferous, perennial, twining, sometimes prostrate, or semierect shrub.*
➤ *Root: Woody, slender, aromatic, and cylindrical in shape, externally dark brown and internally yellowish-brown in color.*
➤ *Leaves: Simple, opposites, variable shape, from elliptical oblong to linear lanceolate, 5 to 10 cm long.*
➤ *Flower: Greenish-yellow to greenish-purple outside, dull yellow to light purple inside.*
➤ *Fruits: Two straight, slender, narrowly cylindrical, widely divergent follicles, 10 to 15 cm by 0.5 to 1 cm.*
➤ *Seeds: Seeds many, flat, black.*

Krishna Sariva (*Cryptolepis buchananii* Roem & Schult)

Family: Asclepiadaceae
Hindi name: Kali Anantamool

Distribution

It is found in the deciduous forest of sub-Himalaya tract, Bihar, Odisha, and Varanasi.

Morphology

It is a large, twining, and straggling shrub, 10 to 20 cm long, stems twining together, old stem 2 to 3 cm in diameter.

- **Leaves:** Simple, opposite, thick, glabrous, 3 to 6 cm in length, elliptic oblong, entire margin, mucronate, upper surface smooth, while lower is rough.
- **Flower:** Pedicellate and bracteate, corolla greenish yellow, filament free, anther more or less triangular

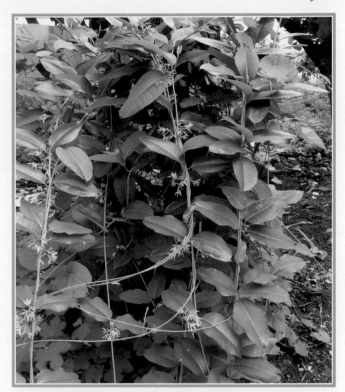

Plant of *Cryptolepis buchananii* Roem & Schult.

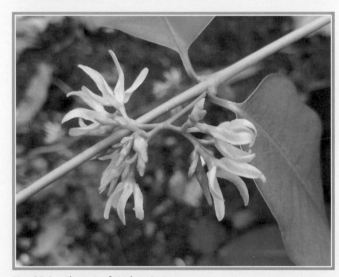

Fig. 85.3 Flowers of Krishna Sariva.

with the connective produced into fleshy apex (**Fig. 85.3**). It is generally known as Jammu patra Sariva.

Phenology

Flowering time: September to December
Fruiting time: January to May

Types

Bhavamishra has described two types of Sariva:

1. Sweta Sariva: *H. indicus* R.Br.
   Family: Asclepiadaceae
2. Krishna Sariva: *C. buchananii* Roem&Schult
   Family: Asclepiadaceae
3. *Ichnocarpus frutescens*
   Family: Apocynaceae
4. Another species: *Decalepis hamiltonii*
   Family: Asclepiadaceae, which falls under Sarivabheda

Bhavamishra has mentioned similar properties and actions for both Sweta and Krishna Sariva.

Rasapanchaka

Guna	Guru, Snigdha
Rasa	Madhur, Tikta
Vipak	Madhur
Virya	Sheeta

Chemical Constituents

The chemical composition of various parts is as follows:

- Root: 2-hydroxy-4benzaldehyde, alpha-amyrinetriterpene, alpha-amyrine, B-amirineacetate, B-amyrine, Beta-amyrin triterpene, B-sitosterol, glucose, hemidesmin 1&2, hemidesmol, hemidesterol, hemidicusin, hexadecanoic acids, lupeol acetate, lupeol octasonate. Its oil contains 80% crystalline matter.
- Stem: Indicine and hemidine, hemidescine, emidine, demicunine, heminine, desinine, indicusin, emisine, desminine steroid, hemisine steroid, hexadecanoic acid, lupanone.
- Leaves: Hemidesminine, hemidesmin 1&2, hyperoside, rutin.
- Flower: Hyperoside, isoquercetin, and rutin (Banerjee and Ganguly 2014).

Identity, Purity, and Strength

- Foreign matter: Not more than 2%
- Ash: Not more than 4%
- Acid-insoluble ash: Not more than 0.5%
- Alcohol-soluble extractive: Not less than 15%
- Water-soluble extractive: Not less than 13%

(Source: The Ayurvedic Pharmacopeia of India 2001)

Karma (Actions)

It is a potent drug for amavishahara, grahi (astringent), shukral (spermatopoetic), sthanyasodhana (purification of breast milk), raktaprasadan (blood purifier), mutrajanana (diuretic), rasayana (rejuvenative), jwarghna (antipyretics), varnya (complexion promoter), kanthya (beneficial for throat), vishaghna (antidote), tonic, aphrodisiac, etc.

- Doshakarma: Tridoshahara
- Dhatukarma: Raktaprasadana, Shukral
- Malakarma: Mutrajanana

Pharmacological Actions

Various pharmacological actions are antienterobacterial, antileprotic, antithrombotic, antiulcer, antiarthritic, anticarcinogenic, antidiarrheal, antihyperlipidemic, anti-inflammatory, antimicrobial, antinociceptive, antioxidant, antipyretic, cytotoxic, hepatoprotective, immunomodulatory, nootropic effect, otoprotective, renoprotective, venum nutrilizaton, wound healing, etc. (Gaurav et al 2009; Sabyasachi et al 2014).

Indications

It is useful in agnimandya (loss of appetite), shwasa (asthma), kasa (cough), sweta pradara (leucorrhea), jwara (fever), kushta (leprosy) and other skin diseases, urticaria, daha (burning sensation), ophthalmopathy, epileptic fits, syphilis, abscess, arsha (hemorrhoids), arthralgia, general debility, and vrana (wounds) (Sharma et al 2000).

Therapeutic Uses

1. **Visham jwara** (intermittent fever): Decoction of Patola, Sariva, Musta, Patha, and Katuki is used to alleviate malaria fever (C.S.Ci. 3.201-203).
2. **Kushta** (leprosy): Bruhati, Ushira, Sariva, Patola, and Katuki are used for drinking, bathing, in ointment, and as paste to cure kushta (C.S.Ci. 7.128).

3. **Vrana** (wounds): Root of Sariva is alone capable for cleansing of all types of wound (VM. 44.33).

4. **Visarpa** (erysipelas): The wise physician should prescribe the decoction of Musta, Sariva, Ushira, and Amalaki for the treatment of visarpa (C.S.Ci. 21.54).

5. **Shwasa** (asthma): Ghee cooked with double quantity of the decoction of Sariva is useful in the treatment of asthma (S.S.U. 51.26).

6. **Raktapitta** (intrinsic hemorrhage): In epistaxis, snuffing should be done with milk or Kamala and Utpala with Sariva (C.S.Ci. 4.101).

7. **Visha** (poisoning): Intake of Madhuka, Kushta, Shirisa, Haridra, Patala, nimba, and Sariva mixed with honey is efficacious in spider poisoning (C.S.Ci. 23.202).

8. **Pregnancy:** The use of Sariva in month to month regimen during pregnancy stabilizes fetus and thus prevents abortion (SS.Sa. 10.60-64).

Officinal Part Used

Root

Dose

Powder: 3 to 5 g
Kalka (paste): 5 to 10 g
Phanta (hot infusion): 50 to 100 mL

Formulations

Sarivadikwath, Sarivadivati, Sarivadyaavaleha, Pindataila, Sarivadyasava.

Substitution and Adulteration

The roots of *C. buchananii* and *I. frutescens* are used as substitutes (Lucas 2013).

Points to Ponder

- *Sariva is of two types: Sweta and Krishna Sariva.*
- *The roots of C. buchananii and I. frutescens are used as substitutes.*
- *Krishna Sariva is known as Jambu patra Sariva.*

Suggested Readings

Banerjee A, Ganguly S. Medicinal importance of *Hemidesmus indicus*: a review on its utilities from Ancient Ayurveda to 20th century. Adv Biores 2014;5(3):208–213

Chatterjee S, Banerjee A, Chandra I. Hemidesmus indicus: a rich source of herbal medicine. Med Aromat Plants 2014;3(4):e155

Chatterjee S, Banerjee A, Chandra I. *Hemidesmus indicus*: a rich source of herbal medicine. Med Aromat Plants 2014;3:e155

Gogte VM. Ayurvedic Pharmacology and Therapeutic Uses of Medicinal Plants. 1st ed. Mumbai: Bhartiya Vidhya Bhavan; 2000:512–513

Gupta NS. The Ayurvedic System of Indian Medicine, Vol. I. New Delhi: Bharatiya Kala Prakashan;2006:96–97

Khare CP. Encyclopedia of Indian Medicinal Plants. New York: Springer; 2004:245-247

Lucas DS, Dravyaguna-Vijnana: Study of Dravya-Materia Medica. Varanasi: Chaukhamba Visvabharati; 2013:275

Panchal GA, Panchal SJ, Patel JA. *Hemidesmus indicus*: a review. Pharmacology 2009;2:758–771

Panchal GA, Panchal SJ, Patel JA. Hemidesmus indicus: a review. Pharmacology 2009;2:758–771

Sharma PC, Yelne MB, Dennis TJ. Database on Medicinal Plants Used in Ayurveda, Vol. I. New Delhi: Central Council for Research in Ayurveda & Siddha; 2000:394-403

Sharma PV. Classical Uses of Medicinal Plants. 1st ed. Varanasi: Chaukhamba Vishvabharati; 2004:391

Sharma PV. Namarupajnanam. 1st ed. Varanasi: Chaukhamba Vishvabharati; 2011:191

The Ayurvedic Pharmacopoeia of India, Part I, Vol. I. 1st ed. New Delhi: Department of Health, Ministry of Health and Family Welfare, Government of India; 2001:142

इन्द्रजम्बूकवत्पत्रासुगन्धाकलघण्टिका।
कृष्णातुशारिवाश्यामागोपीगोपवधूश्चसा॥२०३॥
श्वेतसारिवा-
धवलाशारिवागोपीगोपाकन्याकृशोदरी।
स्फोटाश्यामागोपवल्लीलतास्फोताचचन्दना॥२०४॥
सारिवायुगलंस्वादुस्निग्धंशुक्रकरंगुरु।
अग्निमान्द्यारुचिश्वासकासामविषनाशनम्।
दोषत्रयास्रप्रदरज्वरातीसारनाशनम्॥२०५॥

—B. P. N. Guduchyadi varga

86. Sarpagandha *[Rauvolfia serpentina (L.) Benth. ex]*

Family: *Apocynaceae*

Hindi name: *Chota chand, Dhavalbaruaa, Chandrabhaga, Chadamarava, Harkaichanda, Nai*

English name: *Serpentine root, Rauvolfia root, Serpentina root*

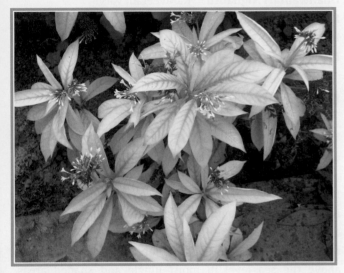

Plant of *Rauvolfia serpentina* (L.) Benth. ex) Kurz.

> *Sarpagandha is one of the popular herbal medicines used in the treatment of high blood pressure, insanity, and schizophrenia, that is why it is known as "Pagalpan ki Buti."*

Introduction

Rauvolfia serpentina (Linn.) Benth. Ex Kurz is a glabrous herb or shrub, belonging to the family Apocynaceae. The genus name was selected in honor of Dr Leonhard Rauwolf of Augsburg, a 16th-century German botanist, physician, and explorer. It was believed that snakes keep away from the scent of this vegetation. According to others, the root of this plant looks like a serpent, but both assumptions look unrealistic and unfounded. The more appropriate reason for this name is that it has therapeutic values that are used in treating the victims of snake bite. There is a popular folklore and belief that before fighting with the cobra, a mongoose first chews the leaf of this herb to gain strength. There is also the belief that it serves as an antidote when its leaves are ground, made a paste, and applied to the toes of snake-bitten victim. It was also used as a medicinal cure for insanity and aptly named as *pagal-ki-dava* (medicine for a mentally disturbed person) in India (Agrawal 2019).

It has been very well described and used by the ancestors of Ayurveda. Acharya Charaka described it as Nakuli, an ingredient of vachadi yoga which is used for the treatment of poisoning. Whereas Sushruta (600 BC) has included it in Aparajita gana and Eksara gana, which are known to treat mental disorders (S.S.U. 60/47) and rat poisoning (S.S.K. 5/84, S.S.K. 7/29), respectively. Vrindamadhav described its use in the treatment of gastroenteritis (visuchika, Vrindamadhava 6/26). In Dhanvantari Nighantu, it is described as Nakuli with other synonyms such as sugandha and katushna and also reported in the treatment of rat poisoning. Bhavaprakash described it as a type of rasna.

This drug is much used in schizophrenia and conditions involving influence of evil spirits (bhutawadha). In modern era, Sarpagandha is used as an effective antihypertensive drug and it is also considered as world's first antihypertensive drug (Singh et al 2015).

Vernacular Names

Sanskrit: Nakuli, Candrika, Chandramarah
Assamese: Arachontita.
Bengali: Chaandar, Chandra, Chotachand
Gujarati: Amelpodee, Sarpagandha
Kannada: Sutranaabhu, Sarpagandhi, Shivanabhiballi, Sutranabi, Patalgaruda, Suvapaval poriyan
Konkan: Patalagarud
Malayalam: Amalpori, Chivanavilpuri, Chivan avelpori, Tulunni, Vantuvala
Marathi: Adkai, Chandra, Harkaya, Harki, Mungusavel, Sapsanda
Oriya: Dhanbarua, Sanochado, Patalagarur
Tamil: Sarppaganti, Chivan melpodi, Sivanamelpodi, Covannamilpori, Savannamilbori
Telugu: Sarpagandhi, Patalagani, Patala garuda, Patalagandhi, Dumparasna
Urdu: Asrel

Synonyms

Bhujangakshi: Mature fruits of this plant look like the eye of a snake.
Dhavalavitapa: The plant purifies the body.
Gandhanakuli: The plant grows in hilly area and it has a peculiar smell.
MahaVirya: It is a potent drug.
Nagasugandha: The plant grows in hilly area and it has a peculiar smell.
Nakuli: The plant easily grows in hilly areas.
Nakulesta: The plant easily grows in hilly areas.
Raktapuspika: It has red-colored flowers.
Sarpagandha: The root of this plant has a peculiar smell which drives away snakes.
Sarpakankalika: The roots of this plant resemble a snake.
Sarpakshi: Mature fruits of this plant look like the eye of a snake.
Sarpangi: The roots of this plant resemble a snake.
Sarpasugandha: The root of this plant has peculiar smell which drives away the snake.
Sumahakanda: The roots have agreeable smell.
Surasa: The plant has exudates or latex.
Swarasa: The plant has exudates or latex.
Vishadamstraka: It has vishaghna property or acts as an antidote.

Vishnasini/Vishaghni: It has vishaghna property or acts as an antidote.
The other synonyms are iswari, ahibhuk, swarasa, sarpadani, vyalagandha, sarpadani, etc.

Classical Categorization

Charak Samhita: Not mentioned in any gana
Sushrut Samhita: Aparajitadi gana, Ekasar gana
Dhanwantari Nighantu: Karaveeradi varga
Kaiyadev Nighantu: Aushadhi varga
Raj Nighantu: Mulakadi varga
Bhavaprakash Nighantu: Haritakyadi varga

Distribution

The plant is found in the tropical Himalayas in lowers hills of Himachal Pradesh, Uttaranchal, Jammu and Kashmir, and at moderate altitude in Sikkim, North Bihar, Patna, Uttar Pradesh, Bhagalpur, Bengal, Konkan, Assam, Burma, Sri Lanka, Andaman, Pegu, Tenasserim, and Deccan Peninsula along with the Ghats of Travancore and Ceylon, Java, and Malay Peninsula. Mostly, it is found at 4,000 feet height above the sea level in moist jungle and shaded areas. Cultivation of Rauvolfia has been started in different areas of India, such as Dehradun, Lucknow, Jammu, and Indore (Nadkarni 2007).

Morphology

It is a small, erect, perennial undershrub of 30 to 40 cm height.

- **Leaves:** Simple, glabrous, in whorls 3–4, rarely opposite, dark green above, pale green below, ecliptic-lanceolate, or obovate, tapering at base, acute apex and entire margin (**Fig. 86.1**).
- **Flowers:** Bisexual, white, often tinged with red color, in 5 to 10 cm long peduncled corymbose cymes, pedicels stout (**Fig. 86.2**).
- **Fruit:** Drupes, ovoid shape, green when unripe and purplish black when fully ripe (**Fig. 86.3**).
- **Roots:** Soft, brownish, tuberous zigzag with irregular nodes, frequently curved and twisted bark pale brown, corky, longitudinally fissured. Dry roots are very hard, tortuous, yellowish brown surface with vertical cracks or wrinkles. Fracture short, irregular, odorless,

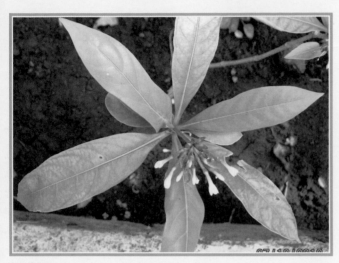

Fig. 86.1 Leaves.

taste very bitter. Dry root when rubbed with water yields a yellowish-tinged paste. In fresh condition, the bark gets easily separated from the woody portion whereas in dry root it doesn't (Vaidyaratnam 2010; Sastry 2008; Gogte 2009; **Fig. 86.4a, b**).

It is propagated through seeds, stem cutting, and root cutting.

Phenology

Flowering time: November to May (almost throughout the year but chiefly during February to May)

Fruiting time: Almost throughout the year

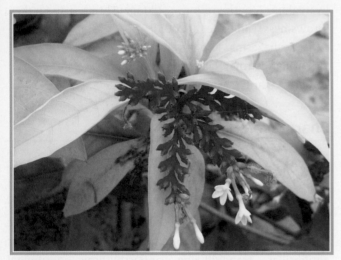

Fig. 86.2 Flowers.

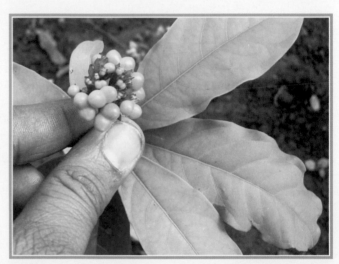

Fig. 86.3 Fruits.

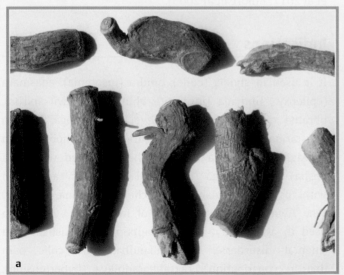

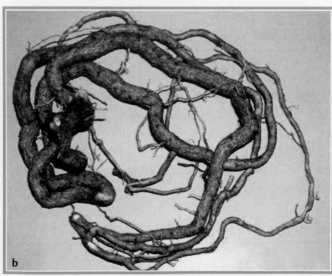

Fig. 86.4 **(a)** Dried roots. **(b)** Root.

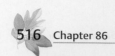

Types

Raj Nighantu has mentioned Nakuli and Gandha nakuli/mahasugandha. The properties of Gandha nakuli are better than Nakuli.

Rasapanchaka

Guna	Ruksha
Rasa	Tikta
Vipaka	Katu
Virya	Ushna
Prabhava	Nidrajanana

Chemical Constituents

R. serpentina is a rich source of different varieties of chemical constituents. Various alkaloids like reserpine, serpentine, serpentinine, ajmalicine, ajmaline, ajmalimine, deserpidine, indobidine, reserpiline, rescinnamine, rescinnamidine, and yohimbine are identified from this plant. The main alkaloid is reserpine. It exerts antihypertensive property by depleting the catecholamine.

Identity, Purity, and Strength

- Foreign matter: Not more than 2%
- Total ash: Not more than 8%
- Acid-insoluble ash: Not more than 1%
- Alcohol-soluble extractive: Not less than 4%
- Water-soluble extractive: Not less than 10%

(Source: The Ayurvedic Pharmacopeia of India 2001)

Karma (Actions)

Actions include deepan (appetizer), pachana (digestive), ruchya (relish), mutral (diuretics), vishaghna (antidote), kamavasadaka, hridavasadaka (cardiac depressant) (The Ayurvedic Pharmacopeia of India 2001), nidrajanana (sedative), mastishkashamaka (peace of mind/brain), sramsana (laxative), krimighna (anthelmintic), raktabharaprashamana (antihypertensive), garbhashayasankochaka (uterine contraction), artavajanana (emmenogague), jwaraghna (antipyretics), tiktapaushtika, tandrakara (drowsiness) (Billore et al 2005).

- Doshakarma: Kapha vatashamaka
- Dhatukarma: Raktabharaprashamana
- Malakarma: Mutral, sramsana

Pharmacological Actions

Antihypertensive, antioxidant, antivenom, hepatoprotective, hypolipidemic, antidiabetic, hypoglycemic, antibacterial, antidiarrheal, anticholinergic, hypotensive, anticontractile, sedative, relaxant, hyperthermic, sympathomimetic, hypnotic, vasodilator, antiemetic, antifibrillar, tranquillizing, antiarrhythmic, antifungal, nematocidal actions are reported with this plant (Chauhan et al 2017; Billore et al 2005).

Indications

It is used in shoola (colic), anidra (insomnia), apasmara (epilepsy), unmada (insanity), bhutabadha (evil spirits), bhrama (vertigo), jvara (fever), krimiroga (worm infestation), madaroga (intoxication), yonishoola (pain in vagina), raktavata (rakta dosha associated with vata dosha), manasaroga (maniacal behavior associated with psychosis), vishuchika (cholera), vrana (wound) (The Ayurvedic Pharmacopeia of India 2001). It is also used in agnimandya (loss of appetite), mastishkavikara (mental disorders), amajavibandhashoola (colic pain due to constipation), raktabharadhikya (hypertension), kashtartava (dysmenorrhea), kashtaprasava (painful labor), pralapa (irrelevantly over talkative), udvega (anxiety), sarpavisha (snake poisoning), bhutonmada (schizophrenia), balatisara (diarrhea in children), netrashukra, shirahshoola (headache; Billore et al 2005).

R. serpentina has an extensive spectrum of valuable therapeutic actions, mainly effective in the treatment of hypertension and psychotic disorders like schizophrenia, anxiety, epilepsy, insomnia, insanity, and also used as a sedative, a hypnotic drug. Extracts of the roots are valued for the treatment of intestinal disorders, particularly diarrhea and dysentery and also as anathematic. Mixed with other plant extracts, they have been used in the treatment of cholera, colic, and fever. The root was believed to stimulate uterine contraction and recommended for the use in childbirth. The juice of the leaves has been used as a remedy for the opacity of the cornea. Rauvolfia's juice and extract obtained from the root can be used for treating gastrointestinal and circulatory diseases. The juice of tender leaves and root extract is used to treat liver pain, stomach pain, dysentery, and to expel intestinal worms (Noce et al 1954; Kirtikar and Basu 1993).

R. serpentina roots are also used to treat hypertension-associated cerebral pain, wooziness, amenorrhea, and oligo-menorrhea in Siddha system of medicine. In Unani system, *R. serpentina* is used as a nervine tonic (Musakkine-Asab), sedative and hypnotic (Musakkin-wo-Munawwim), diuretic (Mudir), and anesthetic (Mukhaddir) (Dey and De 2010).

Therapeutic Uses

1. **Manas roga** (mental disorders): Sarpagandha is included in aparajita gana which is indicated in mental disorder (S.S.U. 60/47).
2. **Visha** (poisoning): It is mentioned in ekasara gana (S.S.Ka. 5/84). Sarpagandha is particularly efficacious in rat poisoning (S.S.Ka. 7/29).
3. **Visuchika** (cholera): Sarpagandha should be taken with warm water (VD. 6/26).
4. **Anidra** (insomnia): Sarpagandha root powder given in doses of 5 g with ghee or rose water at bedtime induces sound sleep and gives relief in panic attacks, palpitation, nervousness, anxiety, and epilepsy.
5. **Unmada** (insanity): One gram of powdered root can be taken thrice with milk in insanity and hysteria.
6. **Uchchraktachapa** (hypertension): Taking half teaspoon full root powder of Sarpagandha twice a day or 2 tablets

of Sarpagandhaghana vati once a day is effective in lowering high blood pressure.
7. **Kandu** (urticaria): One gram of powdered root is taken with water to prevent itching in urticaria.

Officinal Part Used

Root

Dose

Root powder: 3 to 6 g (sedative, insanity); 1 to 2 g (in hypertension).

Formulations

Sarpagandhadi churna, Sarpagandhaghana vati, Sarpagandhayoga, Sarpagandha vati.

Safety and Toxicity Studies

Reserpine is reported to be a cardiovascular depressant with hypnotic activity and it has relatively high toxicity. Minimum therapeutic doses of Reserpine may give rise to nasal congestion, lethargy, drowsiness, peculiar dreams, vertigo, and gastrointestinal symptoms, and sometimes dyspnea and urticarial rash may occur. Higher doses may cause flushing, injection of conjunctivae, insomnia, bradycardia, asthenia, edema, occasionally parkinsonism, and severe mental depression which may lead to suicide. Prolonged previous use of reserpine may cause disturbances in blood pressure during operation under general anesthesia, while some patients may be highly susceptible to a small parental dosage.

The lethal dose of the serpentine group of alkaloids was found to be the same as that of the ajmaline group, *viz.* 0.5 mg/kg of frog. The lethal dose for rat was found to be four times higher (Billore et al 2005).

Substitution and Adulteration

The following plants are used as adulterants and substitutes for Sarpagandha.
- *Rauvolfia canescens* Linn.
- *Rauvolfia. densiflora* Benth. ex Hook.f.

- *Rauvolfia perakensis* King. & Gamble
- *Rauvolfia micrantha* Hook.f.
- *Rauvolfia beddomei* Hook.f.
- *Ophiorrhiza mungos* Linn.
- *Clerodendron* species

The stem of same species is also mixed with roots.

Rauvolfia vomitoria is also a chemotaxonomical substitute to genuine *R. serpentina* (Billore et al 2005).

Points to Ponder

- *Reserpine is the first identified alkaloid from Sarpagandha used in hypertension.*
- *Sarpagandha should be used as a whole. If only alkaloid reserpine is used, it may cause suicidal tendencies.*

Suggested Readings

Agrawal SN. *Rauvolfia serpentina*: A medicinal plant of exceptional qualities. Alt Med Chiropractic OA J 2019;2(2):180016

Ayurvedic Pharmacopoeia of India, Part I, Vol. V. 1st ed. New Delhi: Department of ISM and H, Ministry of Health and Family Welfare, Government of India; 2001:166–167

Billore KV, Yelne MB, Dennis TJ, Chaudhari BG. Database on Medicinal Plants Used in Ayurveda, Vol. 7. New Delhi: CCRAS, Department of AYUSH, Ministry of Health & Family Welfare, Government of India; 2005:386–422

Chauhan S, Kaur A, Pareek RK. Pharmacobotanical and pharmacological evaluation of Ayurvedic crude drug: *Rauwolfia serpentina* (Apocynaceae). Int J Green Pharm 2017;11(4):S688

Chunekar KC. Bhavaprakash Nighantu of Bhavamishra. 3rd ed. Varanasi: Chaukhamba Bharati Academy; 2007:82–85

Dey A, De JN. *Rauwolfia serpentina* (L). Benth. Ex Kurz.: a review. Asian J Plant Sci 2010;9:285–298

Gogte VM. Ayurvedic Pharmacology and Therapeutic Uses of Medicinal Plants: Dravyaguna Vigyan, Part II. New Delhi: Chaukhamba Publication; 2009:510–511

Kirtikar KR, Basu BD. Indian Medicinal Plants. 2nd ed. Calcutta, India: Dehra Dun Publishers; 1993:289

Nadkarni KM. Indian Materia Medica, Vol. I. 1st ed.. Bombay: Popular Prakashan Pvt. Ltd; 2007:1050–1053

Noce RH, Williams DB, Rapaport W. Reserpine (serpasil) in the management of the mentally ill and mentally retarded: preliminary report. J Am Med Assoc 1954;156(9):821–824

Sastri K. Charaka Samhita of Agnivesa of Cakrapanidatta, Part II. Chikitsasthanam. Varanasi: Chaukhambha Sanskrit Sansthan; 2006:582

Sastry JL. Dravyaguna Vijnana, Vol. II. Varanasi: Chaukhamba Orientalia; 2008:334–337

Sharma PV. Dhanvantri Nighantu. Varanasi: Chaukhambha Orientilia; 2005:137

Sharma PV. Dravyaguna-Vijnana (Vegetable Drugs), Vol. II. Varanasi: Chaukhambha Bharti Academy; 2009:36–39

Shastri KA. Susruta Samhita of Maharshi-Susruta, Part II (Uttartantra). Varanasi: Chaukhamba Sanskrit Sansthan; 2004:443

Singh RK, Singh A, Rath S, Ramamurthy A. A review of Sarpgandha: whole herb v/s Reserpine. Its alkaloid in the management of hypertension. Int Ayurv Med J 2015;3(2):565–569

Vaidyaratnam PS. Indian Medicinal Plants, Vol. 4. Hyderabad: Universities Press India Pvt. Ltd; 2010:409–410

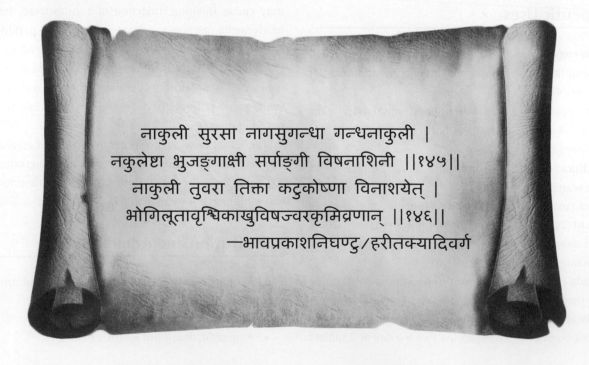

नाकुली सुरसा नागसुगन्धा गन्धनाकुली ।
नकुलेष्टा भुजङ्गाक्षी सर्पाङ्गी विषनाशिनी ॥१४५॥
नाकुली तुवरा तिक्ता कटुकोष्णा विनाशयेत् ।
भोगिलूतावृश्चिकाखुविषज्वरकृमिव्रणान् ॥१४६॥
—भावप्रकाशनिघण्टु/हरीतक्यादिवर्ग

87. Shalaparni [Desmodium gangeticum Linn. DC]

Family:	*Fabaceae*
Hindi name:	*Salvan, shalpan, Sarivan, Gauri, Sar, Salpani, Dinth*
English name:	*Flax weed, flix weed*

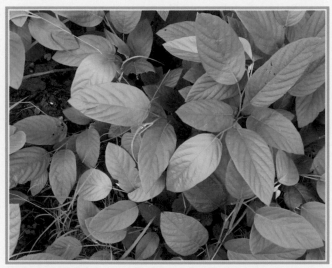

Plant of *Desmodium gangeticum* Linn. DC.

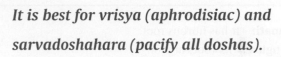

It is best for vrisya (aphrodisiac) and sarvadoshahara (pacify all doshas).

—C.S.Su. 25/40

Introduction

Shalaparni is one of the drugs of Laghupanchamoola and Dashamoola. It is also one of the components of Parnidwaya; Vedic literatures describe its potentiality as regulator of nervous (vata), venous (pitta), and arterial (kapha) systems essential to restore health (Shang-Chih et al 2009). Chatuparni Shalaparni is found widely in Samhitas. It is mainly used in compound form as Panchamoola or Dashamoola and in either Chatuparni or Parnidwaya form.

The genus *Desmodium* is derived from Greek word "Desmos" meaning "bond" or "chain" due to the resemblance of the jointed seed pods to links of a chain. *Desmodium gangeticum* of Fabaceae family, commonly known as Shalaparni, is a perennial, erect, or ascending herb or undershrub 2 to 4 feet in height. It is distributed mainly in tropical and subtropical regions of the world. It is a slender herb with leaves similar to Sala along with long, deep-seated, fibrous, and sweet aroma roots. The drug can be used as rasayana and alleviates cardiac pain and edema. It is Tridoshasamaka in action.

Various ethnomedicinal claims regarding *D. gangeticum* were found from different parts of India, such as Andhra Pradesh, Uttar Pradesh, Madhya Pradesh, West Bengal, Tamil Nadu, and Maharashtra, which shows its availability and popularity among tribal peoples. Ethnomedicinal claims are found mostly in the context of *D. gangeticum* and *D. triflorum*. *Desmodium laxiflorum* is less popular or has less availability as compared to other two species (Singh et al 2015).

Vernacular Names

Bengali: Salpani, Shalpani, Chhalani
Gujarati: Salvan, Shalvan, sameravo, pandadiyo
Kannada: Kadangaa, Maru, Nabiyalabune, Nariyalavona, Bhui, Shevara
Konkani: Salvan

Malayalam: Orila, Pullati

Marathi: Salvan, Ranbhal

Mundari: Oterai

Oriya: Salopornni, Sharpni

Punjab: Shalpurni, Samer, Sarivan

Sanskrit: Vidarigandha, Anshumati, Shalparni, Shaliparni, Somya

Santhal: Tandi Bhedi Janetet

Siddha: Pulladi, Sirupulladi, Moovilai (Root)

Tamil: Orila, Pulladi, Pullati

Telugu: Gitanaram, Kolaka ponna

Tulu: Kolakuponna, Gitanaram

Urdu: Sharpani

Synonyms

Anshumati: It has fibrous root.

Dirghanghri: Its roots are long.

Dirghapatra: It has long leaves.

Guha: The roots are deep seated.

Saumya: It has rasayana properties like that of Soma.

Shalaparni: The leaves look like Sala leaves.

Shoolarogahari: It alleviates cardiac pain.

Shophaghni: It alleviates edema.

Sthira: It gives strength to the body.

Tanwika: It is a slender herb with leaves similar to those of Sala and Guha.

Triparni: It has three leaflets.

Vidarigandha: It bears the smell of Vidarikanda.

Classical Categorization

Charak Samhita: Angamardaprashamana, Shothahara, Balya, Snehopaga, Vayastapana

Sushruta Samhita: Vidarigandhadi, Laghupanchamoola

Astanga Hridaya: Vidaryadi

Dhanwantari Nighantu: Guduchyadi varga

Madanpal Nighantu: Abhayadi varga

Kaiyadev Nighantu: Aushadi varga

Raj Nighantu: Satawahdi varga

Bhavaprakash Nighantu: Guduchyadi varga

Distribution

It is distributed mainly in tropical and subtropical regions of the world. Among 20 to 25 different species, *D. gangeticum* shows highest biodiversity in India. It is found on lower hills and plains throughout India. It is abundantly found in Bihar, Odisha, Madhya Pradesh, Punjab, outer Himalaya, etc. It is also distributed in Sri Lanka, Pakistan, Bangladesh, China, Malaysia, and Australia.

Morphology

It is a perennial, erect, or ascending herb or undershrub 2 to 4 feet in height.

- **Stem:** Angular, woody with numerous prostrate branches.
- **Leaves:** Unifoliate, alternate (6–14 × 2–7 cm) thin lamina, stipulate, petioles 1 to 2 cm long; stipules 6 to 8 mm long, ovate-oblong or rounded in shape, cordate base, acute-acuminate apex, upper surface is glabrous, paler, and clothed with dense, soft, whitish, appressed hair beneath (**Fig. 87.1**).
- **Flower:** Flowers are in large terminal and axillary racemes, usually in small fascicles on a slender rachis; bracts subulate, up to 4 mm, calyx 2 mm long, hairy, corolla 4 to 5 mm long, purple, violet, blue, lilac, or white, with these colors appearing at the same time on the same plant (**Fig. 87.2**).
- **Fruit:** Subfalcate, flat pod, 2 cm by 0.3 cm, slightly indented on the upper and deeply so on the lower

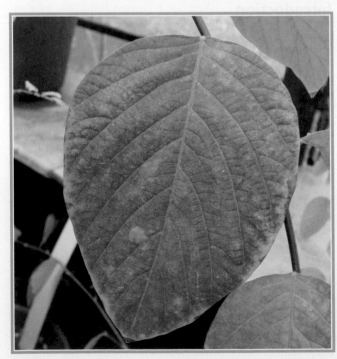

Fig. 87.1 Leaf.

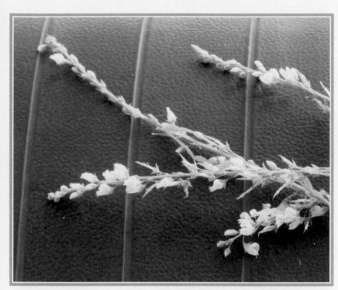

Fig. 87.2 Flower.

suture slightly dehiscent, six to eight jointed. One seeded, more or less straight, or slightly curved above and rounded on the lower (**Fig. 87.3a, b**).

- **Seed:** Compressed, reniform without a strophiole.
- **Root:** Deep rooted, tap root poorly developed, and lateral roots are very strong, nearly cylindrical, light yellow, and smooth (**Fig. 87.4**).

It is propagated through seeds and vegetative methods (Aiyar et al 1957; Anonymous 1956).

Phenology

Flowering time: More or less throughout the year, more so during September to December

Fruiting time: More or less throughout the year, more so during September to December

---

Key Characters for Identification

➤ Perennial, erect, or ascending herb or undershrub 2 to 4 feet in height.

➤ Leaves: Unifoliate, alternate, stipulate ovate-oblong or rounded in shape, cordate base, acute-acuminate apex, upper surface glabrous, with dense, soft, whitish, appressed hair beneath.

➤ Flower: Found in large terminal and axillary racemes, purple, violet, blue, lilac, or white color.

➤ Fruit: Subfalcate, flat pod, 2 cm by 0.3 cm, slightly indented on the upper and deeply so on the lower suture slightly dehiscent, six to eight jointed, one seeded.

➤ Root: Deep rooted, tap root poorly developed, and lateral roots are very strong, nearly cylindrical, light yellow, and smooth.

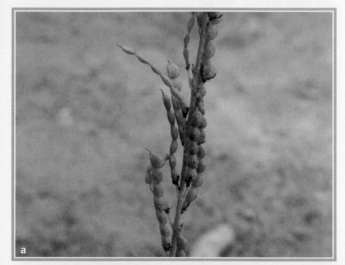

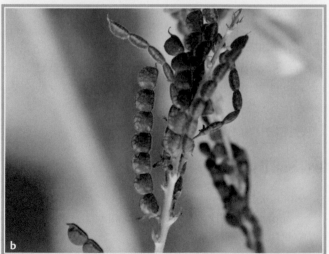

Fig. 87.3 (a) Unripe fruit. (b) Mature fruits

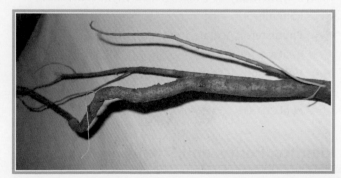

Fig. 87.4 Root.

Types

In Hooker's *Flora of British India* (1879, 1999 [reprint]), 49 species of *Desmodium* were recorded. Among which, *D. gangeticum* is an important and well-explored species in Ayurveda. Shah (1978) has recorded 14 species of *Desmodium* in his book *Flora of Gujarat State*, and later on Raghavan et al. (1981) listed 15 *Desmodium* species in their checklist of the plants of Gujarat. *Desmodium triflorum* and *Desmodium laxiflorum*. *D. gangeticum* is used by most of the tribal communities of India.

Rasapanchaka

Guna	Guru, Snigdha
Rasa	Madhura, Tikta
Vipak	Madhura
Virya	Ushna

Chemical Constituents

D. gangeticum is rich in flavonoids, alkaloids, pterocarpans, steroids, terpenoids, phenylpropanoids, coumarins, and volatile oil as mentioned below.

- Alkaloids: 5-Methoxy-N, B-carbolinium cation, indole-3-alkalamines, N-dimethyl tryptamine, N-Methyl-H4-Harman, uridine triacetate
- Pterocarpans: Desmocarpin, desmodin, gangetial, gangetin, gangetinin
- Flavonoids: 4,5,7-trihydroxy-8-phenylflavone, 4-0-α-L-rhamnopyranosyl (1-6)-B-d-glucopyronoside, 8-c-prenyl-57, 5-trimethoxy-3, 4-methylenedioxyflavone, rutin, kalmoferol
- Phytosterol: Acetate, lupeol, stigma sterol, α-amyrone, β-sitosterol
- Volatile oil: 1-Tritriacontanol, Aliphatic-β-lactone
- Phenyl propanoids: Chlorogenic acids (Bhattacharjee et al 2013)

Identity, Purity, and Strength

- Foreign matter: Not more than 2%
- Total ash: Not more than 6%
- Acid-insoluble ash: Not more than 2%
- Alcohol-soluble extractive: Not less than 1%
- Water-soluble extractive: Not less than 6%

(Source: The Ayurvedic Pharmacopeia of India 1986)

Karma (Actions)

The drug acts in angamarda prashamana (pacify bodyache), balya (physical strength promoter), bharamhara (relieve vertigo), brumhana (body mass improver), rasayana (rejuvenation), santapanasini (antipyretics), sarvadosahara (pacify tridosha), shothahara (reduce edema), vatadoshajit (pacify vatadosha), vishaghna (antidote), vrushya (aphrodisiac), etc.

- Doshakarma: Tridoshahara
- Dhatukarma: Balya, Brumhana, Vrushya
- Malakarma: Mutral

Pharmacological Actions

Various pharmacological actions are antiamnesic (nootropic), antidiabetic, anti-inflammatory, antinociceptive, antioxidant, antiulcerative, cardioprotective, central nervous system (CNS) activity, immunomodulatory, renal protective, and wound healing (Vaghela et al 2013; Vedpal et al 2016).

Indications

It is useful in arsha (piles), atisara (diarrhea), chhardi (diarrhea), hridroga (heart disease), jwara (fever), kasa (cough), krimi (worm infestation), kshaya (emaciation), prameha (diabetes), shoola (colic pain), shopha (edema), shosha (emaciation), shwasa (asthma), trisna (thirst), visha (poisoning), vishama jwara (intermittent fever).

Therapeutic Uses

External Use

1. **Ardita vata** (hemicrania): Juice of Shalaparni should be applied locally or snuffed to alleviate hemicranias (A.H.U-24/10, GN-3/1/63).
2. **Sukhaprasavadhana** (for easy delivery): Application of the Shalaparni root paste on navel, pelvis, vulva, etc. expels the confounded fetus (V.M-65/13).

3. **Diseases of eye:** Shalaparni root combined with rock salt and marica and rubbed with sour gruel in a copper vessel should be used as collyrium; it destroys pila (VM. 61.246).

Internal Use

1. **Hritshoola** (cardiac pain): Shalaparni boiled with milk is efficacious in cardiac pain (C.S.Ci-28/96).
2. **Raktapitta** (hemorrhage): Shalaparni with mudga rasa in ahara (C.S.Ci. 4/46).
3. **Vatarakta** (gout): Shalaparni, Prisniparni, and both types of Brihati are pounded with milk and mixed with tarpana (yavasakyu) and applied externally in gout (S.S.Ci-5/10).

Officinal Parts Used

Roots and whole plant

Dose

Powder: 5 to 10 g
Decoction: 50 to 100 mL

Formulations

Agasthya rasayana, Anutaila, Brahachchhagaladya ghrita, Chitrakaharitaki, Chyavanprash, Dashamoola kwatha, Dashamoola taila, Dashamool arishta, Mahanarayana taila, Mooshikadya taila, Shalparnyadi kvatha, Vayuchchhaya surendra taila, Vyaghri taila.

Toxicity/Adverse Effects

The aqueous extract of root was found to be nontoxic in acute toxicity studies. Gangetina pterocarpene from hexane extract of root is nontoxic up to an oral dose of 7 g/kg in mice (Ghosh and Anandakumar 1983).

Substitution and Adulteration

Desmodium latifolium DC is often used as a substitute for *D. gangeticum* in some parts of Travancore and Cochin (Kirubha et al 2011).

Points to Ponder

- It is best for vrishya and sarvadoshahara (*C.S.Su. 25/40*).
- Sushrut's first gana is Vidarigandhadi (according to name of Shalaparni (Syn-Vidarigandha).

Suggested Readings

Anonymous. Dhanvantari Nighantu (Priyavrat Sharma, ed.). 4th ed. Varanasi: Chaukhambha Orientalia; 2005

Anonymous. The Wealth of India, Vol. III. New Delhi: CSIR;1956:41

Bhattacharjee A, Shashidhara SC, Saha S. Phytochemical and ethno-pharmacological profile of *Desmodium gangeticum* (L.) DC.: a review. Int J Biomed Res 2013;4(10):507–515

Bhavamishra BN. edited by Pandit Shri Brahma Sankar Mishra with the Vidyotani Hindi Commentary, 11th ed. Varanasi: Chaukhambha Sanskrit Sansthan; 2004.

Ghosh D, Anandakumar A. Anti-inflammatory and analgesic activities of gangetin: a pterocarpanoid from *Desmodium gangeticum*. Int J Pharmacol 1983;15:391–402

Kaiydeva A, Nighantu K. Aushadhi varga/20 (Priyavrat Sharma, ed.). 2nd ed. Varanasi: Chaukhambha Orientalia; 2006:1979

Kirubha VT, Jegadeesan M, Kavimani S. Studies on *Desmodium gangeticum*: a review. J Chem Pharm Res 2011;3(6):850–855

Kritikar KR, Basu BD. Indian Medicinal Plants, Vol. I. Dehradun, India: International Book Distributors; 1974:759–760

Lai SC, Peng WH, Huang SC, et al. Analgesic and anti-inflammatory activities of methanol extract from *Desmodium triflorum* DC in mice. Am J Chin Med 2009;37(3):573–588

Lucas DS. Dravyaguna-Vijnana: Study of Dravya-Materia Medica. Varanasi: Chaukhamba Visvabharati; 2013:109

Madanapala A. Madanapala Nighantu (Pandit Hariharprasad Trivedi, ed.). Varanasi: Chaukhambha Krishnadas Academy; 2009

Narayana Aiyar K, Namboodiri AN, Kolammal M. Pharmacognosy of Ayurvedic Drugs, Series 1, No. 3. Trivandrum: The Central Research Institute; 1957:97–100.

Raghavan RS, Wadhwa BM, Ansari MY, Rao SR. A checklist of the plants of Gujarat. Rec Botan Surv India 1981;XXI(2):37

Shah GL. Flora of Gujarat State, Vol. 1. Gujarat: Sardar Patel University; 1978:204–211

Shang-Chih L, Wen-Huang P, Shun-Chieh H, et al. Analgesic and antiinflammatory activities of methanol extract from Desmodium triflorum DC in mice. Am J Chin Med 2009;37(3):573–588

Sharma PV. Classical Uses of Medicinal Plants. 1st ed. Varanasi: Chaukhamba Vishvabharati; 2004:365

Sharma PV. Namarupajnanam. 1st ed. Varanasi: Chaukhamba Vishvabharati; 2011:181.

Singh S, Parmar N, Patel B. A review on Shalparni (*Desmodium gangeticum* DC.) and Desmodium species (*Desmodium triflorum* DC. & *Desmodium laxiflorum* DC.): ethnomedicinal perspectives. J Med Plant Stud 2015;3(4):38–43

The Ayurvedic Pharmacopoeia of India, Part I, Vol. III. 1st ed. New Delhi: Department of Health, Ministry of Health and Family Welfare, Government of India; 1986:179.

Tripathi I, ed. Narhari Pandita, Raja Nighantu. 4th ed. Varanasi: Chowkhambha Krishnadas Academy; 2006:12

Vaghela B, Buddhadev S, Shukla L. Pharmacological activities of *Desmodium gangeticum*: an overview. Pharma Sci Monitor 2013; 4(4):264–278

Vedpal, Dhanabal SP, Dhamodaran P, Chaitnya MVNL, Duraiswamy B, Jayaram U, Srivastava N. Ethnopharmacological and phytochemical profile of three potent *Desmodium* species: *Desmodium gangeticum* (L.) DC, *Desmodium triflorum* Linn and *Desmodium triquetrum* Linn. J Chem Pharm Res 2016;8(7):91–97

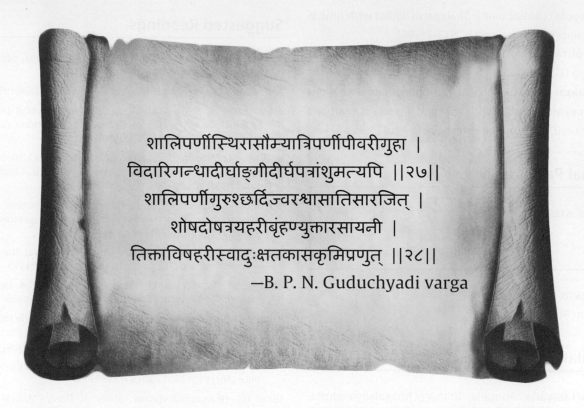

शालिपर्णीस्थिरासौम्यात्रिपर्णीपीवरीगुहा |
विदारिगन्धादीर्घाङ्गीदीर्घपत्रांशुमत्यपि ||२७||
शालिपर्णीगुरुश्छर्दिज्वरश्वासातिसारजित् |
शोषदोषत्रयहरीबृंहण्युक्तारसायनी |
तिक्ताविषहरीस्वादुःक्षतकासकृमिप्रणुत् ||२८||
—B. P. N. Guduchyadi varga

88. Shallaki [Boswellia serrata Roxb.]

Family:	*Burseraceae*
Hindi name:	*Salai guggul, Madi, salai, saler, salga, salhe, sali, anduk, gugal, halar, kundur, loban, lobhan, luban, salaga, salai, salar, salaran, salhe, sel-gond, vellakkunturukkam, labana*
English name:	*Indian olibanum, Indian frankincense*

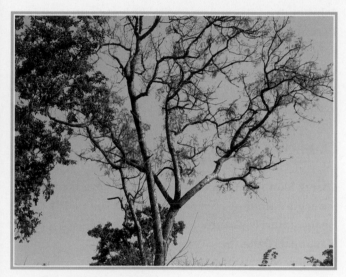

Tree of *Boswellia serrata* Roxb.

> *The fresh gum obtained from the tree is hot dry with a pleasant flavor and slightly bitter taste. It is the "frankincense" of ancient Egyptians, Greeks, and Romans who used it as prized incense, fumigant, as well as a multipurpose aromatic. It is generally used in making incense powder and sticks.*

Introduction

Shallaki is not mentioned in the Vedic literatures but is explained in Charaka Samhita, Sushruta Samhita, and other Samhitas and Nighantus of Ayurveda. Acharya Charaka has advised its use in the treatment of shvasa, kasa, hikka (C.S.Ci. 17/117), vatavyadhi (Bala Taila—C.S.Ci. 28/156), and gulma–ashmari (C.S.Ci. 26/64-65). He has also used it in dhoomvarti (C.S.Su. 5/20-24). Acharya Sushruta has prescribed it in the treatment of puadansha (S.S.Ci. 19/14), pittabhishyanda (S.S.U. 10/4), pakvatisara (S.S.U. 40/19), raktatisara (S.S.U. 40/22), and shvasa–hikka (S.S.U. 51/12). Acharya Bhela has recommended it in the treatment of vata-vyadhi (rasna taila and mulaka taila—Bh.S.Ci. 26). Acharya Harita has also used it in the treatment of vatavyadhi (kalka, kwatha, and mahabala taila—Ha. S. 3rd sthana/chapter 23). Shallaki is described in Chakradatta, particularly in the treatment of vata vyadhi (Prasarani taila, kalka paka, and maha sugandha taila—vata vyadhi chikitsa).

Boswellia serrata is one of the medicinal plants of Burseraceae family. In the plant kingdom, Burseraceae family is characterized with 17 genera and 600 species widespread in all tropical regions. Genus *Boswellia* contains about 25 known species. Most of them occur in Arabia, north eastern coast of Africa, and India (Siddiqui 2011).

The word "olibanum" (Indian frankincense tree) is derived from the Arabic al-Luban which means milk. The word also comes from the Arabic term for oil of Lebanon since Lebanon was the place where the resin was sold and traded with Europeans. The English word is derived from old French frankincense (i.e., high-quality incense) and is used in incense and perfumes (Frankincenses, 2013). "Gajabhakshya," a Sanskrit name sometimes used for Boswellia, suggests that elephants enjoy this herb as a part of their diet (Sharma et al 2012; Upaganlwar and Ghule 2009).

B. serrata is derived from *Boswellia* which is named after Dr Boswel and *Serrata* means saw. The *leaves* of this plant are eaten by elephant that's why it is called Shallaki. Its exudate is known as Kunduru. The first terpenoid, boswellic acid, was isolated from B. serrata Roxb. in 1898.

Vernacular Names

Arabic: Baslaj, Kundur, Laban

Assamese: Sallaki

Bemba: Kundru

Bengali: Luban, salai, salgai

Chinese: Fan Fan Hun Hsiang, Chi ye ru xiang shu

Cutch: Saliyaguggul

French: Arbre à encens de l'Inde, boswellie, encens d'Inde, Franc Encens

German: Indischer Weihrauch

Gujarati: Gugal, saleda, dhup, shaledum, saladi, gugal, saledhi

Italian: Incenso indiano

Japanese: Furankinsensu

Kannada: Madimar, chilakdupa, tallaki, maddi

Kashmiri: Kunturukkam, samprani

Konkani: Lobhan

Malayalam: Salai, kungilyam

Marathi: Salai cha dink, Salai, Dhupali, Dhupsali, Kurunda, Salaphali

Oriya: Salai

Persian: kundru, gandha firoza, loban

Pharmacopoeial: Olibanum Indicum, Gummi Boswellii

Punjabi: Salaigonda

Roman: Safiroos

Sanskrit: Sallaki, kunduru, agavrttika, ashvamutri, asraphala, bahusrava, gajabhaksha, gajabhaksya, gajapriya, gajasana, gajashana, gajavallabha, gandhamula

Spanish: Incienso indio, Asbol, Dol incienzo

Sri Lankan: Kundirikkan

Tamil: Attam, Kunduru, Kungali, Parangisambrani, kungli, kundrikam, gugulu, morada, kundurukam

Telugu: Anduga, kondagugitamu

Trade names: Salai, kundur luban, lobhan, salakhi, dupa, guggul, kaadar, salai guggul

Unani: Kundur

Urdu: Kundar, kundur, loban, lobana, sat loban

Synonyms

Gajabhakshya: Its leaves are eaten by elephant.

Kunduru: Its exudate is known as Kunduru.

Susrava: It produces profuse aromatic exudation.

Srava: It produces profuse aromatic exudation.

Mocha: It produces profuse aromatic exudation.

Surabhi: It produces aromatic exudation.

Surabhisrava: It produces profuse aromatic exudation.

Sallaki: Its leaves are eaten by elephant.

Ashvamutri: Its exudate smells like horse's urine.

Tyasraphala: Its fruit are triangular in shape.

Bahusrava: It produces profuse aromatic exudation.

Hladani: It has pleasant exudates.

Maheruna: Its leaves are eaten by elephant.

Vanya: It is a wild plant.

Classical Categorization

Charak Samhita: Purishavirajaniya, Kashaya skand

Sushruta Samhita: Nyagrodhadi, Eladi, Lodhradi

Dhanwantari Nighantu: Chandanadi varga

Madanpal Nighantu: Vatadi varga

Kaiyadev Nighantu: Aushadhi varga

Raj Nighantu: Amradi varga

Bhavaprakash Nighantu: Vatadi varga

Distribution

This tree is commonly found in West Asia, Oman, Yemen, South Africa, Southern Arabia, and many parts of India. In India, it is found in Western Himalaya, Rajasthan, Gujarat, Maharashtra, Madhya Pradesh, Bihar, Odisha, Jharkhand, and Chhattisgarh (Sunnichan et al 1998; Upadhayay 2006).

Morphology

It is a medium- to large-sized, deciduous tree, up to 18 m in height. Tree produces exudates after three years.

- **Bark:** Papery, pinkish, or light buff colored, smooth, which peels off in thin papery pieces leaving greenish bark on the trunk; young shoots are pubescent (**Fig. 88.1**).

- **Leaves:** The leaves are alternate, imparipinnate, 20 to 35 cm long, exstipulate, crowded at the end of the branches. The leaflets are 2.5 to 6.3 cm long, sessile, ovate serrate, opposite, and mostly pubescent with simple hairs (**Fig. 88.2**).
- **Flowers:** Small, white, in axillary racemes or panicles; calyx is small, capsular, and five- to six-lobed. The petals (three to five) are free or rarely connate, deciduous, imbricate or valvate, 0.5 to 0.8 cm long, oblong-ovate with basal disk. Stamens are many or twice as many as the petals, inserted at the base or margin of the disk equal or unequal, filament free, rarely connate at the base, zero staminodes. Anthers are usually with versatile ovary, having two free ovules (very rarely one) in each cell (**Fig. 88.3**).
- **Fruit:** Trigonous drupe, splitting along three valves, scarlet red when young, turns white at maturity (**Fig. 88.4**).

- **Oleo-resin:** Oleo-resin exudes as colorless semifluid liquid which gradually becomes whitish to golden yellow and solidifies slowly with time. Its color varies from golden brown to reddish brown, greenish yellow or dull yellow to orange, and it occurs in small, ovoid, fragrant tears. Fracture is brittle, and fractured surface is waxy and semitranslucent. Its taste is agreeable, and aromatic with characteristic balsamiferous aroma (**Fig. 88.5**).

It is propagated through seeds and root suckers.

Phenology

Flowering time: March to April
Fruiting time: April to May

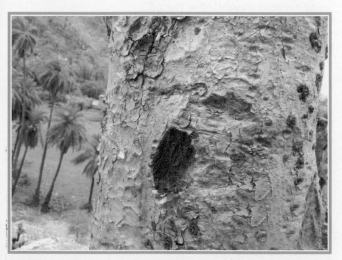

Fig. 88.1 Bark.

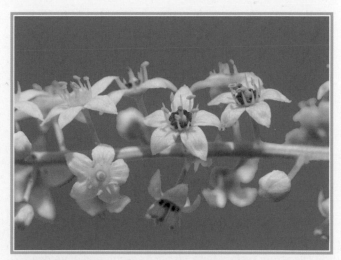

Fig. 88.3 Flowers.

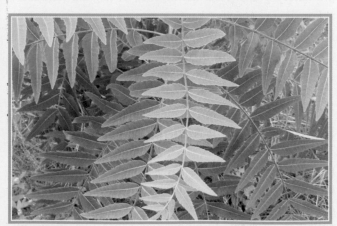

Fig. 88.2 Leaves.

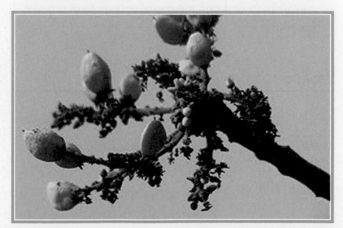

Fig. 88.4 Fruit.

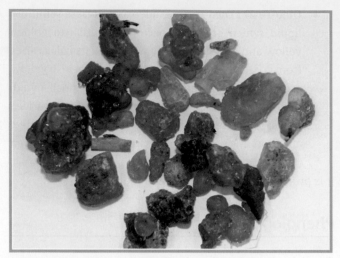

Fig. 88.5 Exudate.

Key Characters for Identification

➤ It is a medium-sized, moderate-to-large branching deciduous tree reaching up to the height of 14 to 18 m and has 1.0 to 1.5 m girth with a spreading flat crown.

➤ Leaves: Alternate, compound, imparipinnate, crowded at the end of branches, leaflets opposite, ovate or ovate-lanceolate shape, serrated margin.

➤ Flowers: Hermaphrodite, small, white in axillary racemes; petals three to five, free or rarely connate, deciduous, imbricate, or valvate.

➤ Fruits: Trifid, drupe, 1.25 cm long trigonous, splitting in three valves, suspended by woody disk. Seeds are heart shaped, attached to the inner angle of the fruit, lanciniate radical, compressed, and multified cotyledons.

➤ Oleo-gum resin: Moist, viscid, fragrant, and of golden color when freshly exudated and solidifies to brownish yellow tears or drops and crusts, varying from pea size to walnut size.

Rasapanchaka

Guna	Laghu, Ruksha (Gum resin: Teekshna
Rasa	Kashaya, Tikta, Madhura (Gum resin: Katu, Tikta)
Vipaka	Katu
Virya	Sheeta

Chemical Constituents

The oleo-gum resins contain 30 to 60% resin, 5 to 10% essential oils, boswellic acid, monoterpenes (α-thujene), α-phellandrene, limonene, diterpenes (incensole, incensole oxide), triterpenes (α- and β-amyrins), and tetracyclic triterpenic acids. Besides boswellic acid, several other triterpenoids have also been isolated from the gum resin; these compounds include α-amyrins, 11-keto-a-boswellic acid, 3'-hydroxyl urs-9, 11-dien-24-oic acid, 3'-acetoxy urs-9, 11-dien-24-oic- acid.

The essential oil of *B. serrata* predominantly comprised monoterpenoids, of which pinene (73.3%) was the major constituent. Other monoterpenoids identified included: pinene (2.05%), cis-verbenol (1.97%), trans-pinocarveol (1.80%), borneol (1.78%), myrcene (1.71%), verbenone (1.71%), limonene (1.42%), thuja-2,4(10)-diene (1.18%), and p-cymene (1.0%), while copaene (0.13%) was the only sesquiterpene identified in the oil.

Identity, Purity, and Safety

- Foreign matter: Not more than 5%
- Total ash: Not more than 10%
- Acid-insoluble ash: Not more than 8%
- Alcohol-soluble extractive: Not less than 45%
- Water-soluble extractive: Not less than 28%

(Source: The Ayurvedic Pharmacopeia of India 1999)

Karma (Actions)

It includes vatahara (pacify vata), varnya (complexion promoter), grahi (fecal astringent), vishaghna (antidote), shlesmahara (pacify kapha), rasayana (rejuvenation), jantuhara (anthelmintic), kusthaghna (antidermatitis).

- Doshakarma: Kaphapittashamaka
- Dhatukarma: Rasayana
- Malakarma: Mutral

Pharmacological Actions

It is reported to have many pharmacological actions like antiobesity, antihyperlipidemia, diuretic, emmenagogue, anti-inflammatory, analgesic, antipyretic, antiatherosclerotic, thrombolytic, concoctive, desiccant, antiarthritic, antitumor and anticarcinogenic, carminative, stomachic, resolvent, astringent, nervine, cardiac tonic, expectorant, alternative, antidiabetic, antitoxin, expectorant, antioxidant, antidiarrheal, immunomodulator, antiseptic, antimicrobial, antibacterial, diaphoretic, and liver stimulant (Anonymous 1988; Hakeem 1311; Ghani 1920, Atal et al 1980, 1981; Dastur 1864).

Indications

It is used in chhardi (vomiting), kasa (cough), raktapitta (hemorrhage), arsha (piles), atisaara (diarrhea), vrana (wound), vyanga (black mole), shiroroga (diseases of head), raktapitta (hemorrhage), drishtiroga (eye diseases), kantha roga (throat disorders), sidhma (a type of skin disease), mutrashotha, udavartta (retention of feces, urine, and flatus), mutraghata (anuria/oliguria), suryavartta (frontal sinusitis), ardhava bhedaka (hemicrania).

The gum resin of Shallaki has been used as incense in religious and cultural ceremonies since time immemorial. The gummy resin and bark have been used in traditional medicine as an effective remedy for rheumatoid arthritis, osteoarthritis, joint disorders, inflammatory conditions, diarrhea, dysentery, skin diseases, mouth sores, bronchitis, asthma, cough, vaginal discharges, foul smelling ulcers, hair-loss, jaundice, and hemorrhoids. The essential oil of gum-resin is used in aromatherapy, paints, and varnishes.

Therapeutic Uses

External Use

1. **Upadansha** (venereal wound): Venereal wound should be washed regularly with the decoction of the leaves of Jambu, Amra, Nimba, Sweta girikarnika, and Mashaparni; barks of Shallaki, Badari, Bilva, Palasa, Tinisha, and Ksirivriksha along with Triphala (S.S.Ci. 19/42,43).
2. **Vrana** (wound): Powder of Shallaki fruit or ash of flax should be applied to the wound and bandaged (S.S.Su. 25/28).
3. **Pittabhishyanda** (Conjunctivitis): The exudates of Palasa or Shallaki mixed with sugar and honey should be applied to eyes in conjunctivitis caused by pitta (S.S.U. 10/7).

4. **Measles**: Paste prepared by mixing Kunduru, Raal, and Gandhak is applied locally in measles, pruritis, erysipelas, and ringworm infections.

Internal Use

1. **Atisara** (diarrhea): Decoction of the barks of Badari, Arjuna, Jambu, Amra, Sallaki, and Vetasa mixed with sugar and honey checks diarrhea (S.S.Ut. 40/96). Barks of Priyala, Salmali, Plaksa, Shallaki, and Tinisa are pressed in milk and added to honey. It checks diarrhea with blood (S.S.U. 40/119, VM. 3/4).
2. **Svasha** (bronchial asthma): Smoke should be inhaled with Turushka, Shallaki, Guggulu, and Padmaka mixed with ghee (S.S.U. 51/52).
3. **Arthritis:** Daily intake of Kunduru powder mixed with Ashwagandha, Shunthi, and Haridra is a sure shot remedy in decreasing the intensity of pain and inflammation of joints in rheumatoid arthritis, osteoarthritis, and other joint diseases.
4. **Raktapitta** (hemorrhage): Bark decoction or powder with goat milk or rice water is given in epistaxis, traumatic injury, bleeding diarrhea, dysentery, hematemesis, and internal hemorrhage.
5. **Bhagna** (fracture): Daily consumption of Shallaki powder mixed with Guggulu and Asthishrunkla fastens the healing process in bone fracture and dislocation.

Officinal Parts Used

Bark and gum resin

Dose

Gum: 1 to 3 g
Bark decoction: 50 to 100 mL

Formulations

Vidangadi kvatha, Sarjyadi kvatha, Karanjadi ghrita, Karpuradyarka, Balarka rasa, Yakuti, Kunkumadya taila, Mahanarayana taila, Pushyanuga curna.

Toxicity/Adverse Effects

Its excessive oral intake with wine may be fatal (Sina 1998).

> **Points to Ponder**
>
> - *The exudate of Shallaki is known as Kunduru.*
> - *The first terpenoid, boswellic acid, was isolated from B. serrata Roxb. in 1898.*

Suggested Readings

Anonymous. Wealth of India, Vol. I. New Delhi: CISR;1988:203–208

Atal CK, Gupta OP, Singh GB. Salai guggal: an anti-arthritic and anti-hyperlipidaemic agent. Br J Pharm 1981;74:203

Atal CK, Singh GB, Batra S, Sharma S, Gupta OP. Salai guggalex: *Boswellia serrata* a promising antihyperlipidemic and antiarthritic agent. Indian J Pharm 1980;12:56

Cooke T. Flora of Presidency of Bombay. Vol. I. London: Taylor & Francis; 1903:197–198

Dastur JF. Medicinal Plants of India and Pakistan. Mumbai: Treasure House of Books, D.B. Taraporevala Sons and co. Ltd;1864:89–90

Frankincenses (2013 January 15) Available from http://en.wikipedia org/wiki/frankincense, page was last modified on 10 Jan. 2013

Ghani N. Khazainul-Advia, Vol. VI. Lucknow: Naval Kishore Publication; 1920:865–867

Hakeem A. Bustanul—Mufradat. Lucknow: Idarah Taraqqui Urdu Publication; 1311:56, 261, 286

Kirtikar KR, Basu BD. Indian Medicinal Plants. 2nd ed. Dehradun: International Book Distributors; 1995:Vol. I:521–523, 526–528; Vol. IV:2435–2437

Sharma S, Thawani V, Hingorani L, Shrivastava M, Bhate VR, Khiyani R. Pharmacokinetic study of 11-Keto β-Boswellic acid. Phytomedicine 2004;11(2-3):255–260

Siddiqui MZ. *Boswellia serrata*, a potential antiinflammatory agent: an overview. Indian J Pharm Sci 2011;73(3):255–261

Sina I. Al Qanoon fit Tibb (Trans: English). Vol. 2. New Delhi: Jamia Hamdard; 1998:399–400

Sunnichan VG, Shivanna KR, Mohan Ram HY. Micropropagation of gum karaya (*Sterculia urens*) by adventitious shoot formation and somatic embryogenesis. Plant Cell Rep 1998;17(12):951–956

The Ayurvedic Pharmacopoeia of India, Part I, Vol. IV. New Delhi: Department of Indian System of Medicine and Homeopathy, Ministry of Health and Family Welfare; 1999:50

Upadhayay, A. Gums and resins NTFP unexplored. Community Forestry 2006:15–20. Available at http://www.banajata.org/pdf/articles/GumsResinsNTFPUnexplored.pdf

Upaganlwar A, Ghule B, Pharmacological activities of *Boswellia serrata* Roxb mini review. Ethnobot Leafl 2009;13:766–774

Warrier PK, Knambia VP, Ramankutty C. Indian Medicinal Plants: A Compendium of 500 Species. Chennai: Orient Longman Publisher; 1997:Vol. I:297–300; Vol II:164–172; Vol III:431–443

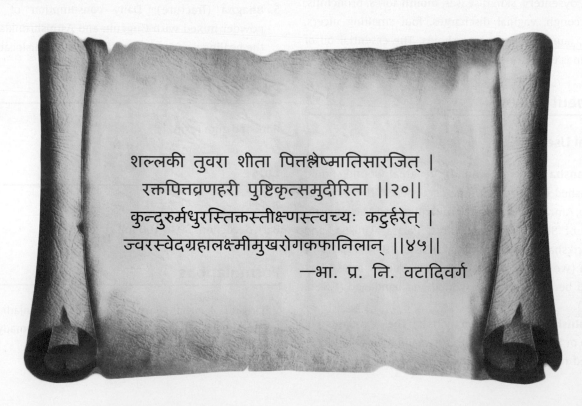

शल्लकी तुवरा शीता पित्तश्लेष्मातिसारजित् ।
रक्तपित्तव्रणहरी पुष्टिकृत्समुदीरिता ॥२०॥
कुन्दुरुर्मधुरस्तिक्तस्तीक्ष्णस्त्वच्यः कटुर्हरेत् ।
ज्वरस्वेदग्रहालक्ष्मीमुखरोगकफानिलान् ॥४५॥
—भा. प्र. नि. वटादिवर्ग

89. Shalmali *[Shalmalia malabaricum (DC.) Schott & Endl.]*

Family: *Bombacaceae*

Hindi name: *Semal, Semar, Semal, Semar, Shimal, Nurma, Deokapas, Huttain*

English name: *Silk cotton tree, Kapok tree*

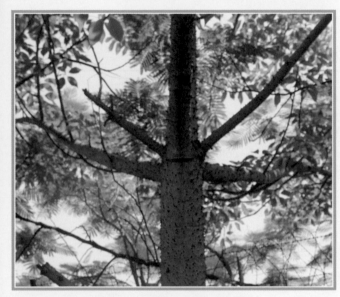

Plant of *Salmalia malabaricum* (DC.) Schott & Endl.

> In Mahabharata, it is narrated that Pitamaha, after having created the world, reposed under the tree Shalmali, and in the code of Yajnavalkya, it is mentioned as one of the trees of the infernal regions (Yamadruma), because it makes a great show of flowers, but produces no fruit fit to eat.
>
> —Dymock et al (1890)

Introduction

Bombax ceiba Linn. or *Salmalia malabarica* (DC.) Schott & Endl is a large, deciduous tree, commonly known as silk cotton tree, Indian red Kapok tree, Semal, Shimul, Shalmali, etc.; it is a member of family Bombacaceae. Mocharasa is the gum of the tree *Bombax malabaricum*. The gum is also known as supari ka phul (*Areca catechu*) in allusion to the fact that children masticate the blunt thorns of this plant and the flower buds are known as semargulla. Seeds are covered with fine cotton hairs and these hairs are used for stuffing pillows and are called sembhal ki rooae.

Shalmali is placed among the five sacred plants of "Panchwati" and is an important multipurpose tree providing medicine, food, fodder, and fiber. Almost all the parts of the plant, i.e., bark, gum, leaves, fruit, flower, thorns, seeds are used medicinally.

This plant has lot of commercial value. The wood is used in the manufacture of matches. The cotton from the fruits of this plant is used commercially for stuffing pillows and mattresses (Bhattacharjee 2000). The floss is also used as an insulating material for refrigerators, sound-proof covers, and walls. Young roots, tender leaves, flower buds, fleshy calyces, and gum are eaten. In Uttar Pradesh, flower buds are consumed as a vegetable. Roots are roasted over the fire and eaten like sweet potatoes. Leaves and younger twigs are used as fodder (Anonymous 1999).

Vernacular Names

Assamese: Simalu, Semul

Bengali: Shimool, Simul

Gujarati: Shemalo

Kannada: Kempuburunga

Malayalam: Mullulavamarum, Samparuthi, Mullilavu

Marathi: Shembalsavari, Sanvar, Katesavar

Punjabi: Simble

Sanskrit: Moca, Shalmali, Chirajivika, Picchila, Kukkuti, Raktapushpaka, Kantakadruma, Bahuvirya, Tulavriksha
Tamil: Elavam
Telugu: Buruga, Mandlaboorugachettu, Kondaburaga
Urdu: Sembhal

Synonyms

Chirajivika: The tree has a long life.
Kantakadhya: It has hard conical thorns.
Kukkuti: Flowers are red in color.
Manadruma: It is a very tall tree.
Mocha: It has exudates.
Picchila: It has shiny juice or resin.
Purani: It has resinous exudates.
Puranii: The plant lives for many years.
Raktapuspa: This is a tree with beautiful red flowers.
Shalmali: It is a handsome tall tree.
Sthirayu: The plant lives for many years.
Tulaphala: The fruits yield cotton.
Vahavirya: An efficacious drug used in many disorders.

Classical Categorization

Charak Samhita: Purishavirajaniya, Shonitasthapana, Vedanasthapana, Kashayaskanda
Sushruta Samhita: Priyangwadi
Astanga Hridaya: Priyangwadi
Dhanwantari Nighantu: Amradi varga
Madanpal Nighantu: Vatadi varga

Kaiyadev Nighantu: Aushadhi varga
Raj Nighantu: Shalmalyadi, Moolakadi, Amradi varga
Bhavaprakash Nighantu: Vatadi varga

Distribution

Bombax ceiba is widely found in temperate Asia, tropical Asia, Africa, and Australia. In India, it can be found at altitudes up to 1,500 m. In peninsular India, the tree is very commonly seen in the dry and moist deciduous forests and also near rivers.

Morphology

A tall, deciduous tree, reaching up to a height of 30 to 40 m with horizontal spreading branches and buttressed at the base.

- **Bark:** Ash colored or silvery gray studded with numerous conical spines (**Fig. 89.1**).
- **Leaves:** Palmate with about five to seven leaflets radiating from a central point. Leaflets are lanceolate, acute, shiny smooth surface, dark green upper surface, and light green beneath (**Fig. 89.2**).
- **Flowers:** Red orange in color, bunched at the tip of leafless branches (**Fig. 89.3**).
- **Fruit:** Capsulated, oblong-ovoid in shape, 5 to 7 cm in length, divided into five compartments, unripe green soft, fully ripe blackish brown and hard, containing cotton-like fibers and several black-colored seeds (**Fig. 89.4a, b**).

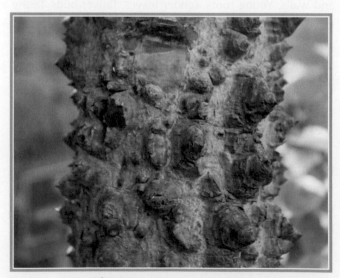

Fig. 89.1 Stem with spine.

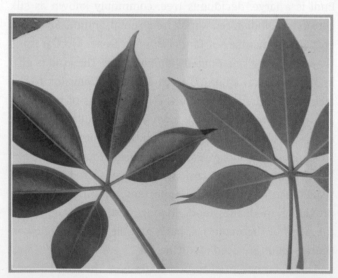

Fig. 89.2 Leaves.

- **Exudate:** A brownish-yellow colored extract known as mocharasa seeps out through the broken crevices of the trunk.

It is propagated through seeds, root, and stem cutting.

Phenology

Flowering time: January to March

Fruiting time: March to May

In February, *B. ceiba* begins dropping all of its leaves. It is time for flowering and follows a sensational display of large, silky, red flowers at the tips of bare branches. In May, white, cottony strands, from opened fruits, float downward, settling on the ground, houses, and whatever else is in their way. New leaves do not appear until almost all the flowers have fallen. Even without its flowers, *B. ceiba* is still an impressive tree. It displays prickly branches arranged in horizontal tiers. Trunk is rough, straight, and spiny with buttress roots. The trunks of the oldest specimens lose much of their spines. *B. ceiba* is rare in cultivation and always impresses tourists and first-time viewers.

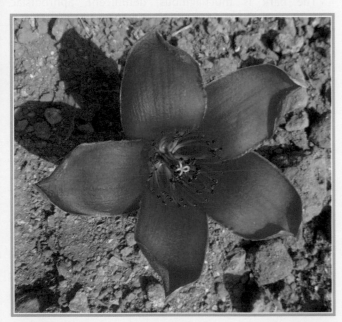

Fig. 89.3 Flower.

Key Characters for Identification

➤ *The plant grows up to 30 to 40 m height and has large spreading branches with young stems covered with stout and hard prickles.*

➤ *Bark: Pale ash to silver gray in color and 1.8 to 2.5 cm thick.*

➤ *Leaves: Large, palmate, glabrous, 13 to 15 cm long, 7 to 10 cm wide and leaflets three to seven, entire, and lanceolate. In winter session, the leaves usually drop and at the time of flowering appear again.*

➤ *Flowers: Large in diameter, red in color, and numerous with copious nectar.*

➤ *Fruits: Brown in color, capsule-like, 5 to 7 cm in length, filled with numerous, black, irregular obovoid-shaped seeds.*

➤ *Seeds: Black, smooth, embedded in white wool.*

➤ *Gummy exudate obtained from the bark is sold in the market as "semul gum," "mocharasa," or "suparika phula."*

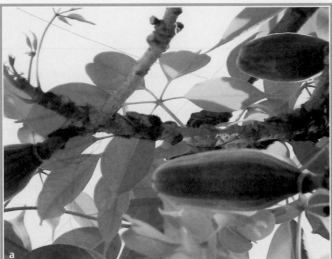
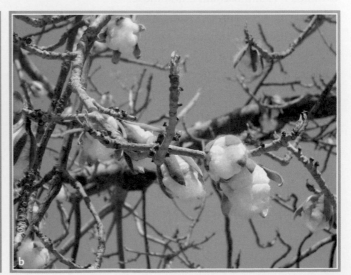

Fig. 89.4 (a) Fruits. (b) Fruits with cotton.

Types

Sembhal tree is of two types. One has prickles and is called Kanti Sembhal. Second type has no prickles. First variety has bluish bark and conical projection in fresh bark with better pharmacological actions (Khan 2014; Lubhaya 1977).

Rasapanchaka

Guna	Laghu, Snigdha, Pichchhila
Rasa	Madhura, Kasaya, Tikta
Vipaka	Madhura (mocharasa: Katu vipaka)
Virya	Sheeta

Chemical Constituents

Leaves contain flavonol C-glycoside shamimin. Root bark contains lactone, 5-isopropyl-3-methyl-2, 4, 7 trimethoxy-8, 1- naphthalene carbolactone together with naphthoquinone, 8-formyl-7-hydroxy-5-isopropyl-2-methoxy3methyl 1,4 naphthoquinone, Hemigossypol-6-methyl ether, isohemigossypol-l-methyl ether. Stem bark contains shamimicin, and (3,4-dihydroxyphenyl)-3,4-dihydro-3,7-dihydroxy-5-O-xylopyranosyloxy-2H-1-benzopyran along with lupeol was isolated. Flowers have hentriacontane and gossypol, polysaccharide, 4(1-4)-β-linked D-galactopyranose and 2 (1-3)-β-linked larabinopyranose units with β-linked D-galactose and α-linked L-rhamnose and L-arabinose.

Seeds possess palmitic acid, tannin and lupeol.

Gum consists of tannic acid, gallic acid, catechins, starch, protein, etc. (Faizi and Ali 1999; Rastogi and Mehrotra 1990; Sankaram et al 1981; Saleem et al 2003).

Identity, Purity, and Safety

- Foreign matter: Not more than 1%
- Total ash: Not more than 13%
- Acid-insoluble ash: Not more than 2%
- Alcohol-soluble extractive: Not less than 2%
- Water-soluble extractive: Not less than 7%

(Source: The Ayurvedic Pharmacopoeia of India 2001)

Karma (Actions)

It has rasayana (rejuvenative), raktapittahara (reduce hemorrhage), shukral (spermatopoetic) actions. Mocharasa (exudate) is grahi (astringent), vrisya (aphrodisiac), and dahashamak (pacify burning sensation). Its flower is raktasthambhan (hemostatic) and its kanda (root) has malarodha (constipation), daha and santapahara (reduce burning sensation and temperature) actions.

The bark is mucilaginous, demulcent, aphrodisiac, diuretic, tonic (balya, brimganiya), slightly astringent, and emetic. Gum is astringent, cooling, aphrodisiac, hemostatic, stimulant, antiseptic, expectorant. Flowers are laxative, diuretic, astringent, absorbent (grahi).

- Doshakarma: Vatapittashamaka, kaphakarak
- Dhatukarma: Balya, brimhana
- Malakarma: Grahi

Pharmacological Actions

It is reported to have actions like analgesic, antioxidant, antiangiogenic, hypoglycemic, hypotensive, anthelmintic, antiangiogenic, antidiabetic, antidiarrheal, antidysenteric, antifilarial, antipyretic, antimicrobial, antibacterial, anti-paralytic, aphrodisiac, astringent, cardioprotective, cardiotonic, demulcent, diuretic, emetic, hemostatic, antihemolytic, hepatoprotective, hepatocuritive, laxative, restorative, stimulant, and tonic (Maurya et al 2018).

Indications

Its bark is used for fomenting and healing wounds and skin eruptions. Gum is used for treating diarrhea, dysentery, hemoptysis, menorrhagia, influenza, burning sensation, and piles. Flowers are good for skin diseases, bleeding disorders, diarrhea, chronic inflammations, and wounds. Semal musali are used traditionally as an aphrodisiac, nutritive, restorative, and sexual stimulant drug in impotency, spermatorrhea, and frequent nocturnal seminal emission.

Therapeutic Uses

External Use

1. **Vyanga** (freckles): Sharp horns of Shalmali powdered with milk should be applied to face. It makes the face clean and smooth (VM. 57/38).
2. **Vrana** (wound): Shalmali bark, Bala root, etc. should be applied to the wound. It removes burning sensation (CS. Ci. 25/63).
3. **Padadaha** (burning sensation in feet): Application of the paste of Shalmali bark removes burning sensation of feet (RM. 23/1).
4. **Snayuka Roga** (guinea worm): Guinea worm is destroyed by application of the paste of Shalmali bark (VM. 55/19).

Internal Use

1. **Atisara** (diarrhea)
   - Enema of the petioles or exudation of Shalmali boiled in milk and added with ghee is useful in diarrhea with tenesmus (C.S.Si. 10/36).
   - Cold infusion of Shalmali petioles kept overnight should be taken after adding Madhuka and honey (S.S.U. 40/98).
   - Slimy enema made of Shalmali petioles by closed heating should be given (S.S.UT. 40/141,142).
2. **Raktapitta** (intrinsic hemorrhage)
   - One should take flowers of Kobidara, Kasmarya, and Shalmali (C.S.Ci. 4/39).
   - Powder of Shalmali flowers should be taken with honey (CD. 9/27).
   - In hemorrhage from the lower passages, goat's milk cooked with crushed fresh Shalmali petioles, added with ghee and cooled should be given as enema (C.S.Si. 7/60).
3. **Pleeha Vriddhi** (splenomegaly)
   - Flowers of Shalmali well steamed should be kept overnight and then taken after mixing Rajika powder. It reduces spleen (BP.Ci. 33/18).
4. **Vajikarana** (aphrodisiac): Shalmali (tuber) is used with cow milk as aphrodisiac (HS. 3.47.15, VD. 20.17.23).
5. **Pradara** (menometrorhagia)
   - Vegetables and Shalmali flowers cooked with ghee and rock salt check bleeding (BPN. 9.51).
   - Shalmalighrita (BS.Striroga 77-78).

6. **Raktarsha** (bleeding piles): The gum (2 g) mixed with cow's milk (30 mL) and water (30 mL) is reported to cure bleeding piles (Anonymous 2000).

Officinal Parts Used

Bark, resin, leaves, flower, thorns

Dose

Root powder: 5 to 10 g
Flower juice: 10 to 20 mL
Gum: 1 to 3 g

Formulations

Shalmali ghrita, Chandanaasava, Himasagar taila

Toxicity/Adverse Effects

The pollens of the plant were reported to cause pollen allergy (seasonal pollen fever, seasonal asthma, and rhinitis) in Pondicherry area and asthma or seasonal rhinitis in Kolkata and neighboring areas (Anonymous 2000). The methanolic extract of defatted stem bark of *B. ceiba* showed adverse effects on heart, liver, and kidneys of mice at the dose of 1,000 mg/kg/d (Anonymous 2008).

Substitution and Adulteration

The various substitutes of mocharasa (*Bombax malabaricum*) are gum of *Butea frondosa*, gum of *Pistacia lentiscus*, stem bark of *Punica granatum*). It is a valuable substitute for gum Kino (*Eucalyptus resinifera*) and red gum of *Eucalyptus camaldulensis* (Anonymous 1997; Fazalullah 1918; Hakeem 1922; Nabi 1958; Usmani 2008; Khory and Katrak 1985).

Moringa oleifera and *Eriodendron anfractuosum* are used as adulterants.

Points to Ponder

- *Young roots of Shalmali tree are known as Semal Musali/Semal Kanda.*
- *Mocharasa is the gum of the tree Shalmali. The gum is also known as Supari ka phul.*

Suggested Readings

Anonymous. Quality Standards of Indian Medicinal Plants, Vol. 5. New Delhi: Indian Council of Medicinal Research; 2008:125–133

Anonymous. Standardization of Single Drugs of Unani Medicine, Vol. III. New Delhi: Central Council for Research in Unani Medicine; 1997:218–222

Anonymous. The Wealth of India: A Dictionary of Indian Raw Materials and Industrial Products, Vol. IX: Rh-So. New Delhi: National Institute of Science Communication, Council of Scientific & Industrial Research; 1999:177–183

Bhattacharjee SK. Handbook of Aromatic Plants. Jaipur: Pointer Publishers; 2000:61

Chavan MS, Beldal B, Londonkar RL. Review on ethnobotany phytoconstituents and phytopharmacology of *Bombax ceiba* Linn. Int J Pharm Biol Sci 2019;9(1):1061–1066

Dymock W, Warden CJH, Hooper D. Pharmacographia Indica, Vol. I. Pakistan: The Institute Of Health and Tibbi Research, Hamdard National Foundation; 1890:215–218

Faizi S, Ali M. Shamimin: a new flavonol C-glycoside from leaves of *Bombax ceiba*. Planta Med 1999;65(4):383–385

Fazalullah MM. Makhzanul Mufradat Maroof ba Jameul Advia. Lucknow: Matba Aam Mufeed Press; 1918:234

Hakeem HA. Bustanul Mufradat Jadeed. Darya Ganj, New Delhi: Idara Kitab-ush-Shifa; 1922:561

Khan A. Muheet-e-Azam, Vol. 3. Urdu Translation. New Delhi: Central Council for Research in Unani Medicine; 2014:252–254

Khory HK, Katrak NN. Materia Medica of India and Their Therapeutics. 3rd ed. Delhi: Neeraj Publishing House; 1985:103–104

Lubhaya HR. Goswami Bayanul Advia, Vol. II. New Delhi: Goswami Pharmacy; 1977:21–23

Maurya SK, Verma NK, Verma DK. *Bombax ceiba* Linn.: a review of its phytochemistry and pharmacology. Curr Res J Pharm Allied Sci 2018;2(3):14–23

Nabi MG. Makhzanul Mufradat Wa Murakkabate Azam Al-maroof ba Khwasul Advia. Narayan Das Jungli Mill, Ballimaran, Delhi: Jayyed Barqi Press; 1958:197

Rastogi RP, Mehrotra BN. Compendium of Indian Medicinal plants, Vol. 2. New Delhi: PID; 1990:104

Reddy VBM, Reddy KM, Gunasekar D, Murthy MM, Caux C, Bodo B. A new sesquiterpene lactone from *Bombax malabaricum*. Chem Pharm Bull (Tokyo) 2003;51(4):458–459

Saleem R, Ahmad SI, Ahmed M, et al. Hypotensive activity and toxicology of constituents from *Bombax ceiba* stem bark. Biol Pharm Bull 2003;26(1):41–46

Sankaram AVB, Reddy NS, Shoolery JN. New sesquiterpenoids of Bombax malabaricum. Phytochemistry 1981;20:1877

The Ayurvedic Pharmacopoeia of India. Part I, Vol. III. New Delhi: Department of AYUSH, Ministry of Health and Family Welfare, Government of India; 2001

The Wealth of India: A Dictionary of Indian Raw Materials and Industrial Products, Vol. I. New Delhi: National Institute of Science Communication, Council of Scientific & Industrial Research; 2000:145.

The Wealth of India: Raw Materials, Vol. I: A-Ci, New Delhi: NISCAIR, CSIR; 2004

Usmani MI. Tanqeehul Mufradat. Azamgarh: Ibn Sina Tibbiya College; 2008:234–235

Warier PK. Indian Medicinal Plants: A Compendium of 500 Species, Vol. 2. 4th ed. Chennai: Orient Longman Private Limited; 1994:104, 133, 224, 289

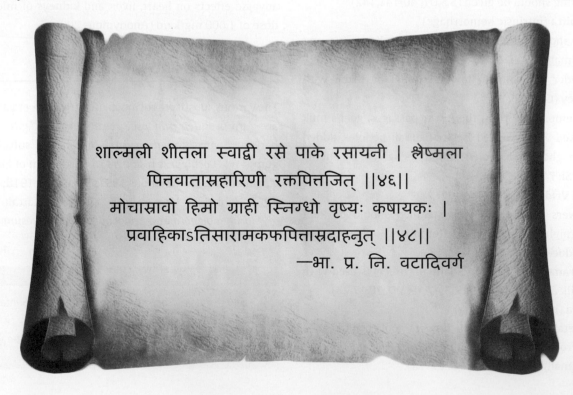

शाल्मली शीतला स्वाद्वी रसे पाके रसायनी । श्रेष्मला
पित्तवातासहारिणी रक्तपित्तजित् ॥४६॥
मोचास्रावो हिमो ग्राही स्निग्धो वृष्यः कषायकः ।
प्रवाहिकाऽतिसारामकफपित्तास्रदाहनुत् ॥४८॥
—भा. प्र. नि. वटादिवर्ग

90. Shankhapushpi *[Convolvulus pluricaulis Chois.]*

Family:	Convolvulaceae
Hind name:	Shankhapuspi, Shyamakranta, Syamakranta, Vishnukranta, Shannkhavalli, Shankhahuli
English name:	Speed wheel

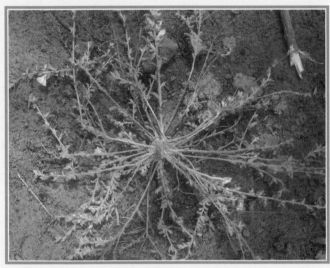

Plant of *Convolvulus pluricaulis* Chois.

The herb induces a feeling of calm and peace, good sleep, and a relief in anxiety, stress, and mental fatigue.

Introduction

The flowers of *Convolvulus pluricaulis* Chois are like Shankha and white in color; hence, it is called Shankhapushpi. Shankhapushpi (*C. pluricaulis* Choisy) is an extremely versatile plant. From ancient times Shankhapushpi has been commonly prescribed as nootropic (*medhya*), rejuvenator, nervine tonic in epilepsy, insanity, brain tonic, memory-enhancing drug, and possesses a wide range of therapeutic attributes. *Shankhapushpi*, with flowers shaped like a *Shankha* (conch), is one of Lord Shiva's sacred instruments often used in rituals. It is considered *Medhya Rasayana* (memory enhancer) in *Ayurvedic* texts. *Evolvulus alsinoides* Linn. of Convolvulaceae family is also considered as a source plant of Shankhapushpi in the southern part of India.

In Brihatrayee, Shankhapushpi is used as a vital ingredient in various memory enhancer formulations along with other therapeutic attributes. Moreover, Charaka has mentioned the medhya guna (nootropic property) of Shankhapushpi as "Medhya Visheshena cha Shankhapushpi." Sushruta has considered Vegavati herb similar to Shankhapushpi in the context of Divya aushadhi (divine herb). Commentators like Vagabhatta, Arunadatta, and Hemadri have not commented regarding Shankhapushpi, but Indu has attributed the synonym Supushpi to it (Paradakara 2010). Chandra has also named Shankhapushpi as Shankhakusuma (Acharya 2002).

Vernacular Names

Bengali: Shankhapuspi, Barabhutra
Gujarati: Shankhavali
Kannada: Bilikantisoppu, Shankhapushpi, Shankhauli, Vishnukarandi, Vishnukranti
Malayalam: Krsna kranti, Vishnukranthi
Marathi: Sankhahuli, Shankhavela, Sankhapuspi
Oriya: Sankhapuspi, Krishna-enkranti
Punjabi: Ksirapuspi, Sankhapuspi, Sankhahuli
Sanskrit: Sankhpuspi, Sankhahva

Tamil: Kakattam, Kakkanangudi, Karakhuratt, Sanghupushpam, Vishnu Kanthi, Vishnukranti, Vishnukkiranti

Telugu: Vishnukranthi, Vishnukranthi, Erravishnukarantha

Tibetan: Khalsa pus syi (d), Sa nkhapu spa

Urdu: Sankhali

Synonyms

Sankhapuspi: The flowers are like Shankha and white in color.

Shankhahwa: All the synonyms of Shankha are used for this plant.

Mangalyakusum: Auspicious plant.

Tilaki: Plants with attractive flowers.

Shankhakusuma: The flowers are like Shankha and white in color.

Medhya: It has medhya properties.

Vanavilasini: The place where flowers look attractive.

Classical Categorization

Charak Samhita: Not mentioned in any gana

Susruta Samhita: Not mentioned in any gana

Astanga Hridaya: Not mentioned in any gana

Dhanwantari Nighantu: Guduchyadi varga

Madanpal Nighantu: Abhayadi varga.

Kaiyadev Nighantu: Aushadi varga

Raj Nighantu: Guduchyadi varga

Bhavaprakash Nighantu: Guduchyadi varga

Distribution

It is commonly found on sandy or rocky land under xerophytic conditions and extensively grows on wasteland of Punjab, Bihar, Haryana, Delhi, or Chhota Nagpur in India. It is also found in Sri Lanka, Tropical Africa, and Southeastern Asia (Austin 2008; Cramer 1981).

Morphology

It is a perennial herb that seems like morning glory. Its branches that spread on the ground are more than 30 cm long.

- **Leaves:** Elliptic in shape, linear-oblong small and sub-sessile, 0.8 to 3 cm long, 1.5 to 6 mm broad, wedge-shaped at the base. Velvety/hairy at alternate position with flowers or branches (**Fig. 90.1**).

- **Flowers:** Inflorescence of axillary, solitary, sessile, calyx of five ovate-lanceolate hairy sepals, color is pale pink, five-lobed, stamens are five with filaments of various size ovary seated on a cup-shaped disc (**Fig. 90.2**).

- **Fruit:** Subglobose-ellipsoid, glabrous capsule, two-celled and four-valved; seeds are four, small, glabrous.

Phenology

Flowering time: March to April
Fruiting time: April to May

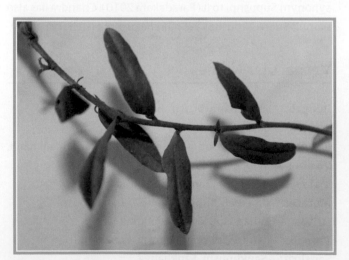

Fig. 90.1 Leaves.

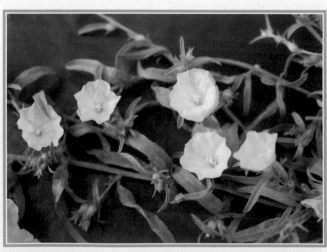

Fig. 90.2 Flower.

Key Characters for Identification

➤ It is a perennial herb spread on the ground, 30 cm long.

➤ Leaves: Elliptic in shape, linear-oblong, small, and subsessile.

➤ Flowers: Inflorescence of axillary, solitary, sessile, calyx of five ovate-lanceolate hairy sepals, color is pale pink/whitish/bluish like a Shankh, five-lobed, stamens are five with filaments of various size ovary seated on a cup-shaped disc.

➤ Fruit: Subglobose-ellipsoid capsule, two-celled and four-valved; seeds are four in number and are smaller in size.

➤ Root: Woody (**Fig. 90.3**).

Types

Dhanvantari Nighantu has mentioned the property of Shankhapushpi under the name of Shankhini (like a conch shell; Tripathi 2008). In contrast, Kaideva Nighantu describes Shankhapushpi and Shankhini as two different plants and suggests they should always be used in fresh state. Raktapushpa and Nilapushpika are two types of Shankhapushpi as per Kaiyadeva Nighantu (Sharma 2006). Raja Nighantu has mentioned Vishnukranti as a variety of Shankhapushpi, while this name is also used as a synonym of Aparajita (*Clitoria ternatea*).

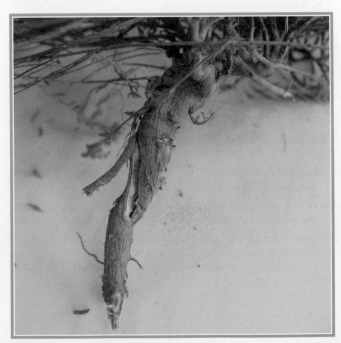

Fig. 90.3 Root.

Rasapanchaka

Guna	Snigdha, Pichhila
Rasa	Kashaya, Katu, Tikta
Vipak	Madhura
Virya	Ushna

Chemical Constituents

The chemical constituents present in this plant are as follows:

- Alkaloids: Convolamine, convoline, convolidine, convolvine, confoline, convosine, shankhapusphine
- Carbohydrates: D-Glucose, maltose, rhamnose, sucrose
- Phenols/glycosides/triterpenoids: Scopoletin, β-sitosterol, ceryl, alcohol, 20-oxodotriacontanol, Tetra triacontanoic acid, 29-oxodotriacontanol
- Flavonoids: Kaempferol
- Steroids: Phytosterols (Debjit et al 2012)

Identity, Purity, and Strength

- Foreign matter: Not more than 2%
- Total ash: Not more than 17%
- Acid-insoluble ash: Not more than 8%
- Alcohol-soluble extractive: Not less than 6%
- Water-soluble extractive: Not less than 10%

(Source: The Ayurvedic Pharmacopeia of India 2001)

Karma (Actions)

The drug is very useful in learning memory and behavioral improvement along with the properties like ayusya (long life), medhya (intellect promoter), balya (enhance physical strength), deepan (digestive), kantiprada (complexion promoter), kaphahara (antitussive), mohanasaka (remove confusion), pittahara (pacify pitta dosha), rasayana (rejuvenative), smritiprada (memory enhancer), vishagarbha, vrushya (aphrodisiac; The Ayurvedic Pharmacopoeia of India 2001).

- Doshakarma: Tridoshahara
- Dhatukarma: Vrushya (aphrodisiac), rasayana (rejuvenative)
- Malakarma: Sara

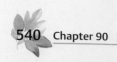

Pharmacological Actions

The pharmacological actions of the drug are analgesic, adaptogenic, anthelmintic, antibacterial, anticonvulsing, antidepressant, antidiabetics, antifungal, anti-inflammatory, antimicrobial, antioxidant, antistress, antiulcer, antiulcerogenic, anxiolytic, brain tonic, central nervous system (CNS) depressant, diuretic, hypoglycemic, hypolipidemic, hypotensive, muscle relaxant, neuroleptic, psychostimulant, sedative, spasmolytic, tranquilizing, and reduction in spontaneous motor activity (Hetal et al 2014).

Indications

It is used in mental disorders, epilepsy, bhutabadha (evil spirit), kushta (skin disease), krimi (worm infestation), visha (poisoning), and to improve memory. It is mainly used in the treatment of disorders such as hypertension, anxiety, neurosis, and stress. It is considered as the best medhyarasayana drug. It is used in memory loss, Parkinson syndrome, and Alzheimer disease. It also works as psychostimulant and tranquilizer.

Therapeutic Uses

1. **Insanity and epilepsy**: Old ghee processed with juice of Brahmi, Vacha, Kusta, and Shankhapushpi is used in insanity and epilepsy (C.S.Ci. 10/25).
2. **Intellect-promoting Rasayana**: Paste of Shankhapushpi is considered the best intellect-promoting drug (C.S.Ci. /3/31).
3. **High blood pressure:** Fresh juice of Shankhapushpi (10–20 mL) is taken twice daily for some days to get rid of high blood pressure.
4. **Bed urination in child**: Two grams of Shankhapushpi and 1 g of black sesame is given with milk to check bed urination problem in children.

Officinal Part Used

Whole plant

Dose

Powder: 3 to 8 g
Paste: 10 to 20 g
(Source: The Ayurvedic Pharmacopoeia of India 2001)

Formulations

Agastyaharitaki rasayana, Brahma rasayana, Brahmi ghrita, Brahmi vati, Gorocanadi vati, Manasmitra vataka, Shankhapushpi taila, Shankhapushpi panak, Shankhapushpi rasayana, Soma ghrita.

Toxicity/Adverse Effects

No toxicity of *C. pluricaulis* is so far reported. Sedative effect was observed in mice at doses more than 200 mg/kg, and moderate to marked decrease in locomotor activity was observed for approximately 12 hours by lethal dose (LD50) of the whole extract of *C. pluricaulis* (Pawar et al 2001).

Substitution and Adulteration

Following plants are used as a substitute of *C. pluricaulis*:
- *Convolvulus microphyllus* Sceb.
- *Evolvulus alsinoides* Linn.
- *Canscora decussata* Schult.

> **Points to Ponder**
> - *Shankhapushpi is the best medhya drug as per Acharya Charak.*

Suggested Readings

Acharya YT. Sushruta Samhita. 7th ed. Varanasi: Chaukhambha Orientalia; 2002:186, 385–542, 506, 770

Austin DF. *Evolvulus alsinoides* (Convolvulaceae): an American herb in the Old World. J Ethnopharmacol 2008;117(2):185–198

Bhowmik D, Kumar KPS, Paswan S, Srivatava S, Yadav APD, Dutta A. Traditional Indian herbs Convolvulus pluricaulis and its medicinal importance. J Pharmacognosy Phytochemistry 2012;1(1):44–51

Bhowmik D, Sampath Kumar KP, Paswan S, Srivatava S, Yadav A, Dutta A. Traditional Indian herbs *Convolvulus pluricaulis* and its medicinal importance. J Pharmacogn Phytochem 2012;1(1):44–51

Cramer LH. Gentianaceae. In: Dassenayake MD, Fosberg FR, eds. A Revised Handbook to the Flora of Ceylon. New Delhi: Amarind Publishing Co; 1981:55–78

Hetal A, Sharma R, Vyas M, Prajapati PK, Dhiman K. Shankhapushpi (*Convolvulus pluricaulis* Choisy): validation of the ayurvedic therapeutic claims through contemporary studies. Int J Green Pharm 2014;8:193–200

Lucas DS. Dravyaguna-Vijnana: Study of Dravya-Materia Medica. Varanasi: Chaukhamba Visvabharati; 2013:286

Paradakara HS. Astanga Hridaya. 4th ed. Varanasi: Chaukhambha Sanskrita Sansthana; 2010:597–927

Pawar SA, Dhuley JN, Naik SR. Neuropharmacology of an extract derived from *Convolvulus microphyllus*. Pharm Biol 2001;39:253–258

Sharma PV. Classical Uses of Medicinal Plants. 1st ed. Varanasi: Chaukhamba Vishvabharati; 2004:352

Sharma PV. Kaiyadev Nighantu. 2nd ed. Varanasi: Chowkhamba Orientalia; 2006:622

The Ayurvedic Pharmacopoeia of India, Vol. 2. Delhi: Ministry of Health and Family Welfare, Department of Indian Systems of Medicine and Homeopathy, Controller of Publications; 2001:147–149

Tripathi H. Dhanwantari Nighantu. 1st ed. Varanasi: Chowkhamba Bharti Academy; 2008:16

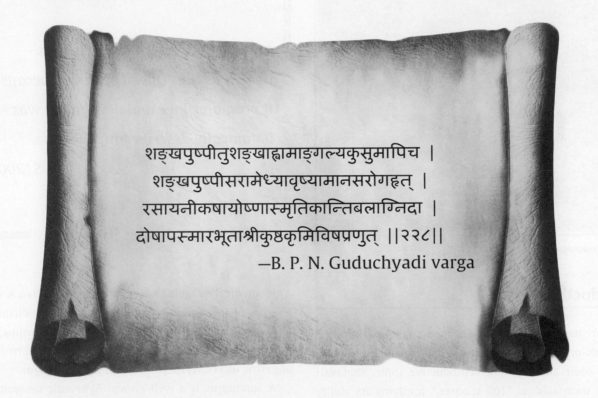

शङ्खपुष्पीतुशङ्खाह्वामाङ्गल्यकुसुमापिच |
शङ्खपुष्पीसरामेध्यावृष्यामानसरोगहृत् |
रसायनीकषायोष्णास्मृतिकान्तिबलाग्निदा |
दोषापस्मारभूताश्रीकुष्ठकृमिविषप्रणुत् ||२२८||
—B. P. N. Guduchyadi varga

91. Shatavari *[Asparagus racemosus Willd.]*

Family:	*Liliaceae*
Hindi name:	*Shatavar, Shatmuli*
English name:	*Wild Asparagus*

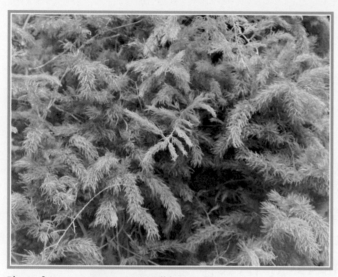

Plant of *Asparagus racemosus* Willd.

> *In Ayurveda, this amazing herb is known as the "Queen of herbs," because it promotes love and devotion. It was botanically described in 1799.*
>
> —US (2009)

Introduction

Shatavari means "a woman who possesses one hundred husbands or acceptable to many." It is considered both a general tonic and a female reproductive tonic. Shatavari may be translated as "100 spouses," implying its ability to increase fertility and vitality. Shatavari is the main Ayurvedic rejuvenative tonic for the female, as is *Withania* for the male. Shatavari has been mentioned in Ayurvedic texts. It is known for its phytoestrogenic properties and is extensively used in combating menopausal symptoms and increasing lactation (Sabnis et al 1968; Mitra et al 1999).

Charaka has included this drug in balya and vayasthapana varga. Sushruta included it in vidharigandhadi and kantaka panchamula. Acharya Kashyapa has dedicated a whole chapter to shathavari in kalpasthana with the tittle shatapushpa shatavari adhyaya.

Its medical usage has been reported in Indian & British Pharmacopeias and in traditional system of medicine such as Ayurveda, Unani, and Siddha. Shatavari, according to the main Ayurvedic texts, is used for prevention and treatment of gastric ulcers, dyspepsia, and as a galactagogue.

A. racemosus is a well-known Ayurvedic rasayana that prevents aging, increases longevity, imparts immunity, improves mental function and vigor, and adds vitality to the body. It is also used in nervous disorders, dyspepsia, tumors, inflammation, neuropathy, and hepatopathy.

Vernacular Names

Assamese: Satmull
Bengali: Satamuli, Satmuli, Shatamuli
Gujarati: Ekalkanto, Satavari
Kannada: Callagadda

Kashmiri: Sejnana

Madhya Pradesh: Narbodh, Satmooli

Malayalam: Satavari, Satavali

Marathi: Asvel, Shatmuli, Satavari

Oriya: Chhotaru, Mohajolo, Sotabori

Rajasthani: Norkanto, Satawar

Tamil: Kilavari, Satavali

Telugu: Satavari, Callagadda

Urdu: Satawari

Synonyms

Abhiru: It makes free from external invasion.

Atirasa: Its tuberous roots contain more juice.

Bahusuta: It has many succulent roots or tubers.

Durmara: The plants don't perish easily; it has a long span of life.

Dwipishatru: It is antagonistic to tikshna substance as it is predominant in watery elements.

Indivari: That which benefits many people.

Narayani: It is of saumya nature.

Phanijivhaparni: The leaves are like the tongue of snakes.

Pivari: The tubers are stout and succulent.

Rushyaprokta: The drug is recommended by sages.

Shatavari: It has many succulent roots or tubers.

Shatapadi: it has many succulent roots or tubers.

Shatavirya: It produces multifold actions and is useful in many disorders.

Sukshmapatra: The leaves are thin or linear cladodes.

Swadurasa: It is sweet in taste (madhura rasa).

Urdhwakantaka: It has recurved spines.

Vari: It is one of best medicines.

Classical Categorization

Charak Samhita: Balya, Vayahsthapana, Madhura skanda

Sushruta Samhita: Vidarigandhadi, Varunadi, Kantaka panchmool, Vatasanshamana

Astanga Hridaya: Vidaryadi, Varunadi, Pittashamana

Dhanwantari Nighantu: Guduchyadhi varga

Madanpal Nighantu: Abhayadhivarga

Kaiyadev Nighantu: Aushadhi varga

Raj Nighantu: Shatvhadi varga

Bhavaprakash Nighantu: Guduchyadi varga

Distribution

It is widely distributed across the globe and its distribution ranges from tropical Africa, Java, Australia, Sri Lanka, Southern parts of China, and India, but it is mainly cultivated in India (Kirtikar and Basu 1985).

Morphology

It is an armed highly branched climber growing to 1 to 2 m in height. Stem is woody terete with recurved spines. Its young stem is delicate, brittle, and smooth.

- **Leaves:** Reduced to minute chaffy scales (known as cladodes) and spines. Cladodes are acicular, two to six in number, falcate, and finely acuminate (**Fig. 91.1**).
- **Flowers:** White, fragrant in simple or branched raceme arising from the axil of the thorns (**Fig. 91.2**).
- **Fruits:** Globular or three-lobed pulpy berries, ripe berries are orange and red, and dry berries are black colored and single seeded (**Fig. 91.3a, b**).
- **Roots:** Stout root stock bearing numerous succulents, fusiform or finger-shaped cluster of tuberous roots, which are nearly 30 to 100 cm long and 1 to 2 cm thick. Unpeeled roots are cream, light-brown colored, wrinkled surface, with scars and protuberance of lateral rootlets (**Fig. 91.4a, b**).

It is propagated through seeds and division of tuberous roots.

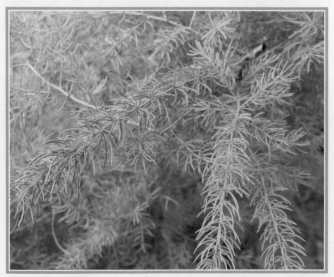

Fig. 91.1   Leaves.

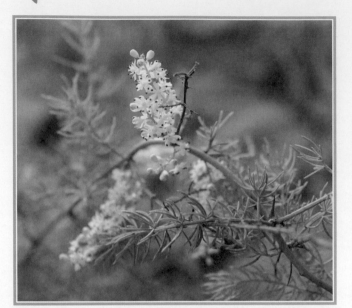

Fig. 91.2 Flowers.

Phenology

Flowering time: June to August
Fruiting time: October to January

Key Characters for Identification

➤ It is a woody climber plant which is 1 to 2 m in length and readily grows over another plant.
➤ Leaves: Looks like pine needles, uniform and small in size.
➤ Flower: It has a tiny, white-colored flower.
➤ Fruits: Globular berries, ripe berries are orange and red and dry berries are black colored.
➤ Roots: The roots of the plant have a finger-like structure and are clustered in nature, nearly 30 to 100 cm long and 1 to 2 cm thick.

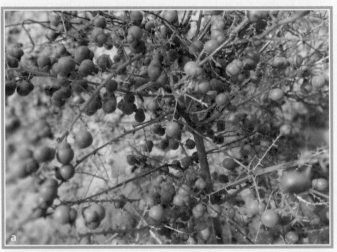

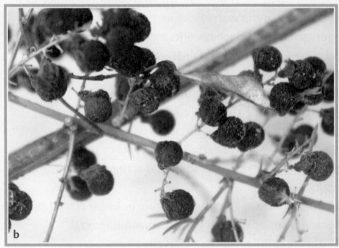

Fig. 91.3 (a) Unripe fruits. (b) Mature fruits.

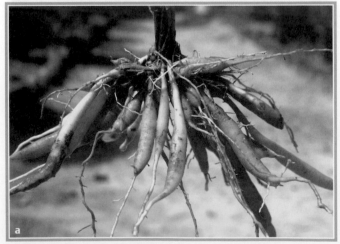

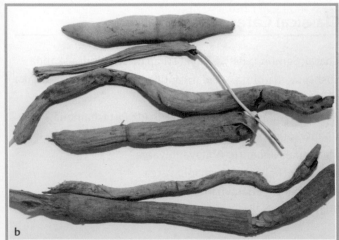

Fig. 91.4 (a) Fresh roots. (b) Dry roots.

Types

According to Nighantukaras it is of two varieties: Shatavari and Maha Shatavari.

Shatavari is *A. racemosus* and Maha Shatavari is *A. sarmentosa* Linn.

Rasapanchaka

Guna	Guru, Snigdha
Rasa	Tikta, Madhura
Vipaka	Madhura
Virya	Sheeta

Chemical Constituents

Root contains steroidal glycosides such as shatavarins I-IV, sarsapogenin, sitosterol, asparagamine A, steroids, saponins, polycyclic alkaloids, proteins, and high level of minerals.

Flowers contain β-sitosterol, sarsasapogenins, diogenins, and asparamins A & B.

Leaves possess diosgenin and quercetin 3-glucuronide.

Fruits are comprised of sitosteral, stigmasterol, saraspogeninsitostererol-B-D glucoside, stigmasterol glucoside, two spirostonalic and furostanolic saponins, and sapogenin (Malhotra 1985).

Identity, Purity, and Safety

- Foreign matter Not more than 1%
- Total Ash Not more than 5%
- Acid-insoluble ash Not more than 0.5%
- Alcohol-soluble extractive Not less than 10%
- Water-soluble extractive Not less than 45%

(Source: The Ayurvedic Pharmacopeia of India 2004)

Karma (Actions)

The roots of this herb is described as balya (strength promoting), shukral (increases semen), stanyakari (galactogogue), medhya (intellect promoting), rasayana (immunomodulator), netrya (eye tonic), vrisya (aphrodisiac), pustivardhaka (nutritive), atisarajit (reduces diarrhea), shotahara (reduces swelling) in Ayurveda.

- Doshakarma: Vatapittashamaka
- Dhatukarma: Stanyavardhaka, Sukravardhaka, Vrisya
- Malakarma: Atisarajit

Pharmacological Actions

It has nematocidal, anticancer, antidysenteric, antifungal, gastric-sedative, antibacterial, antiabortifacient (shatavarin I), antioxytoxic (shatavarin IV), antiviral, diuretic, galactagogue, antiamoebic, spasmodic to uterus, hypoglycemic, phagocytic, hypotensive, anticoagulant, and enzymatic actions (Sharma et al 2000). Besides this it has antioxidant, antiulcer, antitussive, adaptogenic, diuretic, antistress, uterine tonic, antispasmodic, and hepatoprotective properties.

Indications

It is indicated in kshaya (debility), grahani (sprue), gulma (abdominal lump), shotha (swelling), agnimandhya (loss of appetite), raktavikara (blood disorders), rakthapitta (hemorrhagic disorders), arshas (piles), artavakasaya (amenorrhea), amlapitta (hyperacidity), atisara (diarrhea), raktapitta, vatarakta (gout), visarpa (erysipelas), parinama shoola (colic pain), mutrarakta (bleeding during urination), vatajvara (fever due to vata), svarabheda (hoarseness of voice), naktandhya (nightblindness), sutika roga (puerperal diseases), stanya dosha, stanya kshaya (reduction of breast milk).

Root powder is widely used in dyspepsia, hyperacidity, burning micturition, thirst, gonorrhea, nervous disorders, diarrhea, dysentery, tumors, inflammations, hyperdipsia, neuropathy, hepatopathy, cough, bronchitis, leucorrhea, stress, ulcer, fatigue, abortion, general debility, and certain infectious diseases (Sairam et al 2003).

Therapeutic Uses

External Use

Visarpa (erysipelas): Tubers of Shatavari and Vidari mixed with washed ghee should be used as paste (C.S.Ci. 21/84).

Internal Use

1. **Raktapitta** (intrinsic hemorrhage): Shatavaryadi ghrita is given in raktapitta (C.S.Ci. 4.95-96). Milk processed with Shatavari and Goksura or with four-leaved herbs affects hemorrhage particularly of the urinary tract (C.S.Ci. 4.85). Milk processed with Shatavari reduces hemorrhage (BP.Ci. 9.43).

2. **Atisara** (diarrhea): In diarrhea predominant in vata, one should take Shatavari ghrita (AS.Ci. 11.25). Paste of Shatavari should be taken with milk, keeping on milk-diet in diarrhea with blood (CS.Ci. 19.75; also AH.Ci. 9.88; VM. 3.42).

3. **Arsha** (piles): Paste of Shatavari root should be taken with milk (SS.Ci. 6.13).

4. **Svarabheda** (hoarseness of voice): The patient should take powder of Kakolyadi drugs or Shatavari or Bala mixed with honey and ghee (S.S.U. 53.l4).

5. **Kasa** (cough): For the well-being of those suffering from cough, ghee cooked with Shatavari and Nagabala should be administered (S.S.U. 52/47).

6. **Paittik shula** (biliary colic): Shatavari juice mixed with honey should be taken in the morning. It alleviates burning sensation and pain and all disorders of pitta (VM. 26.21, BS.Shula 32, SG.2.1.15).

7. **Vatarakta** (gout): Shatavari ghrita is given (VM. 23.25).

8. **Timir** (defect of vision): Payasa prepared with Shatavari removes the defect of vision (S.S.U. 17.49). In night blindness tender leaves of Shatavari cooked in ghee should be taken (A.H.U. 13/89).

9. **Visha** (poisoning): In case of poisoning, juice of Shatavari mixed with ghee and honey is useful (S.S.Ka. 1.68).

10. **Pittala yonivyapad** (disorder of female genital tract): Shatavari is the main drug in brihat Shatavari ghrita (CS.Ci. 30/64-68) which is useful in disorder of female genital tract caused by pitta.

11. **As rasayana** (rejuvenation): Those who take ghee cooked with paste and decoction of Shatavari with sugar do not suffer in any type of diseases (A.H.U. 39/157).

12. **As Vajikarana** (aphrodisiac): Shatavari ghrita (C.S.Ci. 2.3.18) and powder of Shatavari and Uchata mixed with sugar should be taken with mild warm milk (S.S.Ci. 26/34). Shatavari taken with milk also acts as aphrodisiac (VJ. 5.5).

13. **Apasmara** (epilepsy): Shatavari taken with milk is useful in epilepsy (CS.Ci. 10/64).

14. **Jwara** (fever): Juice of Guduchi and Shatavari in equal quantity mixed with jaggery is taken. It alleviates fever caused by vata (SS.U. 39/174).

15. **Mutrakuchhra** (dysuria): Powder of Shatavari should be taken with cold water (HS.3.29.6).

16. **Stanyavardhanam** (galactopoietic): Shatavari pounded and taken increases the flow of breast milk (YR.P. 427).

Officinal Part Used

Tuberous roots

Dose

Powder: 3 to 6 g
Juice: 10 to 20 mL

Formulations

Shatavariyadi Ghrita, Phala Ghrita, Puga khanda, Erand paka Narayani Taila, Shatavari Taila, Shatavari Modaka, Shatavari Mandura, Shatavaryadi Kwatha, Mahanarayana Taila, Shatavari Chinnaroohadi Kashaya, Shatavaryadi Churna, Shatavari Guda.

Toxicity/Adverse Effects

In Ayurveda, *A. racemosus* has been described as absolutely safe even for long-term use, and during pregnancy and lactation. Systemic administration of higher doses of all extracts did not produce abnormality in behavior pattern of mice and rat (Jetmalani et al 1967). LD_{50} of the product lactate has not been assessed since it did not produce mortality even up to oral dosage of 64 g/kg (Narendranath et al 1986).

Substitution and Adulteration

The roots of *Asparagus sarmentosus* Linn., *Asparagus curillus* Ham., *Asparagus filicinus* Ham., and *Asparagus sprengeri* Regel are also being sold in the name of Shatavari in Indian market (Sharma et al 2000).

Points to Ponder

- *It is considered both a general tonic and a female reproductive tonic.*
- *It has both stanyajanana and shukrajanana properties.*
- *Root of Shatavari is used in the absence of Meda and Mahameda (Bhavaprakash).*

Suggested Readings

Chawla A, Chawla P, Mangalesh, Roy RC. *Asparagus racemosus* (Willd): biological activities & its active principles. Indo-Global J Pharm Sci 2011;1(2):113–120

Department of Agriculture, USA. *Asparagus* racemosus information from NPGS/GRIN. Germplasm resources information network; 2009

Jetmalani MH, Sabins PB, Gaitonde BB. A study on the pharmacology of various extracts of Shatavari: *Asparagus racemosus* (Willd). J Res Indian Med 1967;2:1–10

Kirtikar KR, Basu BD. Indian Medicinal Plants. Dehradun: Bishen Singh Mahendra Pal Singh; 1985

Malhotra SC. Phytochemical Investigations of Certain Medicinal Plants Used in Ayurveda. New Delhi: CCRAS; 1985:470

Mitra SK, Gopumadhavan S, Venkataranganna MV, Sarma DNK, Anturlikar SD. Uterine tonic activity of U-3107: a herbal preparation in rats. Indian J Pharmacol 1999;31:200–203

Narendranath KA, Anuradha V, Mahalingam S, Rao S. Effect of herbal galactagogue (Lactare): a pharmacological and clinical observation. Med Surg 1986;26:19–22

Sabnis PB, Gaitonde BB, Jetmalani M. Effects of alcoholic extracts of *Asparagus racemosus* on mammary glands of rats. Indian J Exp Biol 1968;6(1):55–57

Sairam K, Priyambada S, Aryya NC, Goel RK. Gastroduodenal ulcer protective activity of *Asparagus racemosus*: an experimental, biochemical and histological study. J Ethnopharmacol 2003;86(1):1–10

Sharma PC, Yelne MB, Dennis TJ. Database on Medicinal Plant Used in Ayurveda, Vol. 1. New Delhi: CCRAS; 2000:418

Sharma PV. Charaka Samhita. Varanasi: Chaukhambha Orientalis; 2001:7–14

The Ayurvedic Pharmacopoeia of India, Part I, Vol. IV. 1st ed. New Delhi: Department of Health, Ministry of Health and Family Welfare, Government of India; 2004:108

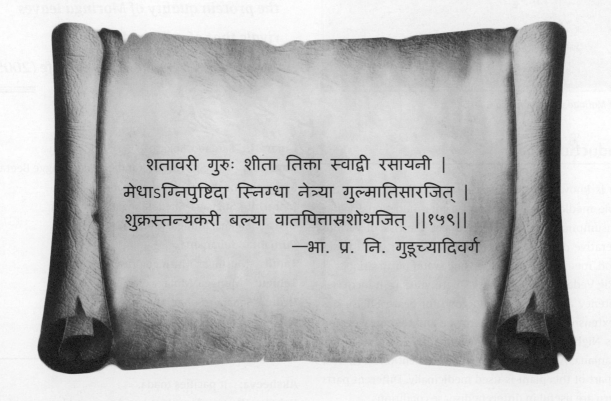

शतावरी गुरुः शीता तिक्ता स्वाद्वी रसायनी ।
मेधाऽग्निपुष्टिदा स्निग्धा नेत्र्या गुल्मातिसारजित् ।
शुक्रस्तन्यकरी बल्या वातपित्तास्रशोथजित् ॥१५९॥
—भा. प्र. नि. गुडूच्यादिवर्ग

92. Shigru [Moringa pterygosperma Gaertn.]

Synonym:	*Moringa oleifera Lamk.*
Family:	*Moringaceae*
Hindi name:	*Sahijan, Shobhanjan, Munga*
English name:	*Drumstick tree, Horse radish tree*

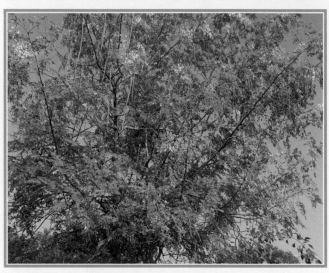

Plant of *Moringa pterygosperma* Gaertn.

> *"Ounce-for-ounce, Moringa leaves contain more vitamin A than carrots, more calcium than milk, more iron than spinach, more vitamin C than oranges, and more potassium than bananas," and the protein quality of Moringa leaves rivals that of milk and eggs.*
>
> —*Trees for Life (2005)*

Introduction

Shigru is known as the miracle vegetable because it has multiple medicinal benefits and a high nutritional value. Its consumption in daily diet reduces the risk of various degenerative diseases. It is used for a number of purposes like food, medicine, dye, fodder, and water purification.

In Rig Veda, we come across Shigru vraksha. It increases the potency and is considered good for heart. Shigru has been extensively used in Brihatrayee and Laghutrayee and various Nighantus. Various synonyms like Krishnagandha, Shobhanjana, Aksheeva, etc. have been mentioned. Almost every part of this plant is used medicinally. Different parts of Shigru are useful in different disease conditions.

Vernacular Names

Assamese: Saijna, Sohjna
Bengali: Sajina, Sajna
Gujarati: Sargavo, Sekato
Kannada: Neegge, Nugge Kand Chakke, Nugge Beeta
Malayalam: Muringa, Tiksnggandha
Marathi: Shevaga, Shegatabeeja, Segat Sala
Oriya: Sajana, Munga, Munika
Punjabi: Sohanjana
Tamil: Muringai, Muringai Virai
Telugu: Munaga, Mulaga
Urdu: Sahajan, Sohanjana

Synonyms

Aksheeva: It pacifies mada.
Bahalapallava: The plant has dense and luxuriant foliage.
Bahumoola: It has many roots.
Ghanachhada: The plant has luxuriant foliage.
Haritashaka: The leaves and fruits are used as green vegetable.
Krushnagandha: It has pungent smell and taste.

Mochaka: It is useful in many diseases or that which removes diseases.

Mulakaparni: The pungent smell is present from mula to patra.

Murangi: It is also known as murangi.

Shigru: It has tikshna guna.

Shobhanjana: That which gives attractive look or a beautiful tree.

Tiksnagandha: It has strong smell.

Tiksnamula: The mula have pungent smell.

Vidradhighna: Shigru possesses antibiotic property and is useful in infective disorders like abscess.

Classical Categorization

Charak Samhita: Krimighna, Swedopaga, Shirovirechanopaga, Katu skandha

Sushruta Samhita: Varunadi, Shirovirechana

Astanga Hridaya: Varunadi, Shyamadi, Shirovirechana

Dhanwantari Nighantu: Karaveeradi varga

Madanpal Nighantu: Shakavarga

Kaiyadev Nighantu: Aushadhi varga

Raj Nighantu: Moolakadi varga

Bhavaprakash Nighantu: Guduchyadi varga

Distribution

It is a beautiful tree found wild in sub-Himalayan range and nowadays commonly cultivated throughout India.

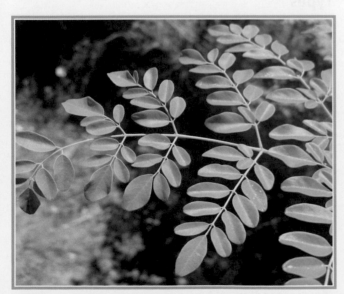

Fig. 92.1 Leaves.

Morphology

It is an evergreen, fast-growing, deciduous tree that grows up to a height of 10 to 12 m. It has a spreading open crown of drooping, fragile branches, feathery foliage of tripinnate leaves, and thick corky whitish bark.

- **Leaves:** Compound, imparipinnate, usually tripinnate up to 45 cm long, leaflets 1 to 2 cm long, the lateral elliptic, the terminal obovate and slightly longer than the lateral ones, entire margin, round or blunt apex, finely hairy and green (**Fig. 92.1**).
- **Flowers:** White fragrant, in large puberulous pinnacles, calyx lobes linear-lanceolate reflexed, puberulous outside. Petals spathulate veined. Stamens 5 fertile, alternating with five to seven antherless ones, filaments villors at the base. Ovary oblong, villous style is cylindric (**Fig. 92.2**).
- **Fruits:** Pods are pendulous, immature pods are green in color and turns brown on maturity, 30 to 45 cm in length, triangular, ribbed, split open longitudinally when dry (**Fig. 92.3**).
- **Seeds:** White trigonous, 25 to 30 in number, with winged angles (**Fig. 92.4**).
- **Bark:** Whitish grey, thick, soft fissured, warty, or corky and rough (**Fig. 92.5**). When incised, it exudates a gum which is initially white and turns reddish-brown on exposure (**Fig.92.6**).

It is propagated through seeds and stem cutting.

Phenology

Flowering time: January to May
Fruiting time: May to December

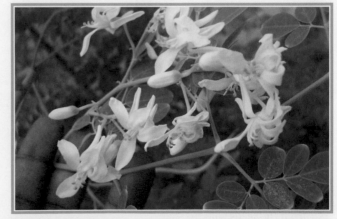

Fig. 92.2 Flowers.

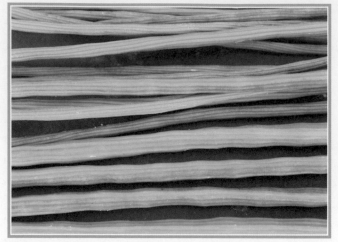

Fig. 92.3 Fruits.

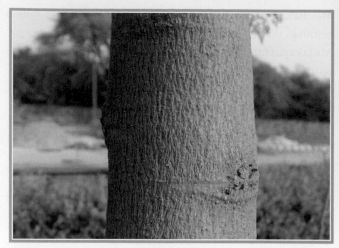

Fig. 92.5 Stem.

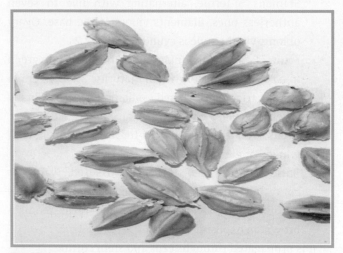

Fig. 92.4 Seeds.

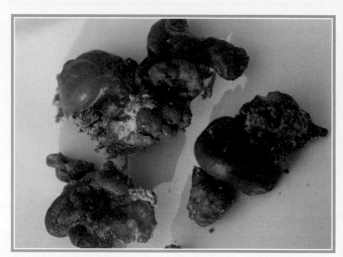

Fig. 92.6 Gum.

Key Characters for Identification

➤ *It is a fast-growing, deciduous tree, about 10 m in height.*

➤ *Bark: Thick, soft, corky, deeply fissured, young part tomentose.*

➤ *Leaves: Usually tripinnate, rachis is slender, thickened, and articulate at the base and with a gland at the articulation.*

➤ *Flowers: White, fragrant, axillary, bisexual, borne on large drooping 10 to 25 cm long panicles.*

➤ *Fruit: Pod, pendulous green, up to 45 cm long, nine-ribbed.*

➤ *Seeds: Three-angled, with the angles winged and bitter in taste.*

➤ *Beeja taila/benp oil/moringa oil: The oil is extracted from the seeds.*

Types

According to Brihatrayees, Bhaishajya Ratnavali, Kashyup Samhita, Dhanvantari Nighantu, Kaiyadeva Nighantu, Shaligrama Nighantu, Shigru is of two types:

• Madhu Shigru (Rakta Shigru)
• Shigru (Shweta Shigru)

According to Raj Nighantu, it is of three types:

• Rakta Shigru
• Shweta Shigru
• Neela Shigru

According to Bhavaprakash Nighantu, it is of three types:

• Rakta Shigru
• Krishna Shigru
• Shweta Shigru

Rasapanchaka

Guna	Laghu, Ruksha, Teekshna
Rasa	Katu, Tikta
Vipaka	Katu
Virya	Ushna

Chemical Constituents

The plant contains moringine, moringinine, pterygo-spermine (antibiotic), indole acetonitrile, bayrenol, flavonoids, polysaccharides, proteins, essential amino acids, minerals, vitamins, fatty acids, and spirochin.

Identity, Purity, and Safety

For Root Bark

- Foreign matter: Not more than 2%
- Total ash: Not more than 18%
- Acid-insoluble ash: Not more than 10%
- Alcohol-soluble extractive: Not less than 3%
- Water-soluble extractive: Not less than 11%

For Seeds

- Foreign matter: Not more than 2%
- Total ash: Not more than 5%
- Acid-insoluble ash: Not more than 0.8%
- Alcohol-soluble extractive: Not less than 12%
- Water-soluble extractive: Not less than 24%

For Stem Bark

- Foreign matter: Not more than 2%
- Total ash: Not more than 11%
- Acid-insoluble ash: Not more than 1%
- Alcohol-soluble extractive: Not less than 1%
- Water-soluble extractive: Not less than 5%

(Source: The Ayurvedic Pharmacopeia of India 2004)

Karma (Actions)

The main actions of Shigru are cakshusya (beneficial for vision), deepana (appetizer), pachana (digestive), pittakara (aggravate pitta), hridya (cardiotonic), vatakaphahara (pacify vata and kapha), medohara (antiobesity), samgrahi (fecal astringent), krimighna (anthelmintic), shotha hara (reduce swelling), swedajanaka (diaphoretic), vishaghna (antidote), sukrala (spermopoetic), shophaghna (anti-inflammatory), rochana (relish), and shoolahara (anticolic).

- Doshakarma: Kaphavatashamaka
- Dhatukarma: Sukrala
- Malakarma: Grahi, swedajanana

Pharmacological Actions

Its roots and bark are bitter, anti-inflammatory, anti-biotic, antispasmodic, digestive, carminative, anthelmintic, analgesic, diuretic, antibacterial, antifungal, rubefacient, expectorant, antihypertensive, liver, cardiac, and circulatory stimulant and antioxidant. Leaves are anti-inflammatory, antibacterial, analgesic, anthelmintic, and rich in vitamins A and C and iron. Unripe pods are anthelmintic, hematinic, and a rich source of protein. Seeds are bitter, antibiotic, anti-inflammatory, analgesic, purgative, antipyretic, and eye tonic. The gum is diuretic, astringent, and abortifacient.

Indications

It is indicated in vrana vikara (wound), granthi (cyst), gulma (abdominal lump), karnashula (earache), medoroga (obesity), vidradhi (abscess), visarpa (erysipelas), shopha (swelling), krimiroga (worm infestations), pliharoga (spleen disorders), galaganda (goiter), mukhajadya (stiffness of mouth), ashmari (urinary calculus), mutra sharkara, kushta (skin diseases), kshata, antarvidradhi (internal abscess), netraroga (eye diseases), apaci (scrofula), shiraroga (diseases of head), atinidra (over sleeping).

Roots and bark are useful in inflammation, skin diseases, abscess, wounds, ulcers, worm infestation, fever, dyspepsia, anorexia, diarrhea, colic, flatulence, paralysis, amenorrhea, dysmenorrhea, fever, ascites, eye and ear infections, cough, asthma, bronchitis, splenomegaly, arthritis, and gout. Leaves are useful in scurvy, anemia, wounds, diarrhea, tumors, inflammations, and helminthiasis. They are also used as vegetable in preparing soup, salad, and for making tea. Unripe pods are used in liver, spleen disorders, diarrhea, worm infestation, and malnutrition. Seeds are useful in neuralgia, inflammations, diabetes, high blood pressure, fever and conjunctivitis, improving eyesight, arthritis, rheumatism, gout, cramp wounds, and boils. Gum is used in asthma.

Therapeutic Uses

External Use

1. **Visarpa** (erysipelas): Warm paste of Shigru, Karanjabark, dried radish, or Bibhitaka should be applied (A.H.Ci. 18/25).
2. **Apachi** (scrofula): Sobhanjana and Devadaru are pounded together with sour gruel. This paste is applied warm in scrofula (VM. 41/22).
3. **Vidarika** (a swelling in the leg): The paste of Shigru and Devadaru controls vidarika (VM. 57/4).
4. **Vidradhi** (abscess): Fomentations and poultices should be applied with Shigru root (VM. 43.3).
5. **Netra roga** (eye diseases): Washing with juice of Shigru leaves alleviates all diseases of eye (VM. 61.40). Juice of Shigru leaves rubbed well in a copper vessel and fumigated with ghee removes swelling, irritation, watering, and pain (AH.U. 16/37, VM. 61/40).
6. **Kushta** (leprosy): In leprotic wounds, oil of Karanja, Sarsapa, Shigru, or Kasamarda should be applied (S.S.Ci. 9/53).
7. **Sannipatika Bodharnatha** (loss of consciousness): The patient should be given snuff with the juice of Sobhanjana root and Maricha combined. This restores consciousness in conditions like typhoid fever (HS. 3.2.33).
8. **Vatarakta** (gout): Application of the paste of Shigru and Varuna made with sour gruel removes pain in gout (BS. Vatarakta.68).
9. **Dadru** (ring worm): Paste of Shigru root bark eradicates ringworm (BS.Kustha.66).

Internal Use

1. **Hikka and svasha** (hic-cough and asthma): Soup of leaves of Kasamarda and Shigru and dry radish alleviate hic-cough and asthma (CS.Ci. 17/99). Soup of Shigru fruits along with Maricha, salt, and yava kshara checks hic-cough and asthma (CS.Ci. 17/98).
2. **Udara** (abdominal diseases): Soup of Sobhhanjana mixed with Pippali, rocksalt, Chitraka, and oil is useful (SS.Ci. 14/13, VM. 37-46).
3. **Sula** (colic): Pills made of rocksalt, borax, and Shunthi with Shigru juice remove colic (SB.45/14). Decoction of Shunthi and Shigru alleviates colic within 3 days. Colic is also reduced by Agastya bark added with rocksalt and Hingu (VM. 8.21). Decoction of Shigru root added with Maricha, Yavakshara, and honey removes colic caused by kapha.
4. **Shotha** (edema): Shigru is useful in erysipelas, edema, piles, and skin diseases (CS.Su. 1/117).
5. **Snayuka roga** (guinea worm): Paste of the root and leaves of Shigru pounded with sour gruel and added with salt destroys guinea worm (VM. 55/19).
6. **Asmari** (calculus): Soup made of the paste of Shigru root 40 g. Fried in ghee and oil and added with curd scum and salt should be taken after cooling in sufficient quantity (CS.Ci. 26.66.67, AH.Ci. 11/31).
7. **Apachi** (scrofula): The seed of Shigru should be taken as pressed snuff (SS.Ci. 18/23).
8. **Vidradhi** (abscess): Decoction of Shigru mixed with Hingu and rocksalt taken every morning alleviates abscess (VM. 43.3). Intake of juice of Shigru root with honey removes internal abscess (VM. 43/11). For internal abscess, decoction of Punarnava and Varuna or of Shigru added with hingu and rocksalt should be taken (SG. 2.2.128).
9. **Karnashoola** (earache): Juice of Shobhanjana mixed with honey, oil, and rocksalt removes earache (CD. 57/5). Slightly heated juice of Shobhanjana mixed with Til oil should be filled in the ear. It removes earache (VM. 59/6).
10. **Netra roga** (eye diseases): Juice of Shigru leaves mixed with honey removes many diseases of eye caused by doshas separately or jointly (A.H.U. 16/9).
11. **Arsha** (piles): The patient should be given tub bath with the decoction of the leaves of Agnimatha, Shigru, and Asmantaka. It removes pain (CS.Ci. 14/45).
12. **Sirashoola** (headache): Headache is removed by snuff of Shobhanjana mixed with jaggery (HS. 3.40.21).
13. **Krimi roga** (worm infestation): Decoction of Shigru and Vidanga mixed with honey acts as anthelmintic (BS.Krimi.22).
14. **Uragraha** (chest pain): Warm juice of Shigru mixed with Hingu is useful (BS. Urograha.5).

Officinal Parts Used

Root, fruit, seed, bark, leaves, flower

Dose

Bark decoction: 40 to 80 mL
Root powder: 3 to 6 g
Leaf juice: 10 to 20 mL
Seed powder: 1 to 3 g

Formulations

Shigru mool Kwath, Shobhanjanadi lepa, Manikya rasa, Shyamadi churna. Sudarsana churna, shothaghna Lepa, Sarsapadi Pralepa, Sarvajvarahara Lauha, Sarasvata Ghrita, Vastyamayanaka Ghrita, Karpasasthyadi Taila, Kshaara Taila, Vishatinduka Taila, Khanda Lavana, Sveta Karavira Pallavadya taila, Unmad Bhanjana Rasa, Varunadi Kwatha, Shakhotakadi Kashaya, Mustadi kwatha.

Toxicity/Adverse effects

LD_{50} of alcoholic extract of whole plant, excluding root, was 8 mg/kg i.p. in Albino mice (Sharma et al 2005).

Substitution and Adulteration

Not reported (Sharma et al 2005).

Points to Ponder

➤ *Bhavaprakash and Raj Nighantu mention three types of Shigru while other Nighantus have mentioned only two types of Shigru.*
➤ *Rakta Shigru is known as Madhu Shigru.*
➤ *Seeds of Shigru is known as Sweta Maricha or Shigruni.*
➤ *The specific action of Sweta Shigru is dahakarak while Rakta Shigru has deepan and sara properties.*
➤ *Seed of Shigru has chakshusya, vishaghna, and avrisya properties.*

Suggested Readings

Anonymous. The Wealth of India: A Dictionary of Indian Raw Materials and Industrial Products, Vol. VIII. New Delhi: National Institute of Science Communication, Council of Scientific & Industrial Research; 1988:210

Ayurvedic Pharmacopoeia of India, Part 1. New Delhi: Department of I.S.M. & H., Ministry of Health & Family Welfare, Government of India; 2004:110–115

Kirtikar KR, Basu BD. Indian Medicinal Plants, Vol. 1. Dehradun: International Book Distribution; 1999:677–678

Sharma PC, Yelne MB, Dennis TJ. Database on Medicinal Plants, Vol. 2. New Delhi: Central Council for Research in Ayurveda and Siddha; 2005:431

Trees For Life: Moringa Book; 2005. http://www.treesforlife.org/project/moringa/boo k/default.asp

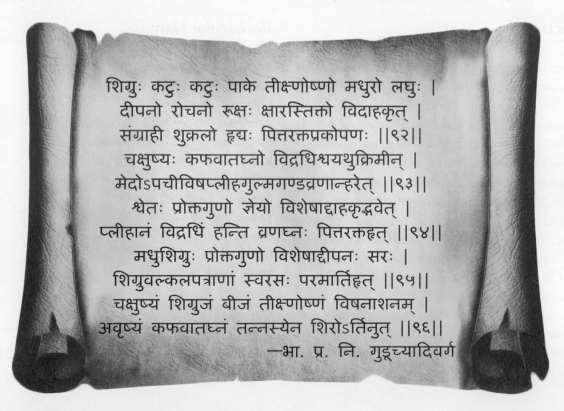

शिग्रुः कटुः कटुः पाके तीक्ष्णोष्णो मधुरो लघुः ।
दीपनो रोचनो रूक्षः क्षारस्तिक्तो विदाहकृत् ।
संग्राही शुक्लो हृद्यः पित्तरक्तप्रकोपणः ॥९२॥
चक्षुष्यः कफवातघ्नो विद्रधिश्वयथुक्रिमीन् ।
मेदोऽपचीविषप्लीहगुल्मगण्डव्रणान्हरेत् ॥९३॥
श्वेतः प्रोक्तगुणो ज्ञेयो विशेषाद्दाहकृद्भवेत् ।
प्लीहानं विद्रधिं हन्ति व्रणघ्नः पित्तरक्तहृत् ॥९४॥
मधुशिग्रुः प्रोक्तगुणो विशेषाद्दीपनः सरः ।
शिग्रुवल्कलपत्राणां स्वरसः परमार्तिहृत् ॥९५॥
चक्षुष्यं शिग्रुजं बीजं तीक्ष्णोष्णं विषनाशनम् ।
अवृष्यं कफवातघ्नं तन्नस्येन शिरोऽर्तिनुत् ॥९६॥
—भा. प्र. नि. गुड्च्यादिवर्ग

93. Shirisha *[Albizia lebbeck (Linn.) Benth]*

Family:	*Fabaceae (Mimosaceae)*
Hindi name:	*Sirish Siris, Shiris*
English name:	*Siris tree, East India Walnut, Lebbeck Tree*

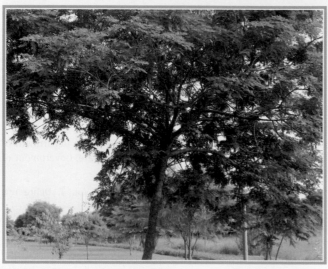

Tree of Albizia lebbeck (Linn.) Benth.

> *Patra (leaves), twak (bark), puspa (flowers), phala (fruits), and moola (roots) of Shirisha are collectively known as panchashairish or panchsarpaka. It has vishaghna properties and cures snake bite and other types of poisoning.*
>
> *—Dhanwantari Nighantu/ Mishrakadi varga/57, 59*

Introduction

Many drugs and formulations have been described as vishaghna (antipoisonous), among which one of the most important and commonly used drug is Shirisha, and it is said to be the best among all the vishaghna (antipoisonous) drugs (Jadavji 2007). In all Samhitas, various yogas (medicinal formulations) containing Shirisha as an ingredient have been mentioned for internal and external uses.

Priyavrat Sharma mentioned in Priya Nighantu that Shirisha or Shukadruma grows wild; it blooms in Vasant ritu (spring); it produces *jhan jhan* (sound produced by an anklet) sound when its fruits are mature and dry. Shirisha is considered as the best vishaghna dravya (antipoison drug; Priya Nighantu/Haritakyadi varga/114).

Shirisha has earned a remarkable reputation in traditional medicines due to its wide use in food, feed, and medicine. It has comprehensively been recommended to remove toxins from the body.

Vernacular Names

Arabic: Sultanatul ashjar
Bengali: Sirish, Siris
Gujarati: Shirish
Kannada: Bagey, Bage Mara, Hombage
Malayalam: Vaka, Nanmenivaka
Marathi: Siris
Oriya: Sersuan, Sirisha
Punjabi: Sirish, Sareehn
Tamil: Vakai
Telugu: Dirisena
Unani: Siras
Urdu: Siris

Synonyms

Bhandila: That which brings happiness in life or is considered as auspicious drug.

Kapitana: It grows wildly.

Lomashapuspaka: The flowers are pubescent.

Mrudupuspa: The flowers are tender and soft.

Shirisha: A beautiful tree to look at.

Shukabhapuspa: Flowers are liked by parrots.

Shukapriya: It is liked by parrots.

Shukapuspa: Flowers of this plant are liked by parrots.

Shukataru: The leaves resemble the color of parrot.

Supuspaka: The flowers are beautiful.

Vishahanta: It is antidote for all types of poisons.

Vishapaha: That which removes poison.

Vruntapuspa: It has round flowers.

Classical Categorization

Charaka Samhita: Vishaghna, Vedanasthapana, Shirovirechana, Kasaya skanda

Sushruta Samhita: Salasaradi

Ashtanga Hridaya: Asanadi

Dhanwantari Nighantu: Amradi varga

Madanpal Nighantu: Vatadi varga

Kaiyadev Nighantu: Aushadhi varga

Raj Nighantu: Prabhadradi varga

Bhavaprakash Nighantu: Vatadi varga

Distribution

It is found throughout India, ascending to 900 m in the Himalayas and also in the Andamans (Kirtikar and Basu 2000).

Morphology

It is a medium to large-sized deciduous tree of about 20 m in height with an umbrella-shaped crown.

- **Stem:** Gray to dark brown bark, rough, irregularly cracked (**Fig. 93.1**).
- **Leaves:** Pinnate compound, bipinnate, leaflets 8 to 18, leaflets oblong, obtuse, midrib divides the lamina in unequal portions (**Fig. 93.2**).
- **Flowers:** Fragrant, cream-colored flowers which develop on lateral stalks in rounded clusters, 5 to 7.5 cm across the many threadlike spreading whitish to yellow stamens with light green tips, borne at the ends of lateral stalks 4 to 10 cm long (**Fig. 93.3**).
- **Fruits:** Flattened pods, 10 to 20 cm long, 3 to 4 cm broad, bluntly pointed, thin, self-dehiscent; immature pods are green turning straw-colored or pale yellow on maturity, usually 6 to 8 months after flowering; smooth shiny surface; reticulate veined above the seed (**Fig. 93.4a, b**).
- **Seeds:** Small, 5 to 12, pale brown, oblong, compressed, smooth with hard testa.

It is propagated by seeds and stem cutting.

Phenology

Flowering time: March to July

Fruiting time: December to May

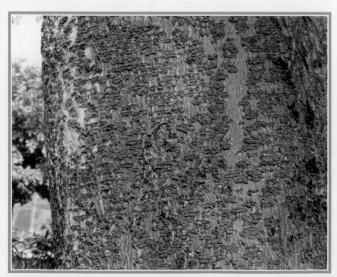

Fig. 93.1 Stem.

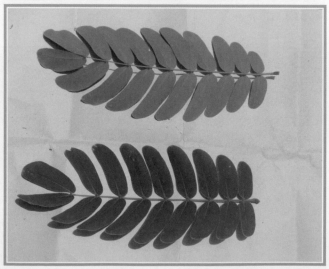

Fig. 93.2 Leaves.

Key Characters for Identification

➤ *A large, deciduous tree gray to dark brown, rough, irregularly cracked bark*

➤ *Leaves: Bipinnate; leaflets 8 to 18, subsessile, obliquely elliptic-oblong or obovate-oblong, midrib divides the lamina in unequal portions*

➤ *Flowers: Greenish-yellow in globose heads*

➤ *Pods: Strap-shaped, 10 to 20 cm long and 3 to 4 cm broad, yellowish-brown when mature*

➤ *Seeds: Six to ten, pale brown*

Types

Albizia odoratissima Benth and *Albizia lucida* Benth are few species of *Albizia*. *A. odoratissima* Benth is considered as Krishna Shirisha (black variety) and another species *Albizia procera* Benth is taken as Sweta Shirisha/Kinihi (white variety) (Sharma 2003; Chunekar 2004).

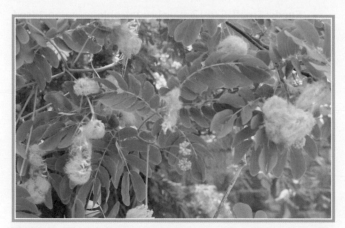

Fig. 93.3 Flowers.

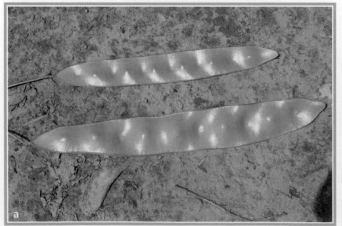

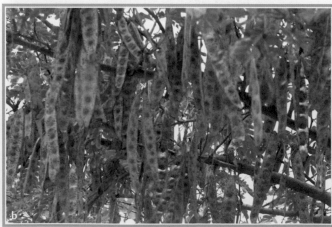

Fig. 93.4 **(a)** Fresh pods. **(b)** Mature pods.

Rasapanchaka

Guna	Laghu, Ruksha, Teekshna
Rasa	Madhura, Tikta, Kashaya
Vipaka	Katu
Virya	Sheeta

Chemical Constituents

Bark contains 7 to 11% tannins; d–catechin, d–leucocyanidin, albigenin, albegenic acid, saponins glycosides, melanoxetin, okanin, phytosterols, triterpenes, albizziagenin, and lebbekanin. Seeds are rich in proteins and amino acids whereas the flowers contain triterpenes and saponins.

Identity, Purity, and Safety

- Foreign matter: Not more than 1%
- Total ash: Not more than 8%
- Acid-insoluble ash: Not more than 1%
- Alcohol-soluble extractive: Not less than 12%
- Water-soluble extractive: Not less than 6%

(Source: The Ayurvedic Pharmacopeia of India 2001)

Karma (Actions)

The main actions are vishaghna (antipoisoning), visarpaghna (antierysipelas), shothaghna (anti-inflammatory), kandughna (antipruritus), kushtagna (antileprotic), twakdoshahara (cure skin diseases), shirovirechana, vrishya (aphrodisiac), varnya (complexion promoter), swasahara (antiasthmatic), and kasahara (anti-cough).

- Doshakarma: Tridoshashamaka
- Dhatukarma: Vrisya, raktashodhak

Pharmacological Actions

Antiprotozoal, hypoglycemic, anticancer, spermicidal, abortifacient, antiasthmatic, antiallergic, analgesic, anti-fertility, antifungal, antiovulatory, antianaphylactic, antibacterial, hypotensive, central nervous system (CNS) depressant, and bronchodilator.

Bark of this plant is anti-inflammatory, antihistaminic, antianaphylactic, antiallergic, antiasthmatic, hepato-protective, antimicrobial, anthelmintic, styptic, and blood purifier. Its root is anticancerous, antispasmodic, cardiac stimulant, and spermicidal.

Indications

It has been used in the treatment of respiratory problems like swasa (bronchial asthma) and kasa (cough) and pratisyaya (cold), in allergic skin conditions, kita dansha (stings of poisonous insects), visha (poisoning), kandu (itching), shotha (inflammations), krimi (intestinal worm), switra (leucoderma), kushta (skin diseases), boils, vicharchika (scabies), visarpa (erysipelas), tumors, dantashoola (toothache), and forstrengthening gums and teeth.

Its leaves are reported to be good for night blindness, syphilis and ulcer cold, cough, and respiratory disorders. The leaves are also used as cattle fodder, mulch, and manure due to high nitrogen content. Its root has spermicidal properties whereas flowers are aphrodisiac and are used for the treatment of spermatorrhea. Seeds are aphrodisiac, astringent, and used as brain tonic as well as for treating gonorrhea and leucoderma.

Therapeutic Uses

External Use

1. **Visphota** (eruptive boils): Shirisha, Udumbara, and Jambu are useful in sprinkling and paste (VM. 55/10).
2. **Kaphaja visarpa** (erysipelas): In erysipelas caused by kapha, flowers of Shirisha mixed with a little ghee should be applied (CS.Ci. 21.91).
3. **Netra roga** (eye disease): The juice of Shirisha mixed with honey should be used as collyrium It alleviates acute conjunctivitis (GN. 33.150).

Internal Use

1. **Hikka and svasha** (hic-cough and asthma): Juice of the flowers of Shirisha or Saptaparna should be taken with Pippali and honey. It is efficacious in predominance of kapha and pitta (CS.Ch. 17/11). Intake of the flowers of Shirisha, Kadali, and Kunda with Pippali followed by rice water alleviates all types of asthma (SS.U. 51/38, AS.Ci. 6.32).
2. **Kushta** (skin diseases): Paste of the bark of Shirisha, flowers of Karpasa, leaves of Aragvaddha and Kakamachi separately alleviate kushta (CS.Ci. 7/96, AH.Ci. 19/63).
3. **Krimi** (worm infestations): Juice of Shirisha and Kinihi mixed with honey should be taken (SU. 54/24, AH.ci. 20/26).
4. **Sthoulya** (obesity): Rubbing with the powder of Shirisha, Lammajaka, Nagakeshara, and Lodhra removes impurities of skin and excessive perspiration (VM. 36.37).
5. **Vrana** (wound): Fruits of Shirisha and Karanja and powders of inorganic substances suppress the excessive granulations in wounds (SS.Su. 37/32).
6. **Shirashoola** (headache): In suryavarta and hemicranias, pressed snuff of the seeds of Shirisha and Mulaka is efficacious (SS.U. 26.31, VM. 62.38).
7. **Mudhagarbha** (difficult labor): As postoperative measure in case of confounded fetus, water processed with Shirisha and Arjuna should be used as intake (SS. Ci. 15/24).
8. **Visha** (poisoning): Shirisha is the best drug for poisoning (CS.SU. 25.40, AH.U. 40.48). Application of the paste of Shirisha and Sinduvara counteracts poison (CS.SU. 3.28). Pancha Shirisha agada (CS.Ci. 23/218) consists of all the five parts of Shirisha. White Maricha soaked in juice of Shirisha flowers for a week acts as good remedy for snake bite and used as snuff, intake, and collyrium (CS.Ci. 23/193, VM. 68.10).
9. **Mushika visha** (rat poisoning): Paste of Shirisha and Ingudi should be taken with honey (SS.KA. 7/12). One should take heart wood, fruit, and bark of Shirisha with honey (SS.Ka. 7.20). Seed and heart wood of Shirisha should be used as snuff for head evacuation (SS.Ka. 7.37).

10. **Kita visha** (insect bite): Decoction of Shirisha mixed with Trikatu, salt, and honey should be taken. It destroys insect poisoning (S.S.KA. 5/81). In predominance of kapha, Shirisha, alone or mixed with Ankola root with rice water, should be given to induce vomiting (A.H.U. 37/76). Shirisha seeds mixed with Pippali powder are impregnated thrice with arka latex. This formulation destroys poison of insects (AH.SU. 37/43).

11. **Vishama jwara** (malarial fever): Paste of Shirisha flowers mixed with Haridra, Daruharidra, and ghee is used as snuff in quartan fever (YR.P. 98).

Officinal Parts Used

Bark, leaves, fruits, seeds

Dose

Bark powder: 3 to 6 g
Decoction: 50 to 100 mL
Seed powder: 1 to 2 g
Leaf juice: 10 to 20 mL

Formulations

Mahashirisha agada, Shirishasava, Shirishadya anjana, Dashanga lepa, Mritasanjivini agada, Pancha shirisha agada, Mahasugandi agada, Ksharagada, Amrita sarpi, Madhukadi yoga.

Toxicity/Adverse Effects

Clinical as well as experimental studies indicated the absence of any serious toxicity.

Substitution and Adulteration

Not reported.

> **Points to Ponder**
>
> - *Shirisha is considered as best vishaghna dravya (C.S.Su. 25/40).*
> - *Patra (leaves), twak (bark), puspa (flowers), phala (fruits), and moola (roots) of Shirish are collectively known as panchashairish or panchsarpaka.*

Suggested Readings

Ayurvedic Pharmacopeia of India, Part I, Vol. 3. 1st ed. New Delhi: Department of AYUSH, Ministry of Health and Family Welfare, Government of India; 2001:291

Chunekar KC. Bhavaprakash, Part I (Vaidhya R, ed.). 11th ed. Varanasi: Chaukhamba Sanskrit Sansthan; 2004:518–519

Jadavji T, ed. Charaka Samhitha, Sutrasthana, Ajjapurishiya adhyaya, 25/16. Reprint edition. Varanasi: Chaukhambha Orientalia; 2007:34

Kirtikar KR, Basu BD. Indian Medicinal Plants, Vol. 4. Allahabad: International Book Distributors; 2000:1311

Sharma PV. Dravyaguna Vigyan, Vol. II. 1st ed. Varanasi: Chaukhambha Bharati Academy; 2003:774

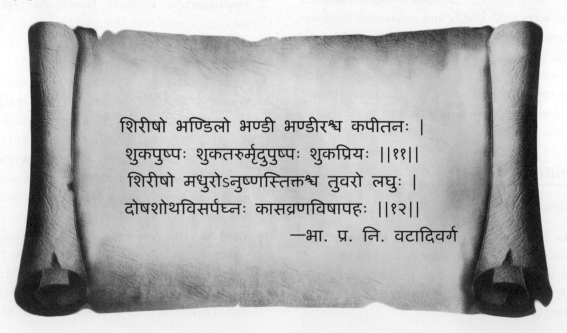

शिरीषो भण्डिलो भण्डी भण्डीरश्च कपीतनः |
शुकपुष्पः शुकतरुर्मृदुपुष्पः शुकप्रियः ||११||
शिरीषो मधुरोऽनुष्णस्तिक्तश्च तुवरो लघुः |
दोषशोथविसर्पघ्नः कासव्रणविषापहः ||१२||
—भा. प्र. नि. वटादिवर्ग

94. Shyonaka *[Oroxylum indicum (Linn.) Vent]*

Family: *Bignoniaceae*

Hindi name: *Arlu, Sonapatha, Shyonak, Tentoo, Patrorna, Putiveriksha, Shallaka, Shuran, Son, Vatuk, Urru, Sauna*

English name: *Oroxylum, Indian trumpet flower, Midnight horror, Broken bones plants*

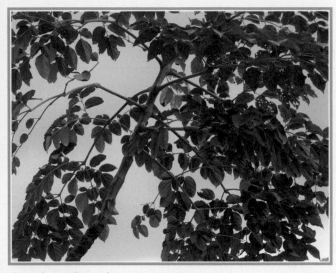

Plant of *Oroxylum indicum* (Linn.) Vent.

Oroxylon refers to the tree Oroxylum indicum (Linn.)Vent, commonly called the tree of Damocles, Indian caper, Indian trumpet flower, Indian trumpet tree. The tree is named as "Tree of Damocles" after an incident depicted in an ancient story by Cicero

Introduction

Oroxylum indicum (L.) Vent. of family Bignoniaceae commonly known as Shyonaka, Sonpatha, or Indian trumpet tree is an important medicinal tree of India and South East Asia. It is small, deciduous, soft-wooded tree up to 40 ft high, branching near top; bark is light brown, usually covered with corky lenticels. This plant is medicinally as well as economically very important and is an endangered tree native to Indian subcontinent. The tree has long fruit pods that are curved downward, hang down from the branches, and look like the wings of a large bird or dangling sickles or sword in the night.

Vernacular Names

Assamese: Kering

Bengali: Sonagachh

Chinese: Butterfly tree

Gujarati: Tentoo

Kannada: Tigudu, Ane-mungu

Konkani: Devamadak

Malayalam: Palagripayanni

Malaysia: Bonglai

Marathi: Tentoo

Nepalese: Tatelo

Oriya: Pamponiya

Punjab: Tatpaling, Talvarphali

Sanskrit: Dirghavrnta, Prthsuimba, Katvanga

Singhala: Totila, Thotila

Tamil: Peruvagai, Cari-konai, Kali-y-utaicci, Puta-pusupam, Achi, Pana, Pei-maram, Venga maram

Telugu: Dundilumu, Gumpena, Pampini, Manduka-paramu, Pampena, Sukanasamu, Nemali, Chettu

Urdu: Sonapatha (Lawania et al 2010; Harminder et al 2011).

Synonyms

Shyonak: It is a drug useful in edema.

Bhalluk: The tree is frequented by bears.

Katambhara: It is useful in vatika disorders.

Shukanasha: The flowers are red in color like beak of parrot.

Kutannata: The leaves look like they are dancing due to wind.

Shoshana: It causes dryness of the body by absorbing accumulated fluid.

Tuntuka: The flowers are bell shaped.

Mayurjangha: The ridges on the leaves are like peacock's leg.

Deerghavrunta: It has long petioles.

Nata: The hanging fruits look like dancing due to wind.

Patrorna: The plant is hairy.

Pruthushimba: The fruits are big, thick, and flat.

Classical Categorization

Charak Samhita: Shothahara, Sheetaprasamana, Anuvasanopaga, Purishasanghrahniya

Sushruta Samhita: Rodhradi, Veeratarvadi, Brihatpanchamoola

Ashtanga Hridaya: Veerataradi, Vatsakadi

Dhanwantari Nighantu: Guduchyadi varga

Madanpal Nighantu: Abhayadi varga

Kaiyadev Nighantu: Aushadi varga

Raj Nighantu: Prabhadradi varga

Bhavaprakash Nighantu: Guduchyadi varga

Distribution

It is a deciduous tree growing throughout the tropical and subtropical region of Asia. It grows at an elevation of 1,200 m mainly in ravines, in damp region, and moist places in the forest. In India, it is found in foothills of Himalaya, Eastern Ghats and Western Ghats, and Northeast India (Kirtikar and Basu 2001).

Morphology

It is a small- to medium-sized deciduous tree up to 12 m in height.

- **Bark:** Light grayish-brown, soft, spongy bark having corky lenticels (**Fig. 94.1**)
- **Leaves:** Very large, 90 to 180 cm long, 2 to 3pinnate, with five or more pairs of primary pinnae, rachis swollen, leaflets 2-pairs ovate-elliptical, acuminate, glabrous, each leaflet 6 to 13 cm by 4 to 10 cm, entire margin (**Fig. 94.2**).
- **Flower:** Inflorescence of large, erect terminal racemes, 30 to 60 cm; flower is large fleshy with unpleasant odor. Flowers are reddish-purple outside and pale pinkish-yellow inside (**Fig. 94.3**).
- **Fruits:** Flat, semiwoody sword-shaped long pod, 30 to 100 cm long and 5 to 10 cm broad tapering at

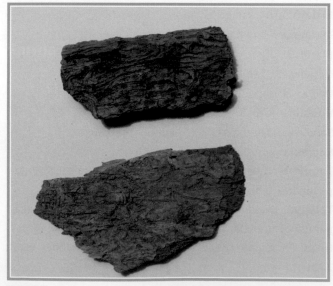

Fig. 94.1 Bark.

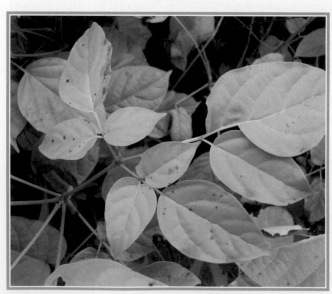

Fig. 94.2 Leaves.

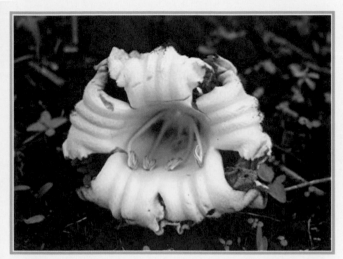

Fig. 94.3   Flower.

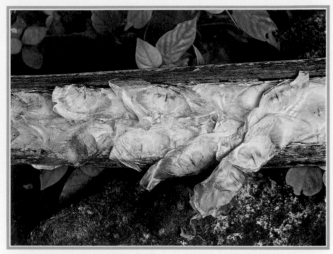

Fig. 94.5   Seeds.

- **Root bark:** Fresh bark is soft and juicy, and on drying the bark shrinks, adheres closely to the wood, and becomes faintly fissure (Dalal and Rai 2004).

It is propagated naturally by seeds.

Phenology

Flowering time: June to July

Fruiting time: November to March

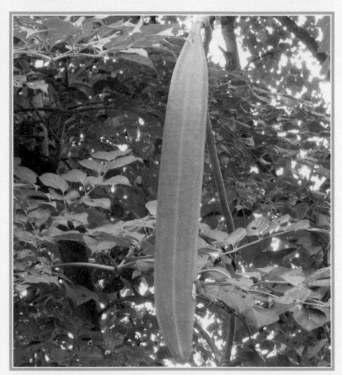

Fig. 94.4   Fruit.

both ends; it curves downward and hangs down from the branches looking like the wings of a large bird or dangling sickles or sword in the night. When the pod bursts open, the seeds flutter to the ground, often traveling some distance, looking like butterflies (**Fig. 94.4**).

- **Seeds:** Numerous, flat, 6 cm long, winged all around except at the base (**Fig. 94.5**).

> ### Key Characters for Identification
>
> ➤ *Small- to medium-sized deciduous tree up to 12 m in height.*
> ➤ *Bark: Light grayish brown, soft, spongy bark with corky lenticels.*
> ➤ *Leaves: Very large, 90 to 180 cm long, 2 to 3 pinnate, rachis swollen, ovate-elliptical, acuminate, glabrous, each leaflet 6 to 13 cm by 4 to 10cm.*
> ➤ *Flower: Inflorescence of large, erect terminal racemes, 30 to 60 cm; flower is large fleshy with unpleasant odor.*
> ➤ *Fruits: Sword-shaped long pod and when the pod bursts open the seeds flutter to the ground, often traveling some distance, looking like butterflies.*
> ➤ *Seeds: Numerous, flat, 6 cm long, winged all around except at the base.*
> ➤ *Root bark: Fresh bark is soft and juicy, and on drying the bark shrinks.*

Rasapanchaka

Guna	Laghu, Rukshya
Rasa	Kasaya, Tikta, Madhur
Vipak	Katu
Virya	Sheeta

Chemical Constituents

- Leaf: Chrysin, oroxylin-A, scutellarin, baicalein, quercetin-3-0-L-arabinopyranoside, 1-(2-hydroxy-methyl) cyclohexane-1,4-diol, apigenin
- Root bark: Chrysin, baicalein biochanin-A, ellagic acid, 2,5-dihydroxy-6, 7-dimethoxy flavone, beta sitosterol, iso-flavone, prunetin
- Stem bark: Ellagic acid, chrysin, baicalein, oxyline-A, scutellarin
- Seeds: Chrysin, baicalein, oroxylin-B
- Fruits: Oroxylin-A, chrysin, ursolic acid, and aloe emodin (Ahad et al 2012)

Identity, Purity, and Strength

- Foreign matter: Not more than 1%
- Total ash: Not more than 5%
- Acid-insoluble ash: Not more than 1%
- Alcohol-soluble extractive: Not less than 20%
- Water-soluble extractive: Not less than 42%

(Source: The Ayurvedic Pharmacopeia of India 2001)

Karma (Actions)

The drug has deepan (appetizer), hridya (cardiotonic), rochan (relish), grahi (digestive and fecal astringent), kasaghna (antitussive), vedanasthapana (analgesic), bastisothahara (reduce inflammation of bladder), stambhana (inhibitory action), sothahara (reduce swelling), vataghna (pacify vata), and kaphaghna (pacify cough) properties. The roots are sweet, astringent, and bitter.

- Doshakarma: Vatakaphahara
- Dhatukarma: Raktastambhak
- Malakarma: Stambhana

Pharmacological Actions

Other pharmacological properties are antimicrobial, antioxidant, anticancer, antimutagenic, immunostimulant, antiproliferative, nephroprotective, photocytotoxic activity, anti-inflammatory, anodyne, aphrodisiac, expectorant, appetizer, carminative, digestive, anthelmintic, constipating, diaphoretic, diuretic, antiarthric, antidiabetic (Ahad et al 2012; Joshi et al 2014).

Indications

It is used in vatatisara (diarrhea with flatus), kasa (cough), aruchi (loss of appetite), basti roga (bladder disease), amavata (rheumatoid arthritis), udara roga (abdominal disease), urustambha (stiffness of thigh), vatavyadhi (neurological disorders), karna roga (ear diseases), shotha (swelling).

Paste of stem bark of this plant is used in scabies locally and arthritis; its bark is used to cure fever, gastritis, hypertension, liver disorder, cancer, and headache. Root bark is used in fever, bronchitis, intestinal worm, vomiting, dysentery, leukoderma, asthma, inflammation, diarrhea, and rheumatism.

Therapeutic Uses

1. **Atisaar** (diarrhea): The juice of Shyonaka obtained by putaka process is used to treat diarrhea (CD. 3.84-85).
2. **Udarroga** (abdominal diseases): Oil processed with alkali of Agnimanth, Shyonaka, Palasa, Tilanala, Vata, Kadali, and Apamarga should be given to alleviate all types of udararoga (C.S.Ci. 13/170-171).
3. **Urusthamba** (stiffness of thigh): Shyonakadi yoga is used in urusthamba (C.S.Ci. 27.56-57).
4. **Karnaroga** (diseases of ear): Shyonaka taila is useful (BS. karnaroga.45).
5. **Vatavyadhi** (neuromuscular diseases): It enters into the formulation of mulaka-taila (CS.Ci. 28.173).
6. **Cyst:** Shyonaka is the main content of Himsradi yoga (SS. Ci. 18.5).
7. **Bhutapasarga** (viral infections): Pellets made of Karanja, Trikatu, roots of Shyonaka, Eranda, Bilva, and two types of Haridra are used as collyrium (SS.U. 60.44).

8. **Nasagata roga** (diseases of nose): For all diseases of nose, Satapushpa, Twak, roots of Bala, Shyonaka, Eranda, and Bilwa with Aragvadha mixed with fat, ghee, and bee wax should be used as smoke (AH.U. 20.7).

Officinal Part Used

Root bark

Dose

Powder: 3 to 6 g
Juice: 10 to 20 mL
Decoction: 50 to 100 mL

Formulations

Amritarista, Brahmarasayan, Brihatpanchamooladikwath, Dantyarista, Dashmoolarista, Dashmoolkwath, Dhanwantarghrita, Narayan taila, Shyonakputapak, Shyonaksiddhaghrita.

Toxicity/Adverse Effects

Both the ethanolic and aqueous extracts of *O. indicum* were safe up to a dose of 5 g/kg BW a day in the acute toxicity tests in the animal model (Tamboli et al 2011).

Aqueous and ethanolic extracts of *O. indicum* stem were administered orally in mice with graded doses (5 mg-3,000 mg/kg BW) and mortality was observed for a period of 72 hours. The administration of aqueous extract did not produce any acute toxic symptoms (100% survival) at doses up to 2,000 mg/kg BW. *O. indicum* is being used as medicinal herb for thousands of years without any known adverse effects. There have been a number of scientific studies conducted to evaluate the toxic effects of the plant. Almost all the studies conducted on *O. indicum* have shown that it is not toxic to humans and experimental animals even up to high doses.

Substitution and Adulteration

Root and bark of *Ailanthus excelsa* Roxb. known as Aralu is commonly used as a substitute in parts of Rajasthan and Gujarat.

> **Points to Ponder**
> - It is one of the ingredients of Brihat panchamoola and dashamoola.

Suggested Readings

Ahad A, Ganai AA, Sareer O, et al. Therapeutic potential of *Oroxylum indicum*: a review. J Pharm Res Opin 2012;2(10):163–172

Dalal NV, Rai VR. In vitro propagation of *Oroxylum indicum* Vent: a medicinally important forest tree. J For Res 2004;9:61–65

Harminder, Singh V, Chaudhary AK. A review on the taxonomy, ethnobotany, chemistry and pharmacology of *Oroxylum indicum* Vent. Indian J Pharm Sci 2011;73(5):483–490

Joshi N, Shukla A, Naiwal TK. Taxonomic and phytomedicinal properties of *Oroxylum indicum* (L.) Vent: a wonderful gift of nature. J Med Plant Res 2014;8(38):1148–1155

Kirtikar KR, Basu BD. Indian Medicinal Plants, Vol. 4. Dehradun: Oriental Enterprises; 2001

Lawania RD, Mishra A, Gupta R. *Oroxylum indicum*: a review. Pharmacol J 2010;2(9):304–310

Lucas DS. Dravyaguna-Vijnana: Study of Dravya-Materia Medica. Varanasi: Chaukhamba Visvabharati; 2013:318

Preety A, Sharma S. A review on *Oroxylum indicum* (L.) Vent: an important medicinal tree. Int J Res Biol Sci 2016;6(1):7–12

Sharma PV. Classical Uses of Medicinal Plants. 1st ed. Varanasi: Chaukhamba Vishvabharati; 2004:381

Sharma PV. Namarupajnanam. 1st ed. Varanasi: Chaukhamba Vishvabharati; 2011:187

Tamboli AM, Karpe ST, Shaikh SA, Manikrao AM, Kature DV. Hypoglycemic activity of extracts of *Oroxylum indicum* (L.) Vent roots in animal models. Pharmacology 2011;2:890–899

The Ayurvedic Pharmacopoeia of India, Part I, Vol. III. 1st ed. New Delhi: Department of Health, Ministry of Health and Family Welfare, Government of India; 2001:210

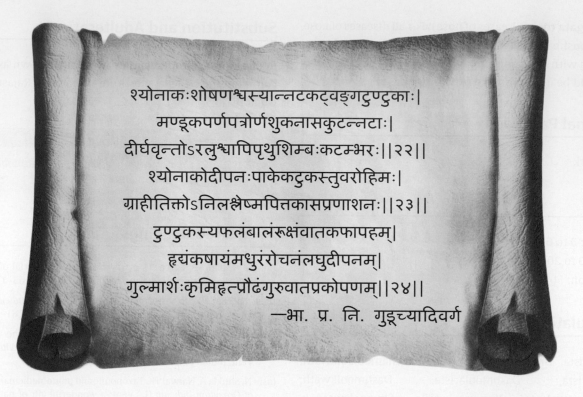

श्योनाकःशोषणश्चस्यान्नटकट्वङ्गटुण्टुकाः।
मण्डूकपर्णपत्रोर्णशुकनासकुटन्नटाः।
दीर्घवृन्तोऽरलुश्चापिपृथुशिम्बःकटम्भरः॥२२॥
श्योनाकोदीपनःपाकेकटुकस्तुवरोहिमः।
ग्राहीतिक्तोऽनिलश्लेष्मपित्तकासप्रणाशनः॥२३॥
टुण्टुकस्यफलंबालंरूक्षंवातकफापहम्।
हृद्यंकषायंमधुरंरोचनंलघुदीपनम्।
गुल्मार्शःकृमिहृत्प्रौढंगुरुवातप्रकोपणम्॥२४॥

—भा. प्र. नि. गुडूच्यादिवर्ग

95. Talisa Patra [*Abies webbiana* Lindl]

Synonym: *Abies spectabilis (D.Don) mirb*

Family: *Pinaceae*

Hindi name: *Talispatra*

English name: *East Himalaya silver fir, Indian silver fir*

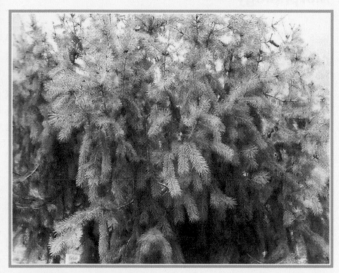
Plant of *Abies webbiana* Lindl.

C-1, i.e., 2-(o-tolylamino) ethanol is a new compound isolated from A. webbiana leaf.

Introduction

Abies webbiana Lindl of Pinaceae family commonly known as Talisa patra is a tall evergreen tree usually stunted and gnarled. It has thick, spreading, horizontal branches of about 60 m height, found in Himalayas at an altitude of 2,800 to 10,000 m. The leaves are beautifully arranged and are parrot green in color and like the leaves of Krisnamusali or are small like the leaves of Amalaki.

It is not described in any mahakashaya of Charaka Samhita but Acharya Charaka has used this plant in treating many diseases. According to Charaka, its decoction is used for kaphaja disorders; Talishadya churna is used in kasa (cough), swasa (asthma), aruchi (anorexia), pleeha vridhi (splenomegaly); kalyanaka ghritam is used in jwara (fever), kasa (cough), vatarakata (gout), pandu (anemia), etc. Sushrut has also mentioned this drug in different contexts like it is used for sirovirachan, ropana (healing) of saddya vrana (acute ulcer); its paste is used in vatarakata; anjana is used in pittabidagdha drishti and mahakalyan ghrita for gulma (abdominal lump), kasa (cough), jwara (fever), swasa (asthma), kshaya (emaciation), unmada (insanity). As per Ashtanga Hridaya, it is used for gurgling in Sarad ritu (autumn), as drinks for garbhasanga (obstructed labor), tejovatyadi ghrita for vatavyadhi (neuromuscular diseases), arsha (piles) and grahani (sprue), roga medicated ghee for shosha, paste for swelling and itching eye, oil for healing of ulcer. Chakra Dutta has used it in rajyakshma (pulmonary tuberculosis) and kasa (cough).

Vernacular Names

Assamese: Talish
Bengali: Talish Pala, Taleesh Patra
Bhutia: Dunshing
Folk: Badar, Chilrow, Morinda, Raisalla, Talispatra
Gujarati: Talish Patra
Kannada: Tales Patra, Talisapathra, Shukodara

Malayalam: Talisapatra, Taleesapatri
Marathi: Laghu Taleespatra
Nepali: Gobray salla
Oriya: Talis
Siddha: Talispatri
Tamil: Talispatra, Taleesapatri
Telugu: Taleesapatri
Unani: Talisapattar
Urdu: Zarnab

Synonyms

Talish: The leaves look like the leaves of Tali.
Ghanachhadam: The leaves are arranged densely.
Patradhya: It has many leaves.
Nilam: The trees are very tall.
Dhatripatra: The leaves are like the leaves of Amalaki.
Nilamber: The trees are tall and beautiful.
Talipatram: The leaves look like the leaves of Tali.
The other synonyms of Talisa patra are Shukodara, Talam, Arkabedha, Karipatra, Talahvayam, etc.

Classical Categorization

Charaka Samhita: Not mentioned in any gana
Sushruta Samhita: Sira virechana
Ashtanga Hridaya: Not mentioned in any gana
Dhanwantari Nighantu: Shatapuspadi varga
Madanpal Nighantu: Pippaladi varga
Kaiyadev Nighantu: Aushadi varga
Raj Nighantu: Pippalyadi varga
Bhavaprakash Nighantu: Karpuradi varga

Distribution

It is a large, tall, evergreen tree found in the Himalayan region from Kashmir to Assam in India and in the state of Sikkim (India), in particular. It is also found in Afghanistan (Hindu Kush range), Tibet (China), Nepal, in Karakoram range, and Bhutan at an altitude of 2,500 to 4,000 m (Anonymous 2004).

Morphology

It is a tall, evergreen, coniferous tree growing up to 60 m with strong horizontally spreading branches, and its young shoots are covered with short brown hair.

- **Leaves:** Simple, densely covering the twigs spreading in all direction. Leaves are flat, 1 to 5.5 cm long, about 2 mm broad; shining, midrib in the upper surface channeled down the middle but raised beneath; with two faint white lines on either side of the midrib beneath, petiole very short; color is grayish-brown; odor is terebinthinate like; taste is astringent (**Fig. 95.1**).
- **Flower:** Monoecious plant as both androecium and gynoecium are found on the same plant.
- **Cones:** Erect, scales thin, breaking away from persistent wood axis when ripe; the carpellary scale is smaller than the placental but occasionally longer and projecting between them, and bluish in color (**Fig. 95.2**).
- **Seeds:** Seeds are winged (Nadkarni et al 1976).

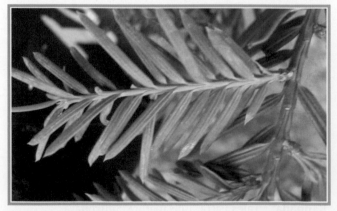
Fig. 95.1   Leaves.

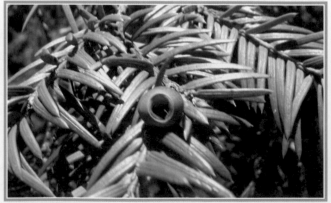
Fig. 95.2   Fruit of *Taxus baccata*.

Phenology

Flowering time: April to June
Fruiting time: August to October

Key Characters for Identification

➤ Tall evergreen tree. Height of the tree is about 60 m.
➤ Leaves: More or less distichously, needle-like, usually flattened.
➤ Cones: Bluish in color.

Types

Abies pindrow Royle is quite similar to A. webbiana. Three plants are considered in the name of Talisa patra:

- *Taxus baccata*: Also identified as Sthauneyaka.
- *A. webbiana*: It is more commonly known by the name Talisa patra.
- *Rhododendron lepidotum*.

Rasapanchaka

Guna	Laghu, Snigdha
Rasa	Tikta, Madhur
Vipak	Katu
Virya	Ushna

Chemical Constituents

- Aminoacid, flavonoids, saponins, tannins, lipids, triterpenoids, and sterol are present.
- Alkaloids are present in leaves of A. webbiana.
- Leaves: Abiesian, n-triacontanol, B-sitosterol, betuloside, bioflavonoid.
- Essential oil from leaves: Alpha-pinene, 1-limonene, deltacarene, dipentene, 1-bornyl acetate, and 1-cardinene.

Identity, Purity, and Strength

- Foreign matter: Not more than 2%
- Total ash: Not more than 6%
- Acid-insoluble ash: Not more than 0.5%
- Alcohol-soluble extractive: Not less than 14%
- Water-soluble extractive: Not less than 15%

(Source: The Ayurvedic Pharmacopeia of India 2004)

Karma (Actions)

According to Ayurveda, the drug has the properties of deepan (appetizer), pachan (digestive), hridya (cardiotonic), swarya (beneficial for voice), vatanuloman (carminative), etc. Various researchers reveal that the drug is aphrodisiac, appetizer, aromatic, astringent, blood purifier, bronchodilator, carminative, decongestant, expectorant, female antifertility, mucolytic, and respiratory tonic in nature.

- Doshakarma: Kaphavatahara
- Dhatukarma: Vajikarana, blood purifier
- Malakarma: Sangahi

Pharmacological Actions

The leaves of this plant have been traditionally used for their carminative, antispasmodic, stomachic, expectorant, antitussive, decongestant, antiseptic, astringent, antispasmodic, antihyperglycemic, female antifertility, febrifuge, and antispasmodic properties (Yadav and Ghosh 2015).

Indications

It is indicated in swasa (chronic obstructive pulmonary diseases), kasa (cough), gulma (tumor), agnimandya (anorexia), amadosha (amoebiasis), hikka (hiccup), chhardi (vomiting), krimi (helminthiasis), and mukharoga (mouth disorders; Ganguly and Kar 1999).

Decoctions of the leaves are useful in cough, phthisis, asthma, chronic bronchitis, and catarrh of the bladder, and other pulmonary infections. Furthermore, leaves of the plant have been used traditionally for its chemotherapeutic efficacies in several ailments like rheumatism, hoarseness, chronic bronchitis, and other pulmonary affections (Anonymous 1976; Kirtikar and Basu 1933; Nadkarni et al 1976; Khare 2007).

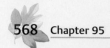

Contraindications

- It should be used cautiously in pitta prakriti people.
- It has antifertility effect.
- Avoid taking the plant in ulcers, acidity, burning sensation, and ulcerative colitis.
- Excess use can cause vomiting, unconsciousness, convulsions and many other side effects.

Therapeutic Uses

1. **Kasa and Swasa** (respiratory disorder): Powder of leaves of Talisa mixed with the juice of leaves of Vasa should be given to treat kaphapittaja kasa. It gives instant relief from asthma, giddiness, and hoarseness of voice (H.S-3/10/27). Talishadi churna and gutika are also used in respiratory diseases (C.S.Ci-8/145to148).
2. **Raktapitta** (intrinsic hemorrhage): Powder of Talisa and juice of Vasa are mixed together and given with honey to cure kaphapittaja kasa, bronchial asthma, hoarseness of voice, and intrinsic hemorrhage (V.M-9/12).
3. **Aruchi** (Anorexia): Pills prepared with powder of Talisa patra, camphor, and sugar candy improve appetite (A.H.Ci-5/49).

Officinal Part Used

Leaves

Dose

Leaf powder: 2 to 3 g

Formulations

Talishadi churna, Drakshadi churna, Talishadi vati, Jatiphaladi churna, Talisadi modak, Bhaskar lavan, Pranada gutika, Vyosadi vati, Kanakasava, Puga khanda.

Toxicity/Adverse Effects

Not reported yet.

Substitution and Adulteration

As per Bhavaprakash, Talisa patra is substituted by Swarna tallish. Talisa patra can be used as substitute in case of Bharangi: *Clerodendrum serratum* .

> **Points to Ponder**
>
> - *Talisa patra is a Himalayan plant.*
> - *Talisadi choorna is a famous medicine used in respiratory tract disorders like cough and asthma.*
> - *Talisa patra is substituted by Swarna tallish.*
> - *Talisa patra can be used as a substitute in case of Bharangi: C. serratum.*

Suggested Readings

Anonymous. The Wealth of India: Raw Materials, Vol. IA. New Delhi: Publication and Information Directorate, CSIR; 1976:16–17

Ayurvedic Pharmacopoeia of India, Part I, Vol. IV. 1st ed. New Delhi: Government of India; 2004:124–125

Ganguly HC, Kar AK. College Botany, Vol. II. Kolkata: Books and Allied (P) Ltd; 1999:1102–1103

Khare CP. Indian Medicinal Plants: An Illustrated Dictionary. Berlin: Springer; 2007:2

Kirtikar KR, Basu BD. Indian Medicinal Plants, Vol. III. 2nd ed. New Delhi: Bishen Singh Mahendra Pal Singh; 1933:2392–2393

Lucas DS. Dravyaguna-Vijnana: Study of Dravya-Materia Medica. Varanasi: Chaukhamba Visvabharati; 2013:408

Nadkarni KM, Nadkarni AK, Chopra RN. Indian Materia Medica, Vol. I. Bombay: Popular Prakashan; 1976:3–4

Sharma PV. Classical Uses of Medicinal Plants. 1st ed. Varanasi: Chaukhamba Vishvabharati; 2004:160

Yadav DK, Ghosh AK. A review of pharmacognostical, phytochemical and pharmacological effect of *Abeis webbiana* Lindl. leaves. World J Pharmaceut Res 2015;4(6):736–740

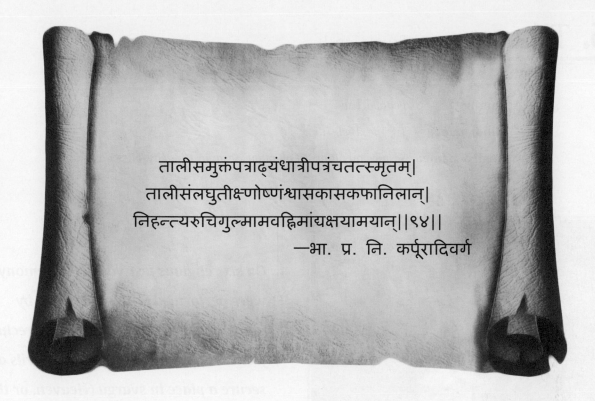

तालीसमुक्तंपत्राढ्यंधात्रीपत्रंचतत्स्मृतम्।
तालीसंलघुतीक्ष्णोष्णंश्वासकासकफानिलान्।
निहन्त्यरुचिगुल्मामवह्निमांद्यक्षयामयान्।।९४।।

—भा. प्र. नि. कर्पूरादिवर्ग

96. Tila [*Sesamum indicum* Linn.]

Family: *Pedaliaceae*

Hindi name: *Til, Tila, Teel, Tili*

English name: *Sesame oil plant, Til oil plant, Sesame, Gingelly-oil Seeds*

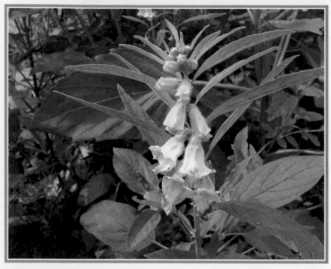

Plant of *Sesamum indicum* Linn.

On six religious festivals, Til ceremony were performed with seeds of Til by which the Hindus hope to obtain recluse from sin and poverty and other evils and secure a place in svarga (Heaven, or the abode of Indra).

Introduction

In Hindu mythology, Til (sesame) seed is symbolic of immortality. According to the Brahma-purana, Til was created by Yama, the "king of death," after prolonged penance. Dymock et al (1893) has described the six acts, namely, (1) holdvartu: bathing in water containing the sesame seeds; (2) filasfia: anointing the body with the pounded seeds; (3) homi: offering of the seeds by burning in homa tila; (4) tila-fadā: offering of the seeds to the dead; (5) tila-bhuj: eating of the seeds ; and (6) tila-vapi: throwing out the seeds.

Til is very well known in northern India. The origin of its use has been lost with time. But evidence of the plant's cultivation goes far back when it was cultivated by the Harappan people about 3,500 years BC. When the Aryans came to India, they followed the same techniques to cultivate the crops of Til (Atharvaveda.I.26.15). Then, it was used as a food in addition as oil or medicine. It is used in

Shraad, Atharvaveda (II.2.13) mentions its use for expiating certain sins, and it is only eaten during the shukla-paksha (full moon days) as a penance (Banerji 1980). Til seeds mixed with rice grain is regarded auspicious (Atharvaveda 18.4.26, 13.3.69, and 11.4.43). De Candolle (1886) was of opinion that India might have received sesame from Malayan and Indonesian regions in pre-Aryan period, possibly, by the South-Indian navigators.

Til is used in various Hindu festivals and ceremonies in different parts of India. Til preparations (mainly of black Til and its laddoos with jaggery) are made in homes and are used in Lohri in Punjab or Bhugga, or Pugga, in the plains of Uttar Pradesh and in western Uttar Pradesh, and in other parts, it is celebrated under the name of Sakat. White Til oil is eaten as an article of food and the black or other forms of seed oil are used for culinary purposes as well as in cosmeceutical and perfumery industry for extraction of perfumes, etc. The black Til seed is the only one used in the sacrificial fire or "havan" and in other religious rites and ceremonies.

In Hindus, during the funeral ceremony in honor of the dead, as a last religious rite, Til seeds are placed in three vessels containing Kusha grass (*Desmostachya bipinnata*) and water. The holy water is sprinkled with the following prayer: "O Tila, sacred to Soma, created by the Gods during the Gosava (the cow-sacrifice, not in practice now), make the dead and us happy!" (Dymock et al 1893). In shraad ceremony (death anniversary of the dead), every Hindu uses the Til seeds with rice and honey in preparing pindas (the funereal cakes) and performs pinda-daan in the last ceremony of the deceased, and on the death anniversary of close relatives and during the Shraad ceremony of mostly mother and father or nearest ones.

In South India, the festivals are the same as in Hindu religion. These are mostly used in paying tribute to dead relatives through a "havan" known as "Tilhāvanam," in which mainly Til seeds are used.

Dymock et al (1893) state that during 19th century the hawkers (street vendors) of Delhi used to sell an aphrodisiac preparation with a street-cry as under "Til, tikhur, alsi, dāna, ghī, śakkar men sāna, khāye buddhe, hoe javāna."

Meaning, Til (*Sesamum indicum*), tikhur (*Curcuma angustifolia*), and alsi, linseed (Flax, *Linum usitatissimum*), dāna or poppy seeds (*Papaver somniferum*), ghee (clarified butter), and sugar are mixed and ground and whosoever, old fellow eats, he speedily becomes young.

It is used in proverbial literature among the people as a symbolic. "Jar Tila," a useless and worthless person is compared to wild Sesame (Jar Tila), which contains no oil. "In Tilon mein tel nahin" meaning there is no good in him. "Til-bhar" means an area or a space equal to "Til-grain." "Tilbhar bhi jagah nahi" means no space left even to the size of a Til. It is said, "Til chor so bajjar chor" meaning, a thief, who can steal a grain of Til would steal a sack. "Til-Til ka hisab" meaning the exact and the final calculation. It is also stated that the word "Taila" in Sanskrit, which stands for oil, is derived from Til. It seems that Til oil is one of the first oil extracted from the seeds by the ancient Hindus. "Tilanjali" also indicates to leave or abandon a thing for ever. The moles of the human body are also called Til in Hindi and Sanskrit.

The festivals like Sattila Ekadashi are celebrated to conserve the germ-plasm (genetical material) available within the country. Further, Sankat-har Chaturthi Puja (Ganesh Chaturdashi), Makar Sankranti, Lohri or Bhugga, or Pugga festivals are the remnant signs to show the importance of Til as an important crop of the past. It is to be noted that Til was included as a cereal under "Saptadhānya," e.g., rice, wheat, barley, black gram or urad (*Phaseolus mungo*), green gram moong (*P. aureus*), Bengal gram, cānā (*Cicer arietinum*), and Til. These are still used in certain pūja and ceremonies like marriage as a "sapta dhānya" (Shah 2013).

Vernacular Names

Afghanistan: Konjele, Kunjit, Til
Africa: Juljulyn
Arabian Countries: Djyldiylan, Duban, Samusam, Simsim
Assamese: Simmasim
Bengali: Tilagachh, Tila
Chinese: Hu ma Zhi or Hei Zhi Ma or Hu-ma
Gujarati: Tall
Japan: Goma
Kannada: Accheellu, Ellu
Malayalam: Achelu, Ellu, Woellu, Yallu, Chitelu, Chitrallu, Ellu, Karellu, Scetel
Marathi: Tila
Oriya: Til
Persia: Kumjad
Punjabi: Til
Sanskrit: Tila
Tamil: Ellu, Hllu, Nuvvulu, Yellu-chedi
Telugu: Tilmi, Nuvvu, Nuvvulu, Polla-nuvullu
Urdu: Kunjad

Classical Categorization

Charaka Samhita: Purishvirajaniya, Swedopaga
Sushruta Samhita: Not mentioned in any varga
Ashtanga Hridaya: Not mentioned in any varga
Dhanwantari Nighantu: Subarnadi varga
Madanpal Nighantu: Dhanya varga
Kaiyadev Nighantu: Aushadhi varga
Raj Nighantu: Shalyadi varga
Bhavaprakash Nighantu: Karpuradi varga

Distribution

It is cultivated throughout India, particularly in Odisha, Andhra Pradesh, Madhya Pradesh, Maharashtra, Uttar Pradesh, Chhattisgarh, Gujarat, and Karnataka. It is also cultivated in other tropical countries like Pakistan and Africa.

Morphology

It is an erect, annual herb 50 to 90 cm in height.

- **Leaves:** Simple, opposite or the upper one alternate 5-10 cm by 2-5 cm. Ovate-elliptic with irregularly toothed or entire margin, acute apex. The lower one is often three-lobed (**Fig. 96.1**).
- **Flowers:** Whitish, pinkish white, axillary, and solitary 2 to 3 cm long, pubescent with a pair of glands at the base (**Fig. 96.2**).
- **Fruits:** Capsular 1 inch, velvety and pubescent, mucronate at first two-celled, afterwards four-celled (**Fig. 96.3**).
- **Seeds:** Numerous, without wings, ovoid, flat, white, brown, or black. It is propagated by seeds (**Fig. 96.4**).

Phenology

Flowering time: August to September and January to February

Fruiting time: November to December and March to April

Key Characters for Identification

➤ *Erect annual herb, 50 to 90 cm in height.*
➤ *Leaves: Simple, opposite, or the upper one alternate 5-10 cm by 2-5 cm. Ovate-elliptical, lower one often three-lobed.*
➤ *Flowers: White, pinkish-white, axillary and solitary 2 to 3 cm long.*
➤ *Fruits: Capsular 1 inch, velvety and pubescent, initially two-celled and then four-celled.*
➤ *Seeds: Numerous, ovoid, flat, white, brown, or black.*

Types

Bhavamishra has mentioned three types of Til in Dhanyavarga of Bhavaprakash Nighantu as per the color of the seed:

- Black: Superior
- White: Medium
- Red variety: Inferior

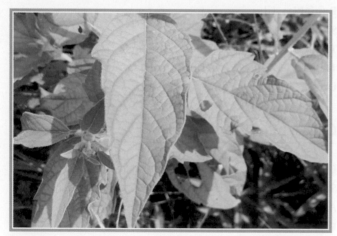

Fig. 96.1 Leaves.

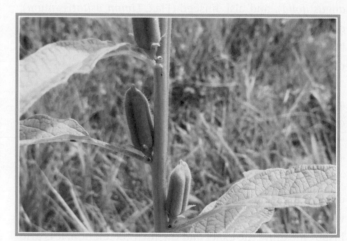

Fig. 96.3 Fruits.

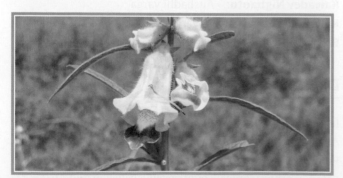

Fig. 96.2 Flower.

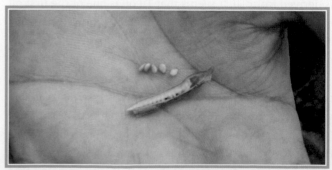

Fig. 96.4 Seeds.

Rasapanchaka

Guna	Guru, Snigdh
Rasa	Katu, Tikta, Madhura, Kasaya
Vipak	Katu
Virya	Ushna

Chemical Constituents

Sesame seeds contain many phytochemically important compounds like flavonoids, phenolic acids, alkaloids, tannins, saponins, steroids, and terpenoids, and minerals like calcium, iron, magnesium, manganese, copper, zinc, and phosphorus. Sesame has compounds like sesamin, sesaminol, gamma tocopherol, cephalin, and lecithin (Neeta et al 2015; Miraj and Kiani 2016).

Seeds: Thelignans, sesamolin, sesamin, pinoresinol, lariciresinol, phospholipids, oleic and linoleic acids, chlorophyll, and sesamol, alphaglobulin, betaglobulin, gamma-tocopherol.

Identity, Purity, and Strength

- Foreign matter: Not more than 2%
- Total ash: Not more than 9%
- Acid-insoluble ash: Not more than 1.5%
- Alcohol-soluble extractive: Not less than 20%
- Water-soluble extractive: Not less than 4%
- Fixed oil: Not less than 35%

(Source: The Ayurvedic Pharmacopeia of India 2004)

Karma (Actions)

Various properties of Tila are agnivardhaka (appetizer), balya (physical strength promoter), bhagna sandhanaka (union of fractured bone), dahanashaka (reduce burning sensation), grahi (fecal astringent), dantya (beneficial for teeth), kesya (hair tonic), medhavardhala (intellect promoter), mrudurechaka (mild laxative), rasayana (rejuvenative), snehana (oleation), sthanya (beneficial for breast milk), sukrala (semen promoter), svarka, twachya (beneficial for skin), vajikara (aphrodisiac), varnya (complexion promoter), visaghna (antidote), vrana samsodhaka (wound healer), mutral (diuretic).

- Doshakarma: Kaphapittahara, vataghna
- Dhatukarma: Vajikarana, balya
- Malakarma: Mutral

Pharmacological Actions

The pharmacological activities of Til are antioxidant, antibacterial, cardiotonic, antidiabetic, hypocholesterolemic, antitumor, antiulcer, anti-inflammatory, and analgesic (Kumar et al 2010).

Indications

It is used in boils, carbuncle, menstrual irregularities, blood dysentery, polyuria, stomach trouble, migraine, skin disease, eye trouble, alopecia, and used as tonic. Sesame oil is important in nutritional, medicinal, and industrial uses. In European countries, it is used as a substitute for olive oil (Kumar et al 2010). It is also used in many industrial products like perfumes, cosmetics, hair oils, soaps, etc.

Sesame is consumed directly as sweetmeat, a "peanut butter-like" product, a candy ingredient, bread condiments, and snack foods. Traditionally, sesame seeds were used in Hindu culture as a "symbol of immortality" and its oil was used widely in prayers and burial ceremony. It was used in traditional Middle Eastern cooking. The nutritious seed cake is used as animal feed and sesame flour (Bedigian 2014). Sesame oil is largely used in southern and Chinese cooking.

Therapeutic Uses

1. **Snehana** (for unction): Among all the oils, Til oil is considered as the best oil for promotion of strength and unction.
2. **Raktaktisara** (diarrhea with blood): Paste of black sesame mixed with 1/5th sugar and taken with goat's milk checks blood immediately (C.S.Ci. 19/34).
3. **Arsha** (piles): Intake of Til and Bhalltaka promotes digestion and destroys piles (S.S.Ci. 6/13).
4. **Vatavyadhi** (diseases of aggravated vata): Old ghee, sesame oil, and mustard oil are useful.

5. **Vranaropana** (wound healing): Paste of Til and Madhuka mixed with ghee are used for healing of wound (S.S.Su. 11/22).

Officinal Parts Used

Seed and oil

Dose

Seed powder: 3 to 6 g
Oil: 10 to 20 mL

Formulations

Laghu-visagarbha oil, Mahamasa oil, Mahanarayan oil, Til-twak, Tiladigutika, Tiladilepa, Tiladimodak, Tila saptakchurna.

Toxicity/Adverse Effects

There are possibilities of allergies to sesame oil; the limit of sensitivity should fall to 5 ppm (Morisset et al 2003).

Points to Ponder

- *Black Tila is considered as best among the three varieties of Tila mentioned by Bhavaprakash.*

Suggested Readings

Banerji SC. Flora and Fauna in Sanskrit Literature. Kolkata: Naya Prokash; 1980

Bedigian D. A new combination for the Indian progenitor of sesame, *Sesamum indicum* L. (Pedaliaceae). Novon 2014;23(1):5–13

De Candolle A. Origin of Cultivated Plants. New York, NY: Hafner Publishing Co; 1886

Dymock W, Hooper D, Warden CJH. Pharmacographica Indica of the Principal Drugs of Vegetable Origin Met with in British India. Kolkata: Thacker, Spink & Co.; 1893

Kumar A, Pal A, Khanum F, Bawa A. Nutritional, medicinal and industrial uses of Sesame (*Sesamum indicum* L.) seeds: an overview. ACS Agric Conspec Sci 2010;75(4):159–168

Lucas DS. Dravyaguna-Vijnana: Study of Dravya-Materia Medica. Varanasi: Chaukhamba Visvabharati; 2013:624

Miraj S, Kiani S. Bioactivity of *Sesamum indicum*: a review study. Der Pharmacia Lettre 2016;8(6):328–334

Morisset M, Moneret-Vautrin DA, Kanny G, et al. Thresholds of clinical reactivity to milk, egg, peanut and sesame in immunoglobulin E-dependent allergies: evaluation by double-blind or single-blind placebo-controlled oral challenges. Clin Exp Allergy 2003;33(8): 1046–1051

Patil NM, Nagpurkar M, Kulkarni B. Comparative qualitative phytochemical analysis of *Sesamum indicum* L. Int J Curr Microbiol Appl Sci 2015;Special Issue 2:172–181

Shah NC. *Sesamum indicum* (Sesame or Til): seeds & oil—an historical and scientific evaluation from Indian perspective. Indian J Hist Sci 2013;48(2):151–174

Sharma PV. Classical Uses of Medicinal Plants. 1st ed. Varanasi: Chaukhamba Vishvabharati; 2004:162

The Ayurvedic Pharmacopoeia of India, Part I, Vol. IV. 1st ed. New Delhi: Department of Health, Ministry of Health and Family Welfare, Government of India; 2004:143

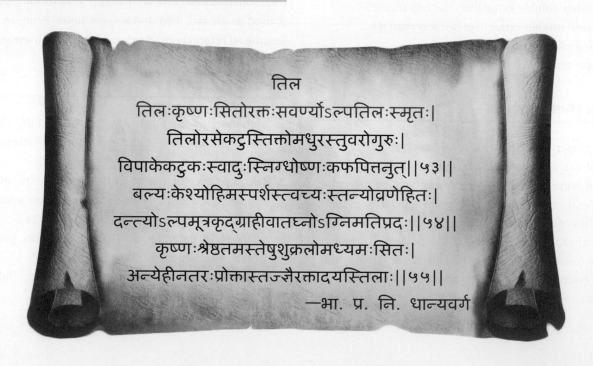

तिल

तिलःकृष्णःसितोरक्तःसवर्णोऽल्पतिलःस्मृतः।

तिलोरसेकटुस्तिक्तोमधुरस्तुवरोगुरुः।

विपाकेकटुकःस्वादुःस्निग्धोष्णःकफपित्तनुत्॥५३॥

बल्यःकेश्योहिमस्पर्शस्त्वच्यःस्तन्योव्रणेहितः।

दन्त्योऽल्पमूत्रकृद्ग्राहीवातघ्नोऽग्निमतिप्रदः॥५४॥

कृष्णःश्रेष्ठतमस्तेषुशुक्लोमध्यमःसितः।

अन्येहीनतरःप्रोक्तास्तज्ज्ञैरक्तादयस्तिलाः॥५५॥

—भा. प्र. नि. धान्यवर्ग

97. Trivrut [*Operculina turpethum* (Linn.) Silva Manso]

Family:	*Convolvulaceae*
Hindi name:	*Nishoth, Nishut, Nishothra, Pithori, Nakpatra*
English name:	*Indian jalap, Turpeth root, transparent wood rose*

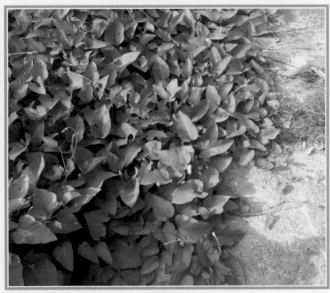

Plant of *Operculina turpethum* Linn.

> *Trivrut is a climber, its roots are reddish (raktanibha), stem is triangular (tripaksha) covered with white hairs, funnel-shaped flowers (antakotarapuspa), white leaves (sweta dala), small globose fruit (kshudra vrita phala), and it is considered as best sukha virechana dravya (purgative drug).*
>
> —Priya Nighantu/Pippalyadi varga/37

Introduction

Charaka has described Trivrut in a separate chapter (kalpa sthan, seventh chapter of Charaka Samhita), including the method of its collection, processing, contraindications, indications, dosage and therapeutic uses, and "one hundred & ten" purgative formulations of Trivrut. The deep-rooted plant grown in ideal land has smooth and straight root which is subjected for medicinal use. Only bark of root (central pith part is not useful) is used for treatment. Various seasonal recipes or purgative yogas (medicinal preparations) of Trivrut are also described by Acharya Charaka (C.S.K. 7/56-59). According to him, Trivrut is best drug for sukha virechan (smooth purgation, C.S.Su. 25/40). Root of Trivrut is best for purgation. Due to its triangular stem, it is called "Trivrut."

Trivrut, the *Operculina turpethum* (Linn.) Silva Manso (Synonyms: *Merremia turpethum* (L)/*Ipomia turpethum* (L)

R.Br/*Convolvulus turpethum* L) of Convolvulaceae family is a large perennial twiner with milky juice and fleshy roots, which are found growing wild nearly throughout the country, ascending to 900 m, and are also occasionally grown in gardens. The roots being fleshy, care is taken in drying as they decay easily; roots, therefore, are cut into pieces and exposed to sun for a day or so, after which it is finally dried in shade.

Vernacular Names

Arabic: Turband, Thurbud
Bengali: Teudi, Tvuri, Dhdhakalami
Chinese: he guo teng
French: Turbith vegetal
German: Turpeth trichterwinde
Gujarati: Kala nasottara
Kannada: Vili Tigade

Malayalam: Trikolpokanna
Marathi: Nisottar
Oriya: Dudholomo
Punjabi: Nisoth
Tamil: Karum Sivadai
Telugu: Tella, Tegada
Urdu: Turbud, Nishoth

Synonyms

Katurana: It shows character of Convolvulaceae.
Kotaravahini: The flowers are funnel shaped.
Nishotha: It is useful in edema.
Nishottra: It relieves the sotha by the action of purgation.
Rechana/Suvaha: With purgative action.
Sarala: The plant has the properties of relieving constipation.
Sarana: It removes constipation by purgative action.
Sarvanubhuti: It is a reputed purgative drug, safe, and effective.
Sweta: The stem is whitish in color.
Trivrut/Trivandi/Triputa: Triangular-shaped stem because of longitudinal furrows.

Classical Categorization

Charaka Samhita: Bhedaniya, Asthapanopaga
Sushruta Samhita: Adhobhagahara, Shyamadi
Ashtanga Hridaya: Shyamadi
Dhanwantari Nighantu: Guduchyadi varga
Madanpal Nighantu: Abhayadi varga

Kaiyadev Nighantu: Aushadi varga
Raj Nighantu: Pippaladi varga
Bhavaprakash Nighantu: Guduchyadi varga

Distribution

This plant is native to Asia (India, Pakistan, Bangladesh, China, Sri Lanka, Myanmar, etc.), Africa, and Australia. It is reported that the plant is found in warmer parts of India up to 900 m.

Morphology

It is a stout perennial climber up to 10 m long with milky exudate.

- **Root:** Fleshy, long, slender (**Fig. 97.1**).
- **Stem:** Long, twisted, pubescent, angled, and winged, which become very tough and brown in old age.
- **Leaves:** Simple, pubescent on both sides, variable in shape, entire margin, subacute or apiculate apex, cordate or truncate at bas e, 5 to 15 cm long × 2 to 7 cm wide (**Fig. 97.2**).
- **Flowers:** White, campanulate, long sepals, borne in cyme of few flowers. Five calyx-lobed funnel-shaped corolla, 5 to 7 cm long and 5 to 6 cm across, white, vivacious purple at the base of the tube within five stamens with long filament (**Fig. 97.2**).
- **Fruits:** Globose capsule 1.5 to 2 cm diameter enclosed by persistent brittle sepals. Contain, normally, four black seeds.

It is propagated by seeds and vegetative method.

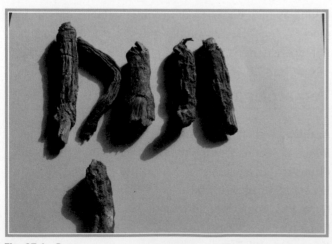

Fig. 97.1 Root.

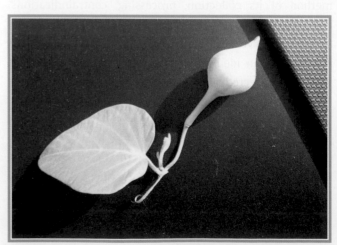

Fig. 97.2 Leaves and flower.

Phenology

Flowering time: October to February
Fruiting time: October to February

Key Characters for Identification

➤ *It is a climber of three-winged, triangular stem with funnel-shaped flower.*
➤ *Root: Fleshy, long, slender.*
➤ *Stem: long, twisted, pubescent, angled, and winged.*
➤ *Leaves: Simple, pubescent on both sides, variable in shape, entire margin, subacute or apiculate apex, cordate or truncate at base.*
➤ *Flower: White, borne in cyme of few flowers. Five calyx-lobed funnel-shaped corolla, 5 to 7 cm long and 5 to 6 cm across, five stamens with long filament.*
➤ *Fruit: Globose capsule enclosed by persistent brittle sepals. It bears four black seeds.*

Types

Trivrut is of two types: (1) Aruna (reddish color root)/Sweta (white root) and (2) Shyam (blackish root) as per the color of the root of the plant (C.S.K/7/7-8). *O. turpethum* is accepted as the botanical source of Aruna variety while that of Shyama is *Ipomoea petaloidea* chois (Srikantha Murty 2008). Aruna or Shweta Trivrut is the best drug used for virechana (therapeutic purgation). It is used in weak person, children, old person for easy purgation (Tripathi 2008). Shyama Trivrut can treat the conditions like intoxication and abdominal tumors due to its drastic purgative action (Nadkarni and Nadkarni 2007). However, Shyama is considered as inferior and can cause fainting, burning sensation, giddiness, confusion, chest pain, and roughness of throat, and hence, it is rarely used in medicine (Srikantha Murty 2008).

Shyama Trivrut

Synonyms

Ardhachandra, Palindi, Sushenika, Masoorvidala, Kali, Kaishika, Kalameshika.

Properties

Less effective (heena guna) in comparison to Aruna variety. It has drastic purgative action (tikshna virechana). It causes murchha (fainting), daha (burning sensation), mada (slight intoxication), bhranti (vertigo/dizziness), and kantha utkarshana (roughness of throat) (B.P.Nighantu Guduchyadi-196).

Rasapanchaka

Guna	Ruksha, Laghu, Tikshna
Rasa	Katu, Tikta
Vipaka	Katu
Virya	Ushna

Chemical Constituents

Root bark is rich in turpeth resin consisting of 10% turpethin.

Other constituents are turpethinic acids-A, B, C, D, and E, scopoletin, botulin, lupiol, Beta-Sitosterol, A and B turpethin, volatile oil, starch, lignen salts, ferric oxide, resin, glycosides, saponin, flavonoids.

Identity, Purity, and Strength

- Foreign matter: Nil
- Total ash: Not more than 10 %
- Acid-insoluble ash: Not more than 1.5 %
- Alcohol-soluble extractive: Not less than 10 %
- Water-soluble extractive: Not less than 8 %

(Source: The Ayurvedic Pharmacopeia of India 2001)

Karma (Actions)

The drug has the properties of jwaraghna (antipyretics), kapha-pittahara (eliminate pita and kaphadosha), vatakarak (aggravate vata dosha), rechan (purgative), sukhavirechanaka (mild purgative), lekhan (scarping), etc.

- Doshakarma: Kaphapittashodhan, vatakarak
- Dhatukarma: Lekhan
- Malakarma: Rechana, Sukhavirecanaka

Pharmacological Actions

The pharmacological actions seen in this drug are anticancer, antidiabetic, anti-inflammatory, antimicrobial, antioxidant, antipyretic, antisecretary, hepatoprotective, ulcer-protective, antibacterial, anti-inflammatory, cathartic, anthelmintic, cardiac depressant and spasmodic to smooth and skeletal muscles, etc. (Bhande et al 2006; Suresh Kumar et al 2006; Prakash et al 2010; Anbuselvam et al 2007).

Indications

Root of Trivrut is used to treat pittajwara (fever caused by pitta), jwara (fever), anorexia, shotha (edema), pandu (anemia), jalodara (ascites), vibandha (constipation), yakrit pleeha vriddhi (hepato-splenomegaly), kamla (hepatitis), udara (abdominal tumors), vrana (wound), krimi (worm infestation), and various skin diseases. It is also used in arsha (piles), sthoulya (obesity), kasa (cough), swasa (asthma), flatulence, vatarakta (gout), amavata (rheumatism), etc.

Contraindications

Trivrut should not be used in pregnancy, in children below 12 years of age, in elderly, physically or mentally weaker persons, and for diarrhea, bleeding per rectum, rectal prolapse, or fecal incontinence. It may act as an abortifacient when used in pregnant ladies. Use in children or in physically or mentally weaker person or overdose of Trivrut may lead to complications like excessive purgative activity, bleeding per rectum, vomiting, abdominal pain, chest pain, dehydration, hypotension, vertigo, confusion, shock, and unconsciousness.

Therapeutic Uses

1. **Fever:** Trivrut with sugar is used in kapha pittaja jwara (fever caused by kapha and pitta) (C.S.Ci. 3/209)
2. **Malaria fever** (vishamjwara): Trivrut is given with honey to get relief from vishamjwara (malaria fever) (V.M.-1/246).
3. **Udavarta and anaha** (reverse peristalsis and constipation): 2 parts Trivrut, 4 parts Pippali, and 5 parts of Haritaki are taken and mixed with jaggery to make pills. This pill is used internally to get relief from constipation and the diseases caused thereby (V.M. 28/6).

4. **Piles:** Trivrut powder is given with Triphala decoction to treat piles by eliminating the impurities through anal orifice (C.S.Ci. 14/66).
5. **Udara roga** (abdominal disorders): Paste of Trivrut should be given with milk (C.S.Ci. 13/69).
6. **Erysipelas** (visarpa): Trivrut is mixed with ghee/milk/hot water/grape juice and given for purgation to alleviate erysipelas (C.S.Ci. 21/64,65).
7. **Vatarakta** (gout): Decoction of Trivrut, Vidari, and Iksuraka destroys vatarakta (BP.Ci. 29.40).
8. **Abscess**: Powder of Trivrut and Haritaki should be taken with ample quantity of honey (SS.Ci. 16.12).
9. **Eye diseases**: Cooked ghee with Trivrut decoction thrice should be given in corneal ulcer (AH.U. 11.30).
10. **Purification of breast-milk:** Trivrut is given with Triphala decoction (CS.Ci. 30.254).
11. **Poison**: Trivrut mixed with equal quantity of tanduliyaka with ghee (AH.U. 37.25).

Officinal Part Used

Root bark

Dose

Powder: 1 to 3 g

Formulations

Abhayadi Modak, Asvagandharista, Avipattikara Churna, ChandraprabhaVati, Haridra Khanda, Hrdyavirecana Leha, Kaisore Guggul, Kalyanak Gud, Mahamanjistadi Kwatha, Manibhadra Guda, Panchasama Churna, Punarnavadi Mandoor, Trivrit Arista, Trivritadi Modak, Trivrutadi Churna, Trivrutadi Ghrita, Trivrutadi Gutika, Trivrutadi Kwatha, Vyosadi Gutika.

Toxicity/Adverse Effects

The effect of the ethanol extract of *O. turpethum* on normal liver functions: it was found to be nontoxic at the dose of 200 mg/kg in rats since the parameters serum glutamic-oxaloacetic transaminase (SGOT), serum glutamic pyruvic transaminase (SGPT), alkaline phosphatase (ALP), and total bilirubin (TBL) were within the normal limits (Kumar et al 2006).

Substitution and Adulteration

Root of *Marsdenia tenacissima* W.A. is sold in the market in the name of safed nishoth (white turpeth). Root of *Argyreia speciosa* sweet is available in the name of nishoth. Stem pieces of *O. turpethum* are also reported to be sold as black nishoth in place of root (Sharma et al 2000).

Points to Ponder

- *Trivrut is best drug for sukha virechan (smooth purgation) (C.S.Su. 25/40).*
- *Charaka has mentioned 110 virechana yoga of Trivrut (C.S.K. 7).*
- *Aruna and Shyama Trivrut are two varieties of Trivrut as per the color of the root.*

Suggested Readings

Anbuselvam C, Vijayavel K, Balasubramanian MP. Protective effect of *Operculina turpethum* against 7,12-dimethyl benz(a)anthracene induced oxidative stress with reference to breast cancer in experimental rats. Chem Biol Interact 2007;168(3):229–236

Bhande RM, Kumar LP, Mahurkar NK, Ramachandra S. Pharmacological screening of root of *Operculina turpethum* and its formulations. Acta Pharmaceut Sci 2006;48:11–17

Harun-or-Rashid M, Gafur MA, Sadik GM, Rahman AA. Antibacterial and cytotoxic activities of extracts and isolated compounds of *Ipomoea turpethum*. Pak J Biol Sci 2002;5(5):597–599

Krishnarajua AV, Raoa TVN, Sundararajua D, Vanisreeb M, Tsayb H, Subbarajua GV. Assessment of bioactivity of indian medicinal plants using brine shrimp (*Artemia salina*) lethality assay. Int J Appl Sci Eng 2005;3(2):12534

Lucas DS. Dravyaguna-Vijnana: Study of Dravya-Materia Medica. Varanasi: Chaukhamba Visvabharati; 2013:290

Nadkarni KM, Nadkarni AK, eds. Indian Materia Medica, Vol. I. Mumbai: Bombay Popular; 2007:691–694

Prakash VB, Mukherjee A. Hepato-protective effect of an Ayurvedic formulation Prak-20 in CCl4 induced toxicity in rats: results of three studies. Int J Pharmaceut Clin Res 2010;2(1):23–27

Sharma PC, Yelne MB, Denni TJ. Database on Medicinal Plants Used in Ayurveda, Vol. 1. New Delhi: Central Council for Research in Ayurveda and Siddha, Department of I.S.M. & H., Ministry of Health & Family Welfare, Government of India; 2000:216–224

Sharma PV. Classical Uses of Medicinal Plants. 1st ed. Varanasi: Chaukhamba Vishvabharati; 2004:179

Sharma PV. Namarupajnanam. 1st ed. Varanasi: Chaukhamba Vishvabharati; 2011:95

Srikantha Murty KR, ed. Bhavaprakasha of Bhavmishra, Vol. I. Varanasi: Chaukhamba Shrikrishna Das; 2008:258–259

Suresh Kumar SV, Sujatha C, Shymala J, Nagasudha B, Mishra SH. Protective effect of root extract of *Operculina turpethum* Linn. against paracetamol induced hepatotoxicity in rats. Indian J Pharm Sci 2006;68(1):32–35

The Ayurvedic Pharmacopoeia of India, Part I, Vol. III. 1st ed. New Delhi: Department of Health, Ministry of Health and Family Welfare, Government of India; 2001:215

Tripathi B, ed. Charaka Samhita of Agnivesha, elaborated by Charaka & Drudhabala, Vol. I. Varanasi: Chaukhamba Surbharti; 2008: 454–455

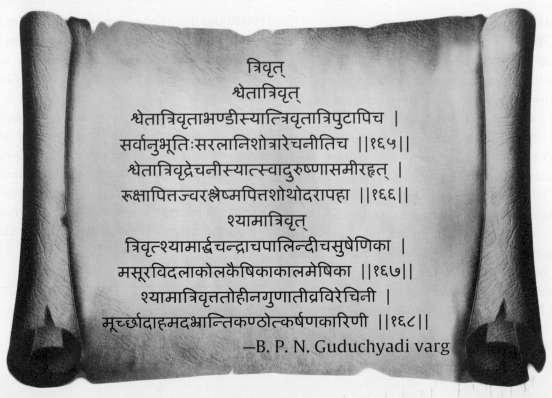

त्रिवृत्
श्वेतात्रिवृत्
श्वेतात्रिवृताभण्डीस्यात्रिवृतात्रिपुटापिच |
सर्वानुभूतिःसरलानिशोत्रारेचनीतिच ||१६५||
श्वेतात्रिवृद्रेचनीस्यात्स्वादुरुष्णासमीरहत् |
रूक्षापित्तज्वरश्लेष्मपित्तशोथोदरापहा ||१६६||
श्यामात्रिवृत्
त्रिवृत्श्यामार्द्धचन्द्राचपालिन्दीचसुषेणिका |
मसूरविदलाकोलकैषिकाकालमेषिका ||१६७||
श्यामात्रिवृत्तोहीनगुणातीव्रविरेचिनी |
मूर्च्छादाहमदभ्रान्तिकण्ठोत्कर्षणकारिणी ||१६८||
—B. P. N. Guduchyadi varg

98. Tulasi *[Ocimum sanctum Linn.]*

Family:	*Lamiaceae*
Hindi name:	*Tulsi*
English name:	*Holy Basil, Sacred Basil*

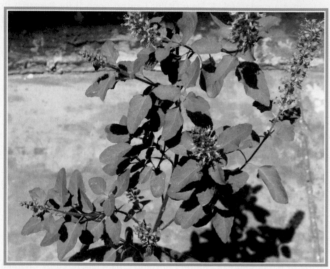

Herb of *Ocimum sanctum* Linn.

> *Tulsi is known as "The Incomparable One," "Mother Medicine of Nature," and "The Queen of Herbs," and is revered as an "elixir of life" that promotes longevity.*
>
> *—Singh et al (2010) and Gupta et al (2002)*

Introduction

Holy basil has a rich and fanciful history known since the Vedic age for its immense curative and multipurpose utility. It has been the "Herb royale" to the French, a sign of love by Italians, and a sacred herb in India.

It is one such medicinal plant having numerous medicinal properties. *O. sanctum* L. (synonym: *O. tenuiflorum* L., Mint Family: Lamiaceae), commonly known as "Holy Basil" in English and "Tulasi" in Hindi and Sanskrit, is a bushy plant with a unique fragrance found in the semitropical and tropical regions of the world. In ancient Hindu scriptures, Tulasi occupies the supreme position among the herbs, so that it is referred to as "Mother." The ancient works of Padma Purana and Tulasi Kavacham describe Tulasi as a protector of life, accompanying human beings from birth to death.

Every part of the Tulasi plant is revered and considered sacred. Even the soil around the plant is holy. The Padma Purana says that a person who is cremated with Tulasi twigs in his funeral pyre gains moksha and a place in Vishnu's abode Vaikuntha. If a Tulasi stick is used to burn a lamp for Vishnu, it is like offering the God lakhs of lamps. If one makes a paste of Tulasi leaves and smears it over his body and worships Vishnu, it is worth several ordinary pujas and lakhs of Godaan (donation of cows). Water mixed with the Tulasi leaves is given to the dying to raise their departing souls to heaven. The presence of Tulasi plant symbolizes the religious bent of a Hindu family. A Hindu household is considered incomplete if it does not have a Tulasi plant in the courtyard (Sen 1993; Khanna and Bhatia 2003).

Vernacular Names

Assamese: Tulasi
Bengali: Tulasi
Gujarati: Tulasi, Tulsi
Kannada: Tulasi, Shree Tulasi, Vishnu Tulasi

Malayalam: Tulasi, Tulasa
Marathi: Tulas
Oriya: Tulasi, Tulsi
Punjabi: Tulasi
Tamil: Tulasi, Thulasi, Thiru Theezai
Telugu: Tulasi
Urdu: Raihan, Tulsi

Synonyms

Apetarakshasi: It repels evil organism.
Bahumanjari: It has numerous spikes in its flower.
Chakrapuspi: Flowers are set densely in a circle.
Devadundubhi: It flower looks like a trumpet.
Gramya: It is a common plant found in every village.
Kayastha: It maintains body by alleviating many disorders.
Putapatri: The leaves of this plant are regarded as sacred.
Shulaghni: It removes colic pain.
Sulabha: It is easily available.
Surabhi: This plant is aromatic. All the parts of this plant have fragrance.
Surasa: Its juice is used to cure many diseases.
Swadugandhichhada: It has sweet aroma.
Tulasi: The leaves of this plant are regarded as sacred.

Classical Categorization

Charaka Samhita: Shwashara
Sushruta Samhita: Surasadi
Ashtanga Hridaya: Surasadi

Dhanwantari Nighantu: Karaveeradi varga
Madanpal Nighantu: Karpooradi varga
Kaiyadev Nighantu: Aushadhi varga
Raj Nighantu: Karaveeradi varga
Bhavaprakash Nighantu: Puspa varga

Distribution

The plant grows all over India up to 2,000 m altitude. It is grown in houses, temples, and gardens. *Ocimum sanctum* is native to India, Iran, and now cultivated in Egypt, France, Hungary, Italy, Morocco, United States. Basil is naturally found wild in the tropical and subtropical regions of the world. Basil thrives in warm and temperate climates (Mandal et al 1993).

Morphology

An erect, aromatic, much branched, soft pubescent, annual herb, 30 to 70 cm high with red or purple subquadrangular hairy branches.

- **Leaves:** Simple, opposite arrangement, 2 to 4 cm long, elliptic-oblong shape, acute or obtuse apex, entire or serrated margin, pubescent on both sides, minutely gland-dotted, petiole slender, hairy and aromatic (**Fig. 98.1a, b**).
- **Flowers:** Tiny, purplish, or crimson in elongate racemes in close whorls. Inflorescence is a long spike or 12 to 14 cm in length (**Fig. 98.2a, b**).

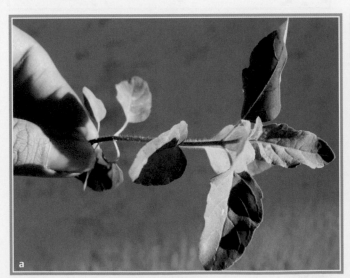
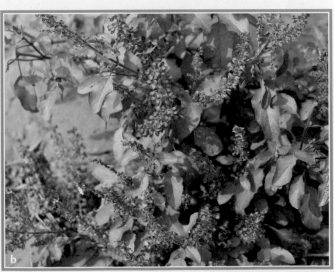

Fig. 98.1 **(a)** Leaves of Rama tulsi. **(b)** Leaves of Shyam or Krishna tulsi.

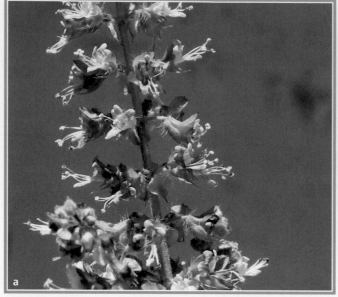

Fig. 98.2 **(a)** Flower of Rama tulsi. **(b)** Flower of Shyam tulsi.

- **Fruit:** Small, smooth nut lets, subglobose or broadly ellipsoid, slightly compressed, pale brown or reddish grey with small black seed (**Fig. 98.3**).

It is propagated through seeds.

Phenology

Flowering time: More or less throughout the year
Fruiting time: More or less throughout the year

Key Characters for Identification

➤ *It is an erect, much branched sub-shrub 30 to 60 cm tall.*
➤ *Leaves: Simple, opposite, green or purple leaves that are strongly scented, usually somewhat toothed, petiole up to 5 cm long.*
➤ *Flowers: Purplish in elongate racemes in close whorls.*
➤ *Fruit: Subglobose or broadly ellipsoid, slightly compressed, pale brown or reddish.*

Types

Three varieties of Tulasi are:
- Rama or Light Tulasi (*O. sanctum*): Tulasi plants with green and slightly sweet leaves. Rama Tulasi is regularly used for worshiping and is more common of the three types.

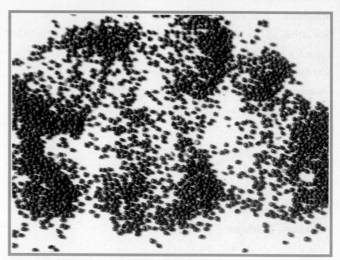

Fig. 98.3 Fruit.

- Shyama/Krishna or Dark Tulsi (*O. sanctum*): Tulasi plants with purple leaves.
- Vana Tulasi (*Ocimum gratissimum*): It is a rare and wild plant.

Rasapanchaka

Guna	Laghu, Ruksha
Rasa	Katu, Tikta
Vipaka	Katu
Virya	Ushna

Chemical Constituents

The plant is rich in essential oil, methyl chavicol, eugenol cineole, mucilage, camphene, methyl ether, β-sitosterol, limonene, β-caryophyllene, carvacrol, and many amino acids.

Some of the most important bioactive phytochemical constituents in plants are alkaloids, flavonoids, phenolics, essential oils, tannins, and saponins (Krishnaiah et al 2009; Pattanayak et al 2010).

Identity, Purity, and Safety

For Leaves

- Foreign matter: Not more than 2%
- Total ash: Not more than 19%
- Acid-insoluble ash: Not more than 3%
- Alcohol-soluble extractive: Not less than 6%
- Water-soluble extractive: Not less than 13%

For Whole Plant

- Foreign matter: Not more than 2%
- Total ash: Not more than 10%
- Acid-insoluble ash: Not more than 1.5%
- Alcohol-soluble extractive: Not less than 4%
- Water-soluble extractive: Not less than 8%

(Source: The Ayurvedic Pharmacopeia of India 1999)

Karma (Actions)

Deepana (appetizer), hridya (cardiotonic), ruchya (relish), kaphavatahara (pacify vata and kapha), pittavardhak (aggravate pitta), durgandhihara (remove foul smell).
- Doshakarma: Kaphavatashamaka, Pittavardhak
- Dhatukarma: Shukrala (seed), raktashodhak
- Malakarma: Mutral (seed), anulomana, swedajanana

Pharmacological Actions

Tulasi has a unique combination of actions that include antimicrobial (including antibacterial, antiviral, antifungal, antiprotozoal, antimalarial, anthelmintic), mosquito repellent, antidiarrheal, antioxidant, anticataract, anti-inflammatory, chemopreventive, radioprotective, hepatoprotective, neuroprotective, cardioprotective, antidiabetic, anti-hypercholesterolemia, antihypertensive, anticarcinogenic, analgesic, antipyretic, antiallergic, immunomodulatory, central nervous system depressant, memory enhancement, antiasthmatic, antitussive, diaphoretic, antithyroid, antifertility, antiulcer, antiemetic, antispasmodic, antiarthritic, adaptogenic, antistress, anticataract, antileukodermal, and anticoagulant activities (Mahajan et al 2013; Mohan et al 2011; Pattanayak et al 2010; Mondal et al 2009).

Indications

It is indicated in ashmari (calculus), shvasa (asthma), chhardi (vomiting), hikka (hic-cough), kasa (cough), krimiroga (worm infestation), kushta (skin diseases), netraroga (eye diseases), parsva shoola (pain in lateral parts).

Different parts of plant have been used in Ayurveda to cure various diseases including common cold, cough, headache, flu, asthma, fever, colic pain, sore throat, bronchitis, hepatic diseases, malaria fever, as an antidote for snake bite, flatulence headaches, fatigue, skin diseases, wound, insomnia, arthritis, influenza, digestive disorders, night blindness, diarrhea. Tulasi acts as an adaptogen that helps the body and mind to encounter different physical, chemical, emotional, and infectious stresses, and restore physiological and psychological functions.

Seeds are mucilaginous and demulcent and are given in disorders of genitourinary system like burning micturition, dysuria, urinary tract infections, etc. Infusion of leaves is used as a stomachic in gastric and hepatic disorders of children. The bruised fresh roots, stems, leaves are applied to bites of mosquitoes. Decoction of root is given as a diaphoretic in malarial fevers. The oil extracted from its leaves is reported to possess antibacterial and insecticidal properties and is effective as mosquitoes repellent.

Therapeutic Uses

External Use

1. **Vrana** (wound): Sprinkling of juice of Surasadi gana drugs or paste of Lasuna (garlic) removes maggots from wound (V.M. 44/44).

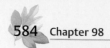

2. **Karnashoola** (earache): Oil cooked with Surasadi gana dravyas should be filled in the ear. It reduces the earache or pain (S.S.U. 21/32).

3. **Netrasotha** (conjunctivitis): Juice of Tulasi mixed with honey is used as collyrium in conjunctivitis (G.N. 3.3.150).

4. **Kushta** (skin disease): Nimbadi pralepa in which Tulasi is one of the ingredients is used locally (G.N. 2.36.141).

5. **Palitya** (graying of hair): Sahacharadi taila is used externally in which Tulasi is one of the ingredients (AH.U. 24/37-38).

6. **Kandu** (urticaria): External application of juice of Tulasi is an excellent remedy for urticaria ((YR.P. 348).

Internal Use

1. **Kasa** (cough): The juice of black Tulasi is taken with honey to cure kaphaja kasa (cough caused by kapha) (C.S.Ci. 18/117).

2. **Pediatric disorders** (fever, cough, etc.): Lavanga, Tulasi leaves, and Tankan are pounded together and given to the child. It alleviates fever, cough, asthma, and abdominal disorders (S.B. 4/1138).

3. **Krimi** (worm infestation): The drugs of surasasdi gana should be taken separately with honey in krimi roga (AH. Ci. 20/27, S.S.Su. 38/18-19).

4. **Vishamajwara** (intermittent fever): Juice of Tulasi or Dronapuspi mixed with Maricha powder should be taken to control intermittent fever (S.G. 2/1/10).

5. **Shirogata visha** (poison located in head): Nasya (snuff) of Bandhuka, Bharangi, and black Tulasi is given in shirogata visha (C.S.Ci. 23/181).

6. **Makkalla** (postpartum pain): Juice of leaves of black Tulasi mixed with honey is given with wine to remove postpartum pain.

7. **Common cold**: Tea prepared by adding four to five leaves of Tulasi, black pepper, and ginger is taken twice daily to relieve the symptoms of common cold, rhinitis, cough, and respiratory infections. Chewing Tulasi leaves daily gives relief in cold, flu, and fever.

8. **Immunity enhancer:** Chewing of 10 to 12 Tulasi leaves daily increases body immunity and the ability to fight against excess emotional or environmental stress.

Officinal Parts Used

Leaves, seed, whole plant

Dose

Juice: 5 to 10 mL
Powder: 1 to 3 g

Formulations

Jwarasamharaka rasa, Tribhuvanakirti rasa, Muktapanchamrita, Mahajwarankusha rasa, Muktadi Mahanjana, Manasamitra Vataka.

Toxicity/Adverse Effects

The fixed oil was well-tolerated up to 30 mL/kg, whereas 100% mortality was recorded with a dose of 55 mL/kg. The LD50 of oil was 42.5 mL/kg. No untoward effect on subacute toxicity was found in the study of *O. sanctum* fixed oil at a dose of 3 mL/kg/d, intraperitoneal for 14 days in rats (Madhuri and Pandey 2007).

Substitution and Adulteration

The leaves of other species of *Ocimum* are often adulterated with the genuine drug.

> **Points to Ponder**
>
> - *Apetarakshasi, Bahumanjari, Chakrapuspi, Devadundubhi are the important synonyms of Tulasi.*
> - *Bhavaprakash mentioned two types of Tulasi: Shukla and Krishna Tulasi.*

Suggested Readings

Gupta SK, Prakash J, Srivastava S. Validation of traditional claim of Tulsi, *Ocimum sanctum* Linn. as a medicinal plant. Indian J Exp Biol 2002;40(7):765–773

Khanna N, Bhatia J. Action of *Ocimum sanctum* (Tulsi) in mice: possible mechanism involved. J Ethnopharmacol 2003;88(2–3):293–296

Krishnaiah D, Sukla AR, Sikand K, Dhawan V. Effect of herbal polyphenols on artherogenic transcriptome. Mol Cell Biochem 2009;278:177–184

Madhuri S, Pandey GP. Studies on oestrogen induced uterine and ovarian carcinogenesis and effect of ProImmu in rats. Int J Green Pharm 2007;1:23–25

Mahajan N, Rawal S, Verma M, Poddar M, Alok S. A phytopharmacological overview on Ocimum species with special emphasis on *Ocimum sanctum*. Biomed Prev Nutr 2013;3:185–192

Mandal S, Das DN, De K, et al. *Ocimum sanctum* Linn: a study on gastric ulceration and gastric secretion in rats. Indian J Physiol Pharmacol 1993;37(1):91–92

Mohan L, Amberkar MV, Kumari M. *Ocimum sanctum* linn. (Tulsi): an overview. Int J Pharm Sci Rev Res 2011;7:51–53

Mondal S, Mirdha BR, Mahapatra SC. The science behind sacredness of Tulsi (*Ocimum sanctum* Linn.). Indian J Physiol Pharmacol 2009;53(4):291–306

Pattanayak P, Behera P, Das D, Panda SK. *Ocimum sanctum* Linn. a reservoir plant for therapeutic applications: an overview. Pharmacogn Rev 2010;4(7):95–105

Sen P. Therapeutic potentials of tulsi: from experience to facts. Drugs News Views 1993;1(2):15–21

Singh N, Hoette Y, Miller R. Tulsi: The Mother Medicine of Nature. 2nd ed. Lucknow: International Institute of Herbal Medicine; 2010:28–47

The Ayurvedic Pharmacopoeia of India, Part 1, Vol. 2. New Delhi: Department of AYUSH, Ministry of Health and Family Welfare, Government of India; 1999:162–167

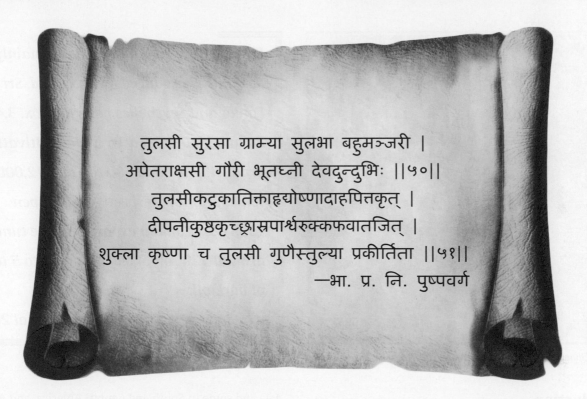

तुलसी सुरसा ग्राम्या सुलभा बहुमञ्जरी |
अपेतराक्षसी गौरी भूतघ्नी देवदुन्दुभिः ||५०||
तुलसीकटुकातिक्ताहृद्घोष्णादाहपित्तकृत् |
दीपनीकुष्ठकृच्छ्रास्रपार्श्वरुक्कफवातजित् |
शुक्ला कृष्णा च तुलसी गुणैस्तुल्या प्रकीर्तिता ||७१||
—भा. प्र. नि. पुष्पवर्ग

99. Tvak [*Cinnamomum zeylanicum* Blume.]

Family:	*Lauraceae*
Hindi name:	*Dalchini*
English name:	*Cinnamon*

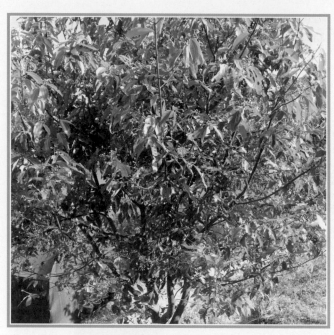

Plant of *Cinnamomum zeylanicum* Blume.

> *Best quality of cinnamon bark, mainly as quills is produced by Sri Lanka. Sri Lanka and Seychelles have approx. 3,400 ha and 24,000 ha area under cultivation producing around 600 ton and 12,000 ton cinnamon, respectively (Coppen 1995). Sri Lankan export is to the tune of around 120 ton of leaf oil and 4 to 5 ton of bark oil.*
>
> *—Ravindran et al 2003*

Introduction

Cinnamon, which is derived from a Greek word that means sweet wood, comes from the inner bark of the tropical evergreen cinnamon tree. *Cinnamomum* (cinnamon) is a genus of the Lauraceae family, many of whose members are used as spices. There are two main varieties of cinnamon: the Ceylon or true cinnamon (*Cinnamomum zeylanicum* Blume) which is grown in Sri Lanka and Southern India and the cassia (*Cinnamomum aromaticum* Ness.) which is grown in China, Indonesia, and Vietnam. *C. zeylanicum* Blume (true cinnamon) provides cinnamon bark of the finest quality and oil of cinnamon whereas *Cinnamomum cassia* provides cassia bark and oil of Cassia (also known as oil of cinnamon).

The genus *Cinnamomum* contains evergreen trees or shrubs belonging to the Lauraceae family containing around 250 species in tropical and subtropical regions, mostly in Asia and some in South and Central America, and Australia (Mabberley 2008). It is indigenous to Sri Lanka, which still produces the largest quantity and best quality, mainly in the form of quills.

IUCN red listed 24 *Cinnamomum* species (Oommen et al 2000). *Cinnamomum* are facing great pressure and threat because of economic activities, especially manual picking of bark and fruits as spice and for their medicinal value. Due to the unregulated use and overexploitation, its number is steadily decreasing. If the necessary conservation measures are not adopted, the species could become extinct.

Vernacular Names

Assamese: Dalcheni
Bengali: Daruchini, Darchini
French: Cammelle

German: Ceylonzeimt/kaneel
Gujarati: Dalchini
Kannada: Dalchini Chakke
Kashmiri: Dalchini, Dalchin
Malayalam: Karuvapatta, Ilavarngathely
Marathi: Dalchini
Oriya: Dalechini, Guda twak
Punjabi: Dalchini, Darchini
Spanish: Canela
Tamil: Lavangapattai, Karuvapattai
Telugu: Lavangapatta, Dalchini chekka
Urdu: Darchini

Synonyms

Bahugandham: The aroma is intense.
Bhringa: It has aromatic smell.
Charmanama: Tvak is the name of the skin or bark. It has leathery leaves.
Chocham: Bark of the plant is useful or prashasta (ideal part).
Darusita: The bark is sweet in taste.
Gudatwak: The bark is sweet like jaggery.
Lataparnanam: Mostly, it grows in lata desha (Eastern Bengal).
Mukhasodhnam: It is mouth refreshing.
Sainhalam: It is common in Simhala country.
Swadi: The bark is sweet in taste.
Swarnabhumikam: It grows in fertile land.
Tanutwak: The thin bark of the stem is useful part.
Twak: The useful part is bark.
Twakswadi: The bark is sweet in taste.
Utkatam: The bark is highly aromatic.

Vanapriyam: It grows wild in forests.
Varangam: Bark is the most useful part of the tree.

Classical Categorization

Charaka Samhita: Not mentioned in any mahakashaya, described in Shiravirechana gana (C.S.Vi. 8/51) and Ushna veerya dravya (Ch.S.Ci. 3/267).
Sushruta Samhita: Eladi gana
Ashtanga Hridaya: Eladigana, Trijataka, Chaturjataka
Dhanwantari Nighantu: Shatpuspadi varga
Madanpal Nighantu: Karpuradi varga
Kaiyadev Nighantu: Aushadhi varga
Raj Nighantu: Pippalyadi varga
Bhavaprakash Nighantu: Karpuradi varga

Distribution

Plant is native to Sri Lanka, found in cultivated and wild form in southern and western India.

Morphology

A moderate-sized evergreen tree, height –8 to 16 m, and 50 cm in diameter.

- **Stem:** Bark reddish brown, 5 mm thick and fragile, fragrant, soft, having numerous small warts (**Fig. 99.1**).
- **Leaf:** Ovate or elliptic-ovate, opposite or subopposite, thick, leathery, hard, coriaceous, 7.5 to 20 by 3.8 to 7.5 cm, subacute or shortly acuminate, glabrous, shining green on upper surface, slightly paler beneath, base acute or rounded, main nerves 3 to 5 from petioles (**Fig. 99.2**).

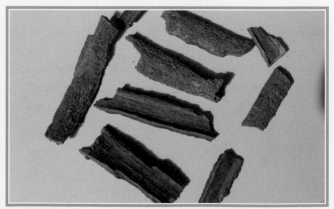

Fig. 99.1 Bark.

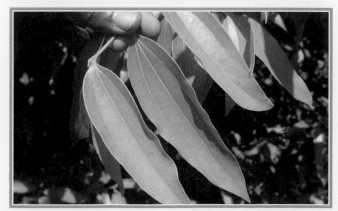

Fig. 99.2 Leaves.

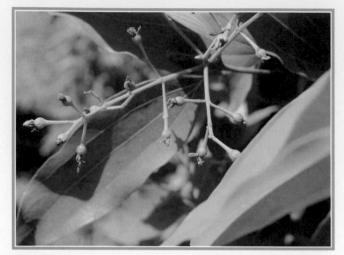

Fig. 99.3 Flowers.

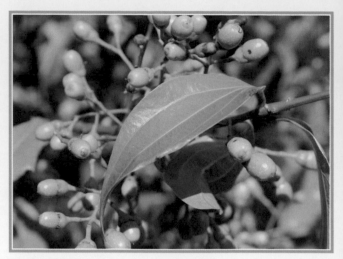

Fig. 99.4 Fruits.

- **Flower:** Numerous, small, in axillary or subterminal silky pubescent lax penducles or cymes, usually longer than leaves (**Fig. 99.3**).
- **Fruit:** Berry, dark purple, having persistent perianth, 1.3 to 1.7 cm long, oblong or ovoid-oblong, minutely apiculate, dry or slightly fleshy (**Fig. 99.4**).
- **Seed:** Single.

It is propagated by seeds, stem cutting, or layering of young shoots.

Phenology

Flowering time: March to May
Fruiting time: March to May

Key Characters for Identification

➤ *An evergreen, moderate-sized tree, 8 to 16 m in height with reddish brown aromatic soft bark with numerous small warts.*

➤ *Leaves: Simple, boat shape, ovate/elliptical ovate, thick, shiny green on upper surface, subacute apex, three to five veined, convergent venation.*

➤ *Flowers: Minute, red colored, in axillary or subterminal cymes or panicles.*

➤ *Fruit: Purple-colored ovoid-shaped berries.*

➤ *Dried bark: One to five mm thick, strongly aromatic, externally dark brown or brownish, and internally reddish brown in color, closely rolled (quill), weak and brittle in fracture.*

Types

The plant drug may be categorized into three kinds based on distribution, occurrence, and native regions, viz. Chinese, Simhali (Sri Lanka), and Indian:

- Siloni Dalchini: *Cinnamomum zeylanicum*
- Bhartiya Dalchini: *C. tamala*
- Chini Dalchini: *C. cassia* (Chunekar and Pandey 2002)

Rasapanchaka

Guna	Laghu, Ruksha, Tikshana
Rasa	Katu, Tikta, Madhur
Vipaka	Katu
Virya	Ushna

Chemical Constituents

The bark yields about 1 to 1.5% oil, which contains 10% cinnamaldehyde, a major constituent comprising 74% of the essential oil of bark; others are eugenol, o–methyl eugenol, benzal dehyde, linalool, benzyl acetate, cinnamic aldehyde, eugenyl acetate, cinnamyl acetate, benzyl benzoate, cinncassiol, easter of butyric acid, mucilage.

Identity, Purity, and Safety

- Foreign matter: Not more than 2%
- Total ash: Not more than 3%
- Acid-insoluble ash: Not more than 2%
- Alcohol-soluble extractive: Not less than 2%
- Water-soluble extractive: Not less than 3%
- Volatile oil: Not less than 1%

(Source: The Ayurvedic Pharmacopeia of India 1989)

Karma (Actions)

Rochan (relish), vishaghna (antidote), mukhashuddhikara (mouth refresher), grahi (astringent), dipana (appetizer), pachana (digestive), krimighna (anthelmintic), utejaka (stimulant), vranaropan (wound healing), Shukral (spermatopoetic), varnya (complexion promoter).

- Doshakarma: Kaphavata shamaka
- Dhatukarma: Shukral
- Malakarma: Grahi

Pharmacological Actions

Cinnamon possesses immunomodulatory, antioxidant, antiviral, lowering blood cholesterol, antimicrobial, lipid-lowering, antihypertension, anti-inflammatory, antitumor, gastroprotective, antidiabetic, neuroprotective, and blood purifying properties (Saeed et al 2018).

Indications

Arsha (piles), hridroga (heart disease), krimiroga (worm infestation), trishna (thirst), kaphanisharak (expectorant), mukhashosha (dryness of mouth), kanthamukharoga (diseases of throat and mouth), pinasa (cold and sinusitis), vastiroga (diseases of bladder), aruchi (loss of appetite), shukra dosha (abnormality of semen), aadhman (flatulence), kandu (itching).

As a stimulant, it is beneficial in preventing cramps of stomach, gastritis, paralysis of tongue. Bark powder is used in chronic cough, asthma, bronchitis, tubercular ulcers, checking nausea, vomiting, diarrhea, and dysentery.

Therapeutic Uses

External Use

1. **Shirashool** (headache): Headache produced by exposure to cold air is readily cured by applying a paste of finely powdered cinnamon mixed in water on the temples and forehead.
2. **Shool and shotha** (pain and inflammation): Two to five drops of cinnamon oil is applied externally in neuralgia, rheumatism, toothache, backache, insect bite, and chronic foul-smelling ulcers.

Internal Use

1. **Mukhasodhana and Rochana** (mouth refreshing and relishing): (1) Tvak, Musta, Ela, Dhanyaka; (2) Musta, Amalaka, Tvak—these are used as mouth freshner. It purifies mouth and improves taste (CS.Ci. 8/137-138).
2. **Shirashoola** (headache): In headache caused by pitta, paste of Tvak, Patra, and Sharkara pounded with rice water should be used as pressed snuff, followed by snuffing of ghee (CS.Ci. 26.178).
3. **Luta visha** (spider poisoning): Equal quantity of Tvak and Shunthi are finely pounded and taken with hot water. It destroys all types of spider poisoning (C.S.Ci. 23/205).
4. **Kasa** (cough): Tvak, Ela, Pippali, Tavakshiri, and sugar successively double in quantity should be powdered and taken in linctus with honey and ghee. It improves voice and alleviates cough, wasting, asthma, chest pain, and kapha (AH.Ci. 5/33-34). Samasarkara churna is also given in kasa (AH.Ci. 5/54/55).

Officinal Parts Used

Bark and oil

Dose

Powder: 1 to 3 g
Oil: 2 to 6 drops

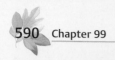

Formulations

Ardrakakhand, Vyaghri haritaki, Chandraprabhavati, Samasarkara churna, Sitopaladi churna, Yavanishadava churna, Shilajatu vataka, Bruhani gutika, Kanakarista, Bala taila, Eladi gutika, Khadiradi gutika, Dadimastaka churna, Talisadi vataka, Talisadi churna, Chaturjataka churna, Lavanbhaskar churna, Vyoshadi gutika, Kanchanar guggulu, Kusmandavaleha Kutajavaleha, Irimedadi taila, Chandanadi taila.

Toxicity/Adverse Effects

Cinnamon has been used in food preparation and as medicinal remedies from ancient period. It is the most commonly and frequently consumed spice and is both safe and relatively inexpensive. The intake of up to 6 g/d of *Cinnamomum cassia* for more than 40 days did not show any adverse effects. The most common adverse effects related to the excessive use of cinnamon were irritation and allergic reaction in skin or mucous membranes.

According to US Food and Drug Administration, cinnamon species including common cinnamon and cassia cinnamon are generally safe and well tolerated in amounts commonly found in food. Cinnamon oil is also recognized as safe and is exempted from toxicity data requirements by the US Environmental Protection Agency.

Substitution and Adulteration

Kabab chini and Kulanjana are substitutes of *C. zeylanicum* (Balkrushna).

> **Points to Ponder**
> - *Twak is a member of trijataka and chaturjatak.*
> - *True cinnamon is mainly procured from Sri Lanka.*

Suggested Readings

Balkrushna A. Ayurveda Jadibuti Rahasya. Haridwar: Divya Prakashan; 2014:165

Chunekar KC, Pandey GS. Bhavaprakash Nighantu of Sri Bhav Misra, Karpuradi varga. Varanasi: Chaukhambha Bharati Academy; 2002:225

Coppen JJW. Flavours and Fragrances of Plant Origin. Rome: FAO; 1995

Mabberley DJ. Mabberley's Plant-Book: A Portable Dictionary of Plants, Their Classifications and Uses. 3rd ed. Cambridge: Cambridge University Press; 2008

Oommen S, Ved DK, Krishnan R. Tropical Indian Medicinal Plants: Propagation Methods. Bengaluru: FRLHT, Foundation for Revitalisation of Local Health Traditions; 2000

Ravindran PN, Nirmal-Babu K, Shylaja M. Cinnamon and Cassia: The Genus *Cinnamomum*. Boca Raton, FL: CRC Press; 2003

Saeed M, Kamboh A, Syed S, et al. Phytochemistry and beneficial impacts of cinnamon (*Cinnamomum zeylanicum*) as a dietary supplement in poultry diets. Worlds Poult Sci J 2018;74(2):331–346

The Ayurvedic Pharmacopoeia of India, Part 1, Vol. 1. New Delhi: Department of AYUSH, Ministry of Health and Family Welfare, Government of India; 1989:113–115

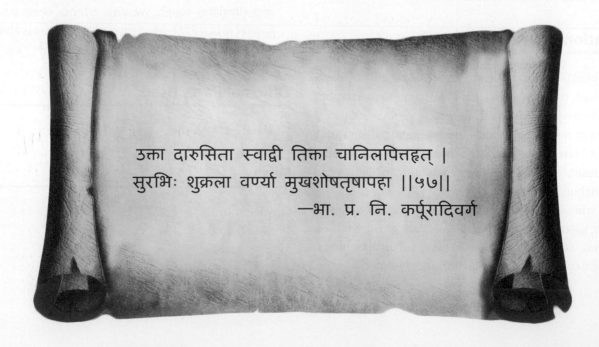

उक्ता दारुसिता स्वाद्री तिक्ता चानिलपित्तहृत् ।
सुरभिः शुक्रला वर्ण्या मुखशोषतृषापहा ॥५७॥
—भा. प्र. नि. कर्पूरादिवर्ग

100. Ushira *[Vetiveria zizanioides (Linn.) Nash]*

Synonym:	*Chrysopogon zizanioides L. Robert*
Family:	*Poaceae/Graminae*
Hindi name:	*Khas, khaskhas, Khasa, Gandar, Bena*
English name:	*Vetiver, Khas khas grass, Cuscus Grass*

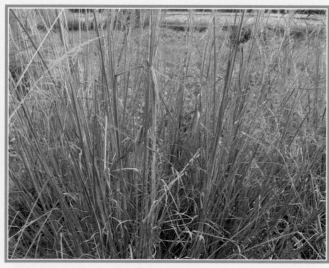

Plant of *Vetiveria zizanioides* (Linn.) Nash.

> *The generic name Vetiveria comes from the Tamil word "vétiver" meaning "root that is dug up." The specific name zizanioides was first given by the Swedish taxonomist Carolus Linnaeus in 1771, meaning "by the river side."*
>
> —*Vietmeyer and Ruskin (1993)*

Introduction

Bhavaprakash Nighantu mentioned that Ushir is the root of Veeran. *Vetiveria zizanioides* (Linn.) Nash, a member of the family Poaceae commonly known as the *Khas-Khas*, *Khas*, or *Khus* grass in India, is a perennial grass with thick fibrous adventitious roots which are aromatic and highly valued. Its root is known as Ushira. It grows in a wide variety of ecological habitats covering all biogeographic provinces of India. No wonder that this is one grass which has been extensively used by almost all the tribes. The oil extracted from the roots is useful in insomnia, depression, anxiety, nervousness, rheumatism, sprain, and headache apart from its use in perfumery and aromatherapy. Two species of *Vetiveria* are found in India, of which *V. zizanioides* is the common source of the well-known oil of Vetiver, which is used in medicine and in perfumery.

Vernacular Names

Assamese: Usir, Virina
Bengali: Venarramula, Khaskhas
Gujarati: Sugandhi Valo, Valo
Kannada: Mudivala, Baladaberu, Lamanch, Bala Deberu
Malayalam: Ramaceam, Vetiver, Lamajja, Ramacham
Marathi: Bala, Vala
Oriya: Ushira, Benachera
Punjabi: Panni, Khas
Sanskrit: Virana, Adhaya, Sevya
Tamil: Vetiver, Vilamichaver
Telugu: Vetivelu, Vettiveru
Urdu: Khas

Synonyms

Amrunala: The stems are like that of Kamala.
Nalada/Sugandhika: It gives pleasant odor.

Samagandhika: Having pleasant odor.

Shitimulakam: The root is sitadravya.

Ushira: It gives complexion.

Vahumulam: It contains many roots.

Varitara/Shishira: Which grow in watery places.

Viranamulaka: Usira is the roots of the plant Virana.

Classical Categorization

Charaka Samhita: Dahaprasamana, Stanyajanana, Chhardinigrahana, Shukrashodhan, Varnya

Sushruta Samhita: Eladi, Sarivadi

Ashtanga Hridaya: Sarivadi

Dhanwantari Nighantu: Chandanadi varga

Madanpal Nighantu: Karpooradi varga

Kaiyadev Nighantu: Aushadi varga

Raj Nighantu: Chandanadi varga

Bhavaprakash Nighantu: Karpuradi varga

Distribution

Vetiver is native to India. The exact location of origin is not precisely known; some say that it is native to northern India; others say that it is native to region around Mumbai (Vietmeyer and Ruskin 1993). As the specific name suggests, Vetiver grows particularly on river banks and in rich marshy soil (Anonymous 1976). This grass grows throughout the plains of India up to an elevation of 1,200 m. It is mainly found in Haryana, Uttar Pradesh, Odisha, Rajasthan, Gujarat, Bihar, and all the South Indian states. This plant survives under long seasonal flooding as well as it tolerates extreme temperature and grows over a wide range of soil pH.

Morphology

It is a perennial, aromatic grass that grows up to 2 m in height.

- **Roots:** Thick, fibrous, adventitious root, aromatic; the roots grow downwards up to 2 to 4 m in depth. Stout and contains oil with fragrance (**Fig. 100.1**).
- **Leaves:** Linear, narrow, erect, grassy, glabrous with scar bid margins, 20 to 60 cm long × 0.5 to 1 cm broad (**Fig. 100.2**).
- **Flower:** Inflorescences is a panicle up to 20 to 45 cm bearing numerous racemes in a whorl on a central axis. Vetiver produces brownish purple-hued flowers. One floret in spike is bisexual, sessile, fruit oblong grain. The other spikelet is pedicelled and staminate. The lower spikelet is reduced to lamina (**Fig. 100.3**).

There are flowering and nonflowering Vetiver plants. The wild-growing variety commonly found in North India is mostly of the former type, whereas in South India both types are found (Anonymous 1976). As not all Vetiver plants flower and the germination rate of the seeds is low, Vetiver propagates itself through axillary shoots (Vietmeyer and Ruskin 1993).

The wild type from North India grows under suitable marshy conditions regularly and sets fertile seeds. The "domesticated" type from South India consists of flowering and nonflowering Vetiver plants (Anonymous 1976). If they flower, they produce no viable seeds. It might be that the seeds are sterile or the conditions for germination are seldom met (Vietmeyer and Ruskin 1993). These Vetiver plants replicate by vegetative propagation via side shoots.

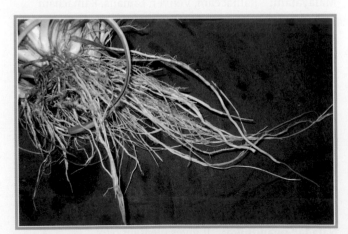

Fig. 100.1 Root.

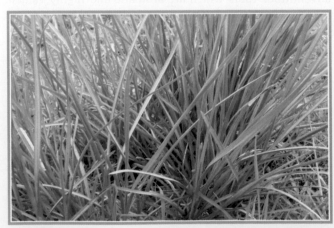

Fig. 100.2 Leaves.

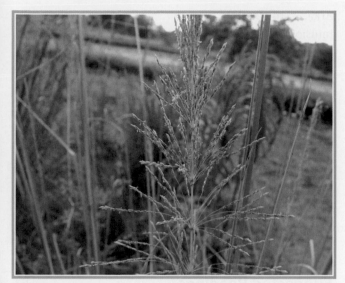

Fig. 100.3 Flowers.

Key Characters for Identification

➤ A densely tufted grass known as virana.
➤ It grows especially on the banks of rivers and in rich marshy soil.
➤ The roots with pleasant odor grow downwards up to 2 to 4 m.
➤ Flowers are brownish-purple-hued.

Rasapanchaka

Guna	Laghu
Rasa	Tikta
Vipak	Katu
Virya	Sheeta

Chemical Constituents

The chemical constituents present in the plant are benzoic acid, b-vetispirene, epizizianal, iso-khusimol, khositone, khusimol, khusimone, prezizaene, ß-Humulene, terpene-4-ol, terpenes, tripene-4-ol, vetivazulene, vetivene, vetivenyl vetivenate, Vetiver oils, vetiverol, vetivone, zizaene, and β-vetivone (Mishra et al 2013).

The main constituents of Vetiver oil are sesquiterpene hydrocarbons such as cadinene, cloven, amorphine aromadendrine, and junipene; alcohol derivatives (vetiverols) such as khusinol, epiglobulol, khusimol, and khusol;

carbonyl derivatives (vetivones) such as α-vetivone and β-vetivone, khusimone.

Identity, Purity, and Strength

- Foreign matter: Not more than 2%
- Total ash: Not more than 9%
- Acid-insoluble ash: Not more than 6%
- Alcohol-soluble extractive: Not less than 4%
- Water-soluble extractive: Not less than 5%
- Volatile oil: Not less than 1%

(Source: The Ayurvedic Pharmacopeia of India 2001)

Karma (Actions)

Pachan (digestive), sthambhana (astringent), jwaraghna (antipyretics), swedapanayana (reduce sweating), dahaprashamana (reduce burning sensation), twakdoshahara (beneficial in skin disease), stanyajanana (galactopoetic), chhardinigrahana (antiemetic), shukrashodhan (purification or bringing normalcy of semen), and varnya (complexion promoter).

Vetiver oil is regarded as stimulant diaphoretic and refrigerant. It is widely used as cooling agent, tonic, and blood purifier. It is used in skin diseases, boils, burns, epilepsy, fever, scorpion sting, snake bites, sore in mouth, headache, toothaches, rheumatism, UTI, hyperacidity, vomiting, erysipelas, wound, burning sensation, and in worms. Leaf paste is used in rheumatism lumango and sprain. Root extract is used for headache and toothache. Vetiver oil possesses sedative property and is used in aromatherapy for relieving stress, anxiety, nervous tension, and insomnia. Roots are used for sharbat or soft drink during seminar and for scenting the cloths.

- Doshakarma: Kaphapittahara
- Dhatukarma: Raktaprasadan, shukrashodhan
- Malakarma: Mutrajanana, swedapanayana

Pharmacological Actions

The various pharmacological actions are as follows: anti-inflammatory, antiseptic, antibacterial, antidepressant, antifungal, antihyperglycemic, antioxidant, antitubercular, aphrodisiac, cicatrisant, hepatoprotective, mosquito repellent, nervine, and sedative (Balasankar et al 2013; Mishra et al 2013).

Indications

It is used for unmada (epilepsy), boils, burns (daha), jwara (fever), trishna (thirst), visha (poisoning), vrana (wound), mada (alcoholism), daurgandhya (bad smell of body), vrikshik danshan (scorpion sting), snakebite, and sores in the mouth. The root extract is useful in headache and toothache. Vetiver oil is regarded as stimulant, diaphoretic, and refrigerant. The paste of leaf when locally applied for rheumatism, lumbago, and sprain gives good relief (Pareek and Kumar 2013).

Therapeutic Uses

1. **Fever:** Shandangapaniya prepared from Musta, Parpataka, Ushira, Chandan, Udichya, and Nagara is used in fever and thirst (C.S.Ci. 3/145).
2. **Intrinsic hemorrhage:** Ushira, Kaliyaka, Lodhra, etc. mixed with equal quantity of sandal wood and sugar taken with rice water alleviate intrinsic hemorrhage, thirst, and burning sensation (C.S.Ci. 4.73-74).
3. **Vomiting**: Ushira and honey is given to check thirst and vomiting (C.S.Ci. 20/32).
4. **Boils:** External application of Ushira destroys boils caused by perspiration (V.M. 11/24).

Officinal Part Used

Root

Dose

Powder: 3 to 6 g
Cold infusion: 25 to 50 mL

Arka: 25 to 50 mL
Infusion: 50 to 100 mL

Formulations

Sadanga Kwatha Churna, Sadangapaniya, Ushiradi choorna, Ushiradikwath, Ushiradi taila, Ushirasava, Yogaraja guggulu.

> **Points to Ponder**
>
> ➤ Ushira is the root of Veeran.
> ➤ Ushira is an ingredient of famous formulation Sadangapaniya used for pipasa and jwara.

Suggested Readings

Anonymous. Vetiveria, Vol. 10. Delhi: Council of Scientific & Industrial Research; 1976

Balasankar D, Vanilarasu K, Selva P, Rajeswari S, Umadevi M, Bhowmik D. Traditional and medicinal uses of Vetiver. J Med Plant Stud 2013;2(3)

Lucas DS. Dravyaguna-Vijnana: Study of Dravya-Materia Medica. Varanasi: Chaukhamba Visvabharati; 2013:290

Mishra S, Sharma SK, Mohapatra S, Chauhan D. An overview on *Vetiveria zizanioides*. Res J Pharmaceut Biol Chem Sci 2013;4(3):777–783

Pareek A, Kumar A. Ethnobotanical and pharmaceutical uses of *Vetiveria zizanioides* (Linn.) Nash: a medicinal plant of Rajasthan. Int J Life Sci Pharma Res 2013;3(4):12–18

Sharma PV. Classical Uses of Medicinal Plants. 1st ed. Varanasi: Chaukhamba Vishvabharati; 2004:444

The Ayurvedic Pharmacopoeia of India, Part I, Vol. III. 1st ed. New Delhi: Department of Health, Ministry of Health and Family Welfare, Government of India; 2001:220

Vietmeyer ND, Ruskin FR. Vétiver Grass: A Thin Green Line Against Erosion. Washington, DC: The National Academies Press; 1993

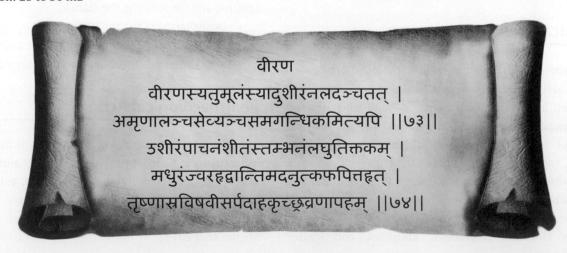

वीरण

वीरणस्यतुमूलंस्यादुशीरंनलदञ्चतत् ।
अमृणालञ्चसेव्यञ्चसमगन्धिकमित्यपि ||७३||
 उशीरंपाचनंशीतंस्तम्भनंलघुतिक्तकम् ।
मधुरंज्वरहृद्दान्तिमदनुत्कफपित्तहृत् ।
तृष्णास्रविषवीसर्पदाहकृच्छ्रव्रणापहम् ||७४||

101. Vacha [*Acorus calamus* Linn.]

Family:	*Araceae*
Hindi name:	*Bach, Ghodvach*
English name:	*Sweet Flag*

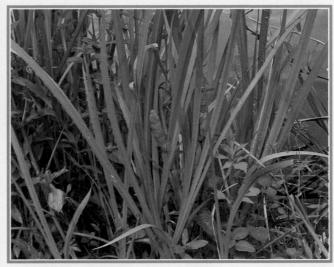

Plant of *Acorus calamus* Linn.

> *Vacha shodhana was first described in Chakradutta followed by Rasa ratnasamuchya.*

Introduction

The plant is designated the name Vacha because of its ability to improve the power of speech. The name "acorus" is derived from the Greek word "acoron," which in turn was derived from "coreon" meaning "pupil," because it was used in herbal medicine as a treatment for inflammation of eye, and the word *calamus* was derived from the Greek word *kalamos*, meaning "reed."

Vacha is one of the oldest herbs used in mental disorders since ages. For the first time, it was described in Atharva Veda. It is widely used in other systems of medicines like Chinese, European, and Greek for many ailments. The native American tribes used it as an anesthetic drug for toothache and headaches. The ancient Chinese used it in swelling and constipation. The Lai people of New Guinea believed that eating the rhizome on the ceremonial day aids in communication with the spirit world. In 1916, it was officially enlisted in the U.S. Pharmacopoeia and National Formulary.

In Ayurvedic system of medicines, Vacha is a popular churna prashana dravya for medha, bala, buddhi vardhan in children (Su.S.Sa. 10/72), (A.H.Sa. 10/72). Charaka has included it in virechan and shirovirechan dravyas (C.S.Vi. 8/150). He also advocated applying its paste locally in kushta, udarshool, and other skin diseases (C.S.Su. 3/4,18,20). Its rhizome is used as an effective antibacterial, antiseptic drug along with Guggulu, Jatamansi, Hingu, Sarshapa, Brahmi in the form of dhupana (fumigation) dravya (S.S.Su./18) (C.S.Sa.8/61). Sushrut used shweta Vacha as rasayana (Su.S.Ci. 28/7) and Vacha as utsadana churna (Su.S.U. 29/5). Acharya sharangdhara describes Vacha as a pramathi and lekhana dravya (Sh.S.P. 4/10,23). Shaligram Nighantu mentioned that on the day of solar or lunar eclipse, if a person eats Vacha churna in a dose of 1 pala he becomes intelligent. It is also advised to eat its rhizome freely during the prevalence of any epidemic disease as it is supposed to be an antidote to poisons.

Vernacular Names

Assamese: Bach
Bengali: Vach, Safed Vach
Gujarati: Vaj, Ghodabaj, Gandhilovaj
Kannada: Baje, Narru Berua, Vaje gida
Kashmiri: Vahi, Mazar posh, Mazarmund
Malayalam: Vayambu
Marathi: Vaca, Vekhandas, Vekhand
Punjabi: Varch, Varaj, Bariboj
Sindhi: Kini kathi
Tamil: Vasambu, Pillai maruntho
Telugu: Vasa, Vadaje
Urdu: Waja-e-Turki

Synonyms

Golomi: The rhizome is studded with minute hairs as present in cow's body.
Jatila: Its rhizome is dense and hairy.
Kshudrapatra: The plant has linear-shaped leaves.
Mangalya: The rhizome is regarded as auspicious.
Shadgrantha: It has six nodes, i.e., more number of nodes.
Shataparvika: It has numerous nodes and internodes.
Ugragandha: It has strong odor or intense smell.

Classical Categorization

Charaka Samhita: Lekhaniya, Triptighana, Arshoghna, Asthapanopaga, Sheetprashamana, Sangya Sthapna, Tiktaskanda
Sushrut Samhita: Pippalyadi, Vachadi, Mustadi
Ashtang Hridaya: Vachadi, Mustadi, Vatsakadi gana
Dhanvantari Nighantu: Shatpushpadi Varga
Madanpal Nighantu: Sunthyadi Varga
Kaiyadev Nighantu: Oushadi varga
Raj Nighantu: Pippalayadi Varga
Bhavaprakash Nighantu: Haritakyadi Varga

Distribution

The plant is native to North America and Northern, eastern Asia, naturalized in Southern Asia and Europe from ancient cultivation. It is found throughout India under cultivation as well as in the wild state, ascending up to an altitude of 2,200 m. It grows vigorously at the waterside in dumpy marshy places such as meadows, edges of lakes, and banks of streams and rivers.

Morphology

The plant is a strongly aromatic gregarious perennial herb of about 2 to 4 feet, arising from a partially underground creeping and branched rhizome. When the older portion of the rhizome decays the branches which get separated becomes independent plant.

- **Leaves:** Strongly aromatic, simple, alternate, distichous, closely arranged, vertically oriented linear to narrowly ensiform, 2 to 3 feet long and ½ to 1 inch broad, occasionally longer and broader, glossy bright green acute tip with a thick and stout midrib (**Fig. 101.1**).
- **Flowering stem:** Scape are one to two in number, arises from the axils of the outer leaves compressed triangular, solid, and spongy, flowering upwards. Inflorescence in a short stumpy spadix, 2 to 3 inch long and 0.5 to 0.75 inch in diameter (**Fig. 101.2**).

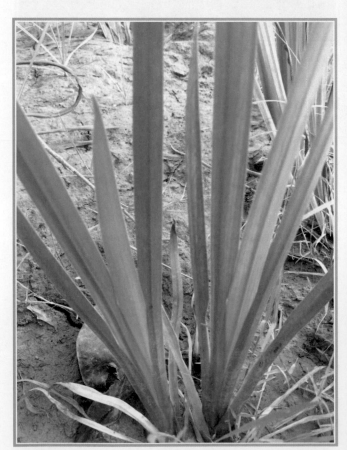

Fig. 101.1 Leaves.

- **Flower:** Small, sessile, bisexual, densely packed so as to form a solid cylindrical tapering blunt spike (spadix) 2 to 4 inch long, often curved.
- **Fruit (usually not seen):** Turbinate, prismatic-clavate, bluntly six-sided, about 0.75 inch in diameter, top pyramidal and few oblong seeds.
- **Rhizomes:** Branched, horizontal, flat, 0.5 to 1 inch thick, aromatic, creeping, with nodes and internodes, upper surface light to dark brown, marked with remnants of leaves, studded with lenticels, lower surface with many rootlets, internally creamy white (**Fig. 101.3a, b**). The plant is propagated by its rhizome.

Phenology

Flowering time: May to June
Fruiting time: May to June

Key Characters for Identification

➤ *An aromatic, evergreen, creeping herb of about 2 to 4 feet.*
➤ *Leaves are simple, distichous, linear to ensiform, glossy, bright green.*
➤ *Flowers are small, sessile, greenish yellow, densely packed to form a solid cylindrical tapering spadix, 2 to 3 inch long.*
➤ *Rhizome is branched, horizontal, creeping, marked with leaf remnants externally brown, internally creamy white.*

Types

- Dhanvantari Nighantu: Two types: Vacha and Shweta vacha
- Raj Nighantu: Three types: Vacha, Shweta vacha, and Kulanjana
- Bhavaprakash Nighantu: Four types:
- Vacha
- Hemavati/Parsikvacha/Swetavacha
- Maha bhari vacha (Kulanjan)
- Dvipantara Vacha (Chopchini)

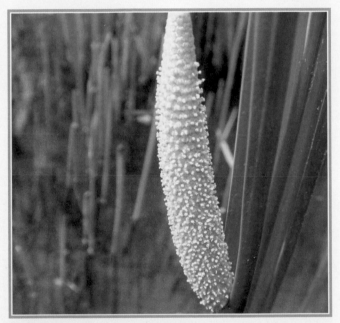

Fig. 101.2 Flower.

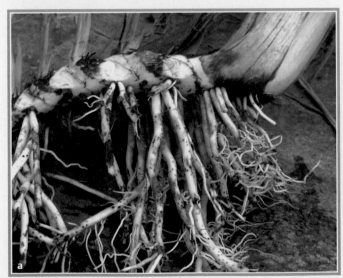

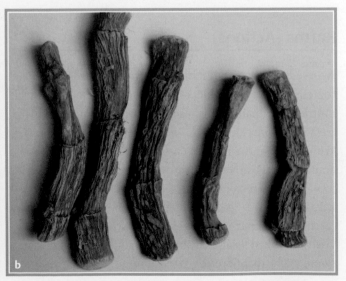

Fig. 101.3 **(a)** Fresh rhizome. **(b)** Dried rhizome.

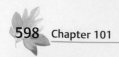

Rasapanchaka

Guna	Laghu, Ruksha
Rasa	Katu, Tikta
Vipaka	Katu
Virya	Ushna

Chemical Constituents

The rhizome contains asarone, β-asarone, calamenol, calamine, calamenone, eugenol, methyl eugenol, α-pinene and camphene, various fatty acids, calamol, acoradin, azulene, two selinane-type sesquiterpenes—acolamone and isoacolamone, sugars, glucosides—acorin, calameon, calamusenone, a flavones—luteolin-6,8-C-diglucoside, new natural products, acoramone, asarylaldehyde, β-asarone, and epoxyisoacoragermacrone (Sharma et al 2000).

Identity, Purity, and Strength

For Rhizome

- Foreign matter: Not more than 1%
- Total ash: Not more than 7%
- Acid-insoluble ash: Not more than 1%
- Alcohol-soluble extractive: Not less than 9%
- Water-soluble extractive: Not less than 16%
- Volatile oil: Not less than 2%

(Source: The Ayurvedic Pharmacopeia of India 1999)

Karma (Actions)

Ayurvedic classics described Vacha as medhya (brain tonic), vamaka (emetic), kanthya (voice promoter), mala, mutra vishodhana (purifies stool urine), sangyasthapana (restore consciousness), vedanasthapana (analgesic), krimighna (anthelmintic), arshoghna (antihemorrhoids), anulomaka (laxative), ayushya (enhances life expectancy), jeevaniya (restorative), jantughna (antibacterial), kasashwasahara (pacify cough and bronchitis), deepan (carminative), pachana (digestive), mutrajanana (diuretic), vrishya (aphrodisiac), akshepashamana (anticonvulsant), swedjanana (diaphoretic), jwaraghna (antipyretic), rasayana

(rejuvinator), rakshoghna (protective), and smritivardhaka (enhances memory).

- Doshakarma: Kapha vatashamaka
- Dhatukarma: Medhya, sangyasthapana, rasayana
- Malakarma: Mala, mutra vishodhana, Swedjanana, mutral

Pharmacological Actions

The rhizome is reported as intellect promoting (medhya), emetic (vamak), sedative, tranquilizer, anticonvulsant, expectorant, carminative, stomachic, anthelmintic, diuretic, antioxidant, anthelminthic, antiproliferative, immunomodulator, anodyne, antispasmodic, anti-inflammatory, antipyretic, antimicrobial, and insecticidal (Gupta et al 2004).

Indications

Vacha is widely used in the treatment of vibandha (constipation), adhamana (flatulence), shool (colic), unmada (insanity), apasmara (epilepsy), hridyaroga (heart diseases), granthi (cystic swelling), shotha (edema), krimi (worm infestation), jwar (fever), atisaar (diarrhea), trishna (thirst), mukharoga (diseases of oral cavity), sandhivata (osteoarthritis), amavata (rheumatoid arthritis), pakshaghata (paralysis), apatantraka (hysteria), agnimandya (loss of appetite), arsha (piles), amajeerna (indigestion), aruchi (unwill to have food), kasa (cough), pratishyaya (common cold), swarbheda (tonsillitis), ashmari (urinary calculus), bhootbadha (microbial infections), grahadosha(Paediatric idiopathic syndrome), kashtaprasava (difficult labor), kashtartava (dysmennorhoea), and medoroga (obesity).

Powdered rhizome is also used for inducing vomiting, in bronchitis, asthma, insomnia, convulsions, hysteria, loss of memory, melancholy, neurosis, dyspepsia, skin diseases, swollen joints, toothache, and filariasis.

Therapeutic Uses

External Use

1. **Vranashodhana** (wound cleansing): Decoction of Vacha mixed with camphor is used for cleansing of wounds and ulcers (S.S.Su. 37/19).

2. **Medoroga** (obesity): The dry powder massage (udvartana) is beneficial in reducing excessive fat.
3. **Tarunyapidika** (acne vulgaris): Local application of Lodhra, Dhanyaka, and Vacha paste removes acne (BS. kustha Ci./45).
4. **Shotha** (inflammatory diseases): Application of Vacha sarsapa paste removes edema (CD. 40/22).
5. **Ardhavabhedaka** (hemicrania): Avpeeda nasya of Vacha and Pippali is advised (S.S.U. 26/33) (VM. 62/38).

Internal Use

1. **Vamanarth** (to induce emesis): One to two grams Vacha powder with lukewarm salt water induces vomiting, relieves phlegm, and eases cough and asthma.
2. **Apasmara** (epilepsy): Purana ghrita prepared with Vacha, Brahmi, Sankhapushpi, and Kushta alleviates epilepsy (C.S.Ci. 10/25). Vacha churna taken with madhu is also recommended in epilepsy (BS. Apasmara ci/37).
3. **Medhya** (memory enhancer): Regular licking of Vacha powder with honey twice a day for 6 months enhances memory in new born.
4. **Atisaar** (diarrhea): One should take water boiled with Vacha and Prativisha to control diarrhea (A.H.Ci. 9/8).
5. **Shool** (colic): Intake of powder prepared with Vacha, Sauvarchal, Hingu, Kushta, Ativisha, Haritaki, and Indrayava alleviates colic immediately (S.S.U. 42/125).
6. **Swasa, Kasa** (asthma and cough): Decoction of Vacha or powder with honey is useful in cough, asthma, bronchitis, dyspepsia, and tertian fever.

Officinal Part Used

Rhizome

Dose

Powder: 125 to 500 mg
For inducing vaman: 1 to 2 g

Formulations

Vachadi churna, Vachyadi ghrita, Saraswataristha, Shisu kalyana ghrita, Brahmi ghrita.

Toxicity/Adverse Effects

The US Food and Drug Administration has considered Vacha unsafe for human consumption because of carcinogenic effect of its content β-asarone. Some adverse effects like disturbed digestion, gastroenteritis, persistent constipation followed by bleeding diarrhea are observed in some cases. Long-term use can cause genotoxicity (Pammel 1994).

Shodhana

Vacha is purified by boiling followed by vashpaswedana (fomentation) in gomutra, mundi kwatha, and panchpallava jala (Tripathi 2010).

Substitution and Adulteration

In local markets, Vacha is available under the name of bach and ghorbach. Rhizomes of *Alpinia galanga*, *Alpinia officinarum*, and *Acorus gramineus Soland* are used as its adulterants (Dey and Das 1982).

Points to Ponder

- *Vacha is a renowned drug in the treatment of vibandha, adhyamana, unmada, apasmara, smritivardhan, swarabheda, grahabadha, and medoroga.*
- *Vacha chatushthya includes Vacha (Acorus calamus L.), Hemavati Vacha (Iris germanica L.), Mahabhari Vacha (Alpinia galanga Willd.), and Dvipanatara Vacha (Smilax china L.).*

Suggested Readings

Dey D, Das MN. Pharmacognostic studies of *Acorus calamus* & its adulterants. Acta Botanica Indica 1982;28–35

Gupta AK, Sharma M, Tandon N. Review on Indian Medicinal Plants, Vol. 1. New Delhi: ICMR; 2004:193–125

Pammel LH. A manual of poisonous plants. 1911. In: Motley TJ, ed. The Ethnobotany of Sweet Flag, *Acorus calamus* (Araceae). Econ Bot 1994;48(4):397–412

Sharma PC, Yelne MB, Dennis TJ. Database on Medicinal Plants Used in Ayurveda, Vol. 1. New Delhi: CCRAS Department of Indian Systems of Medicine and Homeopathy (ISM&H), Ministry of Health and Family Welfare, Government of India; 2000:469–480

The Ayurvedic Pharmacopeia of India, Part I, Vol. 2. New Delhi: Department of AYUSH, Ministry of Health and Family Welfare, Government of India; 1999:178

Tripathi I. Chakrapanidutt's Chakradutta. 2nd ed. Varanasi: Chaukhambha Sanskrit Bhawan; 2010:155

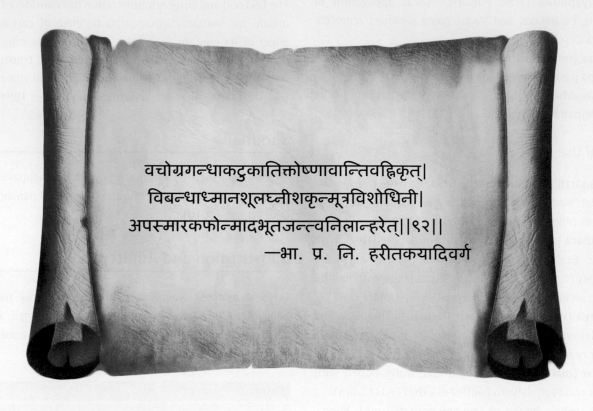

वचोग्रगन्धाकटुकातिक्तोष्णावान्तिवह्निकृत्।
विबन्धाध्मानशूलघ्नीशकृन्मूत्रविशोधिनी।
अपस्मारकफोन्मादभूतजन्त्वनिलान्हरेत्॥९२॥
—भा. प्र. नि. हरीतकयादिवर्ग

102. Varahi *[Dioscorea bulbifera Linn.]*

Family:	*Dioscoreaceae*
Hindi name:	*Barhakand, Zami kanda, Gaithi*
English name:	*Air Potato, Potato Yam*

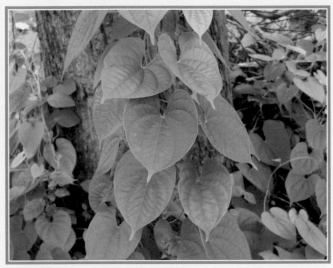

Plant of *Dioscorea bulbifera* Linn.

Diosgenin is the major source for the commercial production of corticosteroids and steroidal contraceptives.

Introduction

Since time immemorial, Varahikand is used as tonic and rejuvenating herb in traditional medicines. It is a prime staple medicinal-food substitute for the rural and tribal people. People follow different traditional practices to make them edible as food supplements. To remove the bitterness, tubers are soaked in water overnight or left overnight in stream and subjected to successive boiling. Tubers are then roasted and cooked as vegetable. In Latin America, the tubers are used to treat diarrhea, dysentery, conjunctivitis, fatigue, and depression. In China, tubers are used in sore throat, rabies, snake poisoning, food poisoning, hepatic fibrosis, gastric and rectal carcinoma, and goiter.

Sushrut for the first time described it as a Rasayana drug and used it for the treatment of Mutraghata and Kushta. Sushrut has included Varahi among the ashtadasha soma sadrishvirya oushada and describes that it has the potency to regenerate and look like a black snake (S.S.Ci. 30/13). Varahyadi ghrita is used for bastikarma in yoni rogas.

Commercially, Varahi is an important drug as it is a good source of starch, used in poultry, livestock feed, and production of yam flour. The steroidal sapogenins and diosgenin are used as precursors for the synthesis of steroidal hormones and contraceptive drugs. Bulbils are used as hunting poison and tubers as fishing poison. But the tubers should be used cautiously as food because they may possess some toxic components such as diosbulbins.

Vernacular Names

Assamese: Kathalu, Patni-alu
Bengali: Ratalu, Banalu
Gujarati: Dukkarkanda, Goradu
Kannada: Kunta Genusu, Heggenusu
Konkani: Kongadde
Malayalam: Varahi, Kattu, Kachil
Marathi: Dukarkanda, Manakund
Oriya: Jhonka alu

Punjabi: Zamin khand
Tamil: Kodikilangu, Pannukilangu
Telugu: Kaya Pendazam, Chedupaddu dumpa

Synonyms

Varda: It enhances physical strength and stamina.
Varahvadana: The tuber externally is rough and resembles the surface of pig.
Grishti: The tuber is irregular in shape.
Charmakaraluka: The surface of the tuber is rough and leathery.

Classical Categorization

Charaka Samhita: Not mentioned
Sushrut Samhita: Not mentioned
Ashtang Hridaya: Not mentioned
Dhanvantari Nighantu: Karviradi varga
Madanpal Nighantu: Abhyadi varga, Shaka varga
Kaiyadev Nighantu: Oushadi varga
Raj Nighantu: Mulakadi varga
Bhavaprakash Nighantu: Guduchyadi varga

Distribution

It is found throughout India ascending up to 1,800 m in the Himalayas, Chota Nagpur Plateau, Bihar, Orissa, and West coast and East coast districts. It is also widely cultivated in the Konkan region.

Morphology

It is a dextrorotatory glabrous climbing herb, 5 to 10 m long with perennial tuberous roots. Stem green, coiled, with longitudinal lines on it (**Fig. 102.1**).

- **Leaves:** Simple, alternate, with 1 to 3 inch long petiole, cordate shape with a deep notch, 2 to 6 inch long, 1 to 4 inch width, prominent 7 to 9 veins, entire margin, acuminate or caudate apex, glaucous surface (**Fig. 102.2**).
- **Flowers:** Separate male and female inflorescence on the same plant. Flowers are axillary, white-colored flowers, pendulous 4 to 10 inch long.
- **Fruits:** Quadrately oblong triquetrous capsule, found attached opposite to petiole. Seeds winged at one end, two per locule (**Fig. 102.3**).
- **Tuber:** Underground, solitary, variable in size, globose-pyriform shape, purplish black externally, internally yellow, clothed with thick fibrous secondary roots, and mucilaginous (**Fig. 102.4**).

The plant is propagated by seed and vegetative methods.

Phenology

Flowering time: August to October
Fruiting time: November to December

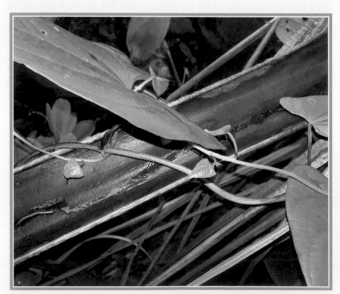

Fig. 102.1 Stem.

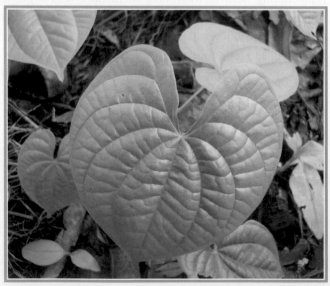

Fig. 102.2 Leaves.

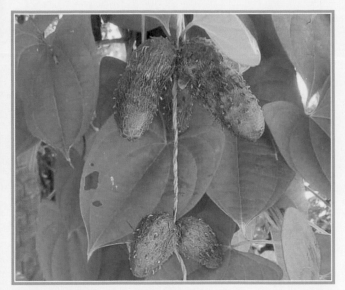

Fig. 102.3 Fruits.

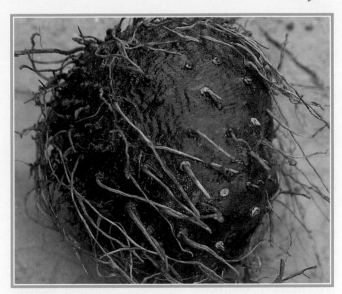

Fig. 102.4 Tuber.

Key Characters for Identification

➤ *A glabrous climbing herb with perennial tuberous roots.*

➤ *Leaves are simple, alternate, cordate shape, with prominent 7 to 9 veins.*

➤ *Flowers are axillary, white, pendulous, male female in separate inflorescence.*

➤ *Fruits are quadrately oblong triquetrous capsule.*

➤ *Tuber is solitary, variable in size, globose, black externally, internally yellow.*

Types

None

Rasapanchaka

Guna	Laghu, Snigdh
Rasa	Madhur, Tikta
Vipaka	Madhur, Kaiyadev N. Katu vipaka
Virya	Sheet

Chemical Constituents

Studies revealed the presence of alkaloids (acetophenone, diosbulbinosides D, G, F, dihydrodioscorine, penogenin), glycosides, proteins, fats, starch, sterols (daucosterol, β-sitosterol, stigmasterol), polyphenols, tannins (catechin, protocatechuic acid, epicatechin), flavonoids (quercetin, kaempferol, myricetin), steroidal sapogenin, spirostane glycosides, cholestane glycosides, diosbulbisin A–D, diosbulbisides A–C, diosgenin, sinodiosgenin, diosbulbins A–P, dioscoreanoside A–K (steroidal saponins), and fatty acids (Galani and Patel 2017).

Identity, Purity, and Strength

- Foreign matter: Not more than 2%
- Total ash: Not more than 6%
- Acid-insoluble ash: Not more than 1%
- Alcohol-soluble extractive: Not less than 3%
- Water-soluble extractive: Not less than 9%

(Source: The Ayurvedic Pharmacopeia of India 2004)

Karma (Actions)

Classical texts have attributed vrishya (aphrodisiac), ayushya (enhances life expectancy), swarya (promotes voice), varnya (complexion promoter), balya (tonic), hridaya (cardiac tonic), rasayana (rejuvinator), agnivardhak (enhances digestive fire), anulomana (laxative), mutral (diuretic), krimighna (anthelmintic), kusthaghna (antidermatosis), and raktashodhaka (blood purifier) properties to it.

- Doshakarma: Kapha vatahara
- Dhatukarma: Rasayana
- Malakarma: Anuloman, mutral

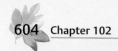

Pharmacological Actions

Several studies suggested its purgative, aphrodisiac, rejuvenating, tonic, anthelmintic, antioxidant, anti-HIV, cardioprotective, neuroprotective, antibacterial, antifungal, anticancer, hepatoprotective, antistress, diuretic, and immunomodulatory properties (Galani and Patel 2017).

Indications

The tuber is used traditionally for the treatment of kushta (skin diseases), prameha (diabetes), and krimi (worm infestation), kandu (pruritus), nadivrana (wounds), klaibya (impotency), daurbalya (general debility), shool (pain), raktavikara (blood-borne diseases), gandmala (goiter). Tuber is also used in hemoptysis, pyogenic infections, scrofula, syphilis, hemorrhoids, flatulence, diarrhea, dysentery, and polyuria.

Therapeutic Uses

External Use

1. **Nadi vrana** (sinus): Tubers are made into decoction, emulsified in oil, then applied on infected ulcers, sinus, and pus pockets (S.S.Ci. 17/36).
2. **Vrana** (wounds): The dried powdered tuber is applied externally on ulcers.

Internal Use

1. **Rasayana** (rejuvenator): Powder of Varahikand mixed with madhu is taken with milk for a month as a health tonic and rejuvenator. During this period, person should take only ghrita, dugdha, and boiled rice in diet (S.S.Ci. 27/11).
2. **Bandhayatva** (infertility): Powder of Vidarikand, Varahikand, Ashwagandha, and Shatavari churna in equal quantity should be taken with milk and ghee twice daily in infertility.
3. **Dourbalya** (debility): Powder of Varahikand, Ashwagandha, Mulethi, Mishri in equal quantity with milk twice daily is used in Dourbalya.

Officinal Part Used

Tuber

Dose

Powder: 3 to 6 g

Formulations

Narasimha churna, Panchnimba churna, Vastyamayantaka ghrita, Shiva gutika.

Toxicity/Adverse Effects

Acute, subacute, and chronic toxicity study of *Dioscorea bulbifera* on mice showed hepatotoxicity, renal toxicity, nausea, abdominal pain, coma, and even death (Li et al 2005; Su et al 2003).

Substitution and Adulteration

Varahikanda is used as a substitute drug for Riddhi and Vriddhi of Ashtavarga (B.P.S. 1/166). Tubers of *Tacca aspera* Roxb. and *Dioscorea pentaphylla* are reported to be used as Varahikand in some regions (Sharma et al 2001).

Points to Ponder

- *Varahikanda is a well-known adaptogenic, reproductive tonic drug.*
- *It is prescribed in infertility, general debility, skin diseases, diabetes, blood-borne diseases, tuberculosis, and tumors.*

Suggested Readings

Galani VJ, Patel DM. A comprehensive phytopharmacological review of *Dioscorea bulbifera* Linn. Int J Environ Sci Natur Res 2017;45(5): 1–11

Li YJ, Liu SM, Luo MM, Liu HF. The express and principle study of liver toxicity of *Dioscorea bulbifera* L. Zhongguo Shiyan Fangjixue Zazhi 2005;11:40–42

Sharma PC, Yelne MB, Dennis TJ. Database on Medicinal Plants Used in Ayurveda. C.C.R.A.S. Department of Indian Systems of Medicine and Homeopathy (ISM&H), Ministry of Health and Family Welfare, Government of India 2001;2:531–536

Su L, Zhu JH, Cheng LB. Experimental pathological study of subacute intoxication by *Dioscorea bulbifera* L. Fa Yi Xue Za Zhi 2003;19(2): 81–83

The Ayurvedic Pharmacopeia of India, Part I, Vol. 4. New Delhi: Department of AYUSH, Ministry of Health and Family Welfare, Government of India; 2004:153

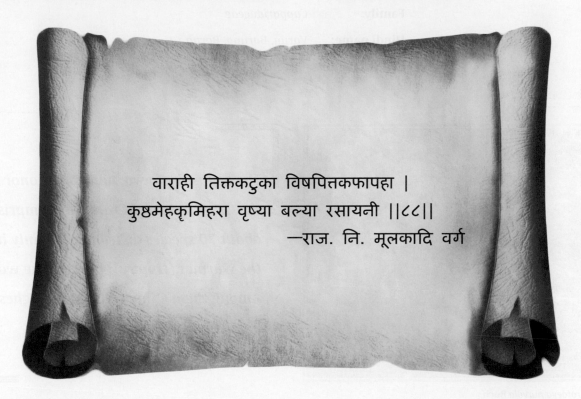

वाराही तिक्तकटुका विषपित्तकफापहा ।
कुष्ठमेहकृमिहरा वृष्या बल्या रसायनी ॥८८॥
—राज. नि. मूलकादि वर्ग

103. Varuna *[Crataeva nurvala Buch.]*

Family: *Capparidaceae*

Hindi name: *Varun, Baruna, Barna*

English name: *Three-leaved creeper*

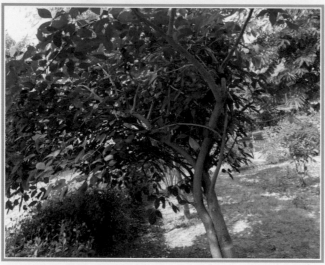

Plant of *Crataeva nurvala* Buch.

The genus Crataeva, named in honor of the Greek botanist Crataevas comprises about 70 species distributed mainly in the warmer (tropical) parts of the world. Among them C. nurvala shows highest biodiversity in India.

Introduction

Crataeva nurvala (*C. nurvala*) Buch-Ham (Family: Capparidaceae), commonly known as Varuna, is an evergreen tree indigenous to India. It is a medium-sized, branched, deciduous plant distributed throughout the river banks of southern India and other tropical, subtropical countries of the world, wild or cultivated. It requires dry, hot climate and shady places to grow effectively. The whole plant possesses high medicinal value and traditionally is used in treating various ailments in human beings. The plant is used internally as well as externally. Varuna is one of the best litholytic herbs and has been used throughout the ages for the treatment of urolithiasis and crystalluria. Varuna is mentioned in Vedic literature, its therapeutic use being known to ancient Ayurvedic physicians, especially as a blood purifier, to maintain homeostasis.

Vernacular Names

Bengali: Varuna

Gujarati: Vayvarno, Varano

Kannada: Bipatri, Mattamavu, Neervalamara, Bitusi, Holenekki, Holethumbe, Maavilanga, Naaram bele, Vitasi, Sethu bandhana, Vaayu varuna, Nervaala

Kashmiri: Kath

Malayalam: Neermatalam

Marathi: Vayavarna, Haravarna, Varon, Karvan, Kumla, Nirvala, Ramala, Varun

Oriya: Baryno

Punjabi: Barna, Barnahi

Tamil: Maralingam, Mavilingam, Narvala, Varanam

Telugu: Ulimidi, Bilvaram, Chinnavulimidi, Maagalingam, Maaredu, Peddamaagalingam, Peddavulimidi, Thellavulimidi

Synonyms

Ashmarighna: It removes urinary calculus.
Bahupushpa: It is covered with flowers.
Kumaraka: The leaflets are glabrous.
Tiktashaka: It is bitter in taste.
Triparna: It has three leaflets
Varun/Varan: It is useful in gulma.
Vruntaphala: Fruits are found on axillary end of leaf.

Classical Categorization

Charaka Samhita: Not mentioned in any varga
Sushruta Samhita: Varunadi
Ashtanga Hridaya: Varunadi
Dhanwantari Nighantu: Amradi varga
Madanpal Nighantu: Vatadi varga
Kaiyadev Nighantu: Aushadi varga
Raj Nighantu: Prabhadradi varga
Bhavaprakash Nighantu: Vatadi varga

Distribution

Varuna is often cultivated throughout India, especially along the streams and river banks. It is distributed in sub-Himalayan tracts and is indigenous to Tamil Nadu, Kerala, and Karnataka. It is found in abundance in Kerala, Madhya Pradesh, Bengal, and Assam.

Morphology

It is moderately sized deciduous tree.

- **Bark:** 5 to 15 mm thickness, outer surface gray to grayish brown, rough, many small and rounded lenticels. Inner surface-smooth, whitish-brown (**Fig. 103.1a, b**).
- **Leaves:** Trifoliate, leaflets ovate, lanceolate or obovate, glabrous on both surfaces (**Fig. 103.2**).
- **Flower:** White to milky-white, 5 to 8 cm in diameter, polygamous, and fragrant in dense terminal corymbs, stamens spreading longer than the petals, gynophore about 5 cm long (**Fig. 103.3**).
- **Fruit:** Fleshy, ovoid berry with a hard rough rind, 2.5 cm in diameter, brown seeds are embedded in the yellow fleshy pulp of the fruit (**Fig. 103.4**).

Phenology

Flowering time: February to April
Fruiting time: June to August

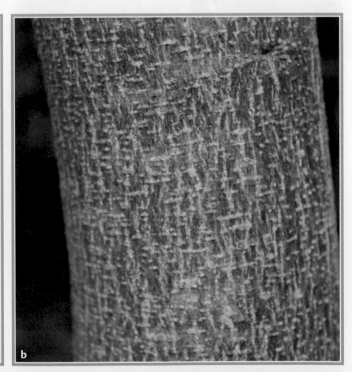

Fig. 103.1 (a) Bark. **(b)** Stem.

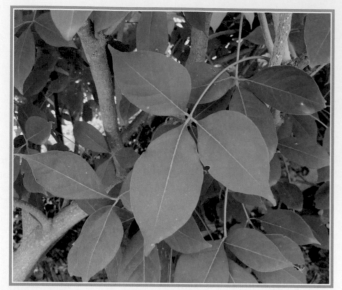

Fig. 103.2 Leaves.

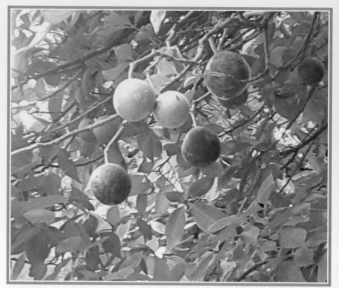

Fig. 103.4 Fruits.

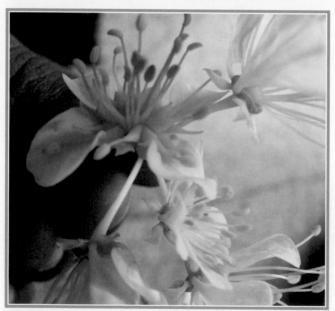

Fig. 103.3 Flower.

Key Characters for Identification

➤ *Moderately sized deciduous tree*
➤ *Bark: 5 to 15 mm thick, grayish brown, rough with many small and rounded lenticels.*
➤ *Leaves: Trifoliate, leaflets ovate, lanceolate or obovate, glabrous on both surfaces.*
➤ *Flower: White or cream colored.*
➤ *Fruit: Fruits have multiple seeds and ovoid berries, 2.5 cm in diameter, and seeds are embedded in the yellow, fleshy pulp of the fruits.*

Rasapanchaka

Guna	Laghu, Ruksha
Rasa	Tikta, Kasaya, Madhura
Vipaka	Katu
Virya	Ushna
Prabhav	Asmarighna

Chemical Constituents

- *C. nurvala* is found to be rich in alkaloids, flavonoids, glucosinolates, phytosterols, saponins, triterpenoids. A wide variety of medicinally important compounds have been reported from *C. nurvala*.
- Fruit: 12-tricosanone, ceryl alcohol, cetyl, friedelin, glucocapparin, n-pentadecane, octanamide, pentadecane, triacontane, triacontanol, β-sitosterol.
- Leaves: Dodecanoic anhydride, glucocapparin , kaempferol-o-α-d-glucoside, L-stachydrine, methyl pentacosanoate, quercitin-3-0-α-D-glucoside.
- Root bark: Alkaloids, betulinic acid, cadabicine diacetate, ceryl alcohol, diosgenin, flavonoids, friedelin, glucosinolates, lupeol and its acetate, phytosterols, quercetin, rutin, saponins, triterpenoids, varunol, and β-sitosterol.
- Stem bark: Betulinic acid, cadabicine diacetate, cadabicine, ceryl alcohol, crataemine, crataenoside,

diosgenin, friedelin, isoquercetin, lupeol and its acetate, quercetin, rutin (Ghani 2003; Khattar and Wal 2013; Bhattacharjee and Shashidhara 2012).

Identity, Purity, and Strength

- Foreign matter: Not more than 2%
- Total ash: Not more than 13%
- Acid-insoluble ash: Not more than 1%
- Alcohol-soluble extractive: Not less than 1%
- Water-soluble extractive: Not less than 8%

(Source: The Ayurvedic Pharmacopeia of India 1990)

Karma (Actions)

Bhedan (cholagogue), deepan (appetizer), laxative, krimighana (anthelmintic), vermicide.

- Doshakarma: Kaphavatahara, Pittavardhaka
- Dhatukarma: Raktashodhak
- Malakarma: Bhedana, Mutral

Pharmacological Actions

The pharmacological actions of *C. nurvala* are analgesic, antiarthritic, antidiabetes, antiarthritic, anticancer, antidiarrheal, antifertility, anti-inflammatory, antinociceptive, antiprotozoal, cardioprotective, hepatoprotective, hyperoxaluria, nephroprotective, urolithic, and wound-healing activities (Khattar and Wal 2013; Bhattacharjee and Shashidhara 2012). Leaves are bitter, acrid, thermogenic, stomachic, depurative, demulcent, anti-inflammatory, tonic, antiperiodic, and expectorant.

Indications

It is used in asmari (urinary calculus), gulma (abdominal lump), mutrakicchra (dysuria), vidradhi (abscess), vatarakta (gout), krimi (worm infestation). The skin, roots, and leaves of Varuna have great medicinal value. The plant is used internally as well as externally. It is externally applied to abscess, boils, carbuncles, and lymphadenopathy. They are used in flatulence, emesis, indigestion, obesity, and are externally applied as poultice over boils, carbuncles, abscess, and scrofula. The decoction of root or bark is beneficial in urinary calculus, dysuria, and cystitis. It is useful in anorexia,

tumors, liver diseases, flatulent, dyspepsia, helminthiasis, gout, internal abscess, and obesity.

Contraindications

No contraindications noted ever.

Therapeutic Uses

1. **Ashmari** (urinary calculus): Decoction of root bark of Varuna is given with jaggery to expel out the calculus and alleviate pain in pelvis (VM-34/26).
2. **Vidradhi** (abscess): Decoction of root of white Punarnava and Varuna should be taken to control the unripe abscess (VM-43/12).
3. **Gandamala** (cervical lymphadenitis): Decoction of Varuna root with honey destroys gandamala even if chronic (VM-41/18).
4. **Visarpa** (erysipelas): Drugs of Varunadi Gana should be given in all measures.
5. **Arsha** (piles): Decoction of Varuna leaves is useful as tub-bath for the patient with piles (ch.ch. 14/45, 46).
6. **Freckles:** Varuna bark pounded with goat's milk destroys freckles (CD. 55.52).
7. **Kikkisa** (striae gravidarum): Kikkisa is destroyed by rubbing of cow-dung at first then anointed with the paste of Varuna leaves (RM. 31.41).
8. **Pediatric disorders:** The Varuna kwatha is sprinkled in child suffering with putana graham (SS.U. 32.3).

Officinal Parts Used

Bark and leaf

Dose

Decoction: 50 to 100 mL
Powder: 1 to 2 g

Formulations

Varunadi taila, Varunadi ghrita, Varunadi kwath, Kanchanara guggulu, Manjistadyarista, Mahamanjishthadyaristha, Ashmarihara kashaya.

Toxicity/Adverse Effects

Topical application of the leaves of *C. nurvala* was reported to cause redness and blistering in rodents. The decoctions of the root bark and stem bark appear to be well tolerated. The LD50 of 50% ethanolic extract of stem bark was found to be more than 1,000 mg/kg i.p. to adult rats (Bhakuni et al 1971). No toxic effects have been seen on the human body with *C. nurvala*.

Substitution and Adulteration

Leaves of *Corchorus capsularis* Linn. (Tiliaceae) are adulterated with leaves of *C. nurvala* Buch. Ham (Sharma et al 2000).

Points to Ponder

- *Varuna is an effective drug for urinary calculus and internal abscess.*

Suggested Readings

Bhakuni DS, Dhar ML, Dhar MM, Dhawan BN, Gupta B, Srimal RC. Screening of Indian plants for biological activity. Indian J Exp Biol 1971;9(1):91–102

Bhattacharjee A, Shashidhara SC, Narayana A. Phytochemical and ethno-pharmacological profile of *Crataeva nurvala* Buch-Hum (Varuna): a review. Asian Pac J Trop Biomed 2012;8:S1162–S1168

Ghani A. Medicinal Plants of Bangladesh with Chemical Constituents and Uses. 2nd ed. Dhaka: Asiatic Society of Bangladesh; 2003:184

Khattar V, Wal A. Utilities of *Crataeva nurvala*. Int J Pharm Pharm Sci 2012;4(Suppl 4):21–26

Lucas DS. Dravyaguna-Vijnana: Study of Dravya-Materia Medica. Varanasi: Chaukhamba Visvabharati; 2013:32

Sharma PC, Yelne MB, Dennis TJ. Database Medicinal Plants Used in Ayurveda, Vol. 2. New Delhi: CCRAS; 2000

Sharma PV. Classical Uses of Medicinal Plants. 1st ed. Varanasi: Chaukhamba Vishvabharati; 2004:338

The Ayurvedic Pharmacopoeia of India, Part I, Vol. I. 1st ed. New Delhi: Department of Health, Ministry of Health and Family Welfare, Government of India; 1990:159

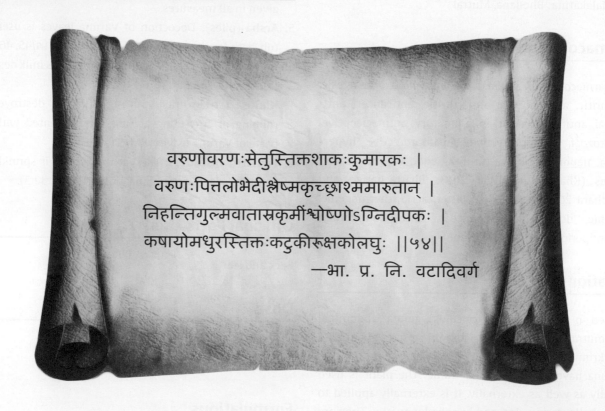

वरुणोवरणःसेतुस्तिक्तशाकःकुमारकः |
वरुणःपित्तलोभेदीश्लेष्मकृच्छ्राश्ममारुतान् |
निहन्तिगुल्मवातास्रकृमींश्चोष्णोऽग्निदीपकः |
कषायोमधुरस्तिक्तःकटुकीरूक्षकोलघुः ||५४||
—भा. प्र. नि. वटादिवर्ग

104. Vasa [*Adhatoda vasica* Nees.]

Family: *Acanthaceae*

Hindi name: *Vasa, Adusa, Arusa*

English name: *Malabar nut, Vasaka*

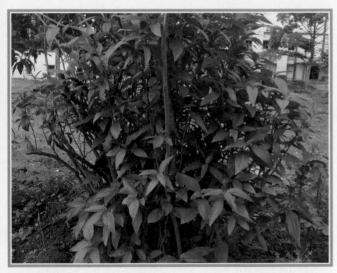

Plant of *Adhatoda vasica* Nees.

Vasa cure kasa and swasa by maintaining the equilibrium of dhosha, dhatu, and malas.

Introduction

Adhatoda vasica (Nees) of family Acanthaceae, known commonly as Malabar nut tree, is a shrub growing throughout the India. It is a well-known drug used for respiratory tract disorders in both Ayurvedic and Unani systems of medicine (Chopra et al 1956; Kapoor 2001). In Ayurvedic preparations, Vasaka leaf juice (Vasa swarasa) is incorporated in more than 20 formulations (Sharma et al 2000). The frequent use of *A. vasica* has resulted in its inclusion in the WHO manual: *The Use of Traditional Medicine in Primary Health Care* (WHO 1990).

Adhatoda is the Malabari name of Vasa and vasica means fragrant or aromatic derived from the Sanskrit name *vasak* (means fragrant).

Vernacular Names

Assamese: Titabahak, Bahak, Vachaka

Bengali: Baksa, Vasaka

Gujarati: Aduso, Ardusi, Adulso

Kannada: Adsale, Adusoge, Atarusha, Adsole, Adasale

Kashmiri: Vasa

Malayalam: Attalatakam, Atalotakam

Marathi: Vasa, Adulsa

Oriya: Basanga

Punjabi: Bhekar, Vansa, Arusa

Tamil: Vasambu, Adathodai

Telugu: Addasaramu

Urdu: Adusa, Basa

Synonyms

Aaatarusha/Atarushaka/Atarusha: The herb is a useful drug which alleviates various diseases.

Bhisangmata: It protects all like a mother .

Dantasatvapradayi: Provides strength to teeth.

Kaphaha: It relieves kapha.

Karkasha: The leaves are minutely pubescent.

Kasanoptatana: It is useful in kasa (cough).

Mata: Supports the patients like a mother.

Raktamutrajit: Relieves the passing of blood in urine or hematuria.

Raktapittaprasadani: It is useful in raktapitta or epistaxis.

Sinhasya: The flowers look like open mouth of a lion.

Sinhika: It is useful in many diseases.

Vajidanta: The flowers are white like the teeth of horse.

Vasadani: It is helpful in the treatment of obesity.

Vasaka/Vasa: The plant grows in plenty and covers the ground with dense foliage.

Vrusha: The flowers have profuse nectar.

Classical Categorization

Charaka Samhita: Tikta skanda

Sushruta Samhita: Tikta skanda, Shakavarga

Ashtanga Hridaya: Viratarvadi gana, Sarivadi gana

Dhanwantari Nighantu: Guduchyadi varga

Madanpal Nighantu: Abhayadi varga

Kaiyadev Nighantu: Aushadhi varga

Raj Nighantu: Shatahwadi varga

Bhavaprakash Nighantu: Guduchyadi varga

Distribution

It is distributed throughout India up to an altitude of 1,300 m especially in sub-Himalayan region.

Morphology

It is a perennial evergreen shrub of 3 to 4 ft in height.

- **Leaves:** Simple, stipulate, 10 to 20 cm long and 3 to 10 cm broad, lanceolate to ovate in shape, alternate, entire margin, acute apex, hairy, light green above, dark below and leathery (**Fig. 104.1**).
- **Flowers:** White with red or yellow barred throats, in short dense axillary peduncle spikes with large bracts (**Fig. 104.2**).
- **Fruit:** Capsules are clavate, longitudinally channeled, 1.9 to 2.2 cm × 0.8 cm and seeds are globular (Anonymous 2005; **Fig. 104.3**).

It is propagated by seeds and stem cutting.

Phenology

Flowering time: Throughout the year

Fruiting time: August to January

Key Characters for Identification
➤ *A perennial evergreen shrub of 3 to 4 ft in height.*
➤ *Leaves: Simple, lanceolate to ovate in shape, alternate, entire margin, hairy, light green above, dark below, and leathery.*
➤ *Flowers: White with red or yellow barred throats.*
➤ *Fruit: Capsules are clavate, longitudinally channeled.*

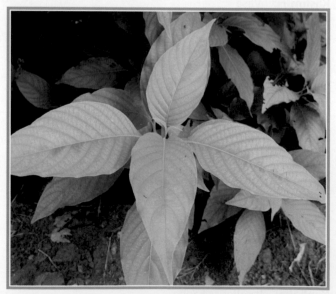

Fig. 104.1 Leaves.

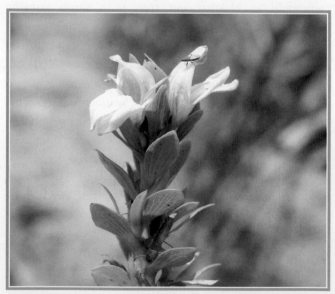

Fig. 104.2 Flowers.

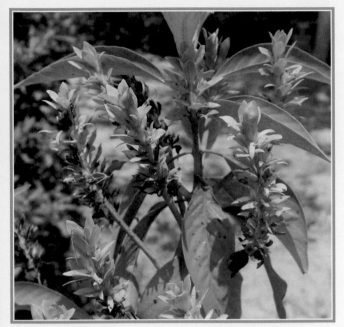

Fig. 104.3 Fruits.

Rasapanchaka

Guna	Ruksha, Laghu
Rasa	Tikta, Kasaya
Vipaka	Katu
Virya	Sheeta

Chemical Constituents

The leaves are the rich source of alkaloids of which vasicine and vasicinone are bioactive. A non-nitrogenous neutral principle, vasakin, vasicinone, two new quinazoline alkaloids, one of which was named as adhvasinone, and two new pyrroloquinoline alkaloids, desmethoxyaniflorine and 7-methoxyvasicinone, were identified from the ethanolic extract of the leaves (Anonymous 2004).

Identity, Purity, and Safety

- Foreign matter: Not more than 2%
- Total ash: Not more than 21%
- Acid-insoluble ash: Not more than 1%

- Alcohol-soluble extractive: Not less than 3%
- Water-soluble extractive: Not less than 22%

(Source: The Ayurvedic Pharmacopeia of India 2004)

Karma (Actions)

The actions of Vasa are hridya (cardiotonic), kaphapittahara (pacify kapha and pitta), raktasangrahika (reduce bleeding), kasaghna (anticough), kushtaghna (cures skin disorder), jvarhara (antipyretic), chhardighna (antiemetic), shoolahara (analgesic).

- Doshakarma: Kaphapittahara
- Dhatukarma: Raktasangrahika

Pharmacological Actions

It also has antitussive, bronchodilator, respiratory stimulant, antibacterial, antiulcer, anti-inflammatory, hepatoprotective, antioxidant, antispasmodic, hypotensive, hypoglycemic, uterine stimulant, antiviral, antiseptic, and antibacterial properties. Vasicine also showed cardiac depressant, uterotonic, and abortifacient activities. Vasicinone showed antianaphylactic, bronchoconstrictor (in vivo), and bronchodilator (in vitro) activities. It is weak cardiac stimulant, antitussive, anticonvulsant, and antiarrhythmic (Sharma et al 2000; Nagarajan et al 2017).

Indications

It is used in svasa and kasa (respiratory diseases like cough and asthma), raktapitta (internal hemorrhage), jvara (fever), chhardi (vomiting), meha (diabetes), kushta (skin diseases), shoola (spasmodic pain), kshaya (tuberculosis), kamala (jaundice), and trishna (thirst). The leaves, flowers, fruits, and roots are extensively used for treating cold, cough, whooping cough, chronic bronchitis, and asthma, as it has sedative, expectorant, and antispasmodic properties. It relieves the irritable cough by its soothing action on the nerves and by liquefying the sputum which makes expectoration easier. It is also used in diarrhea, bleeding dysentery, hemoptysis, bleeding piles, hemorrhage, joint pain, burning sensation, acidity, skin diseases, and vitiated pitta conditions.

Therapeutic Uses

External Use

Tvak roga (skin disease): Tender leaves of Vasa are mixed with Haridra and pounded with cow's urine. Application of this paste destroys scabies in three days (VM.52.40).

Internal Use

1. **Jwara** (fever caused by pitta and kapha): Juice of Vasa leaves mixed with sugar and honey alleviates fever caused by pitta and kapha, intrinsic hemorrhage, and jaundice (As Ci. 1.92; also VM. 1.127). Decoction of Vasa, Kantakari, and Guduchi mixed with honey alleviates fever and cough. Similarly, decoction of Kantakari mixed with Pippali powder checks cough (SG. 2.2.82 also BP.Ci. 1.384). Ghee cooked with Vasa or Bala or Guduchi is useful in chronic fever, edema, and anemia (SS.U. 39.234; also Ah.Ci. 1.93).

2. **Raktapitta** (intrinsic hemorrhage): Vasaghrta is given in raktapitta (CS.Ci. 4.88; AH.Ci. 2.40-42). Vasa is the best remedy for intrinsic hemorrhage (AH.U. 40.49). Juice of Vasa checks intrinsic hemorrhage (AH. Ci. 2.24-25; also VM.9.8). Juice or decoction of Vasa alone or mixed sugar and honey checks hemorrhage immediately as it is an excellent remedy for this (A.H.Ci. 2.24-25; also VM. 9.8). Vasa mixed with Talisa powder and honey should be taken. It alleviates kapha, pitta and cough, bronchial asthma, hoarseness of voice, and intrinsic hemorrhage (VM. 9.12). Haritaki impregnated with juice of Vasa seven times or Pippali taken with honey checks intrinsic hemorrhage immediately (VM. 9.22). Powder of Vasa flower dried in shade should be taken with honey (SB. 4.340).

3. **Kasa and svasa** (cough and asthma): Cold infusion of Vasa checks cough, intrinsic hemorrhage, and fever (SG. 2.4.7). Powder of Haridra cooked with Vasa juice and taken with fatty layer of milk checks dry cough (SB. 4.333). Vasakaghrta is also given in kasa and swasa (SS. U.51.20).

4. **Shosha** (consumption): Vasaghrta (SS.U. 41.43) and Vasavaleha (BP.Ci. 11.55-57) are given to treat shosha.

5. **Gulma** (abdominal lump): Vasaghrta (CS.Ci. 5. 126-27) is administered.

6. **Kushta** (skin diseases): Vasa and Triphala are useful as internal administration, bath, ointment, and paste (CS.Ci. 7.128). Vasa, Kutaja, Saptarna, Karavira, Karanja, Nimba, and Khadira mixed with cow's urine are used as bath, intake, and paste. It cures worm infestation and kushta (CS.Ci. 7.158).

7. **Vatavyadhi** (neuromuscular disease): Vasamuladi taila (CS.Ci. 28.170-71) is useful. One should take decoction of Vasa, Shunthi, and Aragvadha mixed with castor oil. It is useful in sciatica.

8. **Rasayan** (rejuvenation): Oil cooked with the decoction of Vasa root should be taken. It promotes intellect and life span.

9. **Chhardi** (vomiting): Vasa is an excellent remedy for vomiting, cough, and intrinsic hemorrhage (AH.SU. 6.80).

10. **Masurika** (pox): In kapha type, juice of Vasa should be given with honey.

11. **Mutraghata** (retention of urine): Decoction of Duralabha or Vasa should be given (GN. 2.28.32.)

12. **Mukha roga** (disease of mouth): Like rasanjana, semisolid extract of Vasa, Patola, Nimba, Madhuyasti, Irimeda, Khadira, Jati, and Triphala should be prepared and used (AH.U. 22.106).

Officinal Parts Used

Leaves, root, flowers

Dose

Flower/Leaf juice: 10 to 20 mL
Root decoction: 40 to 80 mL or 10 to 20 g of the dried drug for decoction

Formulations

Vasavleha, Vasakhand, KantakariVasa avleha Vasarishta, Vasakantakari leha, Rasnadi Kvatha, Punarnavasava, Ashokarishta, Bhagottara churna, Darvayadi Kvatha, Kumaryasava, Mahatiktaka ghrita, Patangasava, Triphala ghrita, Vasakasava, Adusa kshara, Bhagottara gutika, Devedarvadyarishta, Kanakasava, Kasamrita, Maharasnadi Kvatha, Mahamanjishthadyarishta, Panchatikta ghrita guggulu, Panchatikta ghrita, Vasadhya Ghrita, Mahatriphalaghrita, Vasachandanadi taila, Vasaharitakyavaleha.

Toxicity/Adverse Effects

Vasicinone is reported as safe in mice in acute toxicity study. The acute and chronic toxicity studies revealed the use of vasicine and vasicinone as comparatively safe. The alcoholic extract of leaves is reported to be poisonous to flies, fleas, mosquitoes, centipedes, and other insects (Sharma et al 2000).

Substitution and Adulteration

Another species of Adhatoda like *Adhatoda beddomei* C.B.Cl. is commonly used as substitute in Kerala. *Ailanthus excelsa* Roxb. has been found to be a common adulterant of Vasaka leaves (Sharma et al 2000).

Points to Ponder

- *Vasa is the best medicine for raktapitta.*
- *It is mainly used in kasa, swasa, kshaya, and raktapitta.*
- *The primary alkaloid constituents of Adhatoda are vasicine and vasicinone.*

Suggested Readings

Anonymous. Review on Indian Medicinal Plants, Vol. I. New Delhi: Indian Council of Medical Research; 2004:258

Anonymous. The Wealth of India: Raw Materials, Vol. I. Revised ed. New Delhi: CSIR; 2005:76. Atal

Chopra RN, Nayar SL, Chopra IC. Glossary of Indian Medicinal Plants. New Delhi, India: Council of Scientific and Industrial Research; 1956

Kapoor LD. Handbook of Ayurvedic Medicinal Plants. Boca Raton, FL: CRC Press; 2001:416–417

Nagarajan K, Shanmugham UK, Natarajan K, Thiyagarajan B, Sekkizhar G. Panchatiktam kwatha churna: an Ayurvedic medicine. Int J Curr Res 2017;9(10):59686–59693

Sarita MK, Patil AB. *Adhatoda vasica*: a critical review. Int J Green Pharm 2017;11(4):S654–S662

Sharma PC, Yelne MB, Dennis TJ, eds. Database on Medicinal Plants Used in Ayurveda, Vol. I. New Delhi: Central Council of Research in Ayurveda and Siddha, Department of Indian System of Medicine and Homeopathy, Ministry of Health and Family Welfare (Government of India); 2000:496–509

The Ayurvedic Pharmacopeia of India, Part 1, Vol 1. New Delhi: Department of AYUSH, Ministry of Health & Family Welfare, Government of India; 2004:173–174

World Health Organization. The Use of Traditional Medicine in Primary Health Care: A Manual for Health Workers in South-East Asia. SEARO Regional Health Papers, No 19. New Delhi: World Health Organization; 1990:1–2

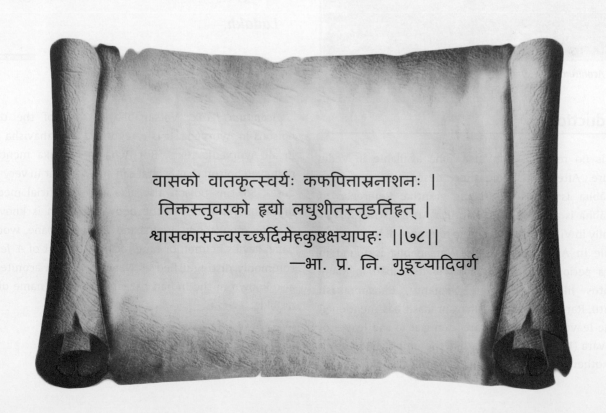

वासको वातकृत्स्वर्यः कफपित्तास्रनाशनः |
तिक्तस्तुवरको हृद्यो लघुशीतस्तृडर्तिहृत् |
श्वासकासज्वरच्छर्दिमेहकुष्ठक्षयापहः ||७८||
—भा. प्र. नि. गुडूच्यादिवर्ग

105. Vatsanabha *[Aconitum ferox Wall.]*

Family:	*Ranunculaceae*
Hindi name:	*Bachnag, Meethavish, Bisa, Teliya Bish*
English name:	*Indian aconite, Monk's hood*

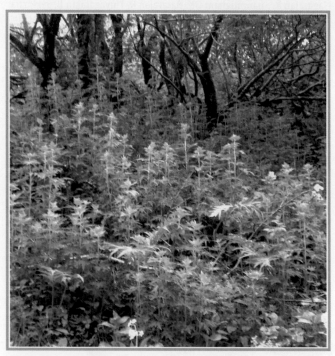

Plant of *Aconitum ferox* Wall.

In the tenth century, the Persian physician Alheroo described the plant under the name bish. Europeans first became aware of Aconitum ferox in the nineteenth century during journeys to Nepal. During the nineteenth century, there was a thriving trade in the root tubers of Aconitum ferox, which were brought from Lhasa via Le (Mustang) to Ladakh.

Introduction

There is no reference of Vatsanābha available in Vedic literature. After the Vedic time, description regarding Vatsanābha is found in Viṣṇus grantha. Reference of Vatsanābha is also found in Kauṭīlya Arthaśāstra (35/12), especially in Viṣavarga. There is no reference of Vatsanābha available in Amarkosha. Use of Vatsanābha is found in Samhita period and it is elaborately described in many Nighantus like Dhanwantari Nighantu, Bhavaprakash Nighantu, Raj Nighantu, etc. Bhavaprakash has mentioned that the leaves of this plant are identical to the leaves of sindhuvara (Nirgundi). It looks like the umbilicus of a calf and no other plant would survive near this plant.

Aconitum ferox (Vatsanabha) is one of the deadly poisons in Ayurveda. It is categorized in mahavisha varga in all Ayurvedic texts. But Acharya Charaka mentioned that even poison that is fatal can act as nectar in very small doses. So, this poison also acts as a beneficial medicine in various ailments of the body. Aconitum is known as aconite, monkshood, wolfsbane, leopard's bane, women's bane, devil's helmet, or blue rocket. The root of *A. ferox* is commonly distinguished as Nepal or Indian aconite. It is also known in the Indian bazaars under the name of Bish or Bikh.

Vernacular Names

Assamese: Mithavish, Bish
Bengali: Kathavish
Gujarati: Vachhanaag, Basanaag
Kannada: Basanalli, Vatsanabha, Vatsanabhi, Vachanaga
Malayalam: Vatsanabhi
Marathi: Bachnaga
Oriya: Tahara, Mahura, Mithvisa
Punjabi: Mitha Visha, Mithatelia
Sanskrit: Amra, Visa Vajranaga, Sthavaravisa, Vatsanagaka
Tamil: Vasanaavi, Vatsanabhi, Nabhi, Vasanabhi
Telugu: Vatsanaabhi, Naabhi
Urdu: Bachnak, Mithalelia, Beesh, Atees

Synonyms

Garala: It leads to death.
Kshveda: It causes mental disorders. This also causes addiction due to its addictive nature.
Vatsanabha: The root resembles the umbilical cord of calf. It causes death to the calf due to accidental ingestion.
Visha: It invades all over the body quickly due to virtue of "Vikāsi" Guṇa.
Amrita: It acts as nectar.
Kalakuṭa: A poison obtained from churning of the ocean as per Hindu mythology, and it was swallowed by Lord Shiva which turned his neck blue.
Mahaushadham: It is reputed drug applicable in numerous disorders.
Sthāvarādhya: A particle vegetable poison.

Classical Categorization

Not mentioned in any Gana of Charaka and Sushrut Samhita. Charaka and Sushruta mentioned it in sthavara visha and kanda visha, respectively.
- Ashtang Hridaya: Viṣopayoga
- Dhanwantari Nighantu: Mishrakadi varga
- Kaiyadev Nighantu: Mishrakadi varga
- Raj Nighantu: Pippaladi varga, Mishrakadi varga
- Bhavaprakash Nighantu: Dhatwadi varga, viṣopviṣādi varga

Distribution

It is distributed in Temperate to Alpine regions of the Himalaya at the altitude of 3,300 to 5,000 m.

Morphology

A biennial herb with tuberous roots, 60 to 90 cm in height with an erect herb. Upper part is finely pubescent.
- **Leaves:** Scattered, up to 20 cm across, orbicular-cordate to reniform, five-pedatipartite to the very base or almost so in the inner, and to 8/9 to 9/10 in the outer incisions, intermediate divisions three-lobed to the middle, outermost two-lobed or two-partite, all further incised, laciniate more or less linear lanceolate and divaricate (**Fig. 105.1**).
- **Flower:** Blue/bluish purple in dense terminal raceme; 10 to 25 cm long; floral leaves are much reduced and pass into trifid or entire and linear-lanceolate bracts. Sepals are blue, hairy, and helmet shaped with a short, sharp beak (**Fig. 105.2**).
- **Fruit:** Oblong, conspicuously reticulate follicles, minute hairy.
- **Seed:** Oblong, obovoid to bipyramidal, winged along the raphe.
- **Root:** Dark brown externally, tuberous, paired, daughter tuber ellipsoid to ovoid oblong, 2 to 4 cm length with filiform root fibers. Fracture is scarcely farinaceous, yellowish. Mother tubers are much shrunk and wrinkled (**Fig. 105.3**; Anonymous 2003).

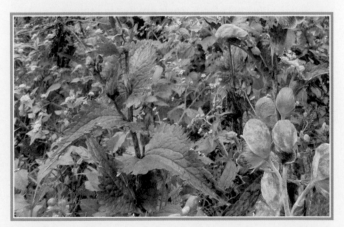

Fig. 105.1 Leaves.

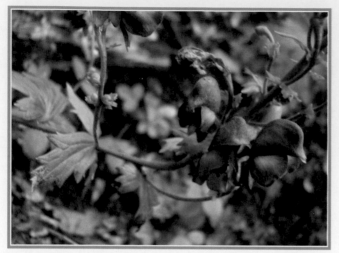

Fig. 105.2 Flowers.

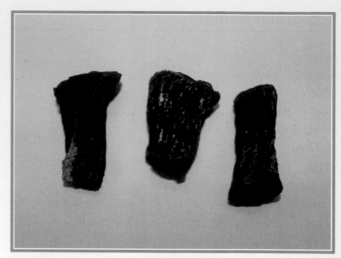

Fig. 105.3 Roots.

Plants are propagated through well-developed tuberous roots, which are planted in the field in the month of December to January (Anonymous 2003).

Phenology

Flowering time: August to November
Fruiting time: August to November

Key Characters for Identification

➤ Stem: erect, 40 to 90 cm high.
➤ Leaves: Scattered, orbicular, cordate to reniform. Palmately five-lobed, blade somewhat fleshy, blade and petiole pubescent.
➤ Inflorescence: Loose raceme, 4 to 10 inch long.
➤ Sepals: Blue in color. Carpels are five in number, conniving and contiguous.
➤ Follicles: Conspicuously reticulate. Seeds are obovoid to bipyramidal, winged along the raphe.
➤ Roots: Paired, biennial, and tuberous. Daughter-tubers are ovoid-oblong to ellipsoid, 2.5 to 4 cm long, about 1 to 1.5 cm thick, with a few filiform root-fibers.

Types

According to Rasashastragrantha and Chikitsagrantha classification, Vatsanabha is of four types according to

Varṇa (cast and color), i.e., Brahmaṇa, Kṣatriya, Vaishya, and Shudra, and are generally of the following colors, respectively, white, red, yellow, and black.

Brāhmaṇa or wise caste Vatsanabha is white or tawny, sweet or salty in taste, and has got hair-like shoots over its body. The Kṣatriya (or warrior class) of the poisons is red in color. The Vaishya (merchant class) is yellow or gray and somewhat sweet in taste. The Shudra (or the agricultural and serving class) is black in color. According to caste properties of poisons, i.e., the Brahmaṇa (white-colored) poison is a curer and preventer of disease and senile decay. The Kṣatriya (red-colored) is used in mercurial operations. The Vaishya (yellow-colored) is a curer of leprosy, and the Shudra (black-colored) is giver of death. The Brahmaṇa variety of poisons is to be used in diseases; the Kṣatriya variety is to be given to a patient who has swallowed some poison; the Vaishya variety is to be used in diseases of minor importance; and the Shudra variety is to be given to a man who has been bitten by a poisonous snake.

Rasapanchaka

Guna	Laghu, Ruksha, Tikshna, Vyavayi, Vikashi
Rasa	Madhura
Vipaka	Madhura
Virya	Ushna

Chemical Constituents

It contains 0.3 to 2% aconite in tubers of fresh plants and 0.2 to 1.2% in the leaves. The highest concentration of aconite is found in winter. Various parts of *A. ferox* have different phytoconstituents.

- Plant: 3-bikhaconitine dichloroethane solvate, 3-bikhaconitine acetone solvate, 14-obenzoyl-8-ethoxy-bikhaconine, 4-O-benzoyl-8-ethoxy-bikhaconine, 14-O-benzoyl-8-methoxy-bikhaconine.
- Root: Indaconitine ($C_{34}H_{47}NO_{10}$), chasmaconitine ($C_{34}H_{47}NO_9$), chasmanthinine, one unidentified alkaloid: base A ($C_{26}H_{43}O_6N$), chasmanine, lycoctonine, pyrosedaconitine, pseudo-aconitine ($C_{36}H_{51}NO_{12}$), delphinie, bikhaconitine ($C_{36}H_{51}NO_{11}$), pyroseudaconitine, isopyroseudaconitine. pyrobikhaconitine, pyrobikhaconine, isopyrobikhaconine; recently two new alkaloids, veratroyl pseudo-aconitine ($C_{34}H_{49}NO_{11}$) and diacetyl pseudo-aconitine ($C_{40}H_{55}NO_4$) (Anonymous 2003; Tsuda and Marion 1963).

Identity, Purity, and Strength

- Foreign matter: Not more than 2%
- Total ash: Not more than 5.5%
- Acid-insoluble ash: Not more than 2%
- Alcohol-soluble extractive: Not less than 8%
- Water-soluble extractive: Not less than 24%

(Source: The Ayurvedic Pharmacopeia of India 1999)

Karma (Actions)

Before shodhan: vyavayi (spreading in the body before digestion), vikashi (sluggish ligament), and pranahara (lethal), agneya (hot), yogavahi (catalyst), madakari (delirium).

After sodhan and rational use: pranada (vitality), rasayana (rejuvenative), tridoshaghna, brahmana (bulk promoting), sukral (spermatopoetic), grahi (astringent).

The root and underground stem are highly toxic, but its toxicity may be reduced by suitable processing of purification and rational use. It has also acted as vedanasthapana (analgesic), sothahara (anti-inflammatory),

deepana (appetizer), pachana (digestive), yakruthejakara (hepatic stimulant), hridya (cardiac tonic), sukrasthambana (semen astringent), mutrala (diuretic), artavajanana (promotes menstruation), amavataghna (antirheumatoid), sandhivatahara (cure osteoarthritis), rasayana (rejuvenative), balya (strength promoter), vyavayi (spreading in the body before digestion), sitahara (control the chill), jwaraghna (antipyretics), swedajana (to induce sweating).

- Doshakarma: Kaphavatashaman, sannipātahara
- Dhatukarma: Sukral, balya, brimhana
- Malakarma: Grahi, swedajanana

Pharmacological Actions

The main pharmacological actions of Vatsanabha are thermogenic, narcotic, anodyne, diaphoretic, diuretics, nervine tonic, expectorant, appetizer, digestive, carminative, cardiotonic, emmenagogue, anaphrodisiac, sedative, febrifuge, hypoglycemic, anti-inflammatory. It is also useful in painful inflammation, bronchitis, hypotension, flatulence, colic, cardiac debility, dysmenorrhea, amenorrhea, spermatorrhea, leprosy, sciatica, paralysis, hepatopathy, splenopathy, diabetes, fever, and debility. It is often used to get relief from nervous and rheumatic pain.

Indications

It is useful in agnimandya (anorexia), swasa (asthma), kasa (cough), (plihodora) splenomegaly, bhagandara (fistula-in-ano), pandu (anemia), vrana (wound), arsha (piles), kushta (skin disease), vatarakta (gout), visarapa (erysipelas), viṣa (poison), netra roga (ocular disorders), vatavyadhi (neurological disorders), shula (colic pain), and gulma (abdominal lump).

Therapeutic Uses

1. **Jeerna jwara** (chronic fever): Vatsanabha, Lodhra, Chandana, Vacha, sugar, ghee, and honey are given with milk to alleviate chronic fever (A.S.U. 48/23).
2. **Shoola** (colic): Equal quantities of Vatsanabha and Pippali are given to treat shoola (R.R.S.).

3. **Shirashoola** (headache): Yastimadhu (1 part) and Vatsanabha (1/4th part) are pounded and administered as nasya in a dose of mustard seed to get relief from headache (Bhavaprakash).

4. **Scorpian bite**: The root paste is used externally to relieve the pain due to scorpion bite.

5. **Jwara** (fever): Root of Vatsanabha is used as an ingredient of mrutunjayarasa which is a very effective medicine for fever (R.T. 24/67).

6. **Prameha** (diabetes): Vatsanabha as a composition of Jaya vati is useful in prameha (RT.24.99).

7. **Rasayana** (rejuvenation): Aindra rasayana (C.S.Ci. 1.3.5) and Amrita rasayana are potent rasayana medicines in which Vatsanabha is the main ingredient.

Officinal Part Used

Roots

Dose

15 mg

Formulations

Amruta rasayana, Anandbhairabh rasa, Hinguleswar rasa, Jaya vati, Jwarmurari, Kaphaketu rasa, Mrityunjaya rasa, Rambana rasa, Tribhuvankirti rasa, Visha taila.

Toxicity/Adverse Effects

Aconite is a fast-acting toxin. Aconite poisoning usually occurs due to ingestion of the wild aconite plant because of misidentification, contamination, adulteration, and misprocessing. The onset of symptoms occurs rapidly within 10 to 20 minutes.

Vatsanābha (*A. ferox* Wall.) is a poisonous plant, though all parts of the plant are poisonous, the root is extremely lethal and contains highly toxic alkaloids like aconitine, pseudaconitine, indaconitine, etc. When taken orally, the toxicity manifests in the form of tingling, numbness, abdominal pain, nausea, vomiting, hypothermia, loss of muscle powder, visual and auditory disturbances, and finally clonic convulsion. Death is caused by myocardial depression or respiratory paralysis.

Singh (2003) estimated that LD50 dose of crude aconite via intraperitoneal (IP) route in Albino mice is 130 mg/kg^2. Thorat and Dahanukar (1991) ascertained the toxicity of crude aconite in mice and reported that the crude drug aconite was toxic to the mice even at a dose as low as 1.3 mg/mouse. 100% mortality resulted when 2.6 mg of crude aconite was administered to each mouse. The median lethal dose of crude aconite was found to be 35 mg/kg as per Sarkar et al (2012).

Treatment

Aconite poisoning needs immediate attention to revive vital function and close monitoring of the blood pressure and cardiac rhythm. Patients must be managed in ICU.

In Ayurveda, Tankan (borax) and ghee or mixture of turmeric juice, borax, and ghee is given to the patient. More quantity of milk is given to the patient to induce vomiting. Strong tea or coffee or tannin acid can be given to precipitate the alkaloid.

Purification

Roots are cut into small pieces and put inside the earthen pot containing cow's urine for 7 days and each day cow's urine is changed. On eighth day, it is removed from the pot and washed with cold water. Then the upper layer of the root is removed and again washed with warm water. After that it is dried in sunlight. The dried pieces are ground to get the powder of Vatsanabha.

Substitution and Adulteration

Various species of Aconitum are used as substitutes and adulterants of *A. ferox*. Few of them are mentioned as under:

- *Aconitum chasmanthum*
- *Aconitum deinorrhizum* Stapf.
- *Aconitum balfourii* Stapf.
- *Aconitum laciniatum* Stapf.
- *Aconitum spicatum*
- *Aconitum falconeri* Stapf.
- *Aconitum heterophyllum* Wall (nonpoisonous)
- *Aconitum palmatum* D.Ron. (nonpoisonous)

Points to Ponder

- *According to Bhavaprakash Nighantu, there are nine varieties of Mahavisha (Vatsanabha, Haridra, Saktuka, Pradipana, Saurastrika, Srngika, Kalakuta, Halahala, and Brahmaputra), out of which Vatsanabha is the most important visha which is used commonly as medicine.*
- *It is purified by dipping it in cow's urine for seven days.*

Suggested Readings

Anonymous. Database on Medicinal Plants Used in Ayurveda, Vol. 8. New Delhi: Documentation and Publication Division, CCRAS; 2003:477

Anonymous. The Wealth of India: Raw Materials, Vol. 1. Revised edition. New Delhi: National Institute of Science Communication and Information Resources, CSIR; 2003:60

Lucas DS. Dravyaguna-Vijnana: Study of Dravya-Materia Medica. Varanasi: Chaukhamba Visvabharati; 2013:3

Sarkar PK. Evaluation of effect of sodhana treatment on pharmacological activities of Aconite. IJPER 2012;46(3):243–247

Sharma PV. Classical Uses of Medicinal Plants. 1st ed. Varanasi: Chaukhamba Vishvabharati; 2004:336

Sheokand A. Vatsanabha (Aconitum Ferox): from visha to amrita. Int J Ayurved Herb Med 2012;2(3):423–426

Singh LB. Poisonous (Visa) Plants in Ayurveda. 2nd ed. Varanasi: Chaukhamba Sanskrit Bhawan; 2003

The Ayurvedic Pharmacopoeia of India, Part I, Vol. II, 1st ed. New Delhi: Department of Health, Ministry of Health and Family Welfare, Government of India; 1999:80

Thorat S, Dahanukar S. Can we dispense with Ayurvedic samskaras? J Postgrad Med 1991;37(3):157–159

Tsuda Y, Marion, L. Pseudaconitine and the stereochemical relationship of the highly oxygenated aconite alkaloids. Can J Chem 1963;41: 1485–1489

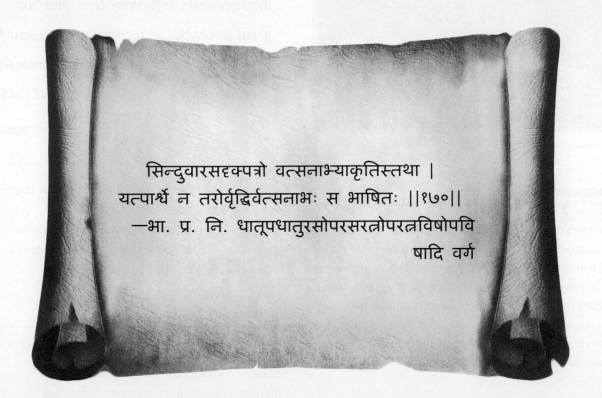

सिन्दुवारसदृक्पत्रो वत्सनाभ्याकृतिस्तथा |
यत्पार्श्वे न तरोर्वृद्धिर्वत्सनाभः स भाषितः ||१७०||
—भा. प्र. नि. धातूपधातुरसोपरसरत्नोपरत्नविषोपवि
षादि वर्ग

106. Vidanga *[Embelia ribes Burm. f.]*

Family:	*Myrsinaceae*
Hindi name:	*Vayavidanga, Bhabhiranga, Baberang, Wawrung, Vayvidamg*
English name:	*Embelia*

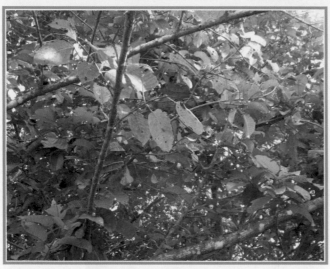

Plant of *Embelia ribes* Burm. f.

> *Embelin has been reported as potentially effective suppressor of tumor cell survival, proliferation, invasion, angiogenesis, inflammation, and has great potential as a therapeutic agent for osteoporosis and cancer-linked bone loss.*
>
> —*Ahn et al (2007)*

Introduction

Embelia ribes Burm. (Myrsinaceae) is a large, woody, tropical forest scandent shrub with slender branches and gland-dotted leaves. It is distributed in moist deciduous forests of the Western Ghats of South India, Jammu & Kashmir, Himachal Pradesh, Uttar Pradesh, Assam, and Maharashtra, and Sri Lanka, Malaya, Singapore, and South China. It is mentioned in ancient classical texts like Charaka Samhita, Sushruta Samhita, and Ashtanga Hridaya as krimighna dravya.

Sushruta recommends using it along with liquorice for strengthening the body and preventing the effect of age. Recent findings also suggest embelin as a novel adjuvant therapeutic candidate for the treatment of hormone-refractory prostate cancer that is resistant to radiation therapy (Dai et al 2011). The berries are used in the preparation of several compositions for ringworm and other skin diseases. The seeds are of high repute as anthelmintic particularly for tapeworms. Pulp of the fruit is purgative. Fresh juice is cooling, diuretic, and laxative.

E. ribes is considered as vulnerable in Karnataka and Tamil Nadu. It is of lower risk (near threatened) in Kerala (Ravikumar and Ved 2000).

Vernacular Names

Assamese: Vidang
Bengali: Vidang, Biranga, Bhai-birrung
Gujarati: Vavading, Vayavadang, Vayvirang
Kannada: Vayuvilanga, Vayuvidanga
Kashmiri: Babading
Malayalam: Vizhalari, Vilal
Marathi: Vavding, Karkannie
Oriya: Bidanga, Vidanga, Baibidanga
Punjabi: Babrung, Vavaring
Tamil: Vayuvilangam, Vayuvidangam, Vellal

Telugu: Vayuvidangalu, Vayu-vilamgam, Vayuvidangamu, Vidanga

Urdu: Baobarang, Babrang

Synonyms

Amogha: It acts without failure.

Bhasmaka: The drugs which destroy worms are known as Jantunashan.

Chitra: The drug which has different seeds.

Chitratandula: Seeds of which are spotted or dotted with another color.

Jantunashan: The drugs which destroy worms are known as Jantunashan.

Kairala: Generally, it is found in Kerala.

Krimighna: It destroys worms.

Tandula: The drugs which destroy thread worms.

Vella: The drug which moves in abdomen or digestive system for curing the diseases is Vella. The drug which promotes elimination of worms is Vella.

Vidanga: Vida means to correct or to cure, that means the drug which cures vahnimaandyam, shoola, adhmana, vibandha, etc. is known as Vidanga.

Classical Categorization

Charaka Samhita: Truptighna, Kushthaghna, Krimighna, Shirovirechana

Sushruta Samhita: Surasaadi, Pippalyadi

Ashtanga Hridaya: Surasaadi, Pippalyadi

Dhanwantari Nighantu: Shatapushpadi varga

Madanpal Nighantu: Sunthyadi varga

Kaiyadev Nighantu: Aushadhi varga

Raj Nighantu: Pippalyadi varga

Bhavaprakash Nighantu: Haritakyadi varga

Distribution

E. ribes is highly restricted to hilly parts of India up to 1,500 m elevation from outer Himalayas to Western Ghats. It is also found in Sri Lanka, Singapore, South China, and Malayan archipelago. It is distributed in moist deciduous forests of the Western Ghats of South India, Jammu & Kashmir, Arunachal Pradesh, Himachal Pradesh, Madhya Pradesh, Uttar Pradesh, Assam, and Maharashtra (Nadkarni 2007;

Shankarmurthy et al 2004; Warrier et al 2001; Anonymous 2005).

Morphology

It is a large, scandent shrub; branches long, slender, flexible, terete with long internodes, the bark studded with lenticels.

- **Leaves:** Coriaceous, 5 to 9 by 2 to 3.8 cm., elliptic or elliptic lanceolate, shortly and obtusely acuminate, entire, shining above, paler, and somewhat silvery beneath; the whole surface is covered with scattered minute reddish sunken gland (conspicuous in the young leaves), base rounded or acute; main nerves are numerous, slender; petioles are 6 to 16 mm long, more or less margined, glabrous (**Fig. 106.1**).
- **Flowers:** Pentamerous, numerous, small, in lax panicled racemes which are terminal and from the upper axils; branches of the panicle often 7.5 to 10 cm long with more or less glandular pubescent; bracts minute, setaceous, deciduous. Calyx is about 1.25 mm long; sepals connate about 1/3rd of the way up, the teeth 5, broadly triangular-ovate, ciliate. Five petals, greenish yellow, free, 4 mm long, elliptic, subobtuse, and pubescent on both sides. Five stamens, shorter than the petals, erect; filaments inserted a little below the middle of the petals.
- **Fruit:** Globose, brownish-black, globular 2 to 4 mm in diameter, warty surface with a beak-like projection at apex, often short, thin pedicel and persistent calyx with usual1y three or five sepals present, pericarp brittle enclosing a single seed (**Fig. 106.2a, b**; Kirtikar and Basu 2006).

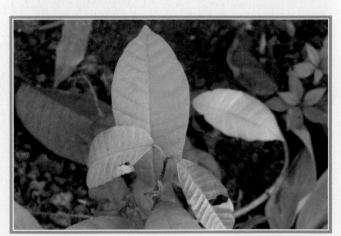

Fig. 106.1 Leaves.

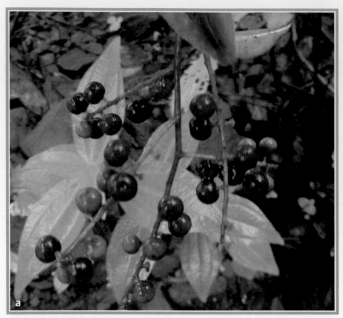
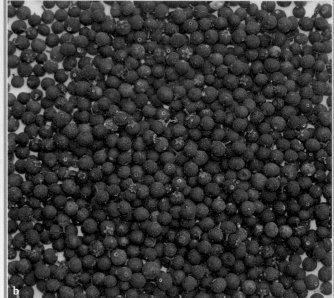

Fig. 106.2 **(a)** Fresh fruits. **(b)** Dry fruits.

Phenology

Flowering time: March to April
Fruiting time: June to October

Key Characters for Identification

➤ *A large, scandent shrub with long slender, flexible, terete branches; bark studded with lenticles.*

➤ *Leaves: Simple, alternate, elliptic-lanceolate, gland dotted, short and obtusely acuminate, entire, shiny above.*

➤ *Flowers: Small, white or greenish, in both terminal and axillary panicles.*

➤ *Fruits: Globose, wrinkled or warty, dull red to nearly black, a short pedicel often present, usually one seeded.*

➤ *Seeds: Globose.*

Rasapanchaka

Guna	Laghu, Ruksha, Tikshna
Rasa	Katu, Kashaya
Vipaka	Katu
Virya	Ushna
Prabhav	Krimighna

Chemical Constituents

Embelin, quercitol, tannin, and an alkaloid christembine are isolated from fruits. The new derivatives of embelin, iodoembelin, and bromoembelin are also isolated from the fruits of Vidanga. The other constituents identified are embolic acid, fatty ingredients, resinoid, and volatile oil (Nadkarni 1976).

Identity, Purity, and Safety

- Foreign matter: Not more than 2%
- Total ash: Not more than 6%
- Acid-insoluble ash: Not more than 1.5%
- Alcohol-soluble extractive: Not less than 10%
- Water-soluble extractive: Not less than 9%

(Source: The Ayurvedic Pharmacopeia of India 1989)

Karma (Actions)

Krimighna (anthelmintic), deepana (appetizer), vishaghna (antidote), rochan (relish), aamahara (digestion), medohara (antiobesity), pramehara (antidibetics).

- Doshakarma: Kapha vatashamaka.
- Dhatukarma: Medohara
- Malakarma: Virechan

Pharmacological Actions

Its actions include nematocidal, estrogenic, hypoglycemic, anthelmintic, antibiotic, antitubercular, anti-implantation, anti-inflammatory, hypotensive, diuretic, hepatoprotective, anticancer, immunostimulant, and antifertility.

Indications

It is used in krimi (worm infestation), krimidanta (dental caries), dantashoola (dental pain), agnimandya (loss of appetite), aruchi (loss of appetite), bhranti (delusion), ajeerna (indigestion), chhardi (vomiting), udarshoola (abdominal pain), gulma (abdominal lump), adhmana (gandamala), kushta (skin disease), vibandha (constipation), arsha (piles), kamala (jaundice), pliha (spleen disease), swasa (asthma), kasa (cough), prameha (diabetes), medoroga (obesity), hridroga (cardiac disease), pratisyaya (rhinitis), kaphavataroga (disease of kapha and vata), rakta vikara (blood disease), shiroroga (disease of head), akshepaka (convulsion), apasmar (epilepsy), pakshaghata (hemiplegia).

Therapeutic Uses

External Use

Vrana (wound): Oil of Karanja, Sarsapa, Shigru, and Koshram should be applied locally (S.S.Ci. 9.52-53).

Internal Use

1. **Krimi** (worm infestation): Vidanga is best drug for worms (C.S.Su. 25/40 & AH.U. 40/49). Vidanga and seeds of Kutaja and palasa should be powdered and taken with sugar. It acts as anthelmintic (BP.Ci. 7/23). Rice scum mixed with Vidanga and Trikatu should be given to destroy worms. It also stimulates digestive power (V.M. 7/3). Warm decoction of Vidanga and Argavadha should be given in worm infestations (A.S.U. 49.91). Paste of Vidanga and Pippali used in non-unctuous enema destroys wound (C.S.Su. 8/10).
2. **Krimija Hridroga** (heart disease caused by worm): Vidanga and Kushta mixed with urine should be taken in krimija hridroga (VM. 31.21).

3. **Kushta** (skin disease): Vidanga, Triphala, and Pippali powder taken with honey destroys kushta, krimi (worms), sinus, and fistula-in-ano (S.S.R. 12/33).
4. **As rasayan** (rejuvenation): Vidanga, Bhallataka, and Shunthi should be given with ghee and honey to prevent old age and diseases (A.H.U. 39/152).
5. **Ardhavabheda** (hemicrania): Vidanga, black Til in equal quantity are pounded together and taken as snuff to alleviate hemicrania (BS.Shiroroga.101).
6. **Kamala** (jaundice): Vadanga and Pippali are used as nasya (snuff) and anjan (collyrium) in kamala (GN. 2.7.52).
7. **Visha** (poisoning): Vidanga root pounded and taken with rice water counteracts snake-poison (GN.7.3.13).

Officinal Parts Used

Fruit, root, leaf

Dose

Powder: 5 to 10 g

Formulations

Vidangarista, Vidanga Lauha, Vidangadi Lauha, Abhayarishtam, Lauhasava, Draksharishtha, Dashamularishtha, Kumari ashava, Pippalyasava Ayaskrithi, Pippallyasavam, Chndraprabha vati, Kankayana vati, Yogaraj guggulu, Kaishore guggulu, Triphala modaka, Ajamodadi churna, Panchnimba churna, Navayas churna, Sudarshan churna, Jatipahladichurna, Narayana churna, Anuthailam, Kachuradithailam.

Toxicity/Adverse Effects

Embelia robusta or *E. ribes* has been reported to possibly cause optic atrophy among the Ethiopian population. It was observed by administering the crude herb in both high doses (5 g/kg/d) and low doses (0.5 g/kg/d), along with regular chick feed. Anatomical evidence of degeneration of ganglion cells was found in retinae exposed to high doses of *E. ribes* but no retinal lesions were detected in chicks following treatment with cumulative doses of less than 5 g/kg/d.

Potassium embelate isolated from *E. ribes* is a safe compound as the results did not indicate adverse effects.

Substitution and Adulteration

E. ribes Burm f. is the original source of Vidanga while two other species of same family (*E. robusta* C.B. Clarke [Syn. *E. tsjeriam–cottam* A. DC.] and *E. acutipetallum* Lam. ExHassk. S.M. & M.R.) are also sold in the name of Vidanga.

E. robusta C.B. Clarke, is sold in the name Vidanga bheda, is a well-known substitute and *M. africana* is known to be used more as an adulterant.

Points to Ponder

- *Vidanga is best drug for worms (C.S.Su. 25/40 & AH.U. 40/49).*
- *E. robusta C.B. Clarke is the substitute and M. africana is known as an adulterant of Vidanga.*
- *As per Bhavaprakash Nighantu, gender of Vidanga is pumlinga (male) and kliba linga.*

Suggested Readings

Ahn KS, Sethi G, Aggarwal BB. Embelin, an inhibitor of X chromosome-linked inhibitor-of-apoptosis protein, blocks nuclear factor-kappaB (NF-kappaB) signaling pathway leading to suppression of NF-kappaB-regulated antiapoptotic and metastatic gene products. Mol Pharmacol 2007;71(1):209–219

Anonymous. Compendium of Medicinal Plants. New Delhi: National Institute of Industrial Research; 2005:110–113

Dai Y, Desano J, Qu Y, et al. Natural IAP inhibitor Embelin enhances therapeutic efficacy of ionizing radiation in prostate cancer. Am J Cancer Res 2011;1(2):128–143

Kirtikar KR, Basu BD. Indian Medicinal Plants, Vol. 2 (Blatter E, Caius JF, Mhaskar KS, eds.). II ed. Dehradun: Bishen Singh, Mahendrapal Singh; 2006:1477–1481

Nadkarni AK. Nadkarni's Indian Materia Medica, Vol. 1. Mumbai: Popular Prakashan; 2007:478

Nadkarni KM. The Indian Materia Medica. Mumbai: Popular Prakashan; 1976:478–480

Ravikumar K, Ved DK. 100 Red Listed Medicinal Plants of Conservation Concern in Southern India. Bangalore: Foundation for Revitalization of Local Health Traditions (FRLHT); 2000:136–141

Shankarmurthy K, Krishna V, Maruthi KR, Rahiman BA. Rapid adventitious organogenesis from leaf segments of *Embelia ribes* Burm.: a threatened medicinal plant. Taiwania 2004;49(3):194–200

The Ayurvedic Pharmacopoeia of India, Part 1, Vol. 1. 1st ed. New Delhi: Department of AYUSH, Ministry of Health and Family Welfare, Government of India; 1989:175–177

Warrier PK, Nambiar VPK, Ganapathy PM. Some Important Medicinal Plants of the Western Ghats, India: A Profile. Canada: International Development Research Centre (IDRC); 2001:139–156

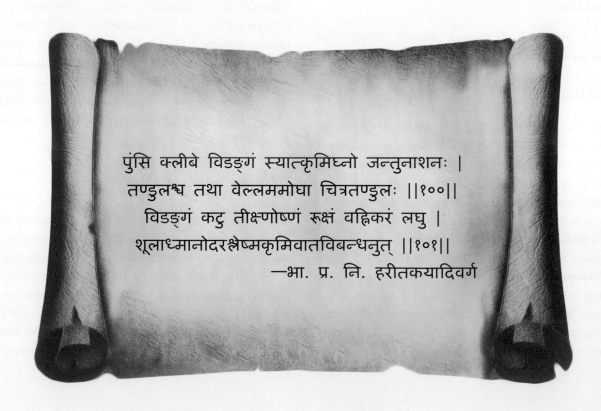

पुंसि क्लीबे विडङ्गं स्यात्कृमिघ्नो जन्तुनाशनः |
तण्डुलश्च तथा वेल्लममोघा चित्रतण्डुलः ||१००||
विडङ्गं कटु तीक्ष्णोष्णं रूक्षं वह्निकरं लघु |
शूलाध्मानोदरश्लेष्मकृमिवातविबन्धनुत् ||१०१||
—भा. प्र. नि. हरीतकयादिवर्ग

107. Vidari *[Pueraria tuberosa (Roxb. ex. Willd.)]*

Family: *Fabaceae*

Hindi name: *Bidari*

English name: *Indian Kudju*

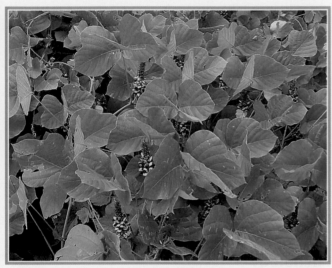

Plant of *Pueraria tuberosa* (Roxb. ex. Willd.).

> *Vidarikanda is a fast growing vine and because of this nature the plant has acquired the name "Mile a minute vine or Foot a night vine."*

Introduction

In Sanskrit, the word "Vidari" means the one which emerges/bursts out itself. The plant has been given the name Vidarikanda because when the size of the tuber becomes extremely large it emerges out of the ground. The plant's tuber is widely used in ethnomedicine as well as in traditional systems of medicine since ages. Charaka, Sushrut, and Ashtang all described it as a rasayana (rejuvenator) drug. Bhavamishra used it as a substitute drug for ashtavarga plants. Its tubers work on plasma, blood, muscles, and reproductive system. Charaka and Ashtang have kept it under shaka varga (C.S.Su. 27/118; A.H.Su. 6/85) whereas Sushrut described it in kanda varga (S.S.Su. 46/301). Ashtang Hridaya has used it in preparation of many vrishya yogas (A.H.U. 40/13-26). Charaka has recommended using it as Vataraktahara paste. In folklore medicine, tubers and leaves of Vidarikanda are used as vegetables.

Vernacular Names

Assamese: Bhedeleton, Bhuikumra

Bengali: Vidari, Bhumikusmanda, Bhuinkumra

Gujarati: Vidarikanta, Bhonykoru, Eagio, Bhoikolu, Sakharvel

Kannada: Nelagumbala Gudde, Gumadi belli, Nelagumbula, Gumadigida

Malayalam: Mudakku

Marathi: Bhuikohala, Ghodvel

Oriya: Bhuiankakharu

Tamil: Nilapoosani

Telugu: Nelagummuda, Darigummadi

Synonyms

Gajavajipriya: The tuber is eaten by elephant and horses.

Ikshugandha: The tuber has aroma like the sugarcane.

Ksheershukla: Internally, the tuber is milky white in appearance.

Bhumikushmanda: The size of the tuber is big like that of Kushmanda.

Shuklakanda: The cut pieces of tuber are white colored.

Sita: The potency of the tuber is sheeta.

Swadukanda: The tuber is sweet in taste.

Vrishyakanda: The tuber is aphrodisiac in action.

Classical Categorization

Charaka Samhita: Balya, Brihganiya, Varnya, Kanthya, Snehopaga, Madhura skanda

Sushrut Samhita: Vidarigandhadi, Vallipanchmool, Pittasansamana

Ashtang Hridaya: Vidaryadi gana

Dhanvantari Nighantu: Guduchyadi varga

Madanpal Nighantu: Abhyadi varga

Kaiyadev Nighantu: Oushadi varga

Raj Nighantu: Moolakadi varga

Bhavaprakash Nighantu: Guduchyadi varga

Distribution

It is found throughout India. It grows well in the hilly forests of Himalaya, Sikkim, Kumaun, Mount Abu, Kerala, Deccan plateau, Western Ghats, and Central India.

Morphology

It is a large, spreading, perennial twiner with a large tuberous root. Young branches are gray pubescent.

- **Leaves:** Pinnately trifoliate with petiole 10 to 20 cm long. The leaflets are 12 to 20 cm long, 11 to 18 cm broad. The terminal leaflet broadly ovate, equal sided, acuminate. The lateral leaflet is ovate-oblong, very oblique, acuminate, silky pubescent below, glabrescent above, stipules small (**Fig. 107.1**).
- **Flowers:** Inflorescence is terminal raceme or panicle. Pedicel 2 to 3 mm long, flowers bisexual, blue-purple in color, usually appears when the plant is leafless (**Fig. 107.2**).
- **Fruit:** Linear, flat, jointed pods about 2 to 5 cm long, with long silky bristly brown hairs. Seeds are three to six in numbers.
- **Tubers:** Globose, pot-like or variable in shape and size, externally rough, dark brown, internally white, starchy, and mildly sweet like madhuyashti (**Fig. 107.3**).

The plant is propagated by its tuber.

Phenology

Flowering time: March to April
Fruiting time: April to May

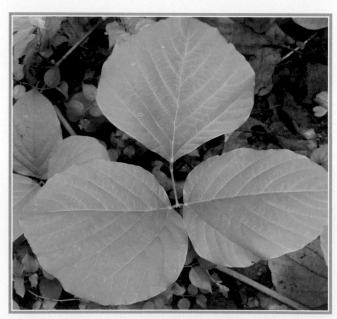

Fig. 107.1 Leaves.

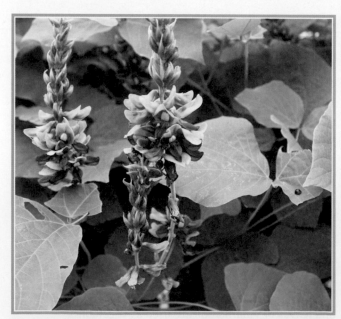

Fig. 107.2 Flowers.

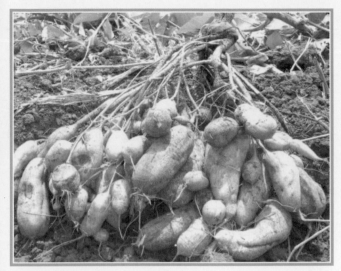

Fig. 107.3 Tuber.

> [!box]
> ### Key Characters for Identification
>
> ➤ *A large, spreading, perennial twiner with a tuberous root.*
> ➤ *Leaves are pinnately trifoliate, terminal leaflet is broadly ovate, and lateral leaflet is ovate-oblong, oblique.*
> ➤ *Flowers are blue-purple, and occur in terminal raceme inflorescence.*
> ➤ *Fruits are linear, flat, jointed pods, studded with brown hairs.*
> ➤ *Tubers are variable in shape and size, externally rough, and dark brown internally white.*

Rasapanchaka

Guna	Guru, Snigdha
Rasa	Madhura
Vipaka	Madhura
Virya	Sheeta

Chemical Constituents

The active constituents present in the tuber are pterocarpan-tuberosin, pterocarpanone-hydroxytuberosone, 2 pterocarpenes-anhydrotuberosin and methyl anhydrotuberosin, coumestan tuberostan, puerarostan,

isoflavonoids—puerarone, puerarin, genistein, daidzein, and tuberosin. It also contains β-sitosterol, stigmasterol, carbohydrates, sugar, protein, and crude fibers (Venkataratnam and Venkataraju 2009; Kirtikar and Basu 1933).

Identity, Purity, and Strength

- Foreign matter: Not more than 2%
- Total ash: Not more than 17%
- Acid-insoluble ash: Not more than 4.4%
- Alcohol-soluble extractive: Not less than 4%
- Water-soluble extractive: Not less than 24%

(Source: The Ayurvedic Pharmacopeia of India 1999)

Karma (Actions)

Classical texts attributed brihmaniya (weight promoter), stanaya (galactogogue), shukral (spermetogenesis), swarya (improves voice), mutral (diuretic), balya (tonic), varnya (complexion promoter), rasayana (rejuvinator), and jeevaniya (nutrient) properties to its tuber. The flowers have madhura rasa, madhura vipaka, sheet virya, virshya, guru, and pittaghna properties.

- Doshakarma: Pitta vataraktashamaka
- Dhatukarma: Balya, brihmaniya, Rasayana
- Malakarma: Mutral

Pharmacological Actions

Scientific researches proved its tuber as a restorative tonic, galactagogue, antiaging agent, antioxidant, spermatogenic, immunity booster, diuretic, aphrodisiac, hypoglycemic, hypolipidemic, antimicrobial, anti-inflammatory, cardioprotective, expectorant, and febrifuge (Bilore et al 2004).

Indications

Ayurvedic classics advocated using Vidari kanda in daha (burning sensation), raktapitta (bleeding disorders), dourbalya (general debility), sosha (emaciation), and angamarda (fatigue). It stimulates milk production in nursing mothers, increases shukra dhatu, and gives physical strength to the body. In traditional system of medicines, tubers are used for treatment of diabetes, acidity, urinary disorders, intermittent fever, dyspepsia, hepatosplenomegaly, cardiac debility, cough, tuberculosis, leprosy, erysipelas, menopausal syndrome, sexual debility, spermatorrhea, and infertility (Warrier et al 1997).

Therapeutic Uses

External Use

Visarpa (erysipelas): Shatavari and Vidarikanda powder added with shatadhauth ghrita should be applied locally in affected areas (C.S.Ci. 21/84).

Internal Use

1. **Mutra kricchta** (dysuria): Regular intake of ghrita and dugdh processed with Vidarikanda increases urine output and removes discoloration (C.S.Ci. 18/154).
2. **Kshayaj kasa** (cough): Vidarikand, Mulethi, Shunthi, and Bala are made into powder and are taken daily with madhu in Kshayaj Kasa (C.S.Ci. 18/154) (A.H.Ci. 3/153).
3. **Vrishya** (aphrodisiac): Intake of powder of Vidarikanda impregnated with its own juice mixed with madhu and ghrita acts as vrishya (S.S.Ci. 26/23).
4. **Klaibyta** (impotency): Vidarikand, Kapikachu seeds, Ashwagandha mool, Shatavari mool, and Bala mool are made into powder. Take 1 tsf of this powder twice daily with milk to treat impotency.
5. **Stanyajanan** (inducing lactation): Intake of Vidarikanda powder with Shatavari along with milk twice daily increases flow of breast milk (CD. 63/51).
6. **Amalpitta** (acidity): Take 10 g Vidarikanda powder or juice with 2 tsf madhu, on empty stomach, every morning and evening to control hyperacidity.
7. **Medhya** (memory booster): Take half tablespoonful of Vidarikand powder with Brahmi or Mandookparni swaras twice daily to reduce anxiety and enhance memory.
8. **Visham jwara** (malarial fever): Take juice of Vidarikanda and Ikshu mixed with madhu, ghrita, taila, and dugdh to alleviate visham jwara (CD. 1/218).

Officinal Part Used

Tuber

Dose

Powder: 3 to 6 g.

Formulations

Shatavari ghrita, Marma gutika, Puga khanda, Vidaryadi churna, Vidaryadi kwath, Vidaryadi.

Toxicity/Adverse Effects

Not reported.

Substitution and Adulteration

Vidarikanda is used as a substitute drug for Jivak and Rshabhaka of Ashtavarga (B.P.S. 1/166). In some markets, Ksheer Vidari roots, i.e., *Ipomea digitata* roots are sold as Vidari.

> ### Points to Ponder
>
> - *Vidarikanda is a renowned rejuvenator, aphrodisiac, strength promoting, adaptogenic drug.*
> - *Folklore women take Vidari and Shatavri powder to increase milk production in lactating mothers.*

Suggested Readings

Bilore KV, Yelne MB, Dennis TJ, Chaudari BG. Database on Medicinal Plants Used in Ayurveda, Vol. 6. 1st ed. New Delhi: Central Council for Research in Ayurveda And Siddha; 2004:442

Kirtikar KR, Basu BD. Indian Medicinal Plants, Vol. 1. Reprinted edition. Allahabad: LM Basu Publishers; 1933:792–793

The Ayurvedic Pharmacopeia of India, Part I, Vol. 2. New Delhi: Department of AYUSH, Ministry of Health and Family Welfare, Government of India; 1999:184.

Venkataratnam K, Venkataraju RR. Preliminary phytochemical and antimicrobial properties of *Pueraria tuberosa* (Willd.) DC: a potential medicinal plant. Ethnobotan Leafl 2009;13:1051–1059

Warrier PK, Nambiar VPK, Raman K. Indian Medicinal Plants, Vol. 4. Kottakkal, Kerala: Orient longman; 1997:360.

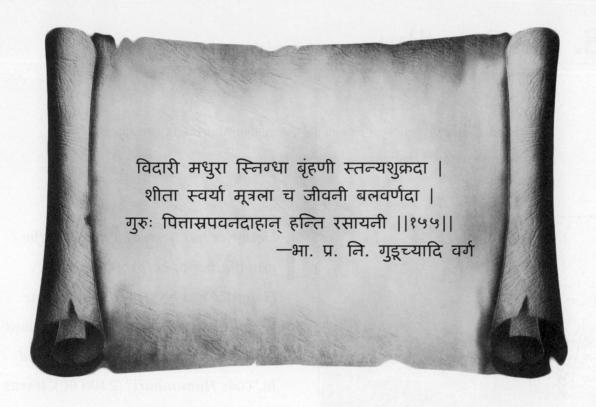

विदारी मधुरा स्निग्धा बृंहणी स्तन्यशुक्रदा ।
शीता स्वर्या मूत्रला च जीवनी बलवर्णदा ।
गुरुः पित्तास्रपवनदाहान् हन्ति रसायनी ।।१५५।।

—भा. प्र. नि. गुडूच्यादि वर्ग

108. Yastimadhu *[Glycyrrhiza glabra Linn.]*

Family: *Fabaceae*

Hindi name: *Mulhatti, Jethimadh, Jethimadhu, Mulethi, Muleti, Mulathi*

English name: *Liquorice, Sweet wood, Licorice root*

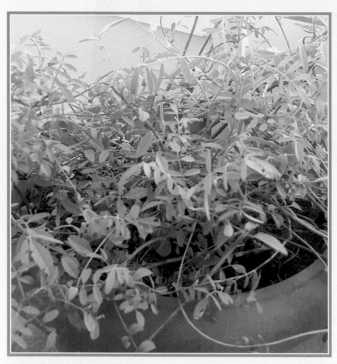

Plant of *Glycyrrhiza glabra* Linn.

> *Liquorice has been described as "the grandfather of herbs" (Ody 2000). Liquorice has been used in medicine for more than 4,000 years. The earliest record of its use in medicine is found in "code Humnubari" (2100 BC). It was also considered as one of the significant plants mentioned in Assyrian herbal (2000 BC). Hippocrates (400 BC) mentioned its use as a remedy of ulcers and quenching of thirst.*

Introduction

Glycyrrhiza glabra Linn. is derived from Glycyrrhiza and Glabra. Glycyrrhiza (Glykas means sweet and Rhiza means root) and Glabra means smooth and hairless.

The reference of Yashtimadhu has been made in it by the term "Madugha." In Atharva veda the meaning of "Madugha" is taken as Yashtimadhu where in the drug is used in the form of Lepa. The meaning of the term "Madugha" is taken as "Jayesthi Madhuka" by the commentator of Kaushiksutra also. In the Bhashya of Atharva veda, Sayana has referred to this as "Madhuk Vriksha" or "Yashtimadhuka."

In Samhitakala, Acharya Charaka dealt with Yashtimadhu in various contexts. In the very first chapter of the Charaka Samhita, Klitaka has been mentioned as being of two types, viz., Anupa and Sthalaja under Phalini varga. Commentator Chakrapani has attempted to equate these types as being that of Yashtimadhu. In another context regarding ingredients of Brihat Shatavarighrita, the word "Dwiyasthimadhukaih" is found. It is also mentioned in many contexts in Sushruta Samhita, Ashtanga Hridaya, and other samhitas. Almost every Nighantu and chikitasa granthas mentioned about Yastimadhu.

Yastimashu is mentioned highest times (11 times) in dashemani of Charaka samhita. This drug is best for chakshushya (eye sight promoter), vrishya (aphrodisiac and fertility promoter), keshya (hair growth promoter), kanthya (voice promoter), varnya (complexion promoter), virajaneeya (antiseptic), and ropana (healing) actions (C.S.Su. 25/40). It has medhya rasayan action when powder of this drug is given with milk (C.S.Ci. 1/3/30).

Bhavamishra referred Yastimadhu with a synonym Klitaka and mentioned two of its varieties based on the ecological distribution. He attributed sukrala (spermatopoetic) activity in addition to chakshushya, balya, vrishya, keshya, swarya, vranasothahara properties. Bhavamishra recorded analgesic activities of Yastimadhu on administration in the form of nasyakarma to relieve all types of headaches. He also described that Yastimadhu relieves cough immediately. Vangasen has reported antiepileptic activity in combination with Kushmanda Swarasa. Sodhala described its aphrodisiac activities, while author of Vaidya manorama confirms the galactagogue activity of Yastimadhu. Chakradutta suggested its application on ulcers due to injury for relieving pain (Anilkumar et al 2012).

The Roman writers referred to it as *Radix dulcis* (Chopra and Chopra 1958). In old Chinese pharmacy, it was considered to belong to drugs of the first class and it has rejuvenating property when consumed for long periods (Vispute and Khopade 2011). It is the most prescribed herb after Ginseng in Chinese medicine (Shah 1995) used for ailments related to spleen, liver, and kidney (Shibata 2000). Historically, the dried rhizome and root of this plant were employed medicinally by the Egyptian, Chinese, Greek, Indian, and Roman civilizations as an expectorant and carminative (Anonymous 2005).

Vernacular Names

Afghanistan: Makk, Sus, Zaisi
Arabic: Aslussus
Assamese: Jesthimadhu, Yeshtmadhu
Bengali: Jaishbomodhu, yashto madhu, Jai-shbomodhu
Bihari: Muraiti
Burmese: Noekhuju, Noe-khiyu, Noe-khiyu-asui
Chinese: Kan ts'ao
French: Racinedouce, Reglisse, Bois doux
German: Lackrizen, Suesshdz
Gujarati: Jethimadha, Jethimard
Kannada: Yashti madhuka, Atimadhura, Jesthamadhu, Madhuka
Kashmiri: Multhi

Malayalam: Atimadhuram, Irattimadhuram, Yashtimadhukam
Marathi: Jeshtamadha
N.W.P.: Mulethi
Oriya: Jaatimadhu
Persian: Bikhe-mahak
Punjabi: Jethimadh, Muleti
Sanskrit: Jalayasti, Klitaka, Madhuka, Madhusrava, Madhuyashti, Yashti, Yashtyawa, Yastika, Yashtimadhuka, Yashtimadhu, Yashtikam, Madhukam, Madhuyashtika, Laksmana
Singapore: Ati-maduram, Veimi
Tamil: Atimadhuram, Adimadhuram, Athimathurappal
Telugu: Yashti-madhukam, Atimadhuramu
Turkish: Meyan, Megarkoku
Urdu: Mitilakdi, Asailasoos, Mulethi

Synonyms

Klitaka: It cures male infertility.
Klitanaka: It is found in terrestrial.
Madhuka: It is sweet like honey.
Yastimadhu: The stem (stick) and roots are sweet in taste.
Yastimadhuka: The stem (stick) and roots are sweet in taste.
Madhurvalli: It is a sweet creeper.
Madhusrava: Its taste is sweet.
Madhurlata: It is a sweet creeper.

Classical Categorization

Charaka Samhita: Jivaniya, Sandhaniya, Varnya, Kanthya, Kandugna, Snehopaga, Vamanopaga, Asthapanopaga, Mutravirajaneeya, Angamardprashamana, Shonitasthapana
Sushruta Samhita: Haridradi, Anjanadi, Brihatyadi, Ambasthadi, Kakolyadi, Nyagrodhadi, Sarivadi, Utapaladi
Ashtanga Hridaya: Vamana, Anjanadi, Niruhana, Aragwadhadi, Pittagna, Haridradi, Sarivadi, Ambasthadi, Padmakadi, Nyagrodhadi
Dhanwantari Nighantu: Guduchyadi varga
Madanpal Nighantu: Abhayadi varga
Kaiyadev Nighantu: Aushadhi varga
Raj Nighantu: Pipalyadi varga
Bhavaprakash Nighantu: Haritkyadi varga

Distribution

It is distributed in the subtropical and warm temperature regions of the world chiefly in the Mediterranean countries, south Europe, Asia Minor, Egypt, Turkistan, Iran, Siberia, Persia, Arab countries, and Afghanistan. In India, it is reported to be cultivated in Baramulla, Srinagar, Jammu, Dehradun, and Delhi (Sharma et al 2005).

Morphology

A perennial herb with a thick rootstock.

- **Root:** Long, straight, cylindrical, slightly tapering, smooth, flexible, about ½ inch in diameter, red or orange-brown on the surface, pale yellow within (**Fig. 108.1**).

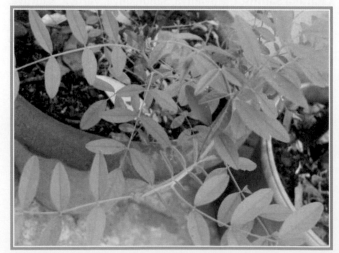

Fig. 108.1   Root.

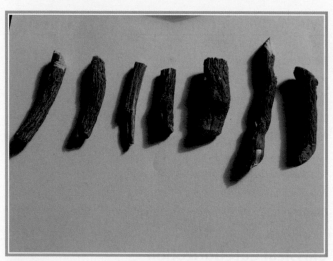

Fig. 108.2   Leaves.

- **Stems:** 2 to 4 feet or more high, erect, stiff, solid, strongly striates, shortly pubescent, and branched.
- **Leaves:** Alternate, spreading, large, stalked, with very minute deciduous stipules, impairipinnate, leaflets opposite in four to seven pairs and a terminal one, shortly stalked, oblong-oval or ovate, obtuse, entire, smooth, except when young, dark green on both sides, glutinous beneath; rachis stout, not furrowed, thickened below (**Fig. 108.2**).
- **Flowers:** Very shortly stalked, erect raceme, which is 1 to 3 inches long and long-stalked, but falling short of the leaves; bracts linear, acute. Calyx tubular, cut about half way down into five unequal teeth, the lowest one is longest and the upper two are connate, pubescent and glandular, green. Petals papilionaceous, pale lilac, the wings darker; 10 stamens, 9 united into a sheath, the vexillary one free, anther-cells confluent at the top. Ovary sessile with several ovules, stigma capitate (**Fig. 108.3**).
- **Pods:** Linear-oblong, compressed, about 1 inch long, pointed, smooth, pale brown indehiscent, containing two to five seeds.
- **Seeds:** Roundish-quadrangular, compressed, about 1/8 inch wide, smooth, dark brown.

It is propagated from cuttings of younger parts of rhizome, as well as from suckles and seeds.

Phenology

Flowering time: August to February
Fruiting time: August to February

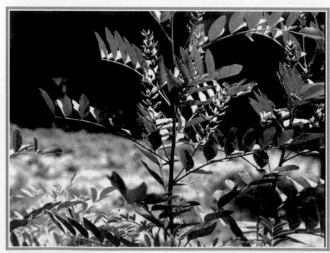

Fig. 108.3   Flowers.

Key Characters for Identification

➤ *A perennial herb with a thick rootstock.*

➤ *Root: Long, straight, cylindrical, red or orange-brown on the surface, pale yellow within.*

➤ *Stems: 2-4 feet or more high, strongly striates.*

➤ *Leaves: Alternate, impairipinnate, leaflets opposite in 4-7 pairs and a terminal one, shortly stalked, oblong-oval or ovate, obtuse, entire.*

➤ *Flowers: Very shortly stalked, erect raceme, calyx tubular, petals papilionaceous, pale lilac, the wings darker; 10 stamens, 9 united into a sheath, the vexillary one free.*

➤ *Pods: Linear-oblong, compressed, about 1 inch long, pointed, smooth, pale brown indehiscent, containing two to five seeds.*

Types

Acharya Charaka has described two types of Yastimadhu: Jalaja yastimadhu (aquatica) and sthalaja (terrestrial). Jalaja variety is also known as Madhoolika.

As per habitat it is of three types:

• Mishri: It is considered as best variety. More sweet in taste.

• Arabi: Medium variety. Medium sweetness.

• Turki: Worst/poor variety. Lesser sweetness.

• As per botanical sources, it is of three types:

• *G. glabra* Regel & Herd: Also known as Spanish liquorice

• *G. glabra* var, glandulifera Waldst. & Kit: Russian liquorice

• *G. glabra* var.violacea Bioss: Persian liquorice (Sharma 2009).

Rasapanchaka

Guna	Guru, Snigdha
Rasa	Madhura
Vipaka	Madhura
Virya	Sheeta

Chemical Constituents

Root: Glycyrrhizin, prenylated biaurone, licoagrone; 7-acetoxy-2- methyl-isoflavone, 7-methoxy-2- methyliso-flavone and 7-hydroxy-2 methyl isoflavone; 4- methyl coumarin, liqcoumarin; isoflavone, glyzaglabrin (7,2'-dihydroxy 3',4' methylenedihydroxy isoflavone); quercetin, quercetin-3-glucoside, kaempferol, astragalin, liquiritigenin, and isoliquiritigenin.

Root and other parts: Include a flavanone rhamnogluco-side, chalcone glucosides, trans-isoliquiritigenin-4-D-glucopyranoside (isoliquiritin) and trans-isoliquiritigenin-4-Dglucopyranoside (neoisoliquiritin); licuraside, liquir-itoside, rhamnoliquiritin,triterpenoid, liquoric acid, licoflavonol, glyzarin, glyzaglabrin, licoisoflavones A, B, and licoisoflavon, glycyrin, sugars, and aspargin (Sharma et al 2005).

Identity, Purity, and Safety

• Total ash: Not more than 10%
• Acid-insoluble ash: Not more than 2.5%
• Alcohol-soluble extractive: Not less than 10%
• Water-soluble extractive: Not less than 20%

(Source: The Ayurvedic Pharmacopeia of India 1989)

Karma (Actions)

Dahashamaka (reduce burning sensation), keshya (hair tonic), vedanasthapana (analgesic), shothahara (reduce swelling), nadibalya (nervine tonic), medhya (intellect promoter), chhardinigrahana (antivomiting), trishnanigrahana (antithirst), vatanulomana (carminative), mridurechana (laxative), shonitasthapana (striptics), kaphanissaraka (antitussive), kanthya (beneficial for throat), mootrala (diuretics), mootravirajaneeya (normalize the urine color), shukravardhaka (spermatogenesis), varnya (complexion promoter), kandughna (antipruritus), jwarashamaka (antipyretics), jeevaneeya (vitality), sandha-neeya (reunion of bone), rasayana (rejuvenative), balya (strength promoter), chakshushya (beneficial for vision).

• Doshakarma: Vatapittashamaka
• Dhatukarma: Shonitasthapana (striptics), shukra-vardhaka (spermatogenesis)

- Malakarma: Mridurechana (laxative), mootrala (diuretics), mootravirajaneeya (normalize the urine color)

Pharmacological Actions

Antiulcer, antioxidant, wound healing, anti-*Helicobacter pylori*, antistaphylococcal, alleviates symptoms of functional dyspepsia, smooth muscle depressant, antimicrobial, hypolipidemic, antiantherosclerotic, antiviral, hypotensive, hepatoprotective, antiexudative, choleretic effect, spasmolytic, antidiuretic, antiulcer, antimutagenic, antipyretic, anti-inflammatory, antinociceptive, and expectorant.

Indications

It is used in netra roga (eye disease), shwasa (asthma), kasa (cough), raktapitta (hemorrhage), swarabheda (hoarseness of voice), khalitya (baldness), palitya (premature greying of hair), amlapitta (hyper acidity), vatavikara (neuromuscular disease), vatarakta (gout), amavata (rheumatoid arthritis), shiroroga (diseases of head), vamana (vomiting), trishna (thirst), vibandha (constipation), udarashoola (abdominal pain), paittika apasmara (epilepsy caused by pitta), hikka (hic-cough), raktavikara (diseases of blood), raktalpata (anemia), yakshma (consumption), urogata vrana (chest injury), urahkshata (pulmonary trauma), vranashotha (wound), shastrabhighataja vrana (incised wound), visha (poisoning), parshwashoola (pleurisy), mootrakrichchhra (dysuria), paittika prameha (diabetes caused by pitta), shukrameha (spermaturia), varnavikara (discoloration of skin), kandu (itching), charma roga (skin diseases), jeerna jwara (chronic fever), samanya daurbalya (general debility).

Therapeutic Uses

External Use

1. **Arsha** (piles): After application of Kshara, Ghrita mixed with Yashtimadhu should be applied on hemorrhoides (S.S.Ci. 6.4).
2. **Visarpa** (erysipelas): The affected part should be sprinkled with Ghrita-scum, cold milk, and decoction of Madhuka or Panchavalkala (C.S.Ci. 21.94; also AH.Ci. 18.21).

3. **Shopha** (edema caused by marking nut): Edema is destroyed by application of the paste of Yashtimadhutaila and milk mixed with butter (Vrunda Madhava.39.18).
4. **Sadyavarna** (accidental wound): Pain of the accidental wound is removed by applying locally warm Ghrita mixed with Yashtimadhu (SS.SU. 5.42; Vrunda Madhava. 45.1).
5. **Vrana** (wound): Paste of Madhuka mixed with Nimba leaves acts as wound cleanser (C.S.Ci. 25.85). Paste of Madhuka and Tila mixed with Ghrita helps in wound healing (Vrunda Madhava. 44.33).
6. **Bhagandar** (fistula-in-ano): The wound should be sprinkled with Madhukataila (S.S.Ci. 8.18).
7. **Dagdha** (burn): Ghrita mixed with Madhuka pacifies burns caused by alkali (S.S.Su. 11.19).
8. **Palitya** (premature graying of hairs): Yashtimadhutaila is used to prevent and cure palitya (SG.S. 2.9.153).
9. **Netra roga** (eye diseases): After scarification of lid, the same sprinkled with the decoction of Madhuka or milk boiled with Chandana (AH.U. 9.18). Bathing with Madhuka and Amalaka pacifies Pitta and alleviates defects of vision (Bangasena.Netraroga. 288). In Upapkshma, sprinkling with Ghrita cooked with Madhuka removes pain immediately (Bangasena. Netraroga. 558). In corneal opacity, one of the following four is used with honey as collyrium Makshika, Madhuka (extract), Bibhitaka seed, and rocksalt (Vrunda Madhava. 61.96).
10. **Karna roga** (eye diseases): Milk processed with Draksha and Yashtimadhu should be used for filling the ear in diseases caused by pitta (Bangasena.Karnaroga).

Internal Use

1. **Shosha** (consumption): In case of pain in head, sides, and shoulders, the parts should be sprinkled with milk and decoction of Madhuka (C.S.Ci. 8.85).
2. **Swarabheda** (hoarseness of voice): Payasa (rice-milk) prepared with Yashtimadhu and mixed with Ghrita should be taken (SS.U. 53.13).
3. **Hridroga** (heart disease): Paste of Yashtimadhu and Katuka should be taken with sugar water (C.S.Ci. 26). Enema of oil cooked with Madhuka and mixed with honey should be given (SS.U. 43.17).
4. **Apasmara** (epilepsy): Ghrita 640 g is cooked with the paste of Madhuka 80 g and Amalaka juice 10.24 L. It is a

good remedy for epilepsy caused by Pitta (C.S.Ci. 10.31). Madhuka pounded with Kushmanda juice should be taken for three days. It alleviates epilepsy (BP.Chi. 23.17).

5. **Hikka** (hic-cough): Pressed snuff of Madhuka mixed with honey or Pippali mixed with fine sugar should be used (SS.U. 50.16; also Vrunda Madhava.12.3).
6. **Trishna** (thirst): Thirst caused by wasting is quenched with Ghrita extracted from milk meat-soup or decoction of Madhuka (SS.U. 48.28).
7. **Pandu** (anemia): One should take decoction of Madhuka or powder of the same with honey (SS.U. 44.20; also Gadanigraha. 2.7.33).
8. **Mutraghata** (retention of urine): Madhuka, Darvi, and seeds of Ervaru should be taken with rice water (AS. Chi. 13.4). Paste of Madhuka and Kumkuma is kept in water mixed with jaggery for whole night and taken in morning. It removes all urinary disorders (KK. 17.64).
9. **Vatarakta** (gout): In Vatarakta predominant in Vata, goat milk mixed with half oil and Madhuka 10 g should be given (S.S.Ci. 5.7).
10. **Vradna** (scrotal enlargement): Unctuous enema should be given with oil cooked with Yashtimadhu (S.S.Ci. 19.7).
11. **Raktapradar** (menometrorrhagia): One affected with the disease should take Madhuka 10 g mixed with sugar 10 g and pounded with rice water (BP.Ci. 68.13).
12. **Sthanyajana** (for promoting lactation): Cow's milk mixed with Yashimadhu and sugar promotes lactation (Vaidyamanorama.13.45).
13. **Vrisya** (as aphrodisiac): Madhuka powder 10 g mixed with Ghrita and honey followed by intake of milk makes a man sexually potent (C.S.Ci. 2.3.19; also AS.U. 50.43).
14. **Medhya rasayana** (as intellect-promoting rasayana): Intake of Madhuka powder with milk acts as rasayana particularly intellect-promoting (C.S.Ci. 1.3.30-31).
15. **Raktapitta** (intrinsic hemorrhage): Paste of Yashtimadhu 10 g should be taken (SS.U. 45.22). Emesis should be given mixed with Madhuka and honey (SS.U. 45). Yashtimadhu and Chandana pounded with milk should be taken with the same. It controls hematemesis (CD. 15.25).
16. **Garbhasrava** (wasting of fetus): Milk processed with Sarkara, Kasmarda, and Madhuka promotes growth of fetus (C.S.Ci. 28.96).
17. **Hemicrania:** Madhuka mixed with honey should be used as pressed snuff (SS.U. 26.33).
18. **Shirashoola** (all headaches): Yashtimadhu 1 g and aconite 250 mg are pounded finely and mixed with mustard powder. Put in the nostrils it removes all types of headache (BP.Chi. 62.59-60).
19. **Sheetapitta** (urticaria): Madhuka mixed with sugar should be used (CD. 51.3).
20. **Udavarta caused by retention of urine:** In such condition, sugar, sugarcane juice, milk, Draksha, and Yashtimadhu should be given (BhP.Chi. 31-25).

Officinal Part Used

Root

Dose

Powder: 3 to 5 g

Formulations

Yashtyadi churna, Sudarshana churna, Saraswata churna, Medhya rasayana, Kalyanavaleha, Dashamularistha, Angamardaprashamana kashaya, Brihat ashwagandha ghrita, Brihachchhagaladya ghrita, Shatavaryadi ghrita, Mahatiktaka ghrita, Mahamayurakghrita, Phala ghrita, Ashwagandhadi ghrita, Panchagya ghrita, Vridhihara lepa, Yashtimadhvadya taila, Guduchyadi taila, Maha mashadi taila, Mahanarayana taila, Pippalyadi taila, Irimedhada taila, Jatyadi taila, Pinda taila, Chandanadi taila, Mayura ghrita, Vyaghri taila, Kubjaprasarani taila, Yasthimadhukadi taila.

Toxicity/Adverse Effects

LD50 of glycyrrhizin and glycyrrhizin-thiamine HCl in rats is reported to be 1.94 and 0.764 g/kg s.c., respectively. Liquiritoside, a root flavonoside, is a low toxic substance.

Consumption of liquorice 10-45 g/ day is reported to cause raised blood pressure, together with a block of aldosterone/ renin axis and electrocardiogram changes (Sharma et al 2005).

Substitution and Adulteration

Roots of *Glycyrrhiza uralensis* Fisch. (Manchurian liquorice) and *Abrus precatorius* Linn. are often adulterated with liquorice. Stem pieces of *G. glabra* are also sold in place of root (Sharma et al 2005).

Points to Ponder

- *Yastimashu is mentioned highest times (11 times) in dashemani of Charaka Samhita.*
- *This drug is best for chakshusya, vrisya, keshya, kanthya, varnya, virajanita, and ropan as per Acharya Charaka (C.S.Su. 25/40).*
- *It has medhya rasayan action when powder of this drug is given with milk (C.S.Ci. 1/3/30).*

Suggested Readings

Anilkumar D, Joshi H, Nishteswar K. Review of *Glycyrrhiza glabra* (Yastimadhu): a broad spectrum herbal drug. Pharma Sci Monitor: Int J Pharmaceut Sci 2012:3171–3195

Anonymous. *Glycyrrhiza glabra:* Monograph. Altern Med Rev 2005;10(3):230–237

Chopra RN, Chopra IC. Indigenous Drugs of India. 2nd ed. Kolkata: Academic Publishers; 1958:183–187

Chunekar KC, Hota NP. Plants of Bhavaprakash. New Delhi: National Academy of Ayurveda; 1999:382

Datta C. Chakradatta of Shri Chakrapani Datta with the Padarthabodhini Hindi Commentary by Vd. Ravidatta Shastri. Reprint. Varanasi: Chaukhambha Surbharti Prakashan; 2006:160

Gogate VM. Ayurvedic Pharmacology & Therapeutic use of Medicinal Plants (Dravyaguna Vignyan). Mumbai: Bharatiya Vidya Bhavan; 2000:457

Kirtikar KR, Basu BD. Indian Medicinal Plant, Vol. 1. 2nd ed. Dehradun: International Book Distributer; 1975:727

Nadkarni AK. Indian Materia Medica, Vol. I. Mumbai: Popular Prakashana; 2007:582

Ody P. The Complete Guide Medicinal Herbal. London: Dorling Kindersley; 2000:75

Shah BG. Nighantu Adarsha: Purvatdha (Vol. I).1st ed. Jamnagar: Gujarat Ayurved University; 1995:502–509

Sharma P. Classical Uses of Medicinal Plant. Varanasi: Chaukhambha; 2004:284–287

Sharma PC, Yelne MB, Dennis TJ. Database on Medicinal Plants Used in Ayurveda. New Delhi: Documentation and Publication Division, Central Council for Research in Ayurveda & Siddha; 2005:561

Sharma PV. Dravyaguna Vijnana, Vol. 2. Varanasi: Chaukhambha Bharti Academy; 2009:253–257

Shibata S. A drug over the millennia: pharmacognosy, chemistry, and pharmacology of licorice. Yakugaku Zasshi 2000;120(10):849–862

Sodhala. Sodhala Nighantu (Sharma PV, Baroda JAN, eds.). Oriental Institute; 1978:19

The Ayurvedic Pharmacopoeia of India, Part 1, Vol. 1. 1st ed. New Delhi: Department of AYUSH, Ministry of Health and Family Welfare, Government of India; 1989:127–128

The Wealth of India: A Dictionary of Indian Raw materials and Industrial Products, Vol. 3. New Delhi: NISCIR; 2002:195-198

Vangasena, by Bopadeva, commented by Shaligram. Mumbai: Khemraj Shrikrishnadas Prakashan; 1996

Vispute S, Khopade A. *Glycyrrhiza glabra* Linn.: "Klitaka": a review. Int J Pharma Bio Sci 2011;2(3):42

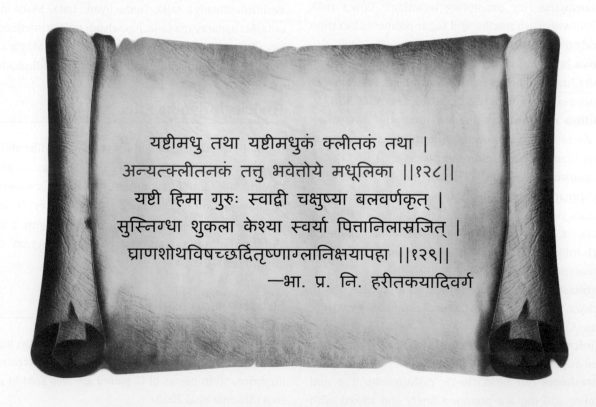

यष्टीमधु तथा यष्टीमधुक् क्लीतकं तथा |
अन्यत्क्लीतनकं तत्तु भवेत्तोये मधूलिका ||१२८||
यष्टी हिमा गुरुः स्वाद्वी चक्षुष्या बलवर्णकृत् |
सुस्निग्धा शुक्ला केश्या स्वर्या पित्तानिलास्त्रजित् |
घ्राणशोथविषच्छर्दितृष्णाग्लानिक्षयापहा ||१२९||
—भा. प्र. नि. हरीतकयादिवर्ग

109. Yavani [Trachyspermum ammi Linn.]

Synonym: Carum copticum Benth. Et.Hook.f.

Family: Apiaceae

Hindi name: Ajwain

English name: Bishop's weed, Carum, Lovage

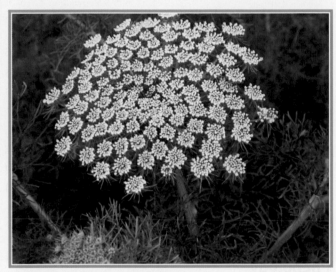

Plant of *Trachyspermum ammi* Linn.

> *An ideal authentic sample of Yavani should contain thymol in the range of 35 to 60%.*

Introduction

Since time immemorial, ajowain has been used as an important constituent of human diet. It is general belief that vata aggravating food should be prepared by tadka with ghrita and ajowain. Besides being an important ingredient of Indian kitchen spices, ajowain has multifold medicinal uses. Ayurveda texts have also mentioned a plant Ajmoda which is almost similar to Yavani in properties and action. To avoid any ambiguity, it is advised to use Yavani for oraland Ajmoda for external application as medicinal purpose. Yavani is an ingredient of Chaturbeej, a famous formulation containing four seeds used in vata diseases, indigestion, flatulence, colic, and backache (B.P.S. 2/98). Charaka has mentioned it in harita and aharayogi varga (C.S.Su. 27/70,307).

Apart from medicinal and culinary use, Yavani and its essential oil have diverse industrial applications. The oil and seeds are used as preservatives, flavoring agent, and for the manufacture of essential oil in perfumery, toothpaste, mouthwashes, antiseptic solutions, and in bakery industry.

Vernacular Names

Arabian: Kamue muluki, Talib-el-khubz, Kamunemaluki

Bengali: Yamani, Yauvan, Yavan, Javan, Yavani, Yoyana

Gujarati: Ajma, Ajmo, Yavan, Javain

Kannada: Oma, Yom, Omu

Kashmiri: Kath, Jawind

Malayalam: Omam, Ayanodakan

Marathi: Onva, Owa, Vova

Oriya: Juani

Persian: Zinian, Nankhwah, Nankhah

Punjabi: Lodhar, Javaina

Tamil: Omam

Telugu: Vamu

Urdu: Ajwan

Synonyms

Ajmodika: The plant resembles Ajmoda in properties and actions.

Brahmadarbha: It is considered as the favorite herb of Lord Brahma.

Dipya: The plant has carminative action.

Dipyaka: The fruits are used to enhance digestive fire.

Ugragandha: The plant especially the fruits are strong smelling.

Yavanika: A small herbaceous plant like that of yava.

Classical Categorization

Charaka Samhita: Shoolaprasasmana
Sushrut Samhita: not mentioned
Ashtang Hridaya: not mentioned
Dhanvantari Nighantu: Shatpushpadi varga
Madanpal Nighantu: Sunthyadi varga
Kaiyadev Nighantu: Oushadi varga
Raj Nighantu: Pippalayadi varga
Bhavaprakash Nighantu: Haritakyadi varga

Distribution

The plant is native to Egypt and cultivated in Mexico, Costa Rica, North-East Africa, Europe, Iraq, Iran, India, Afghanistan, Pakistan, and Baluchistan. It is cultivated in warm and dried regions of India like Rajasthan, Haryana, Punjab, Gujarat, Maharashtra, Madhya Pradesh, Chhattisgarh, and Andhra Pradesh.

Morphology

It is an erect, aromatic, profusely branched, annual herb, 60 to 90 cm tall. Branches are many, striated, hairy all over.

- **Leaves:** Bi or tripinnately compound-decompound, alternate, 2 to 5 cm long, leaflets variously dissected, linear or thread-like (**Fig. 109.1**).
- **Flowers:** Inflorescence compound umbel with 16 umbellets, each containing up to 16 flowers, flowers actinomorphic, white, male and bisexual, petals bilobed, five corolla and five stamens (**Fig. 109.2**).
- **Fruits:** Highly aromatic, consists of two mericarps, grayish brown, ovoid, compressed, about 2 mm long and 1.5 mm wide, five ridges and six vittae in each mericarp, cremocarp with a persistent stylopodium (**Fig. 109.3**).

The plant is propagated by seeds.

Phenology

Flowering time: December to February
Fruiting time: December to February

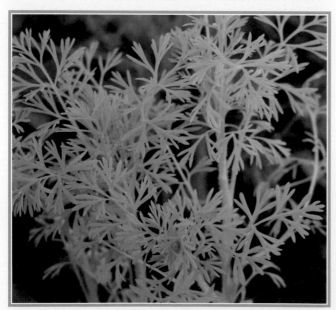

Fig. 109.1 Leaves.

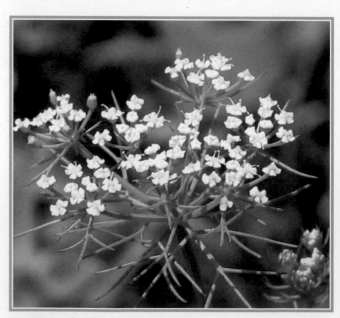

Fig. 109.2 Flowers.

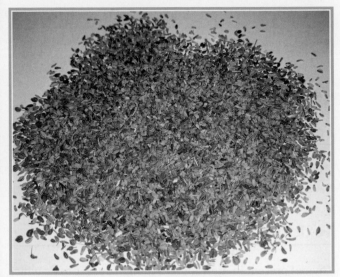

Fig. 109.3 Fruits.

Key Characters for Identification

➤ *It is an erect, aromatic, profusely branched annual herb of 60 to 90 cm height.*

➤ *Leaves are alternate, 2 to 5 cm long, bi to tripinnately compound.*

➤ *Flowers are scented white, occurs in compound umbel inflorescence.*

➤ *Fruits are grayish brown, ovoid, compressed, about 2 mm long, aromatic, with two mericarps.*

Rasapanchaka

Guna	Laghu, Ruksha, Tikshana
Rasa	Katu, Tikta
Vipaka	Katu
Virya	Ushna

Chemical Constituents

The plant mainly contains essential oil, volatile oils, fiber (12%), carbohydrates (25%), tannins, saponins, glycosides, flavonoids, protein (17%), fat, minerals like calcium, phosphorous, iron, cobalt, copper, iodine, manganese, thiamine, riboflavin, and nicotinic acid. The chief active constituents of volatile oil are thymol (40–50%). The nonthymol fraction consists of γ-terpinene, para-cymene,

α- and β-pinene, steroptin, dipentene, cymone, myrcene, thymine, styrene, β-phyllanderene, limonene, carvacrol, and carvone (Chopra 1982; Nagalakshmi 2000).

Identity, Purity, and Strength

- Foreign matter: Not more than 5%
- Total ash: Not more than 9%
- Acid-insoluble ash: Not more than 0.2%
- Alcohol-soluble extractive: Not less than 2%
- Water-soluble extractive: Not less than 13%
- Volatile oil: Not less than 2.5%

(Source: The Ayurvedic Pharmacopeia of India 1989)

Karma (Actions)

Ayurvedic classics attributed deepana (carminative), pachan (digestive), rochana (relish), anulomana (laxative), shoolaprashamana (analgesic), krimighna (anthelmizntic), vishaghna (antidote to toxin), shothaghna (anti-inflammatory), jantughna (antibacterial), hridayottejaka (cardiac stimulant), jwaraghna (antipyretic), shleshmaputihara (pacify foul odour due to kapha), swasahara (antiasthmatic), mutral (diuretic), stanyanashana (reduces lactation), garbhashayottejaka (uterine stimulant), swedajanana (diaphoretic), and sheetaprashamana (calefacient).

- Doshakarma: Vata kaphashamaka, pittavardhaka
- Dhatukarma: Shukranashaka, shoolaghna, shothaghna
- Malakarma: Anulomana, mutral, swedajanan

Pharmacological Actions

Scientific research studied revealed that Yavani possesses stimulant, antispasmodic, anthelmintic, analgesic, anti-inflammatory, diuretic, antibacterial, insecticidal, antifungal, germicidal, aphrodisiac, antitussive, detoxification, antioxidant, antihypertensive, hepatoprotective, bronchodilator, antilithiasis, abortifacient, antiplatelet-aggregatory, nematocidal, and galactagogue properties (Jeet et al 2012).

Indications

In traditional medicines, Yavani is prescribed to be used in treatment of udar roga (abdominal disorders), aanaah (tympanitis), adhyamana (flatulence), shool (pain), gulma (abdominal tumors), pleeha (splenomegaly), krimi roga (worm infestation), chardi (vomiting), vata arsha (piles), vrana (wounds), sheetpitta (urticaria), sandhishool (joint pain), dantashool (toothache), udarshool (abdominal cramps), jeerna kasa (chronic cough), swasa (bronchitis), hridya daurbalya (cardiac debility), mutraghata (urinary obstruction), and kastaartava (dysmenorrhea).

Therapeutic Uses

External Use

1. **Dantashool** (toothache): Yavani and Vacha should be pressed under teeth to get relief in toothache (H.S. 3/6/11).
2. **Visha** (poisoning): Washing the affected part with the decoction of Yavani beeja alleviates the pain caused by scorpion's bite.
3. **Vatavyadhis** (neuromuscular diseases): Yavani taila or beeja kalka is used for local application in paralysis, palsy, tremor, and neuralgic pain. In asthma, hot and dry fomentation of the fruits is applied on chest.

Internal Use

1. **Gulma** (abdominal lump): Powder of Yavani mixed with bida lavan should be taken with takra to allievate gulma, agnimandhya, aruchi, and adhyamaan (C.S.Ci. 5/168) (VM. 30/21).
2. **Arsha** (piles): Saturated drink of buttermilk added with Bhallataka or Bilva and Shunthi or Chitraka and Yavani should be given in arsha (C.S.Ci. 14/70); powdered Yavani, Shunthi, Patha, Dadima, and guda with salted Takra are also beneficial (C.S.Ci. 14/19).
3. **Shoola** (pain): Yavani, rocksalt, Haritaki, and Shunthi churna in equal quantity alleviate udarshool (VM. 26/39).
4. **Aruchi** (loss of appetite): Yavani shadava 20 mL twice daily is used in loss of appetite and indigestion (C.S.Ci. 8/141-45).
5. **Udarda** (urticaria): Intake of Yavani with guda keeping on wholesome diet for a week cures urticaria.

Officinal Part Used

Fruits

Dose

Powder: 1 to 3 g

Oil: 1 to 3 drops

Ark: 20 to 40 mL

Formulations

Yavanishadava, Chaturbeej churna, Yavanikadi ghrita, Yavanarka, Vaisvanara churna, Agnimukh churna, Lohasava.

Toxicity/Adverse Effects

Thymol present in Ajowain taila in high dose is toxic which may lead to fatal poisoning (Billore et al 2005).

Substitution and Adulteration

Market sample of Yavani includes fruits of Ajmoda, vanya ajowain, stem pieces, earthy matter, and oil extracted from fruits of Yavani and Ajmoda (Billore et al 2005).

Points to Ponder

- *Yavani is the drug of choice for gastrointestinal disorders like loss of appetite, dyspepsia, indigestion, abdominal distention, and spasmodic pain.*
- *Ajwain taila is a potent antibacterial, antiseptic, analgesic, antibiotic, and wound-healing agent.*

Suggested Readings

Billore KV, Yelne MB, Dennis TJ, Chaudhari BG. Database on Medicinal Plants Used in Ayurveda, Vol. 7. New Delhi: CCRAS Department of Indian Systems of Medicine and Homeopathy (I. S. M. & H.), Ministry of Health and Family Welfare, Government of India; 2005:496–505

Chopra RN. Chopra's Indigenous Drug of India. 2nd ed. Calcutta: Academic Publishers; 1982

Jeet K, Devi N, Thakur N, Tomar S, Shalta L, Thakur R. *Trachyspermum ammi* (Ajwain): a comprehensive review. Int Res J Pharm 2012;3(5):133–138

Nagalakshmi S. Studies on chemical and technological aspects of ajowain (*Trachyspermum ammi* syn. *Carum copticum*). J Food Sci Technol 2000;37:277–281

The Ayurvedic Pharmacopeia of India. Part I, Vol. 1. New Delhi: Department of AYUSH, Ministry of Health and Family Welfare, Government of India; 1989:171

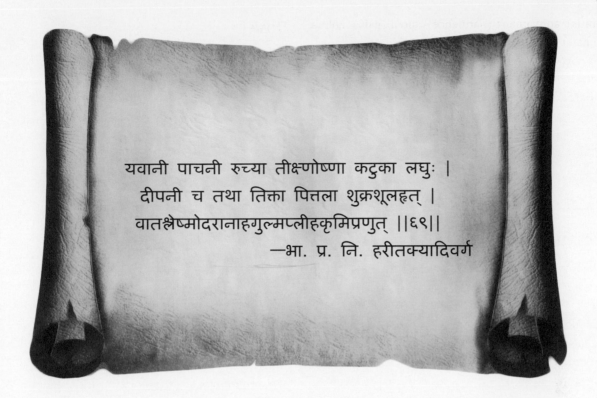

यवानी पाचनी रुच्या तीक्ष्णोष्णा कटुका लघुः ।
दीपनी च तथा तिक्ता पित्तला शुक्रशूलहृत् ।
वातश्लेष्मोदरानाहगुल्मप्लीहकृमिप्रणुत् ।।६९।।
—भा. प्र. नि. हरीतक्यादिवर्ग

Part II

Nondetailed Plants

110. Agastya *[Sesbania grandiflora (L.) Pers.]*

Family:	*Leguminoceae*
Hindi name:	*Basna*
English name:	*The Sesban*
Synonyms:	*Munidruma, Vangasena, Muniputri*

Morphology

It is a fast-growing deciduous legume tree of 10 to 15 m height (**Fig. 110.1**).

Key Characters for Identification

➤ *Leaves: Abruptly pinnate, leaflets are deciduous, linear, and oblong (**Fig. 110.2**)*
➤ *Flowers: Fleshy and showy; petals are white, pink, or red in color (**Fig. 110.3**)*
➤ *Fruits: Pods are long, flat, nontorulose, and septate with swollen margin (**Fig. 110.4 [a, b]**)*
➤ *Seeds: 15–50 in number and pale in color*

Rasapanchaka

Guna	Laghu, Ruksha
Rasa	Katu
Vipaka	Katu
Virya	Ushna
Doshakarma	Kapha-pittahara, vatakaraka

Officinal Parts Used

Patra (leaves) and pushpa (flower)

Dose

Infusion: 10 to 20 mL
Decoction: 50 to 100 mL

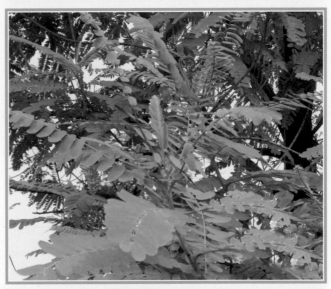

Fig. 110.1 Plant of *Sesbania grandiflora* (L.) Pers.

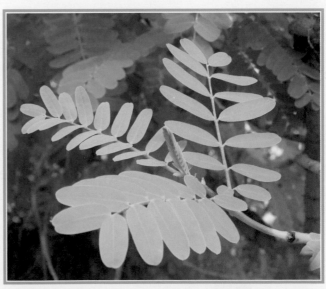

Fig. 110.2 Leaves.

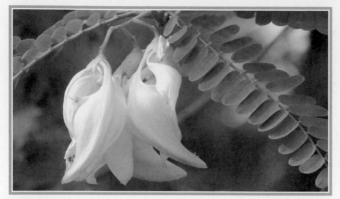

Fig. 110.3 Flower.

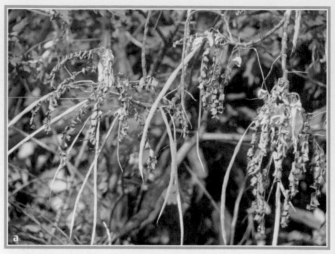

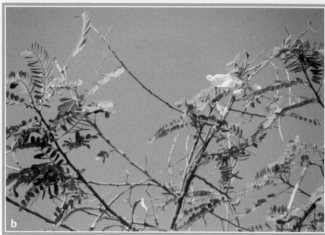

Karma (Actions)

Krimighna (anthelmintic), vishaghna (antidote), medhya (intellect promoter), rochaka (relish), shothhara (anti-inflammatory), shleshmnisaraka (antitussive), vedanasthapana (analgesic), and chakshushya (beneficial for vision).

Indications

Apasmara (epilepsy), naktandhya (night blindness), vatarakta (gout), jwara (fever), pratishyay (cold and coryza), kshaya (emaciation), gulma (abdominal lump), and shool (colic pain).

Fig. 110.4 **(a, b)** Fruits.

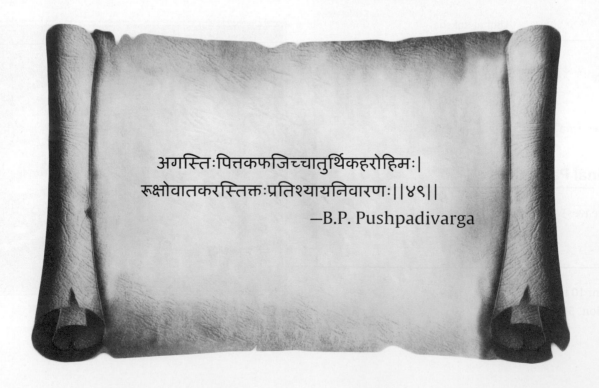

अगस्तिःपित्तकफजिच्चातुर्थिकहरोहिमः।
रूक्षोवातकरस्तिक्तःप्रतिश्यायनिवारणः।।४९।।
—B.P. Pushpadivarga

111. Ajamoda [Apium graveolens Linn.]

Family:	*Umbelliferae*
Hindi name:	*Ajwain*
Synonyms:	*Mayuro, Deepyak, Karavi, Brahmakusha, Kharashwa, Lochmastaka*

Morphology

It is an erect annual or biennial aromatic herb of 2 to 3 feet (**Fig. 111.1**).

Key Characters for Identification

➤ *Leaves: Radical, pinnate with deeply lobed segments, coarsely toothed at apex*
➤ *Inflorescence: Umbel rays with white small flowers* (**Fig. 111.2**)
➤ *Fruit: A cremocarp with two mericarps 1 to 1.5 mm long and with narrow ridges* (**Fig. 111.3 [a, b]**)

Rasapanchaka

Guna	Laghu, ruksha
Rasa	Katu, tikta
Vipaka	Katu
Virya	Ushna
Doshakarma	Kapha-vatahara

Officinal Parts Used

Seed, fruit, root

Dose

Seed powder: 1 to 3 g

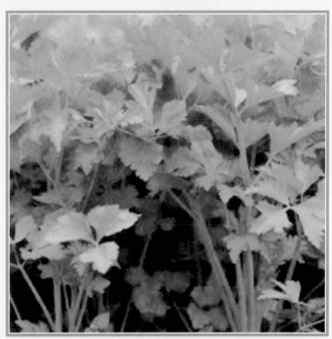

Fig. 111.1 Herb of *Apium graveolens* Linn.

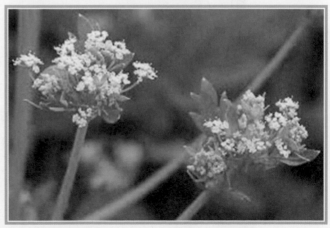

Fig. 111.2 Flowers.

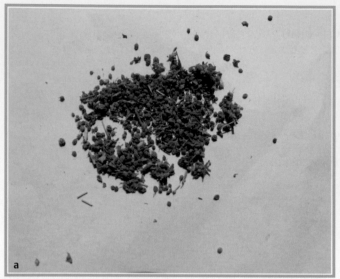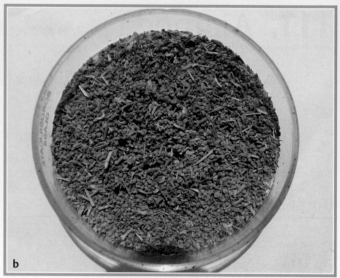

Fig. 111.3 **(a, b)** Fruits.

Karma (Actions)

Deepana (appetizer), balya (physical strength promoter), mutrala (diuretic), hridya (cardiotonic), vrishya (aphrodisiac), vataanulomaka (carminative), and uttejaka (stimulant).

Indications

Udarshoola (abdominal pain), hikka (hic-cough), adhymana (constipation), krimi (worm infestation), udararoga (abdominal disease), sandhishoth (edema in joints), nashtaartava (amenorrhea), netramaya (eye diseases), chhardi (vomiting), and bastiruja (pain in bladder region).

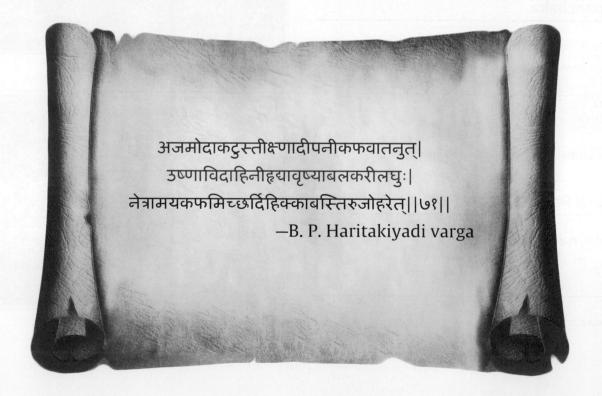

अजमोदाकटुस्तीक्ष्णादीपनीकफवातनुत्।
उष्णाविदाहिनीहृद्यावृष्याबलकरीलघुः।
नेत्रामयकफमिच्छर्दिहिक्काबस्तिरुजोहरेत्।।७१।।
—B. P. Haritakiyadi varga

112. Akarkarabh [*Anacyclus pyrethrum DC.*]

Family:	*Asteraceae*
Hindi name:	*Akarkara*
English name:	*Pellitory root*
Synonyms:	*Akallaka, Kallaka*

Morphology

It is a diffuse perennial herb of 1 foot.

Key Characters for Identification

➤ *Roots: Fusiform, fleshy, and very pungent*
➤ *Leaves: Radical, stalked, and smooth* (**Fig. 112.1**)
➤ *Flowers: White in color, purpe beneath* (**Fig. 112.2**)

Rasapanchaka

Guna	Tikshna, ruksha
Rasa	Katu
Vipaka	Katu
Virya	Ushna
Doshakarma	Kapha vaatshamaka

Officinal Part Used

Mool (root)

Dose

Powder: 0.5 to 1 g

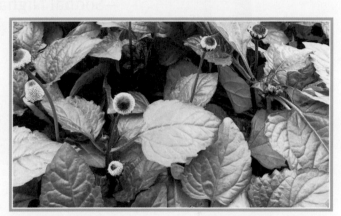

Fig. 112.1 Leaves.

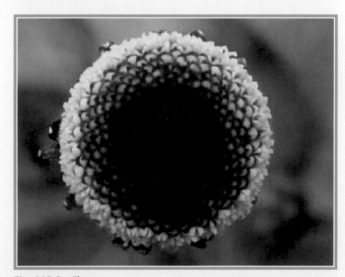

Fig. 112.2 Flower.

Karma (Actions)

Balya (promote physical strength), uttejaka (stimulant), shothahara (reduce swelling), Krimighna(anthelmintic), vajikaran (aphrodisiac), shukrastambhan (reduce ejaculation of semen), and kanthya (beneficial for throat).

Indications

Shotha (swelling), vataroga (neuromuscular disease), dhvajabhang (erectile dysfunction), phirangroga (syphilis), pratisyay (sinusitis), dantakrimi (dental caries), and apasmara (epilepsy).

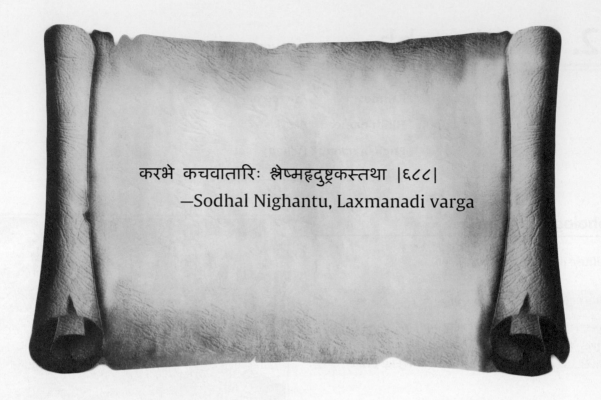

करभे कचवातारिः श्लेष्महृद्दुष्ट्रकस्तथा ।६८८।
—Sodhal Nighantu, Laxmanadi varga

113. Amlavetasa *[Garcinia pedunuculata Roxb.]*

Family:	*Guttiferae*
Hindi name:	*Amalvet*
English name:	*Mangosteen*
Synonyms:	*Chakru, Shatvedhi, Sahastranut*

Morphology

It is a tall deciduous tree of about 20 m height with separate male and female plants (**Fig. 113.1**).

Key Characters for Identification

➤ *Leaves: Lanceolate with prominent midribs (**Fig. 113.2**).*
➤ *Flower: Male flowers are light green in sparsely flowered panicles, and female flowers are solitary.*
➤ *Fruit: Globose, 8 to 10 cm in diameters with fleshy aril (**Fig. 113.3**).*

Rasapanchaka

Guna	Laghu, Ruksha, Tikshna
Rasa	Amla
Vipaka	Amla
Virya	Ushna
Doshaghanta	Kaphavatashamak, Pittavardhak

Officinal Part Used

Phal (fruit)

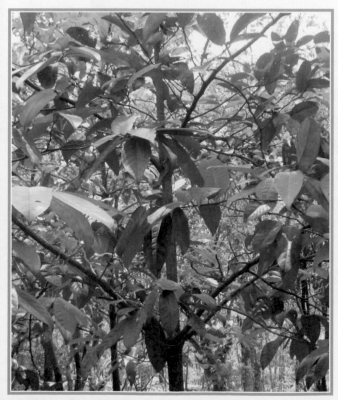

Fig. 113.1 Plant of *Garcinia pedunuculata* Roxb.

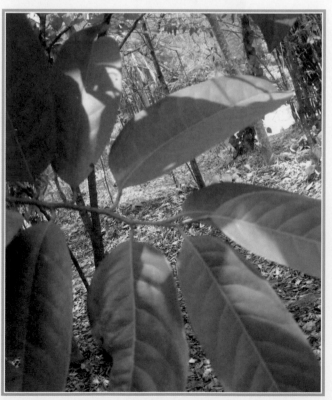

Fig. 113.2 Leaves.

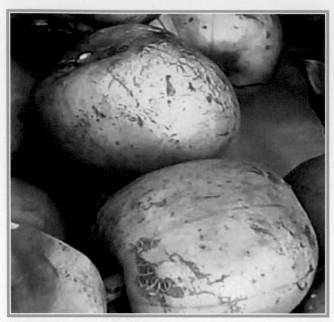

Fig. 113.3 Fruits.

Dose

Swarasa: 5 to 10 mL

Karma (Actions)

Ruchikar (relish), deepan (appetizer), bhedana (purgative), anulomana (laxative), hridya (cardiac tonic), shwasahara (antiasthmatic)

Indications

Amaatisara (diarrhea), pliharoga (diseases of spleen), ajeerna (indigestion), arsha (piles), ashmari (calculus), shool (pain), gulma (abdominal tumor), udavarta (flatulence), hikka (hiccough), aanaah (gas or bloating), aruchi (distaste), vaman (vomiting), kasa (cough), shwasa (asthma).

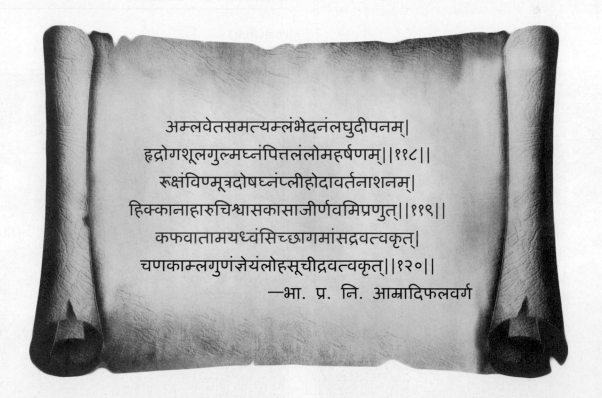

अम्लवेतसमत्यम्लंभेदनंलघुदीपनम्।
हृद्रोगशूलगुल्मघ्नंपित्तलंलोमहर्षणम्।।११८।।
रूक्षंविण्मूत्रदोषघ्नंप्लीहोदावर्तनाशनम्।
हिक्कानाहारुचिश्वासकासाजीर्णवमिप्रणुत्।।११९।।
कफवातामयध्वंसिच्छागमांसद्रवत्वकृत्।
चणकाम्लगुणंज्ञेयंलोहसूचीद्रवत्वकृत्।।१२०।।
—भा. प्र. नि. आम्रादिफलवर्ग

114. Amra *[Mangifera indica Linn.]*

Family:	*Anacardiaceae*
Hindi name:	*Aam, Ambi*
English name:	*Mango*
Synonyms:	*Atisorabh, Madhduta, Maakanda, Rasala, Choot, Sahakar, Kamang*

Morphology

It is a medium-to-large evergreen tree with juicy stone fruits and a doom-shaped crown (**Fig. 114.1**).

Key Characters for Identification

➤ *Bark: Rough, thick, and dark gray* (**Fig. 114.2**)
➤ *Leaves: Simple, linear-oblong, or elliptic-lanceolate, acute, and acuminate* (**Fig. 114.3**)
➤ *Flowers: Reddish-white or yellowish-green* (**Fig. 114.4**)
➤ *Fruits: Fleshy drupes, green, orange, yellow, or red in color*
➤ *Seed: Solitary and encased in a hard-compressed fibrous endocarp*

Rasapanchaka

Guna	Laghu, ruksha (kacha phal)/guru, snighdha (pakwa phal)
Rasa	Amla (kacha phal)/Kasaya, madhura (pakwa phal)
Vipaka	Amla
Virya	Ushna
Doshakarma	Kaphapittashamaka

Officinal Parts Used

Bark, leaf, flower, seed, fruit

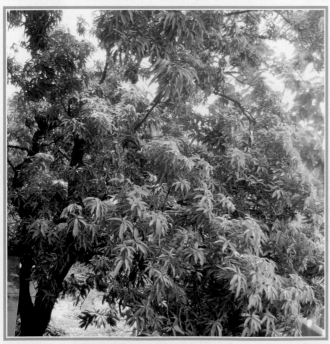

Fig. 114.1   Plant of *Mangifera indica* Linn.

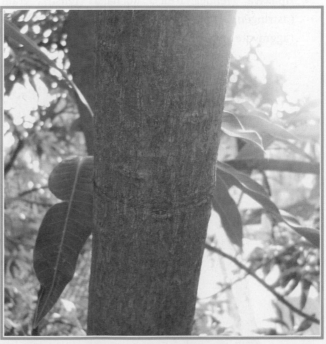

Fig. 114.2   Bark.

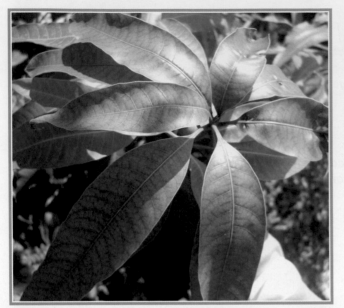

Fig. 114.3 Leaves.

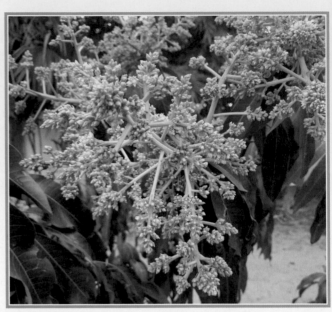

Fig. 114.4 Flowers.

Dose

Powder: 3 to 6 g
Decoction: 50 to 100 mL
Juice: 10 to 20 mL

Karma (Actions)

- **Apakwa** (tender fruit): Rochaka (relish), grahi (astringent), bhedana (laxative), tridoshkaraka (aggravate vata, pitta, and kapha)

- **Pakwa** (mature fruit): Vrishya (aphrodisiac), hridya (cardio tonic), varnya (complexion promoter), balya (increase physical strength), pittashamaka (pacify pitta).

Indications

Chhardi (vomiting), atisaara (diarrhea), prameha (diabetes), trishna (thirst), mukhpaka (stomatitis), raktasrava (bleeding), daha (burning), and aruchi (anorexia).

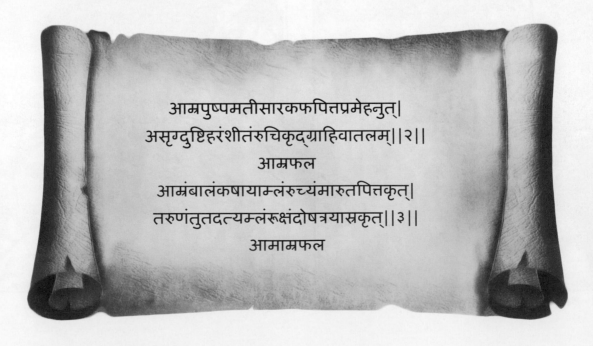

आम्रपुष्पमतीसारकफपित्तप्रमेहनुत्।
असृग्दुष्टिहरंशीतंरुचिकृद्ग्राहिवातलम्॥२॥
आम्रफल
आम्रंबालंकषायाम्लंरुच्यंमारुतपित्तकृत्।
तरुणंतुतदत्यम्लंरूक्षंदोषत्रयास्रकृत्॥३॥
आमाम्रफल

आम्रमामंत्वचाहीनमातपातिविशोषितम्।
अम्लंस्वादुकषायंस्याद्भेदनंकफवातजित्॥४॥

पक्वाम्रफल

पक्वंतुमधुरंवृष्यंस्निग्धंबलसुखप्रदम्।
गुरुवातहरंहृद्यंवर्ण्यंशीतमपित्तलम्।
कषायानुरसंवह्निश्लेष्मशुक्रविवर्धनम्॥५॥
तदेववृक्षसम्पक्वंगुरुवातहरंपरम्।
मधुराम्लरसंकिञ्चिद्ध्वेत्पित्तप्रकोपणम्॥६॥
आम्रंकृत्रिमपक्वञ्चतद्ध्वेत्पित्तनाशनम्।
रसस्याम्लस्यहीनस्तुमाधुर्याच्चविशेषतः॥७॥
चोषितंतत्परंरुच्यंबल्यंवीर्यकरंलघु।
शीतलंशीघ्रपाकिस्याद्वातपित्तहरंसरम्॥८॥
तद्रसोगलितोबल्योगुरुर्वातहरःसरः।
अहृद्यस्तर्पणोऽतीववृंहणःकफवर्धनः॥९॥
तस्यखण्डंगुरुपरंरोचनंचिरपाकिच।
मधुरंवृंहणंबल्यंशीतलंवातनाशनम्॥१०॥
वातपित्तहरंरुच्यंवृंहणंबलवर्धनम्।
वृष्यंवर्णकरंस्वादुदुग्धाम्रंगुरुशीतलम्॥११॥

—B. P. N. Amradiphala varga

115. Amragandhi Haridra [*Curcuma amada Roxb.*]

Family:	*Zingiberaceae*
Hindi name:	*Amahaldi*
English name:	*Mango ginger*
Synonyms:	*Padmpatra, Darvibheda, Aamragandha, Surbhidaru, Karpura*

Morphology

It is an evergreen ginger-like herb whose rhizome tastes like raw mango.

Key Characters for Identification

➤ *Leaves: Long, petiolate, oblong lanceolate, tapering at both ends, and glabrous (***Fig. 115.1***)*
➤ *Flowers: Spikes in the center of the tuft of leaves, white or pale yellow in color (***Fig. 115.2***)*
➤ *Rhizome: Smells like a raw mango; dried and fresh rhizomes are shown in ***Fig. 115.3*** and ***Fig. 115.4***

Rasapanchaka

Guna	Laghu, ruksha
Rasa	Tikta, madhura
Vipaka	Katu
Virya	Sheeta
Doshakarma	Kapha pittashamaka, Vatavardhaka

Officinal Part Used

Rhizome

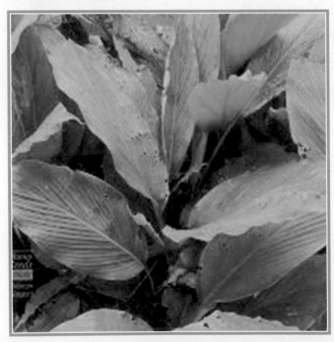

Fig. 115.1 Leaves.

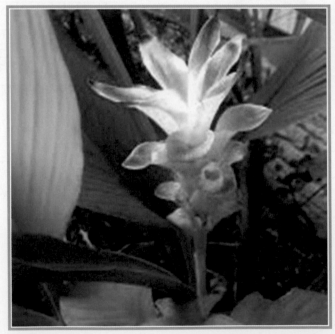

Fig. 115.2 Flower.

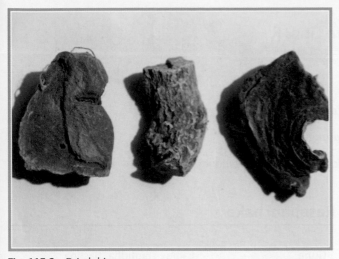

Fig. 115.3 Dried rhizome.

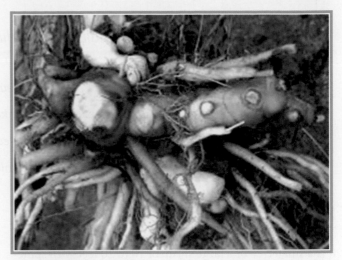

Fig. 115.4 Fresh rhizome.

Dose

Powder: 2 to 4 g
Juice: 5 to 10 mL

Karma (Actions)

Kandughna (antipruritus), krimighna (anthelmintic), deepana (appetizer), grahi (faecal astringent), shothahara (reduce swelling), and vishaghna (antidotes).

Indications

Krimiroga (worm infestations), kandu (pruritus), shivitra (leukoderma), meha (diabetes), aruchi (anorexia), jwara (fever), and sheetpitta (urticaria).

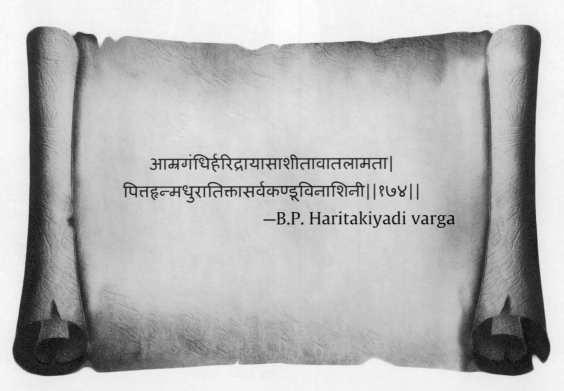

आम्रगंधिर्हरिद्रायासाशीतावातलामता।
पित्तहृन्मधुरातिक्तासर्वकण्डूविनाशिनी।।१७४।।
—B.P. Haritakiyadi varga

116. Ankola [*Alangium salivifolium* Linn. F.]

Family:	*Alangiaceae*
Hindi name:	*Ankol, Ankota*
English name:	*Sage leaved alangium*
Synonyms:	*Deerghakilak, Nikochaka, Guptsneha*

Morphology

It is a small tree or a large shrub of 10 to 20 feet with spine-scent branches. Bark is shown in **Fig. 116.1**.

Key Characters for Identification

➤ *Leaves: Alternate, usually unequal at the base* (**Fig. 116.2**)
➤ *Flowers: White or yellowish-white, axillary* (**Fig. 116.3**)
➤ *Fruits: One- to two-seeded berries crowned by the calyx lobes, yellowish or red when ripe* (**Fig. 116.4**)

Rasapanchaka

Guna	Laghu, snighdha, tikshna
Rasa	Katu, kashaya
Vipaka	Katu
Virya	Ushna
Doshakarma	Kapha-vatahara

Officinal Parts Used

Root and root bark

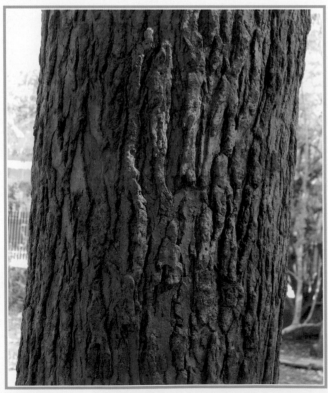

Fig. 116.1 Bark.

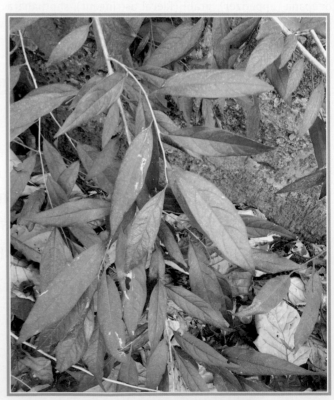

Fig. 116.2 Leaves.

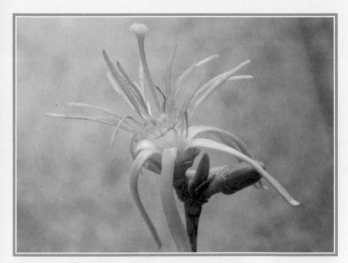

Fig. 116.3 Flowers.

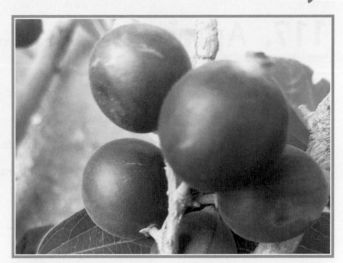

Fig. 116.4 Fruits.

Dose

Powder: 1 to 2 g

Karma (Actions)

Mool (root): Vishaghna (antidotes), rechana (laxative), vedanasthapana (analgesic), shothahar (reduce swelling), krimighna (anthelmintic).

Indications

- **Mool** (root): Visha (poisoning), visharpa (erysipelas), krimi (worm infestation), shoola (colic pain), shopha (inflammation), grahabadha (involvement of evil spirit), atisara (diarrhea)
- **Phal** (fruit): Daha (burning sensation), kshaya (emaciation), raktavikara (blood diseases).

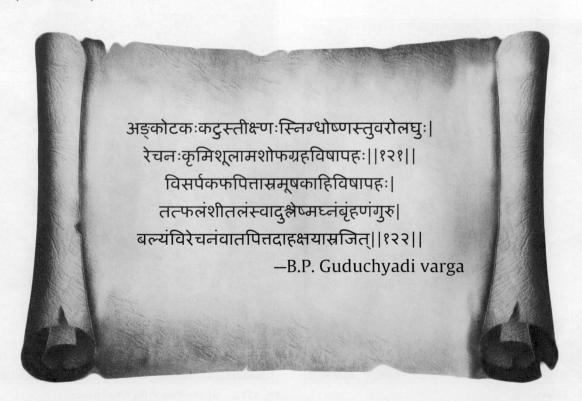

अङ्कोटकःकटुस्तीक्ष्णःस्निग्धोष्णस्तुवरोलघुः।
रेचनःकृमिशूलामशोफग्रहविषापहः॥१२१॥
विसर्पकफपित्तास्रमूषकाहिविषापहः।
तत्फलंशीतलंस्वादुश्लेष्मघ्नंबृंहणंगुरु।
बल्यंविरेचनंवातपित्तदाहक्षयास्रजित्॥१२२॥

—B.P. Guduchyadi varga

117. Aprajita *[Clitoria ternatea Linn.]*

Family:	*Fabaceae*
Hindi name:	*Aprajita*
English name:	*Winged leaves clitoria/Butterfly bean*
Synonyms:	*Vishnukranta, Asphota, Girikarni*

Morphology

It is a beautiful perennial twining climber with terete stem and branches.

Key Characters for Identification

➤ *Leaves: Compound, imperipinnate, 5–7 subcoriaceous leaflets, elliptic, oblong* (**Fig. 117.1**)
➤ *Flowers: Blue or white, solitary, axillary, or in fascicles* (**Fig. 117.2a and b**)
➤ *Fruits: Flattened pods* (**Fig. 117.3**)
➤ *Seeds: 6–10 in number, smooth, yellowish brown* (**Fig. 117.4**)

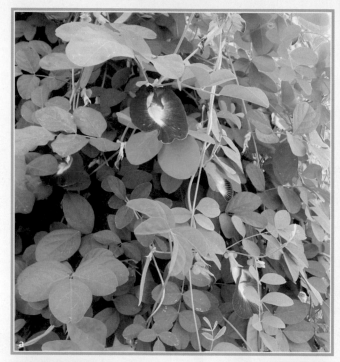

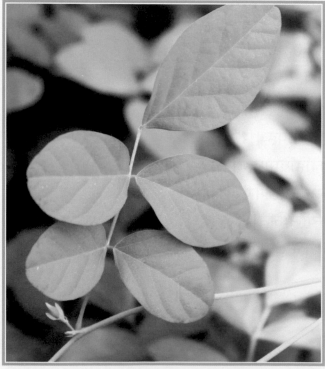

Fig. 117.1 Leaves.

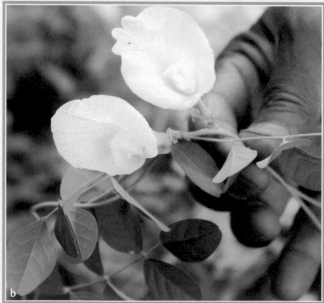

Fig. 117.2 (a) Blue flower. (b) White flower.

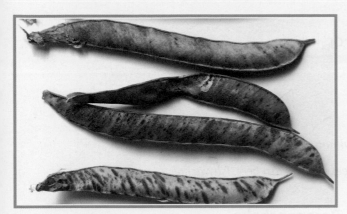

Fig. 117.3 Fruits.

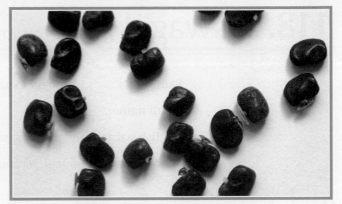

Fig. 117.4 Seeds.

Rasapanchaka

Guna	Laghu, ruksha
Rasa	Katu, tikta, kashaya
Vipaka	Katu
Virya	Sheeta
Doshakarma	Tridoshashamaka

Officinal Parts Used

Root, seed, leaves

Dose

Seed powder: 1 to 3 g
Root powder: 1 to 3 g

Karma (Actions)

Bhedan (purgative), medhya (intellect promoter), smritiprada (memory enhancer), chakshusya (beneficial for vision), kanthya (voice promoter), mutral(diuretics), vishaghna (antidotes), kushtghna (antipruritus), krimighna (anthelmintic), sothaghna (antiinflamatory), and vedanasthapan (anodynes).

Indications

Ardhavbhedaka (hemicrania), unmada (insanity), twak roga (skin diseases), kustha (skin diseases including leprosy), shotha (swelling/inflammation), vrana (wound), visha (poisoning), netraroga (eye diseases), and sukrameha (polyurea with semen).

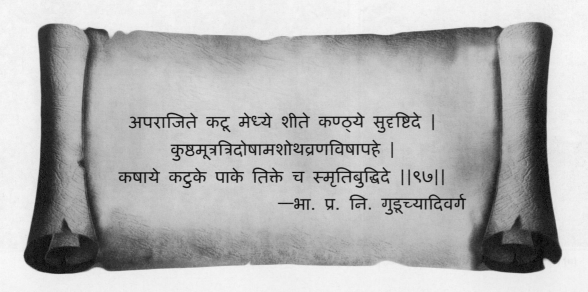

अपराजिते कटू मेध्ये शीते कण्ठ्ये सुदृष्टिदे |
कुष्ठमूत्रत्रिदोषामशोथव्रणविषापहे |
कषाये कटुके पाके तिक्ते च स्मृतिबुद्धिदे ||९७||
—भा. प्र. नि. गुडूच्यादिवर्ग

118. Aswagol [*Plantago ovata Forsk.*]

Family:	*Plantaginaceae*
Hindi name:	*Isabgol*
English name:	*Spogel seeds, psyllium seeds*
Synonyms:	*Isadgol, Sheetabeej, Ashwakarn beej, Ishwarbol*

Morphology

It is a hairy annual herb without stem (**Fig. 118.1a, b**).

Key Characters for Identification

➤ *Leaves: Simple, filiform, acuminate, entire, or distantly toothed* (**Fig. 118.2**)
➤ *Flower: Small, cylindrical, or with ovoid spikes* (**Fig. 118.3**)
➤ *Fruit: Ellipsoid obtuse capsule, the upper half coming off as a blunt conical lid*
➤ *Seed: Smooth, yellowish-brown, ovoid-oblong, boat shaped*

Rasapanchaka

Guna	Guru, snighdha, picchila
Rasa	Madhura
Vipaka	Madhura
Virya	Sheeta
Doshakarma	Vatapittashamak

Officinal Parts Used

Seed and seed covering (husk)

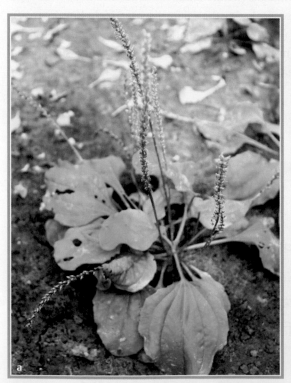
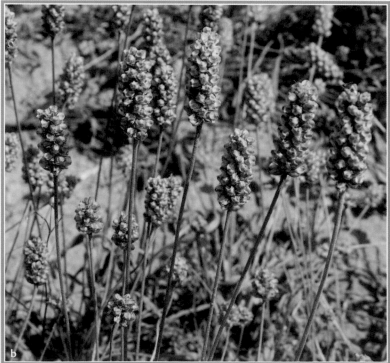

Fig. 118.1 **(a)** Plant of *Plantago ovata* Forsk. **(b)** Dried plant.

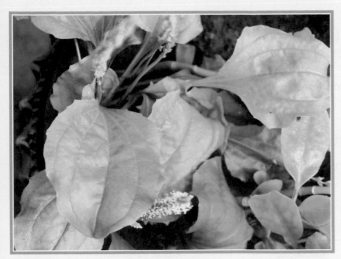

Fig. 118.2 Leaves.

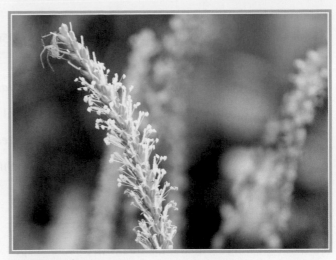

Fig. 118.3 Flower.

Dose

Seed husk: 5 to 10 g

Karma (Actions)

Snehan (oleation), dahaprashman (reduce burning sensation), balya (enhance physical strength), brihmaniya (bulk promoting), shothahara (antiinflamatory), vrishya (aphrodisiac), kaphanisarak (antitussive), mutrajanan (diuretics), and jwaraghna (antipyretics).

Indications

Mutradaha (burning micturition), mutrakricchta (dysuria), mada (slight intoxication), trishna (thirst), vibandh (constipation), atisara (diarrhea), pravahika (dysentric), dourbalya (weakness), jwara (fever), and kasa (cough).

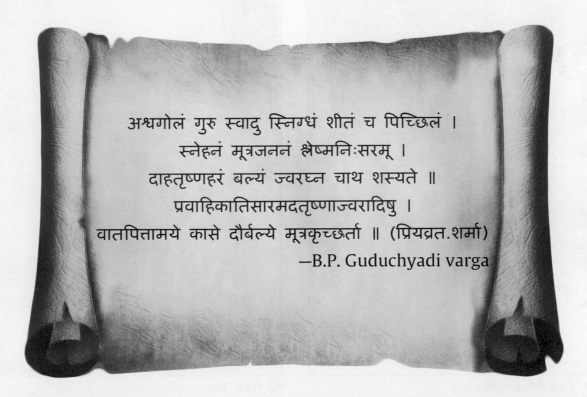

अश्वगोलं गुरु स्वादु स्निग्धं शीतं च पिच्छिलं ।
स्नेहनं मूत्रजननं श्लेष्मनिःसरम् ।
दाहतृष्णहरं बल्यं ज्वरघ्न चाथ शस्यते ॥
प्रवाहिकातिसारमदतृष्णाज्वरादिषु ।
वातपित्तामये कासे दौर्बल्ये मूत्रकृच्छर्ता ॥ (प्रियव्रत.शर्मा)
—B.P. Guduchyadi varga

119. Ashvatha *[Ficus religiosa Linn.]*

Family:	*Moraceae*
Hindi name:	*Pipal*
English name:	*Sacred fig*
Synonyms:	*Bodhidru, Chalpatra, Gajashan*

Morphology

It is a fast-growing deciduous tall tree with cordate-shaped leaves and with few or no aerial roots (**Fig. 119.1**). Bark is shown in **Fig. 119.2**.

Key Characters for Identification

➤ *Leaves: Long petiole, ovate, cordate, shiny leaves, the apex is linear lanceolate tail about half long as the main portion of the blade (**Fig. 119.3**)*
➤ *Fruit: Occurring in pairs, axillary, depressed globose, smooth, purplish when ripe*

Rasapanchaka

Guna	Guru, ruksha
Rasa	Kashaya, madhura
Vipaka	Katu
Virya	Sheeta
Doshakarma	Pitta-kaphahara

Officinal Parts Used

Bark, fruit, latex, tender leaves

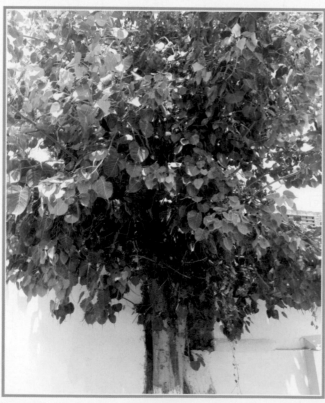

Fig. 119.1   Plant of *Ficus religiosa* Linn.

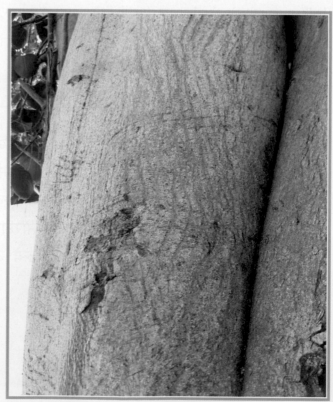

Fig. 119.2   Bark.

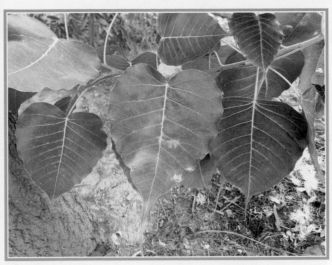

Fig. 119.3 Leaves.

Dose

Powder: 3 to 6 g
Decoction: 50 to 100 mL

Karma (Actions)

Varnya (complexion promoter), stambhaka (astringent), yonivishodhana (purification of vagina), vranaropaka (wound healing), and mutrasangrahniya(urinary astringent).

Indications

Vrana (wound), raktavikara (diseases of blood), yoniroga (diseases of female genital organ), daha (burning sensation), prameha (diabetes), raktapitta(hemorrhage), atisaar (diarrhea), and chhardi (vomiting).

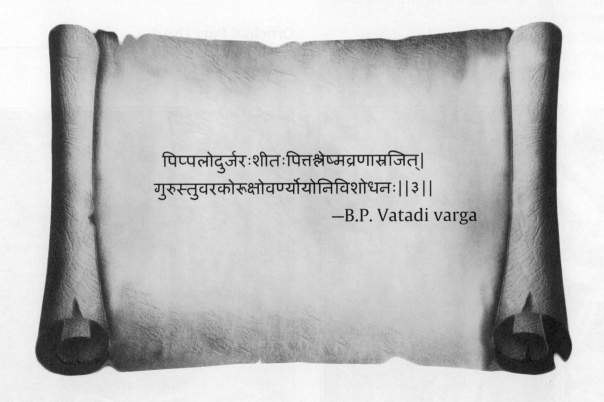

पिप्पलोदुर्जरःशीतःपित्तश्लेष्मव्रणास्रजित्।
गुरुस्तुवरकोरूक्षोवर्ण्यायोनिविशोधनः।।३।।
—B.P. Vatadi varga

120. Asthishrunkhala *[Cissus quadrangularis Linn.]*

Family:	*Vitaceae*
Hindi name:	*Hadjod*
English name:	*Devil's backbone, Veldt Grape*
Synonyms:	*Vajravalli, Hadjoda, Granthimaan, Vajrangi, Asthisanhari*

Morphology

It is a succulent thick green climbing herb with quadrangular stems (**Fig. 120.1**).

Key Characters for Identification

➤ *Leaves: Simple, broadly reniform, entire or toothed, rounded, cuneate at the base (**Fig. 120.2**)*
➤ *Tendrils: Simple, slender and leaf opposed, some aerial roots arise from nodes*
➤ *Flower: Small, greenish hooded at the apex*
➤ *Fruit: Ovoid or globose, red berries*
➤ *Seeds: Ellipsoid*

Rasapanchaka

Guna	Laghu, ruksha
Rasa	Madhura
Vipaka	Katu
Virya	Ushna
Doshakarma	Kapha vatashamaka

Officinal Part Used

Stem

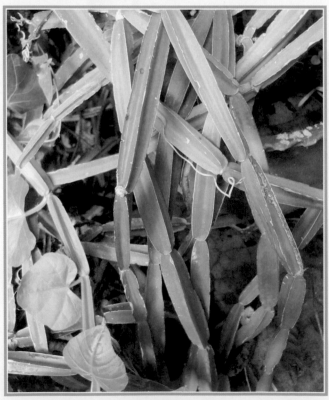

Fig. 120.1 Plant of *Cissus quadrangularis* Linn.

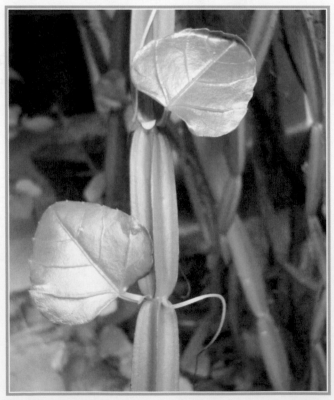

Fig. 120.2 Leaves.

Karma (Actions)

Snehan (oleation), shukranashak (spermicidal), achakshushya (not beneficial for vision), kaphanisaraka (antitussive), mutral (diuretics), balya (physical strength promoter), anulomana (laxative), hridya (cardio tonic) (pushpa), and virechaka (laxative) (taila).

Indications

Vibandh (constipation), arsha (piles), kasa (cough), kushtha (skin disease), bastishoth (cystitis), hridroga (heart diseases), vranashotha (inflammatory wound), vatarakta (gout), and dourbalya (weakness).

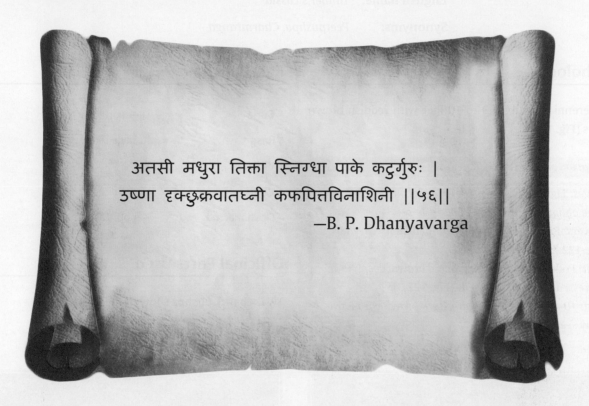

अतसी मधुरा तिक्ता स्निग्धा पाके कटुर्गुरुः |
उष्णा वृक्छुक्रवातघ्नी कफपित्तविनाशिनी ||५६||
—B. P. Dhanyavarga

122. Avartaki *[Cassia auriculata* Linn.]

Family:	*Leguminosae (Caesalpinioideae)*
Hindi name:	*Tarvar*
English name:	*Tanner's cassia*
Synonyms:	*Peetpushpa, Charmranga*

Morphology

It is a perennial shrub of 3 to 10 feet with reddish brown branches (**Fig. 122.1**).

Key Characters for Identification

➤ *Leaves: Eight to twelve pairs of leaflets and a pair of large obliquely cordate stipules at base*
➤ *Flowers: Bright yellow subterminal axillary corymbs* (**Fig. 122.2**)
➤ *Fruit: Pods, flat, thin, papery, pale brown, deeply depressed between the seeds* (**Fig. 122.3**)
➤ *Seed: 10–20 per pod, obovate, dark brown with hard shiny seed coat*

Rasapanchaka

Guna	Laghu, ruksha
Rasa	Kasaya, tikta
Vipaka	Katu
Virya	Sheeta
Doshakarma	Kaphpittashamaka

Officinal Parts Used

Twak (bark), pushpa (flower), beej (seeds)

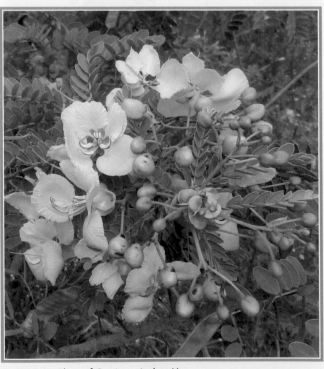

Fig. 122.1　Plant of *Cassia auriculata* Linn.

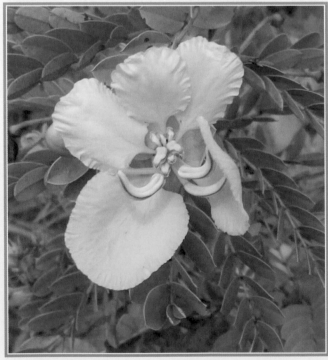

Fig. 122.2　Flower.

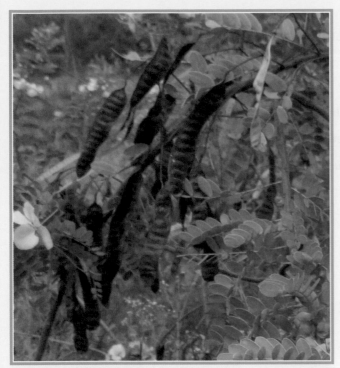

Fig. 122.3 Fruits.

Dose

Flower juice: 10 to 20 mL
Seed powder: 3 to 6 g
Decoction: 50 to 100 mL

Karma (Actions)

Stambhan (astringent), krimighna (anthelmintic), kusthaghna (antipruritus), and mutrasangrahaniya (urinary astringents).

Indications

Prameha (diabetes), atisara (diarrhea), mukhpaka (stomatitis), raktapitta (internal hemorrhage), kustha (skin diseases), krimi (worm infestation), pradar (menometrorrhagia), vrana (wound), and netraabhishyandi (conjunctivitis).

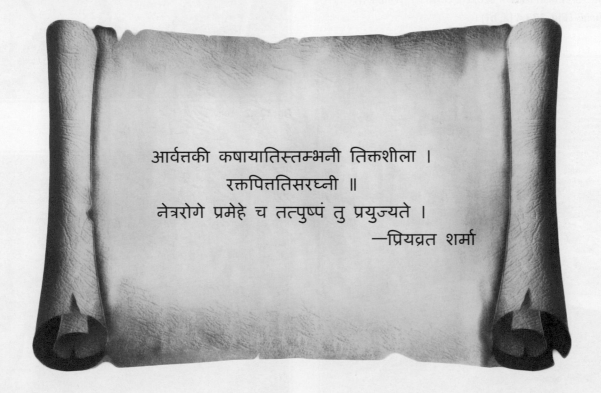

आर्वत्तकी कषायातिस्तम्भनी तिक्तशीला ।
रक्तपित्ततिसरघ्नी ॥
नेत्ररोगे प्रमेहे च तत्पुष्पं तु प्रयुज्यते ।
—प्रियव्रत शर्मा

123. Avartani *[Helicteres isora Linn.]*

Family: *Malvaceae*

Hindi name: *Marodphali*

English name: *Indian screw tree*

Synonyms: *Murva, Avartamala*

Morphology

It is a deciduous large shrub or a small tree of 5 to 8 m with spirally twisted follicular fruits (**Fig. 123.1**).

Key Characters for Identification

➤ *Leaves: Simple, alternate, obovate, and serrated* (**Fig. 123.2**)
➤ *Flower: Red in color and axillary* (**Fig. 123.3**)
➤ *Fruit: Greenish brown beaked, cork-screw–like five follicles* (**Fig. 123.4 [a, b]**)

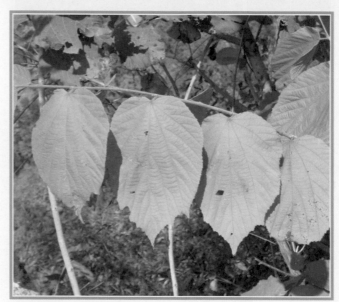

Fig. 123.2 Leaves.

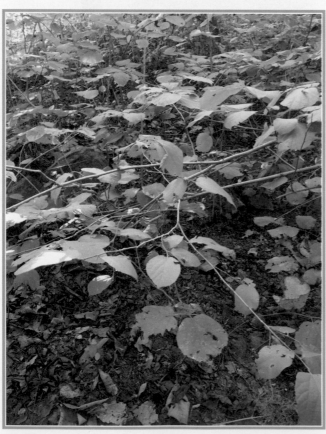

Fig. 123.1 Plant of *Helicteres isora* Linn.

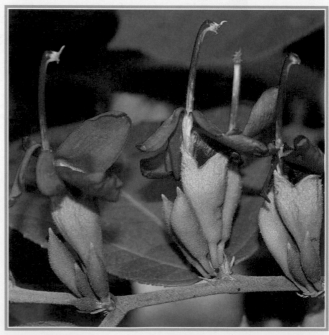

Fig. 123.3 Flower.

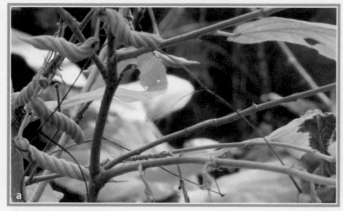 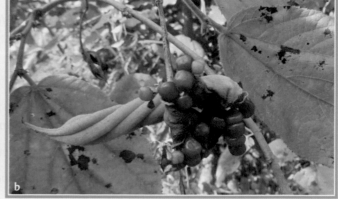

Fig. 123.4 (a, b) Fruit.

Rasapanchaka

Guna	Laghu, ruksha
Rasa	Kashaya
Vipaka	Katu
Virya	Sheeta
Doshakarma	Kaphpittashamaka

Officinal Parts Used

Mool (root), twak (bark), phal (fruit)

Dose

Fruit powder: 3 to 6 g
Decoction: 50 to 100 mL

Karma (Actions)

Raktstambhak (hemostatics), vranropan (wound healing), krimighna (anthelmintic), grahi (faecal astringent), mutrasangrahniya (urinary astringent), and shoolprasasmana (antispasmodic).

Indications

Raktasrava (hemorrhage), udarshool (abdominal pain), aanaah (obstruction/constipation), prameha (diabetes), krimi (worm infestation), vrana (wound), atisara (diarrhea), pravahika (dysentery), and raktapitta (internal hemorrhage).

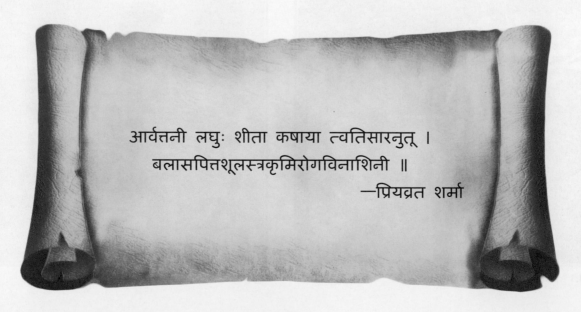

आर्वत्तनी लघुः शीता कषाया त्वतिसारनुतू ।
बलासपित्तशूलस्त्रकृमिरोगविनाशिनी ॥
—प्रियव्रत शर्मा

124. Babbula *[Acacia arabica* Willd.*]*

Family:	*Mimosoideae*
Hindi name:	*Babool, Kikar*
English name:	*Babul, Indian Gum Arabic tree*
Synonyms:	*Yugmakantak, Sookshmapatra, Kinkiraat, Kinkirath, Speetaka, Abhashatpadmodani, Malaphal*

Morphology

It is a perennial tree of medium height, with black rough fissured bark and a pair of long spines in the axil (**Fig. 124.1**).

Key Characters for Identification

➤ *Bark: Black, rough, and longitudinal fissured*
➤ *Leaves: Bipinnate with spinescent stipules*
➤ *Flower: Golden–yellow color, crowned in long-peduncled globose head*
➤ *Fruit: Whitish pod, flat, containing 8–12 seeds* (**Fig. 124.2**)
➤ *Gum: Different shape and size, red or light yellow, tasteless and odorless, soluble in double quantity water* (**Fig. 124.3**)

Rasapanchaka

Rasapanchaka	Twak	Niryasa
Guna	Guru, ruksha	Snigdha
Rasa	Kasaya	Madhura, kashaya
Vipaka	Katu	Madhura
Virya	Sheeta	Sheeta
Doshakarma	Kapha pittashamaka	Vata pittashamaka

Officinal Parts Used

Twak (bark), phal (fruit), niryasa (exudate)

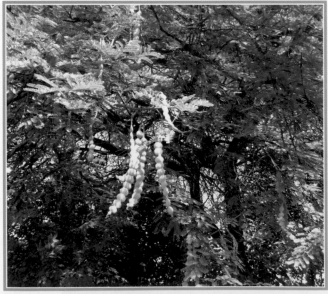

Fig. 124.1   Plant of *Acacia arabica* Willd.

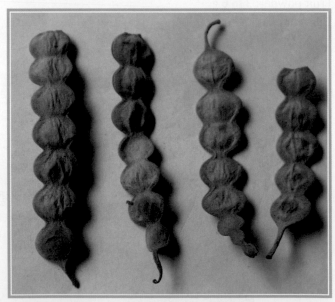

Fig. 124.2   Fruits.

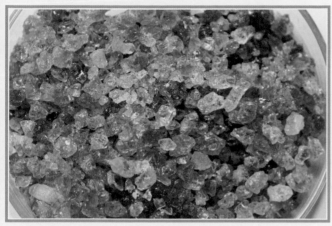

Fig. 124.3 Gum.

Dose

Bark decoction: 50 to 100 mL
Fruit powder: 3 to 6 g
Gum: 3 to 6 g

Karma (Actions)

Sangrahi (appetizer and fecal astringent), stambhak (astringent), vranaropaka (wound healing), krimighna (anthelmintic), kusthaghna (antileprotic), and vishaghna (antidote).

Niryasa

Balya (promote physical strength), vrishya (aphrodisiac), snehan (oleation), and mutral (diuretics).

Indications

Kustha (skin disease), krimi (worm infestation), visha (poisoning), atisara (diarrhea), pravahika (dysentric), asthibhagna (bone fracture), pradar (menometrorrhagia), gudabhransh (rectal prolapse), mukhpaka (stomatitis), prameha (diabetes), raktapitta (hemorrhage), and dourbalya (weakness).

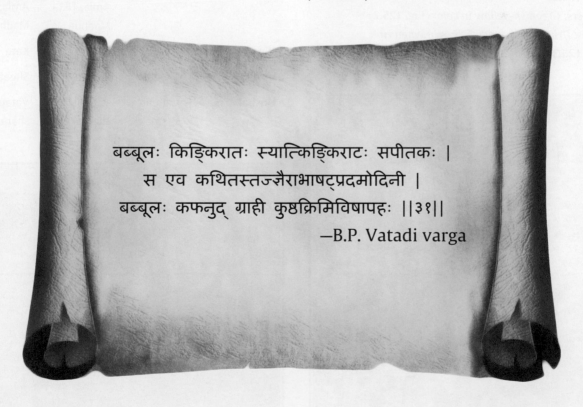

बब्बूलः किङ्किरातः स्यात्किङ्किराटः सपीतकः |
स एव कथितस्तज्ज्ञैराभाषट्प्रदमोदिनी |
बब्बूलः कफनुद् ग्राही कुष्ठक्रिमिविषापहः ||३१||

—B.P. Vatadi varga

125. Badara *[Ziziphus jujube Linn.]*

Family:	*Rhamnaceae*
Hindi name:	*Ber*
English name:	*Plum*
Synonyms:	*Badari, Ajapriya, Kuha, Koli, Ubhaykantaka, Vishama*
Types:	*Sovir, Kola, Karkandhu*

Morphology

It is a medium-height tree growing from 7 to 10 m with spine on the branches (**Fig. 125.1**).

Key Characters for Identification

➤ *Leaves: Alternate, ovate to ovoid-lanceolate* (**Fig. 125.2**)
➤ *Flowers: Greenish-yellow in color* (**Fig. 125.2**)
➤ *Fruits: Drupe, dark reddish-brown when ripe* (**Fig. 125.3**)

Rasapanchaka

Rasapanchaka	Sovir	Karkandhu	Kola
Guna	Guru	Guru	Snigdha, Guru, Pichhal
Rasa	Madhura	Kasaya, Amla, Tikta, Madhur	Kasaya, Amla, Madhur
Vipaka	Madhura	Katu	Katu
Virya	Sheeta	Sheeta	Sheeta
Doshakarma	Vatapitta-shamaka	Vatapitta-shamaka	Vatapitta-shamaka

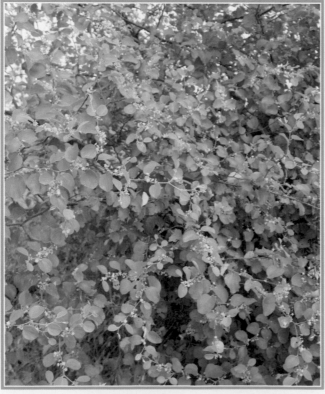

Fig. 125.1   Plant of *Ziziphus jujube* Linn.

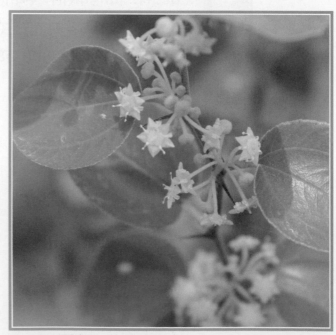

Fig. 125.2   Leaves and flowers.

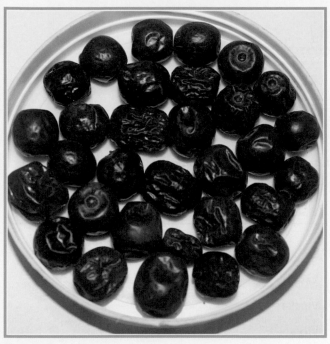

Fig. 125.3 Fruits.

Officinal Parts Used

Phal (fruit), mool (root), patra (leaves)

Dose

Decoction: 50 to 100 mL
Fruit paste: 5 to 10 g

Karma (Actions)

Rochana (relish), sangrahi (astringent), hridya (cardiotonic), sarak (laxative), bhedan (purgative), brihmaniya (bulk promoting), shukral (spermatogenesis), snehana (oleation), and shramhara (antifatigue).

Indications

Hikka (hic-cough), atisara (diarrhea), pradara (menometrorrhagia), kshay (consumption/tuberculosis), daha (burning sensation), trishna (thirst), jwar (fever), and raktaroga (blood disorders).

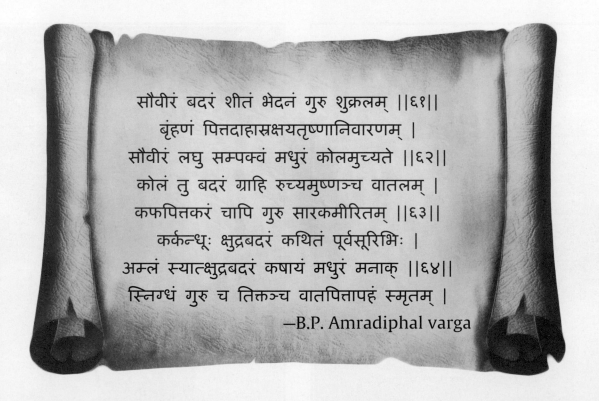

सौवीरं बदरं शीतं भेदनं गुरु शुक्रलम् ||६१||
बृंहणं पित्तदाहास्रक्षयतृष्णानिवारणम् |
सौवीरं लघु सम्पक्वं मधुरं कोलमुच्यते ||६२||
कोलं तु बदरं ग्राहि रुच्यमुष्णञ्च वातलम् |
कफपित्तकरं चापि गुरु सारकमीरितम् ||६३||
कर्कन्धूः क्षुद्रबदरं कथितं पूर्वसूरिभिः |
अम्लं स्यात्क्षुद्रबदरं कषायं मधुरं मनाक् ||६४||
स्निग्धं गुरु च तिक्तञ्च वातपित्तापहं स्मृतम् |

—B.P. Amradiphal varga

126. Bakula [*Mimusops elengi* Linn.]

Family:	*Sapotaceae*
Hindi name:	*Moulasiri*
English name:	*Spanish cherry*
Synonyms:	*Sthirapushp, Chirpushpa, Madhugandha, Sinhkesar*

Morphology

It is a medium-sized evergreen tree (**Fig. 126.1**) with dark gray fissured bark (**Fig. 126.2**) and dense spreading crown.

Key Characters for Identification

➤ *Leaves: Oblong, glabrous with way margins* (**Fig. 126.3**)
➤ *Flower: White fragrant and axillary* (**Fig. 126.4**)
➤ *Fruit: Ovoid or ellipsoid berries*
➤ *Seeds: One to two ovoid in number, compressed, grayish-brown, and shiny*

Rasapanchaka

Guna	Guru
Rasa	Kasaya, katu
Vipaka	Katu
Virya	Anushna
Doshakarma	Pitta kaphashamaka

Officinal Parts Used

Twak (bark), pushpa (flower), phal (fruits)

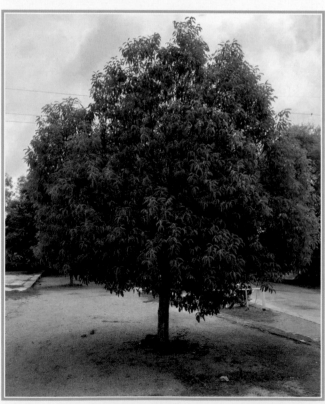

Fig. 126.1 Plant of *Mimusops elengi* Linn.

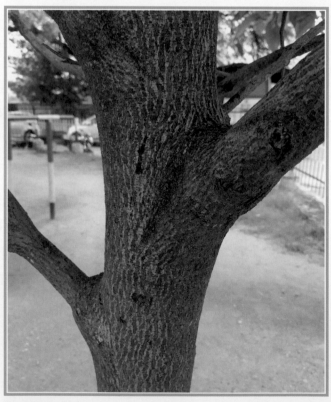

Fig. 126.2 Bark.

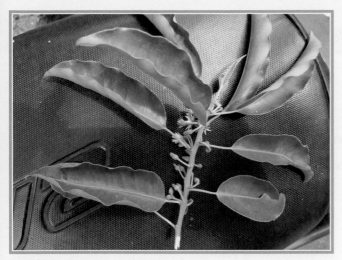

Fig. 126.3 Leaves.

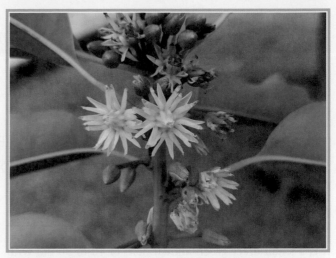

Fig. 126.4 Flowers.

Dose

Flower powder: 1 to 2 g
Bark decoction: 50 to 100 mL

Karma (Actions)

Raktapittahara (subside rakta and pitta), dantyadadhyakar (provide strength to teeth), stambhan (astringent), sangrahi (fecal astringent), krimighna (anthelmintic), hridya (cardiotonic), shothahar (reduce swelling), jwaraghna (antipyretic), and vishaghna (antidote).

Indications

Dantaroga (diseases of teeth), shirashool (headache), atisara (diarrhea), krimi (worm infestation), pradar (menometrorrhagia), shukrameha (spermatorrhea), bastishotha (inflammation in bladder), puyameha (pyorrhea), and shivitra (vitiligo).

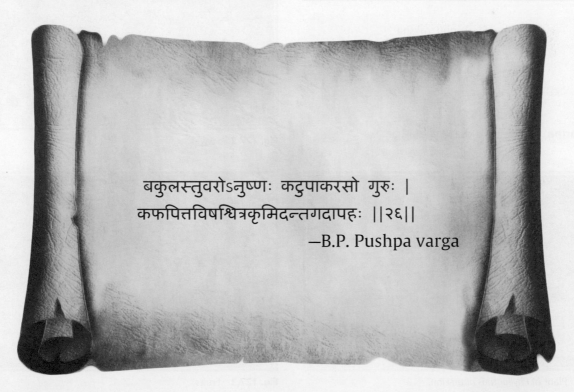

बकुलस्तुवरोऽनुष्णः कटुपाकरसो गुरुः |
कफपित्तविषश्चित्रकृमिदन्तगदापहः ||२६||
—B.P. Pushpa varga

127. Bhumyamlaki *[Phyllanthus niruri Linn.]*

Family:	*Euphorbiaceae*
Hindi name:	*Bhumi-Amla*
English name:	*Stonebreaker, seed under leaf*
Synonyms:	*Bhudhatri, Tamlaki, Shiva, Bahupatra, Bahuphala, Bahuvirya*

Morphology

It is a small erect green annual herb of 10 to 30 cm with pinnate compound leaves (**Fig. 127.1**).

Key Characters for Identification

➤ *Leaves: Numerous, subsessile, elliptic oblong, obtuse, acute stipules present (**Fig. 127.2**)*
➤ *Flower: Yellow in colour, numerous, axillary, male flowers (1–3 in number), female flower (solitary)*
➤ *Fruit: Capsules, depressed, globose, smooth, scarcely lobed (**Fig. 127.3**)*

Rasapanchaka

Guna	Laghu, ruksha
Rasa	Tikta, kasaya, madhur
Vipaka	Madhur
Virya	Sheeta
Doshakarma	Kapha pittashamaka

Officinal Part Used

Panchang (whole plant)

Dose

Powder: 3 to 6 g
Juice: 10 to 20 mL

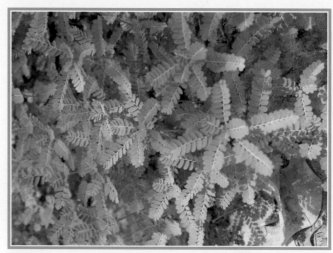

Fig. 127.2 Leaves.

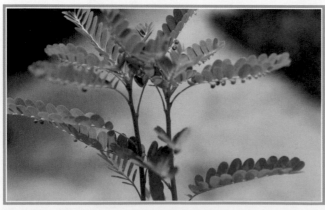

Fig. 127.1   Plant of *Phyllanthus niruri* Linn.

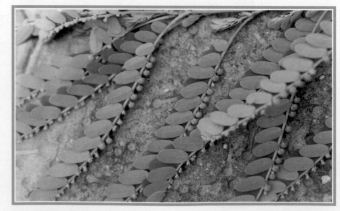

Fig. 127.3 Fruits.

Karma (Actions)

Kasahara (expectorant), shwasahara (antiasthmatic), trishnanigrahan (antithirst), shothahara (anti-inflammatory), kusthghna (antileprotic), jwaraghna (antipyretic), and vishaghna (antidote).

Indications

Prameha (diabetes), pipasa (thirst), kandu (pruritus), kasa (cough), visham jwara (intermittent fever), kamala (jaundice), yakrit pleeha vriddhi (hepatosplenomegaly), mutradaha (burning micturition), and vranashotha (inflammation).

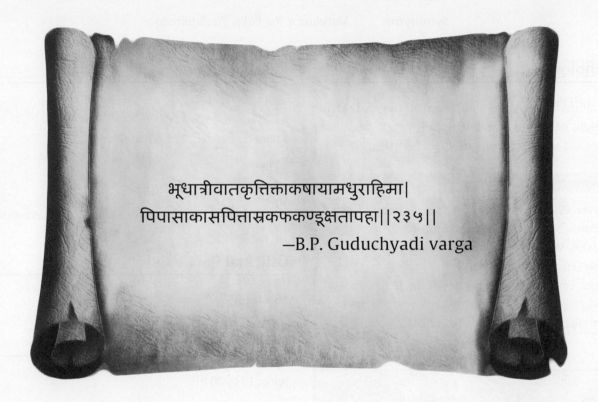

भूधात्रीवातकृत्तिक्ताकषायामधुराहिमा।
पिपासाकासपित्तास्रकफकण्डूक्षतापहा॥२३५॥
—B.P. Guduchyadi varga

128. Beejpura *[Citrus medica Linn.]*

Family: *Rutaceae*

Hindi name: *Bijora nimbu*

English name: *Citron, lemon*

Synonyms: *Matulunga, Ruchaka, Phalapuraka*

Morphology

It is an aromatic, evergreen shrub or small tree that reaches to a height of approximately 8 to 15 feet. It has thorny branches and smooth yellowish-brown bark (**Fig. 128.1**).

Key Characters for Identification

➤ *Leaves: Oblong or elliptic with acute or rounded apex, coriaceous, and pellucid (***Fig. 128.2***)*
➤ *Flowers: White tinged with pink, scented, in axillary cyme (***Fig. 128.3***)*
➤ *Fruits: Large berries, oblong or globose, fleshy, thick rind, rough, irregular, or warted yellow when ripe and contains few smooth seeds (***Fig. 128.4***)*

Rasapanchaka

Guna	Laghu, ruksha
Rasa	Amla
Vipaka	Amla
Virya	Ushan
Doshakarma	Vatashamak, pittakaphavardhak

Officinal Part Used

Phal (fruit)

Dose

Juice: 10 to 20 mL

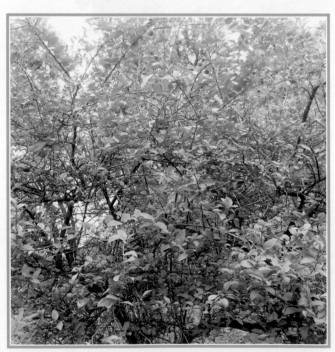

Fig. 128.1   Plant of *Citrus medica* Linn.

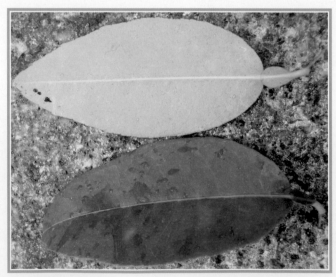

Fig. 128.2   Leaves.

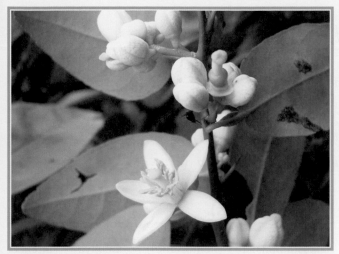

Fig. 128.3 Flowers.

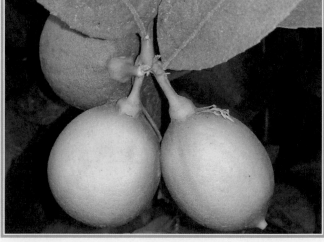

Fig. 128.4 Fruits.

Karma (Actions)

Deepana (appetizer), pachana (digestive), rochana (relish), hridya (cardiotonic), grahi (astringent), and krimighna (anthelmintic).

Indications

Chhardi (vomiting), udarshool (spasmodic pain), aruchi (anorexia), ajirna (indigestion), vishuchika (cholera), trishna (thirst), shrama (tireness), raktapitta (internal bleeding), shwasa (asthma), and kasa (cough).

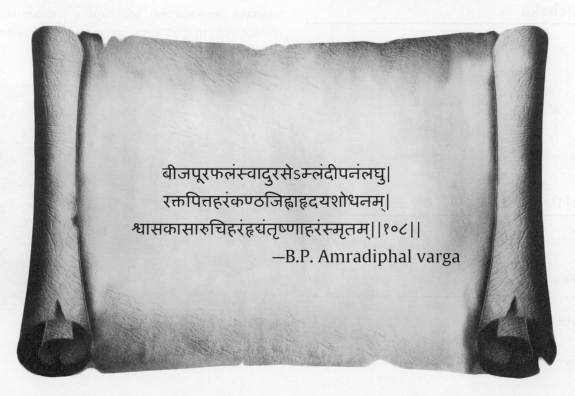

बीजपूरफलंस्वादुरसेऽम्लंदीपनंलघु।
रक्तपित्तहरंकण्ठजिह्वाहृदयशोधनम्।
श्वासकासारुचिहरंहृद्यंतृष्णाहरंस्मृतम्।।१०८।।

—B.P. Amradiphal varga

129. Bol *[Commiphora myrrha Nees.]*

Family:	*Burseraceae*
Hindi name:	*Hirabol*
English name:	*Gum myrrh*
Synonyms:	*Gandhrasa, Pinda, Prana, Goparasa*

Morphology

It is a sturdy, spiny, glabrous shrub or small tree that reaches up to a height of 4 m.

Key Characters for Identification

➤ *The gum resin exudate from wounds in the stem is pale yellow at first and later solidifies to brown–black* (**Fig. 129.1**)

Rasapanchaka

Gun	Laghu, ruksha
Rasa	Madhura, tikta, katu
Vipaka	Katu
Virya	Sheeta
Doshakarma	Tridoshashamaka

Officinal Part Used

Niryas (exudate)

Dose

Powder: 1 to 2 g

Karma (Actions)

Raktastambhaka (hemostatics), medhya (intellect promoter), deepan (appetizer), pachana (digestive), shothahara (antiinflamatory), vedanasthapan (anodynes/analgesic), and garbhasayashodhak (uterine cleansing).

Indications

Daha (burning sensation), sweda (sweating), jwara (fever), apasmara (epilepsy), kustha (skin diseases), anartava (amenorrhea), mukhapaka (stomatitis), pradar (menometrorrhagia), kasa (cough), swasha (asthma), and vrana (wound).

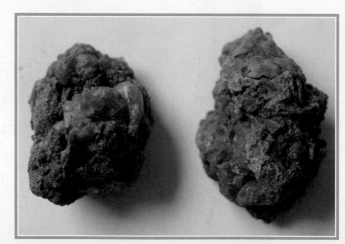

Fig. 129.1 Gum resin exudate.

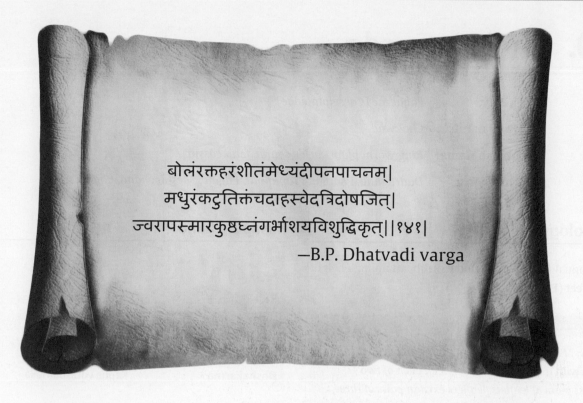

बोलंरक्तहरंशीतंमेध्यंदीपनपाचनम्।
मधुरंकटुतिक्तंचदाहस्वेदत्रिदोषजित्।
ज्वरापस्मारकुष्ठघ्नंगर्भाशययविशुद्धिकृत्।।१४१।
—B.P. Dhatvadi varga

130. Chakramarda *[Cassia tora Linn.]*

Family:	*Fabaceae (Caeselpinoidae)*
Hindi name:	*Chakwad*
English name:	*Ring worm plant, Sickle senna, fetid cassia*
Synonyms:	*Dadrughna, Padmat, Prapunnat, Edgaja, Meshlochana, Chakri*

Morphology

It is an annual fetid herb or undershrub, attaining a height of 1 to 3 feet (**Fig. 130.1**).

Key Characters for Identification

➤ *Leaves: Pinnately compound, rachis grooved in three pairs with a conical gland between each of two lowest pairs of leaflets, leaflets exist in pairs of three, obovate-oblong, membranous, base somewhat oblique* (**Fig. 130.2**)
➤ *Flowers: Axillary, found in pairs, yellow in color* (**Fig. 130.3**)
➤ *Fruits: 4–8 inches long and thin pods, have pointed tips, are initially green, and turn to brown at maturity* (**Fig. 130.4**)
➤ *Seeds: Hard, flat-thin, rounded gray seeds, 20–30 seeds per pod* (**Fig. 130.5**)

Rasapanchaka

Guna	Laghu, ruksha
Rasa	Katu
Vipaka	Katu
Virya	Ushna
Doshakarma	Kapha vatashamaka

Officinal Parts Used

Beej (seeds) and patra (leaves)

Dose

Seed powder: 1 to 3 g
Leaf juice: 5 to 10 mL

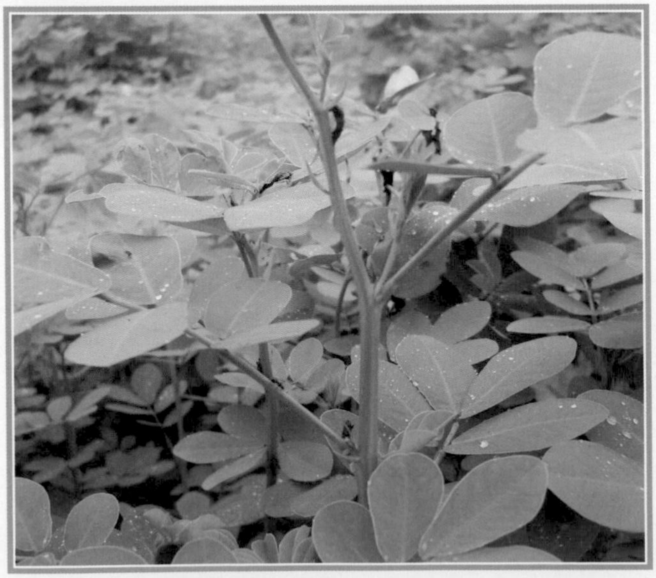

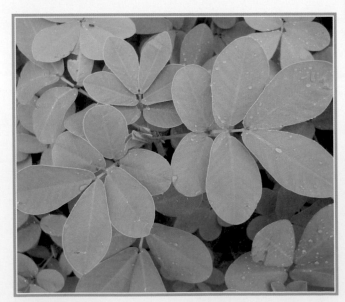

Fig. 130.1 Plant of *Cassia tora* Linn.

Fig. 130.2 Leaves.

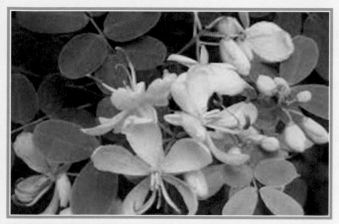

Fig. 130.3 Flowers.

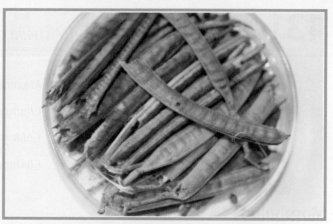

Fig. 130.4 Pods.

Karma (Actions)

Kushthghna (antileprotic), vishaghna (antidote), lekhana (scraping), yakrit uttejaka (hepatic stimulant), and hridya (cardiotonic).

Indications

Kustha (skin diseases), kandu (pruritus), dadru (tinea corporis), visha (poisoning), krimi (worm infestation), kasa (cough), gulma (abdominal lump), and medoroga (obesity).

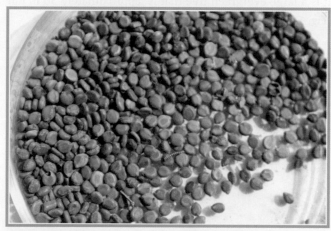

Fig. 130.5 Seeds.

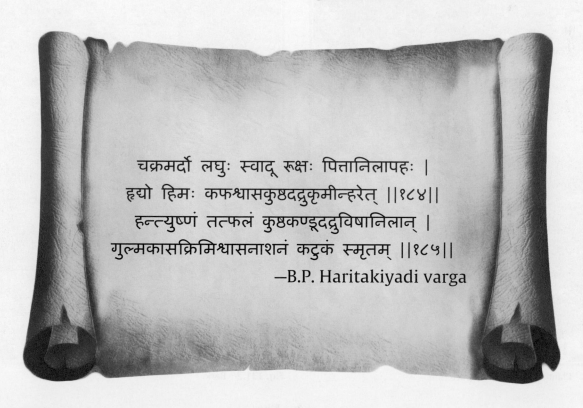

चक्रमर्दो लघुः स्वादू रूक्षः पित्तानिलापहः |
हृद्यो हिमः कफश्वासकुष्ठदद्रुकृमीन्हरेत् ||१८४||
हन्त्युष्णं तत्फलं कुष्ठकण्डूदद्रुविषानिलान् |
गुल्मकासक्रिमिश्वासनाशनं कटुकं स्मृतम् ||१८५||
—B.P. Haritakiyadi varga

131. Champaka *[Michelia champaca Linn.]*

Family:	*Magnoliaceae*
Hindi name:	*Champa*
English name:	*Golden champa*
Synonyms:	*Champeya, Hempushp, Gandhphali*

Morphology

It is a large evergreen tree that is approximately 30 m tall (**Fig. 131.1**). The bark of the plant is shown in **Fig. 131.2**.

Key Characters for Identification

➤ *Leaves: Simple, alternate, lanceolate, entire, and glabrous* (**Fig. 131.3**)
➤ *Flower: Yellowish to orange, solitary, and fragrant* (**Fig. 131.4**)
➤ *Fruit: Capsule contains 1–12, brown, fleshy, aril seeds*

Rasapanchaka

Guna	Laghu, ruksha
Rasa	Katu, tikta, kashaya
Vipaka	Katu
Virya	Sheeta
Doshakarma	Kaphapittashamaka

Officinal Parts Used

Twak (bark) and pushpa (flower)

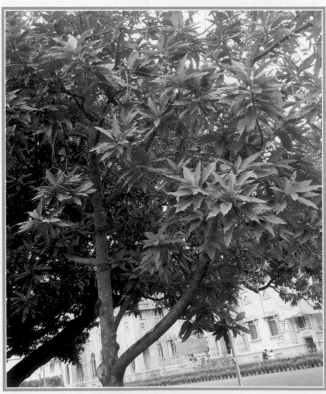

Fig. 131.1　Plant of *Michelia champaca* Linn.

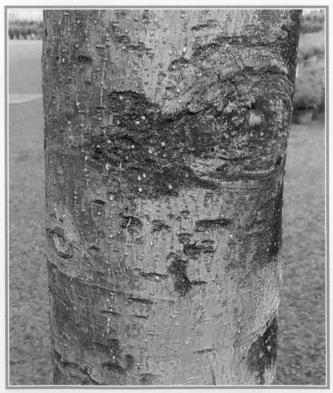

Fig. 131.2　Bark.

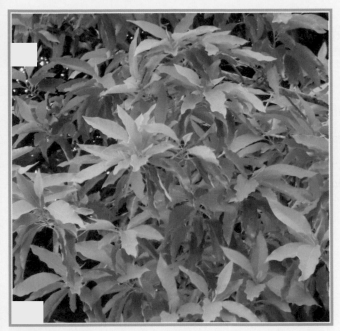

Fig. 131.3 Leaves.

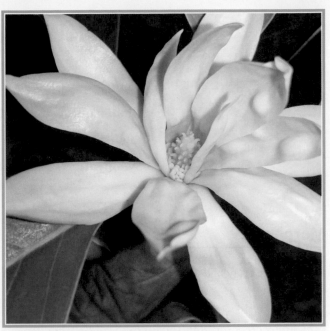

Fig. 131.4 Flower.

Dose

Powder: 3 to 6 g
Decoction: 50 to 100 mL

Karma (Actions)

Krimighna (anthelmintic), dahaprashmana (cooling effect/antiburning), kusthaghna (antipruritus), jwaraghna (antipyretics), raktashodhaka (blood purifier), and vranashodhana (wound cleansing).

Indications

Krimi (worm infestation), mutrakricha (dysuria), raktavikar (blood diseases), mutratisar, yoniroga (diseases of female genital organ), vrana (wound), visha (poisoning), kustha (skin diseases), and kandu (pruritus).

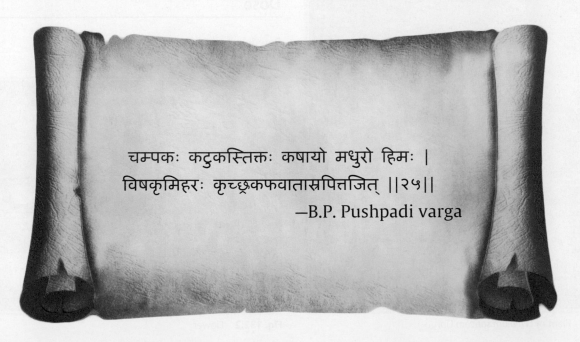

चम्पकः कटुकस्तिक्तः कषायो मधुरो हिमः |
विषकृमिहरः कृच्छ्रकफवातास्रपित्तजित् ||२५||
—B.P. Pushpadi varga

132. Chandrashura [*Lepidium sativum* Linn.]

Family: *Cruciferae*

Hindi name: *Haalo, Chanshur*

English name: *Garden cress*

Synonyms: *Chandrika, Charmhantri, Pashumehankarika, Nandini, Bhadra, Vaaspushpa, Suvaasra, Karvi*

Morphology

It is an erect branched glabrous herb of about 60 cm height (**Fig. 132.1**).

Key Characters for Identification

➤ *Leaves: Entire or variously lobed, lower petiolate, upper sessile.*
➤ *Flower: Small, long raceme, and white in color* (**Fig. 132.2**).
➤ *Fruit: Obovate, small pods, notched at the apex with two seeds per pod.*
➤ *Seeds: Small, slimy, brown* (**Fig. 132.3**).

Rasapanchaka

Guna	Laghu, Ruksha, Tikshna (Whole plant)
Guna	Snigdha, Pichhal (Seed)
Rasa	Katu, Tikta
Vipaka	Katu
Virya	Ushna
Doshakarma	Kapha vatashamaka

Officinal Part Used

Seed

Dose

Powder: 1 to 3 g

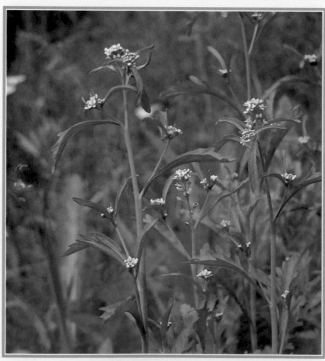

Fig. 132.1   Plant of *Lepidium sativum* Linn.

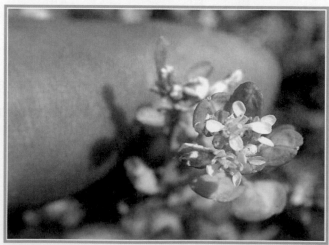

Fig. 132.2   Flower.

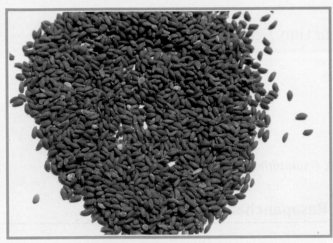

Fig. 132.3 Seeds.

Karma (Actions)

Balya (strength promoting), pushthivardhak (nourishing), rasayana (rejuvenative), stanyajanan (galactogouge), anuloman (laxative), shoolprasasman (antispasmodic), krimighna (anthelmintic), hikkanigrahan (anti-hic-cough).

Indications

Hikka (hic-cough), atisara (diarrhea), vatavyadhi (neurological disorders), vatarakta (gouts), katishool (backache), kasthaartava (dysmenorrhea), sootika roga (puerperal disease), shukradourbalya (deficiency of semen).

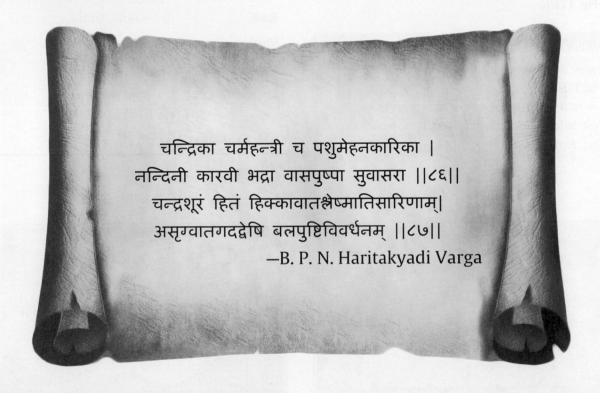

चन्द्रिका चर्महन्त्री च पशुमेहनकारिका |
नन्दिनी कारवी भद्रा वासपुष्पा सुवासरा ||८६||
चन्द्रशूरं हितं हिक्कावातश्लेष्मातिसारिणाम्|
असृग्वातगदद्वेषि बलपुष्टिविवर्धनम् ||८७||
—B. P. N. Haritakyadi Varga

133. Changeri [*Oxalis corniculata* Linn.]

Family:	*Oxalidaceae*
Hindi name:	*Teen pattiyan*
English name:	*Indian sorrel*
Synonyms:	*Amlapatrika, Chukrika, Dantasatha, Ambastha, Amlalonika*

Morphology

It is an annual or short-lived perennial herb with creeping stem (**Fig. 133.1**).

Key Characters for Identification

➤ *Leaves: Alternate, long petiolate, and trifoliate* (**Fig. 133.2**).
➤ *Flower: Axillary and yellow in color* (**Fig. 133.3**).
➤ *Fruit: Subcylindrical capsule containing numerous tiny black seeds.*

Rasapanchaka

Guna	Laghu, Ruksha
Rasa	Kashya, Amla
Vipaka	Amla
Virya	Ushna
Doshakarma	Kaphavatahara

Officinal Part Used

Whole plant

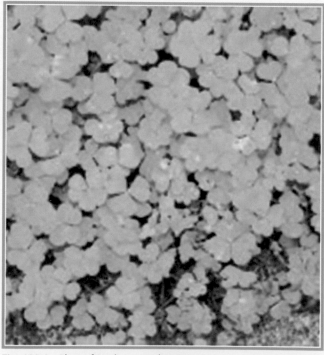

Fig. 133.1 Plant of *Oxalis corniculata* Linn.

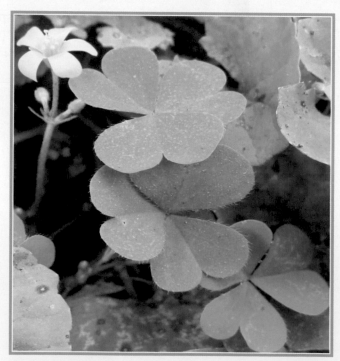

Fig. 133.2 Leaves.

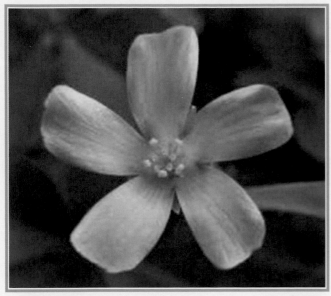

Fig. 133.3 Flower.

Dose

Fresh juice: 5 to 10 mL

Karma (Actions)

Deepana (appetizer), grahi (astringent), ruchya (relish), hridya (cardiotonic), jwaraghna (antipyretics), vishaghna (antidotes).

Indications

Atisara (diarrhea), kushta (skin diseases), arsha (piles), grahani (sprue), gudabhransh (rectal prolapse), raktsrava (hemorrhage).

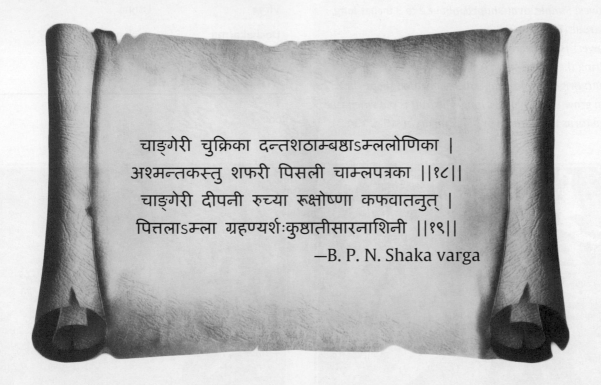

चाङ्गेरी चुक्रिका दन्तशठाम्बष्ठाऽम्ललोणिका ।
अश्मन्तकस्तु शफरी पिसली चाम्लपत्रका ॥१८॥
चाङ्गेरी दीपनी रुच्या रूक्षोष्णा कफवातनुत् ।
पित्तलाऽम्ला ग्रहण्यर्शःकुष्ठातीसारनाशिनी ॥१९॥
—B. P. N. Shaka varga

134. Chavya [Piper chaba Hunter]

Family:	Piperaceae
Hindi name:	Chabh
English name:	Long pepper root
Synonyms:	Chavika moola, Gajapippalimoola, Chavika, Ushna

Morphology

It is a climbing glabrous creeper with bright red fruiting spike (**Fig. 134.1**).

Key Characters for Identification

➤ *Leaves: Simple, oval-shaped, about 2 to 3 inches long, lustrous (***Fig. 134.2***).*
➤ *Flower: The flowers are monoecious and blossom during the monsoon.*
➤ *Fruit: Bright red fruiting spike, elongated shape that can grow up to 3 inches long. The fruit is red when ripe, and turns dark brown or black on drying (***Fig. 134.3***).*

Rasapanchaka

Guna	Laghu, Ruksha
Rasa	Katu
Vipaka	Katu
Virya	Ushna
Doshakarma	Kaphavatahara

Officinal Part Used

Root

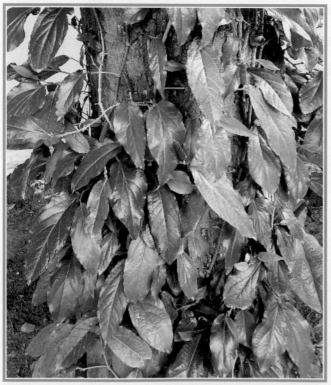

Fig. 134.1   Plant of *Piper chaba* Hunter.

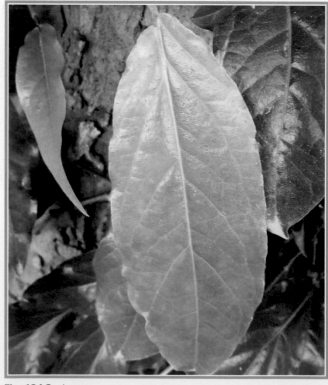

Fig. 134.2   Leaves.

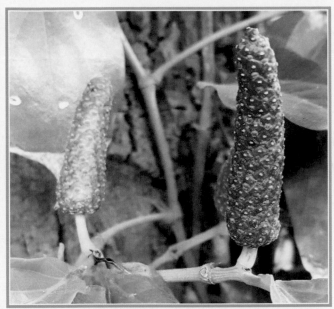

Fig. 134.3 Fruits.

Dose

Powder: 1 to 2 g

Karma (Actions)

Deepana (appetizer), pachana (digestive), bhedana (laxative), shoolprasasmana (antispasmodic).

Indications

Arsha (piles), krimi (worm infestation), kasa (cough), shwasa (asthma), agnimandh (loss of appetite), udarroga (abdominal diseases), pleharoga (splenomegaly), gulma (abdominal distention).

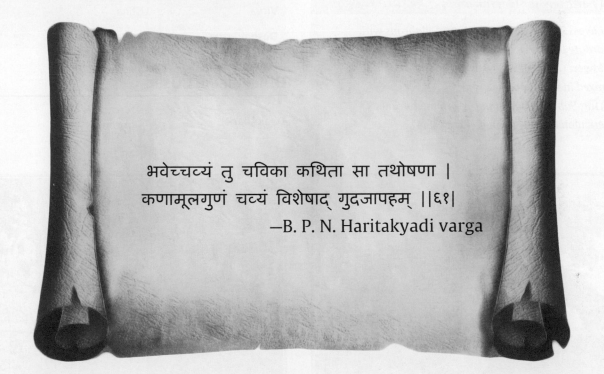

भवेच्चव्यं तु चविका कथिता सा तथोषणा |
कणामूलगुणं चव्यं विशेषाद् गुदजापहम् ||६१|

—B. P. N. Haritakyadi varga

135. Chirbilva *[Holoptelea integrifolia Planch.]*

Family: *Ulmaceae*

Hindi name: *Puti karanj, Chirbil*

English name: *Indian Elm, Jungle cork tree*

Synonyms: *Karanji, Udkirya, Shadgrantha, Hastivaruni, Markati, Vayasi*

Morphology

It is a medium-sized deciduous tree (**Fig. 135.1**) growing to a height of 10 to 15 m characterized with pale white bark (**Fig. 135.2**).

Key Characters for Identification

➤ *Leaves: Simple, alternate, elliptic, glabrous with cordate base (***Fig. 135.3***).*

➤ *Flower: Greenish yellow, male and hermaphrodite mixed in short raceme.*

➤ *Fruit: Suborbicular samara with membranous reticulately veined wings (***Fig. 135.4***).*

Rasapanchaka

Guna	Tikta, Kashaya
Rasa	Tikta
Vipaka	Katu
Virya	Ushna
Doshakarma	Kapha pittahara

Officinal Part Used

Twak (bark)

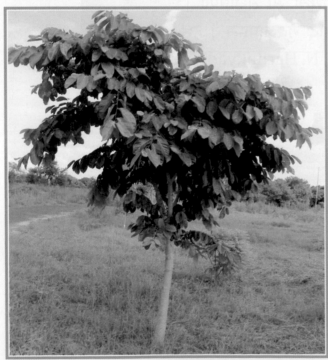

Fig. 135.1 Plant of *Holoptelea integrifolia* Planch.

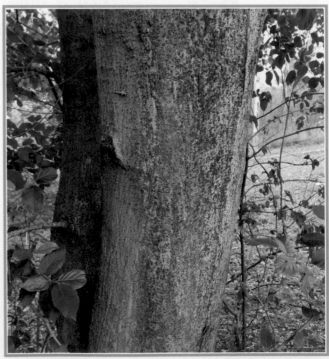

Fig. 135.2 Bark.

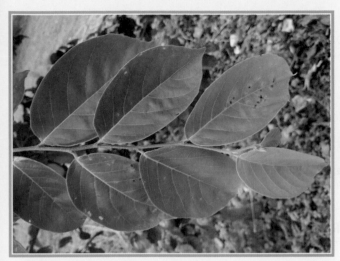

Fig. 135.3 Leaves.

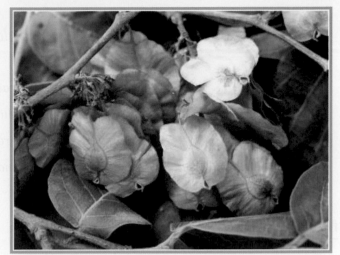

Fig. 135.4 Fruit.

Dose

Decoction: 50 to 100 mL

Karma (Actions)

Deepana (appetizer), lekhana (fat reducing/scraping), bhedana (purgative), krimighna (anthelmintic), stambhana (astringent), shothahara (swelling reducing).

Indications

Krimiroga (worm infestation), kushta (skin diseases), prameha (diabetes), medoroga (obesity), raktarsha (bleeding piles), vranashotha (inflamed wounds).

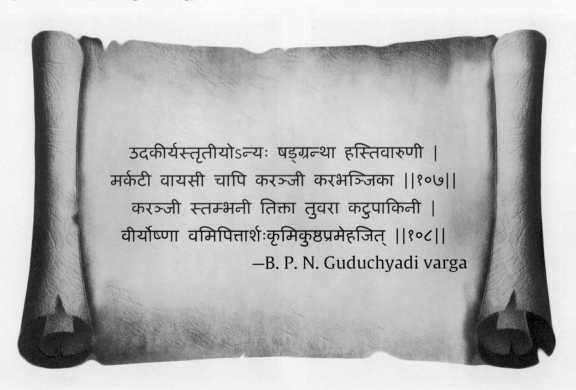

उदकीर्यस्तृतीयोऽन्यः षड्ग्रन्था हस्तिवारुणी ।
मर्कटी वायसी चापि करञ्जी करभञ्जिका ॥१०७॥
करञ्जी स्तम्भनी तिक्ता तुवरा कटुपाकिनी ।
वीर्योष्णा वमिपित्तार्शःकृमिकुष्ठप्रमेहजित् ॥१०८॥
—B. P. N. Guduchyadi varga

136. Chopachini [*Smilax glabra* Roxb.]

Family:	*Liliaceae*
Hindi name:	*Chobchini*
English name:	*China root*
Synonyms:	*Dvipanatar vacha, Madhusnuhi*

Morphology

It is a hard, tendril climber with cordate-shaped leaves and prickles on the stem (**Fig. 136.1**).

Key Characters for Identification

➤ *Leaves: Simple, alternate, elliptic, rounded at base, prominently nerved (**Fig. 136.2**).*
➤ *Flower: Many, small, white in umbels.*
➤ *Fruit: Red berries.*
➤ *Rhizome: Thick and tuberous.*

Rasapanchaka

Guna	Laghu, Ruksha
Rasa	Tikta
Vipaka	Katu
Virya	Ushna
Doshakarma	Tridoshaghna

Officinal Part Used

Tuber

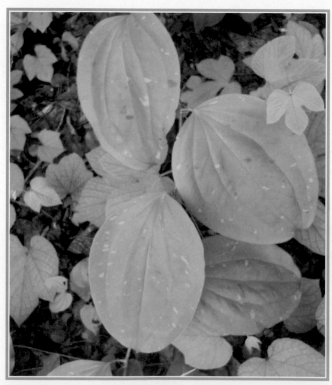

Fig. 136.1 Plant of *Smilax glabra* Roxb.

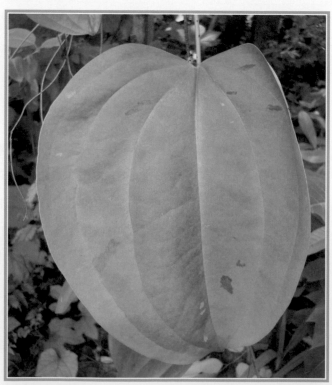

Fig. 136.2 Leaf.

Dose

Powder: 3 to 6 g

Karma (Actions)

Swedana (sweating), deepana (appetizer), uttejaka (stimulant), balya (tonics), shoolprasasman (antispasmodic), shothhara (reduce swelling).

Indications

Phirangroga (syphilis), vatavyadhi (neuromuscular disease), unmada (insanity), apasmar (epilepsy), kushta (skin diseases), adhyaman (flatulence), vibandh (constipation), puyameha (gonorrhea).

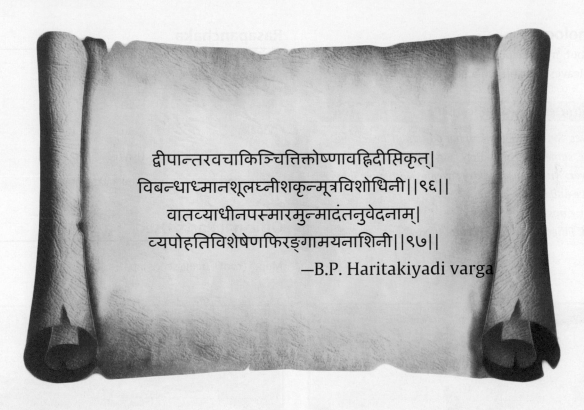

द्वीपान्तरवचाकिञ्चित्तिक्तोष्णावह्निदीसिकृत्।
विबन्धाध्मानशूलघ्नीशकृन्मूत्रविशोधिनी॥९६॥
वातव्याधीनपस्मारमुन्मादंतनुवेदनाम्।
व्यपोहतिविशेषेणफिरङ्गामयनाशिनी॥९७॥
—B.P. Haritakiyadi varga

137. Danti *[Baliospermum montanum (Wild) Muell]*

Family:	*Euphorbiaceae*
Hindi name:	*Danti*
English name:	*Red Physic nut, Wild castor*
Synonyms:	*Udumbarparni, Erandphala, Sheeghra, Nikumbha, Mukulaka*

Morphology

It is a stout, monoceious undershrub up to 3 m high, with toothed leaves and stiff branches (**Fig. 137.1**).

Key Characters for Identification

➤ *Leaves: Simple, toothed, upper one small, lower one large, sometimes palmately (**Fig. 137.2**).*
➤ *Flower: Numerous, axillary racemes with male flowers above and female below.*
➤ *Fruit: Capsule and obovoid.*
➤ *Seed: Ellipsoid, smooth and mottled.*

Rasapanchaka

Guna	Guru, Tikshna
Rasa	Katu
Vipaka	Katu
Virya	Ushna
Doshakarma	Kapha vatahara

Officinal Parts Used

Moola (root), beej (seeds), patra (leaves)

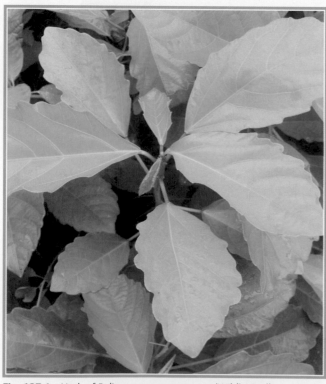

Fig. 137.1 Herb of *Baliospermum montanum* (Wild) Muell.

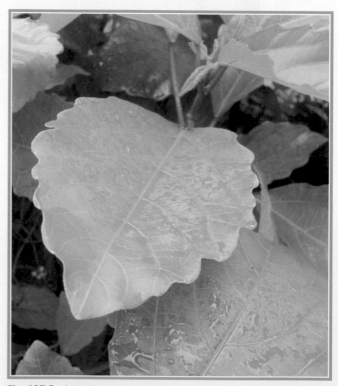

Fig. 137.2 Leaves.

Dose

Root powder: 1 to 3 g
Seed powder: 125 to 250 g
Leaf decoction: 40 to 80 mL

Karma (Actions)

Vedanasthapana (analgesic), shothahara (anti-inflammatory), deepan (appetizer), virechana (purgative), krimighna (anthelmintic), shwasahara (antiasthmatic).

Indications

Arsha (piles), ashmari (calculus), shoola (spasmodic pain), kushta (skin diseases), kandu (pruritus), udar-roga (abdominal diseases), shoth (inflammation), krimi (worm infestation), vrana (wound), gulma (abdominal lump).

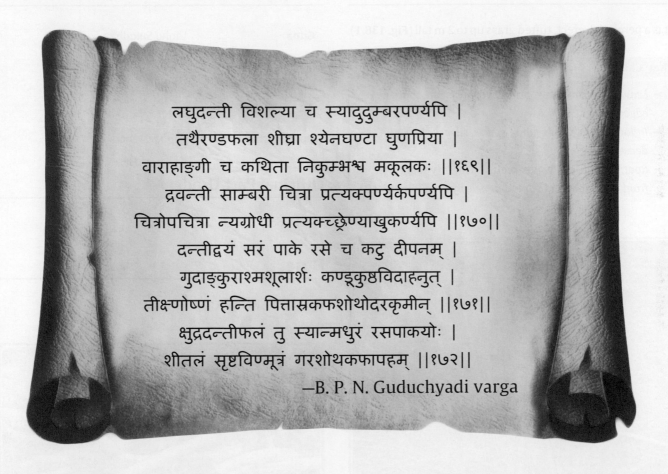

लघुदन्ती विशल्या च स्यादुदुम्बरपर्ण्यपि |
तथैरण्डफला शीघ्रा श्येनघण्टा घुणप्रिया |
वाराहाङ्गी च कथिता निकुम्भश्च मकूलकः ||१६९||
द्रवन्ती साम्बरी चित्रा प्रत्यक्पर्ण्यर्कपर्ण्यपि |
चित्रोपचित्रा न्यग्रोधी प्रत्यक्च्छ्रेण्याखुकर्ण्यपि ||१७०||
दन्तीद्वयं सरं पाके रसे च कटु दीपनम् |
गुदाङ्कुराश्मशूलार्शः कण्डुकुष्ठविदाहनुत् |
तीक्ष्णोष्णं हन्ति पित्तास्रकफशोथोदरकृमीन् ||१७१||
क्षुद्रदन्तीफलं तु स्यान्मधुरं रसपाकयोः |
शीतलं सृष्टविण्मूत्रं गरशोथकफापहम् ||१७२||

—B. P. N. Guduchyadi varga

138. Darbh [*Imperata cylindrica* Linn.]

Family:	*Poaceae*
Hindi name:	*Darbha*
English name:	*Cogan grass*
Synonyms:	*Deerghapatra, Kshurpatra*

Morphology

It is a perennial, erect, tufted grass up to 2 m tall (**Fig. 138.1**).

Key Characters for Identification

➤ *Leaves: Narrow, long, prominently nerved, sharp-edged margin.*
➤ *Inflorescence: It has many spikes, silver-white, and densely silky.*
➤ *Root: Cylindrical, white, many secondary roots arise from main root and spread in nearby area* (**Fig. 138.2**).

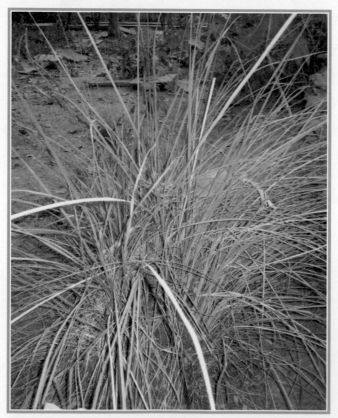

Fig. 138.1 Grass of *Imperata cylindrica* Linn.

Rasapanchaka

Guna	Laghu Snigdha
Rasa	Madhura, Kashaya
Vipaka	Madhura
Virya	Sheeta
Doshakarma	Kaphavatahara

Officinal Part Used

Mool (root)

Dose

Decoction: 10 to 20 mL

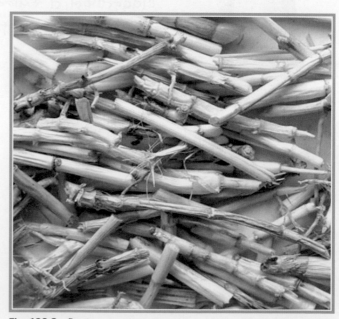

Fig. 138.2 Roots.

Karma (Actions)

Rasayana (rejuvenative), vamaka (induce vomiting), mutravirechaniya (diuretic), kushthaghna (antileprotic), pipasahara (reduce thirst).

Indications

Ashmari (urinary calculus), daha (burning sensation), jwara (fever), trishna (thirst), mutrakricchta (dysuria), raktapitta (bleeding disorders), bastishoola (pain in urinary tract), pradara (excessive vaginal discharge).

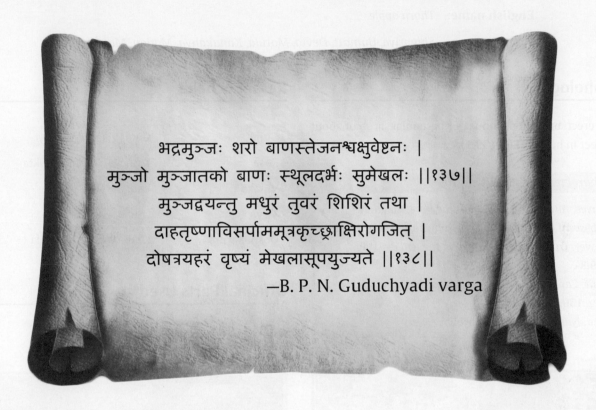

भद्रमुञ्जः शरो बाणस्तेजनश्चक्षुवेष्टनः |
मुञ्जो मुञ्जातको बाणः स्थूलदर्भः सुमेखलः ||१३७||
मुञ्जद्वयन्तु मधुरं तुवरं शिशिरं तथा |
दाहतृष्णाविसर्पाममूत्रकृच्छ्राक्षिरोगजित् |
दोषत्रयहरं वृष्यं मेखलासूपयुज्यते ||१३८||
—B. P. N. Guduchyadi varga

139. Dhatura *[Dhatura metel Linn.]*

Family:	*Solanaceae*
Hindi name:	*Dhatura*
English name:	*Thorn apple*
Synonyms:	*Shivpriya, Unmatt, Devta, Matula, Kanakahva, Madan, Mahamohi*

Morphology

It is an erect, branched, annual, or perennial shrub of about 3 to 4 feet in height (**Fig. 139.1**).

Key Characters for Identification

➤ *Leaves: Alternate, unequal at the base, minutely pubescent on both surfaces, wavy margin (**Fig. 139.2**).*
➤ *Flower: Large, white, solitary in the leaf axil (**Fig. 139.3**).*
➤ *Fruit: Capsule, globose, covered with slender spines (**Fig. 139.4**).*
➤ *Seed: Numerous blackish brown.*

Rasapanchaka

Guna	Guru, Vikashi, Vyavayi
Rasa	Kashaya, Madhura, Tikta
Vipaka	Katu
Virya	Ushna
Doshakarma	Kapha vatahara, Pittala

Officinal Parts Used

Moola, beeja, patra, pushpa, phala

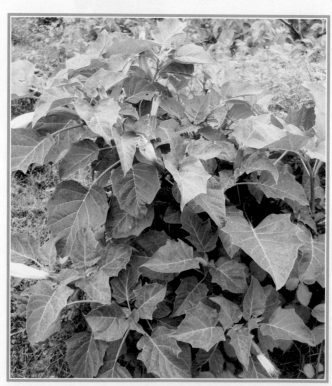

Fig. 139.1 Plant of *Dhatura metel* Linn.

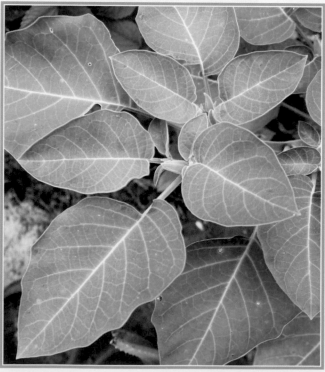

Fig. 139.2 Leaves.

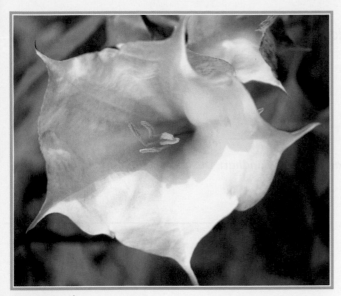

Fig. 139.3 Flower.

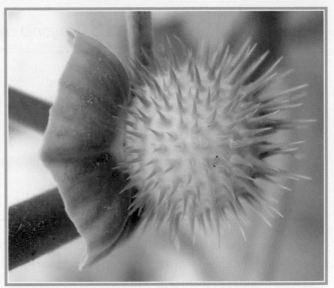

Fig. 139.4 Fruit.

Dose

Root powder: 125 to 250 m
Seed powder: 60 to 120 m
Leaf powder: 1 to 3 g

Karma (Actions)

Deepana (appetizer), madakari varnya (complexion promoter), vedanahara (analgesic), kandughna (antipruritus), krimighna (anthelmintic), vishaghna (antidotes).

Indications

Krimi (worm infestation), kushta (skin diseases), kandu (pruritis), shoola (pain), vrana (wound), jwara (fever), yukaliksha (head lice), visha (poisoning), shwasa (asthma).

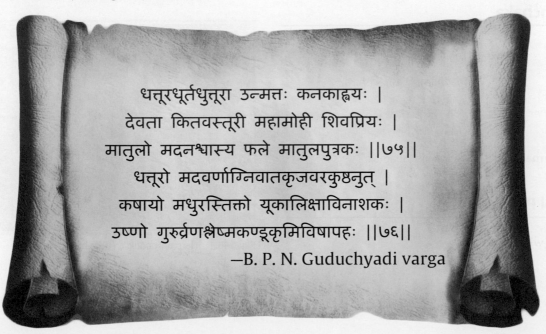

धत्तूरधूर्तधुत्तूरा उन्मत्तः कनकाह्वयः |
देवता कितवस्तूरी महामोही शिवप्रियः |
मातुलो मदनश्चास्य फले मातुलपुत्रकः ||७५||
धत्तूरो मदवर्णाग्निवातकृजवरकुष्ठनुत् |
कषायो मधुरस्तिक्तो यूकालिक्षाविनाशकः |
उष्णो गुरुर्व्रणश्लेष्मकण्डूकृमिविषापहः ||७६||
—B. P. N. Guduchyadi varga

140. Dhanvyas *[Fagonia cretica Linn.]*

Family:	*Zygophyllaceae*
Hindi name:	*Dhamasa*
English name:	*Khorasan thorn*
Synonyms:	*Dhanwayas, Duralabha, Samudranta, Gandhari, Dushparsha, Ananta*

Morphology

It is a procumbent branched herb up to 1 to 3 feet tall, with woody stem and sharp thorns. The small branches are thick and have nodules in them (**Fig. 140.1**).

Key Characters for Identification

➤ *Leaves: Opposite, shrunken, leaflets three to four, entire, linear, or ovate with acute apex.*
➤ *Thorn: Thick and strong (**Fig. 140.1**).*
➤ *Flowers: Violet to light violet, star-shaped, five-narrow petal.*
➤ *Fruits: Plant has large number of small fruits near thorns, divided in to five segments.*
➤ *Plant has sweet, bitter, sharp, and sour taste according to different stages of growth and parts.*

Rasapanchaka

Guna	Laghu, Sara
Rasa	Madhura, Tikta, Kashaya
Vipaka	Madhura
Virya	Ushna
Doshakarma	Kapha pittashamaka

Officinal Part Used

Panchang (whole plant)

Dose

Powder: 5 to 10 g
Decoction: 40 to 80 mL

Karma (Actions)

Dahaprasasmana (cooling effect), vranaropana (wound healing), raktastambhaka (hemostatic), raktaprasadana (blood purifier), mutral (diuretics).

Indications

Vrana (wound), daha (burning sensation), chhardi (vomiting), kasa (cough), jwara (fever), mutrakricchta (dysuria), raktavikara (blood disease), kushta (skin disease), visarpa (erysipelas), medoroga (obesity), trishna (thirst).

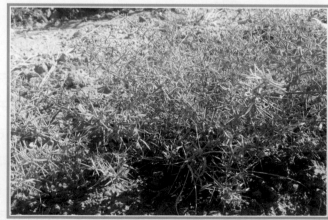

Fig. 140.1 Herb of *Fagonia cretica* Linn.

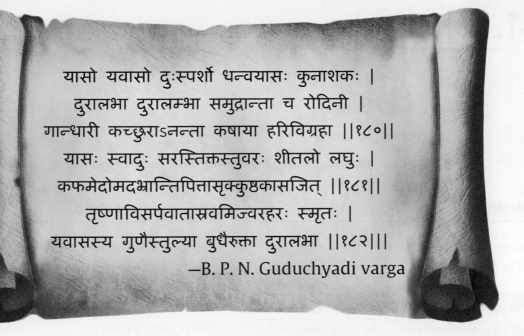

यासो यवासो दुःस्पर्शो धन्वयासः कुनाशकः |
दुरालभा दुरालम्भा समुद्रान्ता च रोदिनी |
गान्धारी कच्छुराऽनन्ता कषाया हरिविग्रहा ||१८०||
यासः स्वादुः सरस्तिक्तस्तुवरः शीतलो लघुः |
कफमेदोमदभ्रान्तिपित्तासृक्कुष्ठकासजित् ||१८१||
तृष्णाविसर्पवातास्रवमिज्वरहरः स्मृतः |
यवासस्य गुणैस्तुल्या बुधैरुक्ता दुरालभा ||१८२||

—B. P. N. Guduchyadi varga

141. Dhanyaka *[Coriandrum sativum Linn.]*

Family:	*Umbelliferae*
Hindi name:	*Dhaniya*
English name:	*Coriander*
Synonyms:	*Dhanya, Dhana, Dhenuka, Kutnnati, Chatra, Kushtumbru, Vitunnaka*

Morphology

It is a green, soft annual aromatic herb with decompound leaves (**Fig. 141.1**).

Key Characters for Identification

➤ *Leaves: Decompound, sub-sessile, imparipinnate.*
➤ *Flower: Small, white, or pinkish purple; compound, terminal umbels.*
➤ *Fruit: Yellowish-brown, globular, and ribbed, separating into two halves, each containing a seed* (**Fig. 141.2**).

Rasapanchaka

Guna	Laghu, Snigdha
Rasa	Kashaya, Tikta, Katu
Vipaka	Madhur
Virya	Ushna
Doshakarma	Tridoshahara

Officinal Part Used

Panchang (whole plant)

Dose

Leaves paste: 5 to 10 g

Karma (Actions)

Vatanulomana (carminative), pachana (digestive), deepana (appetizer), rochana (relish), grahi (astringent), jwaraghna (antipyretics), vrishya (aphrodisiac), dahashamaka (cooling effect), mutral (diuretics).

Indications

Trishna (thirst), jwara (fever), daha (burning sensation), vaman (vomiting), kasa (cough), shwasa (asthma), krimiroga (worm infestation).

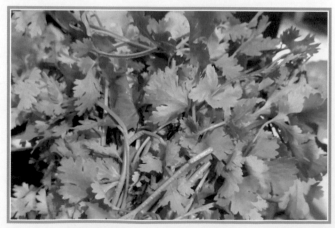

Fig. 141.1   Plant of *Coriandrum sativum* Linn.

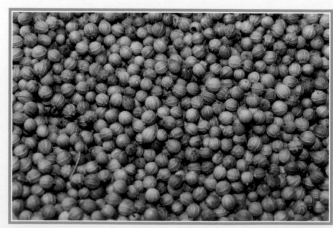

Fig. 141.2   Fruits.

धान्यकं धानकं धान्यं धाना धानेयकं तथा |
कुनटी धेनुका छत्रा कुस्तुम्बुरु वितुन्नकम् ||७७||
धान्यकं तुवरं स्निग्धमवृष्यं मूत्रलं लघु |
तिक्तं कटूष्णवीर्यञ्च दीपनं पाचनं स्मृतम् ||७८||
ज्वरघ्नं रोचकं ग्राहि स्वादुपाकि त्रिदोषनुत् |
तृष्णादाहवमिश्वासकासकार्श्यक्रिमिप्रणुत् |
आर्द्रन्तु तद्गुणं स्वादु विशेषात्पित्तनाशि तत् ||७९||

—B. P. N. Haritakyadi

142. Draksha *[Vitis vinifera Linn.]*

Family: *Vitaceae*

Hindi name: *Angoor*

English name: *Grapes*

Synonyms: *Swaduphala, Madhurasa, Mrudvika, Gostani*

Morphology

It is a woody, tendril climber with palmate-lobed leaves (**Fig. 142.1**).

Key Characters for Identification

➤ *Leaves: Simple, orbicular-cordate, irregularly toothed* (**Fig. 142.2**).
➤ *Flower: Small, green in leaf-opposed, panicle cymes.*
➤ *Fruit: Bluish black, purplish or greenish berries, ovoid to globose* (**Fig. 142.3**).
➤ *Seed: Two to four with a discoidal tubercle on the back.*

Rasapanchaka

Guna	Guru, Sara
Rasa	Madhura, Kashaya
Vipaka	Madhura
Virya	Sheeta
Doshakarma	Tridoshahara

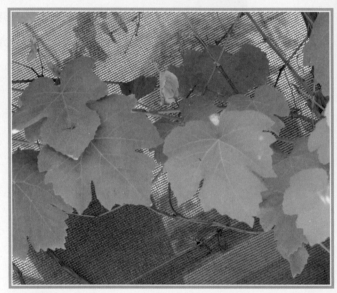

Fig. 142.2 Leaves.

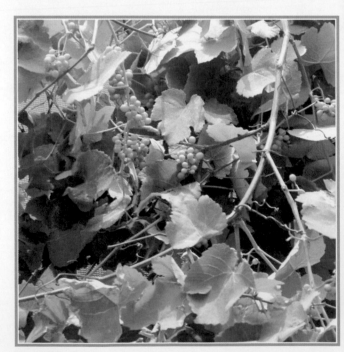

Fig. 142.3 Fruits.

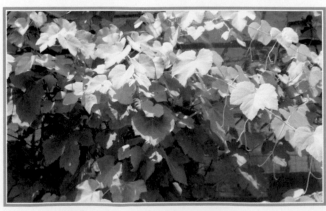

Fig. 142.1 Climber of *Vitis vinifera* Linn.

Officinal Part Used

Phala (fruits)

Dose

Juice: 20 to 40 mL

Karma (Actions)

Chakshushya (beneficial for vision), brihmaniya (bulk promoting), pushtikara (nourishing), swarya (beneficial for voice), hridya (cardio tonic), vrishya (aphrodisiac), rochaka (relish), srishtavinnamutrakara (formation of urine and stool).

Indications

Trishna (thirst), mutrakricchta (dysuria), raktapitta (bleeding disorders), shwasa (asthma), jwara (fever), kamala (jaundice), daha (burning sensation), shosha (emaciation), madatyaya (alcoholism), sanmoha (derillium).

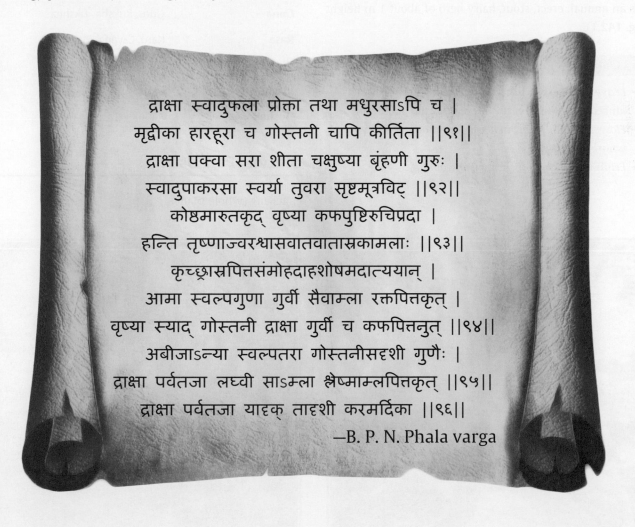

द्राक्षा स्वादुफला प्रोक्ता तथा मधुरसाऽपि च |
मृद्वीका हारहूरा च गोस्तनी चापि कीर्तिता ||९१||
द्राक्षा पक्वा सरा शीता चक्षुष्या बृंहणी गुरुः |
स्वादुपाकरसा स्वर्या तुवरा सृष्टमूत्रविट् ||९२||
कोष्ठमारुतकृद् वृष्या कफपुष्टिरुचिप्रदा |
हन्ति तृष्णाज्वरश्वासवातवातास्रकामलाः ||९३||
कृच्छ्रास्रपित्तसंमोहदाहशोषमदात्ययान् |
आमा स्वल्पगुणा गुर्वी सैवाम्ला रक्तपित्तकृत् |
वृष्या स्याद् गोस्तनी द्राक्षा गुर्वी च कफपित्तनुत् ||९४||
अबीजाऽन्या स्वल्पतरा गोस्तनीसदृशी गुणैः |
द्राक्षा पर्वतजा लघ्वी साऽम्ला श्लेष्माम्लपित्तकृत् ||९५||
द्राक्षा पर्वतजा यादृक् तादृशी करमर्दिका ||९६||

—B. P. N. Phala varga

143. Dronpushpi *[Leucas cephalotes Spreng]*

Family:	*Labiatae*
Hindi name:	*Guma*
English name:	*Spider wort*
Synonyms:	*Phalepushpa, Drona*

Morphology

It is an annual, erect, stout, hairy herb of about 1 m height (**Fig. 142.1**).

Key Characters for Identification

➤ *Leaves: Subsessile, linear or oblong or linear-lanceolate, obtuse, entire or crenate, and pubescent.*
➤ *Flower: White, small, in dense terminal or axillary whorls (**Fig. 142.2**).*
➤ *Fruit: Nutlet, smooth, brown, and oblong.*

Rasapanchaka

Guna	Guru, Ruksha, Tikshna
Rasa	Katu, Lavana, Madhura
Vipaka	Katu/Madhura
Virya	Ushna
Doshakarma	Kapha vatashamaka

Officinal Part Used

Panchang (whole plant)

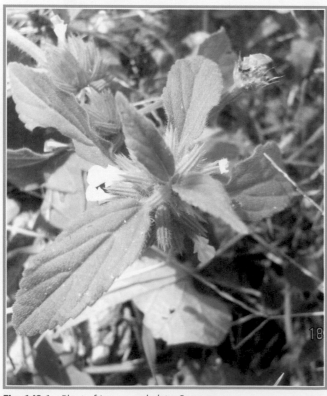

Fig. 143.1   Plant of *Leucas cephalotes* Spreng.

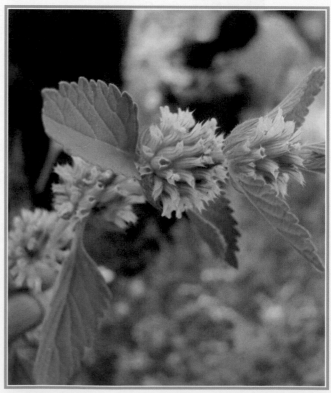

Fig. 143.2   Flower.

Dose

Fresh juice: 10 to 20 mL

Karma (Actions)

Deepana (appetizer), bhedana (purgative), rochana (relish), jwaraghna (antipyretics), krimighna (anthelmintic), shothaghna (reduce swelling).

Indications

Kamala (jaundice), agnimandya (loss of appetite), tamak shwasa (asthma), prameha (diabetes), krimi (worm), shotha (inflammation), visham jwara (intermittent fever).

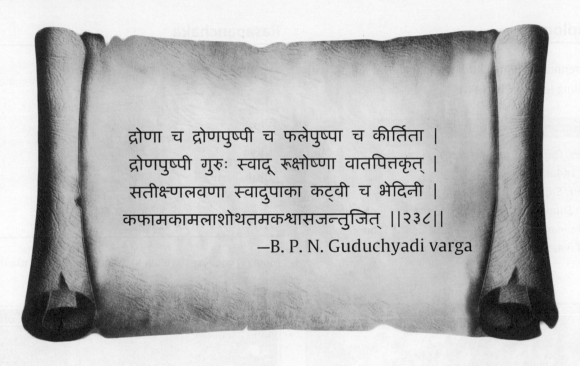

द्रोणा च द्रोणपुष्पी च फलेपुष्पा च कीर्तिता ।
द्रोणपुष्पी गुरुः स्वादू रूक्षोष्णा वातपित्तकृत् ।
सतीक्ष्णलवणा स्वादुपाका कट्वी च भेदिनी ।
कफामकामलाशोथतमकश्वासजन्तुजित् ॥२३८॥
—B. P. N. Guduchyadi varga

144. Gandhaprasharni *[Paederia foetida Linn.]*

Family:	*Rubiaceae*
Hindi name:	*Gandhaprasharni*
English name:	*Skunk vine*
Synonyms:	*Rajbala, Prasarini, Bhadraparni, Pratapani, Sarni, Saarani*

Morphology

It is a perennial twining climber of about 7 m length with foul smelling leaves (**Fig. 144.1**).

Key Characters for Identification

➤ *Leaves: Opposite, margin entire, purple beneath* (**Fig. 144.2**).
➤ *Flower: Small, white with pale violet spot.*
➤ *Fruit: Subovoid, slightly compressed, and glabrous.*
➤ *Whole plant is covered with pubescence; it has a fetid smell when crushed.*

Rasapanchaka

Guna	Guru
Rasa	Tikta
Vipaka	Katu
Virya	Ushna
Doshakarma	Kapha vatahara

Officinal Parts Used

Moola (root), patra (leaves), panchang (whole plant)

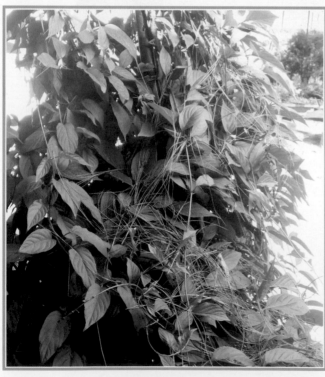

Fig. 144.1 Plant of *Paederia foetida* Linn.

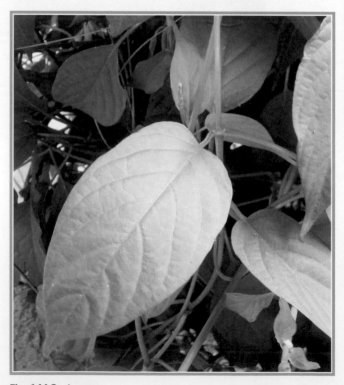

Fig. 144.2 Leaves.

Dose

Decoction: 50 to 100 mL
Juice: 10 to 20 mL

Karma (Actions)

Balya (tonics), vrishya (aphrodisiac), sandhanakara (union of fractured bones).

Indications

Amavata (arthritis), arsh (piles), sotha (inflammation), vatarakta (gout), mutrakricchta (dysuria).

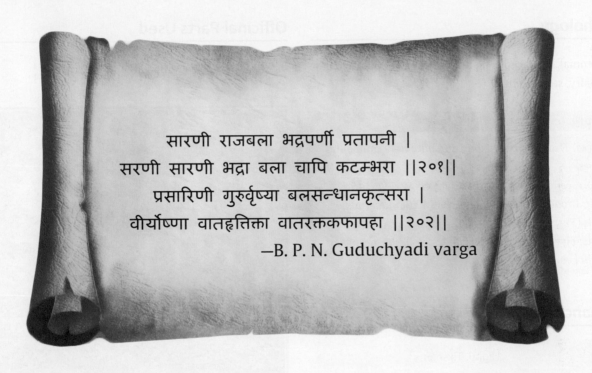

सारणी राजबला भद्रपर्णी प्रतापनी |
सरणी सारणी भद्रा बला चापि कटम्भरा ||२०१||
प्रसारिणी गुरुवृष्या बलसन्धानकृत्सरा |
वीर्योष्णा वातहृत्तिक्ता वातरक्तकफापहा ||२०२||
—B. P. N. Guduchyadi varga

145. Garjar *[Daucas carota Linn.]*

Family:	*Umbelliferae*
Hindi name:	*Gajar*
English name:	*Carrot*
Synonyms:	*Swadumool, Narangvarnak, Raktakanda, Rasalu*

Morphology

It is a biennial, herbaceous plant of about 30 to 60 cm height with a hairy, stout stem.

Key Characters for Identification

➤ *Leaves: Triangular to oblong and pinnately compound leaves.*
➤ *Inflorescence: Umbel, whitish, or yellow (**Fig. 145.1**).*
➤ *Fruit: Broad, including the prickles with numerous seeds (**Fig. 145.2**).*
➤ *Roots: Five to 30 cm long, cylindrical, fleshy, orange or red in color (**Fig. 145.3**).*

Rasapanchaka

Guna	Laghu, Tikshan
Rasa	Madhura, Tikta
Vipaka	Madhura
Virya	Ushna
Doshakarma	Kapha vatahara

Officinal Parts Used

Beeja (seeds), moola (root)

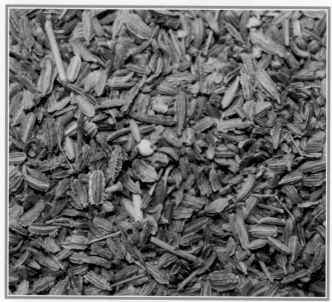

Fig. 145.2 Seeds.

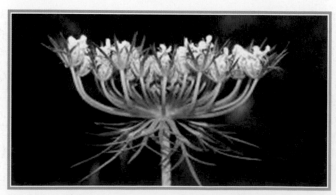

Fig. 145.1 Flower.

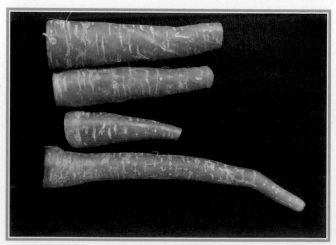

Fig. 145.3 Roots.

Dose

Root juice: 20 to 40 mL
Seed powder: 3 to 6 g

Karma (Actions)

Chaksusya (beneficial for vision), deepana (appetizer), sangrahi (fecal astringent), krimighna (anthelmintic), balya (increase physical strength), vajikara (aphrodisiac).

Indications

Netraroga (eye disease), atisara (diarrhea), arsh (piles), grahani (sprue), rakta pitta (bleeding disorders), shwasa (asthma).

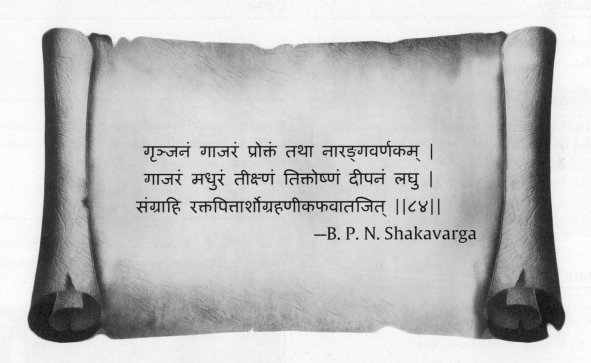

गृञ्जनं गाजरं प्रोक्तं तथा नारङ्गवर्णकम् |
गाजरं मधुरं तीक्ष्णं तिक्तोष्णं दीपनं लघु |
संग्राहि रक्तपित्तार्शोग्रहणीकफवातजित् ||८४||

—B. P. N. Shakavarga

146. Gojihva [*Onosma bracteatum* Wall.]

Family:	*Boraginaceae*
Hindi name:	*Gajwan*
English name:	*Cow's Tongue, Sedge*
Synonyms:	*Kharaparni, Gojika, Darvika, Goji*

Morphology

It is a perennial, hairy herb 20 to 40 cm tall with radical leaves (**Fig. 146.1**).

Key Characters for Identification

➤ *Leaves: Radical, 15 cm long and 3cm wide, petiolate, obovate-oblong, hairy on upper surface and soft on lower side.*
➤ *Flower: Found in bunch, violet color, hairy, 6 to 7 cm in diameter.*
➤ *Fruit: 3 to 15 cm, ovate, and pointed.*

Rasapanchaka

Guna	Laghu, Snigdha
Rasa	Madhura, Tikta
Vipaka	Madhura
Virya	Sheeta
Doshakarma	Kaphapittahara

Officinal Parts Used

Patra (leaves), pushpa (flower), mool (root)

Dose

Leaf and flower powder: 3 to 6 g

Karma (Actions)

Grahi (astringent), mutral (diuretics), hridya (cardiotonics), kasaghna (antitussive), pramehaghna (antidiabetes), jwaraghna (antipyretics)

Indications

Kasa (cough), prameha (diabetes), vrana (wound), raktavikara (diseases of blood), jwara (fever), daha (burning sensation).

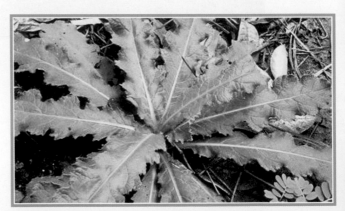

Fig. 146.1 Plant of *Onosma bracteatum* Wall.

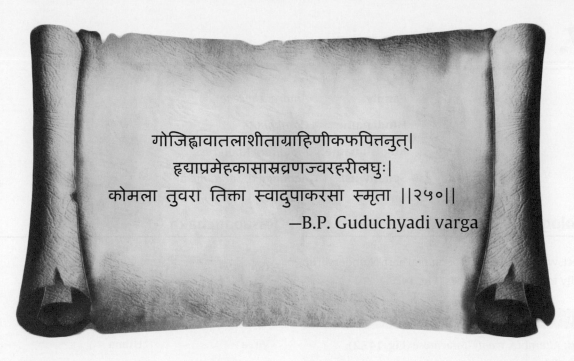

गोजिह्वावातलाशीताग्राहिणीकफपित्तनुत्।
हृद्याप्रमेहकासास्त्रव्रणज्वरहरीलघुः।
कोमला तुवरा तिक्ता स्वादुपाकरसा स्मृता ||२५०||
—B.P. Guduchyadi varga

147. Gorakshganja *[Aerva lanata (Linn) Juss]*

Family: *Amaranthaceae*

Hindi name: *Gorakhbuti*

English name: *Mountain Knotgrass*

Synonyms: *Aadanpaki, Satkabhedi*

Morphology

It is an erect, woody, prostrate, perennial herb or undershrub with woolly tomentose branches (**Fig. 147.1**).

Key Characters for Identification

➤ *Leaves: Alternate, wooly-tomentose* (**Fig. 147.2**).
➤ *Flower: Greenish white, minute, borne in axillary panicles* (Fig. **147.3**).
➤ *Fruit: Greenish, roundish, compressed.*
➤ *Seed: Kidney shaped in shiny black color.*

Rasapanchaka

Guna	Laghu, Tikshna
Rasa	Tikta, Kashaya
Vipaka	Katu
Virya	Ushna
Doshakarma	Kapha vatashamaka

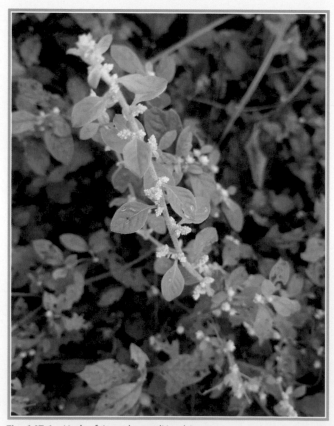

Fig. 147.1   Herb of *Aerva lanata* (Linn.) Juss.

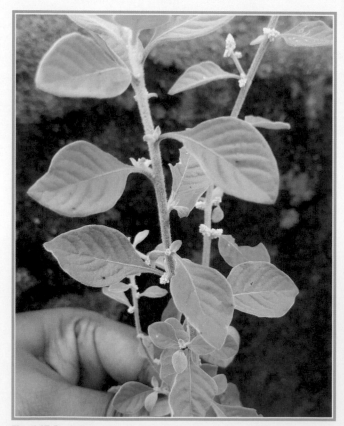

Fig. 147.2   Leaves.

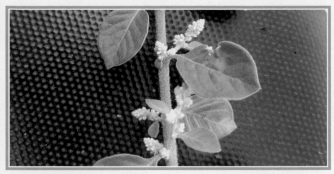

Fig. 147.3 Flower.

Official Part Used

Moola (roots)

Dose

Decoction: 50 to 100 mL

Karma (Actions)

Ashmaribhedana (breaking of urinary calculus), krimighna (anthelmintic), mutral (diuretic), vedanasthapana (analgesic), shothahara (anti-inflammatory).

Indications

Shotha (inflammation), mutrakricchta (dysuria), ashmari (calculus), tamak shwasa (bronchial asthma).

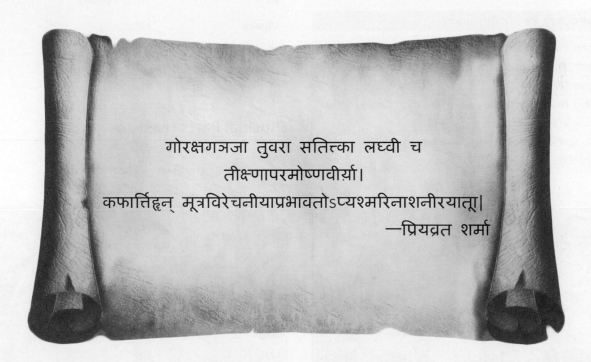

गोरक्षगञ्जा तुवरा सतित्का लघ्वी च
तीक्ष्णापरमोष्णवीर्या।
कफार्त्तिहृन् मूत्रविरेचनीयाप्रभावतोऽप्यश्मरिनाशनीरयात्तु।
—प्रियव्रत शर्मा

148. Gunja *[Abrus precatorius Linn.]*

Family:	*Fabaceae*
Hindi name:	*Ghunghchi, Ratti*
English name:	*Jequirity*
Synonyms:	*Kakantika, Raktika, Kakadani, Kakapilu, Angaarvalli*

Morphology

It is a slender, perennial climber with pinnate compound leaves (**Fig. 148.1**).

Key Characters for Identification

➤ *Leaves: Pinnate, compound, leaflets oblong.*
➤ *Flower: Pink, clustered on tubercles, pedunculate raceme (**Fig. 148.2**).*
➤ *Fruit: 1 to 2 inch oblong pods with pointed ends, occurs in bunch (**Fig. 148.3**).*
➤ *Seed: Scarlet with a black spot or sometimes pure white (**Fig. 148.4**).*

Rasapanchaka

Guna	Laghu, Ruksha
Rasa	Tikta, Kashaya
Vipaka	Katu
Virya	Ushna
Doshakarma	Vata pittahara

Officinal Parts Used

Moola (root), patra (leaves), beeja (seeds).

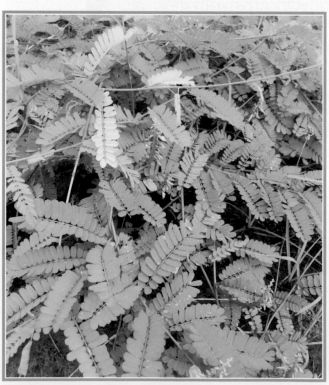

Fig. 148.1   Plant of *Abrus precatorius* Linn.

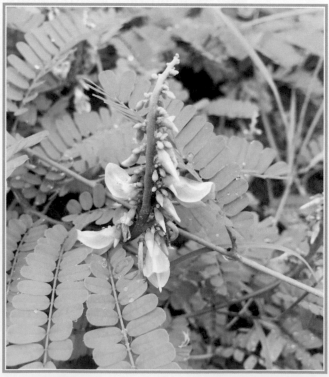

Fig. 148.2   Flowers.

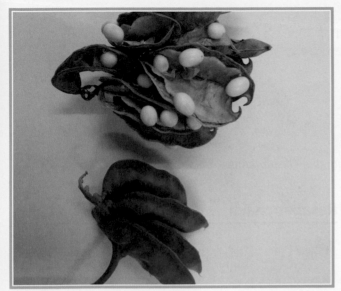

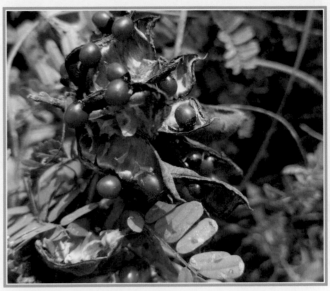

Fig. 148.3 Fruit and seeds.

Fig. 148.4 Seeds.

Dose

Seed powder: 60 to 180 mg
Root powder: 1 to 3 g

Karma (Actions)

Keshya (hair tonic), vranaropan (wound healing), kusthaghna (antidermatosis), mutral (diuretics), balya (tonic), vajikara(aphrodisiac), garbhanirodhaka (seeds prevent conception), krimighna(anthelmintic), kandughna (antipruritus), garbhanirodhaka (beej).

Indications

Vrana (wound), jwara (fever), mukhasosha (dryness in mouth), bhram (giddiness), shwasa (asthma), trishna (thirst), madanashaka (alleviates intoxication), netraroga (eye diseases), kandu (pruritis), krimi (worm infestation), indralupta (baldness), kusta (skin disease), vrana (wound).

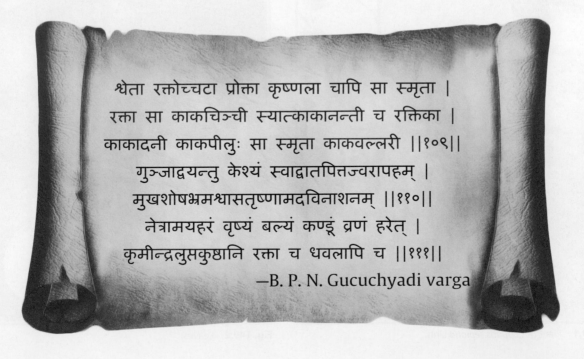

श्वेता रक्तोच्चटा प्रोक्ता कृष्णला चापि सा स्मृता ।
रक्ता सा काकचिञ्ची स्यात्काकानन्ती च रक्तिका ।
काकादनी काकपीलुः सा स्मृता काकवल्लरी ||१०९||
गुञ्जाद्वयन्तु केश्यं स्वाद्वातपित्तज्वरापहम् ।
मुखशोषभ्रमश्वासतृष्णामदविनाशनम् ||११०||
नेत्रामयहरं वृष्यं बल्यं कण्डूं व्रणं हरेत् ।
कृमीन्द्रलुप्तकुष्ठानि रक्ता च धवलापि च ||१११||

—B. P. N. Gucuchyadi varga

149. Hinsra *[Capparis sepiaria Linn.]*

Family:	*Capparidaceae*
Hindi name:	*Hinsra*
English name:	*Wild caper bush, Horse gram*
Synonyms:	*Kanthari, Gridhranakhi, Dupradharsha, Tikshankantaka, Kantha, Kruragandha*

Morphology

It is a much branched woody, thorny shrub of about 5 m height (**Fig. 149.1**).

Key Characters for Identification

➤ *Leaves: Elliptic, ovate or obovate, apically rounded, obtuse or retuse, basally rounded or subcordate; petiole 2 to 5 mm long, pubescent or glabrescent* (**Fig. 149.2**).
➤ *Flowers: In racemes or scattered in upper leaf axils* (**Fig. 149.3**).
➤ *Fruit: Globose, up to more than 1 cm in diameter, usually reddish.*

Rasapanchaka

Guna	Laghu, Ruksha
Rasa	Katu, Tikta
Vipaka	Katu
Virya	Ushna
Doshakarma	Kapha vatahara

Officinal Parts Used

Moola (root) and patra (leaves)

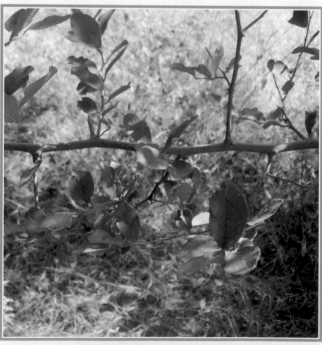

Fig. 149.1 Plant of *Capparis sepiaria* Linn.

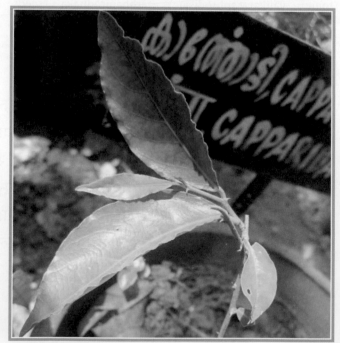

Fig. 149.2 Leaves.

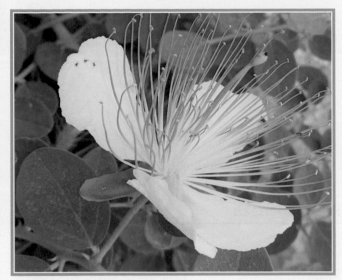

Fig. 149.3 Flower.

Dose

Decoction: 50 to 100 mL

Karma (Actions)

Deepana (appetizer), ruchya (relish), shothahara (reduce swelling), vishaghna (antidote), rujahara (analgesic).

Indications

Rakta-granthi (tumors of accumulated blood), shopha (inflammations), vatavyadhi (neuromuscular diseases), snayukaroga (dracunculiasis), shlipada (filariasis), arbuda (tumors).

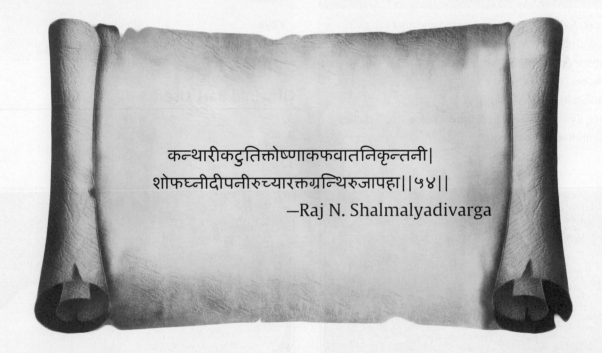

कन्थारीकटुतिक्तोष्णाकफवातनिकृन्तनी।
शोफघ्नीदीपनीरुच्यारक्तग्रन्थिरुजापहा॥५४॥
—Raj N. Shalmalyadivarga

150. Hribera *[Pavonia odorata Willd.]*

Family: *Malvaceae*

Hindi name: *Sugandhbala, Netrabala*

English name: *Fragrant swamp mallow*

Synonyms: *Ambu, Ambunamaka, Bala, Balaka, Udichya, Barhishta, Harivera*

Morphology

It is a straight, branched, annual herb of 1 to 3 feet. The plant is entirely covered with pubescent short hair (**Fig. 150.1**).

Key Characters for Identification

➤ *Leaves: Simple, alternate, ovate shape, three to five lobed, stellate hairy surface*
➤ *Flowers: Light pink or white, clustered at the end of the branches (**Fig. 150.2**)*
➤ *Fruit: Small, oval to spherical*
➤ *Roots: Cylindrical, twisted, brown color, 7 to 8 inches long with many root hairs.*

Rasapanchaka

Guna	Laghu, Ruksha
Rasa	Tikta
Vipaka	Katu
Virya	Sheet
Doshakarma	Kapha pittashamaka

Officinal Part Used

Roots

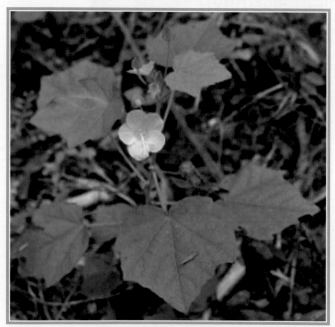

Fig. 150.1 Plant of *Pavonia odorata* Willd.

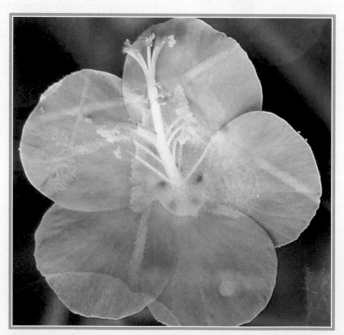

Fig. 150.2 Flower.

Dose

Powder: 3 to 6 g

Karma (Actions)

Deepan (carmina), pachan (digestive), snehan (emolient), vataanulomaka (facilitates downward displacement of vata), balya (tonic), jwarghna (antipyretic), trishnanigrahan (pacify thirst).

Indications

Raktapitta (bleeding disorders), aruchi (distaste), hrillasa (nausea), visarpa (erysipelas), hridyaroga (heart diseases), jwar (fever), daha (burning sensation), trishna (thirst), atisaar (diarrhea), vaman (vomiting), vranashoth (inflamed wounds).

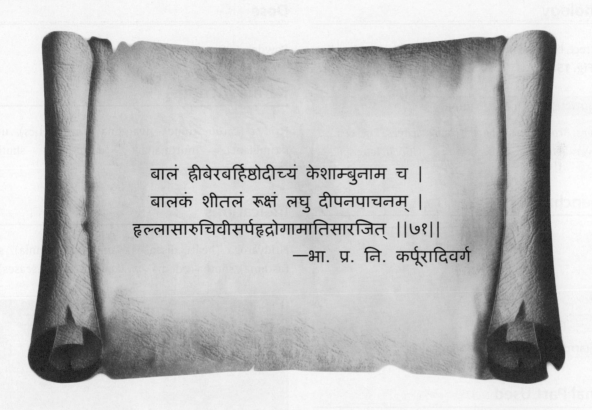

बालं ह्रीबेरबर्हिष्ठोदीच्यं केशाम्बुनाम च ।
बालकं शीतलं रूक्षं लघु दीपनपाचनम् ।
हृल्लासारुचिवीसर्पहृद्रोगामातिसारजित् ।।७१।।
—भा. प्र. नि. कर्पूरादिवर्ग

151. Hrutpatri *[Digitalis purpurea Linn.]*

Family:	*Scrophulariaceae*
Hindi name:	*Hritpatri*
English name:	*Digitalis, Foxglove*
Synonyms:	*Tilapushpi, Hritapatri*

Morphology

It is an erect, biennial herb with hairy, lance-shaped, radical leaves (**Fig. 150.1**).

Key Characters for Identification
➤ *Leaves: Broad, lance-shaped, radical leaves (**Fig. 150.2**).*   ➤ *Flower: Bell-shaped, purple pink or white in long spikes.*

Rasapanchaka

Guna	Laghu, Ruksha
Rasa	Tikta
Vipaka	Katu
Virya	Sheeta
Doshakarma	Kapha vatashamaka

Officinal Part Used

Patra (leaves)

Dose

Powder: 500 mg

Karma (Actions)

Hridya (cardio tonic), jwarghna (antipyretics), uttejaka (stimulant), mutrajanan (diuretics), shothahara (anti-inflammatory).

Indications

Hridyaroga (heart diseases), anidra (insomnia), shwasa (asthma), shotha (edema), twaka roga (skin diseases).

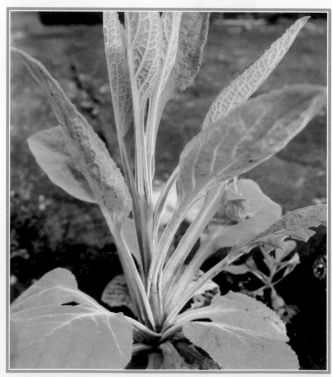

Fig. 150.2 Leaves.

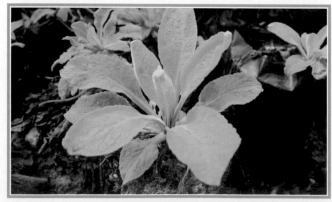

Fig. 150.1 Plant of *Digitalis purpurea* Linn.

152. Ikshu *[Saccharum officinarum Linn.]*

Family: *Graminae*

Hindi name: *Inkh, Ganna*

English name: *Sugarcane*

Synonyms: *Dirghachchhada, Bhurirasa, Gudhamoola, Asipatra, Madhutruna*

Morphology

This perennial plant grows in clumps consisting of a number of strong unbranched stems (**Fig. 152.1**).

Key Characters for Identification

➤ *Stems: The stems vary in color, being green, pinkish, or purple, and can reach 5 m in height and 20 to 45 mm in diameter. They are jointed, with nodes being present at the bases of the alternate leaves. The internodes contain fibrous white pith immersed in sugary sap* (**Fig. 152.2**).

➤ *Leaves: Leaves are arching and linear or lanceolate, about 70 to 150 cm long, 3 to 6 cm wide. Leaves are large with conspicuous midrib and sharply toothed leaf margin. Leaf sheath is loose, mostly glabrous while being slightly hairy at the mouth. Ligule possesses small hair too.*

➤ *Flowers: Flowers are plumelike and usually whitish gray. Panicle is large (50–100 cm long), often hairless but pilose at nodes.*

➤ *Fruits: Seed is oblong and small (about 1.5 mm long).*

Rasapanchaka

Guna	Guru, Snigdha
Rasa	Madhur
Vipaka	Madhur
Virya	Sheeta
Doshakarma	Pittaghna, Kaphavardhak

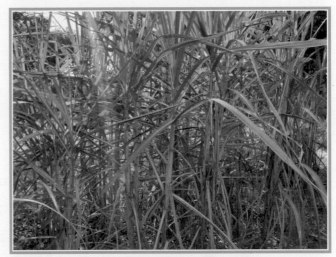

Fig. 152.1 Plant of *Saccharum officinarum* Linn.

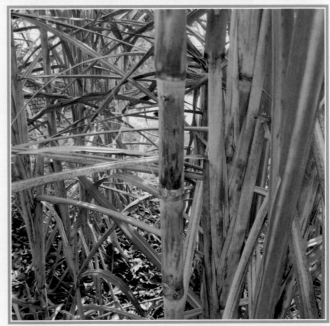

Fig. 152.2 Stem.

Officinal Part Used

Root

Dose

Juice: 200 to 400 mL

Karma (Actions)

Balya (provide physical strength), vrisya (aphrodisiac), shukrashodhak (purify semen), mutral (diuretics), sara (carminatives), kanthya (beneficial for throats), shramahara (antifatigue).

Indications

It cures raktapitta (bleeding disorders), gulma (abdominal lumps), udara (abdominal diseases), kamala (jaundice), pandu (anemia), mutra kshaya (scanty urination).

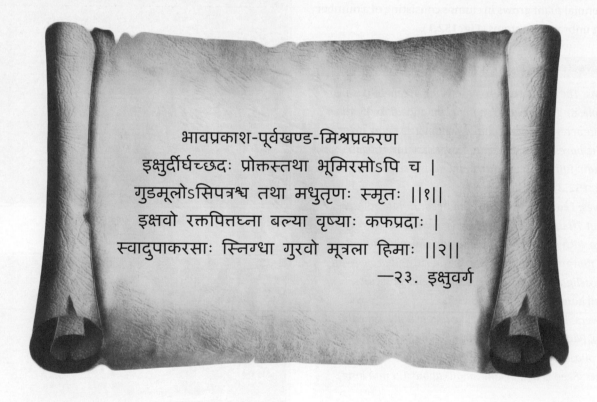

भावप्रकाश-पूर्वखण्ड-मिश्रप्रकरण

इक्षुर्दीर्घच्छदः प्रोक्तस्तथा भूमिरसोऽपि च ।
गुडमूलोऽसिपत्रश्च तथा मधुतृणः स्मृतः ।।१।।
इक्षवो रक्तपित्तघ्ना बल्या वृष्याः कफप्रदाः ।
स्वादुपाकरसाः स्निग्धा गुरवो मूत्रला हिमाः ।।२।।

—२३. इक्षुवर्ग

153. Indravaruni *[Citrullus colocynthis* (Linn.) Schrad.]

Family:	*Cucurbitaceae*
Hindi name:	*Indrayan, Katu Indrayan*
English name:	*Colocynth, Bitter Apple*
Synonyms:	*Indravaruni, Indravalli, Indravarunikaa, Gavakshi, Chitra, Indraasuri, Mrigakshi, Mrigairvaaru, Vishala, Vishalyka, Gavadani, Mahaphala*

Morphology

It is a spreading creeper with a yellow-colored flower (**Fig. 153.1**).

Key Characters for Identification

➤ *Leaves: Ovate or narrowly triangular, coardate at the base, deeply divided*
➤ *Flowers: Yellow in color (***Fig. 153.2***)*
➤ *Fruits: Round, shaped like the eye ball of cow with white or dark green colors (***Fig. 153.3***)*
➤ *Seeds: Not marginal*

Rasapanchaka

Guna	Laghu, Ruksha
Rasa	Katu, Tikta
Vipaka	Katu
Virya	Ushna
Doshakarma	Kaphapittahara

Officinal Parts Used

Fruit and root

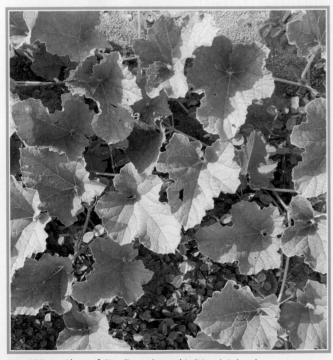

Fig. 153.1 Plant of *Citrullus colocynthis* (Linn.) Schrad.

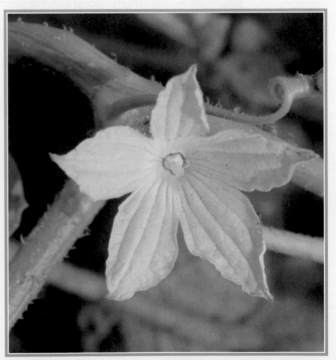

Fig. 153.2 Flower.

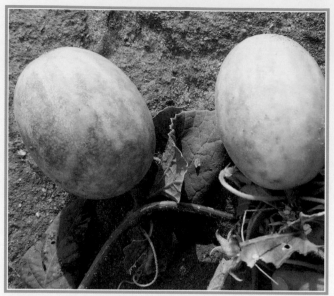

Fig. 153.3 Fruit.

Dose

Dried fruit powder: 125 to 500 mg
Root powder: 1 to 3 g

Karma (Actions)

Rechana (purgative), garbhapatana (abortifacient).

Indications

Kamala (jaundice), plihodara (splenomegaly), krimi (worm infestation), kushta (skin disease), prameha (diabetes), shwasa (asthma), kasa (cough), gulma (abdominal lump), granthi (cyst), vrana (wound), mudhagarbha, gandamala (goiter), visha (poisoning).

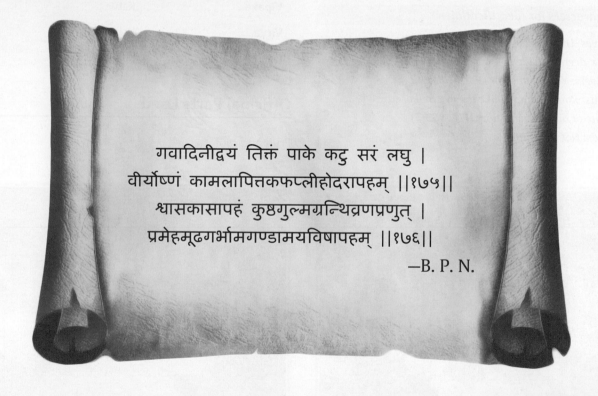

गवादिनीद्वयं तिक्तं पाके कटु सरं लघु ।
वीर्योष्णं कामलापित्तकफप्लीहोदरापहम् ॥१७५॥
श्वासकासापहं कुष्ठगुल्मग्रन्थिव्रणप्रणुत् ।
प्रमेहमूढगर्भामगण्डामयविषापहम् ॥१७६॥

—B. P. N.

154. Ingudi [Balanites aegyptiaca (Linn.) Delile]

Family:	Balanitaceae (Simarobaceae)
Hindi name:	Hingarnber, Hingota
English name:	Desert date, soap berry tree or bush, thorn tree, Egyptian myrobalan, Egyptian balsam, and Zachum oil tree
Synonyms:	Tiktaka, Tapasadruma, Angaravriksha

Morphology

It is a small tree/bush plant with strong, very sharp spines, and greenish-white flowers.

Key Characters for Identification

➤ *Leaves: Ovate, puberulous, entire, coriaceous leaflets.*
➤ *Flowers: Flowers are in close cymes, small, white or greenish-white in color, with fragrance.*
➤ *Fruits: Fruits are ovoid-oblong drupe, hard, olive green in color when young and yellow when mature* (**Fig. 154.1** *and* **Fig. 154.2**).
➤ *Seed: Single-seeded.*

Rasapanchaka

Guna	Laghu, Snigdha
Rasa	Katu, Tikta
Vipaka	Katu
Virya	Ushna
Doshakarma	Kaphavata shamak

Officinal Parts Used

Bark, fruit, seed, leaves

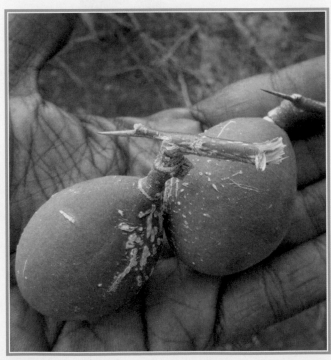

Fig. 154.1 Young fruit.

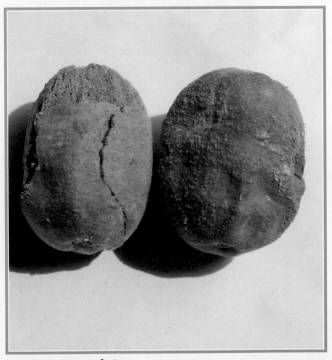

Fig. 154.2 Mature fruit.

Dose

Decoction: 50 to 100 mL
Fruit pulp: 3 to 6 g
Seed powder: 3 to 6 g

Karma (Actions)

Rasayana (rejuvenation), vishaghna (antidote), krimighna (anthelmintic), vrana ropan (wound healing).

Indications

Kushta (skin disease), krimi (worm infestation), visha (poisoning), vataroga (disease of vata), vrana (wound), svitra (leukoderma), shola (colic pain).

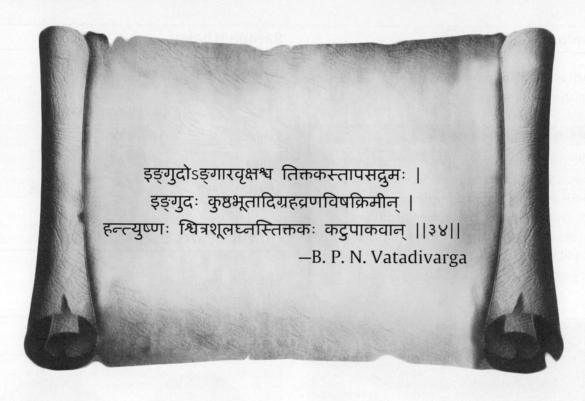

इङ्गुदोऽइङ्गारवृक्षश्च तिक्तकस्तापसद्रुमः |
इङ्गुदः कुष्ठभूतादिग्रहव्रणविषक्रिमीन् |
हन्त्युष्णः श्वित्रशूलघ्नस्तिक्तकः कटुपाकवान् ||३४||

—B. P. N. Vatadivarga

155. Irimeda *[Acacia farnesiana (L.) Willd.]*

Family:	*Mimosaceae*
Hindi name:	*Gandha babool, Gandha khair, Gandha kikar*
English name:	*Cassie flower, Cassie Absolute, Sweet Acacia*
Synonyms:	*Vit khadira, Kalaskandha, Arimedaka*

Morphology

It is a small tree or large shrub with 2.5 m height (**Fig. 155.**1).

Key Characters for Identification

➤ *Leaves: Alternate, bipinnate compound, 4 to 6 cm long, petiole with minute gland* (**Fig. 155.2**).
➤ *Flowers: Bright yellow, globose, calyx about 0.2 cm long, corolla 0.3 cm long.*
➤ *Fruits: Slightly curved, cylindrical, swollen, dark brown pods* (**Fig. 155.3**).
➤ *Seeds: Seeds are in two rows, embedded in white pulp, globose.*

Rasapanchaka

Guna	Laghu, Ruksha
Rasa	Tikta, Kashaya
Vipaka	Katu
Virya	Ushna
Dosha karma	Kaphavatashamaka

Officinal Part Used

Bark

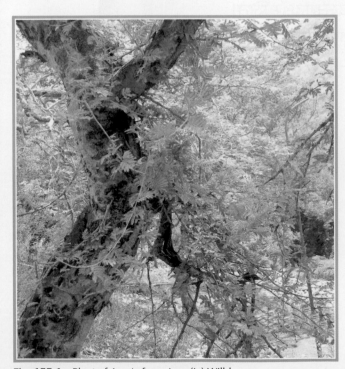

Fig. 155.1　Plant of *Acacia farnesiana* (L.) Willd.

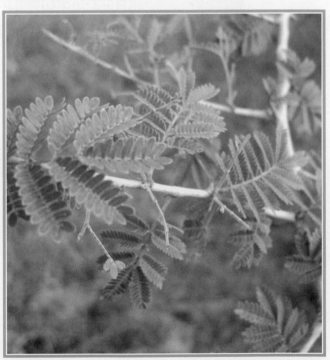

Fig. 155.2　Leaves.

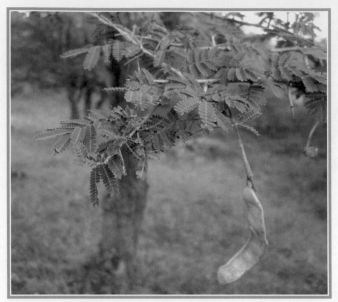

Fig. 155.3 Pod.

Dose

Decoction: 50 to 100 mL
Powder: 1 to 3 g

Karma (Actions)

Pachana (digestive), kushtaghna (antidermatosis), vishaghna (antidotes), kandughna (antipruritics).

Indications

Kandu (pruritis), visha (poison), kapharoga (diseases of aggravated kapha dosha), krimi (worm infestation), kushta (skin diseases), vrana (wounds), mukhadanta roga (diseases of oral cavity and tooth).

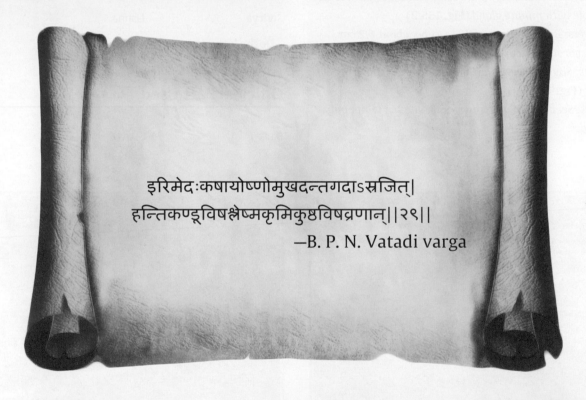

इरिमेदःकषायोष्णोमुखदन्तगदाऽस्रजित्।
हन्तिकण्डूविषश्लेष्मकृमिकुष्ठविषव्रणान्॥२९॥
—B. P. N. Vatadi varga

156. Ikshvaku *[Lagenaria siceraria (Molina) Standley or Lagenaria vulgaris Ser.]*

Family:	*Cucurbitaceae*
Hindi name:	*Kasvi Lauki, Kadva Tumba, Kadva Dudhya*
English name:	*Bitter bottle gourd, bottle gourd*
Synonyms:	*Katutumbi, Mahaphala, Tumbi*

Morphology

It is a tendrillar climber up to 10 m long, and its stem is soft, hairy, and angular (**Fig. 156.1**).

Key Characters for Identification

➤ *Leaves: Alternate, petiolate, broadly ovate-suborbicular, petiole with two glands.*
➤ *Flowers: Monoecious, solitary, axillary, three stamen, anther slightly fused (**Fig. 156.2**).*
➤ *Fruits: Fruits are of various shapes, very long, and club shaped or bottle shaped (**Fig. 156.3a, b**).*

Rasapanchaka

Guna	Laghu, Ruksha
Rasa	Tikta
Vipaka	Katu
Virya	Sheeta
Doshakarma	Pittahara

Officinal Parts Used

Fruit, leaf, root, seed

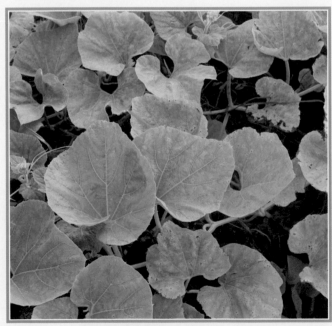

Fig. 156.1   Climber of *Lagenaria siceraria* (Molina) Standley.

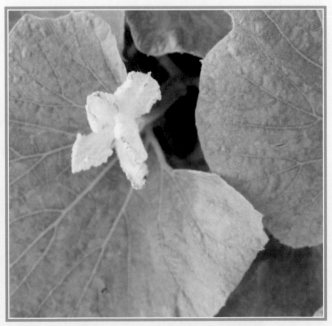

Fig. 156.2   Flower.

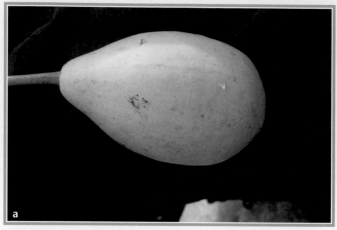
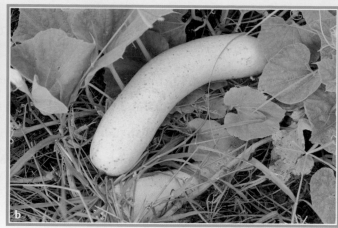

Fig. 156.3 **(a)** Club-shaped fruit. **(b)** Bottle-shaped fruit.

Dose

Juice: 10 to 20 mL

Karma (Actions)

Vamak (induce vomiting), hridya (cardio tonic), vishaghna (antidote), jwarahara (antipyretics), kasahara (anticough), swashara (antiasthmatic).

Indications

Vatapitta jwara (fever caused due to vatapitta), kasa (cough), vishvikar (poisoning), shwasa (asthma), vrana (wound).

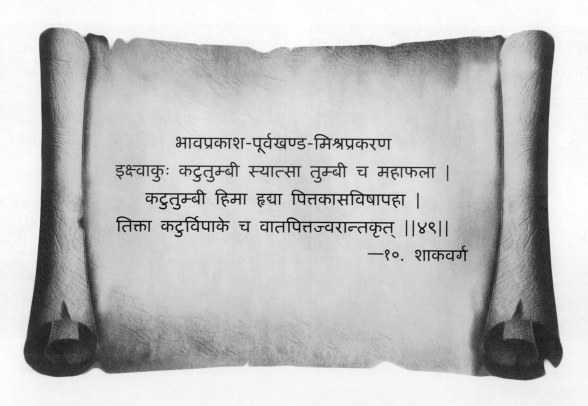

भावप्रकाश-पूर्वखण्ड-मिश्रप्रकरण

इक्ष्वाकुः कटुतुम्बी स्यात्सा तुम्बी च महाफला |

कटुतुम्बी हिमा हृद्या पित्तकासविषापहा |

तिक्ता कटुर्विपाके च वातपित्तज्वरान्तकृत् ||४९||

—१०. शाकवर्ग

157. Ishwari *[Aristolochia indica Linn.]*

Family: *Aristolochiaceae*

Hindi name: *Ishwar mool, Rudrajata*

English name: *The Indian Birth wort*

Synonyms: *Gandhanakuli, Nakuli, Naagadamani, Arkamoola*

Morphology

It is an aromatic perennial twinner, with herbaceous stem and branches (**Fig. 157.1**).

Key Characters for Identification

➤ *Leaves: Alternate, simple petiolate, variously shaped, three-nerved from base (**Fig. 157.2**).*
➤ *Flowers: Greenish and purplish shade, streaks outside and vinaceous purple inside (**Fig. 157.3**).*
➤ *Fruits: A globose, slightly oblong capsule, hanging like an inverted umbrella (**Fig. 157.4**).*
➤ *Seeds: Numerous, ovate, and somewhat cordate, flat, winged, aromatic, and bitter.*
➤ *Root/Rhizomes: Long and thick.*

Rasapanchaka

Guna	Laghu, Ruksha
Rasa	Tikta, Katu, Kasaya
Vipaka	Katu
Virya	Ushna
Doshakarma	Kaphavatahara

Officinal Parts Used

Root and leaf

Dose

Powder (root): 1 to 3 g
Leaf juice: 5 to 10 mL

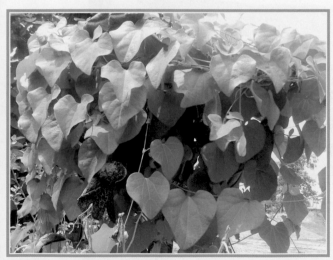

Fig. 157.1 Climber of *Aristolochia indica* Linn.

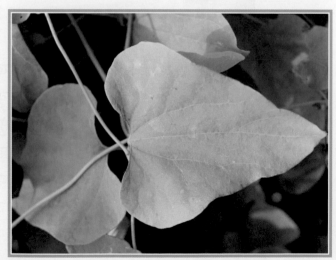

Fig. 157.2 Leaves.

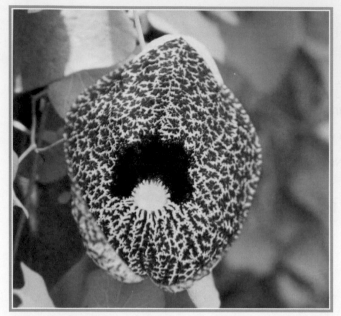

Fig. 157.3 Flower.

Karma (Actions)

Vishaghna (antidote), krimighna (anthelmintic), jwaraghna (antipyretics).

Indications

Sarpavisha (snake poisoning), jwara (fever), akshuvisha (rat poisoning), krimi (worm infestation), vrana (wound), amavata (rheumatoid arthritis), scorpion bite.

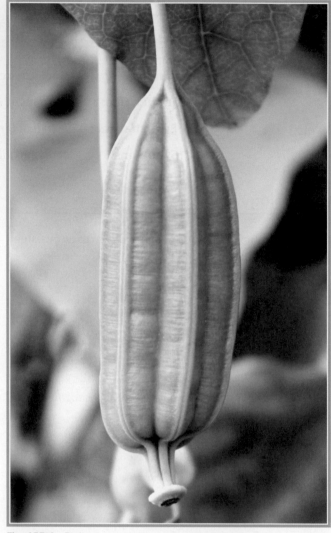

Fig. 157.4 Fruit.

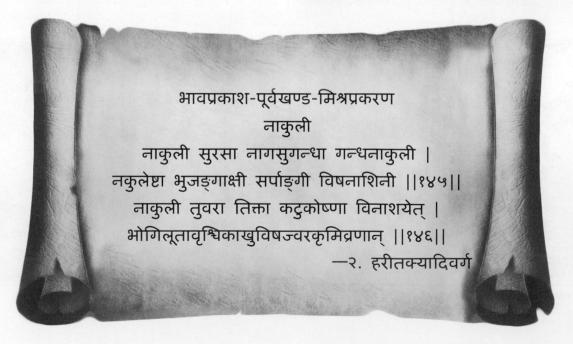

भावप्रकाश-पूर्वखण्ड-मिश्रप्रकरण

नाकुली

नाकुली सुरसा नागसुगन्धा गन्धनाकुली ।

नकुलेष्टा भुजङ्गाक्षी सर्पाङ्गी विषनाशिनी ॥१४५॥

नाकुली तुवरा तिक्ता कटुकोष्णा विनाशयेत् ।

भोगिलूतावृश्चिकाखुविषज्वरकृमिव्रणान् ॥१४६॥

—२. हरीतक्यादिवर्ग

158. Japa [*Hibiscus rosa-sinensis* Linn.]

Family:	*Malvaceae*
Hindi name:	*Japa*
English name:	*Rose-of-China, Shoe flower, Chinese Hibiscus*
Synonyms:	*Japaa, Javaa, Odrapushpa, Rudrapushpa*

Morphology

It is a shrub or small tree, 2 to 4 m high generally, with profuse branches (**Fig. 158.1**).

Key Characters for Identification

➤ *Leaves: Simple, alternate, glabrous, petiolate, lamina ovate with dentate margin (**Fig. 158.2**).*
➤ *Flowers: Axillary, solitary, with a log pedicle, five clawed, crimson colored (**Fig. 158.3a, b**).*
➤ *Fruits: Fruit setting is rare.*

Rasapanchaka

Guna	Laghu, Ruksha
Rasa	Kasaya, Tikta
Vipaka	Katu
Virya	Ushna
Doshakarma	Kaphavatahara

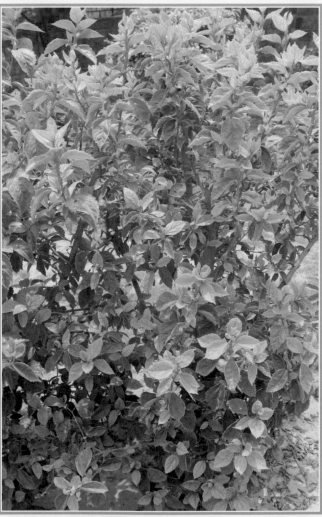

Fig. 158.1 Plant of *Hibiscus rosa-sinensis* Linn.

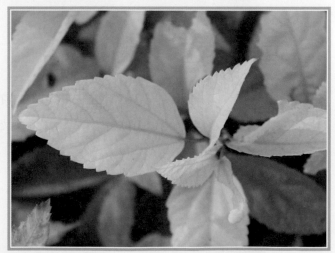

Fig. 158.2 Leaves.

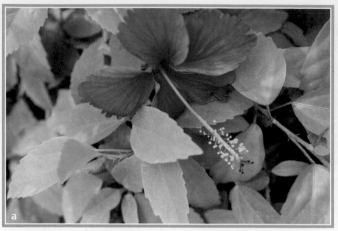 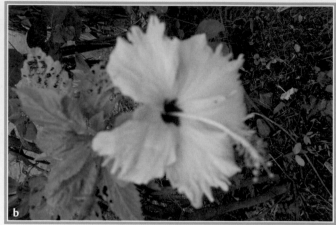

Fig. 158.3 **(a)** Red-colored flower. **(b)** Creamish-colored flower.

Officinal Part Used

Flower

Dose

Powder: 5 to 10 g

Karma (Actions)

Stambhana (astringent/inhibitory process/obstructive process), garbhanirodhaka (prevent conception), keshya (hair tonic), hridya (cardiotonic).

Indications

Raktatisara (hemorrhagic diarrhea), arshas (hemorrhoids), hridroga (heart disease), raktapradara (metrorrhagia), indralupta (alopecia), daha (burning sensation).

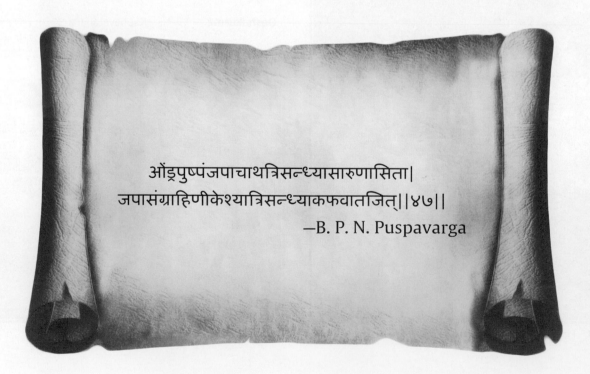

ओंड्रपुष्पंजपाचाथत्रिसन्ध्यासारुणासिता।
जपासंग्राहिणीकेश्यात्रिसन्ध्याकफवातजित्।।४७।।

—B. P. N. Puspavarga

159. Jati *[Jasminum grandiflorum Linn. or Jasminum officinale Linn.]*

Family:	*Oleaceae*
Hindi name:	*Chameli*
English name:	*Spanish Jasmine, Italian Jasmine*
Synonyms:	*Malati, Chetika, Sumana*

Morphology

It is a straggling and climbing shrub with white color, scented flower (**Fig. 159.1**).

Key Characters for Identification

➤ *Leaves: Opposite, imparipinnate, paired leaflets, glabrous subsessile, ovate (**Fig. 159.2**).*
➤ *Flowers: Flowers are sweet-scented and yellow in color (**Fig. 159.3**).*
➤ *Fruit: A two-lobed glabrous, smooth, shining, and black berry.*
➤ *Seed: One seeded.*

Rasapanchaka

Guna	Laghu
Rasa	Tikta, Kasaya
Vipaka	Katu
Virya	Ushna
Doshakarma	Tridoshahara

Officinal Parts Used

Leaf, root, flower

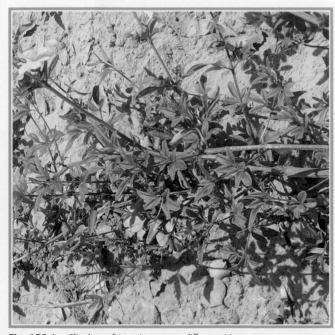

Fig. 159.1 Climber of *Jasminum grandiflorum* Linn.

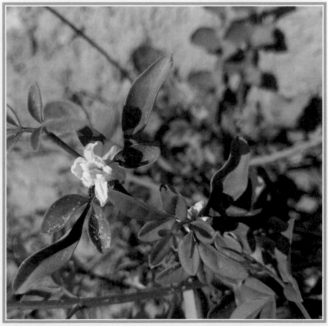

Fig. 159.2 Leaves.

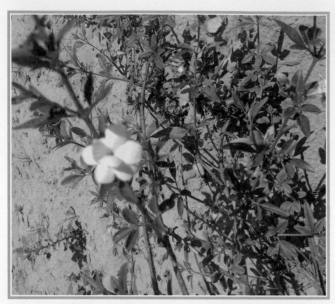

Fig. 159.3 Flower.

Dose

Powder: 1 to 3 g
Decoction: 159 to 100 mL

Karma (Actions)

Ropana (wound healing), vishahara (antidote), vranashodhana (wound cleansing).

Indications

Siroroga (diseases of head), netraroga (eye diseases), mukharoga (mouth diseases), dantashoola (dental pain), kushta (skin disease), visha (poisoning), vrana (wound), vatarakta (gout).

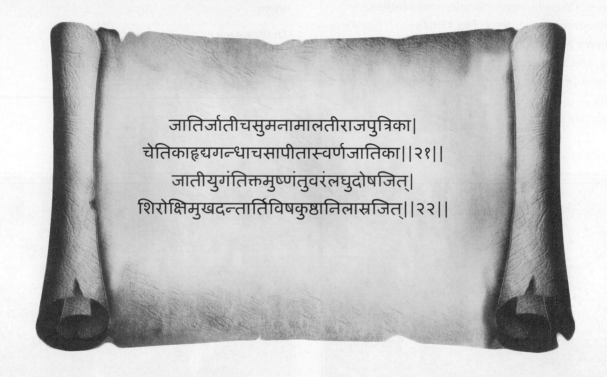

जातिर्जातीचसुमनामालतीराजपुत्रिका|
चेतिकाह्वयगन्धाचसापीतास्वर्णजातिका||२१||
जातीयुगंतिक्तमुष्णंतुवरंलघुदोषजित्|
शिरोक्षिमुखदन्तार्तिविषकुष्ठानिलास्रजित्||२२||

160. Jivanti [*Leptadenia reticulata* (Retz.) Wt.et.Arn*]

Family:	*Asclepiadaceae*
Hindi name:	*Dodisag*
English name:	*Leptadenia*
Synonyms:	*Jivani, Jiva, Payansvini, Shakashresta, Jeevaniya, Madhusrava*

Morphology

It is a perennial, straggling, and climbing shrub, 5 to 10 m or more long, with profuse branches (**Fig. 160.1**).

Key Characters for Identification

➤ *Leaves: Simple, opposite, grayish green; lamina ovate, apex acute (**Fig. 160.2**).*
➤ *Flowers: Greenish yellow, inflorescence of lateral-subaxillary, short paniculate.*
➤ *Fruits: A pair of cylindrical follicles, with each tapering to an obtuse beak (**Fig. 160.3**).*
➤ *Seeds: Seeds are many, narrowly ovate-oblong, and acute with a tuft long white coma.*

Rasapanchaka

Guna	Laghu, Ruksha
Rasa	Madhura
Vipaka	Madhura
Virya	Sheeta
Doshakarma	Tridoshahara

Officinal Parts Used

Root and leaf

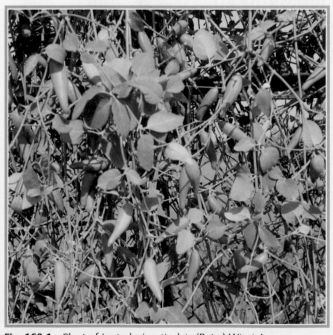

Fig. 160.1   Plant of *Leptadenia reticulata* (Retz.) Wt.et.Arn

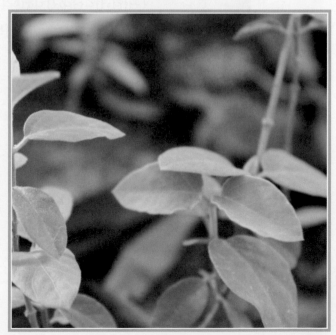

Fig. 160.2   Leaves.

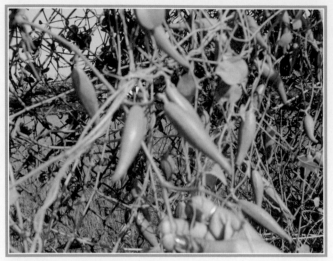

Fig. 160.3 Fruit.

Dose

Decoction: 50 to 100 mL
Powder: 3 to 6 g

Karma (Actions)

Grahi (astringent), balya (strength promoter), rasayana (rejuvenation), chakshusya (beneficial for eyes).

Indications

Grahani (sprue), atisara (diarrhea), pandu (anemia), raktapitta (bleeding disorders).

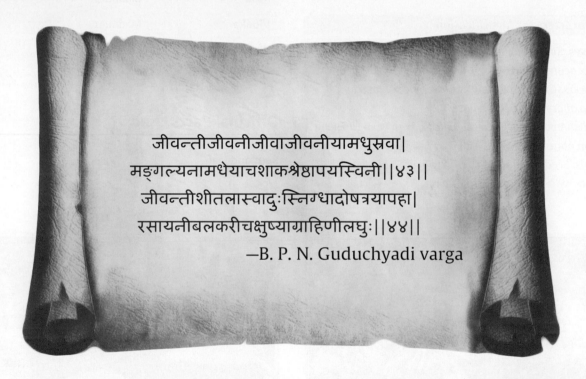

जीवन्तीजीवनीजीवाजीवनीयामधुस्रवा।
मङ्गल्यनामधेयाचशाकश्रेष्ठापयस्विनी।।४३।।
जीवन्तीशीतलास्वादुःस्निग्धादोषत्रयापहा।
रसायनीबलकरीचक्षुष्याग्राहिणीलघुः।।४४।।
—B. P. N. Guduchyadi varga

161. Kadali *[Musa paradisiaca Linn.]*

Family:	*Musacaceae*
Hindi name:	*Kela*
English name:	*Banana, Plantain Tree*
Synonyms:	*Varana, Mocha, Ambusara, Amshumatiphala*

Morphology

It is a tree-like plant, 2 to 6 m tall, aerial parts annual (**Fig. 161.1**).

Key Characters for Identification

➤ *Leaves: Oblong green, up to 3 m long and 65 cm broad* (**Fig. 161.2**).
➤ *Flowers: Unisexual, 3 to 4.5 cm long, in two rows under each bract* (**Fig. 161.3**).
➤ *Fruits: Oblong, hard and green when young, yellow or greenish-yellow and fleshy when fully ripe* (**Fig. 161.4**).
➤ *Root/Rhizomes: Large perennial, stoloniferous, cylindric trunk.*

Rasapanchaka

Guna	Guru, Snigdha
Rasa	Madhura
Vipaka	Madhura
Virya	Sheeta
Doshakarma	Pitta Vatahara

Officinal Parts Used

Fruit, flower, tuber

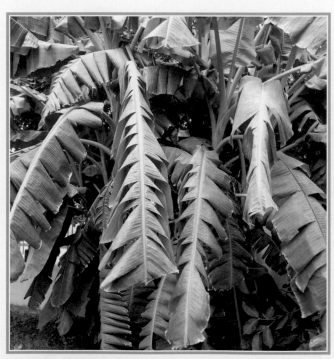

Fig. 161.1 Plant of *Musa paradisiaca* Linn.

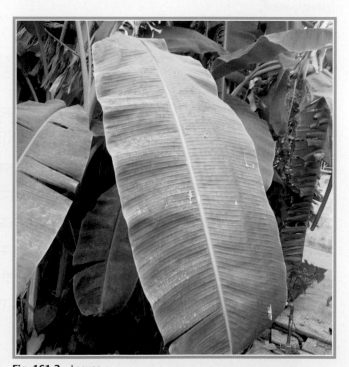

Fig. 161.2 Leaves.

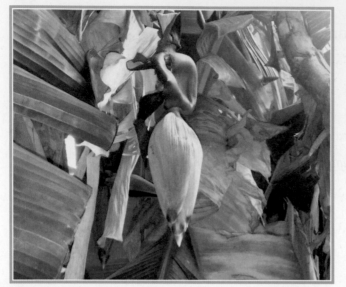

Fig. 161.3 Flower.

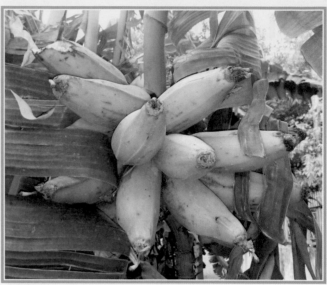

Fig. 160.4 Fruits.

Dose

Powder: 1 to 2 g
Juice: 10 to 20 mL

Karma (Actions)

Vrishya (aphrodisiac), brimhana (bulk promoting), kaphakarak (aggravate kaphadosha), visthambhi (constipative).

Indications

Trishana (thirst), daha (burning sensation), raktapitta (bleeding disorders), prameha (diabetes), netraroga (eye diseases), amlapitta (hyper acidity), kshaya (decay), kshata (cachexia due to chest injury).

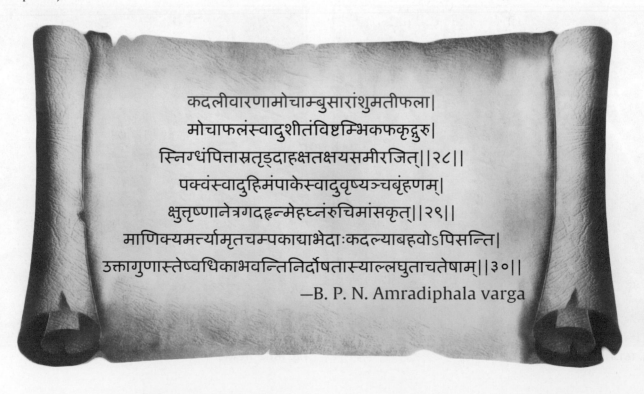

कदलीवारणामोचाम्बुसारांशुमतीफला।
मोचाफलंस्वादुशीतंविष्टम्भिकफकृद्गुरु।
स्निग्धंपित्तासतृड्दाहक्षतक्षयसमीरजित्॥२८॥
पक्वंस्वादुहिमंपाकेस्वादुवृष्यञ्चबृंहणम्।
क्षुत्तृष्णानेत्रगदहृन्मेहघ्नंरुचिमांसकृत्॥२९॥
माणिक्यमर्त्यामृतचम्पकाद्याभेदाःकदल्याबहवोऽपिसन्ति।
उक्तागुणास्तेष्वधिकाभवन्तिनिर्दोषतास्याल्लघुताचतेषाम्॥३०॥

—B. P. N. Amradiphala varga

162. Kadamba *[Anthocephalus cadamba* (Roxb.) Miq]

Family:	*Rubiaceae*
Hindi name:	*Kadamba*
English name:	*Wild anchora, burf lower, Kadam tree*
Synonyms:	*Neepa, Vrittapushpa, Halipriya, Priyako*

Morphology

It is a tree, 10 to 25 m high, straight trunk with smooth dark gray bark, with horizontal branches (**Fig. 162.1**).

Key Characters for Identification

➤ *Leaves: Simple, opposite, lamina entire, glabrous above, hairy beneath* (**Fig. 162.2**).
➤ *Flowers: Orange colored, round, sweet-scented* (**Fig. 162.3**).
➤ *Fruits: Numerous, forming a globose, fleshy mass, orange yellow when ripe* (**Fig. 162.4**).
➤ *Seed: Seeds are minute.*

Rasapanchaka

Guna	Guru, Ruksha
Rasa	Tikta, Kashaya
Vipaka	Katu
Virya	Sheeta
Doshakarma	Tridoshahara

Officinal Parts Used

Bark and fruit

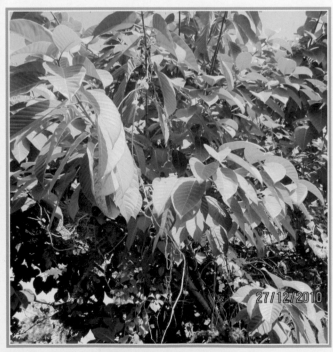

Fig. 162.1 Tree of *Anthocephalus cadamba* (Roxb.) Miq.

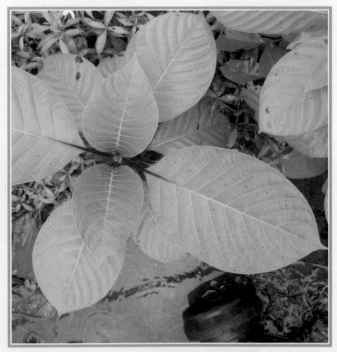

Fig. 162.2 Leaves.

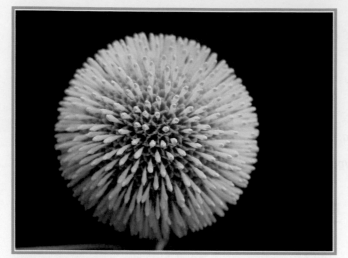

Fig. 162.3 Flower.

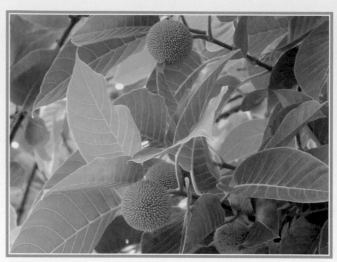

Fig. 162.4 Fruits.

Dose

Powder: 3 to 6 g
Juice: 10 to 20 mL

Karma (Actions)

Vedanasthapana (analgesic), shukra-shodana (semen purification), sara (flowing in nature/carminative), stanyajanak (galactopoietic), shukral (spermatogenic).

Indications

Daha (burning sensation), kasa (cough), visha (poisoning), shopha (edema), vrana (wound).

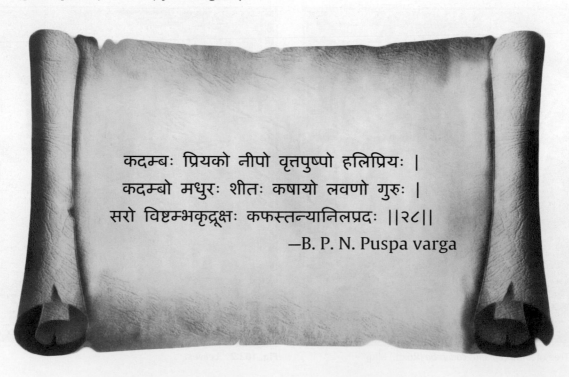

कदम्बः प्रियको नीपो वृत्तपुष्पो हलिप्रियः |
कदम्बो मधुरः शीतः कषायो लवणो गुरुः |
सरो विष्टम्भकृद्रूक्षः कफस्तन्यानिलप्रदः ||२८||
—B. P. N. Puspa varga

163. Kaidarya [*Murraya koiengii* (Linn.) Spreng]

Family:	*Rutaceae*
Hindi name:	*Kadipatta, Meethanimb*
English name:	*Curry leaf*
Synonyms:	*Kaitarya, Surabhinimb*

Morphology

It is a spreading shrub or a small tree, reaching up to 6 m in height with white color flower (**Fig. 163.1**).

Key Characters for Identification

➤ *Leaves: Aromatic, alternate, imparipinnately compound (**Fig. 163.1**).*
➤ *Flowers: White, five oblong petals, ten stamens; ovary two-celled each with ovule (**Fig. 163.2**).*
➤ *Fruits: Sub-globose, green when young and black through vinaceous purple when ripe (**Fig. 163.3**).*
➤ *Seed: One to two seeded.*

Rasapanchaka

Guna	Laghu, Ruksha
Rasa	Kashaya, Tikta
Vipaka	Katu
Virya	Ushna
Doshakarma	Vatahara

Officinal Part Used

Leaves

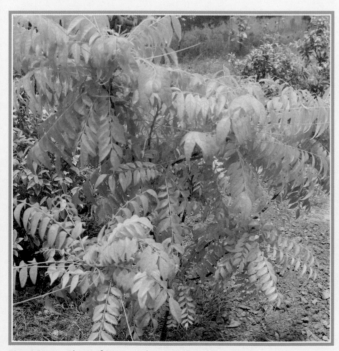

Fig. 163.1 Plant of *Murraya koiengii* (Linn.) Spreng.

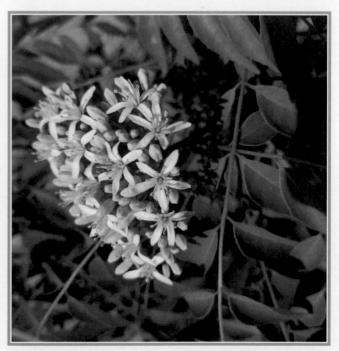

Fig. 163.2 Flowers.

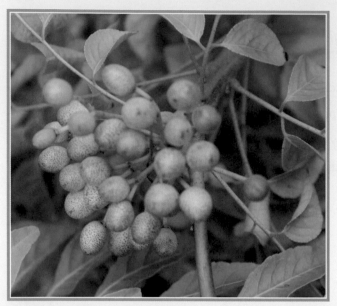

Fig. 163.3 Fruits.

Dose

Fresh leaves juice: 10 to 20 mL
Decoction: 50 to 100 mL

Karma (Actions)

Deepan (appetizer), pachan (digestive), rochan (taste enhancer), vatahara (pacify vatadosha).

Indications

Agnimandya (low digestion/loss of appetite), ajirna (dyspepsia), pravahika (dysentery), atisara (diarrhea), chhardi (vomiting), prameha (diabetes), sadyovrana (traumatic wound), burns, graying of hair.

164. Kakamachi *[Solanum nigrum Linn.]*

Family:	*Solanaceae*
Hindi name:	*Makoye*
English name:	*Black nightshade*
Synonyms:	*Kakahwa, Vayasi, Dwankshamachi*

Morphology

It is an erect, annual–biennial herb, 0.35 to 1.25 m high, profusely divaricately branched (**Fig. 164.1**).

Key Characters for Identification

➤ *Leaves: Simple, alternate, thin, ovate, margin entire, unequal sided, dentate (**Fig. 164.2**).*
➤ *Flowers: White flowers on drooping pedicles, with three to eight-flowered cymes (**Fig. 164.3**).*
➤ *Fruits: A globose berry, which is green when young and almost black when mature (**Fig. 164.4**).*
➤ *Seeds: Seeds are many, discoid, about 0.15 cm in diameter, and minutely pitted.*

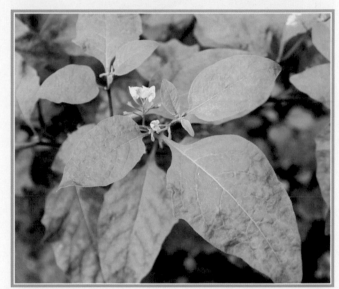

Fig. 164.2 Leaves.

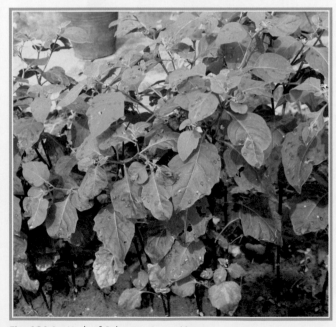

Fig. 164.1 Herb of *Solanum nigrum* Linn.

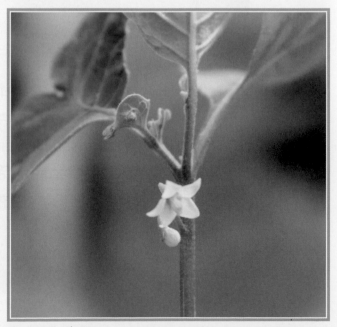

Fig. 164.3 Flower.

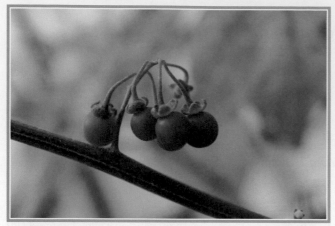

Fig. 164.4 Fruits.

Rasapanchaka

Guna	Laghu, Snigdha
Rasa	Tikta
Vipaka	Katu
Virya	Ushna
Doshakarma	Tridoshahara

Officinal Parts Used

Fruit and whole plant

Dose

Powder: 1 to 3 g (fruit)
Juice: 10 to 20 mL

Karma (Actions)

Bhedana (purgative), vrishya (aphrodisiac), swarya (beneficial for voice), rasayana (rejuvenative), shukrada (spermatogenetic), chakshusya (beneficial for vision).

Indications

Shotha (edema), kushta (skin diseases), urustambha (stiffness of thigh), arsha (piles), prameha (diabetes), hikka (hic-cough), chhardi (vomiting), jwara (fever), hridroga (heart disease).

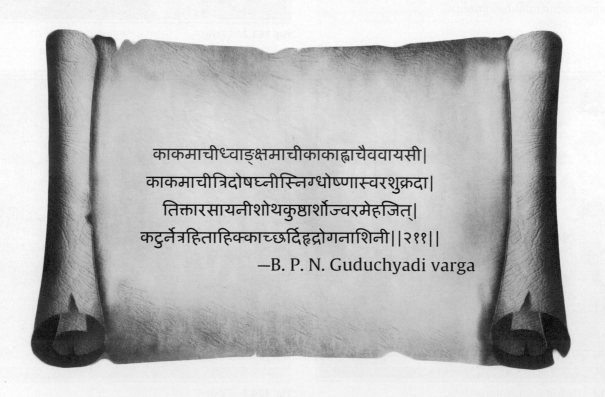

काकमाचीध्वाङ्क्षमाचीकाकाह्वाचैववायसी।
काकमाचीत्रिदोषघ्नीस्निग्धोष्णास्वरशुक्रदा।
तिक्तारसायनीशोथकुष्टार्शोज्वरमेहजित्।
कटुर्नेत्रहिताहिक्काच्छर्दिहृद्रोगनाशिनी।।२११।।
—B. P. N. Guduchyadi varga

165. Kamal [*Nelumbo nucifera* Gaertn.*]

Family:	*Nelumbonaceae*
Hindi name:	*Kamal*
English name:	*Sacred Lotus, Indian Lotus*
Synonyms:	*Padma, Aravinda, Rajeev, Pushkara, Shatapatra, Nalinda, Pankeruha*

Morphology

It is an aquatic herb with rose-colored or white-colored flower (**Fig. 165.1**).

Key Characters for Identification

➤ *Leaves: Float above water, are orbicular, entire, and radially nerved, and the petiole is cylindrical.*
➤ *Flowers: Solitary, rose colored or pure white, and dry and fall off early (**Fig. 165.2a, b**).*
➤ *Fruits: A nutlike carpel sunk in the torus, ellipsoid, and smooth with hard coat (**Fig. 165.3**).*
➤ *Root/Rhizomes: Root stock is tuberous, with irregular shape and round raised tubercle (**Fig. 165.4**).*

Rasapanchaka

Guna	Laghu, Snigdha
Rasa	Tikta, Madhura, Kashaya
Vipaka	Madhura
Virya	Sheeta
Doshakarma	Kapha Pittahara

Officinal Parts Used

Flower, seed, root

Dose

Powder: 3 to 6 g
Root juice: 10 to 20 mL

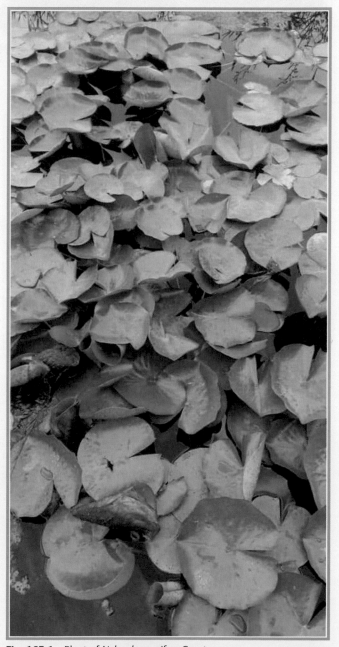

Fig. 165.1 Plant of *Nelumbo nucifera* Gaertn.

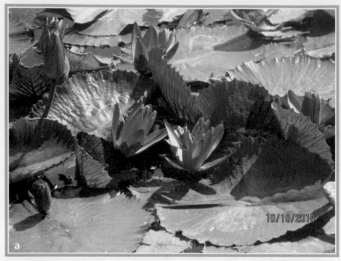

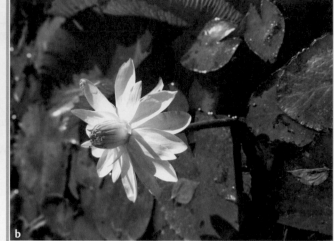

Fig. 165.2 **(a)** Red flower. **(b)** White flower.

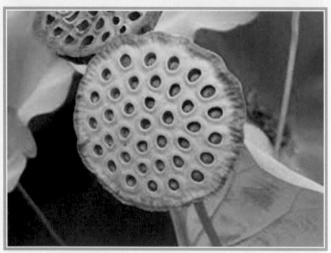

Fig. 165.3 Fruit.

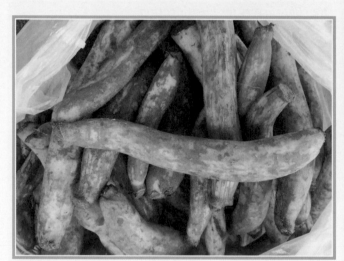

Fig. 165.4 Root.

Karma (Actions)

Varnya (complexion promoter), vrishya (aphrodisiac), grahi (digestive and fecal astringent), mutra-virajaneeya (urine color restoring).

Indications

Daha (burning sensation), trishna (thirst), arshas (piles), raktapitta (bleeding disorders), visarpa (erysipelas), mutrakricchra (dysuria).

वापुंसिपद्मंनलिनमरविन्दंमहोत्पलम्।
सहस्रपत्रंकमलंशतपत्रंकुशेशयम्।।१।।
पङ्केरुहंतामरसंसारसंसरसीरुहम्।
बिसप्रसूनराजीवपुष्कराम्भोरुहाणिच।।२।।
विशेषतःसितंपद्मंपुण्डरीकमितिस्मृतम्।
रक्तंकोकनदंज्ञेयंनीलमिन्दीवरंस्मृतम्।।३।।
कमलंशीतलंवर्ण्यमधुरंकफपित्तजित्।
तृष्णादाहास्रविस्फोटविषवीसर्पनाशनम्।।४।।
धवलंकमलंशीतंमधुरंकफपित्तजित्।
तस्मादल्पगुणंकिञ्चिदन्यद्रक्तोत्पलादिकम्।।५।।
मूलनालदलोत्फुल्लफलैःसमुदितापुनः।
पद्मिनीप्रोच्यतेप्राज्ञैर्बिसिन्यादिचसास्मृता।।६।।
पद्मिनीशीतलागुर्वीमधुरालवणाचसा।
पित्तासृक्कफनुद्रूक्षावातविष्टम्भकारिणी।।७।।
संवर्तिकानवदलंबीजकोशस्तुकर्णिका।
किञ्जल्कःकेसरःप्रोक्तोमकरन्दोरसःस्मृतः।
पद्मनालंमृणालंस्यात्तथाबिसमितिस्मृतम्।।८।।
संवर्तिकाहिमातिक्ताकषायादाहतृट्प्रणुत्।
मूत्रकृच्छ्रगुदव्याधिरक्तपित्तविनाशिनी।।९।।
पद्मस्यकर्णिकातिक्ताकषायामधुराहिमा।
मुखवैशद्यकृल्लघ्वीतृष्णाऽस्रकफपित्तनुत्।।१०।।
किञ्जल्कःशीतलोवृष्यःकषायोग्राहकोऽपिसः।
कफपित्ततृषादाहरक्तार्शोविषशोथजित्।।११।।
मृणालंशीतलंवृष्यंपित्तदाहास्रजिद्गुरु।
दुर्जरंस्वादुपाकञ्चस्तन्यानिलकफप्रदम्।
संग्राहिमधुरंरूक्षंशालूकमपितद्गुणम्।।१२।।
स्थलकमल-
पद्मचारिण्यतिचराऽव्यथापद्माचशारदा।
पद्मानुष्णाकटुस्तिक्ताकषायाकफवातजित्।
मूत्रकृच्छ्राश्मशूलघ्नीश्वासकासविषापहा।।१३।।

— B. P. N. Puspa varga

166. Kankola *[Piper cubeba* Linn. f.]

Family:	*Piperaceae*
Hindi name:	*Kabab chini, Sheetal chini*
English name:	*Cubebs, Tailed pepper*
Synonyms:	*Koshaphala, Kolaka, Gondha Maricha*

Morphology

It is a large perennial climber (**Fig. 166.1**).

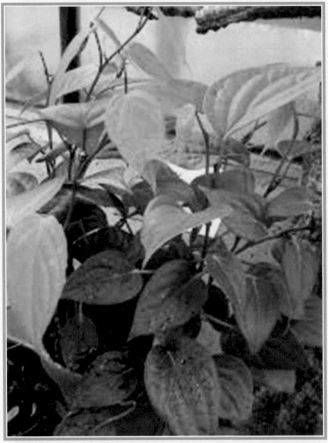

Fig. 166.1 Climber of *Piper cubeba* Linn. f.

Key Characters for Identification

➤ *Leaves: Simple, glabrous, ovate-oblong with cordate base, petiolate.*
➤ *Flowers: Flowers are unisexual, dioecious, minute, and densely arranged on peduncle.*
➤ *Fruits: A globose drupe, 6 to 8 mm in diameter with a stalk of 5 to 10 mm* (**Fig. 166.2**).
➤ *Seed: Fruits are collected and dried to obtain seeds, and seeds are spicy, aromatic, slight bitter, and acrid.*

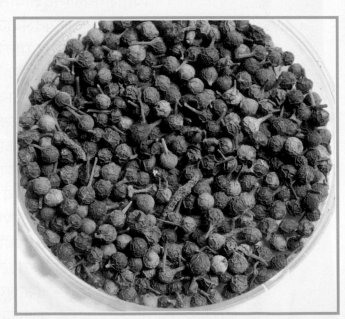

Fig. 166.2 Fruits.

Rasapanchaka

Guna	Laghu, Tikshna
Rasa	Tikta
Vipaka	Katu
Virya	Ushna
Doshakarma	Kaphavatashamaka

Officinal Part Used

Fruit

Dose

Powder: 1 to 3 g
Oil: 1 to 3 drops

Karma (Actions)

Dipana (appetizer), pachan (digestive), ruchya (taste enhancer), vrishya (aphrodisiac), hridya (cardiotonic).

Indications

Aruchi (loss of appetite), aasyadaurgandhya (foul smell in mouth), kaphavataroga (diseases of kapha and vata), kasa (cough), shwasa (asthma), trishna (thirst), hridroga (heart disease), andhatwa (blindness).

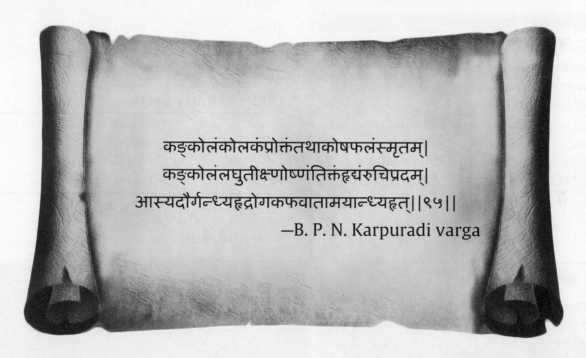

कङ्कोलंकोलकंप्रोक्तंतथाकोषफलंस्मृतम्।
कङ्कोलंलघुतीक्ष्णोष्णंतिक्तंहृद्यंरुचिप्रदम्।
आस्यदौर्गन्ध्यहृद्रोगकफवातामयान्ध्यहृत्।।९५।।
—B. P. N. Karpuradi varga

167. Karanja *[(Pongamia pinnata (Linn.) Pierre) or Syn-Pongamia glabra Vent.]*

Family:	*Fabaceae*
Hindi name:	*Karanj*
English name:	*Pongam Tree, Hongay Oil Tree*
Synonyms:	*Naktamala, Chirabilva, Karaja, Ghritapoorna*

Morphology

It is a medium-sized deciduous tree 8 to 20 m high, with spreading branches, and grayish brown bark and tubercle (**Fig. 167.1a, b**).

Key Characters for Identification

➤ *Leaves: Alternate, imparipinnate, leaflets opposite with an odd one, ovate* (**Fig. 167.2**).
➤ *Flowers: White with purple tinge or purple, turning bluish at length* (**Fig. 167.3**).
➤ *Fruits: Woody, flattened, indehiscent pod, glabrous oblong, falcate* (**Fig. 167.4**).
➤ *Seed: Solitary, reniform, flat, reddish brown* (**Fig. 167.5**).

Rasapanchaka

Guna	Laghu, Tikshna
Rasa	Tikta, Katu, Kashaya
Vipaka	Katu
Virya	Ushna
Doshakarma	Kaphavatahara

Officinal Parts Used

Bark, leaf, seed

Dose

Powder: 1 to 3 g
Juice: 10 to 20 mL

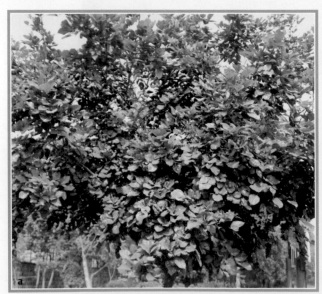
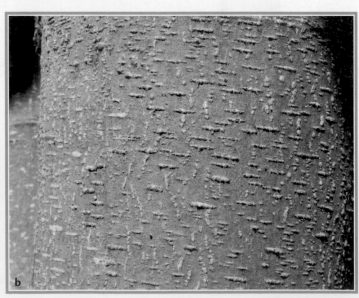

Fig. 167.1 **(a)** Plant of *Pongamia pinnata* (Linn.) Pierre. **(b)** Bark.

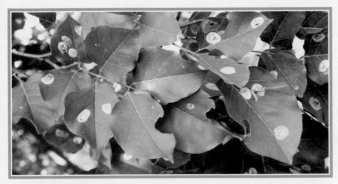

Fig. 167.2 Leaves.

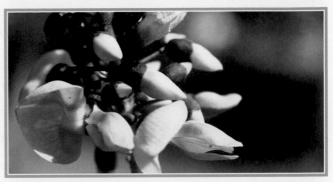

Fig. 167.3 Flower.

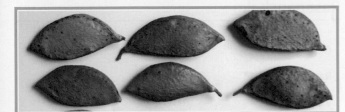

Fig. 167.4 Fruits.

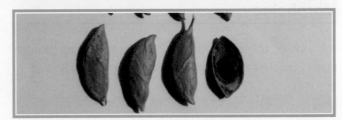

Fig. 167.5 Seeds.

Karma (Actions)

Deepana (appetizer), pachana (digestive), krimighna (anthelmintic), kandughna (antipruritus).

Indications

Arshas (piles), kushta (skin disease), granthi (cysts), visarpa (erysipelas), gulma (abdominal lump), yoniroga (vaginal disease), dushtavrana (infected wound), shotha (inflammation), udavarta (retention of feces, urine, and flatus).

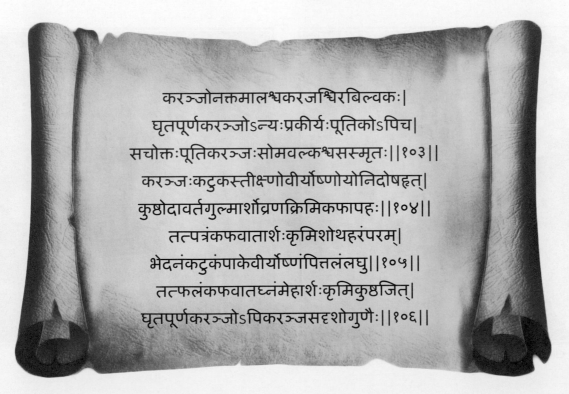

करञ्जोनक्तमालश्चकरजश्चिरबिल्वकः।
घृतपूर्णकरञ्जोऽन्यःप्रकीर्यःपूतिकोऽपिच।
सचोक्तःपूतिकरञ्जःसोमवल्कश्चसस्मृतः॥१०३॥
करञ्जःकटुकस्तीक्ष्णोवीर्योष्णोयोनिदोषहृत्।
कुष्ठोदावर्तगुल्मार्शोव्रणक्रिमिकफापहः॥१०४॥
तत्पत्रंकफवातार्शःकृमिशोथहरंपरम्।
भेदनंकटुकंपाकेवीर्योष्णंपित्तलंलघु॥१०५॥
तत्फलंकफवातघ्नंमेहार्शःकृमिकुष्ठजित्।
घृतपूर्णकरञ्जोऽपिकरञ्जसदृशोगुणैः॥१०६॥

168. Karavellaka [*Momoradica charantia* Linn.]

Family:	*Cucurbitaceae*
Hindi name:	*Karela*
English name:	*Bitter gourd, Balsam Pear*
Synonyms:	*Karavelli, Sushavi, Katilla*

Morphology

It is a weak, tendrillar climber, 2 to 6 m long or more, with many branches that are grooved and hairy (**Fig. 168.1**).

Key Characters for Identification

➤ *Leaves: Alternate, simple, petiolate, ovate lamina orbicular in outline.*
➤ *Flowers: Monoecious, yellow, solitary, axillary, slender* (**Fig. 168.2**).
➤ *Fruits: Oblong, fusiform, pendulous, beaked berry, green colored* (**Fig. 168.3**).
➤ *Seed: Numerous, imbedded in orange-red flesh, compressed, corrugated on margin* (**Fig. 168.4**).

Rasapanchaka

Guna	Laghu, Ruksha
Rasa	Tikta, Katu
Vipaka	Katu
Virya	Ushna
Doshakarma	Kaphapittahara

Officinal Parts Used

Pericarp and whole plant

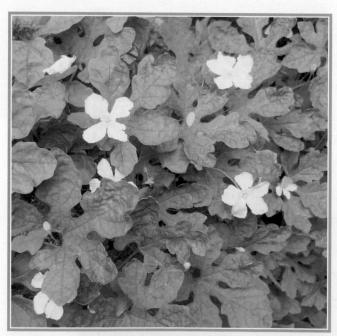

Fig. 168.1 Climber of *Momoradica charantia* Linn.

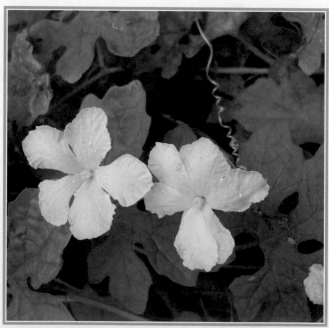

Fig. 168.2 Flowers.

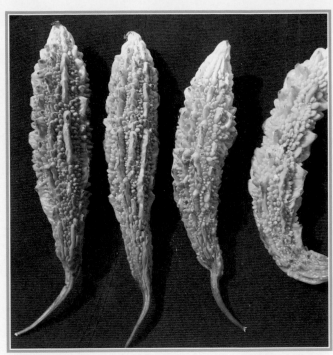

Fig. 168.3 Fruits.

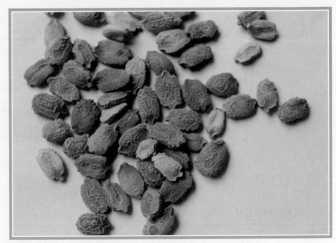

Fig. 168.4 Dry seeds.

Dose

Juice: 10 to 20 mL

Karma (Actions)

Deepan (appetizer), bhedan (purgative), krimighna (anthelmintic), jwaraghna (antipyretics).

Indications

Jwara (fever), pandu (anemia), krimi (worm infestation), prameha (diabetes).

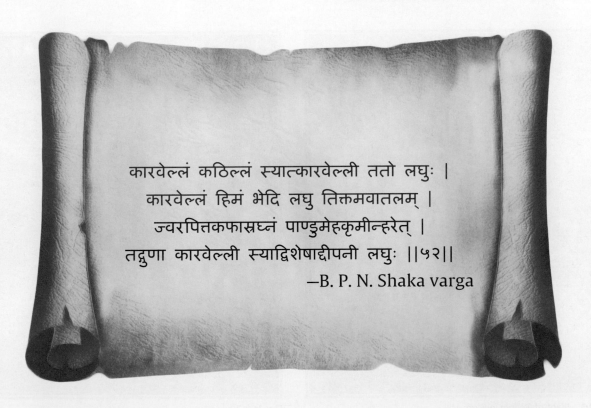

कारवेल्लं कठिल्लं स्यात्कारवेल्ली ततो लघुः ।
कारवेल्लं हिमं भेदि लघु तिक्तमवातलम् ।
ज्वरपित्तकफास्रघ्नं पाण्डुमेहकृमीन्हरेत् ।
तद्गुणा कारवेल्ली स्याद्विशेषाद्दीपनी लघुः ॥५२॥

—B. P. N. Shaka varga

169. Karavira [*Nerium indicum* Mill.]

Family:	*Apocyanaceae*
Hindi name:	*Kaner, Lal Kaner, Saphed Kaner*
English Name:	*Indian Oleander, Sweet-scented Oleander*
Synonyms:	*Ashwamara, Hayamara*

Morphology

It is a shrub or small tree, 2 to 5 m high with profuse straight branching (**Fig. 169.1**).

Key Characters for Identification

➤ *Leaves: Simple, coriaceous, three at each node, linear, oblong, lanceolate (**Fig. 169.2**).*
➤ *Flowers: Pure white to rose red through pink in different plants, sweet scented (**Fig. 169.3**).*
➤ *Fruits: A pair of follicles or solitary on abortion of one carpel, linear, oblong (**Fig. 169.4**).*
➤ *Seed: Many, linear with a tuft of brownish hairs.*

Rasapanchaka

Guna	Laghu, Ruksha
Rasa	Katu, Tikta
Vipaka	Katu
Virya	Ushna
Doshakarma	Kaphavatahara

Officinal Parts Used

Root and root bark

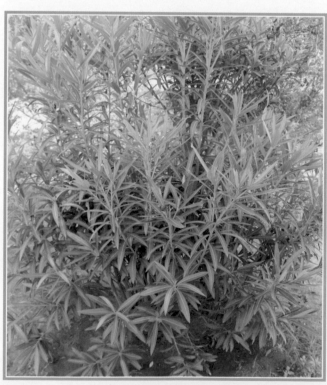

Fig. 169.1 Plant of *Nerium indicum* Mill.

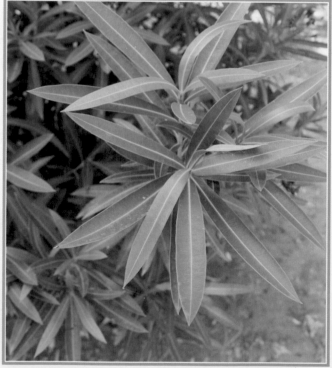

Fig. 169.2 Leaves.

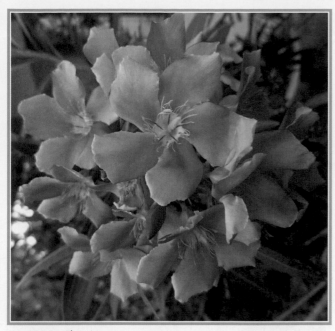

Fig. 169.3 Flowers.

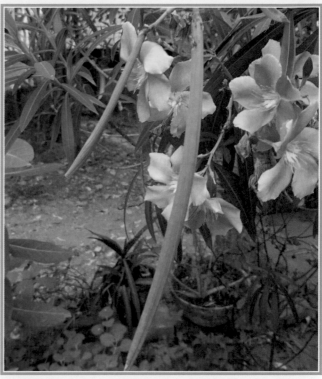

Fig. 169.4 Fruits.

Dose

Powder: 30 to 125 mg

Karma (Actions)

Vranashodhan (wound cleansing), krimighna (anthelmintic), kushtaghna (antileprotic/cure skin problems), kandughna (antipuritus), vishaghna (antidote).

Indications

Kushta (skin disease), upadamsha (syphilis), ashmari (urinary calculus), kandu (itching), palitya (premature graying of hairs), indralupta (alopecia), vrana (wound), visha (poisoning), eye diseases.

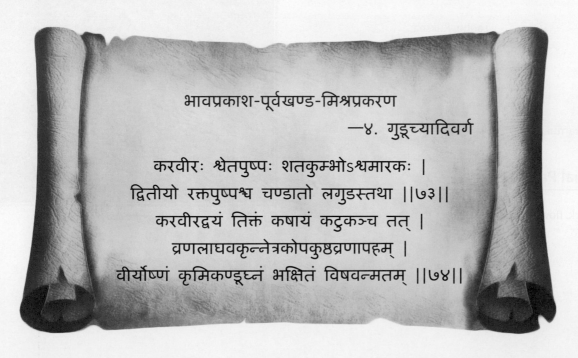

भावप्रकाश-पूर्वखण्ड-मिश्रप्रकरण
—४. गुडूच्यादिवर्ग

करवीरः श्वेतपुष्पः शतकुम्भोऽश्वमारकः |
द्वितीयो रक्तपुष्पश्च चण्डातो लगुडस्तथा ||७३||
करवीरद्वयं तिक्तं कषायं कटुकञ्च तत् |
व्रणलाघवकृन्नेत्रकोपकुष्ठव्रणापहम् |
वीर्योष्णं कृमिकण्डूघ्नं भक्षितं विषवन्मतम् ||७४||

170. Kareera *[Capparis decidua (Forsk.) Edgew.]*

Family:	*Capparaceae*
Hindi name:	*Kareel*
English name:	*Caper berry*
Synonyms:	*Apattra, Nigudha pattra, Marubhuruha, Granthila, Krakaro*

Morphology

It is an erect shrub, 1.5 to 2.5 m high with copious scandent branching, bushy appearance (**Fig. 170.1**).

Key Characters for Identification

➤ *Branches: Glabrous, soft, and thorny. Thorns are straight and found in pairs.*
➤ *Leaves: Found in young shoot only and are simple, alternate, oblong.*
➤ *Flowers: Pedicellate, attractive, red or orange red in color, with many stamens (Fig. 170.2).*
➤ *Fruit: A sub-globose berry, green, which turns bright red on maturity (Fig. 170.3).*
➤ *Seed: Imbedded in white pulp.*

Rasapanchaka

Guna	Laghu, Ruksha
Rasa	Katu, Tikta
Vipaka	Katu
Virya	Ushna
Doshakarma	Kaphavatahara

Officinal Parts Used

Root, bark, flowers

Dose

Decoction: 50 to 100 mL
Powder: 1 to 3 g

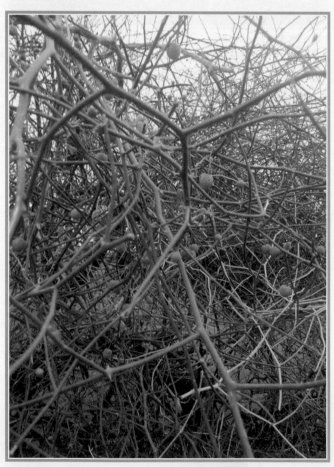

Fig. 170.1 Plant of *Capparis decidua* (Forsk.) Edgew.

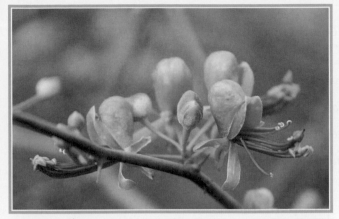

Fig. 170.2   Flower.

Karma (Actions)

Bhedana (purgative), vishaghna (antidote), vranaropan (wound healing), shothaghna (anti-inflammatory), krimighna (anthelmintic).

Indications

Krimi (worm infestation), shotha (edema), vrana (wound), arshas (piles), kaphavataroga (kaphavata disorders), garavisha (poisoning with synthetic or man-made poison).

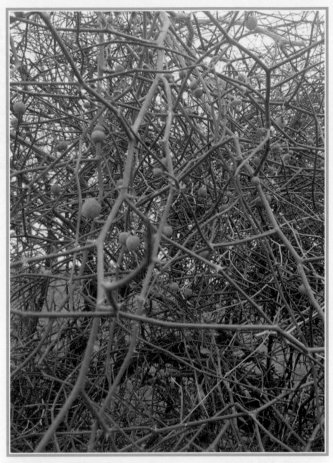

Fig. 170.3   Fruits.

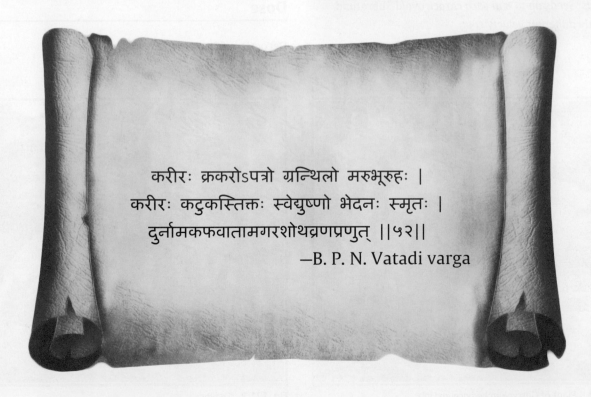

करीरः क्रकरोऽपत्रो ग्रन्थिलो मरुभूरुहः |
करीरः कटुकस्तिक्तः स्वेद्युष्णो भेदनः स्मृतः |
दुर्नामकफवातामगरशोथव्रणप्रणुत् ||५२||
—B. P. N. Vatadi varga

171. Karpasa *[Gossypium herbaceum Linn.]*

Family:	*Malvaceae*
Hindi name:	*Kapas*
English name:	*Cotton, Lavant*
Synonyms:	*Samudranta, Tundikeri*

Morphology

It is a small, erect, annual–perennial shrub 1 to 1.5 m tall (**Fig. 171.1**).

Key Characters for Identification

➤ *Leaves: Alternate, simple, petiolate, lumina ovate-rotund in outline, almost reniform, cordate-auriculate, leathery, blade less than half incised into three to five lobes* (**Fig. 171.2**).

➤ *Flowers: Axillary, solitary, yellow with purple claws, ovate, cordate, acute and shortly toothed* (**Fig. 171.3**).

➤ *Fruits: An ovoid, acute three- to five-valved capsule* (**Fig. 171.4**).

➤ *Seeds: Seeds up to 8 in each carpel, ovoid-subrotund, firmly adherent velvety coat.*

Rasapanchaka

Guna	Laghu, Ruksha (seed-guru)
Rasa	Madhur
Vipaka	Madhur
VIrya	Ushna
Doshakarma	Vatahara

Officinal Parts Used

Root, bark, flower, seed

Dose

Decoction: 50 to 100 mL
Powder: 3 to 6 g

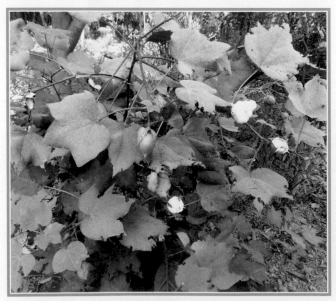

Fig. 171.1　Plant of *Gossypium herbaceum* Linn.

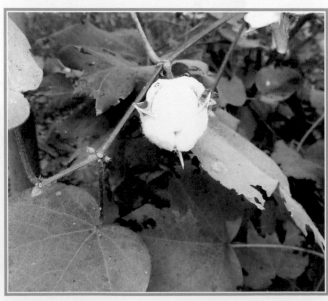

Fig. 171.2　Leaves.

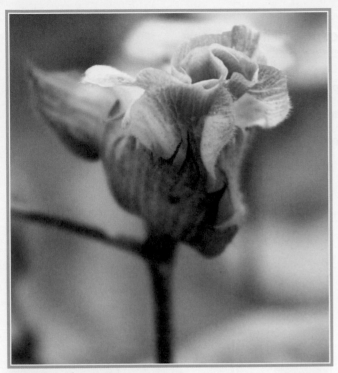

Fig. 171.3 Flower.

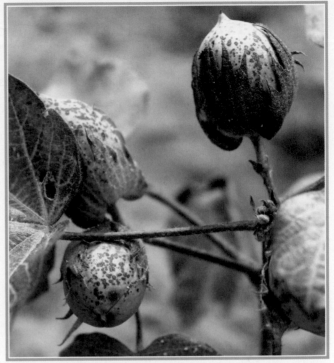

Fig. 171.4 Fruits.

Karma (Actions)

Vatahara (pacify vata dosha), muttral (diuretics), vrishya (aphrodisiac), rakta-vardhaka (aggravate blood), sthanyajanan (galactopoietic), kaphakarak (increase kapha).

Indications

Muttrakricchra (dysuria), karanpeeda (earache/otalgia), anartava (amenorrhea), kashtartava (dysmenorrhea), karna pooya (pus in ear).

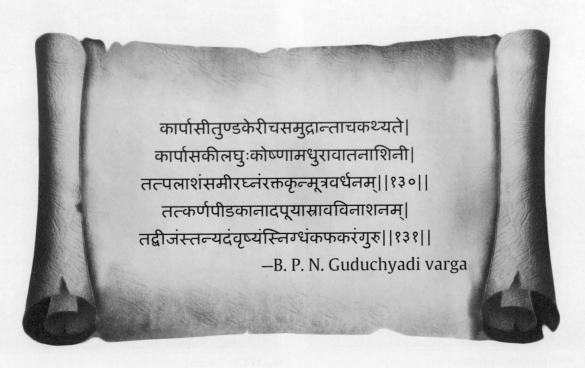

कार्पासीतुण्डकेरीचसमुद्रान्ताचकथ्यते|
कार्पासकीलघुःकोष्णामधुरावातनाशिनी|
तत्पलाशंसमीरघ्नंरक्तकृन्मूत्रवर्धनम्||१३०||
तत्कर्णपीडकानादपूयास्रावविनाशनम्|
तद्बीजंस्तन्यदंवृष्यंस्निग्धंकफकरंगुरु||१३१||

—B. P. N. Guduchyadi varga

172. Kasamarda *[Cassia occidentalis Linn.]*

Family:	*Caesalpinioideae*
Hindi name:	*Kasoundi*
English name:	*Negro coffee*
Synonyms:	*Kasari, Arimarda, Karkasha*

Morphology

It is an erect, annual–biennial herb–undershrub, 0.5 to 1.5 m tall (**Fig. 172.1**).

Key Characters for Identification

➤ *Leaves: Alternate, paripinnately compound, sessile, smooth gland on petiole (**Fig. 172.2**).*
➤ *Flowers: Inflorescence of few flowered, axillary racemes, with yellow and reddish vein (**Fig. 172.3**).*
➤ *Fruits: An elongate, falcate, compressed, shortly stalked, glabrous, and torulose pod (**Fig. 172.4**).*
➤ *Seed: Thirty to 50 in number, compressed, smooth, ovate-cordate in shape (**Fig. 172.5**).*

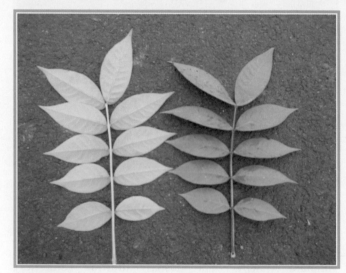

Fig. 172.2 Leaves.

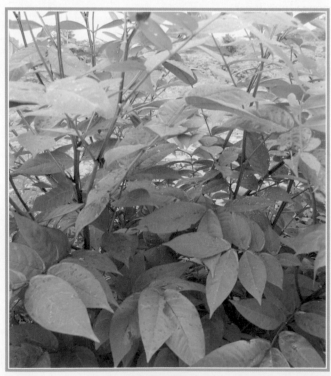

Fig. 172.1 Herb of *Cassia occidentalis* Linn.

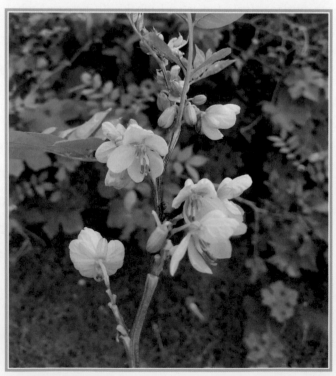

Fig. 172.3 Flowers.

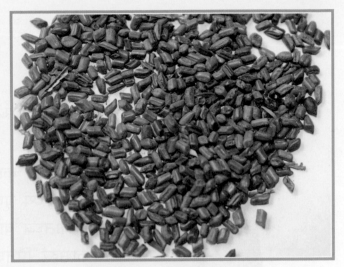

Fig. 172.5 Seeds.

Officinal Parts Used

Root, leaf, seed

Dose

Leaf juice: 10 to 20 mL
Seed powder: 2 to 4 g
Decoction: 50 to 100 mL

Karma (Actions)

Rochan (relish), vrisya (aphrodisiac), pachan (digestive), kantha shodhan (purification of throat), vishaghna (antidote), pittanashana (pacify pitta), grahi (appetizer and fecal astringent).

Indications

Kasa (cough), shwasa (asthma), visha (poison).

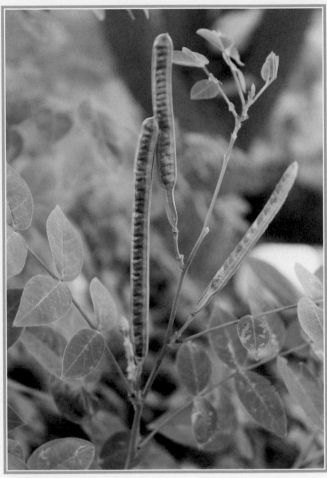

Fig. 172.4 Fruits.

Rasapanchaka

Guna	Laghu, Ruksha
Rasa	Tikta, Madhur
Vipaka	Katu
Virya	Ushna
Doshakarma	Kaphavatahara

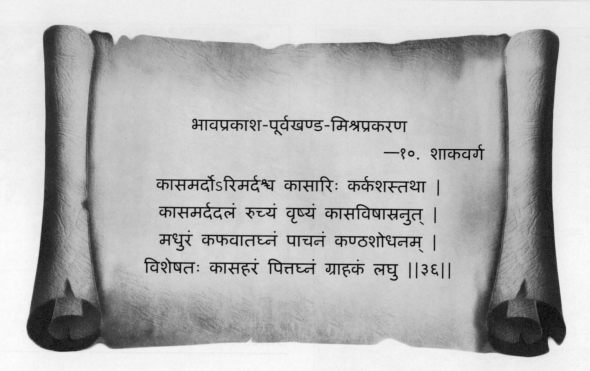

भावप्रकाश-पूर्वखण्ड-मिश्रप्रकरण

—१०. शाकवर्ग

कासमर्दोऽरिमर्दश्च कासारिः कर्कशस्तथा |
कासमर्ददलं रुच्यं वृष्यं कासविषासनुत् |
मधुरं कफवातघ्नं पाचनं कण्ठशोधनम् |
विशेषतः कासहरं पित्तघ्नं ग्राहकं लघु ||३६||

173. Kasha *[Saccharum spontaneum Linn.]*

Family:	*Poaceae*
Hindi name:	*Kasa*
English name:	*Thatch grass*
Synonyms:	*Ikshugandha, potagala, ikshwalika, kashekshu*

Morphology

It is an erect, tufted, perennial grass, 0.75 to 3 m tall (**Fig. 173.1**).

Key Characters for Identification

➤ *Leaves: Linear, flat, acuminate, rough to touch*
➤ *Flowers: Inflorescence of large, silvery hairy, rachis fragile; spikelets sessile (**Fig. 173.2**)*

Rasapanchaka

Guna	Laghu, Snigdha
Rasa	Madhura, Tikta
Vipaka	Madhura
Virya	Sheeta
Doshakarma	Vatapittashamaka

Officinal Part Used

Root

Dose

Decoction: 50 to 100 mL

Karma (Actions)

Mutrala (diuretic), stanya-janana (galactogogue), sara (laxation).

Indications

Muttrakricchra (dysuria), ashmari (calculus), rakta-pitta (bleeding disorders), kshaya (emaciation), pittajaroga (diseases caused by aggravated pitta), daha (burning sensation).

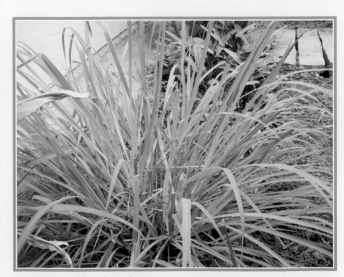

Fig. 173.1   Plant of *Saccharum spontaneum* Linn.

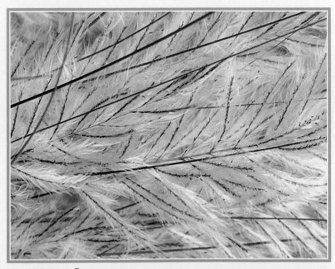

Fig. 173.2   Inflorescence.

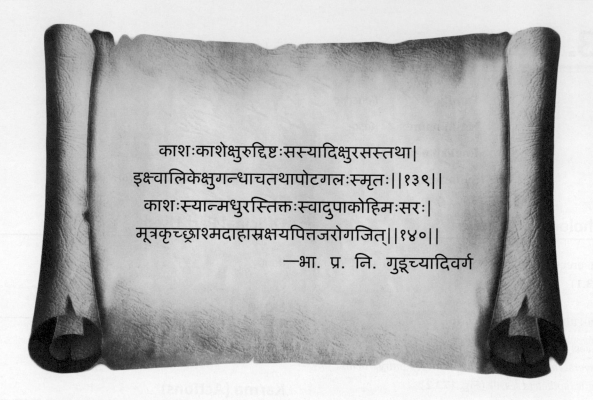

काशःकाशेक्षुरुद्दिष्टःसस्यादिक्षुरसस्तथा।
इक्ष्वालिकेक्षुगन्धाचतथापोटगलःस्मृतः॥१३९॥
काशःस्यान्मधुरस्तिक्तःस्वादुपाकोहिमःसरः।
मूत्रकृच्छ्राश्मदाहास्रक्षयपित्तजरोगजित्॥१४०॥

—भा. प्र. नि. गुडूच्यादिवर्ग

174. Kasani *[Cichorium intybus Linn.]*

Family:	*Asteraceae*
Hindi name:	*Kasani, Chichori*
English name:	*Chicory, Siccory, Endive*

Morphology

It is an annual or perennial herb, 1/3 to 1 m high. It is usually rough and is more or less like a grandular herb (**Fig. 174.1**).

Key Characters for Identification

➤ *Leaves: Simple, alternate, basal leaves lyrate, margin pinnatified, coarsely toothed (***Fig. 174.2***).*
➤ *Flowers: Inflorescence of homogamous, solitary/ clustered, bright blue, bisexual (***Fig. 174.3***).*
➤ *Root/Rhizomes: Brownish, fleshy, and tapering, 10 to 30 cm long.*

Rasapanchaka

Guna	Laghu, Ruksha
Rasa	Tikta
Vipaka	Katu
Virya	Ushna
Doshakarma	Kaphapittahara

Officinal Parts Used

Root, leaf, seed

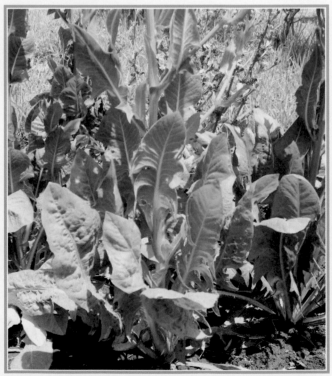

Fig. 174.1   Plant of *Cichorium intybus* Linn.

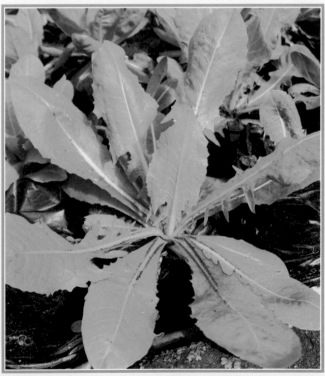

Fig. 174.2   Leaves.

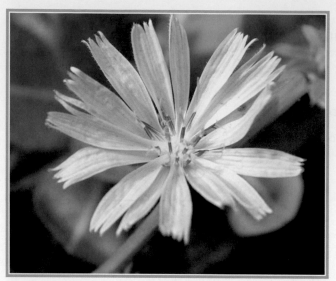

Fig. 174.3 Flower.

Dose

Powder: 3 to 6 g

Juice: 10 to 20 mL

Karma (Actions)

Deepana (appetizer), shothaghna (anti-inflammatory), yakrituttejaka (hepatic stimulant), jwaraghna (antipyretic), hridya (cardiotonic).

Indications

Yakrittroga (hepatic disorder), hridroga (heart disease), muttrakricchra (dysuria), pleehavridhi (splenomegaly).

175. Kataka *[Strychnos potatorum Linn.f.]*

Family:	*Loganiaceae*
Hindi name:	*Nirmali*
English name:	*Clearing NutTree*
Synonyms:	*Payah-prasadi, Chakshushya*

Morphology

It is a tree, 10 to 15 m high (**Fig. 175.1**).

Key Characters for Identification

➤ *Stem: Dark black bark with vertical cracks (**Fig. 175.2**).*
➤ *Leaves: Opposite, simple, subsessile ovate broadly, leathery and glabrous, three-nerved (**Fig. 175.3**).*
➤ *Flowers: Greenish-white, sweet-scented; ovary with two-lobed style.*
➤ *Fruits: A globose berry, which is green, turning black at maturity.*
➤ *Seed: Solitary or two, round, compressed or otherwise subglobose, imbedded in white fleshy pulp, coated with appressed silky hair (**Fig. 175.4**).*

Rasapanchaka

Guna	Guru
Rasa	Tikta, Madhura, Kashaya
Vipaka	Madhura
Virya	Sheeta
Doshakarma	Kaphavatahara

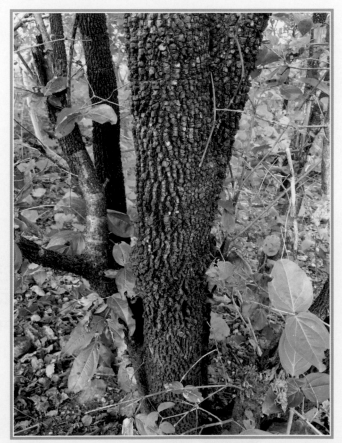

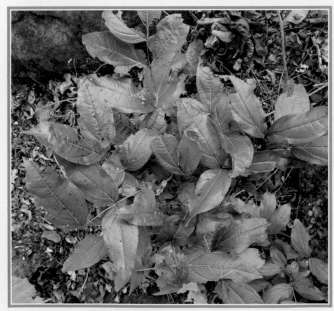

Fig. 175.1 Plant of *Strychnos potatorum* Linn.f.

Fig 175.2 Bark.

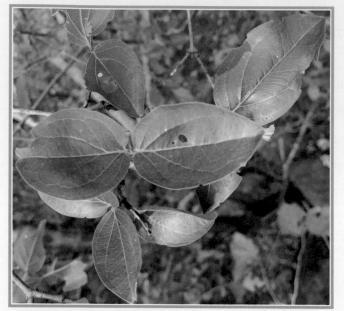

Fig. 175.3 Leaves.

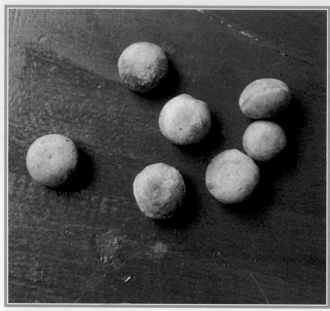

Fig. 175.4 Seeds.

Officinal Part Used

Seed

Dose

Powder: 1 to 3 g

Karma (Actions)

Lekhana (scraping), vishaghna (antidote), payaprasadana (water purification), netrya (beneficial for vision).

Indications

Eye disorders, asmari (urinary calculus), pandu (anemia), shoth (edema), kamala (jaundice), visha (poisoning), kushta (skin disease), prameha (diabetes).

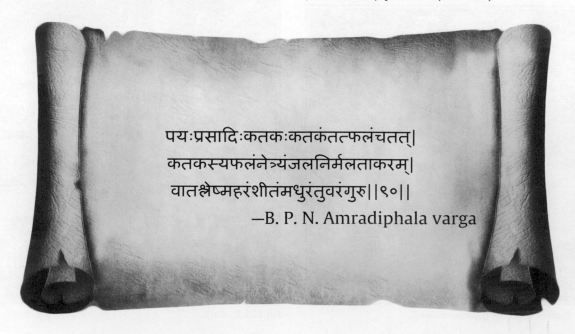

पयःप्रसादिःकतकःकतकंतत्फलंचतत्।
कतकस्यफलंनेत्र्यंजलनिर्मलताकरम्।
वातश्लेष्महरंशीतंमधुरंतुवरंगुरु॥९०॥
—B. P. N. Amradiphala varga

176. Katphala [*Myrica esculenta* Buch.ham Ex.D.Don *or Myrica nagi* Thumb. Hook.f.]

Family:	*Myricaceae*
Hindi name:	*Kebuk, Kemuk*
English name:	*Box myrtle, Bay berry*
Synonyms:	*Somabalka, Kaitarya, Kumbhika, Shreeparnika, Kumudika, Bhadra, Bhadravati*

Morphology

It is a small or moderate tree, 3 to 15 m high. Its bark is rough with deep vertical wrinkles (**Fig. 176.1**).

Key Characters for Identification

➤ *Leaves: Simple, oblong-lanceolate, 9.5 to 15 cm long.*
➤ *Flowers: Inflorescence of axillary spikes with unisexual flowers.*
➤ *Fruits: Fruit a drupe, ellipsoid-ovoid in shape, waxy with black–brown spots.*
➤ *Seed: Nut solitary, rugose.*

Rasapanchaka

Guna	Laghu, Tikshna
Rasa	Katu, Tikta, Kashya
Vipaka	Katu
Virya	Ushna
Doshakarma	Kapha vatashamaka

Officinal Part Used

Bark

Dose

Powder: 3 to 5 g

Karma (Actions)

Kasaghna (expectorant), shwasaghna (antiasthmatic), mehaghna (antidiabetic), jwaraghna (antipyretics).

Indications

Kasa (cough), pratisyaya (common cold), jwar (fever), kushta (skin disease), prameha (diabetes), mukhapaka (stomatitis), tamaka shwasa (bronchial asthma), svarabhanga (hoarseness of voice), agnimandya (loss of appetite), amatisara (diarrhea with ama), aruchi, raktatisara (diarrhea with blood), gidhrasi (sciatica).

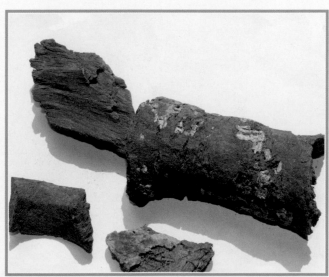

Fig. 176.1 Bark of Katphala (*Myrica esculenta* Buch.ham Ex.D.Don).

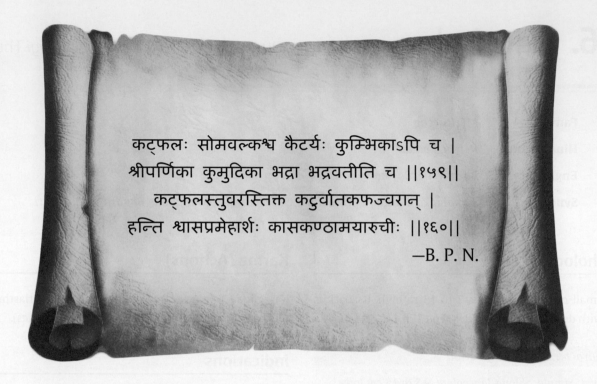

कट्फलः सोमवल्कश्च कैटर्यः कुम्भिकाऽपि च |
श्रीपर्णिका कुमुदिका भद्रा भद्रवतीति च ||१५९||
कट्फलस्तुवरस्तिक्त कटुर्वातकफज्वरान् |
हन्ति श्वासप्रमेहार्शः कासकण्ठामयारुचीः ||१६०||

—B. P. N.

177. Kebuk *[Costus speciosus (Koen.ex.Retz) Sm.]*

Family:	*Zingiberaceae*
Hindi name:	*Kebuk, Kemuk*
English name:	*Crepe ginger*
Synonyms:	*Kemuka*

Morphology

It is an erect, succulent, perennial herb 0.75 to 2.25 m tall; aerial parts are annual with white/red-colored flower (**Fig. 177.1**).

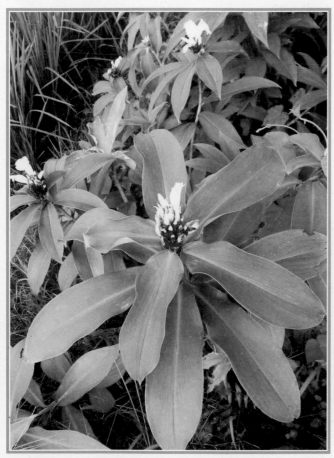

Fig. 177.1 Plant of *Costus speciosus* (Koen.ex.Retz) Sm.

Key Characters for Identification

➤ *Leaves: Simple, entire, spirally arranged, oblong-oblanceolate, with parallel ascending nerves and caudate-acuminate apex (***Fig. 177.2***).*
➤ *Flowers: White, calyx tubular, corolla tube equaling calyx, lips broadly obovate (***Fig. 177.3***).*
➤ *Fruits: An ovoid three-gonous, three-valved, bright red at maturity.*
➤ *Seed: Many, black-and-white aril at fruiting, entire fruiting-spike attains bright red color.*

Rasapanchaka

Guna	Laghu, Ruksha
Rasa	Tikta, Kashya
Vipaka	Katu
Virya	Sheeta
Doshakarma	Kapha pittahara and Vata vardhak

Officinal Part Used

Tuber

Dose

Powder: 3 to 6 g
Juice: 10 to 20 mL

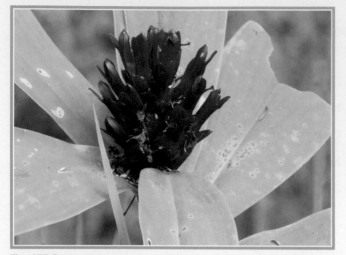

Fig. 177.2 Leaves.

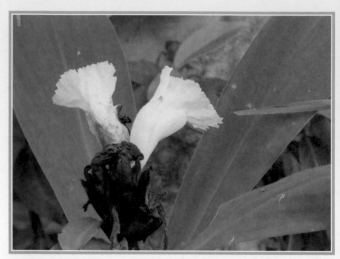

Fig. 177.3 Flower.

Karma (Actions)

Deepan (appetizer), pachan (digestive), hridya (cardiotonic), grahi (fecal astringent), jwaraghna (antipyretics).

Indications

Kasa (cough), jwar (fever), kushta (skin disease), prameha (diabetes), raktavikar (blood-related diseases), shleepada (filaria).

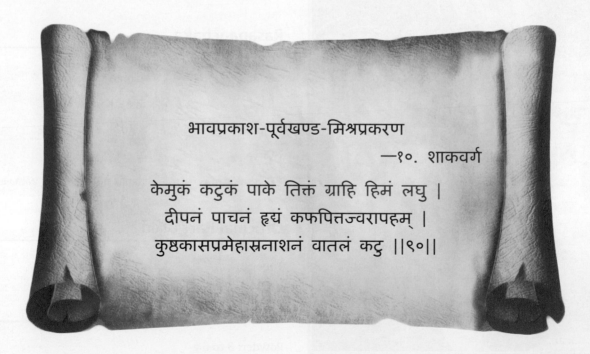

भावप्रकाश-पूर्वखण्ड-मिश्रप्रकरण

—१०. शाकवर्ग

केमुकं कटुकं पाके तिक्तं ग्राहि हिमं लघु ।

दीपनं पाचनं हृद्यं कफपित्तज्वरापहम् ।

कुष्ठकासप्रमेहासनाशनं वातलं कटु ॥९०॥

178. Kharjura *[Phoenix dactylifera Linn.]*

Family:	*Arecaceae*
Hindi name:	*Kharjur*
English name:	*Date Palm*
Synonyms:	*Skandaphala, Bhumikharjurika, Swadi, Duraroha, Mriduchhada*

Morphology

It is a tall palm, reaching a height of 20 to 40 m, with many offshoots from the base of its trunk (**Fig. 178.1**).

Key Characters for Identification

➤ *Leaves: Pinnately compound, grayish, leaflets linear, folded longitudinally.*
➤ *Flowers: Dioecious, sessile on the bends of long, glabrous undulating spikelets.*
➤ *Fruits: A single, oblong, reddish- or yellowish-brown berries, 2.5 to 7.5 cm long, and pulp is fleshy and sweet in taste (*Fig. 178.2a, b*).*
➤ *Seed: One-seeded berry, with longitudinal grove.*

Rasapanchaka

Guna	Guru, Snigdha
Rasa	Madhura
Vipaka	Madhura
Virya	Sheeta
Doshakarma	Vataipitta Shamaka

Officinal Parts Used

Fruit and leaf

Dose

Decoction: 50 to 100 mL

Karma (Actions)

Hridya (cardiotonic), balya (provide physical strength), vrishya (aphrodisiac).

Indications

Raktapitta (bleeding disorders), chardi (vomiting), jwara (fever), atisara (diarrhea), kshaya (emaciation), trishna (thirst), kasa (cough), shwasa (asthma), mada (excitement), murchha (unconsciousness).

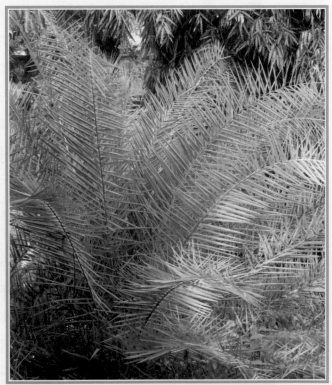

Fig. 178.1　Plant of *Phoenix dactylifera* Linn.

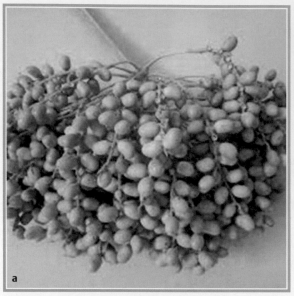
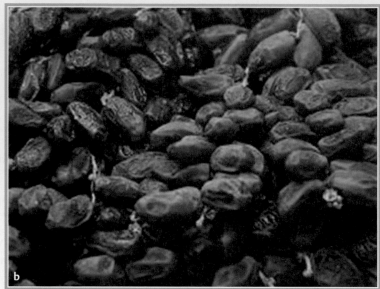

Fig. 178.2 **(a)** Young fruits. **(b)** Mature fruits.

भूमिखर्जूरिकास्वाद्वीदुरारोहामृदुच्छदा।
तथास्कन्धफलाकाककर्कटीस्वादुमस्तका॥९७॥
पिण्डखर्जूरिकात्वन्यासादेशेपश्चिमेभवेत्।
खर्जूरीगोस्तनाकारापरद्वीपादिहागता।
जायतेपश्चिमेदेशेसाच्छोहारेतिकीर्त्यते॥९८॥
खर्जूरीत्रितयंशीतंमधुरंरसपाकयोः।
स्निग्धंरुचिकरंहृद्यंक्षतक्षयहरंगुरु॥९९॥
तर्पणंरक्तपित्तघ्नंपुष्टिविष्टम्भशुक्रदम्।
कोष्ठमारुतहृद्दल्यंवान्तिवातकफापहम्॥१००॥
ज्वरातिसारक्षुत्तृष्णाकासश्वासनिवारकम्।
मदमूर्च्छामरुत्पित्तमद्योद्भूतगदान्तकृत्।
महतीभ्यांगुणैरल्पास्वल्पखर्जूरिकास्मृता॥१०१॥
खर्जूरीतरुतोयंतुमदपित्तकरंभवेत्।
वातश्लेष्महरंरुच्यंदीपनंबलशुक्रकृत्।
सुलेमानीतुमृदुलादलहीनफलाचसा।
सुलेमानीश्रमभ्रान्तिदाहमूर्च्छाऽस्रपित्तहृत्॥१०२॥

—B. P. N. Amradiphala varga

179. Kitmaari *[Aristolochia bracteolata Lamk.]*

Family:	*Aristolochiaceae*
Hindi name:	*Keedmaar*
English name:	*Bracteated Birth wort*
Synonyms:	*Keetari, Dhoomrapatra, Nakuli*

Morphology

It is a prostrate-trailing, ashy, perennial herb, 0.34 to 0.50 m long. It branches from base (**Fig. 179.1**).

Key Characters for Identification

➤ *Leaves: Simple, alternate, broadly ovate-reniform in outline, glabrous, wavy (**Fig. 179.2**).*
➤ *Flowers: Axillary, solitary, pedicellate, revolute lip, striated, stamens and style are 6 in number.*
➤ *Fruits: An oblong-obovoid, 12-ribbed and stalked capsule, dehiscing from base (**Fig. 179.3**).*
➤ *Seed: Many, flat, somewhat cordate, bitter, and aromatic to taste.*

Rasapanchaka

Guna	Laghu, Ruksha
Rasa	Tikta
Vipaka	Katu
Virya	Ushna
Doshakarma	Kapha vatahara

Officinal Parts Used

Root and leaf

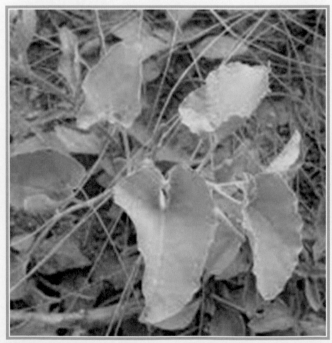

Fig. 179.1   Climber of *Aristolochia bracteolata* Lamk.

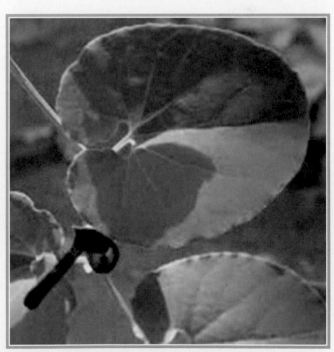

Fig. 179.2   Leaves.

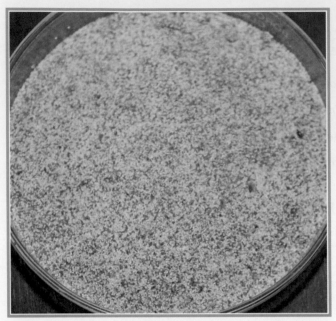

Fig. 179.3 Seeds.

Dose

Decoction: 50 to 100 mL

Powder: 1 to 3 g

Juice: 5 to 10 mL

Karma (Actions)

Rechan (purgative), krimighna (anthelmintic), deepan (appetizer), kasaghna (anticough), shophaghna (antiinflamatory).

Indications

Krimi (worm infestation), vishamajwara (intermittent fever), shotha (sweeling), kastartava (dysmenorrhoea), kasa (cough), jwara (fever).

180. Kokilaksha [Hygrophila schulli (Ham.) Almeida and Almeida or Asteracantha longifolia (Linn.)]

Family: Acanthaceae

Hindi name: Talmakhana

English name: Long-leaved Barleria

Synonyms: Kshuraka, Bhikshu, Kandekshu, Iksshugandha, Kakekshu, Ikshuvalika

Morphology

It is an erect, annual, water-loving herb, which is 75 cm tall with purple-colored flower.

Key Characters for Identification

➤ *Leaves: Simple, sessile, in verticles of 6 at each node, oblong, hispid on both sides, 3.8 cm long (**Fig. 180.1**).*

➤ *Spines: Straight, sharp, yellowish-red spine at the axil of the leaves, 2.5 to 3 cm long (**Fig. 180.2**).*

➤ *Flowers: Bracteates, bracteolate, upper one longer, corolla purple, lips subequal (**Fig. 180.3**).*

➤ *Fruits: An oblong capsule, pointed at apex.*

➤ *Seeds: Seeds 4 to 8 supported by retinacula, orbicular, slimy on wetting, brownish (**Fig. 180.4**).*

Rasapanchaka

Guna	Picchila, Snigdha
Rasa	Madhura, Amla, Tikta
Vipaka	Madhura
Virya	Sheet
Doshakarma	Vatapittahara

Officinal Parts Used

Root, seed, panchang (whole plant), alkali

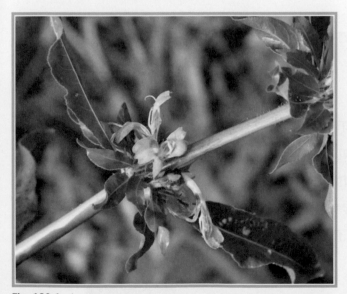

Fig. 180.1 Leaves.

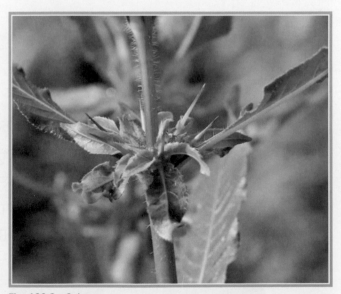

Fig. 180.2 Spines.

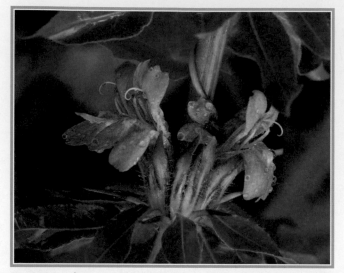

Fig. 180.3 Flowers.

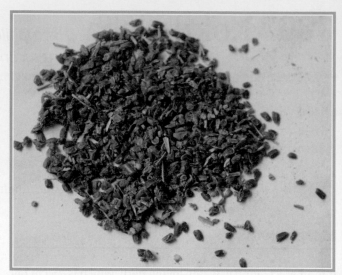

Fig. 180.4 Seeds.

Dose

Decoction: 50 to 100 mL
Powder: 3 to 6 g
Alkali: 1 to 2 g

Karma (Actions)

Deepana (digestive), vrishya (aphrodisiac), vamaka (induce vomiting).

Indications

Vatarakta (gout), amavata (rheumatoid arthritis), shotha (edema), trishna (thirst), ashmari (urinary calculus), netraroga (eye disease).

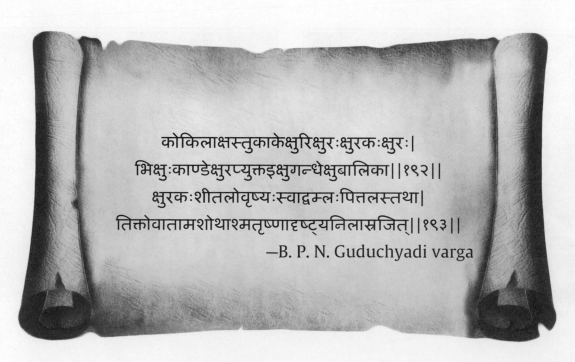

कोकिलाक्षस्तुकाकेक्षुरिक्षुरःक्षुरकःक्षुरः।
भिक्षुःकाण्डेक्षुरप्युक्तइक्षुगन्धेक्षुबालिका॥१९२॥
क्षुरकःशीतलोवृष्यःस्वाद्वम्लःपित्तलस्तथा।
तिक्तोवातामशोथाश्मतृष्णादृष्ट्यनिलास्रजित्॥१९३॥
—B. P. N. Guduchyadi varga

181. Koshataki *[Luffa acutangula* (Linn.) Roxb]*

Family:	*Cucurbitaceae*
Hindi name:	*Tori, Kadva torai*
English name:	*Ridged gourd*
Synonyms:	*Kritavedhana, Mridangaphala, Jalini, Rajakoshataki, Rajimatphala*

Morphology

It is a weak, annual, tendrillar climber (**Fig. 181.1**).

Key Characters for Identification

➤ *Leaves: Alternate, simple, lamina orbicular in outline, white hairy at first (**Fig. 181.2**).*
➤ *Flowers: Monoecious, yellow with male and female varieties.*
➤ *Fruits: Obovoid, green with bitter white flesh inside when young, forming a fibrous and netlike structure at maturity, attached to thick stalk (**Fig. 181.3**).*
➤ *Seed: Many, compressed, obovoid, corrugated, black in color, bitter to taste.*

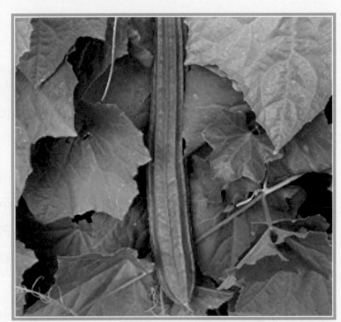

Fig. 181.2 Leaves.

Rasapanchaka

Guna	Laghu, Ruksha
Rasa	Tikta
Vipaka	Katu
Virya	Ushna
Doshakarma	Kaphapitta shamshodhana

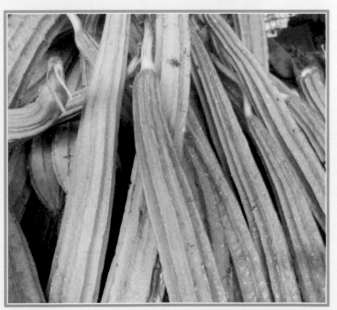

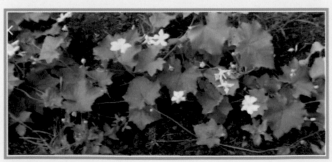

Fig. 181.1 Climber of *Luffa acutangula* (Linn.) Roxb.

Fig. 181.3 Fruits.

Official Parts Used

Fruit, root, leaves

Dose

Powder: 3 to 6 g
Juice: 10 to 20 mL

Karma (Actions)

Deepan (appetizer), vamaka (induce vomiting).

Indications

Jwara (fever), kushta (skin diseases), pandu (anemia), shotha (inflammation), gulma (abdominal distension), garavisha (slow poisons), daha (burning sensation), trishna (thirst), prameha (diabetes).

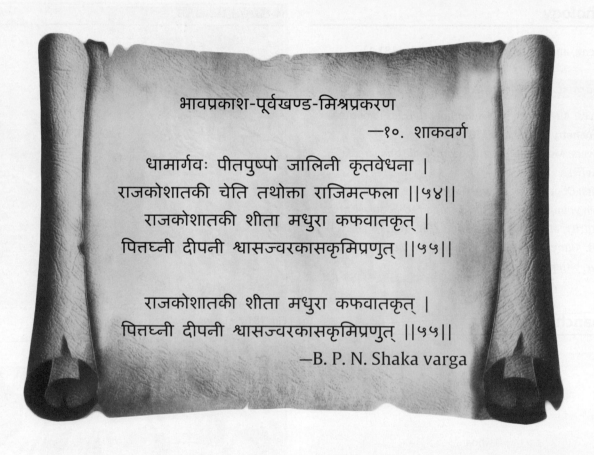

भावप्रकाश-पूर्वखण्ड-मिश्रप्रकरण

—१०. शाकवर्ग

धामार्गवः पीतपुष्पो जालिनी कृतवेधना |
राजकोशातकी चेति तथोक्ता राजिमत्फला ||५४||
राजकोशातकी शीता मधुरा कफवातकृत् |
पित्तघ्नी दीपनी श्वासज्वरकासकृमिप्रणुत् ||५५||

राजकोशातकी शीता मधुरा कफवातकृत् |
पित्तघ्नी दीपनी श्वासज्वरकासकृमिप्रणुत् ||५५||

—B. P. N. Shaka varga

182. Kulattha [Dolichos biflorus non Linn.]

Family:	*Fabaceae*
Hindi name:	*Kulthi*
English name:	*Horse gram*
Synonyms:	*Tamrabeej, Kulatthika*

Morphology

It is a weak, twinning–training, annular herb, with erect branches (**Fig. 182.1**).

Key Characters for Identification

➤ *Leaves: Alternate, petiolate, leaflets stipitate, ovate, entire, acute, unequal sided (**Fig. 182.2**).*
➤ *Flowers: Axillary, solitary or in pairs, softly hairy, pale yellow with purple blotch (**Fig. 182.2**).*
➤ *Fruits: A linear oblong, falcate, pubescent, compressed pod (**Fig. 182.3**).*
➤ *Seed: Up to six in numbers, oblong, reniform, flattened, smooth, brownish, shaded (**Fig. 182.4**).*

Rasapanchaka

Guna	Laghu, Ruksha
Rasa	Kashaya
Vipaka	Katu
Virya	Ushna
Doshakarma	Vata kaphahara

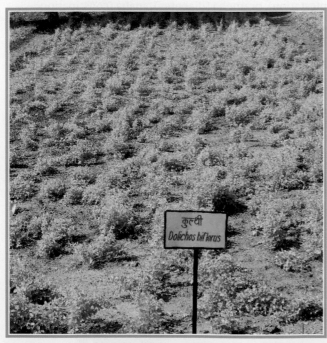

Fig. 182.1   Plant of *Dolichos biflorus* non Linn.

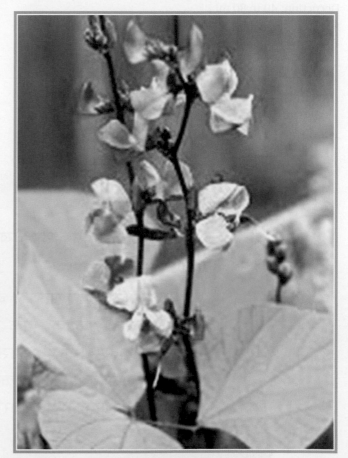

Fig. 182.2   Leaves and flower.

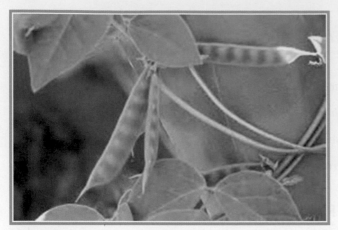

Fig. 182.3 Pods.

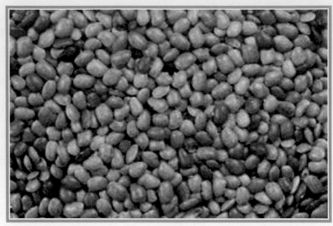

Fig. 182.4 Seeds.

Officinal Part Used

Seed

Dose

Decoction: 40 to 80 mL
Powder: 3 to 6 g

Karma (Actions)

Rakta-Pitta prakopaka (aggravate rakta and pitta), vidahi (burning sensation), medohara (fat reducing), sara (purgative), swedasangrahika (inhibition of sweat), jwarahara (antipyretics), krimighna (anthelmintic).

Indications

Shwasa (asthma), kasa (cough), hikka (hic-cough), ashmari (urinary calculus), peenasa (sinusitis), medoroga (obesity), daha (burning sensation), jwara (fever), krimi (worm infestation), prameha (diabetes), anaha (constipation).

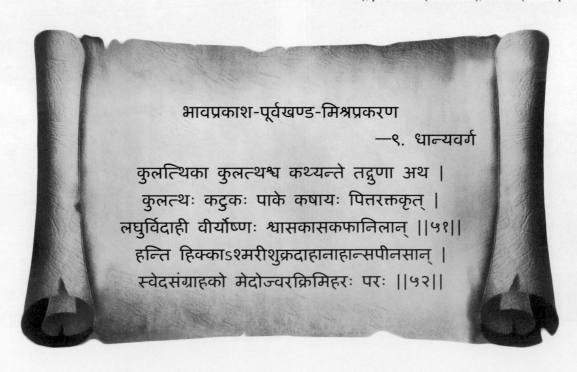

भावप्रकाश-पूर्वखण्ड-मिश्रप्रकरण

—९. धान्यवर्ग

कुलत्थिका कुलत्थश्च कथ्यन्ते तद्गुणा अथ ।
कुलत्थः कटुकः पाके कषायः पित्तरक्तकृत् ।
लघुर्विदाही वीर्योष्णः श्वासकासकफानिलान् ॥७१॥
हन्ति हिक्काऽश्मरीशुक्रदाहानाहान्सपीनसान् ।
स्वेदसंग्राहको मेदोज्वरक्रिमिहरः परः ॥७२॥

183. Kumuda [*Nymphaea nouchali* Burm. f. or *Nymphaea rubra* Roxb.ex Salibs.]

Family:	*Nymphaeaceae*
Hindi name:	*Kumud*
English name:	*Indian Water Lily*
Synonyms:	*Shweta Kuvalaya, Kairava, Utpala*

Morphology

It is an aquatic plant with tuberous root stock and red purplish flower (**Fig. 183.1**).

Key Characters for Identification

➤ *Leaves: Floating, lamina peltate, dentate margin, greenish above purple beneath (**Fig. 183.1**).*
➤ *Flowers: Solitary, red, purplish, pale rose, or white on different plants (**Fig. 183.2**).*
➤ *Fruits: A fleshy, globose, greenish berry, ripening under water, irregular bursting.*
➤ *Seed: Numerous, minute, arillate, and imbedded in soft flesh.*
➤ *Root/Rhizomes: Root stock tuberous, roundish.*

Rasapanchaka

Guna	Snigdha, Picchila
Rasa	Madhura
Vipaka	Madhura
Virya	Sheeta
Doshakarma	Kapha pittahara

Officinal Parts Used

Root, flower, seed

Dose

Powder: 3 to 6 g
Juice: 10 to 20 mL

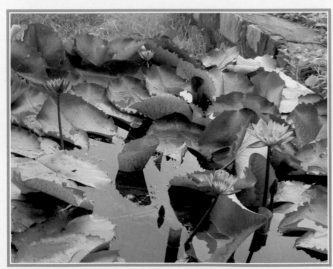

Fig. 183.1 Plant of *Nymphaea nouchali* Burm.f.

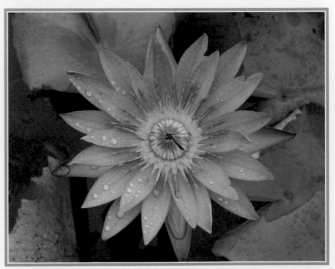

Fig. 183.2 Flower.

Karma (Actions)

Grahi (digestive and fecal carminative), medhya (intellect promoter), mutravirajaniya (normalize the urine color), varnya (complexion promoter), vishaghna (antidote).

Indications

Prameha (diabetes), daha (burning sensation), jwara (fever), trishna (thirst), vispota (blisters), visarpa (erysipelas), raktapitta (bleeding disorders).

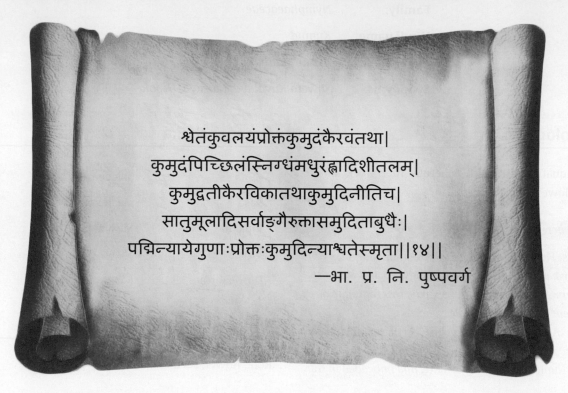

श्वेतंकुवलयंप्रोक्तंकुमुदंकैरवंतथा।
कुमुदंपिच्छिलंस्निग्धंमधुरंह्लादिशीतलम्।
कुमुद्वतीकैरविकातथाकुमुदिनीतिच।
सातुमूलादिसर्वाङ्गैरुक्तासमुदिताबुधैः।
पद्मिन्यायेगुणाःप्रोक्तःकुमुदिन्याश्चतेस्मृता।।१४।।
—भा. प्र. नि. पुष्पवर्ग

184. Kusha *[Desmostachya bipinnata (Linn.) Starf]*

Family:	*Poaceae*
Hindi name:	*Kushaa, Daabh*
English name:	*Halfa grass*
Synonyms:	*Yajnabhushana, Barhi, Kusha, Darbha, Suchyagra*

Morphology

A rhizomatous perennial grass of dry areas with an extensive system of rhizomes: 2 to 3 mm thick and 20 to 30 cm deep (**Fig. 184.1**).

Key Characters for Identification

➤ *Leaves: Coarse, narrow, tough, up to 50 cm long, 3 to 19 mm wide, ligule a very short ring of hairs, 1 to 2 mm. Culms with glossy yellow leaf sheaths at the base, up to 1 m high.*
➤ *Inflorescence: 30 to 60 cm long. Spikelets carried in two dense rows on short branches, 2 to 3 cm long arranged in whorls of 2 to 4 racemes. Individual spikelets 3 to 10 mm long, laterally compressed, comprising up to 14 florets. Glumes one-nerved, 1 to 2 mm long, lemmas 2 to 3 mm long, often purple (**Fig. 184.2**).*
➤ *Seed: Ovoid, 1 mm long, narrow, grooved.*

Rasapanchaka

Guna	Laghu, Snigdha
Rasa	Madhur, Kashaya
Vipaka	Madhura
Virya	Sheeta
Doshakarma	Tridoshahara

Officinal Part Used

Root

Dose

Decoction: 50 to 100 mL

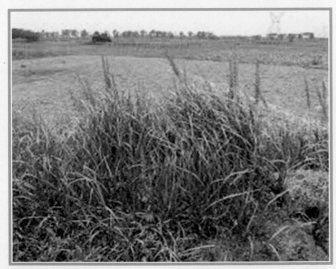

Fig. 184.1   Grass of *Desmostachya bipinnata* (Linn.) Starf.

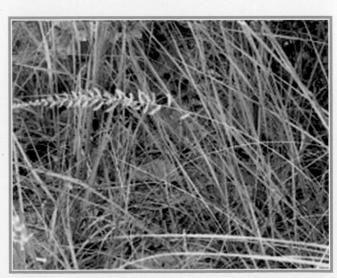

Fig. 184.2   Inflorescence.

Karma (Actions)

Stanyajanana (galactopoietic), mutra-virechaniya (diuretics).

Indications

Mutrkrichha (dysuria), ashmari (urinary calculus), pradara (menometrorrhagia), trishna (thirst), visarpa (erysipelas).

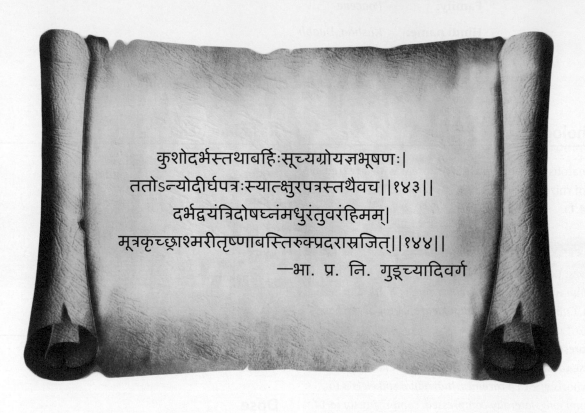

कुशोदर्भस्तथाबर्हिःसूच्यग्रोयज्ञभूषणः|
ततोऽन्योदीर्घपत्रःस्यात्क्षुरपत्रस्तथैवच||१४३||
दर्भद्वयंत्रिदोषघ्नंमधुरंतुवरंहिमम्|
मूत्रकृच्छ्राश्मरीतृष्णाबस्तिरुक्प्रदरास्रजित्||१४४||
—भा. प्र. नि. गुड्डच्यादिवर्ग

185. Kusmanda *[Benincasa hispida* (Thunb.) Cogn.]

Family:	*Cucurbitaceae*
Hindi name:	*Petha*
English name:	*Ash Gourd*
Synonyms:	*Puspaphala, Pitapuspa, Bruhatphala*

Morphology

It is an annual, tendrillar, branched, bristly climber up to 10 m in height. It may spread on the ground (**Fig. 185.1**).

Key Characters for Identification

➤ *Leaves: Hairy, alternate, simple, bristly, lamina broadly ovate-cordate in outline* (**Fig. 185.1**).
➤ *Flowers: Monoecious, axillary, yellow with both male and female varieties* (**Fig. 185.1**).
➤ *Fruits: A pepo, broadly oblong, rounded on both ends and without ribs, hairy* (**Fig. 185.2**).
➤ *Seed: Numerous imbedded in white flesh, ovoid, compressed, and marginate.*

Rasapanchaka

Guna	Laghu, Snigdha
Rasa	Madhur
Vipaka	Madhur
Virya	Sheeta
Doshakarma	Vatapittahara

Officinal Parts Used

Fruit and seed

Dose

Powder: 1 to 2 g

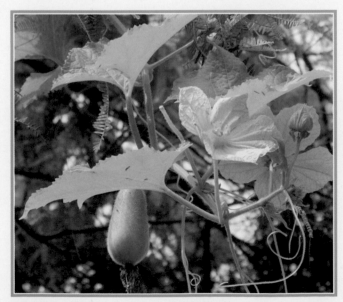

Fig. 185.1   Climber of *Benincasa hispida* (Thunb.) Cogn.

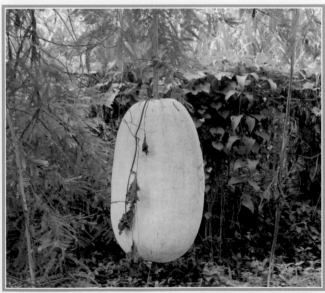

Fig. 185.2   Fruit.

Karma (Actions)

Brimhana (bulk promoting), vrisya (aphrodisiac), medhya (intellect promoter), vasthishodhan (urinary bladder cleansers/diuretics).

Indications

Raktapitta (bleeding disorders), raktavikar (diseases of blood), mutrakuchhra (dysuria), mutraghata (anuria/oliguria), trishna (thirst), apasmar (epilepsy).

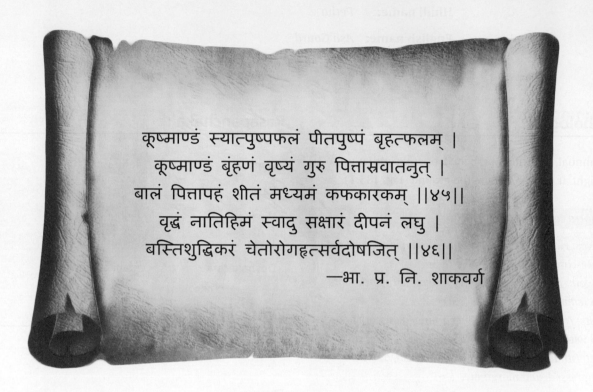

कूष्माण्डं स्यात्पुष्पफलं पीतपुष्पं बृहत्फलम् ।
कूष्माण्डं बृंहणं वृष्यं गुरु पित्तास्त्रवातनुत् ।
बालं पित्तापहं शीतं मध्यमं कफकारकम् ॥४५॥
वृद्धं नातिहिमं स्वादु सक्षारं दीपनं लघु ।
बस्तिशुद्धिकरं चेतोरोगहृत्सर्वदोषजित् ॥४६॥
—भा. प्र. नि. शाकवर्ग

186. Lajjalu *[Mimosa pudica Linn.]*

Family:	*Mimosaceae*
Hindi name:	*Lajwanti, Chhuimui*
English name:	*Touch me Not, Sensitive Plant*
Synonyms:	*Namaskari, Samanga, Shamipatra, Jalakarika, Raktapadi, Khadiraka*

Morphology

It is a perennial, ascending, spreading herb, or undershrub with pink flower (**Fig. 186.1**).

Key Characters for Identification

➤ *Leaves: Alternate, bipinnately compound; pinnae 1 to 2 pairs (**Fig. 186.2**).*
➤ *Flowers: Pink in axillary heads of about 1.5 cm in diameter (**Fig. 186.3**).*
➤ *Fruits: Flat, bristly and prickly along the sutures, brown in color (**Fig. 186.4**).*
➤ *Seed: Ovoid and compressed about 3 mm in diameter.*

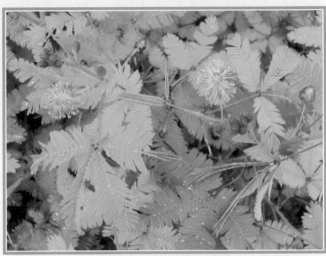

Fig. 186.1 Plant of *Mimosa pudica* Linn.

Rasapanchaka

Guna	Laghu, Ruksha
Rasa	Tikta, Kashaya
Vipaka	Katu
Virya	Sheeta
Doshakarma	Kaphapitta shamaka

Officinal Parts Used

Root and whole plant

Dose

Decoction: 50 to 100 mL
Juice: 10 to 20 mL

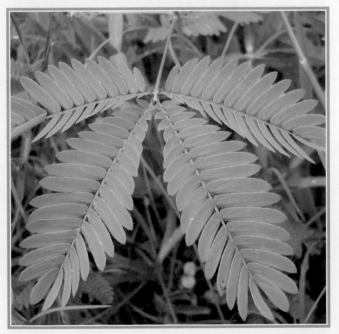

Fig. 186.2 Leaves.

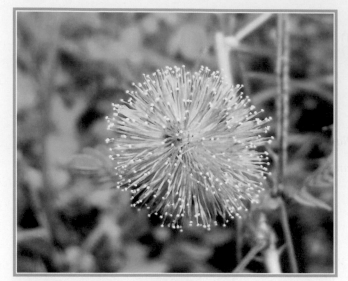

Fig. 186.3 Flower.

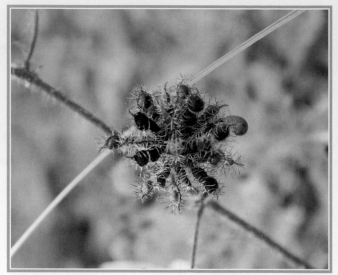

Fig. 186.4 Fruits.

Karma (Actions)

Sandhaniya (union of bone fracture), purisha sangrahaniya (fecal astringent).

Indications

Atisara (diarrhea), raktapitta (bleeding disorders), yoniroga (diseases of vagina), shwasa (asthma), kushta (skin disease), shotha (edema), vrana (wound).

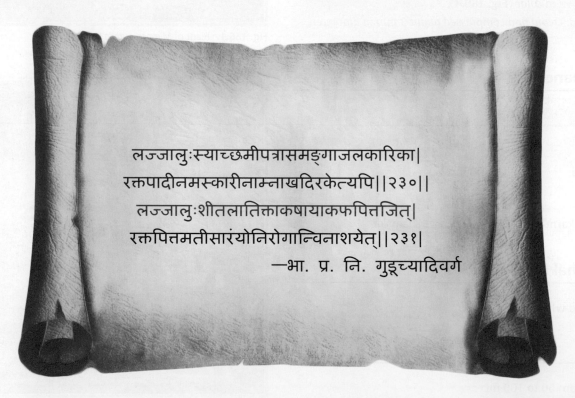

लज्जालुःस्याच्छमीपत्रासमङ्गाजलकारिका।
रक्तपादीनमस्कारीनाम्नाखदिरकेत्यपि॥२३०॥
लज्जालुःशीतलातिक्ताकषायाकफपित्तजित्।
रक्तपित्तमतीसारंयोनिरोगान्विनाशयेत्॥२३१॥
—भा. प्र. नि. गुडूच्यादिवर्ग

187. Langali *[Gloriosa superba Linn.]*

Family: *Liliaceae*

Hindi name: *Kalihari*

English name: *Malabar Glory Lily, Climbing Lily*

Synonyms: *Kalihari, Agnishikha, Sakrapuspi, Vishalya, Garbhanut, Halini, Vahnivaktra*

Morphology

It is a herbaceous climber 2 to 4 m long, perennial, plough-shaped (**Fig. 187.1**).

Key Characters for Identification

➤ *Leaves: Sessile, alternate, opposite, ternate, simple, and with a cordate base* (**Fig. 187.2**).
➤ *Flowers: Yellow or red or orange, axillary, solitary-subcorymbose* (**Fig. 187.3**).
➤ *Fruits: An oblong-ellipsoid, trilocular, torulose capsule of 5 to 6 cm long.*
➤ *Seed: Many, black, globose, and warty.*
➤ *Root/Rhizomes: Cylindrical brown root-stock* (**Fig. 187.4**).

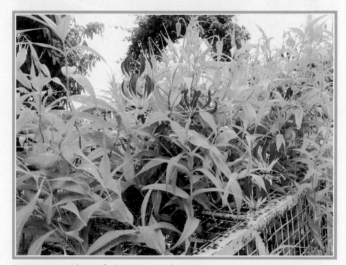

Fig. 187.1 Plant of *Gloriosa superba* Linn.

Rasapanchaka

Guna	Laghu, Tikshna
Rasa	Katu, Tikta
Vipaka	Katu
Virya	Ushna
Doshaghanta	Kaphahara, pittakara

Officinal Part Used

Rhizome

Dose

Powder: 250 to 500 mg

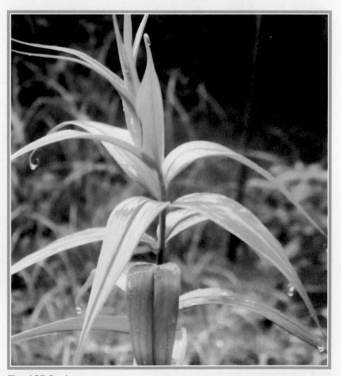

Fig. 187.2 Leaves.

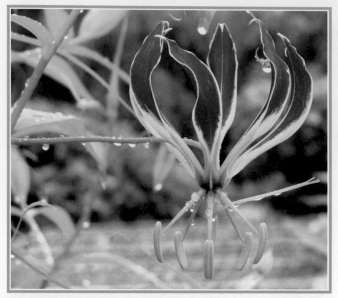

Fig. 187.3 Flower.

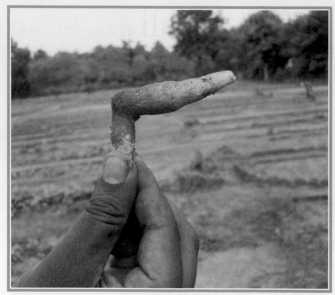

Fig. 187.4 Root.

Karma (Actions)

Sara (flowing in nature/mild purgative), garbhapatan (abortifacient), krimighna (anthelmintic), shoolaghna (antispasmodic).

Indications

Krimi (worm infestation), kushta (skin disease), shopha (edema), arsha (piles), shula (colic pain), vrana (wound).

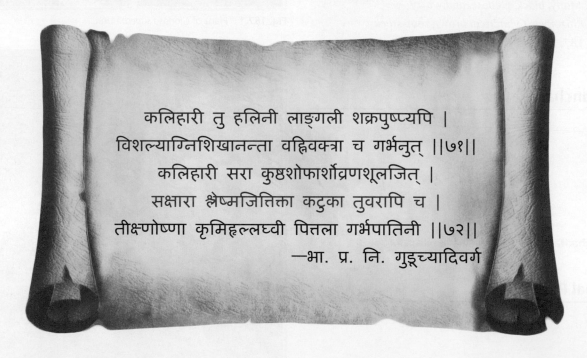

कलिहारी तु हलिनी लाङ्गली शक्रपुष्प्यपि |
विशल्याग्निशिखानन्ता वह्निवक्त्रा च गर्भनुत् ||७१||
कलिहारी सरा कुष्ठशोफार्शोव्रणशूलजित् |
सक्षारा श्लेष्मजित्तिका कटुका तुवरापि च |
तीक्ष्णोष्णा कृमिहृल्लघ्वी पित्तला गर्भपातिनी ||७२||
—भा. प्र. नि. गुडूच्यादिवर्ग

188. Latakaranja *[Caesalpinia bonduc (Linn.) Roxb.]*

Family:	*Caesalpiniaceae*
Hindi name:	*Kantakikaranja*
English name:	*Fever Nut, Physic Nut*
Synonyms:	*Putikaranja, Kantakikaranja, Kuberaksha*

Morphology

It is a profusely spinous, perennial, straggling shrub or climber around 4 to 6 m long (**Fig. 188.1**).

Key Characters for Identification

➤ *Leaves: Alternate, bipinnately compound, paripinnate, very large (***Fig. 188.2***).*
➤ *Flowers: Bright yellow, fulvous hairy, clawed petals, have around 10 free stamens (***Fig. 188.3***).*
➤ *Fruit: A shortly stalked ovate-oblong pod, initially green and turns brown at maturity, is covered with spines (***Fig. 188.4***).*
➤ *Seed: One or two per pod, subglobose-ovoid, hard, grayish (***Fig. 188.5***).*

Rasapanchaka

Guna	Laghu, Ruksha
Rasa	Tikta, Kashaya
Vipaka	Katu
Virya	Ushna
Doshakarma	Tridoshahara

Officinal Parts Used

Seed, leaf, root

Dose

Powder: 1 to 3 g
Juice: 10 to 20 mL

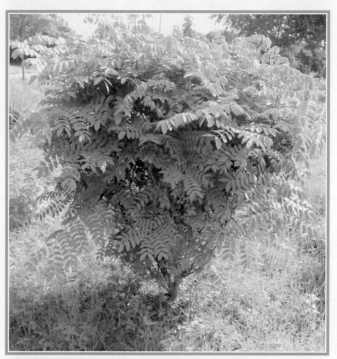

Fig. 188.1 Plant of *Caesalpinia bonduc* (Linn.) Roxb.

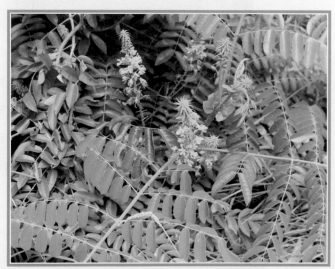

Fig. 188.2 Leaves.

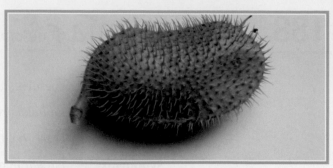

Fig. 188.4 Fruit

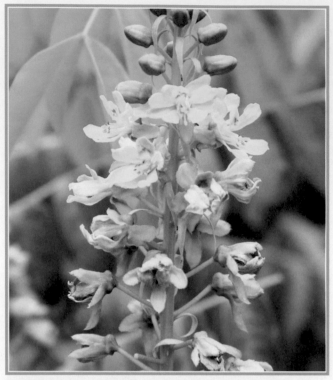

Fig. 188.3 Flower.

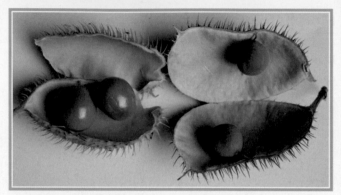

Fig. 188.5 Seeds inside the pod.

Karma (Actions)

Deepana (appetizer), sthambhan (astringent).

Indications

Shoola (colic pain), grahani (sprue), prameha (diabetes), kushta (skin disease), krimi (worm infestation), vishamajwara (intermittent fever), chhardi (vomiting), pittarsha (piles due to pitta).

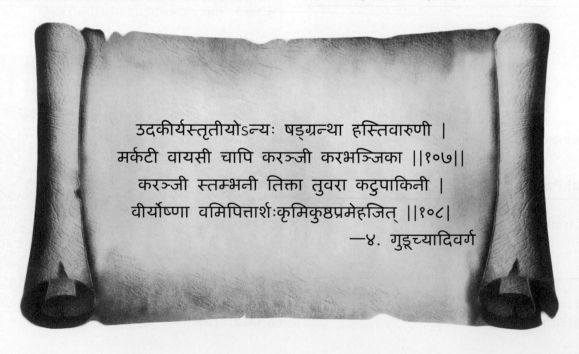

उदकीर्यस्तृतीयोऽन्यः षड्ग्रन्था हस्तिवारुणी ।
मर्कटी वायसी चापि करञ्जी करभञ्जिका ॥१०७॥
करञ्जी स्तम्भनी तिक्ता तुवरा कटुपाकिनी ।
वीर्योष्णा वमिपित्तार्शःकृमिकुष्ठप्रमेहजित् ॥१०८।
—४. गुडूच्यादिवर्ग

189. Latakasturi *[Abelmoschus moschatus (Linn.) Medik.]*

Family:	*Malvaceae*
Hindi name:	*Muskdana, Kasturidana*
English name:	*Musk Mallow, Ambrette Seed*
Synonyms:	*Latakasturika*

Morphology

It is an annual, erect herb or undershrub, 0.75 to 1.5 m tall (**Fig. 189.1**).

Key Characters for Identification

➤ *Leaves: Alternate, simple, polymorphous, dentate margins, bristly, hairy, long petiole* (**Fig. 189.2a, b**)

➤ *Flowers: Yellow with purple cetrate, axillary, solitary with long pedicle*

➤ *Fruits: Oblong lanceolate, 4 to 8 cm long capsule, dehisces into three locules* (**Fig. 189.3**)

➤ *Seed: Many, globose, giving musk-like odor on crushing*

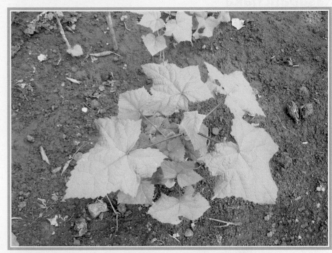

Fig. 189.1 Plant of *Abelmoschus moschatus* (Linn.) Medik.

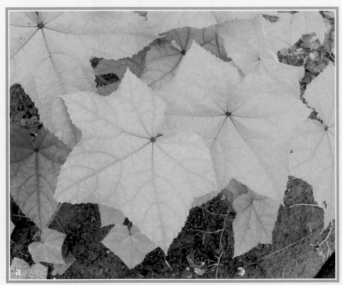
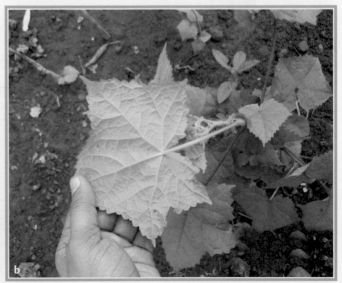

Fig. 189.2 **(a)** Leaves. **(b)** Leaves with hairy long petiole.

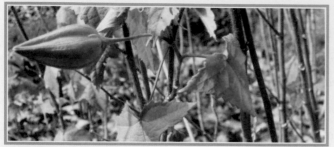

Fig. 189.3 Fruits.

Rasapanchaka

Guna	Laghu, Ruksha
Rasa	Tikta, Madhura
Vipaka	Katu
Virya	Sheeta
Doshakarma	Kaphapittahara

Officinal Part Used

Seed

Dose

Powder: 1 to 3 g

Karma (Actions)

Deepana (appetizer), chakshusya (beneficial for vision), vrishya (aphrodisiac), chhedan (expectorant).

Indications

Mutrakricchra (dysuria), trishna (thirst), mukharoga (disease of mouth), bastiroga (bladder disease).

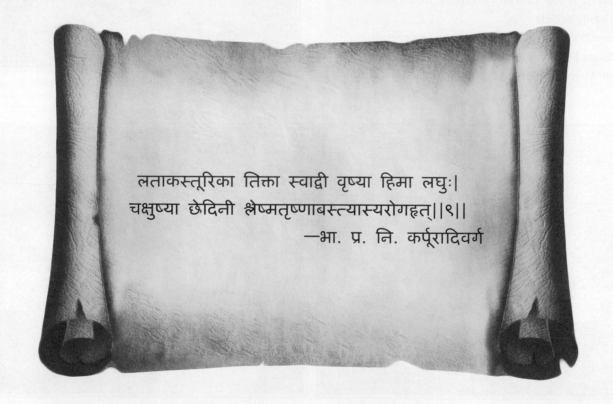

लताकस्तूरिका तिक्ता स्वाद्वी वृष्या हिमा लघुः।
चक्षुष्या छेदिनी श्रेष्मतृष्णाबस्त्यास्यरोगहृत्।।९।।
—भा. प्र. नि. कर्पूरादिवर्ग

190. Madyantika *[Lawsonia inermis Linn.]*

Family:	*Lythraceae*
Hindi name:	*Mehendi*
English name:	*Henna shrub*
Synonyms:	*Modaganti*

Morphology

It is either a large shrub (or sometimes even small), 2 to 8 m tall; twigs spinescent (**Fig. 190.1**).

Key Characters for Identification

➤ *Leaves: Opposite, simple, elliptic-obovate-lanceolate* (**Fig. 190.2**).
➤ *Flowers: Dirty white, sweet-scented, terminal, panicled racemes* (**Fig. 190.3**).
➤ *Fruits: Globose capsules, dehiscing irregularly* (**Fig. 190.4**).
➤ *Seed: Many, trigono-pyramidal in shape.*

Rasapanchaka

Guna	Laghu, Ruksha
Rasa	Tikta, Kashaya
Vipaka	Katu
Virya	Sheeta
Doshakarma	Kaphapittahara

Officinal Parts Used

Flower, leaf, seed

Dose

Powder: 1 to 3 g
Juice: 5 to 10 mL

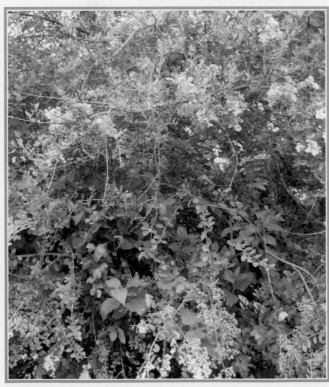

Fig. 190.1   Plant of *Lawsonia inermis* Linn.

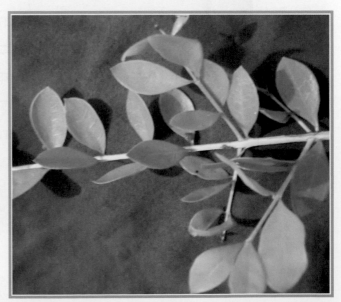

Fig. 190.2   Leaves.

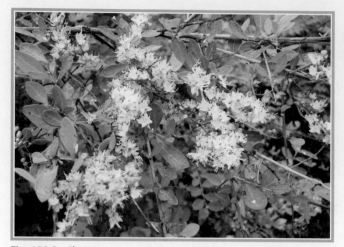

Fig. 190.3 Flowers.

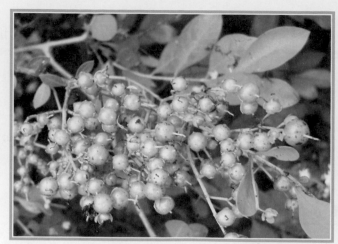

Fig. 190.4 Fruits.

Karma (Actions)

Kandughna (antipruritus), kushtaghna (antileprotic).

Indications

Kushta (skin disease), kandu (pruritus), kamala (jaundice), raktatisara (diarrhea with blood), mutrakrichha (dysuria), apashmar (epilepsy), vrana (wound), hridroga (heart disease), jwara (fever), daha (burning sensation), raktapitta (bleeding disorders), brahma (vertigo).

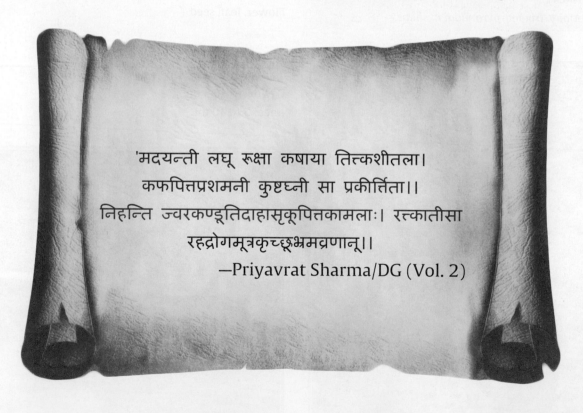

'मदयन्ती लघू रूक्षा कषाया तित्कशीतला।
कफपित्तप्रशमनी कुष्टघ्नी सा प्रकीर्त्तिता॥
निहन्ति ज्वरकण्डूतिदाहासृकूपित्तकामलाः। रत्कातीसा
रहद्रोगमूत्रकृच्छूभ्रमव्रणान्॥
—Priyavrat Sharma/DG (Vol. 2)

191. Mahanimba [*Melia azedarach* Linn.]

Family: *Meliaceae*

Hindi name: *Bakayan*

English name: *Persian Lilac, Bead Tree*

Synonyms: *Mahapichumarda, Vishamustika, Parvatanimba, Ramyaka, Drekka*

Morphology

It is a tree, 10 to 15 m tall. Its trunk is thick, and it has grayish-brown bark with vertical fissures (**Fig. 191.1**).

Key Characters for Identification

➤ *Leaves: Alternate, bipinnately-tripinnately compound, imparipinnate (**Fig. 191.2**).*
➤ *Flowers: Inflorescence in axillary panicled cymes; flowers lilac-bluish white (**Fig. 191.3**).*
➤ *Fruits: Subglobose drupes, greenish, turning pale yellow when ripe (**Fig. 191.4**).*
➤ *Seed: Five-celled, bony, and shallowed furrowed.*
➤ *Bark: Dark grayish brown color with plenty of lenticels (**Fig. 191.5**).*

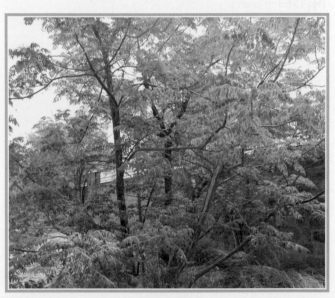

Fig. 191.1 Plant of *Melia azedarach* Linn.

Rasapanchaka

Guna	Laghu, Ruksha
Rasa	Katu, Tikta, Kashaya
Vipaka	Katu
Virya	Ushna
Doshakarma	Kaphapittahara

Officinal Parts Used

Root, leaf, seed

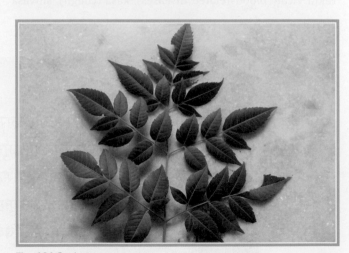

Fig. 191.2 Leaves.

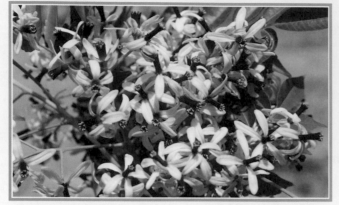

Fig. 191.3   Flowers.

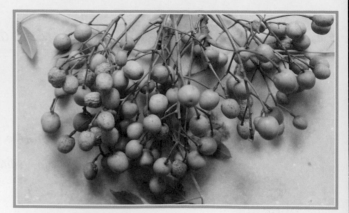

Fig. 191.4   Fruits.

Dose

Decoction: 50 to 100 mL
Powder: 3 to 6 g

Karma (Actions)

Kusthaghna (antileprotic), vranashodhan (wound cleanser), vrananropan (wound healing), krimihara (anthelmintic), raktadoshahara (blood purifier).

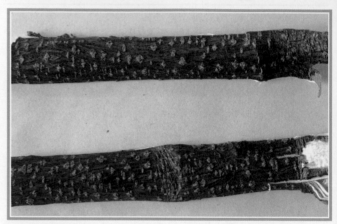

Fig. 191.5   Bark.

Indications

Kushta (skin diseases), hrillasa (nausea), prameha (diabetes), rakta vicar (blood-related diseases), kasa (cough), shwasa (asthma), gulma (abdominal lump), arsha (piles), mushika visha (rat poisoning), chhardi (vomiting), brahma (vertigo).

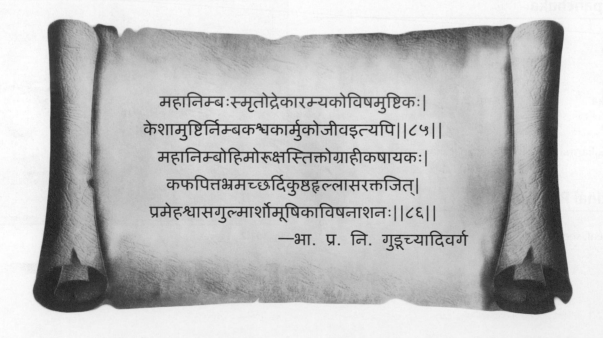

महानिम्बःस्मृतोद्रेकारम्यकोविषमुष्टिकः।
केशामुष्टिर्निम्बकश्चकार्मुकोजीवइत्यपि॥८५॥
महानिम्बोहिमोरूक्षस्तिक्तोग्राहीकषायकः।
कफपित्तभ्रमच्छर्दिकुष्ठहृल्लासरक्तजित्।
प्रमेहश्वासगुल्मार्शोमूषिकाविषनाशनः॥८६॥
—भा. प्र. नि. गुड़ूच्यादिवर्ग

192. Markandika *[Cassia angustifolia Vahl.]*

Family:	*Fabaceae*
Hindi name:	*Sonapatha*
English name:	*Mecca Senna*
Synonyms:	*Bhumivalli, Markandi, Mridurechani, Sonamaki*

Morphology

It is an erect, perennial herb or undershrub, 0.5 to 1.5 m tall (**Fig. 192.1**).

Key Characters for Identification

➤ *Leaves: Alternate, paripinnately compound; leaflets five to eight pairs, elliptic-lanceolate* (**Fig. 192.2**).
➤ *Flowers: Yellow, 1.5 cm across, in terminal racemes* (**Fig. 192.3**).
➤ *Fruits: An oblong, flat, curved pod, greenish-yellow when young, blackish when dry* (**Fig. 192.4**).
➤ *Seed: Four to eight in number, compressed and heart-shaped.*

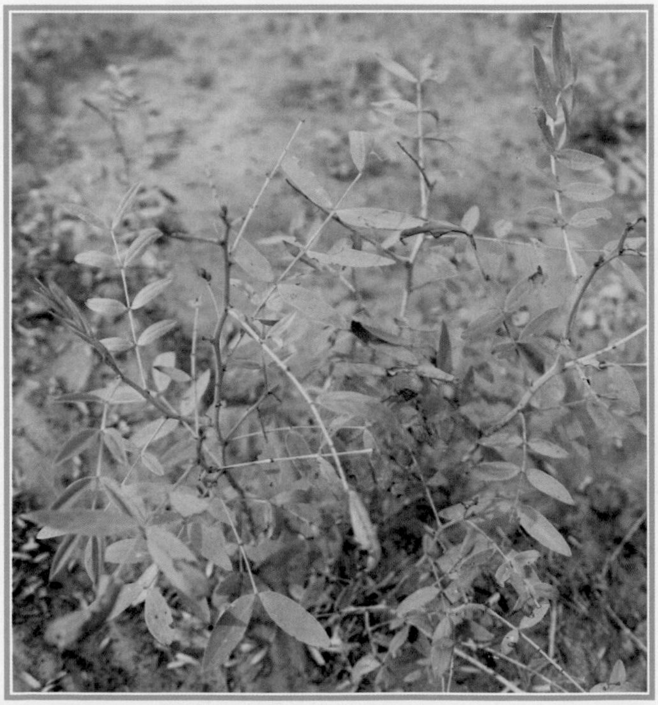

Rasapanchaka

Guna	Ruksha
Rasa	Tikta, Kashaya
Vipaka	Katu
Virya	Ushna
Doshakarma	Vatakaphahara

Officinal Parts Used

Leaf and fruit

Dose

Powder: 3 to 6 g

Fig. 192.1   Plant of *Cassia angustifolia* Vahl.

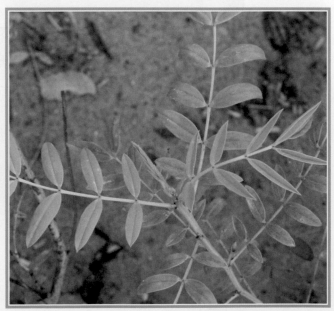

Fig. 192.2   Leaves.

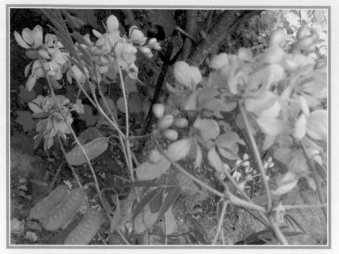

Fig. 192.3 Flowers.

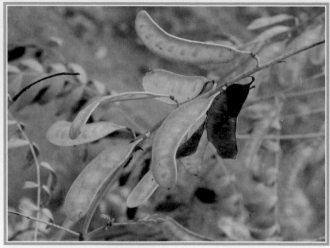

Fig. 192.4 Pods.

Karma (Actions)

Vamak (induce vomiting), rechaka (purgative), kasaghni (anticough).

Indications

Kushta (skin disease), krimi (worm infestation), udara (abdominal diseases), gulma (abdominal lump), kasa (cough), visha (poisoning), durgandha (foul smelling).

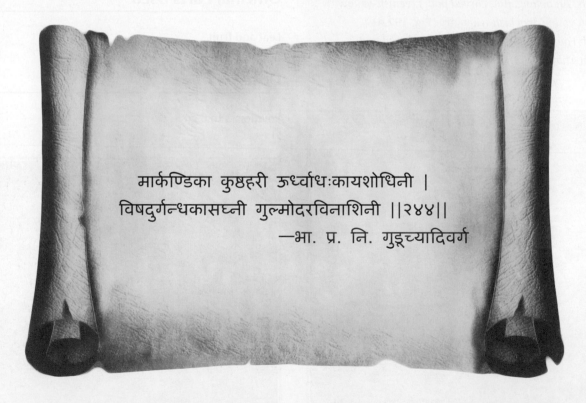

मार्कण्डिका कुष्ठहरी ऊर्ध्वाधःकायशोधिनी ।
विषदुर्गन्धकासघ्नी गुल्मोदरविनाशिनी ।।२४४।।
—भा. प्र. नि. गुडूच्यादिवर्ग

193. Masha *[Phaseolus mungo Linn.]*

Family:	*Fabaceae*
Hindi name:	*Udad, Udid, Urdi*
English name:	*Black gram*
Synonyms:	*Masha*

Morphology

It is an erect, fast-growing, annual, herbaceous legume reaching 30 to 100 cm in height. It has a well-developed taproot and its stems are diffusely branched from the base. Occasionally, it has a twining habit and is generally pubescent.

Key Characters for Identification

➤ *Leaves: The leaves are trifoliate with ovate leaflets, 4 to 10 cm long and 2 to 7 cm wide.*
➤ *Flowers: The inflorescence is borne at the extremity of a long (up to 18 cm) peduncle and bears yellow, small, papilionaceous flowers.*
➤ *Fruits: Cylindrical, erect pod, 4 to 7 cm long × 0.5 cm broad. The pod is hairy and has a short-hooked beak. It contains 4 to 10 ellipsoid, black, or mottled seeds.*

Rasapanchaka

Guna	Snigdha, Guru
Rasa	Madhur
Vipaka	Madhur
Virya	Ushna
Doshakarma	Vatashamak kaphapittakaraka

Officinal Part Used

Seeds

Dose

Powder: 3 to 6 g

Karma (Actions)

Balya (physical strength promoter), vrishya (aphrodisiac), brimhana (bulk promoter), sransan (purgative), tarpan (nourishment), rechan (purgative), mutral (diuretic), sthanyajanana (galactogague), medavardhak (intellect promoter).

Indications

Gudakila (hemorrhoid), ardita (facial paralysis), shwasa (asthma), pakti shola (colic), anidra (insomnia), vatavyadhi (neurological disorders).

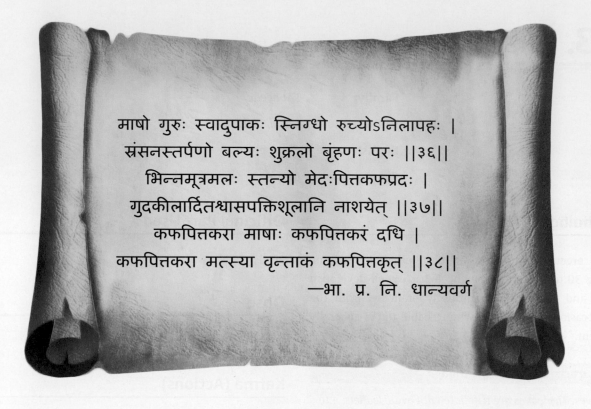

माषो गुरुः स्वादुपाकः स्निग्धो रुच्योऽनिलापहः |
संसनस्तर्पणो बल्यः शुक्लो बृंहणः परः ||३६||
भिन्नमूत्रमलः स्तन्यो मेदःपित्तकफप्रदः |
गुदकीलार्दितश्वासपक्तिशूलानि नाशयेत् ||३७||
कफपित्तकरा माषाः कफपित्तकरं दधि |
कफपित्तकरा मत्स्या वृन्ताकं कफपित्तकृत् ||३८||

—भा. प्र. नि. धान्यवर्ग

194. Mashparni *[Teramnus labialis* (Linn.f.) Spreng.*]*

Family:	*Fabaceae*
Hindi name:	*Mashparni, Mashvan, Banudad, Mashoni, Vana udad*
English name:	*Vogel-Tephrosis, Blue Wiss, Horse vine, Rabbit vine*
Synonyms:	*Mahasaha, Kamboji, Krishnavrinta, Hayapuchikka, Suryasani, Mahasaha, Pandutomasa*

Morphology

It is a perennial, spreading, twining, hairy herb, 2 to 6 m long with red-, pink-, purple-, or white-colored flower.

Key Characters for Identification

➤ *Leaves: Alternate, 3-foliolate, obovate-lanceolate in terminal, lateral ones unequal-sided at base.*
➤ *Flowers: Reddish-purple, 2 to 3 mm long, weak, lax axillary racemes.*
➤ *Fruits: A linear, flat, pod with shortly bent tip.*
➤ *Seed: Five to nine, oblong, and smooth.*

Rasapanchaka

Guna	Laghu, Snigdha
Rasa	Madhura, Tikta
Vipaka	Madhura
Virya	Sheeta
Doshakarma	Vattapittahara

Officinal Parts Used

Whole plant and root

Dose

Decoction: 40 to 80 mL
Powder: 3 to 6 g

Karma (Actions)

Grahi (digestive and fecal astringent), balya (strength promoter), shukral (spermatogenetic), jeevaniya (vitality).

Indications

Shotha (edema), jwara (fever), raktapitta (bleeding disorder), daha (burning sensation), atisara (diarrhea), pravahika (dysentery, vatapitta jvara (fever caused due to vatapitta), shukralpata (semen deficit), raktavikara (blood-related diseases), shirashoola (headache).

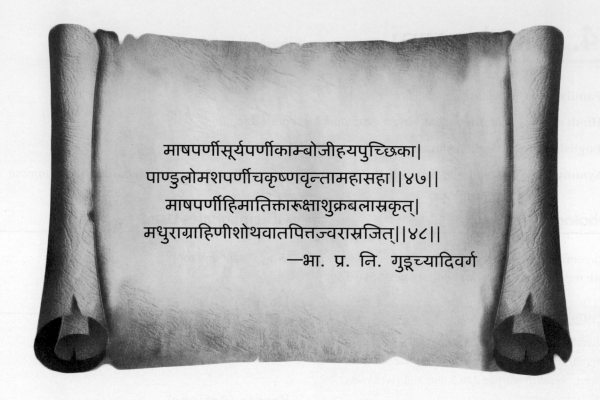

माषपर्णीसूर्यपर्णीकाम्बोजीहयपुच्छिका।
पाण्डुलोमशपर्णीचकृष्णवृन्तामहासहा।।४७।।
माषपर्णीहिमातिक्तारूक्षाशुक्रबलास्रकृत्।
मधुराग्राहिणीशोथवातपित्तज्वरास्रजित्।।४८।।

—भा. प्र. नि. गुड्ूच्यादिवर्ग

195. Matulunga *[Citrus medica Linn.]*

Family:	*Rutaceae*
Hindi name:	*Bijora nimbu*
English name:	*Citron, The lemon of India, Lemon*
Synonyms:	*Bijapura, Ruchak, Phalapurak*

Morphology

It is a straggling bush or small tree, 3 to 4 m high with thorny branches (**Fig. 195.1**).

Key Characters for Identification

➤ *Leaves: Simple, coriaceous, winged petiole, elliptic or oblong, dark green* (**Fig. 195.2**).
➤ *Flowers: Scented, white, occurs in axillary cymes* (**Fig. 195.3**).
➤ *Fruits: Oblong-globose berries, fleshy, rough warty surface, thick rind, yellow when ripe* (**Fig. 195.4**).

Rasapanchaka

Guna	Laghu, Snigdha
Rasa	Amla, Madhur
Vipaka	Amla
Virya	Ushna
Doshakarma	Vatakaphahara

Officinal Part Used

Fruits

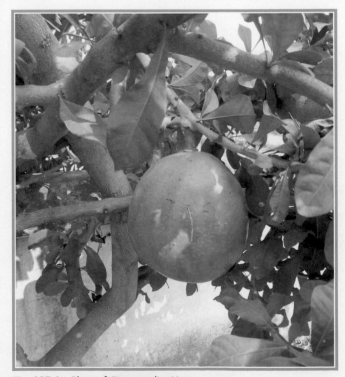

Fig. 195.1　Plant of *Citrus medica* Linn.

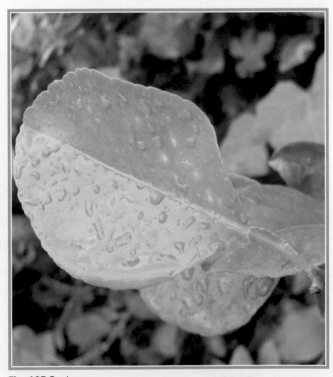

Fig. 195.2　Leaves.

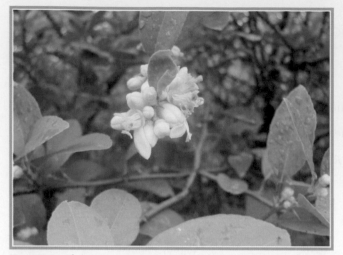

Fig. 195.3 Flower.

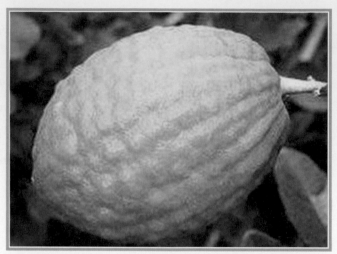

Fig. 195.4 Fruit.

Dose

Powder: 6 to 12 g

Karma (Actions)

Hridya (cardiac tonic), deepan (appetizer), pachan (digestive), kanthashodhan (clearance of throat), jihvashodhan (cleaning/purification of tongue).

Indications

Shwasa (asthma), kasa (cough), raktapitta (bleeding disorders), aruchi (distaste), trishna (thirst), hridayaroga (heart diseases), agnimandya (dyspepsia), chardi (vomiting), krimi (worm infestation), vibandha (constipation), vatikashoola (neuralgic pain), udararoga (abdominal disorders), vishuchika (cholera).

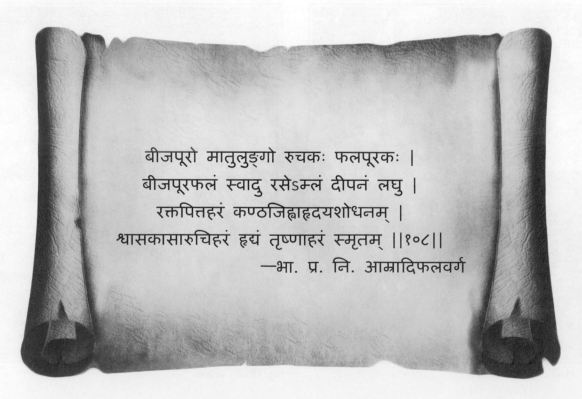

बीजपूरो मातुलुङ्गो रुचकः फलपूरकः |
बीजपूरफलं स्वादु रसेऽम्लं दीपनं लघु |
रक्तपित्तहरं कण्ठजिह्वाहृदयशोधनम् |
श्वासकासारुचिहरं हृद्यं तृष्णाहरं स्मृतम् ||१०८||
—भा. प्र. नि. आम्रादिफलवर्ग

196. Mayaphal [*Quercus leucotrichophora A.Camus or Quercus incana Roxb.*]

Family:	*Fagaceae*
Hindi name:	*Majuphal*
English name:	*Gray Oak, White Oak*
Synonyms:	*Mayuka, Majja Phala, Mayika, Mayiphala, Chhidraphala*

Morphology

Evergreen tree, 15 to 20 m high, all parts coated with white tomentum.

Key Characters for Identification

➤ *Leaves: Alternate, simple, elliptic-lanceolate with serrate margins, acuminate.*
➤ *Flowers: Whitish, monoecious, male in axillary, female solitary or in clusters.*
➤ *Fruits: A conico-ovoid nut, half of it embraced by a cup.*
➤ *Gall: Globose with elevated warts, 10 to 15 mm in diameter, heavy, initially bluish-gray in color and later green, and finally whitish-brown (**Fig. 196.1**).*

Rasapanchaka

Guna	Laghu, Ruksha
Rasa	Kashaya
Vipaka	Katu
Virya	Sheeta
Doshakarma	Kapha pittahara

Officinal Part Used

Gall

Dose

Powder: 1 to 3 g

Karma (Actions)

Grahi (fecal astringent), deepana (appetizer).

Indications

Atisara (diarrhea), grahani (sprue/IBS), pravahika (dysentric), shweta pradara (leucoria), arshas (piles), mukha danta roga (mouth and teeth diseases), yoni kanda (Bartholin cysts or abscess).

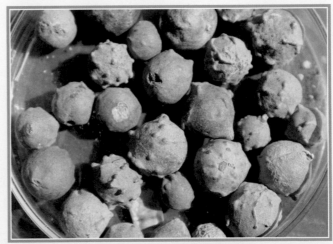

Fig. 196.1 Gall of *Quercus leucotrichophora* A.Camus.

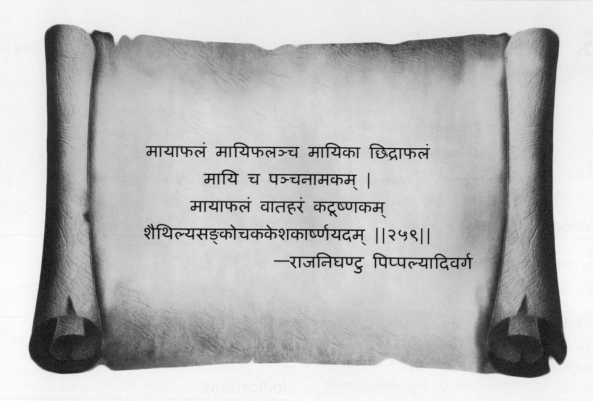

मायाफलं मायिफलञ्च मायिका छिद्राफलं
मायि च पञ्चनामकम् |
मायाफलं वातहरं कटूष्णकम्
शैथिल्यसङ्कोचककेशकार्ष्ण्ययदम् ||२५९||
—राजनिघण्टु पिप्पल्यादिवर्ग

197. Meshashringi *[Gymnema sylvestre (Retz.) R.Br.ex Schult.]*

Family:	*Asclepiadaceae*
Hindi name:	*Gudmar, Meshingi*
English name:	*Periploca of the woods*
Synonyms:	*Vishani, Meshavalli, Ajashringika*

Morphology

It is a perennial climber, 4 to 10 m long; main stem becomes woody on aging, and latex is milky (**Fig. 197.1**).

Key Characters for Identification

➤ *Leaves: Opposite, simple, ovate-lanceolate, thin, less hairy (**Fig. 197.2**).*
➤ *Flowers: Flowers 2 to 3.5 mm across, yellow, star-shaped (**Fig. 197.3**).*
➤ *Fruits: A pair of cylindrical, 4–8 × 0.4–0.7 cm follicles.*
➤ *Seed: Many, flat, ovate with a tuft of long hair at pointed end.*

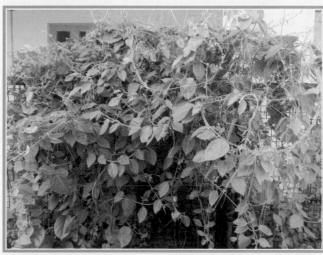

Fig. 197.1   Climber of *Gymnema sylvestre* (Retz.) R.Br.ex Schult.

Rasapanchaka

Guna	Laghu, Ruksha
Rasa	Tikta, Kashya
Vipaka	Katu
Virya	Ushna
Doshakarma	Kaphapittahara

Officinal Parts Used

Root and leaf

Dose

Decoction: 50 to 100 mL
Powder: 3 to 6 g

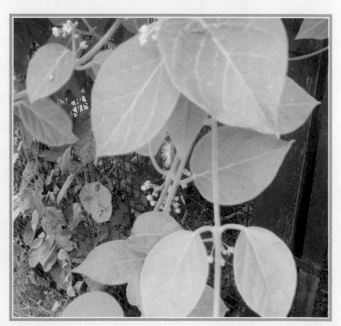

Fig. 197.2   Leaves.

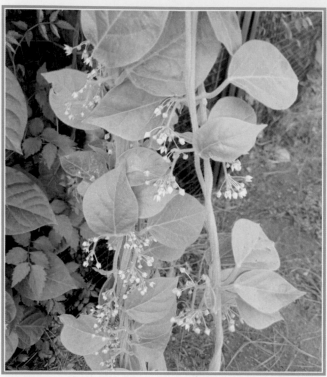

Fig. 197.3 Flowers.

Karma (Actions)

Deepana (appetizer), samsramana (laxative), krimighna (anthelmintic), mehaghna (antidiabetic), kushtaghna (antileprotic).

Indications

Kushta (skin disease), prameha (diabetes), kasa (cough), shwasa (asthma), krimi (worm infestation), vrana (wound), visha (poisoning), akshishoola (ocular pain), pitta vrana (wound due to pain).

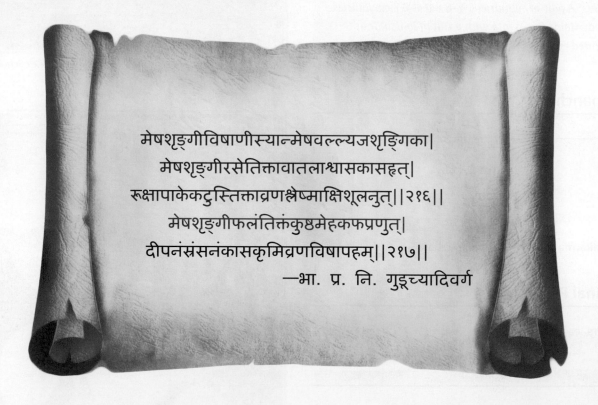

मेषशृङ्गीविषाणीस्यान्मेषवल्ल्यजशृङ्गिका।
मेषशृङ्गीरसेतिक्तावातलाश्वासकासहृत्।
रूक्षापाकेकटुस्तिक्ताव्रणश्लेष्माक्षिशूलनुत्॥२१६॥
मेषशृङ्गीफलंतिक्तंकुष्ठमेहकफप्रणुत्।
दीपनंस्रंसनंकासकृमिव्रणविषापहम्॥२१७॥
—भा. प्र. नि. गुडूच्यादिवर्ग

198. Methika *[Trigonella foenum-graecum Linn.]*

Family:	*Fabaceae*
Hindi name:	*Methi*
English name:	*Fenugreek*
Synonyms:	*Methi, Pittabeeja, Bahuptrika, Bahu beeja, Chandrika, Kairavi, Deepani*

Morphology

It is an aromatic, 30 to 60 cm tall, annual herb (**Fig. 198.1**).

Key Characters for Identification

➤ *Leaves: Trifoliolate, leaflets obovate-oblanceolate with entire margins (**Fig. 198.2**).*
➤ *Flowers: Pale yellow, axillary, solitary, or in pairs.*
➤ *Fruits: An elongate pod with a long beak.*
➤ *Seed: 15 to 20 in number, yellowish or light brown, somewhat quadrangular in outline (**Fig. 198.3**).*

Rasapanchaka

Guna	Laghu, Snigdha
Rasa	Katu
Vipaka	Katu
Virya	Ushna
Doshakarma	Vatakaphashamak

Officinal Parts Used

Seed and whole plant

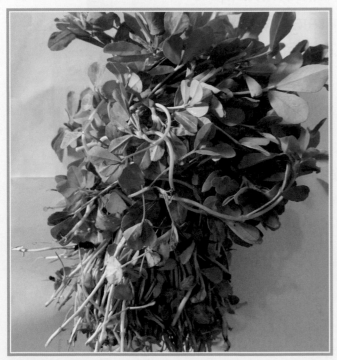

Fig. 198.1 Plants of *Trigonella foenum-graecum* Linn.

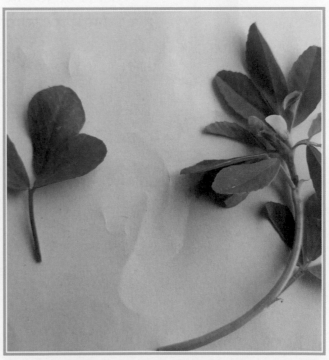

Fig. 198.2 Leaves.

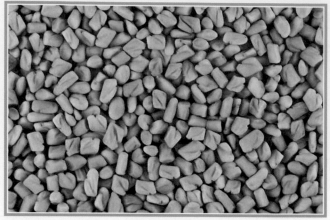

Fig. 198.3 Seeds.

Dose

Powder: 1 to 3 g

Karma (Actions)

Deepan (appetizer), raktapittakarak (aggravate rakta and pitta), kaphahara (pacify kapha), rucya (relish), vatahara (pacify vata dosha).

Indications

Aruchi (distaste), jwara (fever), shoola (pain), grahani (IBS), prameha (diabetes).

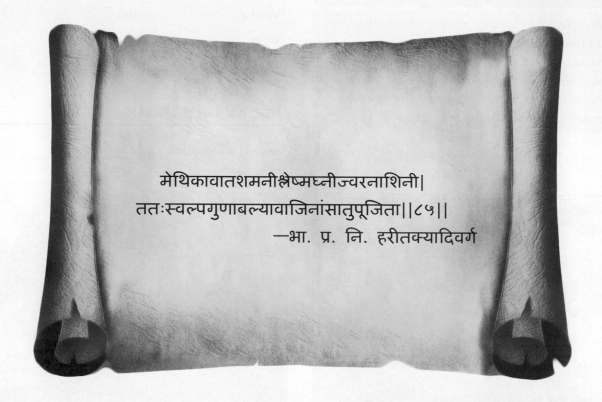

मेथिकावातशमनीक्ष्लेष्मघ्नीज्वरनाशिनी।
ततःस्वल्पगुणाबल्यावाजिनांसातुपूजिता॥८५॥
—भा. प्र. नि. हरीतक्यादिवर्ग

199. Mudgaparni [*Phaseolus trilobus* Ait., non Linn. *or Vigna trilobata* (Linn.) Verdc.]

Family:	*Fabaceae*
Hindi name:	*Mat, Mukni, Jangli mung, Mugavan*
English name:	*Mat Bean*
Synonyms:	*Kshudrasaha, Kakaparni, Suryaparni, Alpika, Saha, Kakamudga*

Morphology

It is a trailing annual-perennial herb; stems are wiry, many from woody root stock, is 0.5 to 1 m long (**Fig. 199.1**).

Key Characters for Identification

➤ *Leaves: Alternate, three-foliate; leaflets 1.5 to 3 cm, three-lobed, entire, glabrous* (**Fig. 199.2**).
➤ *Flowers: Yellow, in subcapitate racemes on a peduncle* (**Fig. 199.3**).
➤ *Fruits: A straight, subcylindric, glabrous, or sparingly hairy pod, 2 to 5 cm long and 3 mm in diameter.*
➤ *Seeds: Six to twelve in number, black coloured, 2 to 2.5 mm long, and truncate at the ends.*

Rasapanchaka

Guna	Laghu, Ruksha
Rasa	Madhura
Vipaka	Madhura
Virya	Sheeta
Doshakarma	Tridoshahara

Officinal Parts Used

Root and whole plant

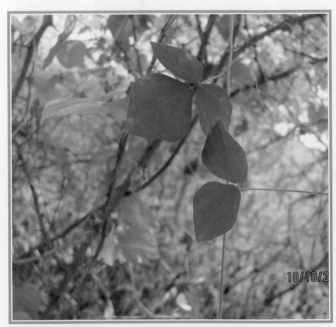

Fig. 199.1 Plant of *Phaseolus trilobus* Ait., non Linn.

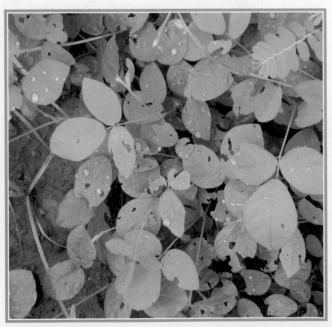

Fig. 199.2 Leaves.

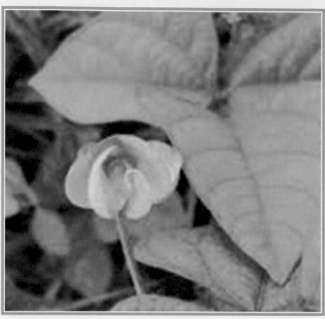

Fig. 199.3 Flower.

Dose

Decoction: 50 to 100 mL
Powder: 3 to 6 g

Karma (Actions)

Shukrajanana (spermatogenesis), chakshushya (beneficial for vision), grahi (digestive and fecal astringent), shothaghni (anti-inflammatory), jwaraghna (antipyretics), jeevaniya (vitality).

Indications

Grahani (sprue), atisara (diarrhea), arshas (piles), jwara (fever), daha (burning sensation), shotha (edema), kashaya (emaciation), vatarakta (gout).

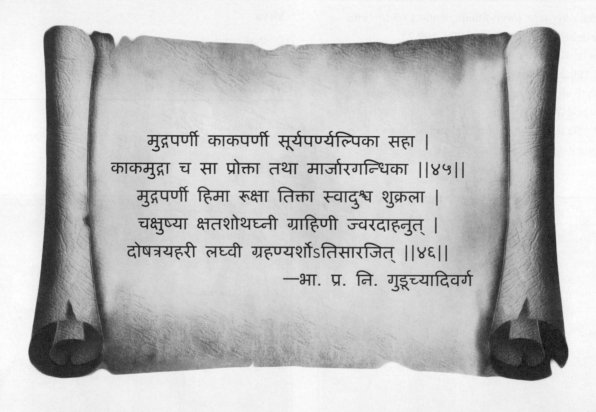

मुद्रपर्णी काकपर्णी सूर्यपर्ण्यल्पिका सहा |
काकमुद्रा च सा प्रोक्ता तथा मार्जारगन्धिका ||४५||
मुद्रपर्णी हिमा रूक्षा तिक्ता स्वादुश्च शुक्रला |
चक्षुष्या क्षतशोथघ्नी ग्राहिणी ज्वरदाहनुत् |
दोषत्रयहरी लघ्वी ग्रहण्यर्शोऽतिसारजित् ||४६||
—भा. प्र. नि. गुडूच्यादिवर्ग

200. Mulaka *[Raphanus sativus Linn.]*

Family:	*Cruciferae*
Hindi name:	*Muli*
English name:	*Radish*
Synonyms:	*Marusambhava, Chanakyamulaka*

Morphology

It is an erect annual-biennial herb, 0.25 to 1 m tall (**Fig. 200.1**).

Key Characters for Identification

➤ *Leaves: Radical, simple; lamina oblanceolate in outline, lyrate with pinnatisect and dentate lobes; cauline leaves linear oblong (**Fig. 200.2**).*

➤ *Flowers: White or tinged with pink, in terminal racemes of 10 to 15 cm long (**Fig. 200.3**).*

➤ *Fruits: An elongate siliqua of 2.5 to 5 cm long and 0.6 to 8 cm thick.*

➤ *Seed: Two to six, ovoid, about 3 mm in diameter, reddish-brown (**Fig. 200.4**).*

➤ *Root/Rhizomes: White, tap root tuberous, fleshy, 15 to 40 cm long and 5 to 10 cm thick (**Fig. 200.5**).*

Rasapanchaka

Guna	Laghu
Rasa	Tikta, Katu
Vipaka	Katu
Virya	Ushna
Doshakarma	Tridoshahara

Officinal Parts Used

Root, seed, leaf

Dose

Decoction: 50 to 100 mL
Juice: 10 to 20 mL

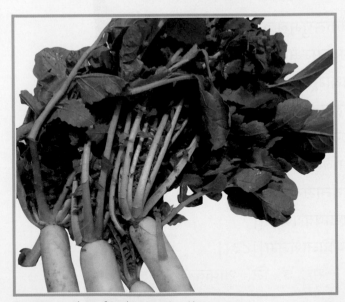

Fig. 200.1   Plant of *Raphanus sativus* Linn.

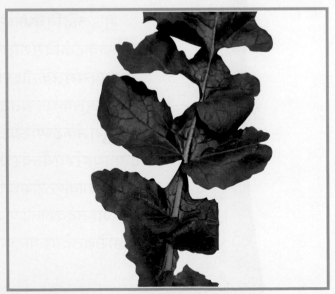

Fig. 200.2   Leaves.

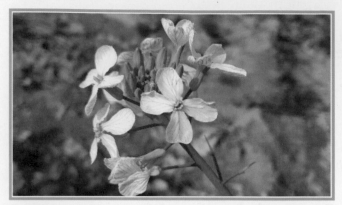

Fig. 200.3 Flowers.

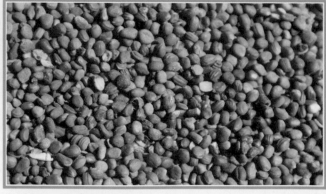

Fig. 200.4 Seeds.

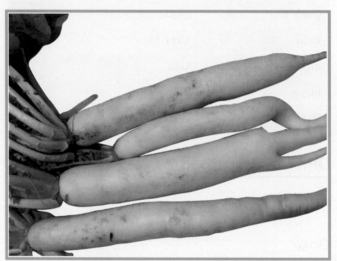

Fig. 200.5 Roots.

Karma (Actions)

Pachan (digestive), deepana (appetizer), grahi (fecal astringent), swarya (beneficial voice).

Indications

Shwasa (asthma), kasa (cough), jwara (fever), arsha (piles), gulma (abdominal lump), shoola (colic pain), nasika-kantha and netra vyadhi (ear-nose-eye disease).

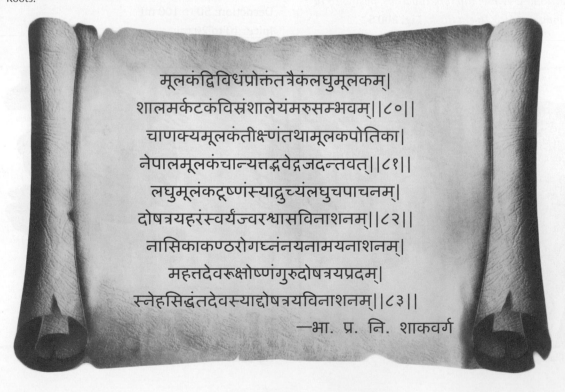

मूलकंद्विविधंप्रोक्तंत्रैकंलघुमूलकम्।
शालमर्कटकंविसंशालेयंमरुसम्भवम्॥८०॥
चाणक्यमूलकंतीक्ष्णंतथामूलकपोतिका।
नेपालमूलकंचान्यत्तद्वेद्रजदन्तवत्॥८१॥
लघुमूलंकटूष्णंस्याद्रुच्यंलघुचपाचनम्।
दोषत्रयहरंस्वर्यंज्वरश्वासविनाशनम्॥८२॥
नासिकाकण्ठरोगघ्नंनयनामयनाशनम्।
महत्तदेवरूक्षोष्णंगुरुदोषत्रयप्रदम्।
स्नेहसिद्धंतदेवस्याद्दोषत्रयविनाशनम्॥८३॥
—भा. प्र. नि. शाकवर्ग

201. Murva *[Marsdenia tenacissima Wight & Arn]*

Family: *Asclepiadaceae*

Hindi name: *Maruabel*

English name: *Rajmahal Hemp*

Synonyms: *Madhurasa, Devi, Morata, Tejani, Sruva, Madhulikha, Madhushreni, Gokarni, Piluparni, Tiktavalli.*

Morphology

It is a perennial straggler, 10 to 30 m long; velvety-hairy, latex milky (**Fig. 201.1**).

Key Characters for Identification

➤ *Leaves: Simple, opposite, broadly ovate, deeply cordate at base, 3 to 6 inch long and 3 to 4 inch wide, velvety-hairy with entire margins, acute-acuminate apex (**Fig. 201.2**).*
➤ *Flowers: Green or yellowish-green with linear corona and erect pollinia.*
➤ *Fruits: A pair of ovate-oblong, divaricate, and terete follicles.*
➤ *Seeds: Many, flat, ovoid with narrowed apex crowned by tuft of dirty white hair.*
➤ *Root: Cylindrical (**Fig. 201.3**).*

Rasapanchaka

Guna	Guru, Ruksha
Rasa	Madhura, Tikta, Kasaya
Vipaka	Katu
Virya	Ushna
Doshakarma	Tridoshahara

Officinal Part Used

Root

Dose

Powder: 3 to 6 g
Decoction: 50 to 100 mL

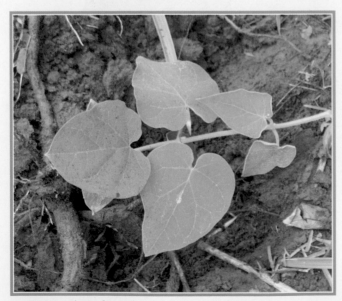

Fig. 201.1   Plant of *Marsdenia tenacissima* Wight & Arn.

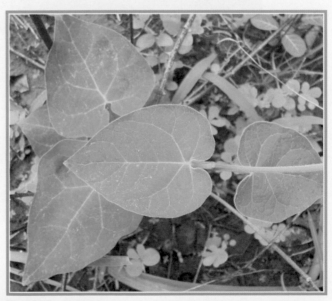

Fig. 201.2   Leaves.

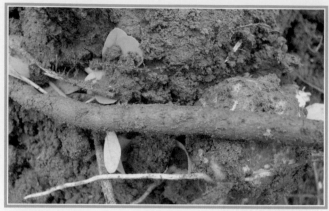

Fig. 201.3 Root.

Karma (Actions)

Sara (flowing in nature/mild purgative), sthanyashodhan (purification of breast milk), hridya (cardiotonic), pramehaghna (antidiabetes), jwaraghna (antipyretics).

Indications

Raktapitta (bleeding disorders), prameha (diabetes), trishna (thirst), hridroga (heart disease), kandu (pruritus), kushta (skin disease), jwara (fever).

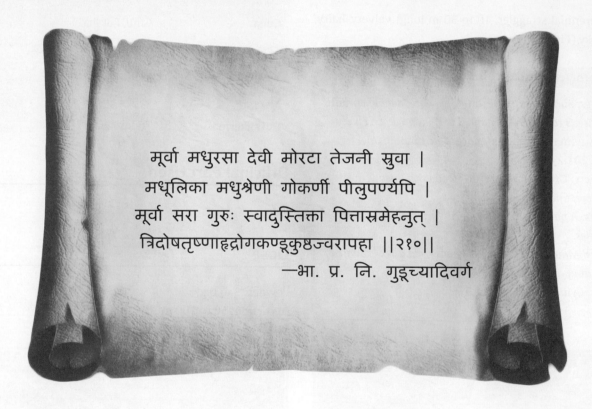

मूर्वा मधुरसा देवी मोरटा तेजनी सुवा |

मधूलिका मधुश्रेणी गोकर्णी पीलुपर्ण्यपि |

मूर्वा सरा गुरुः स्वादुस्तिक्ता पित्तास्रमेहनुत् |

त्रिदोषतृष्णाह्द्रोगकण्डूकुष्ठज्वरापहा ||२१०||

—भा. प्र. नि. गुडूच्यादिवर्ग

202. Nagabala *[Grewia hirsuta Vahl]*

Family:	*Malvaceae , Tiliaceae*
Hindi name:	*Gulshakari, Gudkhandi, Faridbuti*
English name:	*Country mallow*
Synonyms:	*Vishwadeva, Bhumibala*

Morphology

It is an erect-scandent shrub, 1.5 to 4 m high; branches softly pubescent (**Fig. 202.1**).

Key Characters for Identification

➤ *Leaves: 5 to 11 cm × 2.5 cm, alternate, shortly petiolate, lamina oblong-lanceolate with acute apex (**Fig. 202.2**).*
➤ *Flowers: Polygamous, calyx of five sepals and corolla of five petals, white turning yellow, with gland (**Fig. 202.2**).*
➤ *Fruits: Slightly four-lobed, fleshy, wrinkled drupe, sweet tasted, sparsely long hairy (**Fig. 202.3**).*
➤ *Seed: One seeded.*

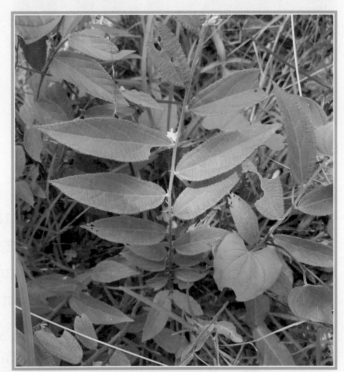

Fig. 202.1 Plant of *Grewia hirsuta* Vahl.

Rasapanchaka

Guna	Guru, Snigdha, Picchila
Rasa	Madhura, Kashaya
Vipaka	Madhura
Virya	Sheeta
Doshakarma	Vatapittahara

Officinal Part Used

Root

Dose

Decoction: 50 to 100 mL
Powder: 3 to 6 g

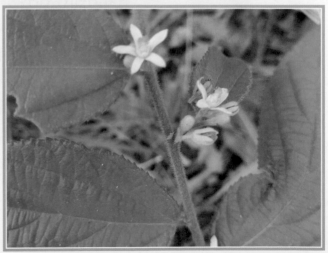

Fig. 202.2 Flowers and leaves.

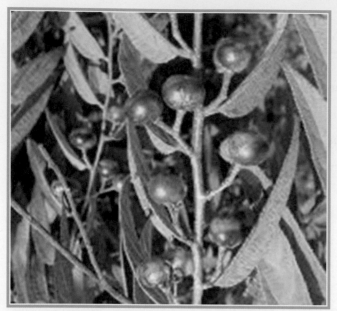

Fig. 202.3 Fruits

Karma (Actions)

Rasayana (rejuvinator), balya (physical strength promoter), grahi (digestive and fecal astringent), ruchya (relish), vranaropana (wound healing).

Indications

Vrana (wound), rajayakshma (tuberculosis), hridroga (heart disease), shwasa (asthma), kasa (cough), amatisara (diarrhea associated with aama), raktapitta (bleeding disorders), netraroga (eye disease), sotha (edema), sukradaurbalya (decreased semen). Nagabala is a controversial plant. The following three plants are considered to be Nagabala.

1. Sida spinosa Linn (Malvaceae)
2. Sida Veroniceaefolia Lam. (Malvaceae)
3. Grewia hirsuta Vahl. (iliaceae).

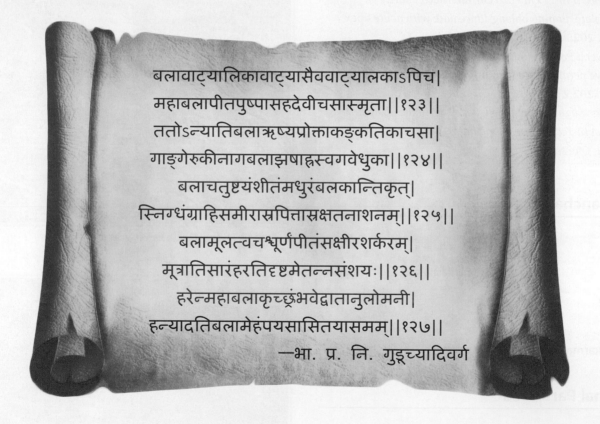

बलावाट्यालिकावाट्यासैववाट्यालकाऽपिच।
महाबलापीतपुष्पासहदेवीचसास्मृता॥१२३॥
ततोऽन्यातिबलाऋष्यप्रोक्ताकङ्कतिकाचसा।
गाङ्गेरुकीनागबलाझषाह्वस्वगवेधुका॥१२४॥
बलाचतुष्टयंशीतंमधुरंबलकान्तिकृत्।
स्निग्धंग्राहिसमीरास्रपित्तास्रक्षतनाशनम्॥१२५॥
बलामूलत्वचश्चूर्णपीतंसक्षीरशर्करम्।
मूत्रातिसारंहरतिदृष्टमेतन्नसंशयः॥१२६॥
हरेन्महाबलाकृच्छ्रंभवेद्वातानुलोमनी।
हन्यादतिबलामेहंपयसासितयासमम्॥१२७॥
—भा. प्र. नि. गुड्ड्च्यादिवर्ग

203. Nala *[Arundo donax Linn.]*

Family:	*Poaceae*
Hindi name:	*Bara nal*
English name:	*Giant reed*
Synonyms:	*Shunyamadhya, Vibhishana, Dhamana, Potagala*

Morphology

It is a perennial grass, 2 to 3 m tall; culms are erect, with often creeping lower part (**Fig. 203.1**).

Key Characters for Identification

➤ *Leaves: Glabrous, linear-lanceolate with cordate base and pointed apex (**Fig. 203.2**).*
➤ *Flowers: Three-flowered, rachilla glabrous; glumes linear lanceolate, one-nerved.*
➤ *Fruits: Caryopsis oblong.*
➤ *Root: Creeping rhizome (**Fig. 203.3a, b**).*

Rasapanchaka

Guna	Guru, Snigdha
Rasa	Madhura, Kashaya, Tikta
Vipaka	Madhura
Virya	Sheeta
Doshakarma	Kaphapittahara

Officinal Part Used

Root

Dose

Decoction: 50 to 100 mL

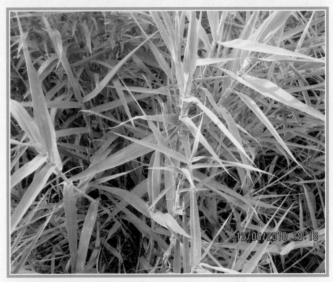

Fig. 203.1 Grass of *Arundo donax* Linn.

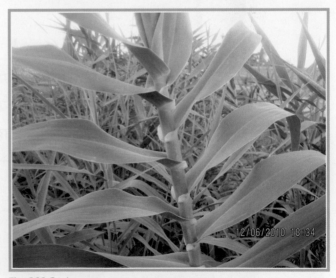

Fig. 203.2 Leaves.

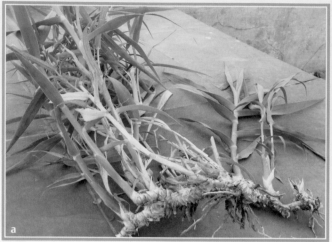
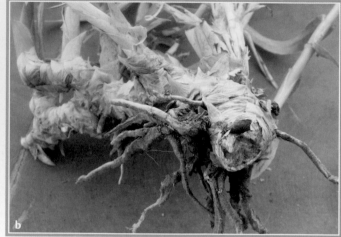

Fig. 203.3 (a, b) Roots.

Karma (Actions)

Vrishya (aphrodisiac), mutrala (diuretics), pittahara (pacify pitta).

Indications

Daha (burning sensation), pittaja vicar (diseases of pitta), raktapitta (bleeding disorders), mutrakricchra (dysuria), visharpa (erysipelas), hridshool (cardiac pain), yonishool (pain in vagina), vastishool (pain in bladder).

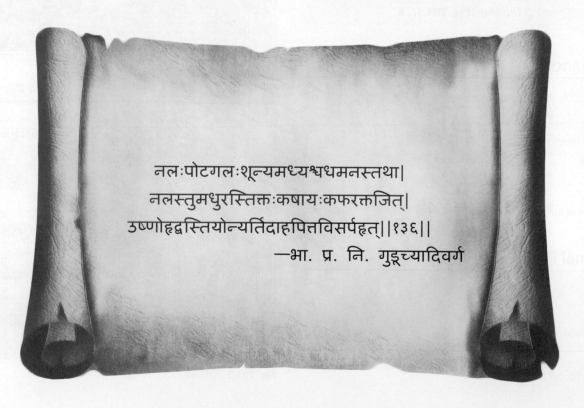

नलःपोटगलःशून्यमध्यश्चधमनस्तथा।
नलस्तुमधुरस्तिक्तःकषायःकफरक्तजित्।
उष्णोहृद्वस्तियोन्यर्तिदाहपित्तविसर्पहृत्।।१३६।।
—भा. प्र. नि. गुडूच्यादिवर्ग

204. Narikel *[Cocos nucifera Linn.]*

Family:	*Arecaceae*
Hindi name:	*Narial*
English name:	*Coconut palm*
Synonyms:	*Dridhaphala, Langali, Tunga, Trinaraja*

Morphology

It is a 15 to 30 m tall tree with unarmed trunk (**Fig. 204.1**).

Key Characters for Identification

➤ *Stem: Straight or curved, marked with ring-like leaf scar, grayish, light brown bark (***Fig. 204.2***).*
➤ *Leaves: Pinnately compound, linear oblong with a flexible midrib, 1.5 to 4.5 m long (***Fig. 204.3***).*
➤ *Flowers: Greenish-yellow, monoecious; spadix interfoliar, boat-shaped.*
➤ *Fruits: Green, yellowish, or orange, 20 to 30 cm long, obovoid-subglobose with thick fibrous covering and a hard, ovoid-ellipsoid shell inside bearing a seed. Endosperm is a layer of white, albuminous matter containing a watery fluid (***Fig. 204.3***).*

Rasapanchaka

Guna	Guru, Snigdha
Rasa	Madhura
Vipaka	Madhura
Virya	Sheeta
Doshakarma	Vatapittahara

Officinal Parts Used

Fruit, flower, oil, alkali

Dose

Fruit: 10 to 20 g
Oil: 10 to 20 drops
Alkali: 1 to 2 g

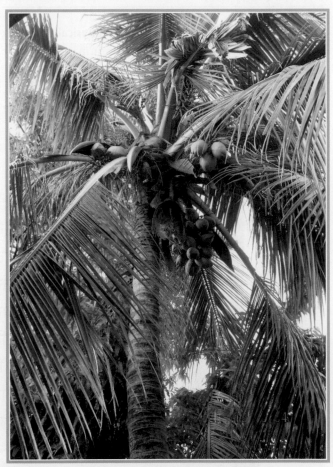

Fig. 204.1 Tree of *Cocos nucifera* Linn.

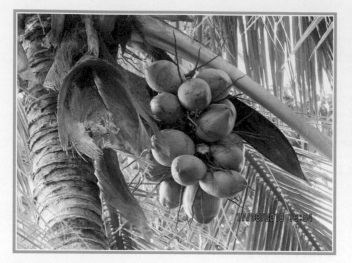

Fig. 204.2 Stem.

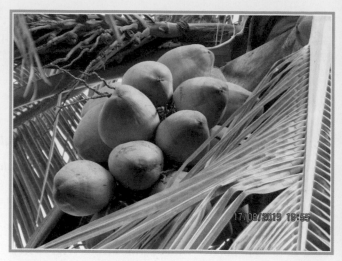

Fig. 204.3 Leaves and fruits.

Karma (Actions)

Brimhana (bulk promoting), balya (physical strength enhancer), vastishodhan (diuretics/urinary bladder cleanser), vrishya (aphrodisiac), mutrala (diuretics), visthambhi (constipation with retention of gases and pain), hridya (cardiotonic), deepan (appetizer), shukral (semen promoting).

Indications

Daha (burning sensation), trishna (thirst), pittajwara (fever due to pitta), raktapitta (bleeding disorders), mutrakricchra (dysuria), pittajavikara (diseases of pitta).

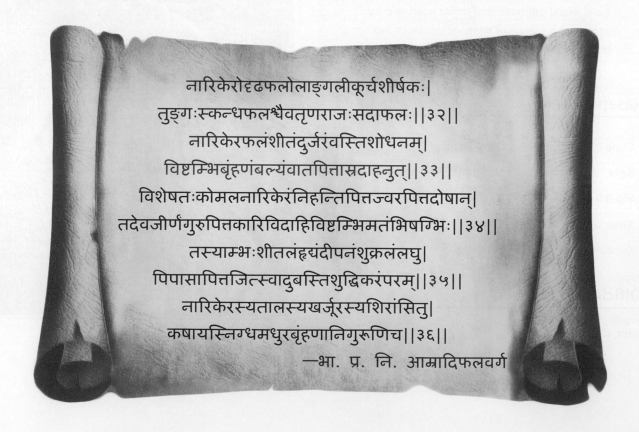

नारिकेरोद्वढफलोलाङ्गलीकूर्चशीर्षकः।
तुङ्गः स्कन्धफलश्चैवतृणराजःसदाफलः॥३२॥
नारिकेरफलंशीतंदुर्जरंवस्तिशोधनम्।
विष्टम्भिबृंहणंबल्यंवातपित्तास्रदाहनुत्॥३३॥
विशेषतःकोमलनारिकेरंनिहन्तिपित्तज्वरपित्तदोषान्।
तदेवजीर्णंगुरुपित्तकारिविदाहिविष्टम्भिमतंभिषग्भिः॥३४॥
तस्याम्भःशीतलंहृद्यंदीपनंशुक्रलंलघु।
पिपासापित्तजित्स्वादुबस्तिशुद्धिकरंपरम्॥३५॥
नारिकेरस्यतालस्यखर्जूरस्यशिरांसितु।
कषायस्निग्धमधुरबृंहणानिगुरुणिच॥३६॥
—भा. प्र. नि. आम्रादिफलवर्ग

205. Nili *[Indigofera tinctoria Linn.]*

Family:	*Leguminosae*
Hindi name:	*Neel*
English name:	*Indigo*
Synonyms:	*Neeli, Neelini, Tooli, Kaladola, Shriphali, Ranjani, Tuttha, Gramina, Neelapuspa, Sharadi, Madhuparnika, Kalkeshi*

Morphology

It is an erect, annual herb or perennial shrub, 0.5 to 1.5 m tall, and is appressedly hairy all over (**Fig. 205.1**).

Key Characters for Identification

➤ *Leaves: Imparipinnately compound; leaflets subopposite, ovate-oblong (**Fig. 205.2**).*
➤ *Flowers: Pink, in axillary, spike-like racemes (**Fig. 205.3**).*
➤ *Fruits: A linear, cylindric pod with thickened sutures, curved at pointed tip.*
➤ *Seed: Eight to ten, about 1 mm long, oblong with truncate ends.*

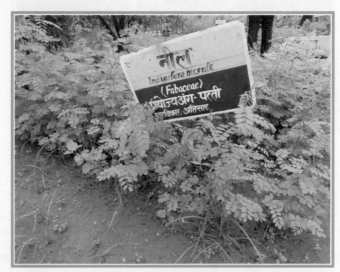

Fig. 205.1 Plant of *Indigofera tinctoria* Linn.

Rasapanchaka

Guna	Laghu, Ruksha
Rasa	Tikta
Vipaka	Katu
Virya	Ushna
Doshakarma	Kaphavatashaman

Officinal Part Used

Whole plant (panchanga)

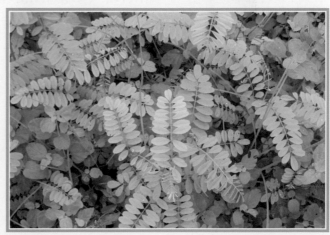

Fig. 205.2 Leaves.

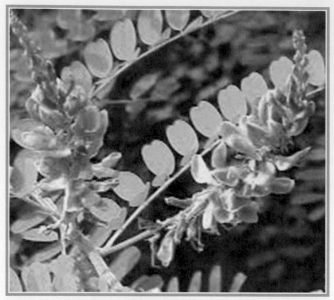

Fig. 205.3   Flower.

Dose

Decoction: 50 to 100 mL

Karma (Actions)

Rechani (purgative), kesya (hair tonic), krimighna (anthelmintic), vishaghni (antidote).

Indications

Moha (confusion), brahma (vertigo/dizziness), udara (abdominal diseases), pliha (splenomegaly), vatarakta (gout), aamavata (rheumatoid arthritis), udavarta (retention of urine, Feces, and flatus), mada (delirium), visha (poisoning), jwara (fever), krimi (worm infestation).

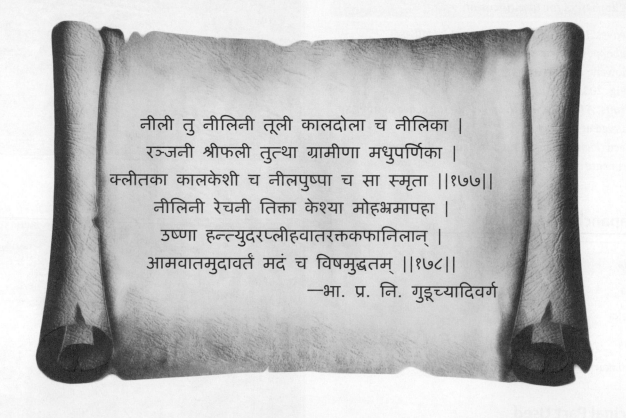

नीली तु नीलिनी तूली कालदोला च नीलिका ।
रञ्जनी श्रीफली तुत्था ग्रामीणा मधुपर्णिका ।
क्लीतका कालकेशी च नीलपुष्पा च सा स्मृता ॥१७७॥
नीलिनी रेचनी तिक्ता केश्या मोहभ्रमापहा ।
उष्णा हन्त्युदरप्लीहवातरक्तकफानिलान् ।
आमवातमुदावर्तं मदं च विषमुद्धतम् ॥१७८॥
—भा. प्र. नि. गुडूच्यादिवर्ग

206. Padmaka [*Prunus cerasoides D.Don.*]

Family:	*Rosaceae*
Hindi name:	*Padmakha, Padmakatha*
English name:	*Bird cherry*
Synonyms:	*Padmagandhi, Padmahwaya*

Morphology

It is a tree, 15 to 20 m tall, and the stem bark is brown, peeling off in horizontal stripes (**Fig. 206.1**).

Key Characters for Identification

➤ *Leaves: Alternate, simple, ovate-elliptic-lanceolate, rounded base, serrate margin (***Fig. 206.2***).*
➤ *Flowers: Pinkish about 3 cm across, in axillary fascicles.*
➤ *Fruits: An ovoid-globose, yellow and red, drupe, 1.5 to 2 cm long; stony solitary, ovoid, rugose, and furrowed (***Fig. 206.3***).*

Rasapanchaka

Guna	Laghu
Rasa	Kasaya, Tikta
Vipaka	Katu
Virya	Sheeta
Prabhav	Vedanasthapan
Doshakarma	Kaphapittashamak, Vatakarak

Officinal Parts Used

Bark and seed

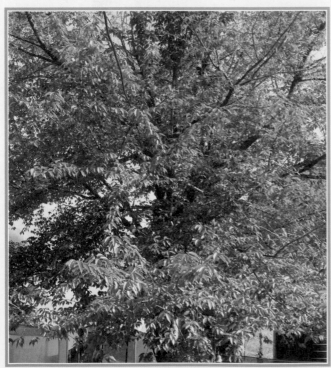

Fig. 206.1   Tree of *Prunus cerasoides* D.Don.

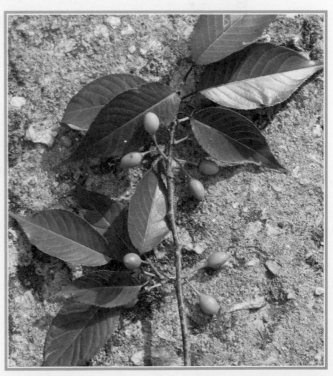

Fig. 206.2   Leaves.

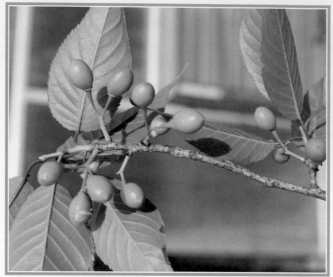

Fig. 206.3 Fruits.

Dose

Powder: 1 to 3 g

Karma (Actions)

Garbhasthapan (maintenance of fetus), vrisya (aphrodisiac), rochan (relish), dahashamak (cooling).

Indications

Visarpa (erysipelas), vispota (blisters), kushta (skin diseases), chhardi (vomiting), vrana (wound), trishna (thirst), jwara (fever), visha (poisoning), moha (confusion), daha (burning sensation), raktapitta (bleeding disorders).

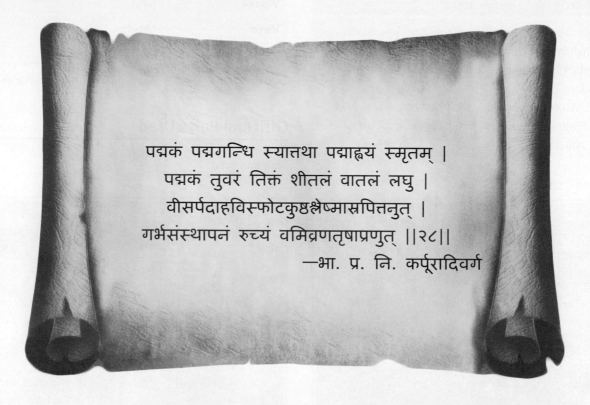

पद्मकं पद्मगन्धि स्यात्तथा पद्माह्वयं स्मृतम् ।
पद्मकं तुवरं तिक्तं शीतलं वातलं लघु ।
वीसर्पदाहविस्फोटकुष्ठश्लेष्मास्रपित्तनुत् ।
गर्भसंस्थापनं रुच्यं वमिव्रणतृषाप्रणुत् ॥२८॥
—भा. प्र. नि. कर्पूरादिवर्ग

207. Palandu *[Allium cepa Linn.]*

Family:	*Liliaceae*
Hindi name:	*Pyaaz*
English name:	*Onion*
Synonyms:	*Yavaneshta, Mukhdushaka, Durgandh*

Morphology

It is a biennial aromatic herb of 2 to 3 feet (**Fig. 207.1**).

Key Characters for Identification

- ➤ *Bulb: The bulbs are composed of shortened, compressed, underground stems surrounded by fleshy modified scale (leaves) that envelop a central bud at the tip of the stem (**Fig. 207.2**).*
- ➤ *Leaves: Basal, hollow, bluish-green leaves, bulb at the base of the plant, linear leaf blade.*
- ➤ *Inflorescence: An umbel.*
- ➤ *Flower: Pink to red, white, 3 to 4.5 mm in length, perianth fusion of petals (**Fig. 207.3**).*
- ➤ *Fruit: Capsule up to 5 mm.*

Rasapanchaka

Guna	Guru, Tikshan, Snigdha
Rasa	Madhur, Katu
Vipaka	Madhur
Virya	Anushna
Doshakarma	Kaphavatahara

Officinal Parts Used

Kanda and beej

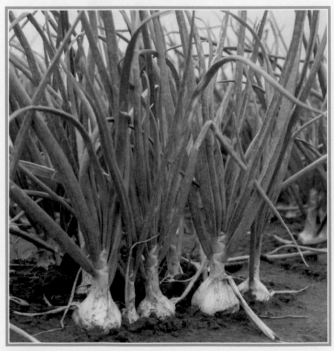

Fig. 207.1 Plant of *Allium cepa* Linn.

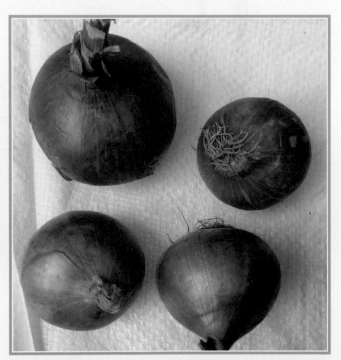

Fig. 207.2 Bulbs.

Dose

Tuber juice: 10 to 30 mL
Seed powder: 1 to 3 g

Karma (Actions)

Vedanasthapak (anodyne), shothhara (anti-inflammatory), vranashoth pachana (induction of suppuration), krimighna (anthelmintic), kandughna (antipruritus), deepan (appetizer), rochan (relish), anuloman (laxative), lekhan (scraping), chhedana (antitussive), kaphanisaraka (removes cough), amedhya (unhealthy for brain), shukrajanan (spermatopoetic), artavajanan (emmenogague), mutrajanan (diuretic).

Indications

Raktasrava (hemorrhage), karnashool (otalgia), krimi (worms), twakroga (skin diseases), adhyaman (flatulence), nadishool (neuritis).

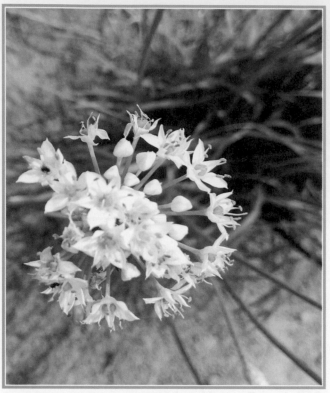

Fig. 207.3 Flowers.

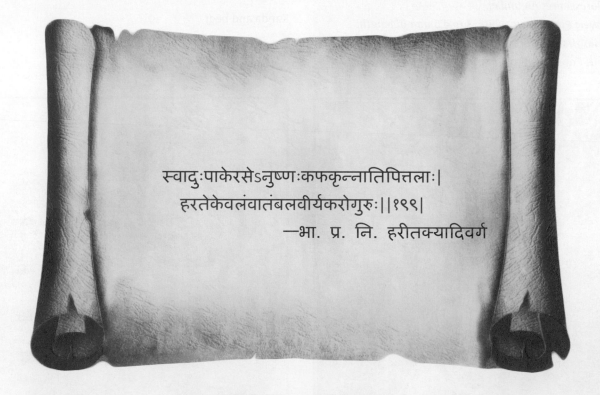

स्वादुःपाकेरसेऽनुष्णःकफकृन्नातिपित्तलाः।
हरतेकेवलंवातंबलवीर्यकरोगुरुः।।१९९।
—भा. प्र. नि. हरीतक्यादिवर्ग

208. Parasikayavani *[Hyoscyamus niger Linn.]*

Family:	*Solanaceae*
Hindi name:	*Khurasani ajwain*
English name:	*Black Henbane*
Synonyms:	*Madakarini, Yavaani, Turushka*

Morphology

It is a small, erect, annual-biennial coarse herb of about 1 m height (**Fig. 208.1**).

Key Characters for Identification

➤ *Leaves: Small, sessile, irregular, oblong, triangular, lanceolate, pale green and brittle, fleshy, entire margin (**Fig. 208.2**).*
➤ *Flower: Crowded at the ends of the stems, deep purple with yellowish streaks (**Fig. 208.3**).*
➤ *Fruit: Bilocular, cylindrical, pyxis, 1.3 cm diameter, enclosed in globose tube of enlarged calyx, lower part membranous, hard top, narrow at a junction of two portion, transverse opening (**Fig. 208.4**).*
➤ *Seed: Numerous brown-colored seeds, 1.5 cm long and 6 mm wide, embryo embedded in an oily endosperm.*

Rasapanchaka

Guna	Guru, Ruksha
Rasa	Tikta, Katu
Vipaka	Katu
Virya	Ushan
Doshakarma	Vaat Shlesmahara

Officinal Parts Used

Beeja (seeds), patra (leaves), pushpa (flowers)

Dose

Powder: 125 mg to 1 g

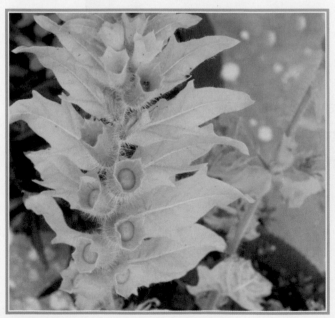

Fig. 208.1   Plant of *Hyoscyamus niger* Linn.

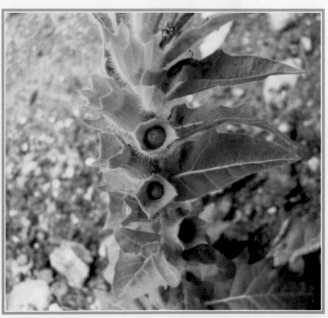

Fig. 208.2   Leaves.

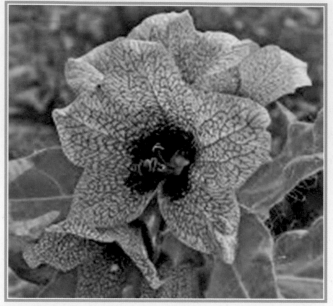

Fig. 208.3 Flower.

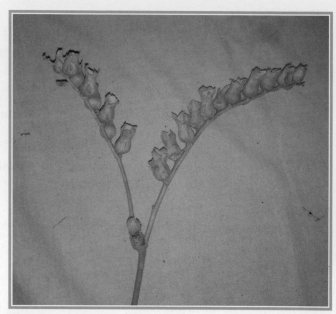

Fig. 208.4 Fruits.

Karma (Actions)

Madakari (delirium), grahi (fecal astringent), deepana (appetizer), pachana (digestive), shukrahara (semen reducing), vedanasthapaka (analgesic), nidrajanak (sleep inducing).

Indications

Krimi (worm infestation), shola (colic pain), gulma (abdominal lump), agnimandya (loss of appetite), pleeharoga (spleen diseases).

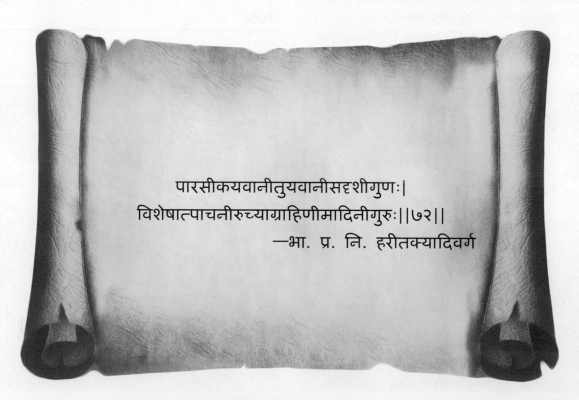

पारसीकयवानीतुयवानीसदृशीगुणः।
विशेषात्पाचनीरुच्याग्राहिणीमादिनीगुरुः॥७२॥
—भा. प्र. नि. हरीतक्यादिवर्ग

209. Parijaat *[Nyctanthes arbor tristris Linn.]*

Family: *Oleaceae*

Hindi name: *Harsingar*

English name: *Night jasmine, Coral jasmine*

Synonyms: *Kharapatraka, Shefalika, Harshringar*

Morphology

It is a profusely branched shrub or small tree (**Fig. 209.1**).

Key Characters for Identification

➤ *Bark: Grey or greenish-white rough bark.*
➤ *Leaves: Simple, opposite, ovate, acute, densely pubescent* (**Fig. 209.2**).
➤ *Flower: Small, white, and bright orange corolla tubes* (**Fig. 209.3**).
➤ *Fruit: Capsule, compressed, separating into two one-seeded segments* (**Fig. 209.4**).

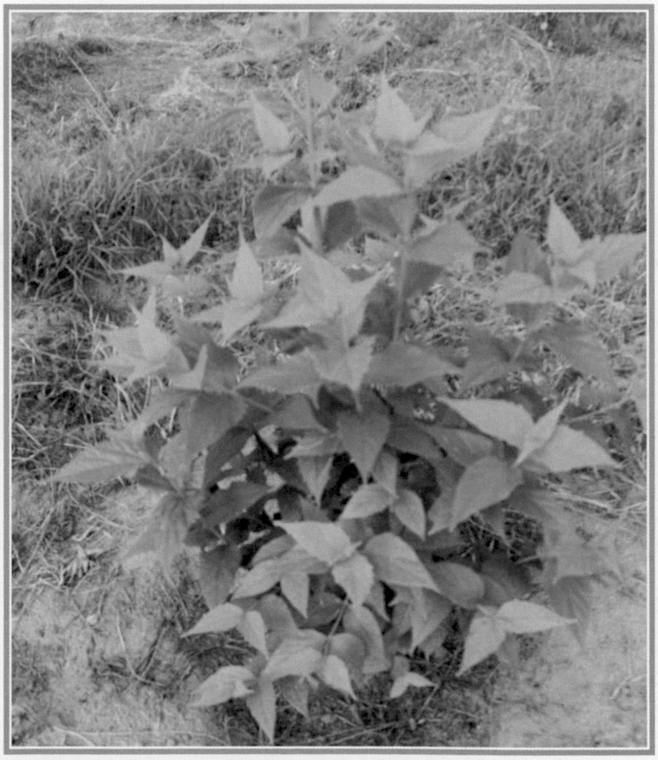

Rasapanchaka

Guna	Laghu, Snigdha
Rasa	Tikta
Vipaka	Katu
Virya	Ushan
Doshaghanta	Kapha-vatahara

Officinal Parts Used

Patra (leaves), twak (bark), moola (root)

Dose

Powder: 1 to 3 g
Juice: 10 to 20 mL
Decoction: 50 to 100 mL

Fig. 209.1 Plant of *Nyctanthes arbor tristris* Linn.

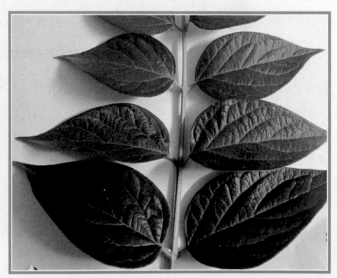

Fig. 209.2 Leaves.

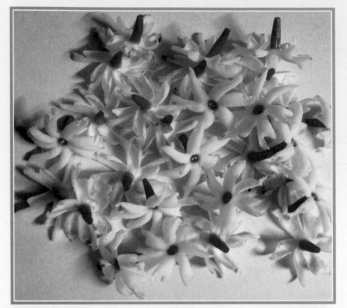

Fig. 209.3 Flowers.

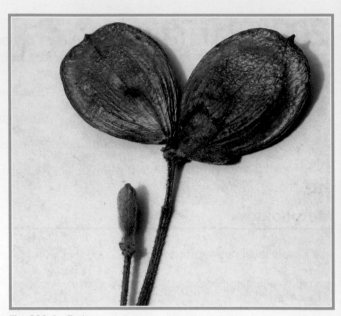

Fig. 209.4 Fruits.

Karma (Actions)

Anulomana (laxative), jwaraghna (antipyretics), krimighna (anthelmintic), yakrit uttejaka (hepatic stimulant), mradu virechak (mild purgative).

Indications

Sandhivaat (osteoarthritis), gridhrasi (sciatica), kasa (cough), shwasa (asthma), jeerna jwar (chronic fever), krimi (worm infestation), pleehavriddhi (splenomegaly).

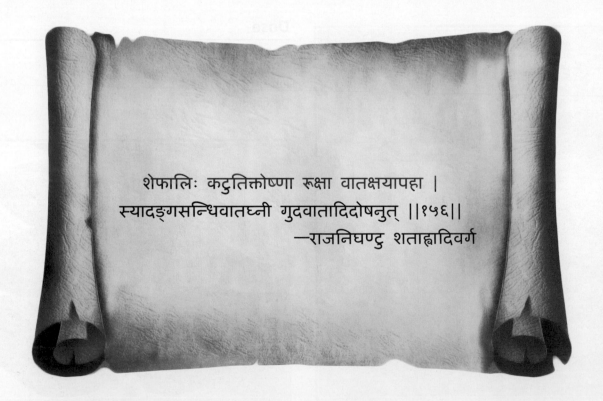

शेफालिः कटुतिक्तोष्णा रूक्षा वातक्षयापहा ।
स्यादङ्गसन्धिवातघ्नी गुदवातादिदोषनुत् ॥१५६॥
—राजनिघण्टु शताह्वादिवर्ग

210. Parisha *[Thepesia populnea (Linn.) Soland. Ex Corr.]*

Family:	*Malvaceae*
Hindi name:	*Paras pipal*
English name:	*Portia tree*
Synonyms:	*Kapichoota, Kamandalu, Kapitana, Gardabhanda, Kandral*

Morphology

It is an evergreen tree of 10 to 20 m height (**Fig. 210.1**).

Key Characters for Identification

➤ *Stem: Cylindrical stem, gray bark, plenty of warts* (**Fig. 210.2**).
➤ *Leaves: Alternate, petiolate, dark green, glossy, blades, cordate, and long petiole* (**Fig. 210.3**).
➤ *Flower: Showy, yellow with maroon to purple in center, solitary in the leaf axils* (**Fig. 210.4**).
➤ *Fruit: A brown, flattened, globose capsule enclosing sticky yellow sap* (**Fig. 210.5**).
➤ *Seed: About 10 hairy seeds.*

Rasapanchaka

Guna	Laghu, Snigdha
Rasa	Amla (fruit), Madhur and Kashaya (majja and pulp), Madhur (root)
Vipaka	Katu
Virya	Sheet
Doshakarma	Kaphakaraka

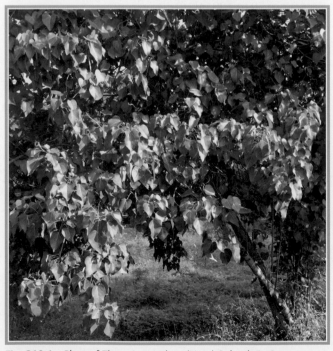

Fig. 210.1　Plant of *Thepesia populnea* (Linn.) Soland. Ex Corr.

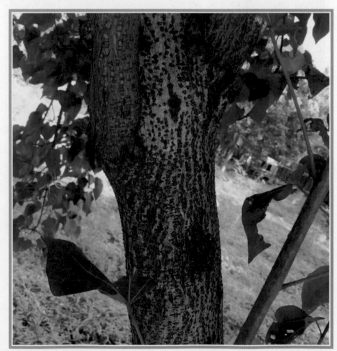

Fig. 210.2　Stem.

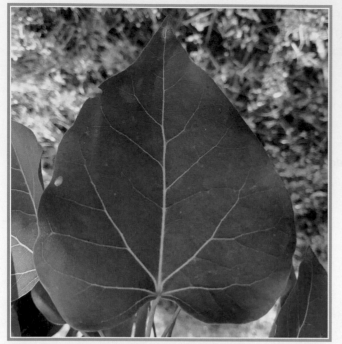

Fig. 210.3 Leaf.

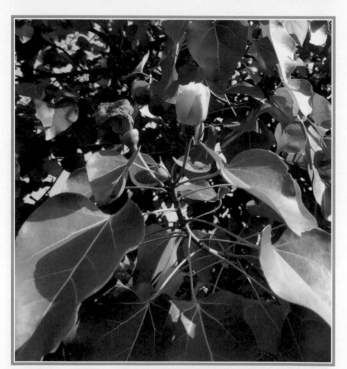

Fig. 210.4 Flower.

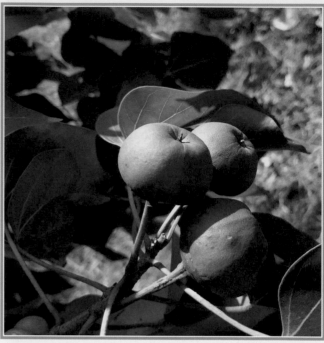

Fig. 210.5 Fruits.

Officinal Part Used

Kanda twak (stem bark)

Dose

Decoction: 50 to 100 mL
Powder: 3 to 6 g

Karma (Actions)

Grahi (fecal astringent), durjar (difficult to digest), krimighna (anthelmintic), mutrasangrahniya (urinary astringent).

Indications

Prameha (diabetes), kushta (skin diseases), kandu (pruritus), yoniroga (diseases of vagina), vrana (wound).

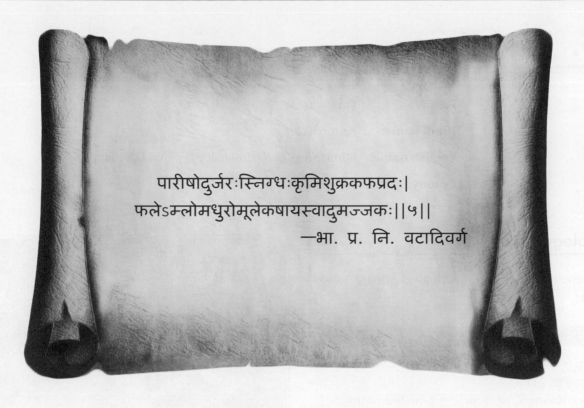

पारीषोदुर्जरःस्निग्धःकृमिशुक्रकफप्रदः।
फलेऽम्लोमधुरोमूलेकषायस्वादुमज्जकः।।५।।

—भा. प्र. नि. वटादिवर्ग

211. Parnabija *[(Bryophyllum pinnatum (Lamk.) Kurz]*

Family:	*Crassulaceae*
Hindi name:	*Pattarchatta*
English name:	*Miracle leaf, Cathedral bell, Air plant, Life plant*
Synonyms:	*Patharchur*

Morphology

It is a perennial erect herb with thick fleshy leaves (**Fig. 211.1**).

Key Characters for Identification

➤ *Leaves: Fleshy, 10 to 20 cm, dentate, ovate, three to five leaflets* (**Fig. 211.2**).
➤ *Flowers: Greenish-red, 5-cm long, bent downward* (**Fig. 211.3**).
➤ *Fruits: Four-angled, contain many seeds.*
➤ *Seeds: Small and smooth.*

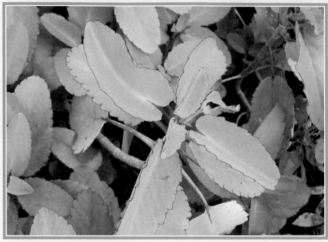

Fig. 211.1 Herb of *Bryophyllum pinnatum* (Lamk.) Kurz.

Rasapanchaka

Guna	Laghu, Ruksha
Rasa	Kasaya, Amla
Vipaka	Madhura
Virya	Sheet
Doshakarma	Vata-pittahara

Officinal Part Used

Patra (leaves)

Dose

Juice: 10 to 20 mL

Karma (Actions)

Raktastambhak (hemostatic), vranaropak (wound healing).

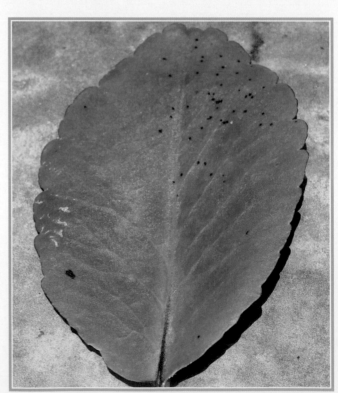

Fig. 211.2 Leaf.

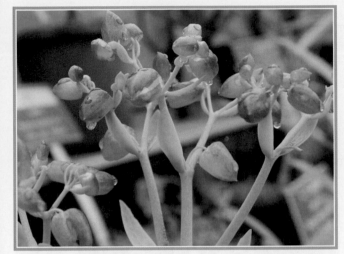

Fig. 211.3 Flower.

Indications

Rakta-pravahika (dysentric with blood), rakta-pradara (metrorrhagia), rakta-arshas (bleeding piles), sadhyavrana (fresh blood).

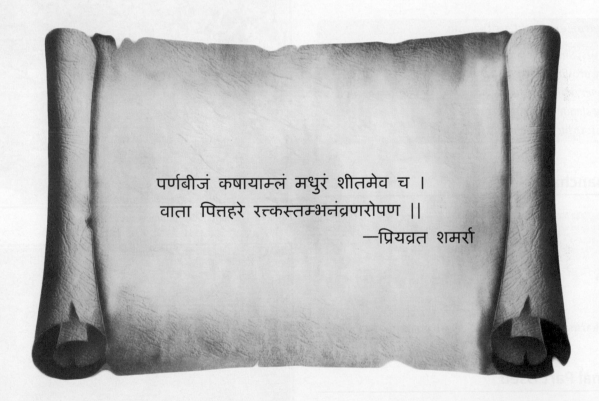

पर्णबीजं कषायाम्लं मधुरं शीतमेव च ।
वाता पित्तहरे रक्तस्तम्भनंव्रणरोपण ॥

—प्रियव्रत शर्मा

212. Paraayavani *[Coleus amboinicus Benth.]*

Family: *Lamiaceae*

Hindi name: *Pattaajwain*

English name: *Country borage*

Synonyms: *Karpuravalli, Yavanigandhaparnika, Patharchur*

Morphology

It is a large succulent aromatic perennial herb with tomentose fleshy stem (**Fig. 212.1**).

Key Characters for Identification

➤ *Leaves: Simple, opposite, broadly ovate, crenate, fleshy, very aromatic (**Fig. 212.2**).*
➤ *Flower: Pale purplish, whorls at distant intervals in a long slender raceme (**Fig. 212.3**).*
➤ *Fruit: Orbicular or ovoid nutlet.*

Rasapanchaka

Guna	Laghu, Ruksha
Rasa	Katu, Tikta
Vipaka	Katu
Virya	Ushan
Doshakarma	Kapha-vatashamaka

Officinal Part Used

Patra (leaves)

Dose

Leaves juice: 5 to 10 mL

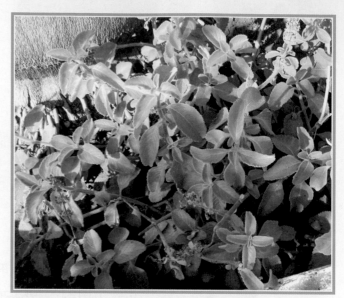

Fig. 212.1 Plant of *Coleus amboinicus* Benth.

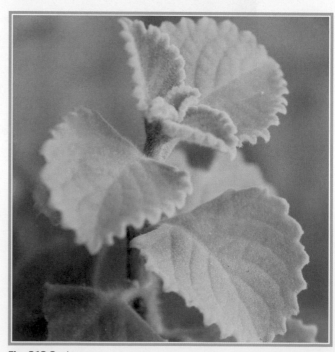

Fig. 212.2 Leaves.

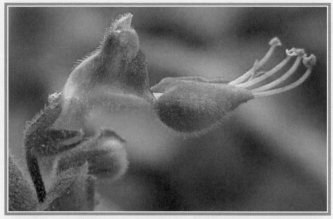

Fig. 212.3 Flower.

Karma (Actions)

Deepan (appetizer), pachana (digestive), ruchya (relish), grahi (astringent), mutral (diuretics), udveshtananirodhi (antianxiety).

Indications

Ashmari (lithiasis), mutrakricchta (dysuria), udarroga (abdominal diseases), krimi (worm), grahani (IBS), agnimandhya (dyspepsia), jwara (fever), yakritroga (liver diseases).

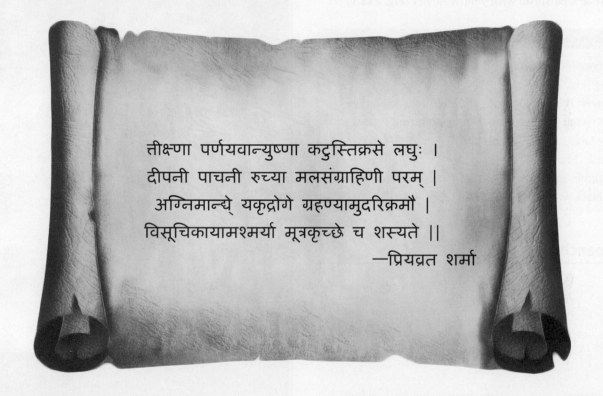

तीक्ष्णा पर्णयवान्युष्णा कटुस्तिक्रसे लघुः ।
दीपनी पाचनी रुच्या मलसंग्राहिणी परम् ।
अग्निमान्द्ये यकृद्रोगे ग्रहण्यामुदरिक्रमौ ।
विसूचिकायामश्मर्या मूत्रकृच्छे च शस्यते ॥

—प्रियव्रत शर्मा

213. Parushaka *[Grewia asiatica Mast. non Linn.]*

Family:	*Tiliaceae*
Hindi name:	*Phalsa*
English name:	*Falsa tree*
Synonyms:	*Parusha, Alpashti, Parapar*

Morphology

It is a small tree/shrub with yellow flower (**Fig. 213.1**).

Key Characters for Identification

➤ *Leaves: Broadly rounded, with a petiole 1 to 1.5 cm long (**Fig. 213.2**).*

➤ *Flower: Produced in cymes of several together, the individual flowers about 2 cm in diameter, yellow, with five large (12 mm) sepals and five smaller (4–5 mm) petals (**Fig. 213.3**).*

➤ *Fruit: An edible drupe 5 to 12 mm in diameter, purple to black when ripe (**Fig. 213.4**).*

Rasapanchaka

Guna	Laghu
Rasa	Kasaya, Amla
Vipaka	Madhur (matured fruit)
Virya	Sheeta
Doshakarma	Vatapittahara but Apakwa fruit Pittakar

Officinal Part Used

Fruit

Dose

Juice: 10 to 20 mL

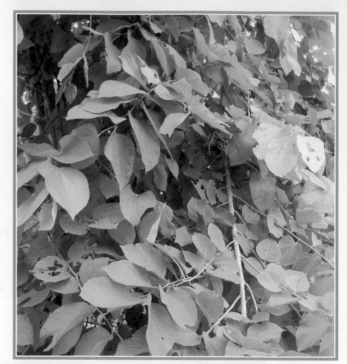

Fig. 213.1 Plant of *Grewia asiatica* Mast.non Linn.

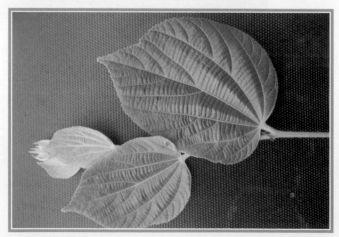

Fig. 213.2 Leaf.

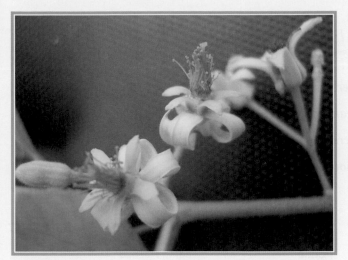

Fig. 213.3 Flower.

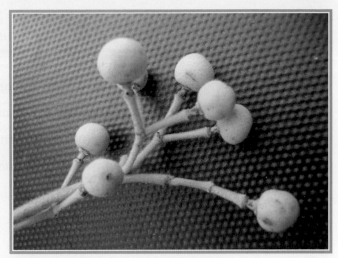

Fig. 213.4 Fruits.

Karma (Actions)

Visthambhi (constipation with retention gases and pain), brimhana (bulk promoting), hridya (cardiotonic), dahashamak (cooling), jwaraghna (antipyretics).

Indications

Pittaja vyadhi (diseases of pitta), daha (burning sensation), jwara (fever), kshaya (emaciation), rakta vikara (blood-related diseases).

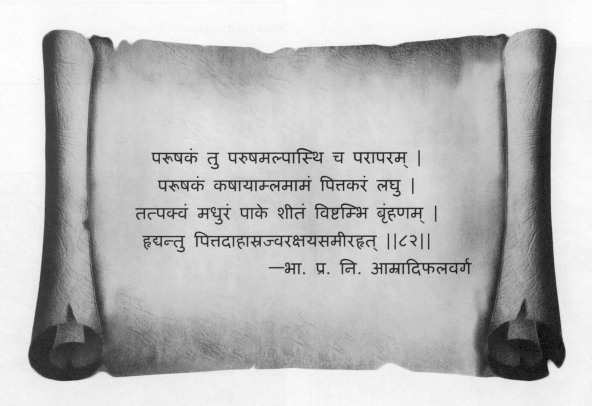

परूषकं तु परुषमल्पास्थि च परापरम् ।
परूषकं कषायाम्लमामं पित्तकरं लघु ।
तत्पक्वं मधुरं पाके शीतं विष्टम्भि बृंहणम् ।
हृद्यन्तु पित्तदाहास्रज्वरक्षयसमीरहृत् ॥८२॥
—भा. प्र. नि. आम्रादिफलवर्ग

214. Patalgarudi *[Cocculus hirsutus (Linn.) Diels]*

Family: *Menispermaceae*

Hindi name: *Jalajamani, Jamtikibel, Farid buti*

English name: *Broom creeper, Ink berry*

Synonyms: *Mahamoola, Chilahinta*

Morphology

It is a perennial, creeping, pubescent herb with soft hairy branches (**Fig. 214.1**).

Key Characters for Identification

➤ *Leaves: Simple, ovate-oblong, alternate, soft villous surface, base subcordate or truncate (**Fig. 214.2**).*
➤ *Flowers: Whitish-pink, male flower small in axillary cymes, female flowers in clusters of three to four.*
➤ *Fruits: Purple black drupe.*

Rasapanchaka

Guna	Laghu, Picchila
Rasa	Tikta
Vipaka	Katu
Virya	Ushan
Doshakarma	Kaphavatahara

Officinal Parts Used

Mool (root) and patra (leaves)

Dose

Decoction: 50 to 100 mL
Juice: 10 to 20 mL

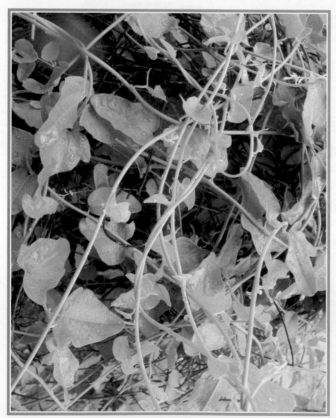

Fig. 214.1 Plant of *Cocculus hirsutus* (Linn.) Diels.

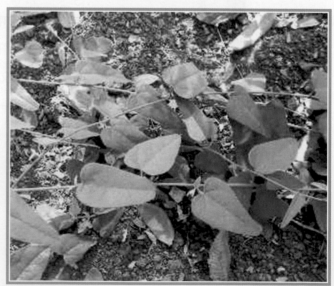

Fig. 214.2 Leaves.

Karma (Actions)

Vrishya (aphrodisiac), vishaghna (antidotes), mutral (diuretics), kushtaghna (antidermatosis), jwaraghna (antipyretics), deepen (appetizer).

Indications

Agnimandya (dyspepsia), kushta (skin diseases), mutra-kricchta (dysuria), shukra-daurbalya (semen debility), sarpavisha (snake poisoning), snayukaroga (dracunculiasis).

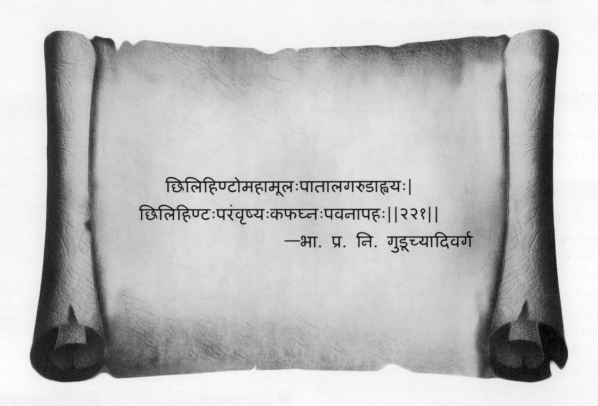

छिलिहिण्टोमहामूलःपातालगरुडाह्वयः।
छिलिहिण्टःपरंवृष्यःकफघ्नःपवनापहः।।२२१।।
—भा. प्र. नि. गुडूच्यादिवर्ग

215. Patha *[Cissampelos pareira Linn.]*

Family:	*Menispermaceae*
Hindi name:	*Patha, Padhi*
English name:	*False Pareira Brava*
Synonyms:	*Ambashtha, Pathika, Rasa, Prachina, Papachelika, Varatikta, Ekashthila*

Morphology

It is a weak perennial climbing shrub of about 3 to 5 m long (**Fig. 215.1**).

Key Characters for Identification

➤ *Leaves: Peltate, 2.5 to 12 cm long, 2.5 to 11.5 cm broad, triangularly broad-ovate, or orbicular, obtuse, mucronate, base cordate, or truncate, tomentose on both sides; petiole pubescent (**Fig. 215.2**).*

➤ *Flowers: Small, pedicels filiform. Male flowers are clustered in the axil of a small leaf; sepals are four in number, obovate-oblong, hairy outside; petals four in number, united to form a four-toothed cup, hairy outside; stamens four, column short, anthers connate, encircling the top of the column. Female flowers are clustered in the axils of orbicular, hoary imbricate bracts, on 5 to 10-cm-long racemes; sepal one, petal one; carpel one, densely hairy; style shortly three-fid (**Fig. 215.3**).*

➤ *Fruit: 4 to 6-mm-long drupe, 3 to 4 mm broad, subglobose, compressed, hairy-pubescent, red when fresh, black when dry.*

➤ *Seeds: Horseshoe-shaped.*

Rasapanchaka

Guna	Laghu, Tikshna
Rasa	Tikta
Vipaka	Katu
Virya	Ushna
Doshakarma	Vaat shleshmhara

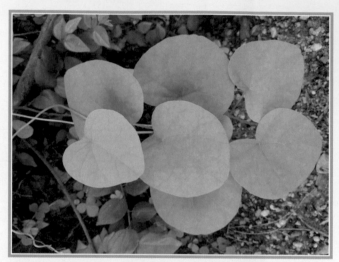

Fig. 215.1   Shrub of *Cissampelos pareira* Linn.

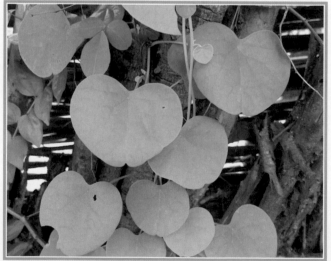

Fig. 215.2   Leaf.

Officinal Parts Used

Root and rhizome

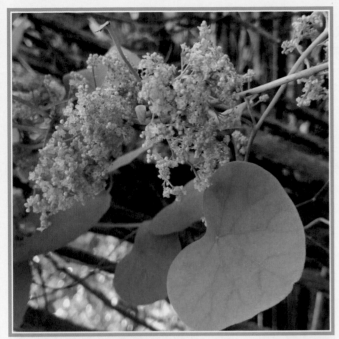

Fig. 215.3 Flowers.

Dose

Decoction: 50 to 100 mL
Powder: 1 to 3 g

Karma (Actions)

Balya (tonic), vishaghna (antidotes), grahi (astringent), sandhaniya (union promoter), stanyashodhana (galacto purifier).

Indications

Shoola (pain), jwara (fever), chardi (vomiting), gulma (abdominal distension), atisara (diarrhea), vrana (wound), kushta (skin diseases), daha (burning sensation), kandu (pruritis), garvisha (artificial poisoning), visha (poisoning), shwasa (bronchitis).

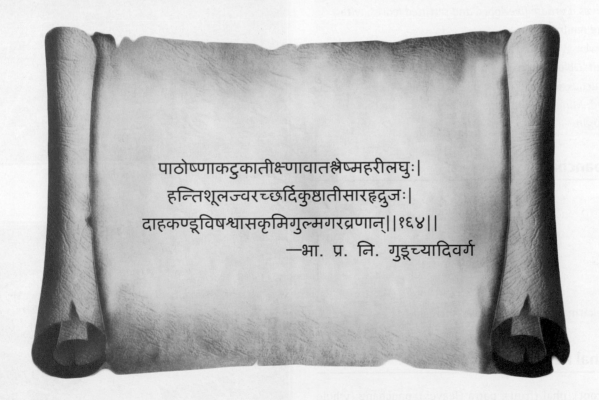

पाठोष्णाकटुकातीक्ष्णावातश्लेष्महरीलघुः।
हन्तिशूलज्वरच्छर्दिकुष्ठातीसारहृद्रुजः।
दाहकण्डूविषश्वासकृमिगुल्मगरव्रणान्।।१६४।।
—भा. प्र. नि. गुडूच्यादिवर्ग

216. Patola *[Trichosanthes dioica Roxb.]*

Family:	*Cucurbitaceae*
Hindi name:	*Parwal*
English name:	*Pointed gourd*
Synonyms:	*Raajiphal, Tiktauttam, Beejgarbh, Karkaschhad, Katuphal, Panduphal*

Morphology

It is a perennial, dioecious climber with rough heart-shaped leaves (**Fig. 216.1**).

Key Characters for Identification

➤ *Stem: Quadrangular, twinning, and striated, sometimes woody or scabrous.*
➤ *Leaves: Cordate five-lobed and serrated leaves, with bifid tendrils.*
➤ *Flower: White and fringed (**Fig. 216.2**).*
➤ *Fruit: Oblong, narrow, pointed at both the ends, glaucous, longitudinal strips mark (**Fig. 216.3**).*
➤ *Seed: Minute, compressed, and corrugate on the margin.*

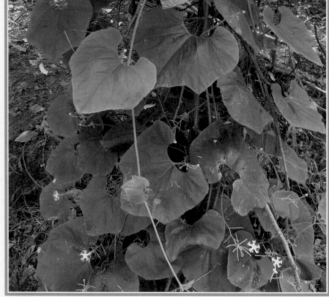

Fig. 216.1 Climber of *Trichosanthes dioica* Roxb.

Rasapanchaka

Guna	Laghu, Snigdh
Rasa	Tikta
Vipaka	Madhura
Virya	Ushna
Doshakarma	Tridoshashamaka

Officinal Parts Used

Mool (root), phal (fruit), patra (leaves), panchang (whole plant)

Dose

Decoction: 40 to 80 mL
Powder: 3 to 6 g

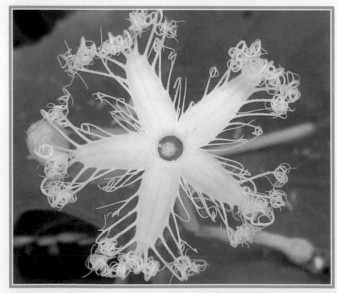

Fig. 216.2 Flower.

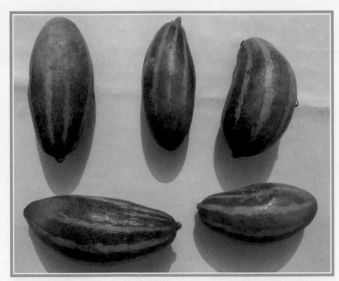

Fig. 216.3 Fruits.

Karma (Actions)

Deepan (appetizer), pachan (digestive), hridya (cardiotonic), vrishya (aphrodisiac), krimighna (anthelmintic), vishaghna (antidote), triptighna (a disease of kapha in which a person feels satisfaction even without having food, the medicine which cures such a feeling is called triptighna), trishna nigrahan (reduces excessive thirst); Root is virechaka (purgative).

Indications

Kasa (cough), jwara (fever), raktvikara (blood diseases), krimi (worm infestation), kushta (skin disease), vrana (wound), kamala (jaundice), shoth (edema).

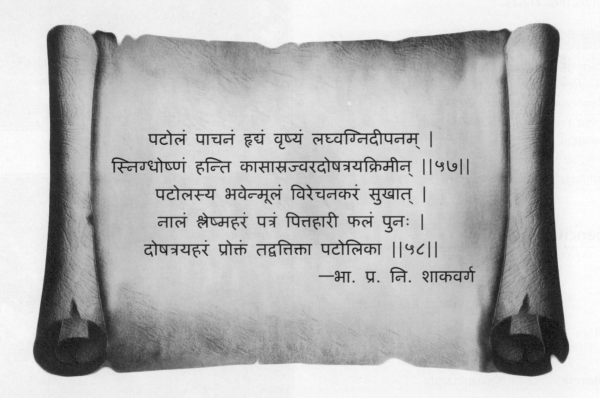

पटोलं पाचनं हृद्यं वृष्यं लघ्वग्निदीपनम् ।
स्निग्धोष्णं हन्ति कासास्रज्वरदोषत्रयक्रिमीन् ॥५७॥
पटोलस्य भवेन्मूलं विरेचनकरं सुखात् ।
नालं श्लेष्महरं पत्रं पित्तहारी फलं पुनः ।
दोषत्रयहरं प्रोक्तं तद्वत्तिका पटोलिका ॥५८॥
—भा. प्र. नि. शाकवर्ग

217. Patrang *[Caesalpinia sappan Linn.]*

Family: *Caesalpiniaceae*

Hindi name: *Patang chandan, Bakamkath*

English name: *Sappan wood*

Synonyms: *Pataranjaka, Raktasaar, Surang, Ranjan, Pattur, Kuchandan*

Morphology

It is a small thorny tree 6 to 8 m in height with hard wood, and brownish-red, prickly stems (**Fig. 217.1**). Young shoots are tomentose, and branches are glabrous covered with short spines (**Fig. 217.2**).

Key Characters for Identification

➤ *Leaves: Alternate, pinnate leaflets, glabrous above, tomentose beneath (**Fig. 217.3**).*
➤ *Inflorescence: Terminal raceme.*
➤ *Flower: Yellow peduncle clothed with a ferruginous tomentum.*
➤ *Fruit: Pod compressed with hard cell and sharp horn containing yellowish-brown seed (**Fig. 217.4**).*

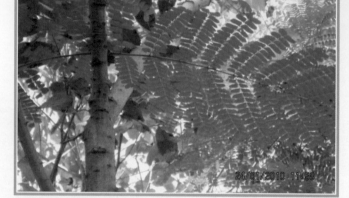

Fig. 217.1 Plant of *Caesalpinia sappan* Linn.

Rasapanchaka

Guna	Ruksha
Rasa	Tikta, Madhura, Kashaya
Vipaka	Katu
Virya	Sheet
Doshakarma	Kaphapittahara

Officinal Part Used

Heartwood

Dose

Decoction: 40 to 80 mL

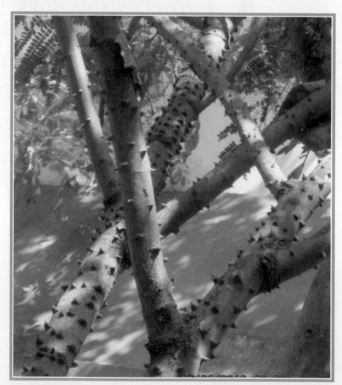

Fig. 217.2 Spinous branches.

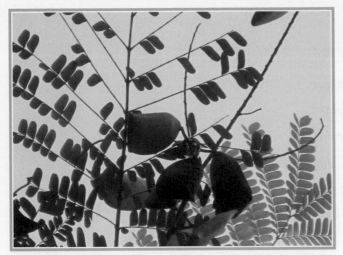

Fig. 217.3 Leaves.

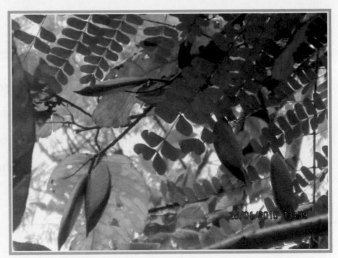

Fig. 217.4 Pods.

Karma (Actions)

Vranaropana (wound healing), dahanashak (reducing burning sensation), sangrahi (absorbent), stambhaka (astringent).

Indications

Jwar (fever), daha (burning sensation), trishna (thirst), vrana (wounds), chardi (vomiting), raktapitta (bleeding disorders), vyanga (acne).

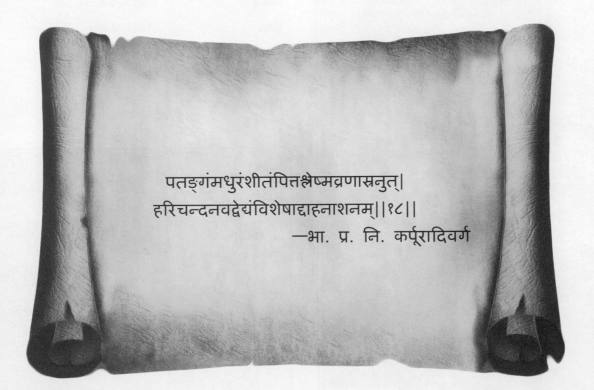

पतङ्गंमधुरंशीतंपित्तश्लेष्मव्रणास्रनुत्।
हरिचन्दनवद्द्रेयंविशेषाद्दाहनाशनम्।।१८।।
—भा. प्र. नि. कर्पूरादिवर्ग

218. Pilu *[Salvadora persica* Linn.*]*

Family: *Salvadoraceae*

Hindi name: *Pilu, Meswak*

English name: *Tooth brush tree*

Synonyms: *Gud phal, Sheetphala, Sanshrani*

Morphology

It is a large much branched evergreen shrub or small tree (**Fig. 218.1**) with short trunk, drooping branches, and soft whitish-yellow wood (**Fig. 218.2**).

Key Characters for Identification

- *Leaves: Ovate, oblong, grayish-green, mucronate at the apex, main nerves five to six pairs.*
- *Flower: Small, greenish-yellow in axillary and terminal compound lax panicles* (**Fig. 218.3**).
- *Fruit: Globose, smooth, red when ripe* (**Fig. 218.4**).

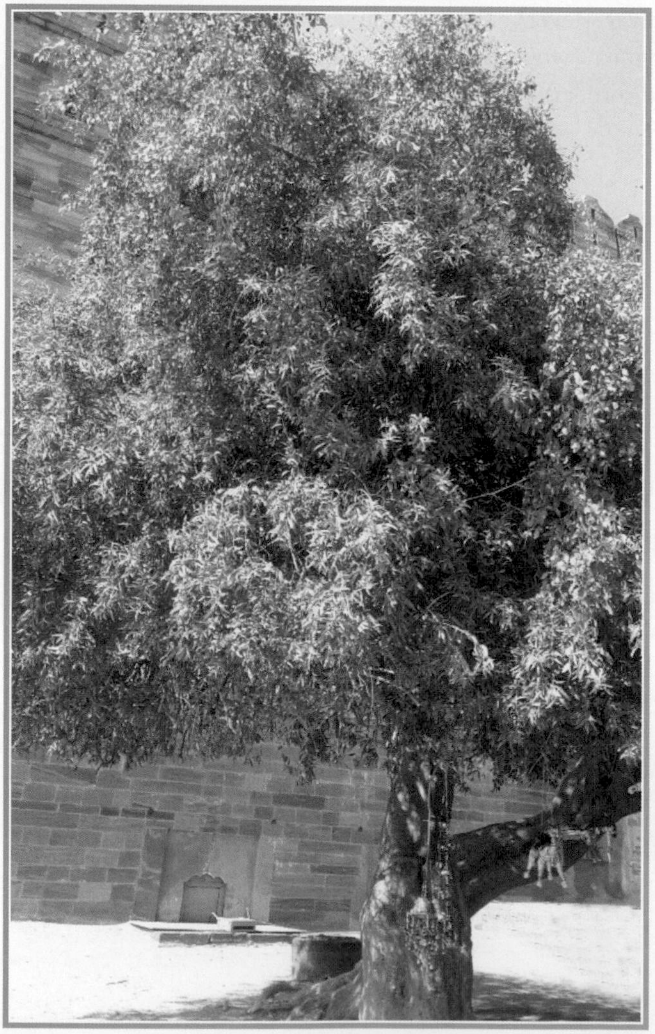

Fig. 218.1 Plant of *Salvadora persica* Linn.

Rasapanchaka

Guna	Laghu, Snigdh
Rasa	Tikta, Madhur
Vipaka	Katu
Virya	Ushna
Doshakarma	Kapha Vatahara

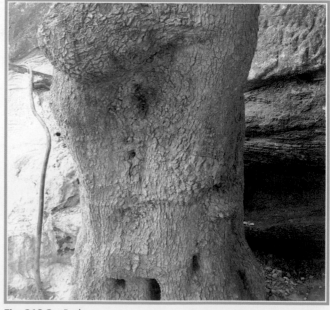

Fig. 218.2 Bark.

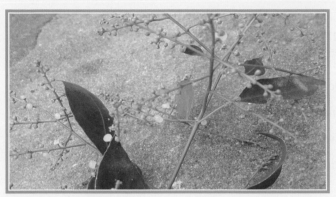

Fig. 218.3 Flowers.

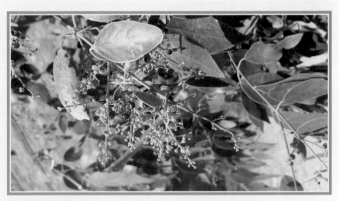

Fig. 218.4 Fruits.

Officinal Parts Used

Phal (fruit), beej (seed), mool (root), twak (bark), patra (leaves)

Dose

Seed powder: 1 to 3 g
Decoction: 50 to 100 mL

Karma (Actions)

Rechak (purgative), krimighna (anthelmintic), bhedan (drastric purgative/braking of hard stool), uttejaka (stimulant), mutrajanan (diuretics), deepan (appetizer), vishaghna (antidotes)

Indications

Arsha (piles), gulma (abdominal distension), raktapitta (bleeding disorders), dantroga (tooth diseases), mutrakricch (dysuria), udarroga (abdominal disorders).

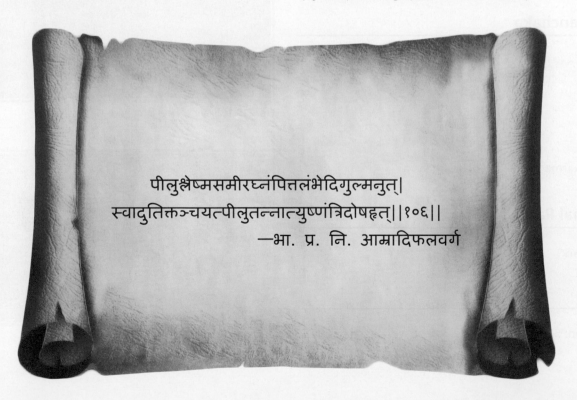

पीलुश्लेष्मसमीरघ्नंपित्तलंभेदिगुल्मनुत्।
स्वादुतिक्तञ्चयत्पीलुतन्नात्युष्णांत्रिदोषहृत्।।१०६।।
—भा. प्र. नि. आम्रादिफलवर्ग

219. Plaksh *[Ficus lacor Buch-Ham]*

Family:	*Moraceae*
Hindi name:	*Pakar, Pakhar*
English name:	*Java fig*
Synonyms:	*Jati, Parkari, Parkati*

Morphology

It is a much branched evergreen medium-sized tree, with aerial roots (**Fig. 219.1**).

Key Characters for Identification

➤ *Bark: Thin, with outer surface cream in color and inner surface reddish-brown* (**Fig. 219.2**).
➤ *Leaves: Simple, alternate, glabrous, ovate-oblong* (**Fig. 219.3**).
➤ *Flower: Receptacle axillary, in pairs, globose, male flower is sessile.*
➤ *Fruit: Globose, yellowish when ripe.*

Rasapanchaka

Guna	Guru, Ruksha
Rasa	Kashaya
Vipaka	Katu
Virya	Sheet
Doshakarma	Kapha pittahara

Officinal Part Used

Twak (bark)

Dose

Decoction: 50 to 100 mL

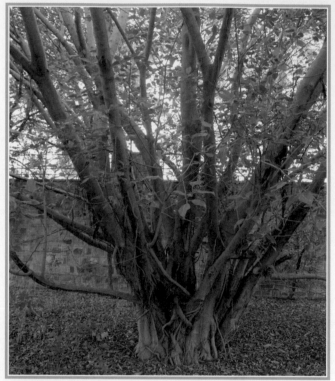

Fig. 219.1 Plant of *Ficus lacor* Buch-Ham.

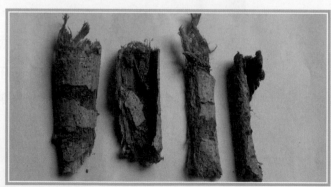

Fig. 219.2 Bark.

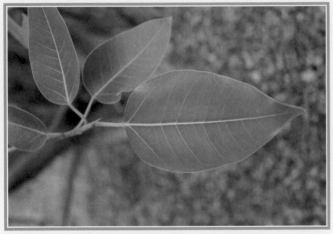

Fig. 219.3 Leaves.

Karma (Actions)

Stambhan (inhibitory action), mutrasangrahniya (urinary astringent), sandhaniya (union promoter), shothhar (reduce swelling), vranaropana (wound healing).

Indications

Rakta pitta (bleeding disorders), yoniroga (vaginal diseases), daha (burning sensation), vrana (wounds), murcha (fainting), mukhapak (stomatitis), pradar (excessive vaginal discharge), prameha (diabetes), atisaar (diarrhea), pravahika (dysentry).

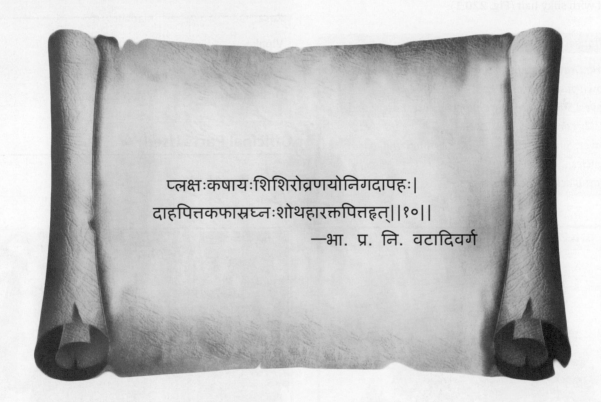

प्लक्षःकषायःशिशिरोव्रणयोनिगदापहः।
दाहपित्तकफास्रघ्नःशोथहारक्तपित्तहृत्॥१०॥
—भा. प्र. नि. वटादिवर्ग

220. Priyala *[Buchanania lanzang Spreng.]*

Family: *Anacardiaceae*

Hindi name: *Chironji*

English name: *Almondette, cuddapah almond*

Synonyms: *Kharaskandh, Bahulvalkal, Tapeshta, Sannkadru, Dhanusthpat, Chaar*

Morphology

It is a medium height tree of about 50 feet, young branches clothed with silky hair (**Fig. 220.1**).

Key Characters for Identification

➤ *Bark: Gray rough fissured bark, exudating reddish-brown gummy resin (***Fig. 220.2***).*
➤ *Leaves: Simple, broadly oblong, obtuse, base rounded, thickly coriaceous (***Fig. 220.3***).*
➤ *Flower: Small, greenish-white, terminal and axillary panicles.*
➤ *Fruit: Black, lenticular drupes.*

Rasapanchaka

Guna	Guru, Snigdha, Sar
Rasa	Madhur
Vipaka	Madhur
Virya	Sheet
Doshakarma	Vatapittashamaka

Officinal Parts Used

Fruit pulp and bark

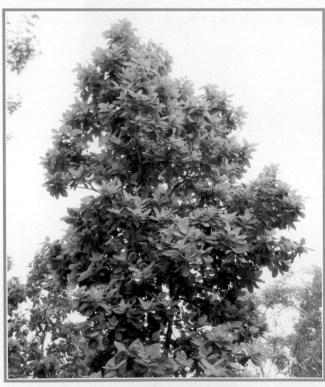

Fig. 220.1 Plant of *Buchanania lanzang* Spreng.

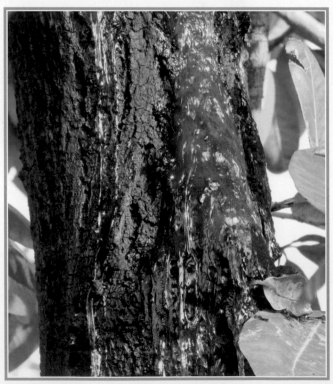

Fig. 220.2 Bark with exudate.

Dose

Decoction: 40 to 80 mL
Pulp powder: 10 to 20 g

Karma (Actions)

Balya (tonics), brihmaniya (bulk promoting), vrishya (aphrodisiac), hridya (cardiac stimulant), atidurjar (difficult to digest), visthambhi (constipative), aamvardhak (increase aam/causes indigestion).

Indications

Daha (burning sensation), jwar (fever), trishna (thirst), rakt pitta (bleeding disorders), kasa (cough).

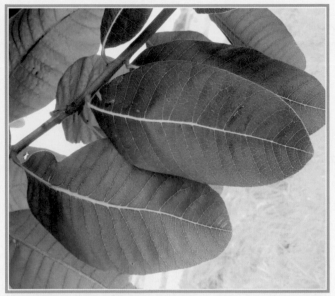

Fig. 220.3 Leaves.

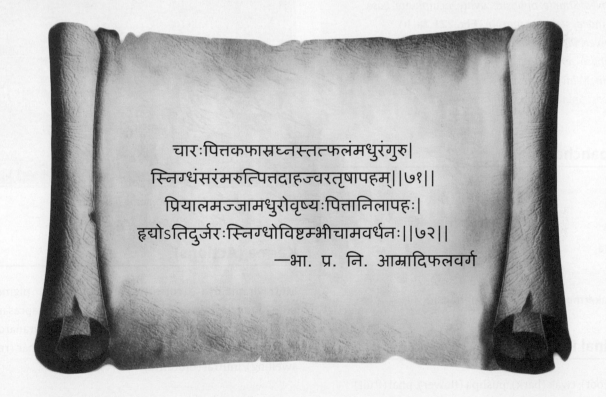

चारःपित्तकफास्रघ्नस्तत्फलंमधुरंगुरु|
स्निग्धंसरंमरुत्पित्तदाहज्वरतृषापहम्||७१||
प्रियालमज्जामधुरोवृष्यःपित्तानिलापहः|
हृद्योऽतिदुर्जरःस्निग्धोविष्टम्भीचामवर्धनः||७२||
—भा. प्र. नि. आम्रादिफलवर्ग

221. Priyangu [*Callicarpa macrophylla* Vahl.]

Family:	*Verbenaceae*
Hindi name:	*Phoolpriyangu*
English name:	*Beauty berry*
Synonyms:	*Phalini, Anganapriya, Gandhphala, Kaanta, Lata, Priya, Vishvaksena, Mahilavaha*

Morphology

It is a deciduous shrub of 4 to 8 feet with soft hairy branches (**Fig. 221.1**).

Key Characters for Identification

➤ *Leaves: Simple, opposite, ovate, acuminate, base rounded, serrated margin* (**Fig. 221.2a, b**).
➤ *Flower: Pinkish-purple colored, axillary, peduncle, globose cymes* (**Fig. 221.3**).
➤ *Fruit: White drupes.*
➤ *Seeds: Small, globose, many* (**Fig. 221.4**).

Rasapanchaka

Guna	Guru, Ruksha
Rasa	Tikta, Kashaya, Madhur
Vipaka	Katu
Virya	Sheet
Doshakarma	Kaphapittahara

Officinal Parts Used

Mool (root), twak (bark), pushpa (flower), phal (fruit)

Dose

Powder: 3 to 6 g

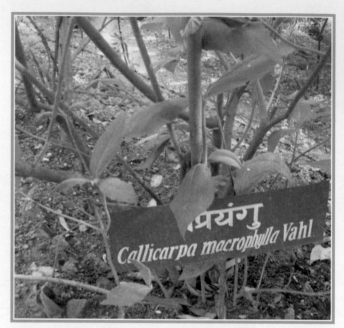

Fig. 221.1 Plant of *Callicarpa macrophylla* Vahl.

Karma (Actions)

Mutraviranjaniya (corrective of urinary pigments), purishsangrahniya (intestinal astringent), dahaprasamana (refrigerant), jwaraghna (antipyretics), vranaropaka (wound healing), vishaghna (antidotes), shothahar (reduce swelling), mutral (diuretics).

Indications

Raktaatisaar (bleeding diarrhea), dourgandhya (foul smell), sweda (perspiration), daha (burning sensation), jwara (fever), gulma (abdominal tumor), trishna (thirst), visha (poisoning), moha (delusion), vaman (vomiting).

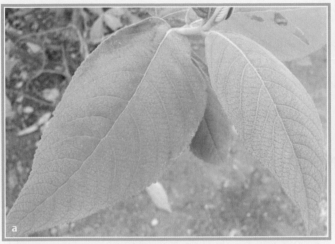

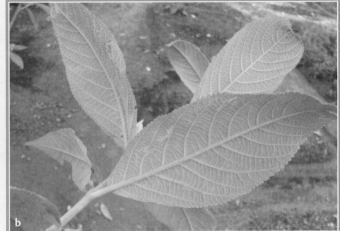

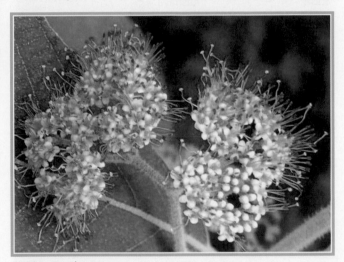

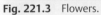

Fig. 221.2 **(a)** Leaves' ventral surface. **(b)** Leaves' dorsal surface.

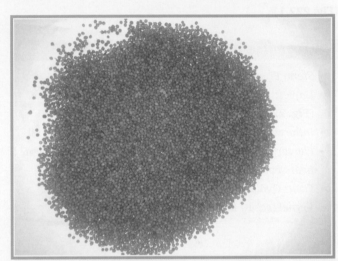

Fig. 221.3 Flowers.

Fig. 221.4 Seeds.

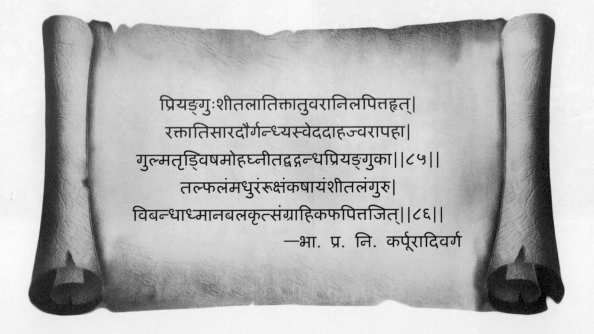

प्रियङ्गुःशीतलातिक्तातुवरानिलपित्तहृत्।
रक्तातिसारदौर्गन्ध्यस्वेददाहज्वरापहा।
गुल्मतृड्विषमोहघ्नीतद्वन्द्वप्रियङ्गुका॥८५॥
तत्फलंमधुरंरूक्षंकषायंशीतलंगुरु।
विबन्धाध्मानबलकृत्संग्राहिकफपित्तजित्॥८६॥
—भा. प्र. नि. कर्पूरादिवर्ग

222. Puga *[Areca catechu Linn.]*

Family:	*Arecaceae*
Hindi name:	*Supari*
English name:	*Betel Nut Palm*
Synonyms:	*Ghorant, Pugi, Guvaak, Kramuka, Pugiphal, Udvega*

Morphology

It is a tall, slender, unbranched tree of 40 to 50 feet, and is surmounted by broad glossy green feather-shaped leaves (**Fig. 222.1**).

Key Characters for Identification

➤ *Stem: Erect, surrounded by a crown of leaves.*
➤ *Leaves: Pinnate, petiole broadly expanded at the base* (**Fig. 222.2**).
➤ *Inflorescence: Spadix incased in a spathe.*
➤ *Flower: Yellowish-white in branched raceme, the plant bears both male and female flowers.*
➤ *Fruit: Ovoid, pericarp hard and fibrous* (**Fig. 222.3**).
➤ *Kernel* (*seed*): *Brown.*

Rasapanchaka

Guna	Guru, Ruksha
Rasa	Kashaya
Vipaka	Katu
Virya	Sheet
Doshakarma	Kaphapittashamak

Officinal Part Used

Fruits

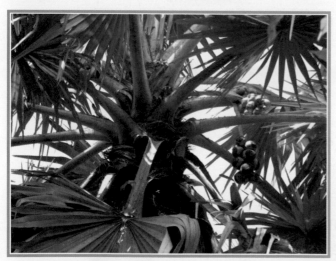

Fig. 222.1 Plant of *Areca catechu* Linn.

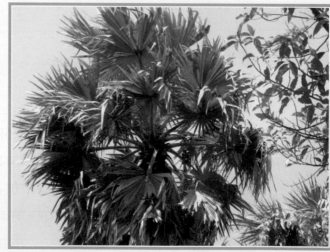

Fig. 222.2 Leaves.

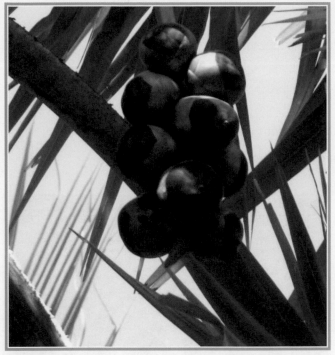

Fig. 222.3 Fruits.

Dose

Powder: 1 to 3 g

Karma (Actions)

Agnideepan (appetizer), rochaka (relish), mohajanak (create confusion), aasyavairasya nashnam (reduce tastelessness of mouth), vikasi (sluggishness of joints and diminishing of ojus), krimighna (anthelmintic), artavapravartaka (induce menstruation), Aadra Puga (fresh fruit of puga), Abhishyandi (blockage of channel), agnishamaka (reduce appetite), drishtihar (reduce the power of vision).

Indications

Raktapravahika (bleeding dysentery), atisaar (diarrhea), krimi (worm infestation), prameha (diabetes), raktasrava (hemorrhage), mukhapaka (stomatitis).

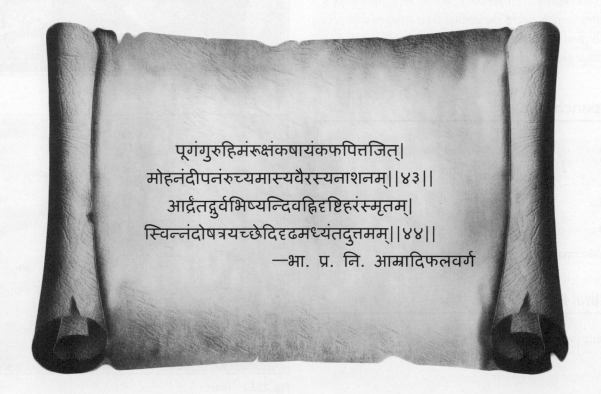

पूगंगुरुहिमंरूक्षंकषायंकफपित्तजित्।
मोहनंदीपनंरुच्यमास्यवैरस्यनाशनम्॥४३॥
आर्द्रंतद्दुर्वभिष्यन्दिवह्निदृष्टिहरंस्मृतम्।
स्विन्नंदोषत्रयच्छेदिदृढमध्यंतदुत्तमम्॥४४॥
—भा. प्र. नि. आम्रादिफलवर्ग

223. Putiha [*Mentha spicata* Linn.]

Family:	*Lamiaceae*
Hindi name:	*Pudina*
English name:	*Spearmint or Garden mint*
Synonyms:	*Rochani, Vahinjanini, Vaktrajadyanishudani*

Morphology

It is a perennial, aromatic herb with creeping rhizome (**Fig. 223.1**).

Key Characters for Identification

➤ Leaves: Smooth, arranged in opposite pairs, oblong to lanceolate/ovate in shape, often downy, have serrated margin, dark green to gray green color (**Fig. 223.2**).
➤ Flower: White to purple color, produced in false whorls called verticillasters, the corolla is two-lipped with four subequal lobes (**Fig. 223.3**).
➤ Fruits: Nutlets, contain one to four seeds.

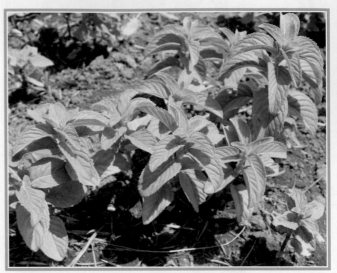

Fig. 223.1 Plant of *Mentha spicata* Linn.

Rasapanchaka

Guna	Laghu, Ruksha, Tikshan
Rasa	Katu
Vipaka	Katu
Virya	Ushna
Doshakarma	Kapha vatahara

Officinal Part Used

Panchang (whole plant)

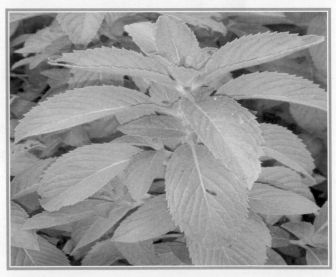

Fig. 223.2 Leaves.

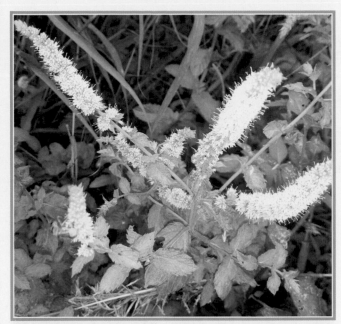

Fig. 223.3 Flowers.

Dose

Leaf juice: 5 to 10 mL
Oil: 1 to 3 drops

Karma (Actions)

Deepana (appetizer), pachana (digestive), udveshtannirodhi (antispasmodic), mutral (diuretics), artavajanan (emmenogague), chhardinigrahan (antiemetic), dourgandhyanashan (removes bad smell), krimighna (anthelmintic).

Indications

Ajeerna (indigestion), vaman (vomiting), shool (pain), adhyaman (flatulence), jwar (fever), krimi (worm infestation), rajorodha (amenorrhea).

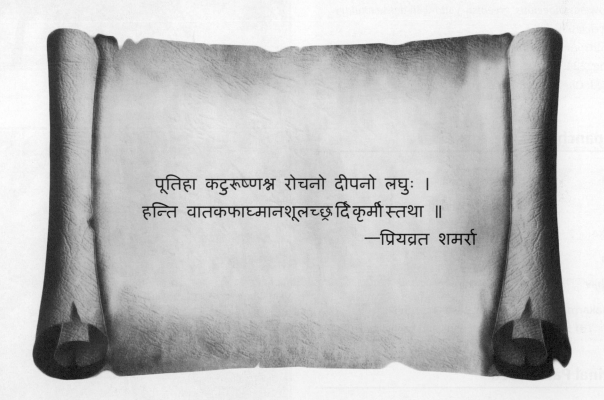

पूतिहा कटुरूष्णश्च रोचनो दीपनो लघुः ।
हन्ति वातकफाध्मानशूलच्छर्दिकृमींस्तथा ॥
—प्रियव्रत शर्मा

224. Putranjiva *[Putranjiva roxburghii Wall.]*

Family:	*Euphorbiaceae*
Hindi name:	*Jiyapota, Putranjiva*
English name:	*Indian Amulet Tree*
Synonyms:	*Garbhakar, Garbhada, Yastipuspa, Arthasadhaka, Shleepadapaha*

Morphology

It is an evergreen tree, 10 to 20 m tall, with gray stem (bark), which is whitish when young (**Fig. 224.1**).

Key Characters for Identification

➤ *Leaves: Alternate, simple, dark green, ovate-lanceolate with serrate, wavy margins (**Fig. 224.2**).*
➤ *Flowers: Dioecious, greenish-yellow, in dense axillary fascicles.*
➤ *Fruits: An ellipsoid drupe, subglobose, endocarp, woody (**Fig. 224.3**).*
➤ *Seed: One-seeded.*

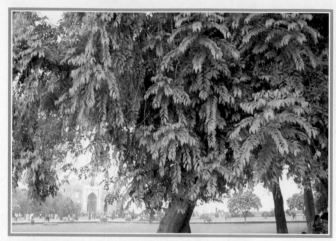

Fig. 224.1 Plant of *Putranjiva roxburghii* Wall.

Rasapanchaka

Guna	Guru, Ruksha
Rasa	Madhur, Katu, Lavana
Vipaka	Madhur
Virya	Sheeta
Prabhav	Garbhakara
Doshakarma	Kaphavatashamak (BPN), Pittashamana and kaphakarak (RN)

Officinal Parts Used

Seed and leaves

Dose

Seed powder: 3 to 6 g
Leaf juice: 10 to 20 mL

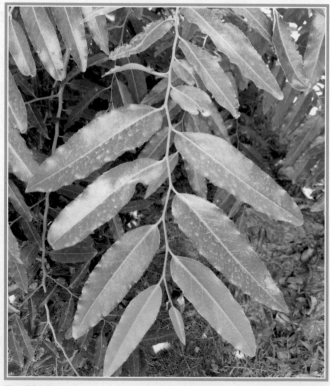

Fig. 224.2 Leaves.

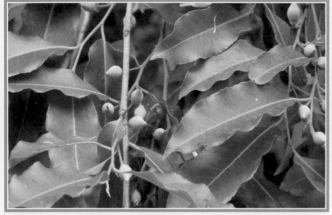

Fig. 224.3 Fruits.

Karma (Actions)

Vrisya (aphrodisiac), chakshusya (beneficial for vision), mutral (diuretics), virechan (purgative), dahashamak (refrigerant), trishnanigrahan (antithirst).

Indications

Daha (burning sensation), trishna (trishna thirst), garbhakar (maintains pregnancy), mutrakrichha (dysuria), vibandha (constipation), netraroga (eye disorders), pratisyaya (common cold), shirashoola (headache).

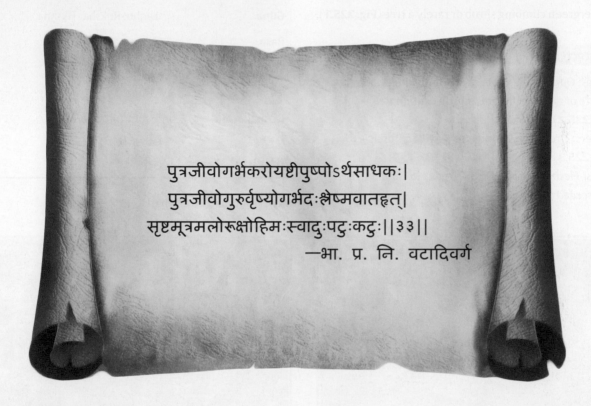

पुत्रजीवोगर्भकरोयष्टीपुष्पोऽर्थसाधकः।
पुत्रजीवोगुरुर्वृष्योगर्भदःश्लेष्मवातहृत्।
सृष्टमूत्रमलोरूक्षोहिमःस्वादुःपटुःकटुः॥३३॥
—भा. प्र. नि. वटादिवर्ग

225. Saptachakra *[Salacia chinensis Linn.]*

Family:	*Hippocrataceae*
Hindi name:	*Saptrangi*
English name:	*Lolly berry*
Synonyms:	*Swarnamoola, Saptrangi*

Morphology

It is an evergreen climbing shrub or rarely a tree (**Fig. 225.1**).

Key Characters for Identification

➤ *Leaves: Opposite, 6 to 11 cm, ovate-oblong-lanceolate, serrate or crenate margin, shortly acuminate* (**Fig. 225.2**).
➤ *Flowers: Greenish-yellow, 6 mm, axillary fascicles* (**Fig. 225.3**).
➤ *Fruits: Fleshy, globose, orange–red color at maturity, one-seeded* (**Fig. 225.4**).

Rasapanchaka

Guna	Laghu, Ruksha, Tikshna
Rasa	Tikta, Kashaya
Vipaka	Katu
Virya	Ushna
Doshakarma	Kapha pittashamak

Officinal Parts Used

Mool (root) and twak (bark)

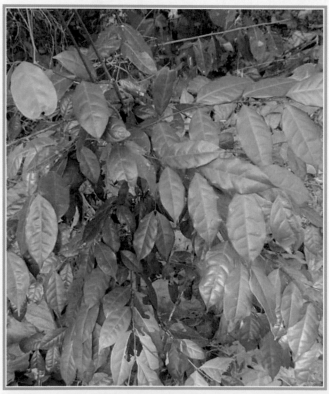

Fig. 225.1 Shrub of *Salacia chinensis* Linn.

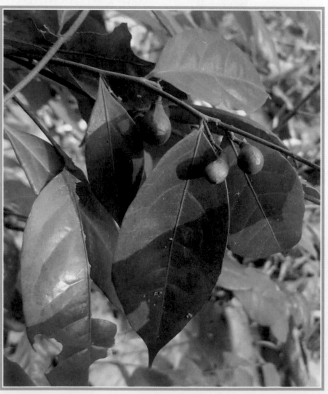

Fig. 225.2 Leaves.

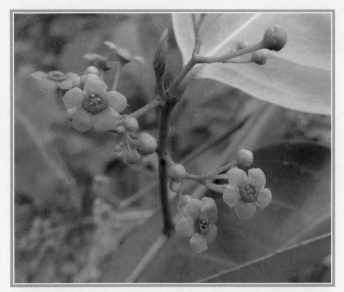

Fig. 225.3 Flowers.

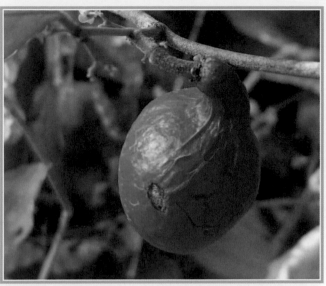

Fig. 225.4 Fruit.

Dose

Powder: 1 to 3 g
Decoction: 50 to 80 mL

Karma (Actions)

Yakrit uttejaka (hepatic stimulant), rechak (purgative), deepan (appetizer), raktashodhaka (blood purifier), mutrasangrahniya (urinary astringent), shothhara (reduces swelling).

Indications

Yakritvriddhi (hepatomegaly), madhumeha (diabetes mellitus), adhyaman (flatulence), rajorodha (amenorrhea), pramehapidika (carbuncles).

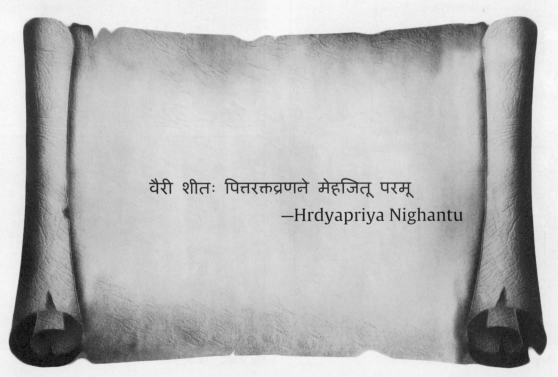

वैरी शीतः पित्तरक्तव्रणने मेहजित् परम्
—Hrdyapriya Nighantu

226. Saptaparna [*Alstonia scholaris* (Linn.) R. Br.]

Family:	*Apocynaceae*
Hindi name:	*Chitwan, Saataun*
English name:	*Dita Bark*
Synonyms:	*Vishaltwak, Sharad,Vishamchad, Bahutwak, Bahuchad, Ayugmpatra*

Morphology

It is a beautiful medium-height evergreen tree (**Fig. 226.1**).

Key Characters for Identification

➤ *Bark: Grayish-brown, rough, lenticellate, abounding in bitter, milky latex (**Fig. 226.2a, b**).*
➤ *Leaves: Four to seven in a whorl, coriaceous, elliptic-oblong, pale beneath (**Fig. 226.3**).*
➤ *Flower: Small, greenish-white, umbel panicle, scented (**Fig. 226.4**).*
➤ *Fruit: Follicles, 30 to 60 cm long (**Fig. 226.5**).*
➤ *Seed: Papillose with brownish hair at each end.*

Rasapanchaka

Guna	Laghu, Snigdh, Sar
Rasa	Tikta, Kashaya
Vipaka	Katu
Virya	Ushna
Doshakarma	Vata kapha shamak

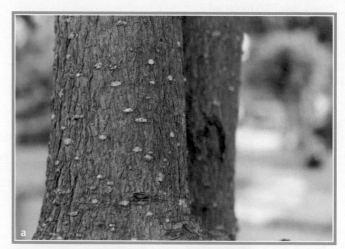

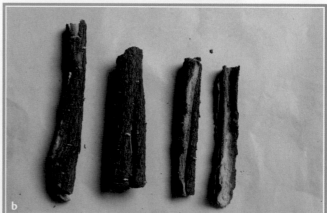

Fig. 226.2 (a, b) Bark.

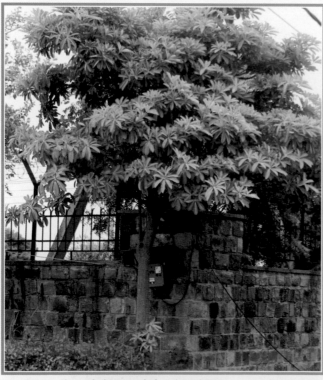

Fig. 226.1 Plant of *Alstonia scholaris* (Linn.) R. Br.

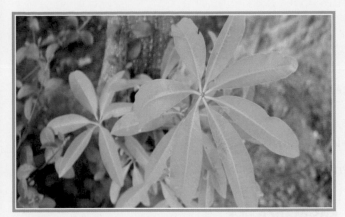

Fig. 226.3   Leaves.

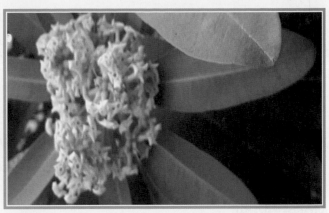

Fig. 226.4   Flower.

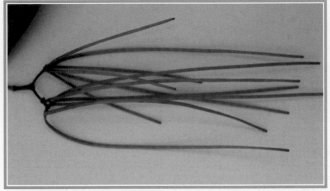

Fig. 226.5   Fruit.

Officinal Parts Used

Twak (bark), ksheer (latex), pushpa (flower)

Dose

Decoction: 40 to 80 mL

Karma (Actions)

Deepan (appetizer), krimighna (anthelmintic), jwaraghna (antipyretics), vranashodhana (wound cleanser), sara (laxative).

Indications

Vrana (wound), krimi (worm infestation), kushta (skin diseases), jeerna jwar (chronic fever), shwasa (asthma), gulma (abdominal distension), grahni (sprue).

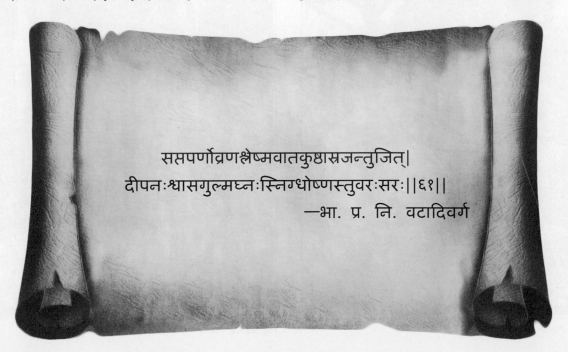

सप्तपर्णोव्रणश्लेष्मवातकुष्ठास्रजन्तुजित्।
दीपनःश्वासगुल्मघ्नःस्निग्धोष्णस्तुवरःसरः॥६१॥
—भा. प्र. नि. वटादिवर्ग

227. Saral *[Pinus longifolia* Roxb.]

Family:	*Pinaceae*
Hindi name:	*Chir*
English name:	*Long-leaved Pine*
Synonyms:	*Peetvriksha, Surbhidaruk*

Morphology

It is a tall tree of about 55 m height with whorled branches (**Fig. 227.1**).

Key Characters for Identification

➤ *Bark: Dark gray or red, deeply fissured, rough, exfoliated bark (***Fig. 227.2***).*
➤ *Leaves: Bundles of three, 20 to 30 cm long, needle-shaped, acicular, triquetrous, bright green (***Fig. 227.3***).*
➤ *Fruit: Male cones 13 mm long, ripe female cones 10 to 20 cm long on short stiff stalk (***Fig. 227.4***).*
➤ *Seed: Membranous and winged.*

Rasapanchaka

Guna	Laghu, Tikshan, Snigdha
Rasa	Katu, Tikta, Madhur
Vipaka	Katu
Virya	Ushna
Doshakarma	Kapha vatashamaka

Officinal Parts Used

Kastha (heart wood), niryasa (exudate), taila (oil)

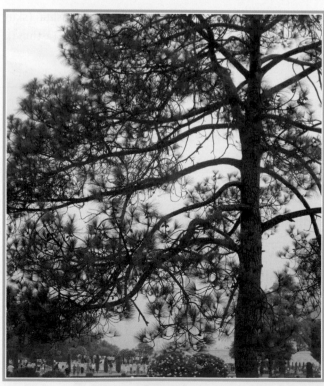

Fig. 227.1 Plant of *Pinus longifolia* Roxb.

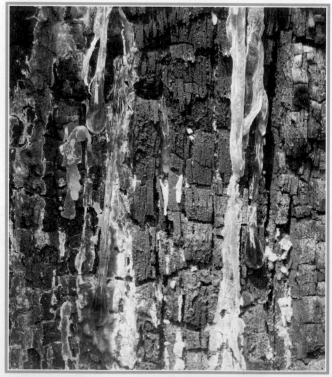

Fig. 227.2 Bark.

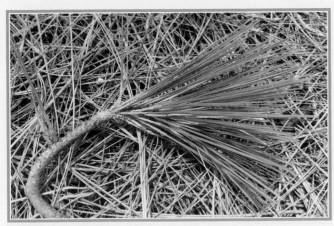

Fig. 227.3 Leaves.

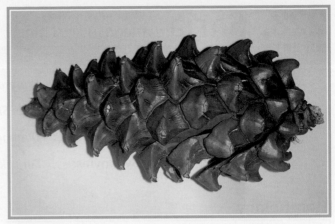

Fig. 227.4 Dried cone.

Dose

Kastha churna: 1 to 3 g

Taila: 1 to 3 drops

Karma (Actions)

Deepan (appetizer), vataanulomaka (carminative), krimighna (anthelmintic), kushtaghna (antipruritus), swedajanan (diaphoretic), mutral (diuretics), uttejaka (stimulant), durgandhhar (remove foul smell).

Indications

Karna, kantha, akshi roga (diseases of eyes, ear, throat), sweda (perspiration), daha (burning sensation), kasa (cough), murccha (fainting), vrana (wounds).

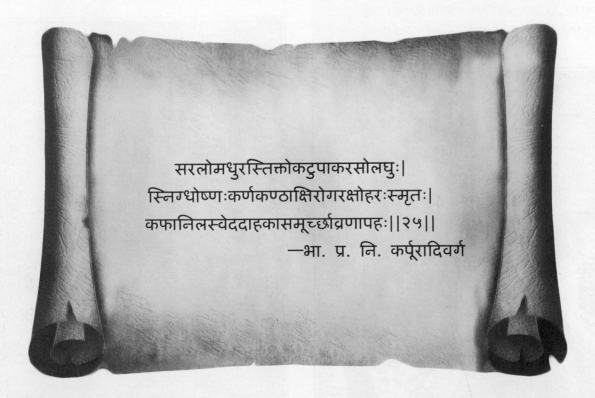

सरलोमधुरस्तिक्तोकटुपाकरसोलघुः।
स्निग्धोष्णःकर्णकण्ठाक्षिरोगरक्षोहरःस्मृतः।
कफानिलस्वेददाहकासमूर्च्छोव्रणापहः।।२५।।
—भा. प्र. नि. कर्पूरादिवर्ग

228. Sarja *[Vateria indica Linn.]*

Family:	*Dipterocarpaceae*
Hindi name:	*Bada Shaal, Chandras*
English name:	*Dammer*
Synonyms:	*Sarjrak, Ajakarna, Marichpatrak*

Morphology

It is a beautiful evergreen tree, and its trunk is about 3 m in girth (**Fig. 228.1**).

Key Characters for Identification

➤ *Bark: Appears rough, whitish to gray, peeling off in thick round flakes.*
➤ *Leaves: Simple, alternate, spiral, stipules caduceus, petiole 2 to 3.5 cm, swollen at apex, apex abruptly acuminate or obtuse, base rounded, margin entire, midrib flat above and curved near margin (**Fig. 228.2**).*
➤ *Flowers: White, fragrant, arranged in panicles.*
➤ *Fruit: Fleshy, wingless, about 50 to 60 mm long.*
➤ *Seed: One large seed which is filled with fat.*

Rasapanchaka

Guna	Snigdha
Rasa	Katu, Tikta, Kashaya
Vipaka	Katu
Virya	Ushna
Doshakarma	Kapha vatahara

Officinal Part Used

Niryaas

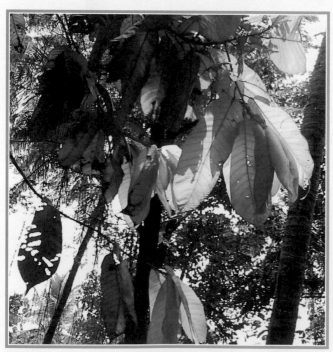

Fig. 228.1 Plant of *Vateria indica* Linn.

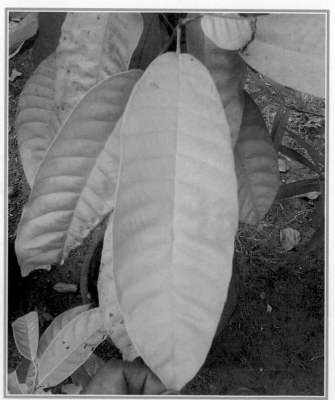

Fig. 228.2 Leaves.

Dose

Powder: 1 to 2 g

Karma (Actions)

Kandughna (antipruritus), kushtaghna (antidermatosis), vranaropaka (wound healing), vedanasthapana (anodynes).

Indications

Pandu (anemia), meha (urinary disorders), kushta (skin diseases), visha (poisoning), vrana (wounds), karnaroga (diseases of ear).

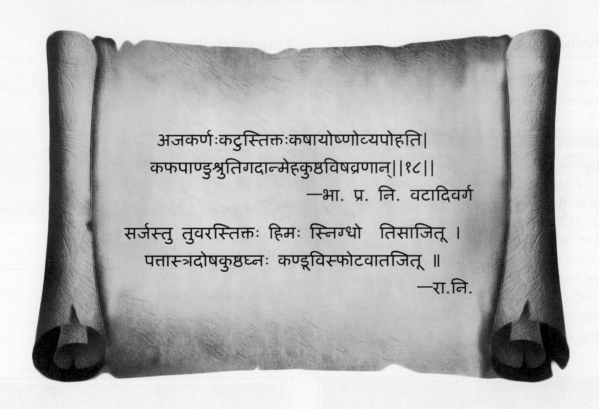

अजकर्णः कटुस्तिक्तः कषायोष्णोव्यपोहति।
कफपाण्डुश्रुतिगदान्मेहकुष्ठविषव्रणान्॥१८॥
—भा. प्र. नि. वटादिवर्ग

सर्जस्तु तुवरस्तिक्तः हिमः स्निग्धो तिसाजितू ।
पत्तास्त्रदोषकुष्ठघ्नः कण्डूविस्फोटवातजितू ॥
—रा. नि.

229. Sarsapa [Brassica campestris var. sarson Prain]

Family:	*Crucifer*
Hindi name:	*Sarso*
English name:	*Yellow Sarson, Mustard*
Synonyms:	*Katuk, Sneha, Tutubha, Kadambak, Siddharth*

Morphology

It is an annual herb of a height of 1 m or more with bright yellow flowers (**Fig. 229.1**).

Key Characters for Identification

➤ *Leaves: Basal leaves long, 6 to 9 cm long, broadly ovate, coarsely dentate, middle leaves oblong, eight-dentate, upper leaves broadly linear, entire (***Fig. 229.2***).*
➤ *Flower: Yellow in raceme (***Fig. 229.3***).*
➤ *Fruit: 6 to 10 cm long pod, siliqua breaking away from below upward, initially green but turns to brown at maturity (***Fig. 229.4***).*
➤ *Seed: Attached to the replum, reddish-brown small globose seed (***Fig. 229.5***).*

Rasapanchaka

Guna	Tikshan, Ruksha (Shaka), Snigdh (Beej, Taila)
Rasa	Katu, Tikta
Vipaka	Katu
Virya	Ushna
Doshakarma	Kapha Vaatghna, Rakta Pittavardhak

Officinal Parts Used

Beej (seed) and taila (oil)

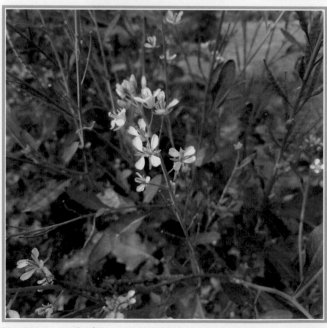

Fig. 229.1 Herb of *Brassica campestris* var. sarson Prain.

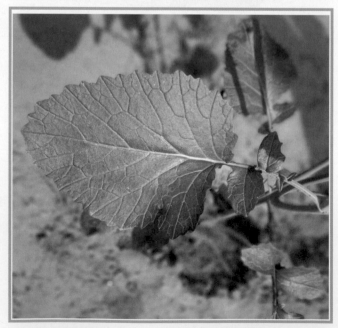

Fig. 229.2 Leaves.

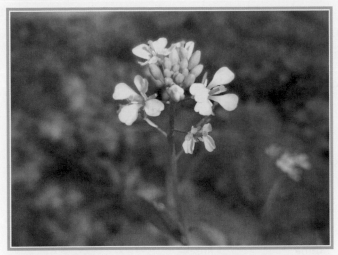

Fig. 229.3 Flowers.

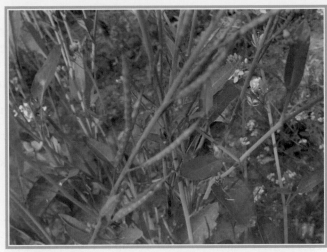

Fig. 229.4 Fruits.

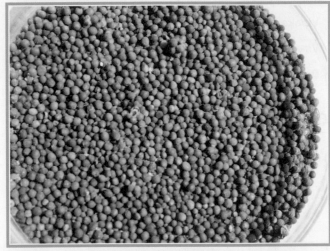

Fig. 229.5 Seeds.

Dose

Beej: 2 to 4 g

Karma (Actions)

Deepana (appetizer), rakshoghna (bacteriological), mutral (diuretic), krimighna (anthelmintic).

Indications

Kandu (pruritus), kushta (skin disease), kostha krimi (abdominal worms), aamavata (rheumatoid arthritis), pleehavriddhi (splenomegaly).

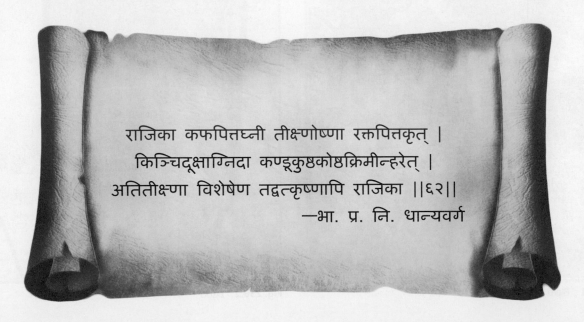

राजिका कफपित्तघ्नी तीक्ष्णोष्णा रक्तपित्तकृत् ।
किन्चिदूक्षाग्निदा कण्डूकुष्ठकोष्ठक्रिमीन्हरेत् ।
अतितीक्ष्णा विशेषेण तद्वत्कृष्णापि राजिका ||६२||
—भा. प्र. नि. धान्यवर्ग

230. Shala *[Shorea robusta Gaertn. f]*

Family:	*Dipterocarpaceae*
Hindi name:	*Sal, Sakhu*
English name:	*The Sal tree*
Synonyms:	*Sarjark, Karshya, Salsaar, Dhupvriksh*

Morphology

It is a large, straight, deciduous tree up to 150 feet high and 15 feet wide (**Fig. 230.1**).

Key Characters for Identification

➤ *Bark: Smooth or longitudinally fissured, reddish-brown or gray bark (***Fig. 230.2***).*
➤ *Leaves: Simple, ovate-oblong, acuminate, coriaceous, glabrous, base cordate (***Fig. 230.3***).*
➤ *Flower: Yellowish, terminal.*
➤ *Fruit: Indehiscent, ovoid with five equal wings with ovoid seeds (***Fig. 230.4***).*
➤ *Exudate: Hard, resinous, creamy yellow colored (***Fig. 230.5***).*

Rasapanchaka

Guna	Ruksha
Rasa	Kashaya (twak), Niryasa (Kashaya, Madhur)
Vipaka	Katu
Virya	Sheet
Doshakarma	Kapha pittashamak

Officinal Parts Used

Twak (bark) and niryasa (exudate, it is known as Raal)

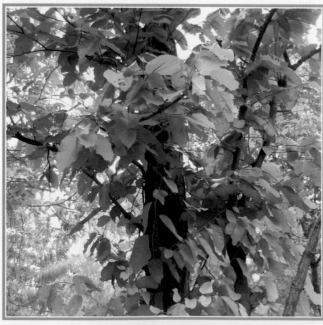

Fig. 230.1   Plant of *Shorea robusta* Gaertn. F.

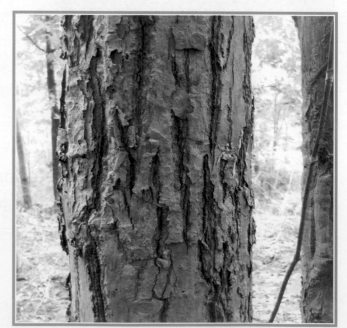

Fig. 230.2   Bark.

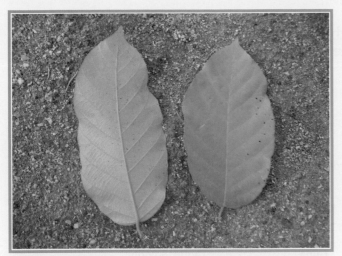

Fig. 230.3 Leaves.

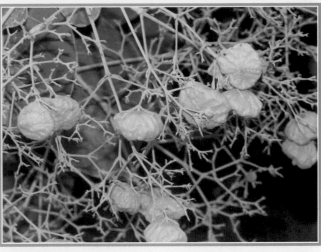

Fig. 230.4 Fruits.

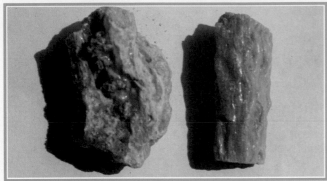

Fig. 230.5 Exudate.

Dose

Decoction: 50 to 100 mL
Niryasa: 1 to 3 g

Karma (Actions)

Vedanasthapana (anodynes), raktastambhak (hemostatics), vranaropana (wound healing), krimighna (anthelmintic), sandhaniya (union promoter), bhagnasandhankrit (union of fractured bone).

Indications

Karnaroga (ear disorders), visha (poisoning), vrana (wounds), vidridhi (abcess), yoniroga (vaginal diseases), kushta (skin diseases), meha (diabetes), pandu (anemia), badhirya (deafness), medoroga (obesity), raktatisaar (diarrhea with blood).

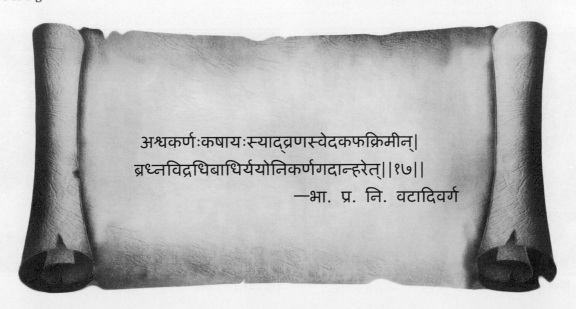

अश्वकर्णःकषायःस्याद्व्रणस्वेदकफक्रिमीन्।
ब्रध्नविद्रधिबाधिर्य्ययोनिकर्णगदान्हरेत्॥१७॥
—भा. प्र. नि. वटादिवर्ग

231. Shara *[Saccharum munja Roxb.]*

Family:	*Poaceae*
Hindi name:	*Sarpat, moonj*
English name:	*Pin red grass*
Synonyms:	*Baan, Tejana, Ikshuveshtan, Bhadramunj, Munj, Munjataka, Sthooldarbh, Sumekhal*

Morphology

It is a tall, thick, perennial grass growing up to 2 m in height (**Fig. 231.1**).

Key Characters for Identification

- ➤ *Roots: Deep and long spreading rhizomes (**Fig. 231.2**).*
- ➤ *Foliage: Leaf blades linear, green with white midrib, margins finely serrated and prickly. Culms (leaf stalks) slender, fibrous with little juice, arranged in small clumps, 1 to 4 m tall, turning brown or black when mature (**Fig. 231.3**).*
- ➤ *Flowers: Spikelets of florets with long silky white hairs, borne in branching panicle inflorescences (20–60 cm tall) that typically tower above the rest of the plant. Plume branches ascending and often tinged reddish or purplish. Blooms toward the end of rainy season in native range.*
- ➤ *Fruits: One-seeded caryopsis grains (1.5 mm), tufted, and dispersed by wind.*

Rasapanchaka

Guna	Laghu, Snigdh
Rasa	Madhur, Tikta
Vipaka	Madhur
Virya	Sheet
Doshakarma	Tridoshahara

Officinal Part Used

Mool (root)

Dose

Decoction: 50 to 100 mL

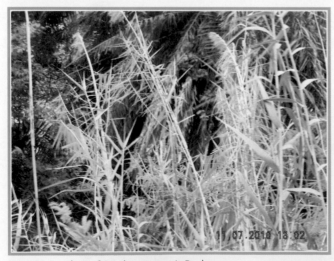

Fig. 231.1 Plant of *Saccharum munja* Roxb.

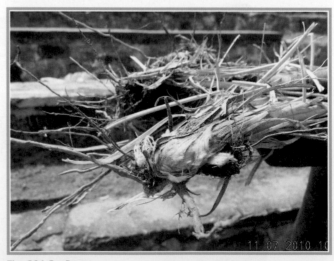

Fig. 231.2 Roots.

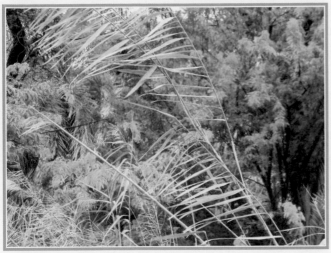

Fig. 231.3 Foliage.

Karma (Actions)

Vrishya (aphrodisiac), dahaprasasman (refrigerant), mutral (diuretics), trishnanigrahan (antithirst), stanyajanan (galactogague), chakshushya (beneficial for vision).

Indications

Ashmari (lithiasis), kasa (cough), trishna (thirst), visarpa (erysipelas), akshiroga (eye diseases), daha (burning sensation), mutrakricchta (dysuria), raktapitta (bleeding disorders).

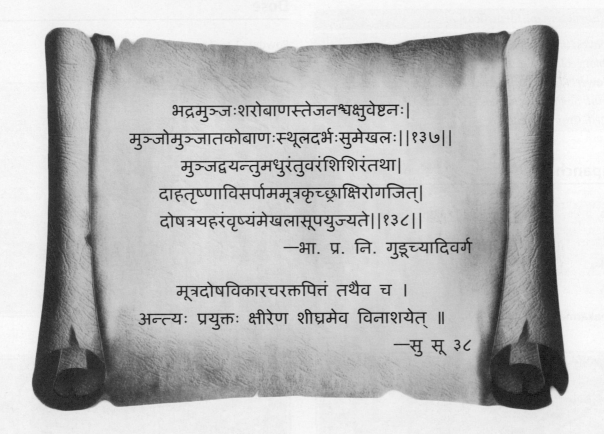

भद्रमुञ्जःशरोबाणस्तेजनश्चक्षुवेष्टनः।
मुञ्जोमुञ्जातकोबाणःस्थूलदर्भःसुमेखलः॥१३७॥
मुञ्जद्वयन्तुमधुरंतुवरंशिशिरंतथा।
दाहतृष्णाविसर्पाममूत्रकृच्छ्राक्षिरोगजित्।
दोषत्रयहरंवृष्यंमेखलासूपयुज्यते॥१३८॥
—भा. प्र. नि. गुडूच्यादिवर्ग

मूत्रदोषविकारचरक्तपित्तं तथैव च।
अन्त्यः प्रयुक्तः क्षीरेण शीघ्रमेव विनाशयेत्॥
—सु सू ३८

232. Sharpunkha *[Tephrosia purpurea (Linn.) Pers.]*

Family:	*Fabaceae*
Hindi name:	*Shara*
English name:	*Wild indigo, purple tephrosia*
Synonyms:	*Pleehashtaru, Pleehaari, Neelvrikshaakriti*

Morphology

It is a branched perennial herb of about 2 to 3 feet, with spreading branches (**Fig. 232.1**).

Key Characters for Identification

➤ *Leaves: Imparipinnate, leaflets 11 to 21, narrow, oblanceolate (**Fig. 232.2**).*
➤ *Flower: Red or purple in extra-axillary raceme.*
➤ *Fruit: Slightly curved pod (**Fig. 232.3**).*
➤ *Seed: Gray smooth.*

Rasapanchaka

Guna	Laghu, Ruksha, Tikshna
Rasa	Tikta, Kashaya
Vipaka	Katu
Virya	Ushna
Doshakarma	Kapha vatashamak

Officinal Part Used

Panchang (whole plant)

Dose

Powder: 1 to 2 g

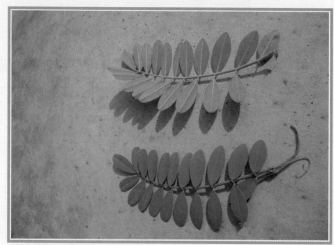

Fig. 232.2 Leaves.

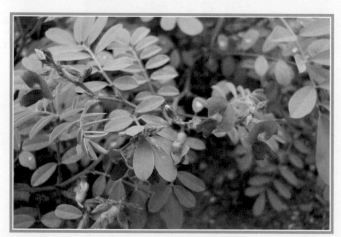

Fig. 232.1 Plant of *Tephrosia purpurea* (Linn.) Pers.

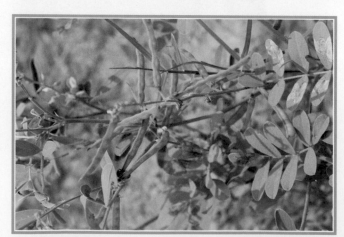

Fig. 232.3 Fruits.

Karma (Actions)

Vishaghna (antidote), vranaropan (wound healing), pittasharaka (cholerative).

Indications

Yakrit-pleeha vriddhi (hepato-splenomegaly), gulma (abdominal distension), vrana (wounds), visha (poisoning), kasa (cough), shwasa (asthma), jwar (fever).

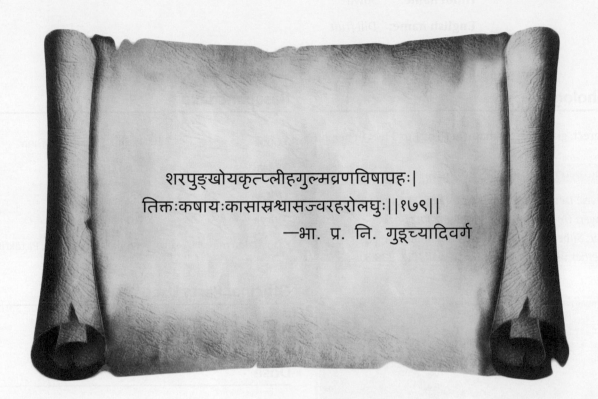

शरपुङ्खोयकृत्प्लीहगुल्मव्रणविषापहः।
तिक्तःकषायःकासास्त्रश्वासज्वरहरोलघुः।।१७९।।
—भा. प्र. नि. गुडूच्यादिवर्ग

233. Shatavah *[Anethum sowa Kurz.]*

Family:	*Umbelliferae*
Hindi name:	*Sowa*
English name:	*Dill fruit*
Synonyms:	*Satvaha, Karvi, Mishi, Shitchatra, Chatra*

Morphology

It is an erect, glabrous, aromatic herb of 1 to 3 feet in height.

Key Characters for Identification

➤ *Leaves: Decompound aromatic* (**Fig. 233.1**).
➤ *Flower: Umbel, pale yellow* (**Fig. 233.2**).
➤ *Fruit: Subelliptical, mericarps remaining joined together with irregular margin wall* (**Fig. 233.3**).

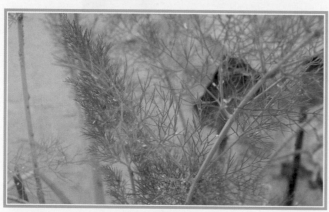

Fig. 233.1 Leaves of *Anethum sowa* Kurz.

Rasapanchaka

Guna	Laghu, Ruksha, Tikshna
Rasa	Katu, Tikta
Vipaka	Katu
Virya	Ushna
Doshakarma	Kapha vatashamak, Pittakrita

Officinal Parts Used

Fruit, seed, oil

Dose

Powder: 1 to 3 g
Oil: 1 to 3 drops
Ark: 20 to 40 mL

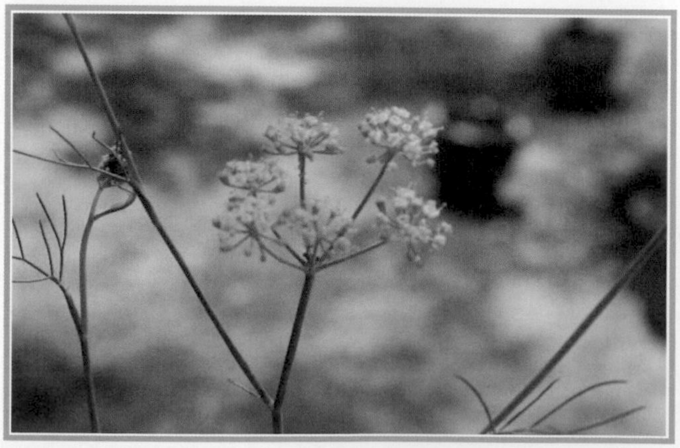

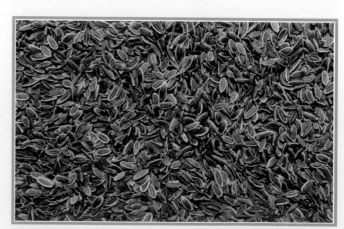

Fig. 233.2 Flowers.

Fig. 233.3 Fruits.

Karma (Actions)

Deepana (appetizer), pachana (digestive), vataanulomaka (carminative), krimighna (anthelmintic), vedanasthapana (anodynes), artavajanan (emmenogague), shothahar (reduces swelling), mutral (diuretics).

Indications

Adhyaman (flatulence), ajeerna (indigestion), udarshool (stomachache), vaman (vomiting), jwar (fever), akshiroga (eye diseases), vrana (wounds), krimi (worm infestation), rajorodha (amenorrhea), yonishool (vaginal pain), mutrakricchta (dysuria).

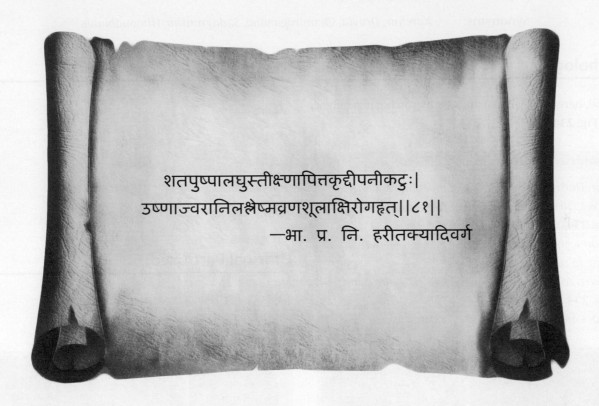

शतपुष्पालघुस्तीक्ष्णापित्तकृद्दीपनीकटुः।
उष्णाज्वरानिलक्ष्लेष्मव्रणशूलाक्षिरोगहृत्।।८१।।
—भा. प्र. नि. हरीतक्यादिवर्ग

234. Shati [Hedychium spicatum Hamitt ex Smith]

Family:	*Scitamineae*
Hindi name:	*Karpurkachari, Gandhpalashi*
English name:	*Spiked ginger lily, Zedoary*
Synonyms:	*Karchur, Dravid, Chandragandha, Sadagrantha, Himoudbhava*

Morphology

It is a tall, perennial, rhizomatous herb growing to a height of 1 m (**Fig. 234.1**).

Key Characters for Identification

➤ *Root: Horizontal root stock and tuberous root fibers.*
➤ *Leaves: 30 cm or more in length, oblong-lanceolate* (**Fig. 234.2**).
➤ *Inflorescence: Spiked, 30 cm long, densely flowered, white in color.*
➤ *Flower: Ascending and dense yellowish-white color* (**Fig. 234.3**).
➤ *Seed: Capsule.*

Rasapanchaka

Guna	Laghu, Tikshan
Rasa	Katu, Tikta
Vipaka	Katu
Virya	Ushna
Doshakarma	Kapha vatashamaka

Officinal Part Used

Tuber

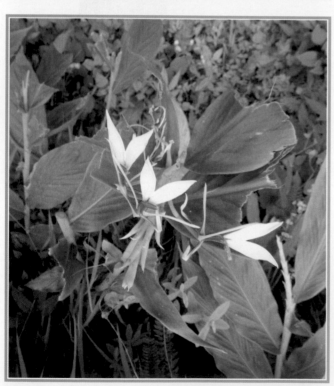

Fig. 234.1 Plant of *Hedychium spicatum* Hamitt ex Smith.

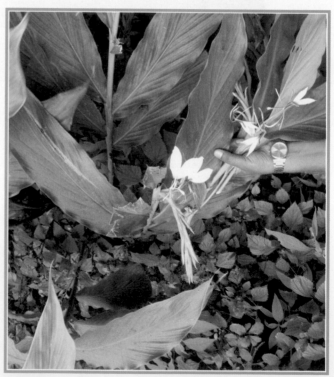

Fig. 234.2 Leaves.

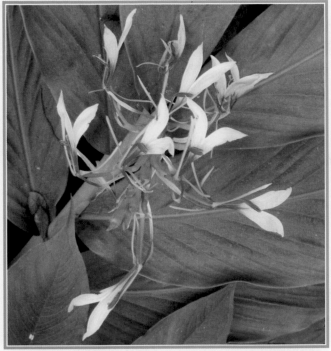

Fig. 234.3 Flowers.

Dose

Powder: 1 to 3 g

Karma (Actions)

Swarya (beneficial for voice), shothahar (anti-inflammatory), sugandhi (freshner), shwasahara (antiasthmatic), hikkanigrahan (anti-hic-cough), krimighna (anthelmintic), jwaraghna (anti-pyretic), hridya (cardiotonic), grahi (digestive and fecal astringent), deepana (appetizer), rochana (relish).

Indications

Kasa (cough), shwasa (asthma), hikka (hic-cough), ajeerna (indigestion), dusthavrana (infected wound), sannipatikjwar (fever with involvement of all doshas), gulma (abdominal lump), krimi (worm infestation), kushta (skin disease).

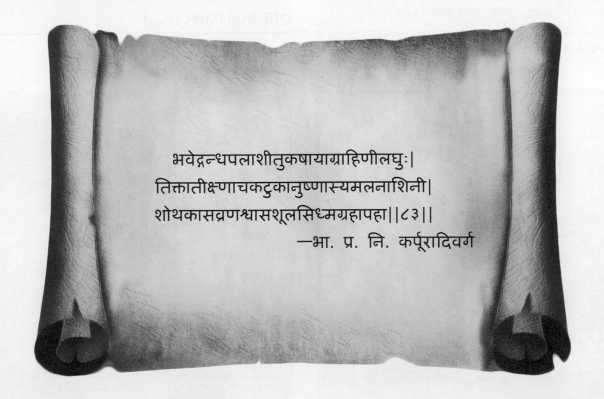

भवेद्रन्धपलाशीतुकषायाग्राहिणीलघुः।
तिक्तातीक्ष्णाचकटुकानुष्णास्यमलनाशिनी।
शोथकासव्रणश्वासशूलसिध्मग्रहापहा॥८३॥
—भा. प्र. नि. कर्पूरादिवर्ग

235. Simshapa *[Dalbergia sissoo Roxb.]*

Family:	*Fabaceae*
Hindi name:	*Sissam*
English name:	*Indian Rosewood*
Synonyms:	*Picchila, Shyama, Krishnasara, Vritapatra, Anupushpaka*

Morphology

It is an evergreen medium-height tree with cracked bark (**Fig. 235.1**).

Key Characters for Identification

➤ *Leaves: Alternate, imparipinnate, rachis zigzag, conspicuously, acuminate.* (**Fig. 235.2**).
➤ *Flower: Pale, yellowish-white, sessile (**Fig. 235.3**).*
➤ *Fruit: Pod, narrow at the base with a long stalk (**Fig. 235.4**).*
➤ *Seed: Pods are one- to four-seeded.*

Rasapanchaka

Guna	Laghu, Ruksha
Rasa	Tikta, Katu, Kashaya
Vipaka	Katu
Virya	Ushan
Doshakarma	Kapha vatahara

Officinal Parts Used

Bark, root, heartwood, leaves

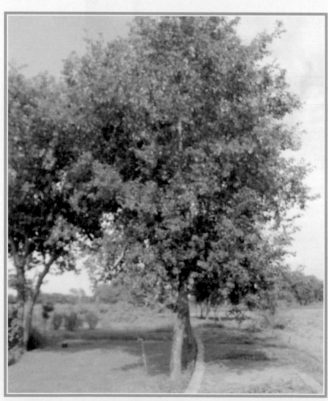

Fig. 235.1 Plant of *Dalbergia sissoo* Roxb.

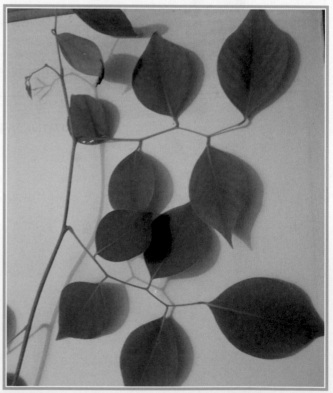

Fig. 235.2 Leaves.

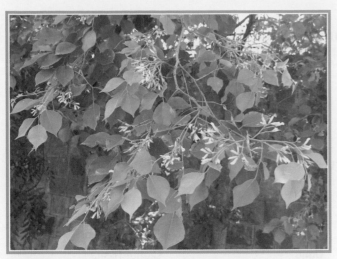

Fig. 235.3 Flowers.

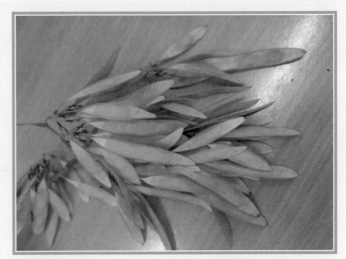

Fig. 235.4 Fruits.

Dose

Decoction: 40 to 80 mL
Powder: 3 to 6 g

Karma (Actions)

Garbhapataka (abortificient), dahaprasamana (refrigerant), kusthaghna (antidermatosis), krimighna (anthelmintic), vranashodhana (wound cleansing)..

Indications

Shosha (emaciation), meda (obesity), kushta (skin diseases), shivitra (leucoderma), vaman (vomiting), krimi (worm infestation), bastiroga (diseases of urinary bladder), vrana (wounds), daha (burning sensation), garbhapataka (abortifacient).

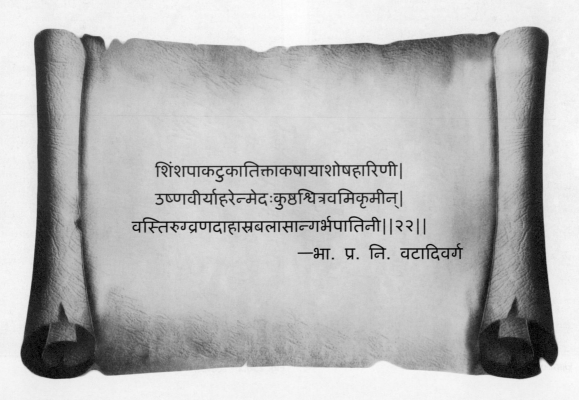

शिंशपाकटुकातित्ताकषायाशोषहारिणी।
उष्णवीर्याहरेन्मेदःकुष्ठश्चित्रवमिकृमीन्।
वस्तिरुग्व्रणदाहास्रबलासान्गर्भपातिनी।।२२।।
—भा. प्र. नि. वटादिवर्ग

236. Snuhi *[Euphorbia nerifolia Linn.]*

Family:	*Euphorbiacea*
Hindi name:	*Sehund, Thuhar*
English name:	*Milk Hedge*
Synonyms:	*Sudha, Samastadugdha, Vajri, Vajradruma, Snuka, Guda*

Morphology

It is an erect, succulent, thorny, milk-exudating shrub of 10 to 15 feet (**Fig. 236.1**).

Key Characters for Identification

➤ *Leaves: Fleshy, deciduous, obovate, spathulate, shortly, acute (**Fig. 236.2**).*
➤ *Flower: Red colored in short cymes (**Fig. 236.3**).*
➤ *Fruit: Tricoccus.*
➤ *Seed: Greenish-brown in colour.*

Rasapanchaka

Guna	Laghu, Tikshan
Rasa	Katu
Vipaka	Katu
Virya	Ushna
Doshakarma	Kaphavata hara

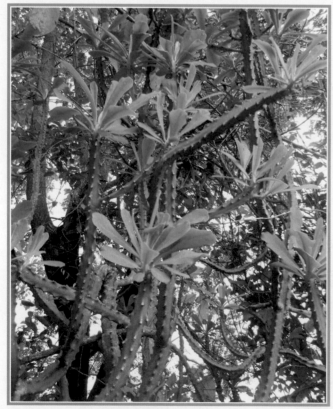

Fig. 236.1 Plant of *Euphorbia nerifolia* Linn.

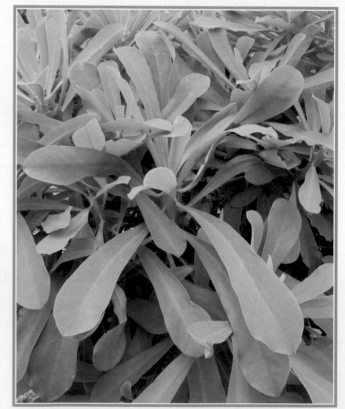

Fig. 236.2 Leaves.

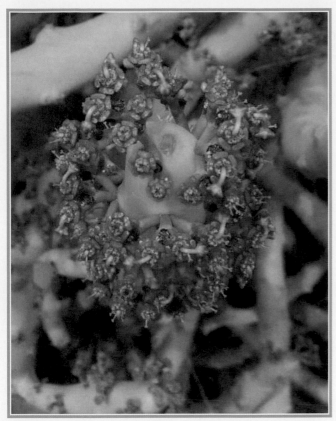

Fig. 236.3 Flowers.

Officinal Parts Used

Mool (roots), patra (leaves), ksheer (latex), kaand (stem)

Dose

Powder: 0.5 to 1 g
Ksheer: 125 to 250 mL
Kaandswaras: 5 to 10 mL

Karma (Actions)

Tikshna virechana (drastic purgatives), deepana (appetizer), shothahar (reduces swelling), vedanasthapana (anodynes).

Indications

Gulma (abdominal tumor), adhyaman (flatulence), arsha (piles), shool (pain), udarroga (abdominal diseases), shotha (inflammation), kushta (skin diseases), visha (poisoning), medoroga (obesity), unmada (insanity), prameha (diabetes), pandu (anemia).

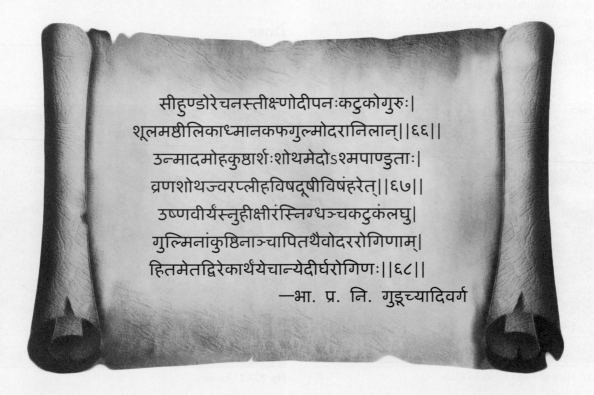

सीहुण्डोरेचनस्तीक्ष्णोदीपनःकटुकोगुरुः।
शूलमष्ठीलिकाध्मानकफगुल्मोदरानिलान्॥६६॥
उन्मादमोहकुष्ठार्शःशोथमेदोऽश्मपाण्डुताः।
व्रणशोथज्वरप्लीहविषदूषीविषंहरेत्॥६७॥
उष्णवीर्यंस्नुहीक्षीरंस्निग्धञ्चकटुकंलघु।
गुल्मिनांकुष्ठिनाञ्चापितथैवोदररोगिणाम्।
हितमेतद्विरेकार्थ्येचान्येदीर्घरोगिणः॥६८॥
—भा. प्र. नि. गुड्ड्च्यादिवर्ग

237. Sringataka *[Trapa bispinosa Roxb.]*

Family: *Trapaceae*

Hindi name: *Singhada*

English name: *Water chestnut*

Synonyms: *Jalphala, Trikonphala*

Morphology

It is an annual, succulent, spongy, aquatic, floating herb (**Fig. 237.1**).

Key Characters for Identification

➤ *Root: Green, photosynthetic, submerged root.*
➤ *Leaves: Simple, alternate, crowded at the upper parts of stem in rosettes, rhomboidal, apex triangular, inciso-serrate in the upper part, green above, reddish-purple beneath, petioles dilated near the apex into a large spongy float (***Fig. 237.2***).*
➤ *Flower: White, axillary, and solitary.*
➤ *Fruit: Obovoid, bony, sharp spinous horn, indehiscent, one-seeded (***Fig. 237.3***).*
➤ *Seed: White, starchy.*

Rasapanchaka

Guna	Guru
Rasa	Madhur, Kashaya
Vipaka	Madhur
Virya	Sheet
Doshakarma	Pittahara

Officinal Part Used

Phal majja (fruit sap)

Dose

Powder: 5 to 10 g

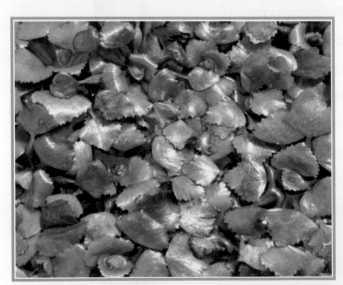

Fig. 237.1 Plant of *Trapa bispinosa* Roxb.

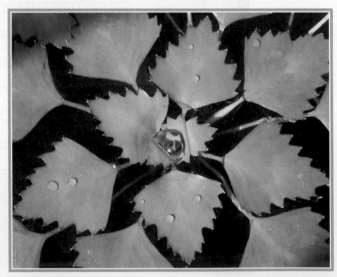

Fig. 237.2 Leaves.

Karma (Actions)

Vrishya (aphrodisiac), grahi (astringent), dahashamak (refrigerant), balya (tonics), paushtika (nourishment), garbhastapaka (establishment of foetus), shramahara (antifatigue), shonitasthapaka (hemostatics), mutral (diuretics).

Indications

Daha (burning sensation), trishna (thirst), jwar (fever), raktapitta (bleeding disorders), garbhapaat (abortion), shukradushti (diseases of impure semen), mutrakricchta (dysuria), pradar (leucorrhea).

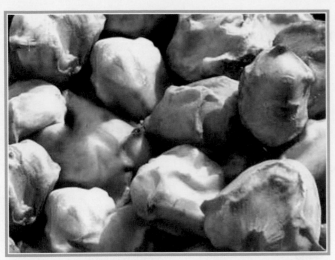

Fig. 237.3 Fruits.

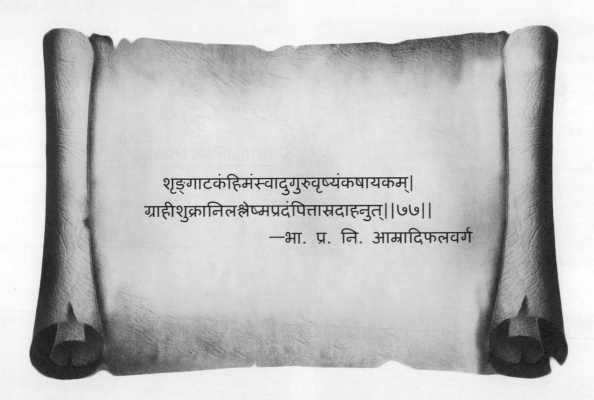

शृङ्गाटकंहिमंस्वादुगुरुवृष्यंकषायकम्।
ग्राहीशुक्रानिलश्लेष्मप्रदंपित्तास्रदाहनुत्॥७७॥
—भा. प्र. नि. आम्रादिफलवर्ग

238. Surana *[Amorphophallus campanulatus Blume]*

Family: *Araceae*

Hindi name: *Jimikand*

English name: *Elephant Foot Yam*

Synonyms: *Kand, Oal, Kandal, Arshoghna*

Morphology

It is a straight, evergreen herb with rhizomatous corm (**Fig. 238.1**).

Key Characters for Identification

➤ *Leaves: Compound, large, solitary, petiole stout, mottled, obovate, acute (**Fig. 238.2**).*

➤ *Corm: Spherical, inverted at the tip, 20 to 30 cm in diameter, depressed dark-brown corm (**Fig. 238.3**).*

➤ *Stem: Cylindrical, 30 to 40 cm long, greenish-white with plenty of white warts (**Fig. 238.4**).*

➤ *Inflorescence: Male and female inflorescence contiguous, neuters absent, appendage of spadix subglobose or amorphous, equaling or longer than the fertile region, spathe campanulate, pointed, strongly and closely veined.*

➤ *Fruit: Obovoid, two- to three-seeded red berries.*

Rasapanchaka

Guna	Katu, Kashaya
Rasa	Laghu, Ruksha, Tikshan
Vipaka	Katu
Virya	Ushna
Prabhav	Arshoghna
Doshakarma	Kapha vatashamak

Officinal Part Used

Kanda (tuber)

Dose

Powder: 3 to 6 g

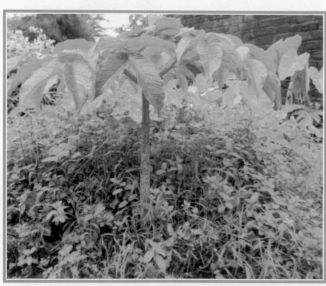

Fig. 238.1 Herb of *Amorphophallus campanulatus* Blume.

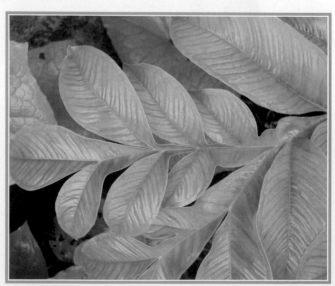

Fig. 238.2 Leaves.

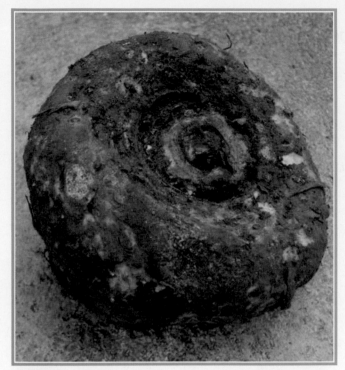

Fig. 238.3 Corm.

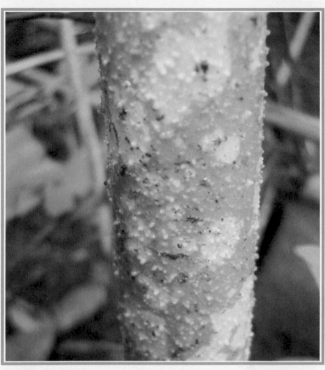

Fig. 238.4 Stem.

Karma (Actions)

Deepana (appetizer), pachana (digestive), vedanasthapana (analgesic), shothhara (anti-inflammatory).

Indications

Arsha (piles), gulma (abdominal lump), pleeharoga (disease of spleen), shool (colic pain), krimi (worm infestation), kasa (cough).

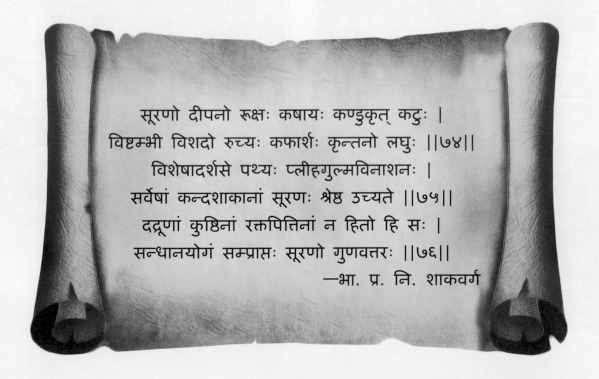

सूरणो दीपनो रूक्षः कषायः कण्डुकृत् कटुः |
विष्टम्भी विशदो रुच्यः कफार्शः कृन्तनो लघुः ||७४||
विशेषादर्शसे पथ्यः प्लीहगुल्मविनाशनः |
सर्वेषां कन्दशाकानां सूरणः श्रेष्ठ उच्यते ||७५||
दद्रूणां कुष्ठिनां रक्तपित्तिनां न हितो हि सः |
सन्धानयोगं सम्प्राप्तः सूरणो गुणवत्तरः ||७६||
—भा. प्र. नि. शाकवर्ग

239. Swarnashiri *[Argemone mexicana Linn.]*

Family: *Papavereceae*

Hindi name: *Satyanashi, Kantella*

English name: *Prickly poppy, Yellow thistle*

Synonyms: *Katuparni, Hemvati, Hemksheeri, Himavati, Himvaha, Peetadugdha, Chok (root).*

Morphology

It is an evergreen, erect, annual, prickly herb of 2 to 3 feet height, with yellow latex (**Fig. 239.1**).

Key Characters for Identification

➤ *Leaves: Simple, sessile, spiny, variegated with white spinous, vein white.*
➤ *Flower: Yellow, terminal on short leafy branches (**Fig. 239.1**).*
➤ *Fruit: Prickly capsule, oblong-ovoid, four to six valves opening (**Fig. 239.2**), and contains many globose black seeds (**Fig. 239.3**).*

Rasapanchaka

Guna	Laghu, Ruksha
Rasa	Tikta
Vipaka	Katu
Virya	Sheet
Doshakarma	Kapha pittahara

Officinal Parts Used

Mool (root), beej (seed), beej taila (seed oil)

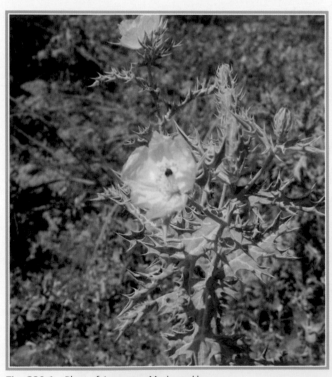

Fig. 239.1 Plant of *Argemone Mexicana* Linn.

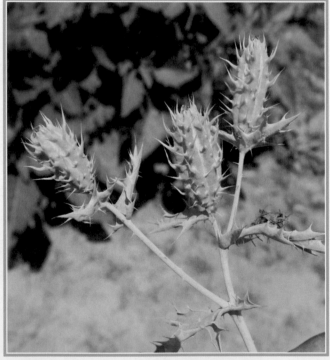

Fig. 239.2 Fruits.

Dose

Powder: 1 to 3 g
Taila: 10 to 30 drops
Ksheer: 5 to 10 drops

Karma (Actions)

Mool (root): Rechana (laxative), bhedana (purgative), kushtaghna (antipruritus), utkleshkar (induce nausea), krimighna (anthelmintic), vishaghna (antidotes).
Ksheer (latex): Krimighna (anthelmintic), vranashodhak (wound cleanser), vranaropaka (wound healing), shothhar (reduce swelling), jwaraghna (antipyretics).

Indications

Visha (poisoning), krimi (worm infestation), kandu (pruritis), kushta (skin diseases), aanaah (flatulence), visarp (erysipelas), phirang (syphilis), updansha (chancre), shotha (inflammation).

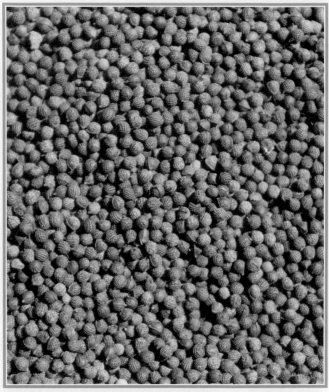

Fig. 239.3 Seeds.

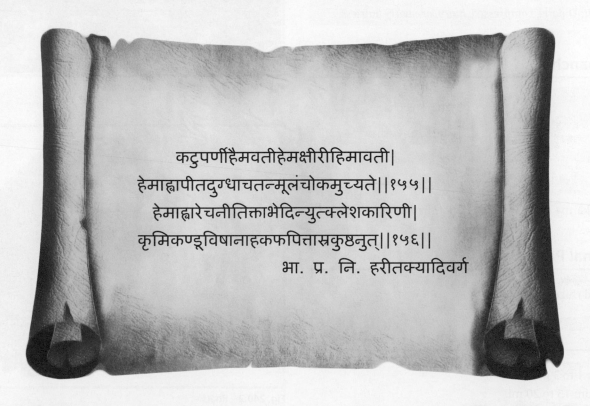

कटुपर्णीहैमवतीहेमक्षीरीहिमावती।
हेमाह्वापीतदुग्धाचतन्मूलंचोकमुच्यते॥१५५॥
हेमाह्वारेचनीतिक्ताभेदिन्युत्क्लेशकारिणी।
कृमिकण्डूविषानाहकफपित्तास्रकुष्ठनुत्॥१५६॥
भा. प्र. नि. हरीतक्यादिवर्ग

240. Tagar *[Valeriana wallichii DC]*

Family:	*Valerianaceae*
Hindi name:	*Sugandbala, Tagar*
English name:	*Indian valerian*
Synonyms:	*Nata, Nahush, Kutila, Vakra, Dand, Hasti, Kalanusarya, Chakra*

Morphology

It is a slightly hairy, tufted perennial herb up to 45 cm in height (**Fig. 240.1**).

Key Characters for Identification

➤ *Root: Thick horizontal root stock (***Fig. 240.2***).*
➤ *Leaves: Basal radical, long stalked, cordate-ovate, toothed, entire.*
➤ *Flower: White or tinged with pink in terminal corymbs, unisexual (***Fig. 240.3***).*
➤ *Fruit: Oblong, compressed, hairy, or nearly hairless.*

Rasapanchaka

Guna	Laghu, Snigdha
Rasa	Tikta, Katu, Kashaya
Vipaka	Katu
Virya	Ushna
Doshakarma	Tridoshashamak

Officinal Parts Used

Root and rhizome

Dose

Powder: 1 to 3 g
Decoction: 15 to 20 mL

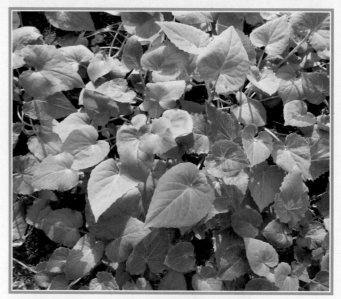

Fig. 240.1 Plant of *Valeriana wallichii* DC.

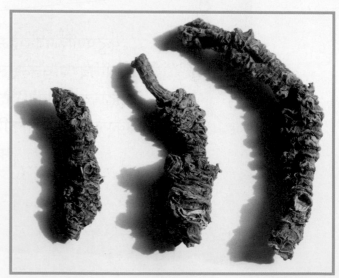

Fig. 240.2 Roots.

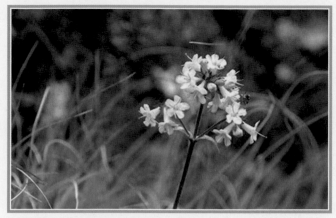

Fig. 240.3 Flowers.

Karma (Actions)

Vatanulomaka (carminative), vedanasthapaka (anodynes), vranaropaka (wound healing), uttejaka (stimulant), udveshtannirodhi (antianxiety).

Indications

Visha (poisoning), apasmaar (epilepsy), aptantrak (hysteria), shool (pain), netraroga (eye diseases), raktagatvata (increased blood pressure), anidra (insomnia), jeerna jwar (chronic fever).

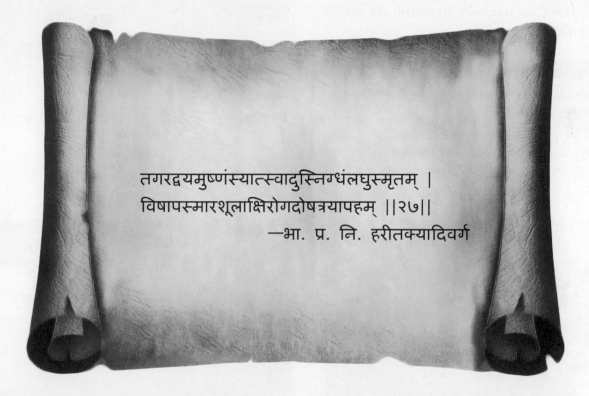

तगरद्वयमुष्णंस्यात्स्वादुस्निग्धंलघुस्मृतम् |
विषापस्मारशूलाक्षिरोगदोषत्रयापहम् ||२७||
—भा. प्र. नि. हरीतक्यादिवर्ग

241. Tailparna *[Eucalyptus globulus Labill.]*

Family: *Myrtaceae*

Hindi name: *Safeda, Niligiri*

English name: *Eucalyptus*

Synonyms: *Tailpatra, Sugandhpatra, Sugandhadhyapatra, Haritparnak*

Morphology

It is an evergreen, tall tree, with erect stem and smooth, peeled bark (**Fig. 241.1**).

Key Characters for Identification

➤ *Bark: Smooth, white–cream colored, peels off in long stripes (**Fig. 241.2**).*
➤ *Leaves: Opposite, alternate.*
➤ *Flowers: Large, white, one to three together in axils.*
➤ *Fruits: Capsule, dehiscent, and contain small seeds.*

Rasapanchaka

Guna	Laghu, Snigdha
Rasa	Katu, Tikta, Kashaya
Vipaka	Katu
Virya	Ushna
Doshakarma	Kapha vatashamak

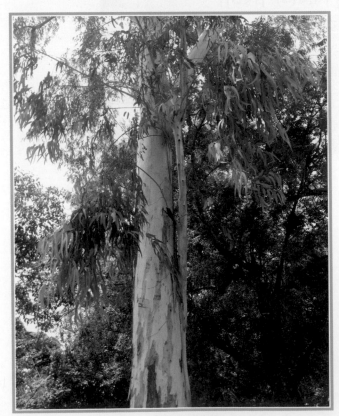

Fig. 241.1 Tree of *Eucalyptus globulus* Labill.

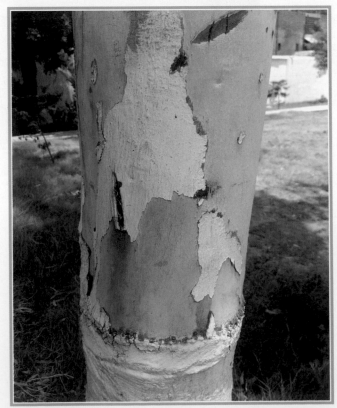

Fig. 241.2 Bark.

Officinal Parts Used

Patra (leaves), niryasa (exudates), taila (oil)

Dose

Powder: 1 to 2 g
Niryasa: 1 to 2 g
Taila: 1 to 3 drops

Karma (Actions)

Putijantu hara (remove putrification and insecticidal), durgandhnashak (remove bad smell), twakraagkarak (causes redness of skin).

Indications

Jeerna kasa (chronic cough), pratishyay (common cold), swarbheda (tonsillitis), vrana (wounds), aamvaat (rheumatoid arthritis).

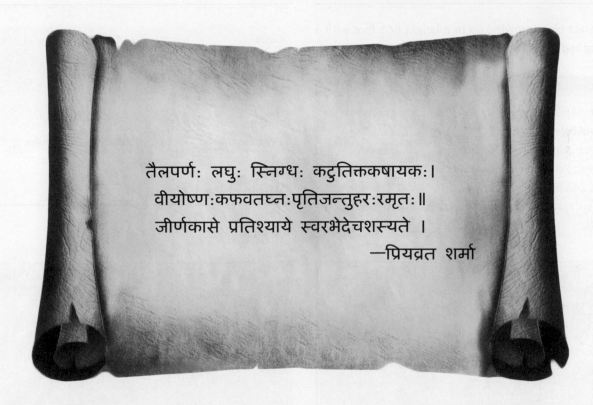

तैलपर्णः लघुः स्निग्धः कटुतिक्तकषायकः।
वीयोष्णःकफवतघ्नःपृतिजन्तुहरःरमृतः॥
जीर्णकासे प्रतिश्याये स्वरभेदेचशस्यते ।

—प्रियव्रत शर्मा

242. Talmuli *[Curculigo orchioides Gaertn.]*

Family:	*Amaryllidaceae*
Hindi name:	*Kali Musali*
English name:	*Musali*
Synonyms:	*Taalmuli, Durnamaari, Vrishya kanda, Maharrusha*

Morphology

It is an erect plant growing up to a height of 1 foot with a sheathing leaf base (**Fig. 242.1**).

Key Characters for Identification

➤ *Root: Short or elongated root-stock bearing several lateral roots (**Fig. 242.2**).*
➤ *Leaves: Simple, sessile, linear or linear-lanceolate.*
➤ *Flower: Yellow, on the bases of the leaves underground (**Fig. 242.3**).*
➤ *Fruit: Capsule, tricarpellary, contains one to four black seeds.*

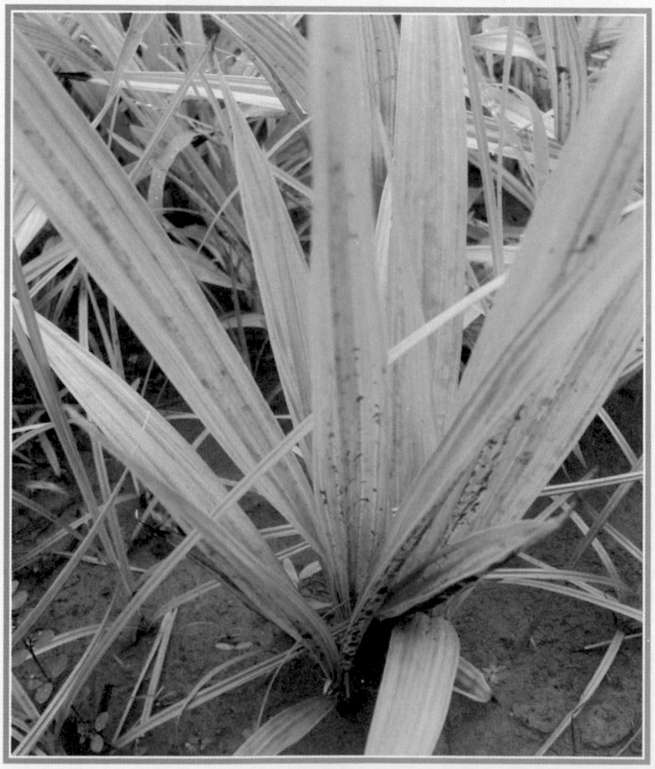

Rasapanchaka

Guna	Guru, Snigdha
Rasa	Madhura
Vipaka	Sheeta
Virya	Madhura
Doshakarma	Vata pittashamaka

Officinal Part Used

Tuberous root

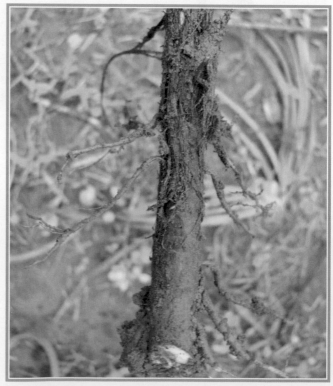

Fig. 242.1   Plant of *Curculigo orchioides* Gaertn.

Fig. 242.2   Root.

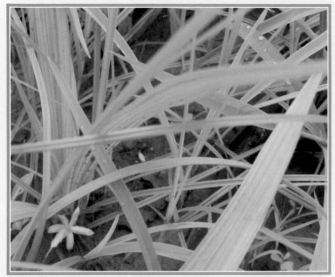

Fig. 242.3 Flower.

Dose

Powder: 3 to 6 g

Karma (Actions)

Snehana (oleation), vrishya (aphrodisiac), balya (tonic), mutral (diuretics), rasayan (rejuvenative), stanyavardhak (promote lactation), brihmaniya (bulk promoting).

Indications

Bandhyatva (infertility), soujaka (gonorrhea), mutrakricchta (dysuria), atyaartava (excessive menstruation), asthibhagna (fracture), dourbalya (general debility).

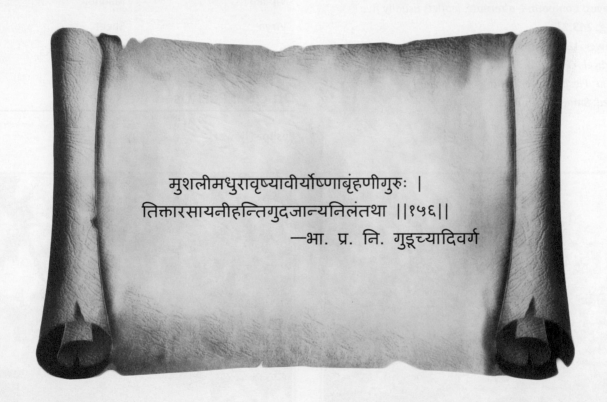

मुशलीमधुरावृष्यावीर्योष्णाबृंहणीगुरुः |
तिक्तारसायनीहन्तिगुदजान्यनिलंतथा ||१५६||
—भा. प्र. नि. गुडूच्यादिवर्ग

243. Taruni *[Rosa centifolia Linn.]*

Family:	*Rosaceae*
Hindi name:	*Gulab*
English name:	*Rose*
Synonyms:	*Shatpatri, Charukeshara, Mahakumari, Lakshapushpa, Atimanjula, Gandhadhya*

Morphology

It is a prickly branched shrub (**Fig. 243.1**).

Key Characters for Identification

➤ *Leaves: Compound, alternate, leaflets usually five* (**Fig. 243.2**).
➤ *Flower: Usually red or pink, fragrant, long slender pedicels (***Fig. 243.3a, b***).*
➤ *Fruit: Fleshy hip-enclosing bony achenes.*
➤ *Seed: Small, pendulous.*

Rasapanchaka

Guna	Laghu, Snigdh
Rasa	Katu, Tikta
Vipaka	Madhur
Virya	Sheet
Doshakarma	Tridoshshamaka

Officinal Part Used

Pushpa (flower)

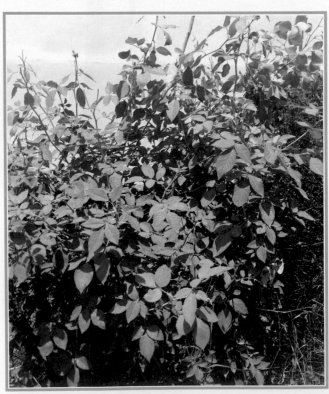

Fig. 243.1 Plant of *Rosa centifolia* Linn.

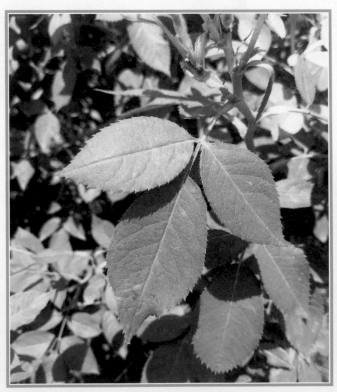

Fig. 243.2 Leaves.

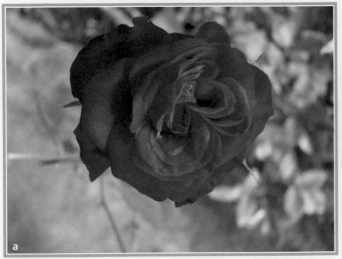
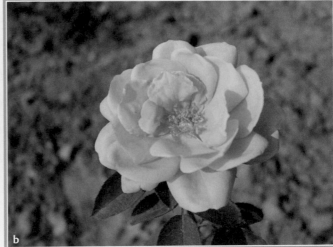

Fig. 243.3 (a, b) Flowers.

Dose

Powder: 1 to 3 g
Ark Gulab: 20 to 50 mL
Gulkand: 10 to 20 mL

Karma (Actions)

Hridya (cardio tonic), grahi (astringent), shukral (sementopoetic), varnya (complexion promoter), pachan (digestive), mrudusarak (smooth purgative), poushtik (nourishment).

Indications

Rakta vikara (diseases related to blood), twak roga (skin diseases), netraroga (eye diseases), sotha (inflammation), mukhavrana (mouth ulcers), jwar (fever), amalpitta (acidity).

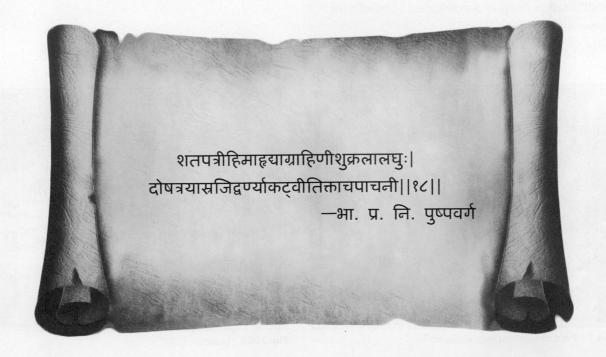

शतपत्रीहिमाहृद्याग्राहिणीशुक्रलालघुः।
दोषत्रयास्रजिद्वर्ण्याकट्वीतिक्ताचपाचनी॥१८॥
—भा. प्र. नि. पुष्पवर्ग

244. Tavakshiri [*Curcuma angustifolia* Roxb.]

Family:	*Scitaminae*
Hindi name:	*Tikhura*
English name:	*East India Arrowroot*
Synonyms:	*Tugaksheeri, Tvaksheeri*

Morphology

It is an evergreen, aromatic, herbaceous plant resembling turmeric in morphology (**Fig. 244.1**).

Key Characters for Identification

➤ *Stems: Stems are usually short, and are replaced by pseudostems formed by leaf sheaths.*
➤ *Leaves: Distichous, simple, leaf sheath open; ligule usually present, leaf blade suborbicular or lanceolate to narrowly strap-shaped, glabrous or hairy, midvein prominent, pinnate, parallel, margin-entire (**Fig. 244.2**).*
➤ *Inflorescence: Terminal on pseudostems or on separate, short, sheath-covered shoots arising from rhizomes, cylindric or fusiform, sometimes globose, raceme, or spike.*
➤ *Flowers: Bisexual, epigenous, zygomorphic.*
➤ *Fruit: Capsule, fleshy or dry, dehiscent or indehiscent, sometimes berry-like.*
➤ *Seed: Small, arillate.*

Rasapanchaka

Guna	Laghu, Snigdh
Rasa	Madhur
Vipaka	Madhur
Virya	Sheet
Doshakarma	Vatapittashamak

Officinal Part Used

Kanda (tuber)

Dose

Kanda churna: 1 to 3 g

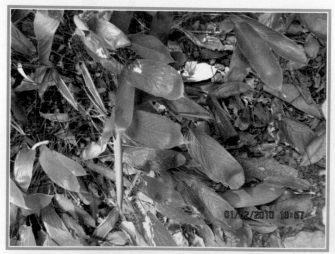

Fig. 244.1 Plant of *Curcuma angustifolia* Roxb.

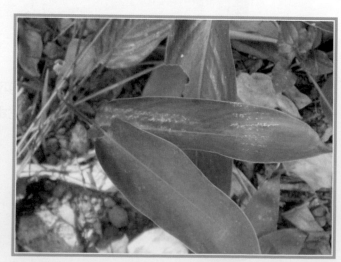

Fig. 244.2 Leaves.

Karma (Actions)

Snehan (oleation), anulomana (laxative), grahi (astringent), vrishya (aphrodisiac), balya (tonics), brihmaniya (bulk promoting), jwaraghna (antipyretic).

Indications

Atisaar (diarrhea), dourbalya (weakness), jwar (fever), kashaya (emaciation), kasa (cough), shwasa (asthma).

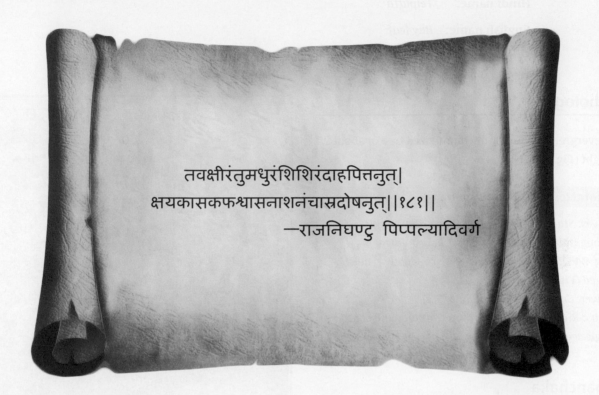

तवक्षीरंतुमधुरंशिशिरंदाहपित्तनुत्।
क्षयकासकफश्वासनाशनंचास्रदोषनुत्॥१८१॥
—राजनिघण्टु पिप्पल्यादिवर्ग

245. Tejpatra [*Cinnamomum tamala* Nees & Eberm]

Family: *Lauraceae*

Hindi name: *Tejpatta*

English name: *Bay leaf*

Synonyms: *Patra, Patrak, Patranamak, Tamalpatra, Taapicch, Kalskandh*

Morphology

It is an evergreen, aromatic, medium-sized tree of about 25 feet height (**Fig. 245.1**).

Key Characters for Identification

➤ *Leaves: Staked, opposite, or subopposite, elliptic-oblong, shining, leathery, entire, long pointed (**Fig. 245.2a**), tender new leaves are slightly reddish tinged (**Fig. 245.2b**).*
➤ *Flower: Small, yellowish (**Fig. 245.3**).*
➤ *Fruits: Ripe fruits are dark purple in color and contain single seed (**Fig. 245.4**).*

Rasapanchaka

Guna	Laghu, Picchila, Kinchit Tikshna
Rasa	Madhura, Katu, Tikta
Vipaka	Madhura
Virya	Ushna
Doshakarma	Kapha vaatshamak

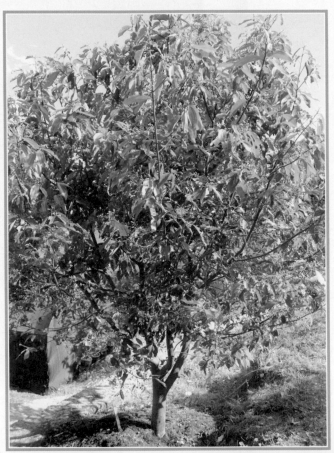

Fig. 245.1   Tree of *Cinnamomum tamala* Nees & Eberm.

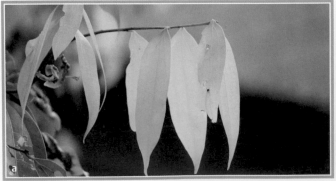
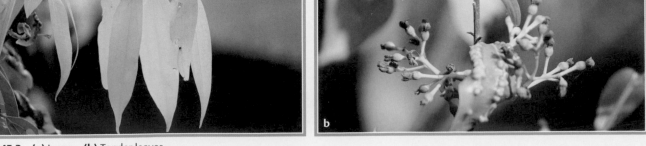

Fig. 245.2   (a) Leaves. **(b)** Tender leaves.

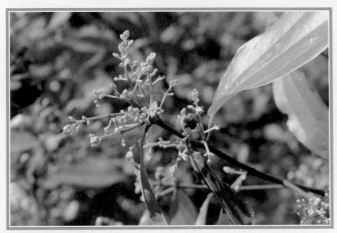

Fig. 245.3 Flowers.

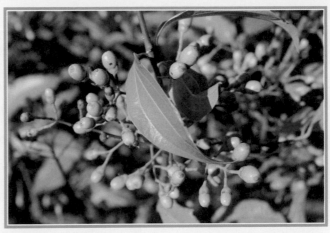

Fig. 245.4 Fruits.

Officinal Part Used

Patra (leaves)

Dose

Powder: 1 to 3 g

Karma (Actions)

Rochaka (relish), deepan (appetizer), swedajanan (diaphoretics), mutrajanan (diuretics), uttejaka (stimulant).

Indications

Arsha (piles), aruchi (distaste), hallash (nausea), peenasa (common cold), udarshool (stomach ache), atisaar (diarrhea).

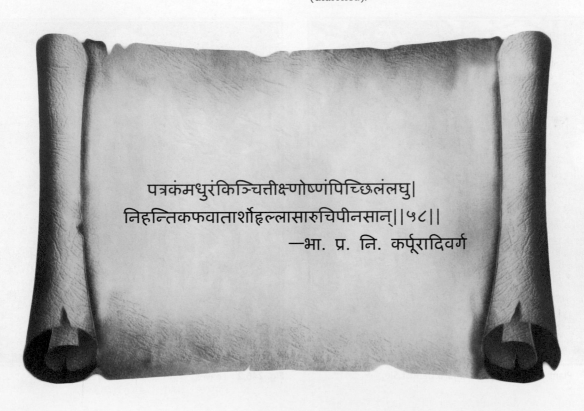

पत्रकंमधुरंकिञ्चित्तीक्ष्णोष्णंपिच्छिलंलघु।
निहन्तिकफवातार्शोहृल्लासारुचिपीनसान्॥७८॥
—भा. प्र. नि. कर्पूरादिवर्ग

246. Tuvraka *[Hydnocarpus laurifolia Dennst.Sle.]*

Family:	*Flacourtiaceae*
Hindi name:	*Chalmogra*
English name:	*Soorty oil tree*
Synonyms:	*Katukapitha, Kushtavairi*

Morphology

It is an evergreen deciduous tree of about 40 to 50 feet height (**Fig. 246.1**).

Key Characters for Identification

➤ *Bark: Pale-brown, rough bark, mottled with white.*
➤ *Leaves: Simple alternate, ovate, oblong, lanceolate, serrate (**Fig. 246.2**).*
➤ *Flower: Small, greenish-white, solitary, unisexual.*
➤ *Fruit: Globose or tomentose berries (**Fig. 246.3**).*
➤ *Seed: 15 to 20 per fruit, obtusely angular, yellowish.*

Rasapanchaka

Guna	Laghu, Snigdh, Tikshan
Rasa	Tikta, Katu, Kashaya
Vipaka	Katu
Virya	Ushna
Doshakarma	Kaphavatashamak

Officinal Parts Used

Seeds and oil

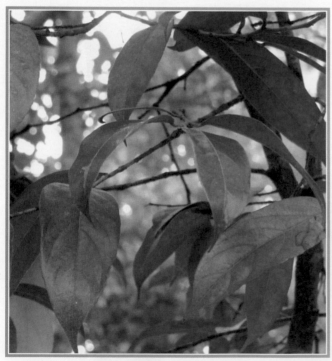

Fig. 246.1 Plant of *Hydnocarpus laurifolia* Dennst.Sle.

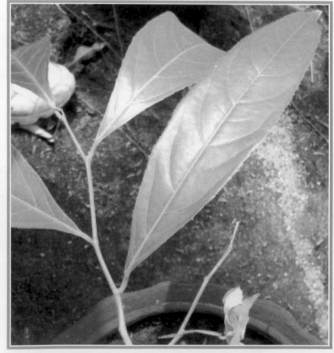

Fig. 246.2 Leaves.

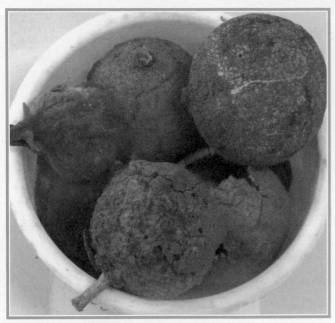

Fig. 246.3 Dried fruits.

Dose

Powder: 1 to 3 g
Oil: 30 to 60 drops

Karma (Actions)

Kushtaghna (antidermatosis), kandughna(antipruritus), krimighna (anthelmintic), vranaropaka (wound healing), vranashodhak (wound cleanser), vamak (induce vomiting), rechak (laxative).

Indications

Vrana (wounds), krimi (worm infestation), kushta (skin diseases), meha (diabetes), jwara (fever), arsha (piles), shopha (swelling).

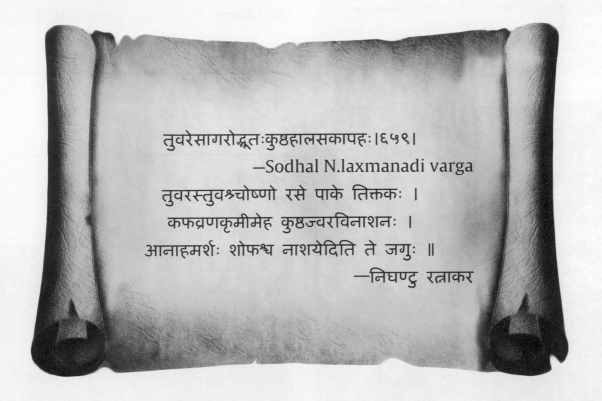

तुवरेसागरोद्भूतःकुष्ठहालसकापहः।६५९।

—Sodhal N.laxmanadi varga

तुवरस्तुवश्चोष्णो रसे पाके तिक्तकः ।

कफव्रणकृमीमेह कुष्ठज्वरविनाशनः ।

आनाहमर्शः शोफश्च नाशयेदिति ते जगुः ॥

—निघण्टु रत्नाकर

247. Udumbar *[Ficus glomerata Roxb.]*

Family:	*Moraceae*
Hindi name:	*Gular*
English name:	*The cluster fig*
Synonyms:	*Yagyang, Sadaphal, Jantuphal, Hemdugdh, Shwetvalkal*

Morphology

It is a much branched evergreen tree of about 60 feet height (**Fig. 247.1**).

Key Characters for Identification

➤ *Leaves: Simple, alternate, petiolate, stipulate, entire lamina, ovate-elliptival, 8–15 × 5–7 cm, acute apex and narrow base (**Fig. 247.2**).*
➤ *Fruits: Globose, green initially and becomes red at maturity, 3 to 5 cm in diameter (**Fig. 247.3a, b**).*

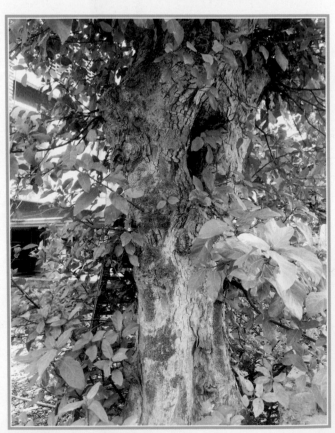

Fig. 247.1 Tree of *Ficus glomerata* Roxb.

Rasapanchaka

Guna	Kashaya, Madhura
Rasa	Guru, Ruksha
Vipaka	Katu
Virya	Sheet
Doshakarma	Kapha pittaghna

Officinal Parts Used

Twak (bark), phal (fruit), ksheer (exudate)

Dose

Powder: 3 to 6 g
Decoction: 50 to 100 mL

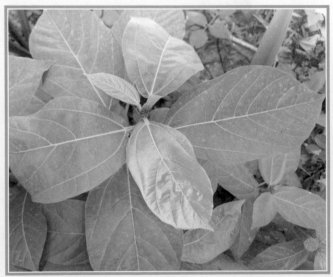

Fig. 247.2 Leaves.

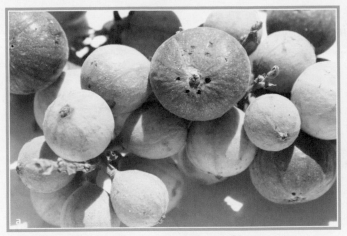

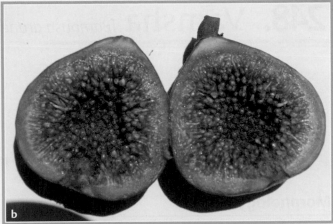

Fig. 247.3 **(a)** Fruits. **(b)** Longitudinal section of fruit.

Karma (Actions)

Stambhana (inhibitory action), sangrahi (astringent), mutrasangrahniya (urinary astringent), varnya (complexion promoter), vranashodhana (wound cleanser), vranaropana (wound healing).

Indications

Mukhapaka (stomatitis), granthi (cystic swellings), raktapitta (bleeding disorders), rakta atisaar (diarrhea associated with blood), prameha (diabetes), daha (burning sensation).

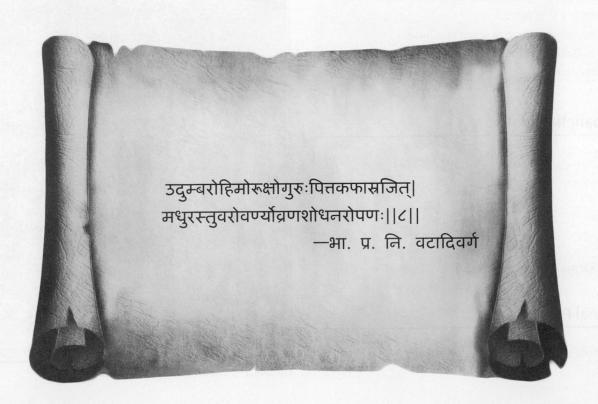

उदुम्बरोहिमोरूक्षोगुरुःपित्तकफास्रजित्।
मधुरस्तुवरोवर्ण्योव्रणशोधनरोपणः॥८॥
—भा. प्र. नि. वटादिवर्ग

248. Vamsha *[Bambusa arundinaceae Willd.]*

Family:	*Poaceae*
Hindi name:	*Bans*
English name:	*Bamboo*
Synonyms:	*Twaksaar, Shatparva, Trinadhwaj, Venu, Yavaphal, Maskar, Tejan, Shubha*

Morphology

It is a straight, unbranched tall tree of 15 to 35 m height, with joint stems (**Fig. 248.1**).

Key Characters for Identification

➤ *Stem: Bright green to brown in color, jointed, hollow from inside (**Fig. 248.2**).*
➤ *Leaves: Leaf sheaths with a short bristly auricle, ligule short (**Fig. 248.3**).*
➤ *Inflorescence: Spikelet glabrous, yellow or yellowish-green in a long panicle.*
➤ *Floral glumes: Three to seven in numbers.*
➤ *Fruit: Oblong grains, beaked by the style base, grooved on one side.*

Rasapanchaka

Guna	Laghu, Ruksha
Rasa	Madhura, Kashaya
Vipaka	Madhura
Virya	Sheeta
Doshakarma	Kapha pittashamak

Officinal Parts Used

Mool (root), phal (fruit), patra (leaves), vanshlochana (exudate)

Dose

Vanshlochana: 1 to 3 g
Decoction: 50 to 100 mL

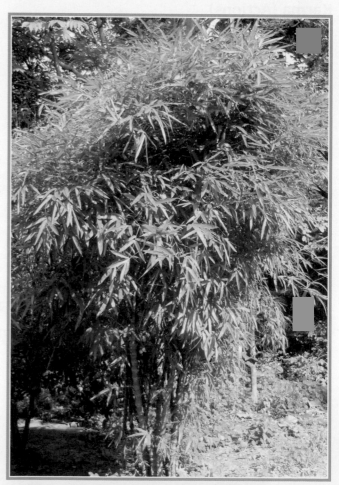

Fig. 248.1 Plant of *Bambusa arundinaceae* Willd.

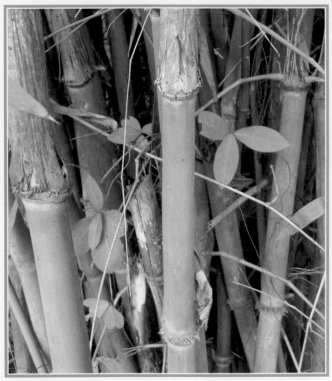

Fig. 248.2 Stem.

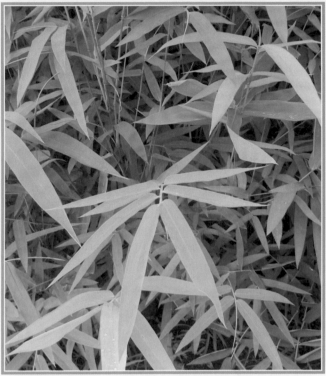

Fig. 248.3 Leaves.

Karma (Actions)

Sara (laxative), bastishodhana (purification of bladder), chhedana (antitussive)..

Indications

Kushta (skin diseases), shwasa (asthma), kasa (cough), raktavikara (diseases related to blood), shoth (inflammation), mutrakricchta (dysuria), prameha (diabetes).

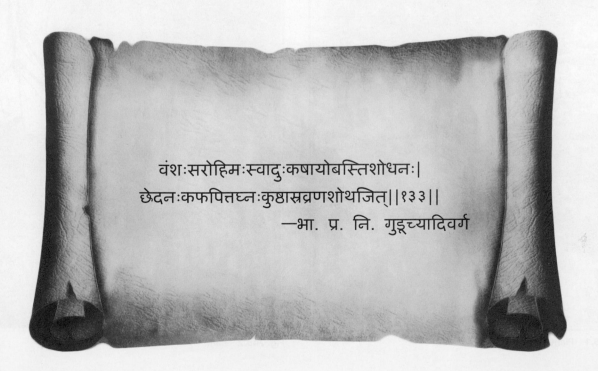

वंशःसरोहिमःस्वादुःकषायोबस्तिशोधनः।
छेदनःकफपित्तघ्नःकुष्ठास्रव्रणशोथजित्।।१३३।।
—भा. प्र. नि. गुडूच्यादिवर्ग

249. Vata *[Ficus bengalensis Linn.]*

Family:	*Moraceae*
Hindi name:	*Bargad, Bad*
English name:	*Banyan*
Synonyms:	*Raktphal, Shringi, Nyaygrodh, Skandhaj, Dhruv, Ksheeri, Vanaspati, Bahupada*

Morphology

It is a much-branched evergreen tree bearing many aerial roots, functioning as prop roots (**Fig. 249.1**).

Key Characters for Identification

➤ *Bark: Greenish-white (***Fig. 249.2***).*
➤ *Leaves: Simple, alternate, stipulate, broadly elliptic to ovate, entire, coriaceous (***Fig. 249.3***).*
➤ *Fruit: Receptacles are axillary, sessile in pairs, globose, brick red when ripe, enclosing male–female and gall flowers, fruits are small, achenes, enclosed in the common fleshy receptacles.*

Rasapanchaka

Guna	Guru, Ruksha
Rasa	Kashaya
Vipaka	Katu
Virya	Sheet
Doshakarma	Kapha pittahara

Officinal Parts Used

Twak (bark), patra (leaves), ksheer (latex), phal (fruits), praroh (arial roots)

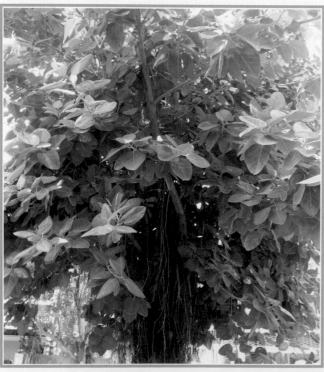

Fig. 249.1 Plant of *Ficus bengalensis* Linn.

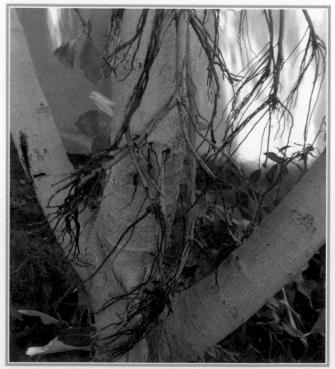

Fig. 249.2 Bark.

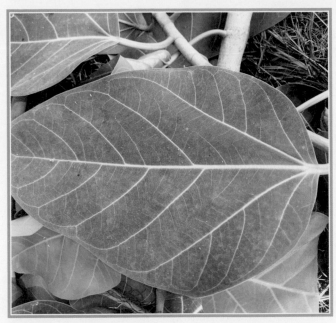

Fig. 249.3 Leaves.

Dose

Powder: 3 to 6 g

Decoction: 50 to 100 mL

Karma (Actions)

Stambhana (inhibitory action), grahi (fecal astringent), mutrasangrahniya (urinary astringent), varnya (complexion promoter), vranaropana (wound healing), vedanasthapana (anodynes).

Indications

Rakta pitta (bleeding disorders), pradar (excessive vaginal discharge), yonidosha (defects of female genital organs), visarpa (erysipelas), daha (burning sensation), vrana (wounds), chardi (vomiting), vyanga (blemishes), madhumeha (diabetes mellitus), atisaar (diarrhea).

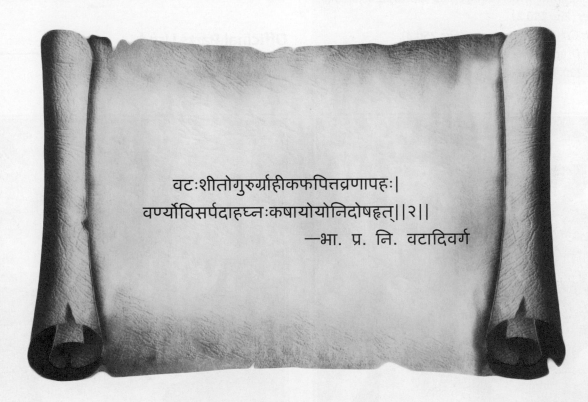

वटःशीतोगुरुर्ग्राही कफपित्तव्रणापहः।
वर्ण्योविसर्पदाहघ्नःकषायोयोनिदोषहृत्।।२।।
—भा. प्र. नि. वटादिवर्ग

250. Vatada [*Prunus amygdalus* Batsch.]

Family:	*Rosaceae*
Hindi name:	*Badam*
English name:	*Almond*
Synonyms:	*Vatavairi, Netroupmamphal*

Morphology

It is a medium-height tree with tufts of leaves at the end of branches (**Fig. 250.1**).

Key Characters for Identification

➤ *Leaves: Simple, alternate, oblong-lanceolate, minutely serrate.*
➤ *Flower: White with red tinge, and appearing before the leaves (**Fig. 250.2**).*
➤ *Fruit: Green velvety drupes (**Fig. 250.3**).*
➤ *Seed: Drupe stones enclose the valuable kernel (**Fig. 250.4**).*

Rasapanchaka

Guna	Guru, Snigdh
Rasa	Madhur
Vipaka	Madhur
Virya	Ushna
Doshakarma	Vataghna

Officinal Parts Used

Beej (seeds) and beej taila (seed oil)

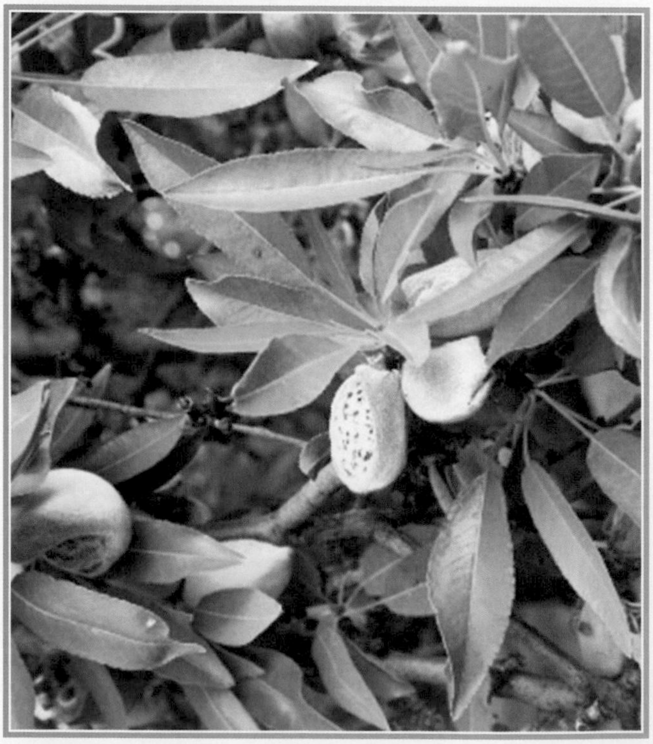

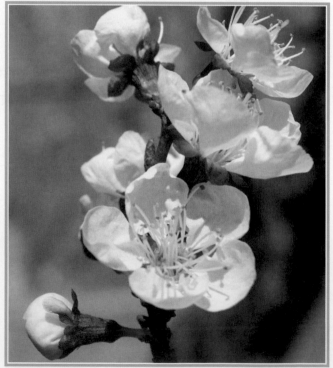

Fig. 250.1 Plant of *Prunus amygdalus* Batsch.

Fig. 250.2 Flowers.

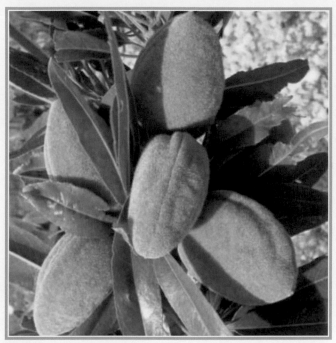

Fig. 250.3 Fruits.

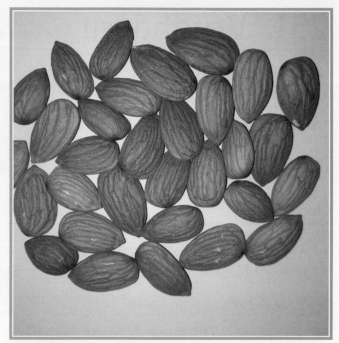

Fig. 250.4 Seeds.

Dose

Beej majja churna (seed pulp powder): 3 to 6 g
Taila (oil): 2 to 10 mL

Karma (Actions)

Vrishya (vrishya), kaphavardhak (aggravate kapha), raktapittavardhak (aggravate rakta and pitta), balya (tonics), brihmanya (bulk promoting), uttejaka (stimulant).

Indications

Shwasa vikara (respiratory infections), mutra dosha (urinary tract infections), madhumeha (diabetes), katishool (backache), shwetpradar (leucorrhea), kshata (accidental wounds), kshaya (emaciation).

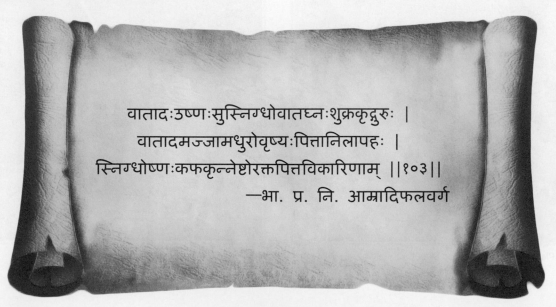

वातादःउष्णःसुस्निग्धोवातघ्नःशुक्रकृद्गुरुः |
वातादमज्जामधुरोवृष्यःपित्तानिलापहः |
स्निग्धोष्णःकफकृन्नेष्टोरक्तपित्तविकारिणाम् ||१०३||
—भा. प्र. नि. आम्रादिफलवर्ग

251. Vrudhdaru *[Argyreia speciosa Sweet.]*

Family: *Convolvulaceae*

Hindi name: *Vidhara, Samudrashosh, Ghavpatta*

English name: *Elephant creeper*

Synonyms: *Aavegi, Chagantri, Vrishyagandhika*

Morphology

It is a large climbing shrub with woody, white, tomentose stem (**Fig. 251.1**).

Key Characters for Identification

➤ *Leaves: Simple, large, ovate, acute, base cordate, glabrous above, white tomentose beneath (**Fig. 251.2**).*
➤ *Flower: Large, purple, silky-pubescent in long-peduncle cymes, with corolla tubular, infundibuliform (**Fig. 251.3**).*
➤ *Fruit: Dry, globose, apiculate (**Fig. 251.4**).*

Rasapanchaka

Guna	Laghu, Snigdh
Rasa	Kashaya, Katu, Tikta
Vipaka	Madhur
Virya	Ushna
Doshakarma	Kapha vatashamaka

Officinal Part Used

Mool (root)

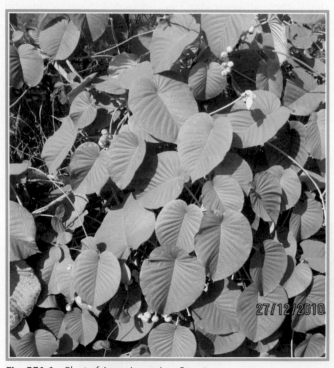

Fig. 251.1 Plant of *Argyreia speciosa* Sweet.

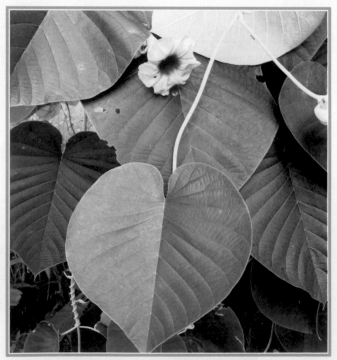

Fig. 251.2 Leaves.

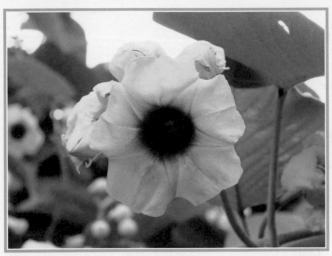

Fig. 251.3 Flower.

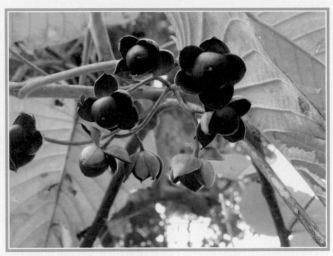

Fig. 251.4 Fruits.

Dose

Powder: 3 to 6 g

Karma (Actions)

Rasayana (rejuvenation), vrishya (aphrodisiac), balya (tonic), agnivardhak (appetizer), medhavardhak (intellect promoter), swarya (voice promoter), kantikara (improve complexion), sara (laxative).

Indications

Aamvata (rheumatoid arthritis), vataarsha (piles), shoth (inflammation), prameha (diabetes), kasa (cough), swarbhed (tonsillitis), vibandh (constipation).

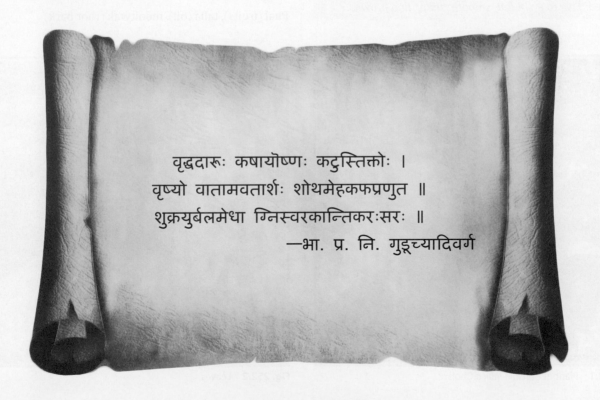

वृद्धदारूः कषायोष्णः कटुस्तिक्तोः ।

वृष्यो वातामवतार्शः शोथमेहकफप्रणुत ॥

शुक्र्युर्बलमेधा ग्निस्वरकान्तिकरःसरः ॥

—भा. प्र. नि. गुडूच्यादिवर्ग

252. Vrukshamla [*Garcinia indica* Chois.]

Family:	*Guttiferae*
Hindi name:	*Kokum*
English name:	*Kokum Butter tree*
Synonyms:	*Tintindik, Chuk, Amlavrikshak*

Morphology

It is a medium-sized evergreen tree with drooping branches (**Fig. 252.1**).

Key Characters for Identification

➤ *Leaves: Opposite, inverted, egg-shaped, oblong to elliptic-lanceolate, narrowed at base, acuminate at apex, shiny, dark green (**Fig. 252.2**).*
➤ *Flowers: Male and female flowers are separate, orange–yellow, with male flower appearing in cluster and female flowers being solitary.*
➤ *Fruit: Berries, spherical, purple or pinkish-orange.*
➤ *Seed: Five to eight flat, smooth, shiny, and brown.*

Rasapanchaka

Guna	Guru, Ruksha
Rasa	Apakwa—Amla, Madhur; Pakwa—Amla, Katu, Kashaya
Vipaka	Amla
Virya	Ushna
Doshakarma	Kaphapittavardhak and kapha vatahara

Officinal Parts Used

Phal (fruits), taila (oil), mooltwak (root bark)

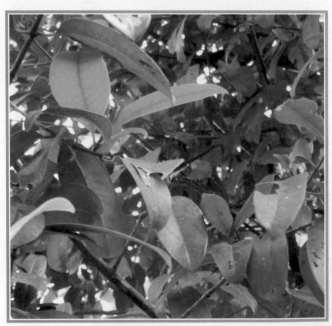

Fig. 252.1 Plant of *Garcinia indica* Chois.

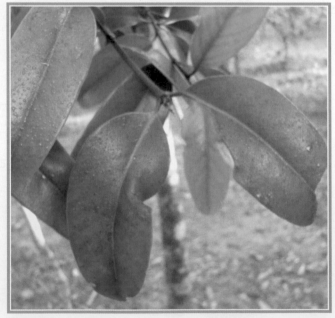

Fig. 252.2 Leaves.

Dose

Phalpanak (fruit juice drink): 10 to 20 mL
Taila (oil): 3 to 5 mL
Decoction: 40 to 80 mL

Karma (Actions)

Deepan (appetizer), rochana (relish), hridya (cardio tonic), grahi (fecal astringent), stambhan (inhibitory action), vranaropana (wound healing).

Indications

Atisaar (diarrhea), raktatisaar (bleeding diarrhea), trishna (thirst), arsha (piles), grahani (sprue), gulma (abdominal tumors), shool (pain), hridyaroga (heart diseases), krimiroga (worm infestation).

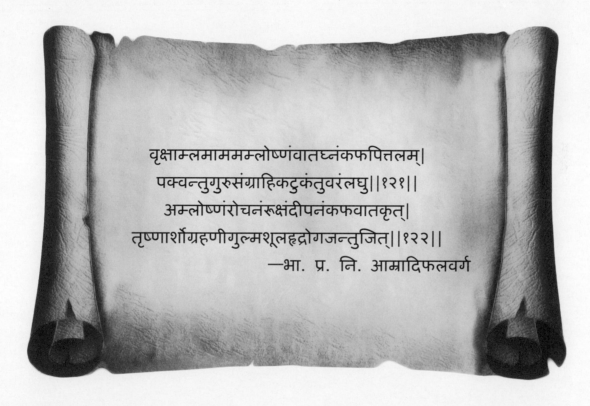

वृक्षाम्लमाममम्लोष्णंवातघ्नंकफपित्तलम्।
पक्वन्तुगुरुसंग्राहिकटुकंतुवरंलघु।।१२१।।
अम्लोष्णंरोचनंरूक्षंदीपनंकफवातकृत्।
तृष्णार्शोग्रहणीगुल्मशूलह्रद्रोगजन्तुजित्।।१२२।।
                    —भा. प्र. नि. आम्रादिफलवर्ग

Part III

Jangama Dravya (Drugs of Animal Origin)

253. Gorochana

Hindi name: *Gorochana*

English name: *Gallstone of cow or bull*

Synonyms: *Gorachana, Rochana, Gopitta, Mangalya, Vandya, Gouri*

Description

It is the bile's stone or collected bile from the gall bladder of cow or bull. It is turbid yellow or grayish-yellow in color with mild fragrance.

Key Characters for Identification

This is the biliary calculus formed in the gall bladder of a cow or bull.
➤ *Color: Turbid yellow/grayish yellow*
➤ *Odor: Mild fragrance*
➤ *Shape: Oval/egg-like*
➤ *Taste: Bitter*

Rasapanchaka

Guna	Laghu, Ruksha
Rasa	Tikta
Vipak	Katu
Veerya	Ushna
Doshakarma	Kaphavata shamaka

Karma (Actions)

Pachana (digestive), vishaghna (antidotes), medhya (intellect promoter), chakshusya (beneficial for vision), anulomana (laxative), lekhan (fat reducing), brain tonic, mitigates kapha, anti-inflammatory.

Indications

Pandu (anemia), kamala (jaundice), switra (leucoderma), agnimandya (loss of appetite), visharoga (poisoning), chakshu roga (eye diseases), unmada (insanity), apasmara (epilepsy), akshepa (convulsion), atisara (diarrhea), garbhasrava (habitual abortion), krimi (worm infestation), edema, piles, and glaucoma (as anjana).

Officinal Part Used

Ox bile or cow's bile

Dose

250 to 750 mg

Therapeutic Uses

1. **Svitra** (leukoderma): Its local application is done in leucodema and piles.
2. **Apasmara** (epilepsy): It give good result when 1.5 to 2 g of Gorachana is used with rose water.
3. **Trachoma:** Its anjana (collyrium) used locally in eye for the diseases of trachoma and for better vision.

Formulations

Balarka rasa, Gorachanadi vati

254. Kasturi

Latin name:	*Moschus moschiferus Linn.*
Family:	*Cervidae*
Hindi name:	*Kasturi*
English name:	*Musk*
Synonyms:	*Kasturika, Mruganabhi, Mrigamadaa, Sahasrabhit, Vedhamukhya*

Description

- Musk is secreted in a small sac of male musk deer. This kind of deer is found in the forests of Kashmir, Nepal, Assam, Bhutan, China Hindukush, as well as in Himalayas at 8,000 to 12,000 ft.
- A musk deer is blue-grayish or black in color. It has no tail or has a very small tail. The height of the deer is about 50 cm. It has a tendency to jump frequently while moving. It is a generally shy animal and prefers to live alone in a calm place.
- It is found in a sac present between prepuce and navel region of a male musk deer. The outer surface is covered with hair.
- It has a very good fragrance which attracts the female deer. The male deer is not aware of this and moves around in search of the source of the smell. The hunters kill the deer and remove the pod from its body.
- A young deer has 1 to 2 ounce of musk. Very young animals do not have musk and old animals produce very little.

Key Characters for Identification

➤ *Color: Blackish brown*
➤ *Consistency: Granular*
➤ *Odor: Penetrating, intensive, and persistent. Its fragrance remains even after diluting it 3,000 times.*
➤ *Taste: Pungent*
➤ *Solubility: Not soluble in water*

Types of Kasturi

As per Bhava Prakash it is of three types.

Types	Color	Quality
1. Kamarupa	Krishna Varna	Superior
2. Nepali	Neela Varna	Medium
3. Kashmeri	Kapila Varna	Inferior

Rasapanchaka

Guna	Guru
Rasa	Katu, Tikta
Vipaka	Katu
Virya	Ushna
Doshakarma	Kapha-vata shamaka

Artificial Kasturi

- Musk ketone
- Musk ambrette
- Musk xylene
- Aldehyde Musk
- Cyano Musk
- Azimido Musk

Karma (Actions)

Shukrala (spermatopoitics), balya (tonics), vishaghna (antidotes), shoshaghna (removes weakness), dourgandha hara (freshner), chakshusya (beneficial for vision), hridya (cardiotonic)

Indications

Visha (poisoning), chhardi (vomiting), sheeta (shivering), shosha (emaciation), mukha dourgandha (foul smell in mouth), shukra dourbalya (less semen), kalasha (leukoderma), kustha (skin disease), kasa (cough), vata vikara (neuromuscular disease), kapha vikara (diseases of kapha), akshepa (convulsions), tasmak swasha (bronchial asthma), unmada (insanity), apasmara (epilepsy), hridayamatiska dourbalya (weakness of heart and brain), pakshaghata (hemiplesia), ardita (facial paralysis), yoshapsmara (hysteria), hikka (hic-cough), hridayspandan (palpitation), kampavata (tremor), shunyata (numbness), jirnakasa (chronic cough)

Officinal Parts Used

Musk

Dose

- 125 to 500 mg
- Tincture: 10 to 30 drops

Therapeutic Uses

1. **Vajikaran** (as aphrodisiac): Musk is given with other drugs for aphrodisiac purposes in semen discharge and impotency.
2. **Hridayadaurbalya** (heart weakness): Chandrodaya and Brihat Kasturi bhairava are given with Bala root in heart weakness.
3. **Convulsions:** Vaidya of South India used it with opium to treat convulsion in children.

Formulations

Apurvamalini vasant rasa, Kasturi bhairava rasa, Mrigamadasava, Amritaprasa ghrita, Kasturi bhusana rasa, Kasuri modak, Rati ballav modak, Brihat chandrodaya makardhwaja

255. Mrigashringa

Hindi name: *Harina Singha*

English name: *Hart's horn*

Scientific name: *Cervus elaphus*

Synonyms: *Enashringa, Mrigavishanika, Harinashringa, Vishana, Shringa*

Description

- Horn of deer is known as mrigashringa and species of deer as Baraha singha.
- The horns that are heavy, solid, nonperforated, and thick are used for medicinal purposes.
- Purified shringa is cut into small pieces and subjected to gajaputa to prepare bhasma (ash/calcined preparation) by incinerating in a round pit of a depth and circumference of 1.25 hand.
- It produces black-colored bhasma.
- This bhasma is mixed with aloe vera juice and then subjected to Gajaputa.
- It produces white-colored bhasma which is used clinically.

Key Characters for Identification

➤ *Horn of deer or species of deer is known as mrigashringa.*

➤ *Heavy, nonperforated, solid, and thick horn are ideal for clinical utility.*

➤ *Fine white-colored ash.*

Rasapanchaka

Guna	Laghu
Rasa	Kasaya
Vipak	Katu
Virya	Ushna
Doshakarma	Kaphavatahara

Karma (Actions)

Kasaghna (antitussive), swashaghna (antiasthmatic), hridya (cardiotonic), shothaghna (reduce swelling), shoolaghna (antispasmodic).

Indications

Parshwashoola (pain inlateral part of chest), kasa (cough), shwasa (asthma), hrid roga (heart disease), hikka (hic-cough), katishoola (pain in waist region/lumbar pain), vatavyadhi (neuromuscular disease), granthishotha (edema with nodules), gridhasi (sciatica), joint pain.

Therapeutic Uses

- Hridshoola: 125 mg of mrigashringa bhasma is given with honey.
- Swasha: Powder of shringa bhasma, badara phala majja, pippali, apamarga bija are mixed and given with honey.

Officinal Parts Used

Mrigashringa bhasma (ash of horn)

Dose

250 mg to 2 g

Formulations

Mrigashringa bhasma

Part IV

Ahara Dravya

256. Aharayogi Varga

Acharya Charak mentions Aharayogi varga among 12 vargas in sutra sthan, 27th chapter of Charak Samhita. The substances/drugs used for processing of food (ahar samskaratha) come under Aharayogi varga. Following are a few of Aharayogi varga.

Sneha Dravya

Taila: Til, erand, sarsapa, priyala, atasi, kusumba taila, vasa, majja, and ghrita are used for processing of food.

Katu Dravya

Shunthi, Pippali, Marich, Hingu, Karavi, Jeerak, Yavani, Dhanyak Tumburu are the katu dravya used for processing and preparation of various types of food. These drugs are laghu, ushna, and katu rasayukta, having deepan, pachan, rochan, and daurgandhya nashan properties.

Lavan and Kshar Dravya

Saindhav, sauvarchal, vid lavan (salt), etc., and yava and sarji kshar (alkali) are used to give proper taste to food. These dravyas have rochan, deepan, vatanuloman properties.

Points to Ponder

- *Acharya Charak has mentioned Aharayogi varga among 12 vargas (C.S.Su. 27).*
- *Aharayogi varga is used for processing of food.*
- *Sneha dravya, katu, lavan, and kshar dravyas are used for processing of food.*

257. Dugdha Varga

Synonyms: *Dugdha, kshira, payah, payas, sthanya, balajeevan*

Properties

- Guna: Guru, snigdha, mridu, pichhila
- Rasa: Madhura
- Vipak: Madhur
- Veerya: Sheeta
- Doshakarma: Vatapittahara, kaphavardhak

Karma (Actions)

Preenanam (nourishment), rasayana (rejuvenation), vajikaran (aphrodisiac), jeevaniya (vitality), snehan (oleation), brimhana (bulk promoting), medhya (intellect promoter), balya (tonics), sandhaniya (union promoter), vayasthapan (antiaging), shramahar (antifatigue), varnya (complexion promoter), mutral (diuretics), stanyajanana (galactogugue), garbhasthapan (establishment of fever), ayushya (long healthy life).

Uses

Jeernajwar (chronic fever), kshaya (decrease/decay), amlapitta (hyperacidity), raktapitta (hemorrhage), parinamashoola (duodenal ulcer), gulma (abdominal lump), atisar (diarrhea), udararoga (abdominal disease), shukradaubalya (deficiency of semen), vibandha (constipation), shopha (swelling), pandu (anemia), shosha (emaciation/tuberculosis), daha (burning sensation).

Milk is best for jeevaniya karma. Acharya Charak also opined that use of milk along with ghee is best for rasayan karma. Cow's milk is heetatama and sheep's milk is Aheetatama.

Ksheerastak

Eight types of milk is mentioned by almost all ancient acharyas:

- Godugdha (cow's milk)
- Ajadugdha (goat's milk)
- Avidugdha (sheep's milk)
- Mahishadugdha (buffalo milk)
- Ustradugdha (camel's milk)
- Hastidugdha (elephant's milk)
- Vadavadugdha (horse's milk)
- Manusha dugdha (women's milk)

Properties of Astadugdha

S. No.	Milk	Guna Karma	Action and Uses
1	Godugdha	Guna: Guru, snigdha Rasa: Madhur, kashaya Vipak: Madhur Virya: Sheeta Doshakarma: Vatapittahara	Ishat abhisyandhi, jeevaniya, medhya raktapittahara, jararoganashak
2	Ajadugdha	Guna: Laghu Rasa: Kasaya, madhur Virya: Sheeta Doshakarma: Vatapittahara	Grahi, raktapitta, atisara, shaya, kasa, visha

S. No.	Milk	Guna Karma	Action and Uses
3	Avidugdha	Guna: Guru, snigdha Rasa: Madhur Virya: Ushna Doshakarma: Kaphapittavardhak	Vatavyadhi, vatarakta, asmarinashak, excessive uses cause hikka and swasa
4	Mahisha dugdha	Guna: Laghu, Ishat ruksha Rasa: Madhur, lavana Virya: Ushna Doshakarma: Kaphavatashamak	Nidrajanana, agnimandyakara, shukrajanana, stanyajanana
5	Ustra dugdha	Guna: Guru, snigdha Rasa: Madhur Vipak: Madhur Virya: Sheeta Doshakarma: Vatapittahara	Deepan, sara, used in anaha, krimi, udara, shopha, arsha, kushta
6	Hasti dugdha	Guna: Guru, snigdha Rasa: Madhur, kasaya Virya: Sheeta Doshakarma: Kaphavardhak	Balya, sthairya kara, chakshusya
7	Vadava dugdha	Guna: Ruksha Rasa: Ishat Amla lavana Virya: Ushna Doshakarma: Vatashamak	Balya. It is used in shosha, shakhagata vata
8	Stree dugdha	Guna: Snigdha Rasa: Madhur Virya: Sheeta Doshakarma: Vatapittahara	Satmya, jeevaniya, brimhana, chakshusya, snehana, deepen, used as nasya in raktapittahara and tarpan in akshishoola

Points to Ponder

- *Godugdha: Dhraroshna hittakar; Mahish dugdha: Dharasheeta heetakara; Avi dugdha: Shrutoshna heetakara, Aja dugdha: Shrutosheeta heetakara*
- *Take milk (1 part) and water (half part) and boil till complete evaporation of water—it becomes Laghutara*
- *Milk boiled without water: Guru, snigdha; Unboiled milk: Guru, abhisyandi; Boiled milk: Laghutara, anabhisyandi*
- *Unboiled human milk is beneficial for health*
- *Morning milk is more guru and sheeta than evening milk*

258. Jala Varga

Water is one of the most important substances for the survival of the members of the animal as well as the plant kingdom. It is a *Mahabhuta* and is essential for basic health as well as for fighting diseases.

Synonyms

Paniya, Salila, Neera, Ambu, Vari, Toya, Paya, Udaka, Ambha, Jeevan, Amrita.

Classification of Jala

1. According to yoni, jala is of two types:
   a. Divya jala
   b. Bhauma jala
2. According to Desha, jala is of three types:
   a. Jangal jala
   b. Anup jala
   c. Sadharana jala
3. According to Tapa, it is of two types:
   a. Sheetal jala
   b. Ushna jala
4. According to Ritu, jala is of six types (as described by Acharya Charak).
   Out of all the types listed under "Ritu (season)," jala of Sharad Ritu (water of autumn season) is considered as Prasastha (best) jala.

According to Yoni

1. Divya jala

It is obtained from the sky. It has six qualities, namely sheeta, suchi, shiva, madhura, vimala, and laghu. It can be divided into four types:
   a. Dhara jala (rain water):
      - Laghu, avyakta rasa, tridosha hara, tarpana, balya, rasayana, pachana, pathya
      - It is of two types:
        ➢ Ganga jala
        ➢ Samudra jala
   b. Kara jala (hail water):
      - Obtained from hail

   - Ruksha, Guru, sheeta, pittashamaka, kapha-vatakara
   c. Haima jala (snowfall water):
      - Water obtained from glaciers
      - Sheeta, Pittahara, Guru, Vata-vardhak
   d. Tushara jala (dew water):
      - Water collected in the form of dew
      - Apathyakara, ruksha, sheeta, vatavardhak, kapha shamak

2. Bhauma jala

When there is scarcity of divya jala, bhauma jala should be used. Acharya Sushruta has described seven types of jala and Acharya Vagabhatta mentioned eight varieties of jala.
   a. Kaupya
   b. Nadeya
   c. Sarasa
   d. Tadaga
   e. Prasravana
   f. Audbhidya
   g. Chauntya
   h. Vandya (Vagabhatta)

According to Desha

1. **Jangala jala** (arid land): Laghu (light), ruksha (nonunctuousness), kapha-pitta shamaka (pacify kapha and pitta dosha), deepana (appetizer), and pathya (healthy)
2. **Anupa jala** (marshy land): Guru (heaviness), snigdha (unctuousness), abhisyandi (channel blocker), kapha vardhak (aggravate kapha dosha), causes agnimandya (loss of appetite), and other diseases
3. **Sadharana jala:** Laghu (lightness), sheeta (cold), madhura (sweet), deepan (appetizer), and tridosha shamaka (pacify vata, pitta and kapha dosha)

According to Tapa

1. **Sheetal jala: Three types**
   a. Ishat sheeta (slightly cold)
   b. Sheeta (cold)
   c. Atisheeta (very cold)

- Uses of Sheetal jala: Pittaja vikara (disease of pitta), bhrama (vertigo/dizziness), murchha (unconsciousness), daha (burning sensation), visha (poisoning), rakta vikara (blood diseases), madatyaya (alcoholism), vamana (vomiting), urdwaga-raktapitta (hemorrage from orifices of upper part of body)
- Contraindication of Sheetal jala: Vata roga (neuromuscular disease), pratisyaya (cold), galagraha (stiffness of mouth), adhmana (distension), kosthavadhhata (constipation), saddya-sudhhi (immediate after purification of body through panchkarma), nawajwara (acute fever), hikka (hic-cough), snehapana (internal oleation)

2. **Ushna jala**
   a. Mild
   b. Moderate
   c. Severe
   - Uses of Ushna jala: Kasa, swasha, jwara, kapha-vata vikara, amadosha, agnimandya, mutraghata, amajirna, vistavdharjirna
   - Contraindication of Ushna jala: Pittaja vikara, those who are eligible for taking Sheetal jala

Paka Period of Jala (Bhava Prakash)

- In general, jala is digested in two yamas (6 hours).
- Shrutasheeta jala is digested in one yama (3 hours).
- Warm water is digested in 0.5 yama (1.30 hour).

Quality of Jala

- Rasa: Ishat kashaya madhura (Susrut-avyakta)
- Guna: Sukshma, vishada, laghu, aruksha, anabhisyandi
- Other qualities: Nirgandhi, suchi, sheeta, hridya, trishnaghna

Dosha of jala: There are six as per Sushruta

1. Sparsha dosha
2. Rupa dosha
3. Rasa dosha
4. Gandha dosha
5. Veerya dosha
6. Vipaka dosha

Purification of Jala

1. Filtration
2. Prasadana
3. Boiling
4. Adhibasana: Adding of fragrance substance like Champa, Nagakeshara
5. Kamalapushpa reduces the bad smells.

Jala Sevana Vidhi

- Quantity: Neither too much nor too less
- Intake of sky water, kaupa or tubewell water in rainy season
- Water should be consumed in less quantity in aruchi, pratisyaya, lala praseka, mandagni, udararoga, kushta, jwara, netra roga, vrana, and madhumeha
- According to Vagabhatta, water should not be given in mandagni
- If water taken
  ➤ Before food: It causes agnimandya and karsha
  ➤ After food: It causes kaphaja vikara and sthaulya
  ➤ Between meals: It causes easy digestion, dhatusamya

Points to Ponder

- *Jala is mainly of two types: Divya and Bhauma.*
- *Divya jala is of four types: Dhara, kara, taushar, and haima.*
- *Dhara jala is considered as best: It is tridoshashamak, avyakta, and rasa yukta, and it has laghu, soumya, rasayan, balya, tarpan, hladi, jeevaniya, pachan properties.*
- *Anshudaka of Sharad Ritu is considered as best for drinking.*

259. Madhu Varga

Latin name:	*Apis mellifera Linn.*
Family:	*Apidae*
Hindi:	*Shahad*
English:	*Honey*
Synonyms:	*Madhu, Makshika, Maadhwika, Kshaudra, Vrungavant, Saradha, Makshikavant, Varati, Vaanta, Pusparasodbhava*

Description

Honey is a secretion deposited in the honey comb by honey bees.

Apis mellifera Linn. of Apidae family and other species of *Apis* from this family collect the nectar of flowers and deposits in the bee hive.

It is viscid, transparent, and yellowish-brown in color.

Geographical Source

It is produced in Africa, Australia, New Zealand, California, and India.

Properties

As per Acharya Charak:
- Guna: Guru, ruksha
- Rasa: Kasaya, madhura
- Vipak: Madhur
- Veerya: Sheeta
- Doshakarma: Kaphapittashamak and Vatavardhak; Tridoshashamak (Sushrut)

Karma (Actions)

Sandhaniya (union promoter), chhedan (antitussive), agnideepan (appetizer), varnya (complexion promoter), balya (tonic), swaryya (beneficial for voice), srotovishodhan (channel cleanser), grahi (astringent), chakshusya (beneficial for vision), lekhan (scarping), vrana shodhan and ropan (wound cleansing and healing), medhya (intellect promoter), vrusya (aphrodisiac), rochan(relish), hridya (cardio tonic), prasadak (purification)

Naveen madhu (Fresh honey)

Brimhaniya (bulk promoting), ishat kasaya (slightly astringent taste), ishat kaphaghna (slighty pacify vatadosha)

Purana madhu (Old honey)

Ati lekhan (scraping), grahi (astringent), medohara (fat reducing), sthaulya nashak (antiobesity)

Uses

Pittashleshma vicar (disease of pitta and kapha), medohara(obesity), prameha (diabetes), hikka (hic-cough), kasa (cough), swasa (bronchial asthma), atisara (diarrhea), chhardi (vomiting), trishna (thirst), krimi (worm infestation), visha (poisoning) (S.S.Su.45/)

Types

Different types of Madhu Varga are listed as follows:

Charak: Four Types	Sushrut: Eight Types
1. Makshik: Taila varna (best)	1. Makshik
2. Bhramar: Sweta varna	2. Bhramar
3. Kshaudra: Kapil varna	3. Kshaudra
4. Paitik: Ghrita varna	4. Paitik
	5. Chhatra
	6. Daala
	7. Aardhya
	8. Audalaka

Properties and Uses of Various Varieties of Madhu

S. No.	Variety	Properties	Uses
1	Makshika	More laghu (light) than kshaudra variety, ruksha	It is used in eye diseases, kamala, arsha, kshata, swasa, kasa, kshaya
2	Bhramar	Guru, pichchhil, abhisyandi, madhur vipak, sheet veerya, mutrajadyakar, Clear-like spatika	It is used in raktapitta
3	Kshaudra	Same as makshika variety	Specifically used in prameha
4	Paitika	Ruksha, ushna, it aggravates pitta, daha, rakta and vata, vidahi	Used in prameha, mutrakrichha, kshata and granthishoshi
5	Chhatra	Kapilpita varna, guru, pichhil, sheeta, madhur vipak, truptikarak	Used in krimi, sweta kushta, raktapitta, prameha, brahma, trusha, moha, and visha
6	Daal	Madhur, kashaya and amla rasa, laghu vipak ruksha, guru in weight, deepaniya, kaphanashak, ruchikar, brimhana	Used in chhardi and prameha
7	Aardhya	Kashaya and tikta rasa, katu vipak, balya, pustikarak, kaphapittahara, chakshushya	Used in eye diseases
8	Audalaka	Kashaya and amla rasa, katu vipak, ushna, pitta karak, ruchya, swarya, kushtaghna, vishaghna	Used in kushta, visha

Precautions During Madhu Sevan

- Honey should not be taken with hot substance or in hot stage or in hot season (sharad, grishma, noon).
- Honey should not be taken with rain water (antariksha jala); it becomes poison.
- Equal quantity of honey and ghee also becomes poison.
- Ajirna (indigestion) obtained due to excess use of honey is a very serious condition like poison because ajirna is always well treated by hot substance but honey is incompatible with hot substance.

- But honey can be used with hot things during vamana procedure because emetic drugs produce the action before digestion.

> ### Points to Ponder
>
> - *Acharya Charak mentioned four types of madhu, whereas Acharya Sushrut and Bhavmishra described eight types of madhu.*
> - *Makshika is the best variety of madhu.*

260. Mamsa Varga

Hindi:	Mamsa, Goshta
English:	Meat
Synonyms:	Pishita, Palala, Amisha, pala, Kravya

Acharya Charak has described Mamsa as the best for brimhana karma (C.S.Su. 25/40). Mamsa is given to increase the mamsa dhatu of the body. Different types of Mamsa with their properties are mentioned in the various Samhita granthas and Nighantus of Ayurveda.

Properties and Actions

- Guna: Guru
- Rasa: Madhur
- Vipak: Madhur
- Virya: Sheeta

Karma (Actions)

Vatashamak (pacify vata dosha), brimhana (bulk promoting), balya (tonics), pustikarak (nourishment), santarpana (nourishment therapy), hridya (cardiotonic)

Classification

Charak Samhita

As per Acharya Charak, it is classified into eight groups according to yoni (sources).

1. Prasaha: cat
2. Bhumishaya: The animals that reside inside burrows, such as mandook, nakula, etc.
3. Anoopamriga: The animals that reside near the Anoop-pradesh or marshy areas, such as gaja, mahisha, etc.
4. Varija: Aquatic animals or the animals that stay in water bodies, such as fish, tortoise.
5. Varicharina/Jalachara: The birds that move or swim in water, such as hamsa, balaaka, etc.
6. Jangala: Those that live in Jangaladesha, such as harina, gokarna, etc.
7. Vishkira: Those birds that use their beaks to gather and pick up food, such as lava, shuka, etc.

8. Pratuda: Those birds that use their beaks to kill small worms and insects and use it as food, such as paravata, kalakantaka, etc.

These eight groups are further classified into two groups according to their guna, such as guru and laghu.

- Guru: The meat of prasaha, bhumishaya, anoopa, jalaja, and jalachara is included in this group. This type of meat has guru, snigdha, madhura, ushna properties and balya, vrishya, vatashamak, and kaphapittavardhak actions.
- Laghu: The meat of jangala, pratuda, and viskira are laghu. This type of meat has properties like kashaya madhur rasa and sheeta virya.

Sushruta Samhita

Acharya Sushruta has classified the mamsa varga into six groups. They are jaleshaya, anoopa, gramya, kravyabhuja, ekashapha, and jangala.

Again these are further divided into two groups: jangala and anoopa. Jangala mamsa is classified into eight types while anoopa mamsa is divided into five types of animals.

- Jangala mamsa: Meat of jangal, viskira, pratuda, guha-shaya, prasaha, parnamriga, vileshaya, and gramya.
- Anoopamamsa: Meat of kulachara, plava, koshastha, paadina, and matsya.

Bhavaprakash

Bhavamishra has followed the classification method of Sushruta. He has described the properties of jangala mamsa and anoopa mamsa.

Jangala mamsa

It has madhura kashaya rasa, laghu and ruksha guna, and has deepan, balya, brimhana actions. It is used in vata vyadhi, badhirya, aruchi, chhardi, prameha, mukharoga, shlipada, galaganda, etc.

Anoopa mamsa

It has madhura rasa, snigdha, guru, and pichhila guna. It decreases agni, kaphakarak, and abhisyandikarak.

Properties and Actions of Different Mamsa

- **Aja mamsa**: Laghu, snigdha, madhura, natiushna, tridoshahara
- **Avimamsa**: Madhur, sheeta, guru, brimhaniya
- **Gomamsa**: Guru, snigdha, kaphapitta vardhak, brimhana, vatashamak, balya, apathya, and is used in pinasa roga
- **Mahisha mamsa**: Snigdha, guru, madhura, ushna, tarpana, vrisya, brimhana, nidrajanana
- **Aswamamsa**: Kashayamadhurarasa, laghu, deepaniya, chakshusya, vatashamak, kaphapittavardhak, balya, brimhaniya
- **Varaha mamsa**: Guru, snigdha, vatashamaka, swedana, shramahara, balya, vrishya, brimhaniya
- **Harinamamsa**: Madhur, laghu, sheeta, vibandhakarak, sangrahi, mutrarodhak, deepaniya, tridoshashamak
- **Mayurmamsa**: Balya, sukral, mamsavridhi, vatashamak, chakshusya, agnivarshak, ayuvardhak, varnya, and swarya
- **Kukkuta mamsa**: Guru, snigdha, ushna, vatashamaka and kaphavardhak, balya, brimhaniya, vrishya, chakshusya
- **Kapota mamsa**: Kashayamadhur, sheeta, raktapittashamak
- **Shasha mamsa**: Laghu, ruksha madhur, kashaya, katuvipaka, sheetavirya, tridoshashamak
- **Manduka mamsa**: Kaphavardhak, balya
- **Kurma mamsa**: Vatashamak, balya, vrishya, mamsa vardhak, chakshusya, medhya
- **Koshastha jantu** (shankha, shukti, shambuka): Madhur, snigdha, sheeta, balya, vatapittashamaka, and kaphavardhak
- **Matsya**: Madhur, snigdha, guru, ushna virya, balya, vrishya, brimhaniya, vatashamak, and kaphapitta vardhak. Rohita matsya is considered as best matsya.
- **Nadeya matsya** (fish of river): Madhur, guru, ushna, vatashamak, raktapittavardhak, balya
- **Samudra matsya** (fish of ocean): Kaphavardhak, ishat pitta vardhak, vatashamak, valya

Testing of Guru and Laghu Quality of Mamsa

Acharya Sushruta has described the following methods to test the heaviness and lightness quality of various meats (S.S.Su. 46/138).

- **Chara**: Jangal mamsa is laghu and anoopa mamsa is guru.
- **Sharira avayava**: Skanda mamsa is laghu and shira mamsa is guru.
- **Swabhava**: Ajamamsa is laghu while mahisha mamsa is guru.
- **Dhatu**: Successive dhatu is guru.
- **Kriya**: Meat of active animal is light in comparison to meat of inactive or less active animal.
- **Linga (sex)**: Meat of male animals is heavy than female ones. In birds, it is opposite.
- **Pramana (size of animal)**: Meat of big animal is heavy than that of small animal.
- **Sanskar (method of processing)**: Method of processing or preparation play a major role in converting heavy meat into light and vice versa.
- **Matra**: More quantity of mamsa causes guruta (heaviness), while small quantity causes laghu (lightness and it digests without difficulties).

Points to Ponder

- *Mamsa is the best for brimhana karma (C.S.Su. 25/40).*
- *Rohita matsya is considered as the best matsya (C.S.Su. 25/38).*
- *Enamamsa is the best among mrigamamsa (C.S.Su. 25/38).*
- *Lava mamsa is the best among bird mamsa (C.S.Su. 25/38).*
- *Godha mamsa is the best among vileshaya mamsa (C.S.Su. 25/38).*
- *Gomamsa (cow's meat) is the worst among mrigamasa (C.S.Su. 25/38).*
- *Kanakapota mamsa is the worst among bird meat (C.S.Su. 25/38).*
- *Bheka (frog's meat) is worst among vileshaya mamsa (C.S.Su. 25/38).*
- *Chilchim mamsa is worst among matsyamamsa (C.S.Su. 25/38).*

261. Phalavarga

Acharya Charak mentioned Draksha first in phalavarga, whereas Acharya Sushrut started with Dadima. Charak mentioned Draksha is the best, however Lakucha, the worst fruit among all. Acharya Sushruta listed the following sequence of fruits with respect to their properties: Amla phala, kashaya phala, madhur phala, shuksha phala, and other fruits.

Amlarasayukta phala

Dadima, amalaka, badara, kola, karkandhu, saubir, sinchitkaa, kapitha, matulunga, amra, amrataka, karamarda, priyala, naranga, jambira, lakucha, bhavya (kamarakh), paravata, vetraphala, prachina amalaka (pani amalaka), chincha, nipa (kadamba), koshamra, amlika are the predominant sour-tasting fruits.

Properties

- Rasa: Amla
- Vipaka: Guru
- Veerya: Ushna
- Doshakarma: Pittala, vataghna, kaphoutkleshakara. The properties and actions of individual fruits are given in **Table 261.1**.

Table 261.1 Properties and Actions of Amlarasayukta Fruits

S. No.	Name of the Fruit	Properties	Actions	Uses
1	Dadima	Kasaya anurasa does not aggravate pitta in large quantity. It is of two types as per the taste of the fruit: Madhur (having sweet taste) and Amla (having sour taste). Madhur dadima is tridoshaghna while amla dadima is vatakapha shamak	Deepaniya, ruchikara, hridya, varcha bibandhakaraka	It is used in hridaya roga, aruchi
2	Amalaki	Amla, madhura, tikta, kashaya, katu rasa, sara	Chakshusya, tridoshaghna, vrishya. Amalaki pacify vatadosha by its amla rasa, pitta by its madhura rasa and sheeta veerya, kapha dosha by its ruksha guna and kashaya rasa	It is best among all fruits
3	Badara	Three types of badara is described by Acharya Sushrut: Karkandhu, Kola, Badara	Young fruits (apakwa phala) aggravate pitta and kapha dosha while mature fruits pacify vata and pitta dosha. Dry fruit has shramaghna (antifatigue), deepan (appetizer), laghu (light) properties. Saubir variety of badara is snigdha (unctuous), sweet and vatapittashamak in nature	Old fruits (dry badara) cure trishna (thirst), shrama (fatigue)

(Continued)

Table 261.1 *(Continued)* Properties and Actions of Amlarasayukta Fruits

S. No.	Name of the Fruit	Properties	Actions	Uses
4	Sinchitika phala (sev)	Kashaya, madhur (sweet)	Sangrahi (fecal astringent), sheeta	
5	Kapittha	Aam kapittha is swarya (beneficial for voice), kaphaghna, grahi (fecal astringent), vatalam while pakwa kapittha (ripen kapittha) is kaphapittahara, Madhur, amlarasayukta, and guru (heavy)	It has trishnaghna (antithirst), kanthashodhan (clear the throat) action. It is used in wasa (asthma), kasa (cough), aruchi (anorexia), trishna (thirst)	
6	Matulunga	Laghu, amla, covering of Matulunga is tikta, durjara (difficult to digest), vatakaphahara, krimighna, mamsa (pulp of matulunga) is swadu, sheeta, guru, snigdha, vatapittashamak, and medhya. Keshar of matulunga is agnideepak, laghu, and sangrahi	Deepan, hridya	Pulp of Matulunga is used in shoola, vata, and kapha roga, chhardi and arochaka.Keshar is used in gulma and arsha. Rasa of matulunga is used in shoola, aruchi, ajirna, vibandha, mandaghni, and kaphavataja roga
7	Amra	Kashaya anurasayuktam, swadu, guru	Bala phala: vatapittakara Baddha keshar: pittala Pakwa phala: hridya, varnakara, ruchya, raktamamsabalaprada, vataghna, brimhana, pitta avirodhi, shukravardhan	
8	Amrataka	Madhur, guru, snigdha	Brimhana, balya, vasthmbhi, vrisya, kaphakarak	
9	Lakucha	Amla	Tridoshakarak, vistambhi, shukranashana	
10	Karamarda	Amla	Ruchya and pittakara	It is used in trishna
11	Priyala	Guru, sheetal	Vatapittahara, vrishya	
12	Bhavya (kamarakh)	Swadu, kashayamla, guru, sheeta	Hridya, asyashodhan, pittashlesmahara, grahi, vistambhi	
13	Paravata	Madhura	Ruchya	It is used in atyghni
14	Neepa (Kadamba)	Garadoshahara		

(Continued)

Table 261.1 *(Continued)* Properties and Actions of Amlarasayukta Fruits

S. No.	Name of the Fruit	Properties	Actions	Uses
15	Prachinaamalaka (pani aamla)	Garadoshahara		
16	Tintidika	Aama phala: vatahara, pittakaphakara Pakwa: grahi, ushna, deepan, ruchya, kaphavatahara		
17	Koshamra	Somewhat less properties in comparison to tintidika		
18	Amlika	Same as tintidika but bhedan (drastic purgative) in nature		
19	Narangphala	Amla, samadhur, vishada, durjara, guru	Hridya, bhaktarochana, vataghna	
20	Jambira (nimbu)	Guru	Vatakaphahara, pittakarak, vibandhaghna	It is used in trishna, shoola, kaphaklesha, chhardi'swasa
21	Eravata and Dantashatha	Amla	Raktapittakarak	

Kashayarasayukta Dravya

Table 261.2 depicts properties and actions of Kashayarasayukta phala, whereas **Table 261.3** shows properties and actions of Madhurrasayukta phala. **Table 261.4 and Table 261.5** depict properties and actions of dry fruits and other fruits, respectively.

Table 261.2 Properties and Actions of Kashayarasayukta Phala

S. No.	Names of the Fruits	Properties	Actions
1	Kshirivriksha phala	Guru, sheeta, kashaya, madhur, amla	Vishtambhi, alpa vataparkopa (less vata aggravative)
2	Jambu	Kashaya	Excessive vatakarak, kaphapitta shamak
3	Rajadana	Snigdha, madhur, kashaya, guru	
4	Todana	Kashaya, madhur, ruksha	Kaphavatashamak
5	Tinduka	Tender fruit is kashaya, and mature fruit is guru in vipaka, madhur	Tender fruit is sangrahi, vataprakopaka, and mature fruit is kaphapittashamak
6	Bakula	Madhur, kashaya, snigdha	Sangrahi, provides strength to the teeth, vishada
7	Dhanwana	Kashaya, sheeta, madhur	Kaphavatashamak

(Continued)

Table 261.2 *(Continued)* Properties and Actions of Kashayarasayukta Phala

S. No.	Names of the Fruits	Properties	Actions
8	Gangeruki	Same as Dhanwana phala	
9	Asmantaka	Same as Dhanwana phala	
10	Phalagu	Madhura, snigdha, guru	Visthambhi, tarpana
11	Parushaka (phalsa)	Tender fruit: excessive sour, slightly sweet, kashaya anurasa, laghu, and pittajanak. Mature fruit: madhur rasa and madhur vipak, sheeta	Tender fruit: vatashamak. Mature fruit: vatapittashamak, raktapittaprashadana
12	Paushkara (Sringataka)	Madhur, guru	Visthambhi, balya, kaphakara
13	Bilwa	Tender fruit: tikshna, snigdha, katutiktakashaya, ushna; Mature fruit: madhur anurasa, guru	Tender fruit: kaphavatahara, sangrahi, deepan; Mature fruit: vidahi, vistambhi, doshakarak, causes puti maruta (foul smell flatus)
14	Bimbi and aswakarna	Kashaya	Sthanyajanana, kaphapittashamak, cures trishna, daha, jwara, raktapitta, kasa, swasa, kshaya

Table 261.3 Properties and Actions of Madhurrasayukta Phala

S. No.	Names of the Fruits	Properties	Actions
1	Tala, narikela, panasa, mocha (kadali)	Madhur in rasa and vipak, snigdha, sheeta	Vatapittahara, balya, brimhana
2	Tala	Fruit of tala is madhur, guru; seed is madhur in vipak	Pittashamak: seed is mutral and vatapittashamak
3	Narikela	Guru, snigdha, madhur, sheeta	Pittashamak, balya, mamsaprada, brimhana, bastishodhan
4	Panasa	Kashaya, snigdha, swadurasa, guru	Vistambhi
5	Mouch (kadali)	Swadu and kashaya rasa, natisheeta, guru	Raktapittahara, vrishya, ruchya, shleshmakara
6	Draksha, gambhari, kharjura, madhookpuspa, etc.	Guru, madhur	Raktapittahara
7	Draksha	Sara, madhur, snigdha, sheeta	Swarya. It is used in raktapitta, jwara, swasa, trishna, daha, kshaya
8	Gambhari	Kashaya	Hridya, mutravarodhanashan, raktapitta and vataroga nashak, kesya, rasayan, medhya
9	Kharjura	Sheetal, guru, madhur in rasa and vipak	Kshatakshaya nashak, hridya, tarpana, raktapittanashak
10	Madhuk	Guru	Brimhaniya, hridya, vatapittashamak

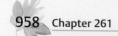

Table 261.4   Properties and Actions of Dry Fruits

S. No.	Names of the Fruits	Properties	Actions
1	Dry fruits: badam, akhrot, abhishuka (kaju), nichula, pichu, nikochaka (pista), urumana (nasapati)	Snigdha, ushna, guru, madhur	Pittakaphahara, brimhana, vatanashak, balya

Table 261.5   Properties and Actions of Other Fruits

S. No.	Names of Fruits	Properties	Actions
1	Lavali phala	Kashaya, slightly tikta (bitter), vishada	Kaphapittahara, ruchikarak, hridya, sugandhi
2	Vasiraphala, sheetapaki (bala phala), bhallatka phala, or nibandhan (pedicel)	Durjara, ruksha, sheetal, madhur vipaka	Visthambhi, vata prakopak, raktapitta prasadan
3	Tanka (neelakapitha)	Sheeta, kashaya, madhur, guru	Vatakarak
4	Inguda	Snigdha, ushna, tikta, madhur	Vatakaphahara
5	Shamiphala	Guru, swadu	Rukshoghna, keshanashak
6	Shlesmataka	Guru, madhur, sheeta	Kaphakarak
7	Karira, akshika, pilu, trinashunya (mallika)	Madhur, tikta, katu, ushna	Kaphavatahara
8	Pilu	Tikta, sara, katu vipaka, tikshna, ushna, katu rasa, snigdha	Pittakara, kaphavatahara
9	Tuvaraka	Kashaya, katu vipak, ushna	Vranakarak, used in krimi, jwara, anaha, prameha, udavarta
10	Karanja, palash, arista (Nimba)	Katu vipaka	Krimighna, pramehaghna, used in kushta, gulma, udara, arsha
11	Ankola	Visra, guru, sheeta	Kaphahara
12	Vidanga	Ruksha, ushna, katu vipaka, laghu, slightly tikta	Vatakaphahara, beneficial in poisoning, krimighna
13	Haritaki (abhaya)	Ushna, sara, kashaya	Vranya, medhya, doshaghna, deepan amla, chakshusya, cures shopha and kushta
14	Aksha (bibhitaki)	Laghu, ushna, ruksha, madhur vipak, kashaya	Bhedan, chakshusya, kaphapittashamak, cures vaiswarya, and krimi
15	Puga	Rukshya, kashaya, slightly madhur, and sara	Kaphapittahara, vakrakledamalapaham
16	Jatikosha (javitri), karpur, jatiphala, kankola, lavang	Tikta, katu, laghu	Kaphahara, trishnashamak, vakrakledadaurgandhanashak

(Continued)

Table 261.5 *(Continued)* Properties and Actions of Other Fruits

S. No.	Names of Fruits	Properties	Actions
17	Karpura	Tikta, surabhi, sheeta, laghu	Lekhan. It is used in trishna, mukhashosha, and vairasya
18	Priyalmajja	Madhur	Vrisya, vatapittashamak
19	Bibhitaki majja	Kashaya	Madakara, kaphavatashama
20	Badara majja	Kashaya, madhur	Vatapittashamak, used in trishna and chhardi
21	Amalaki majja	Same as badara majja	
22	Bijapura and aragvadhamajja and koshamra majja	Madhur vipaka, snigdha	Agnideepak, vatapittahara

General Rules for Selection of Fruits

All fruits are used in mature stage except Bilwa fruit. Apakwa Bilwa fruit (tender fruit) is more beneficial for health than the mature one. Tender bilwa fruit is ushna, deepan, katu, tikta, kashaya rasa. The fruits that are affected by krimi, and over-ripe, unseasonal, and immature fruits should not be used.

> **Points to Ponder**
>
> - *Draksha is the best fruit, and lakucha is the worst fruit among all.*

262. Shakavarga

Acharya Chakrapani mentioned six types of shaka in Dravyaguna sangraha. Bhavaprakash also mentioned the same number of shakavarga as patra, puspa, phala, nala, kanda, and sanswedaja, and these are gurus in successive order. Acharya Charak included patrashaka, kandashaka, and phalashaka in shakavarga, and Acharya Chakrapani included these three prime shakavargas along with pushpashaka in it. Acharya Sushrut mentioned five types of shaka such as puspa, patra, phala, nala, and kanda in shakavarga and is heavier (guru) in successive order.

Satin, vastuka, chuchchu, chilli, balamulak, manduka parni, and jeevanti are considered as ideal (S.S.Su. 46). As per Acharya Charak, Jeevanti is considered as hitatama (best) and sarsapa is the (ahitatama) worst among shaka varga (C.S.Su. 25).

Properties and Actions of Shakavarga

All shakas are vistambhi, guru, and ruksha, and cause sristavinmutramaruta, are purgative, reduce the power of vision, and destroy rakta, blood, intellect, and memory, and cause premature graying of hairs.

Patrashaka

- Vastuka: Laghu, kshariya madhur, katu vipak, krimighna, medha, agni and bala vardhak, rochan, sara, sarvadoshaghna, shukral. It is used in pliha, arsha, raktapitta, and krimi.
- Upodika: Guru, snigdha, pichhila, madhur, kaphavardhak, vatapittashamak, anuloman, vrishya, brimhana, madanashan, and nidrajanana.
- Marisha: Guru, madhur, sheeta, pittashamak and vatakaphavardhak, vistambhi, and raktapittahara. Red part of the plant is kshariya, guru, madhur, and sara.
- Tanduliya: Laghu, ruksha, sheeta, madhur rasa, and madhur vipak, pittakapharaktashamak, sristavinmutra, ruchya, deepan, vishaghna, madahara. It is mainly beneficial in raktapitta and raktarsha.
- Palamkya: Madhur, ruksha, sheeta, kaphashamak, vistambhi.

- Kalambi: Kashaya, madhur, guru, vrisya, stanyajanana, shukrajanana.
- Chanchu: Madhur, pichhila, sheeta, sara, rochana, tridoshahara, balya, vrishya, and medhya.
- Lonika: Ruksha, guru, lavana, vatakaphahara, deepan, arshoghna, vishaghna. The big variety of Lonika has the properties like amla, sara, vatakara, and pittakaphahara and is used in swarabheda, vrana, gulma, kasa, swasa, prameha, shotha, and netraroga.
- Changeri: Amla, ruksha, ushna, kaphavatahsamak, deepan, grahi, and is used in grahani and arsha.
- Chukra: Laghu, amla, ushna, vatashamak and pittakaphashamak, ruchya, deepan, pathya, and is used in vatagulma.
- Hilmochika: Tikta, sheeta, bhedan, kushtaghna, kaphapittashamak.
- Sunishanak: Laghu, sheeta, grahi, chakshusya, medhya, tridoshghna, and it is mainly beneficial in netraroga, raktapitta, arsha, and manas roga.
- Patragobhi: Guru, madhur, ruchikara, durjara, sarak.
- Mulakapatra: Laghu, ushna, ruchikara, pachan, and it is tridoshashamak when processed with Sneha otherwise it is kaphapittakarak.
- Dronapuspi patra: Guru, ruksha, katu, madhur, bhedan, pittakarak, and is used in kamala, shotha, prameha, and jwara.
- Yavani patra: Laghu, katutikta, ushna, vatakapha shamak, and pitta vardhak, ruchikara, and sholaghna.
- Chakramarda patra: Laghu, amla, kaphavatashamak, and is used in various skin diseases like dadru, kandu, kasa, swasa, and krimi.
- Sehunda patra: Tikshna, rechan, and is used in adhmana, gulma, shoola, udara roga, and shotha.
- Parpata patra: Tikta, sheeta, pittashamak, grahi, dahashamak, and is used in jwara, trishna, kaphapitta, and raktaja vicar.
- Patola patra: Laghu, snigdha, ushna, pittashamak, deepan, pachan, vrishyam, and is used in jwara, kasa, and krimi.
- Gojihwapatra: laghu, and it is beneficial in kushta, prameha, raktajavikar, mutrakrichha, and jwara.
- Guduchi patra: Laghu, katu, tikta, kashaya rasa, madhur vipak, ushna virya, jwaraghna, rasayan, grahi,

balya, tridoshahara, and is used in jwara, daha, trishna, prameha, vatarakta, kushta, kamala, and pandu.

- Kasamarda patra: Kaphavatashamak, kanthashodhan, kasahara.
- Sarsapa patra: Guru, ruksha, tikshna, katu, lavana, kshariya, amla vipaka, vidahi, ushna virya, tridosha-kopak, and it is considered as worst among shaka.
- Putiha patra: Ruchikara, deepan, pachan, anuloman, and it is used in adhmana, chhardi, shoola, krimi.
- Nimba: Kaphavatashamak, kustaghna, and it is used in chhardi, hrillasa, vrana, raktavikar.
- Punarnava: Ushna, sara, rasayan, and it is used in kaphavata vicar, arsha, shotha, and udara roga. It is mainly beneficial in shotha.
- Chirabilwa: Sara, deepan, kaphashamak, and is used in gulma.
- Chanaka: Madhur, amla, madhur vipak, durjara, pittashamak, and is used in dantashotha.

Phalashaka

- Kushmanda: It is considered as best among valliphala. In tender stage (balavasta), it is pittashamak, in middle stage it is kaphakarak and mature stage (pakwavasta), it is laghu, ushna, and kshariya. It is sarvadoshahara, deepan, hridya, vastishodhan, hridya, pathya, balya, ruchikara, vrishya, arochakahara. It is used in mutraghata, prameha, mutrakrichcha, ashmari.
- Alabu: Ruksha, sheeta, guru, malabhedan, hridya, pittakaphashamak, vrisya, ruchikar, brimhana.
- Mahakoshataki: Snigdha, raktapittavatashamak.
- Koshataki: Madhura, sheeta, sara, kaphavatakarak, pittashamana, and is used in jwara, kasa, and mandangi.
- Karkati: Ruksha, guru, madhur, sheeta, grahi, pitta-shamak, kaphavatavardhak. Pakwa (mature) karkati is slightly ushna and agni deepak.
- Trapusha: Soft fruit of trapusha is madhur-sheeta and pittashamak while pakwa (mature) fruit is ushna and pittavardhak. Seed of trapusha is mutral, sheeta, ruksha, and it is used in raktapitta and mutrakrichchha.
- Karchari: Tikta, amla, laghu, ushna, tridoshashamak, and it is used in kasa, jwara, and vatavikar.
- Chichinda: Balya, pathya, ruchikara, vatapittashamak, beneficial for shosharoga. Its properties are similar to patola but are fewer than patola.

- Karavellak: Tikta rasa and katu vipak, avatala, deepana, bhedan, kaphapittashamak, and is used in jwara, prameha, pittavikara, raktavikar, krimi, kasa, swasa.
- Patola: Laghu, snigdha, ushna, deepan, pachan, hridya, vrisya, and it is used in kasa, jwara, krimi, and tridoshjavikar.
- Bimbi: Madhur, guru, sheeta, vatapittahara, stambhan, lekhan, ruchikar, vibandha, and adhmanakarak.
- Shimbi: Madhur, guru, sheeta, vatapittashamak, kaphavardhak, balya, adhmanakara.
- Shobhanjana: Madhur, kinchit tikta-katu, ushna, kaphavatashamak, deepan, anuloman. It is used in udarashoola and gulma.
- Vruntaka: Madhur, laghu, ushna, deepan, kapha-pittavardhak. Bala (apakwa) phala: tridoshahara; madhyam phala: pittakarak; and pakwa phala (kathina): vata vardhak.
- Kadali: Apakwa kadali is used as shaka. It is kashaya, guru, sheeta, stambhan, and used in atisara and raktapitta.
- Dindish: Ruchikarak, bhedan, pittashleshmahara, sheeta, vatakarak, ruksha, mutral, and ashmarihara.
- Karkoti: Ruchikara, kinchit tikta, katuvipak, ushnaveerya, kaphavatashamak, deepan, anuloman, raktashodhak, and is used in jwara, kasa, swasa, kasa, kushta, and prameha.
- Shringataka: Guru, madhur, sheeta, pittashamak, vatapittavardhak, vistambhi, stambhana, and vrisya, and is used in raktapitta.
- Jeevanti: Madhur, sheeta, tridoshhara, jeevaniya, chakshusya.
- Bhindika: Madhur, guru, pichhila, sheeta, vatapitta-shamak, kaphavardhak, balya, vrisya.
- Rajamasha: Fresh fruits are used as shaka.
- Gopashimbi: Guru, ruksha, sara, madhur, vatakapha-karak, pittashamak, ruchya, balya
- Pitakushmanda: Koshna, ruksha, guru, madhur, vatakara, kaphaprakopa, vistambhi, malavardhana.
- Raktavrintaka: Similar as the properties of vrintaka. It is specifically balya and jeevaniya.
- Puskarabeeja: Madhur, kashaya, sheeta, guru, pittashamak and kaphavardhak, vistambhi, balya, raktapittaprasadana.

Nalashaka

- Sarsapanala: Tikshna, ushna, vatakaphashamak, twagdoshahara, krimighna, kandughna, dadrughna, ruchikarak, vranadoshahara.
- Mrinala and bisa: Guru, bistambhi, sheeta, avidahi, raktapittaprasadan, durjara, ruksha
- Venukarira: Madhur and kashaya rasa and madhur vipak, kaphavatakarak, vidahi, virukshana.

Kandashaka

- Surana: It is best among kandashaka. It has deepan, ruchya, kaphaghna, vishada, ruksha properties. It is considered as best to use in arsha (piles). It is also used in gudakila.
- Aluka: Madhur, guru, sheeta, vistambhi, sristavinmutra, ruksha, durjara, raktapittashamak, kaphavatakarak, balya, vrishya, swalpa agnivardhak. It is considered as ahitatama (worst) among kandashaka as per Acharya Charak (C.S.Su. 25).
- Alooka: Madhur, ushna, balya, ruchikara, brimhana, vistambhakara, kaphapittakarak.
- Aluki: Snigdha, guru, vistambhi, balya, pittakaphakarak.
- Manakanda: Laghu, sheeta, madhur, raktapittahara, shothakarak.
- Hastikarna: Kashaya, tikta, madhur vipak, ushna, kaphavatashamak. It cures sheetajwara, pandu, shotha, krimi, pliha, anaha, udara, grahani, arsha. It has properties like vanasuran (wild Suran).
- Kaseru: Guru, sheeta, vistambhi.
- Shatavari: Madhur, tikta, hridya, medhya, agni and bala vardhakrasayan, vatapittahara. It cures grahani and arsha. Its ankura (germinated tubers) is tikta and kaphapittahara.
- Kadali: Sheeta, balya, keshya, madhur, ruchya. It cures amlapitta, daha.
- Shalooka: Sheeta, vrishya, pitta shamaka and kaphavata vardhak, guru, durjara, madhur vipak, ruksha, guru, sangrahi, stanyajanana. It has properties like Bisa (bhissanda).
- Granthigobhi: Balya, durjara, grahi, sheeta.

- Salayama: Madhur, laghu, lochana, jwarahara, sara, mridu, deepan, ishat ushna, tridoshashamak, beneficial always for udara roga.
- Sitaluka: Guru, swadu, ishat ushna, vistambhi, vatapittahara, balya, brimhana, kaphakarak.
- Grunjana: Madhur, tikta, tikshna, ushna, deepan, laghu, grahi, vatakaphashamak, used in raktapitta, arsha, and grahani.
- Varahikanda: Katu, tikta, vatakaphashamaka and pittavardhak, balya, rasayana, shukral, ayushya, deepan, and is used in prameha and kushta.
- Moolaka: It is used in vibandha, eye diseases. Tender mooli is tridoshahara, laghu, katu, ushna, pachana, swarya, jwaraghna, swasaghna, nasikakantharogaghna.

Sanswedaja Shaka

Chhatrak: Guru, sheeta, doshala, pichchhila, and it causes chhardi, atisara, jwara, and aamaja vyadhi.

Puspa Shaka

- Agathya puspa: Tiktakashaya rasa, katu vipaka, sheeta veerya, and it is used in chaturthaka jwara, raktandhya, pinasa, kaphapitta, and vatashamak.
- Kadali puspa: Madhur, kashaya, snigdha guru, sheet, vatapitta, rakta pitta, kshaya naashana.
- Shigru puspa: Katu, tikshna, ushna, shotha shamak, krimighna, and it cures vidradhi, gulma, and pliha.
- Shalmali puspa: Kashaya, madhura, sheeta, guru, grahi, vatakarak, and kaphapittashamak. It cures raktaja vicar.

Points to Ponder

- *Jeevanti is considered as hitatama (best) and sarsapa as ahitatama (worst) among shaka varga (C.S.Su. 25/38-39).*
- *Suran is the best kanda shaka. Sringavera is considered as the best kanda, while Aaluka is the worst kanda.*
- *Mridhwika is the best phala (fruit) and Nikucha is the worst one among fruits (C.S.Su. 25/38-39).*
- *Kusmanda is the best among valliphala.*

263. Shami Dhanya Varga

This group includes all the pulses (dicots) which are the major source of protein in vegetarian diet. Vagabhatta has described this group under the name of Shimbi dhanya whereas Sushrut named it as Mudgadi or vaidala varga. In general, all the Shimbi dhanya are ruksha, madhura kashaya rasa, sheeta virya, vata prakopak, achakshushya, avrishya, difficult in digestion, reduces physical strength, and mala mutrabandhaka in properties. Some important Shimbi dhanya along with their properties and actions as described in Brihtrayee are provided in **Table 263.1**.

Table 263.1 Properties of Various Shami Dhanya

S. No.	Names/Varieties	Properties	Actions
1	Mudga (green gram)	Laghu, ruksha, vishad, madhura, kashaya rasa, sheet virya, katu vipaka	Shleshmapittaghna, shoopyautam
2	Masha (black gram)	Guru, snigdha, madhura rasa, ushna virya	Vatahara, param, vrishya, balya, malavardhaka, shukravridhivirekkrita
3	Raj masha	Guru, ruksha, vishad, sara, madhura, kashaya rasa	Ruchya, vatavardhak, kapha, shukra, and amlapittahara
4	Kulathi (horse gram)	Kashaya rasa, amla vipaka, ushna virya	Grahi, vata kaphahara, useful in kasa, swasa, hikka, peenasa, ashmari, arsha, and shukra dosha
5	Makushta	Ruksha, madhura rasa, madhura vipaka sheet virya	Grahi, useful in raktapitta and jwara
6	Chanak, Masoor, Khandika, Harenu	Laghu, ruksha, madhura, kashaya rasa, sheet virya	It is used for soup and lepa in kapha pitta diseases. Out of these, Masoor is sangrahi and Kalaya is param vatavardhaka
7	Tila	Guru, snigdha, madhura, tikta, katu, kashaya rasa, ushna virya, katu vipaka	Vataghna, kapha pittavardhaka, balya, keshya, twachya, medhya, agnivardhak, alpamutrakrit
8	Adhaki		Kaphapittaghna, vatavardhak
9	Avalguja		Kapha vatahara
10	Seeds of Edgaj and Nishpav		Vata pittavardhak
11	Kakandola and Atmagupta	Properties same as Masha	
12	Nishpav (A.H. 6/20)	Guru, sara	Vidahi, vata, pitta, rakta, stanya, mutra vardhaka. Useful in eye diseases, shukra, kapha, shotha, and visha dosha
13	Uma (Alasi) and Kusumbh seed (A.H. 6/24)	Guru, snigdha, madhura, tikta rasa, ushna virya, katu vipaka	Drikashukranashaka

Points to Ponder

- *In Shimbi dhanya, Mudga is given the best category while Masha is inferior, whereas in Shuka dhanya, Rakta shali is stated as the best and Yava is inferior in properties.*

264. Shuka Dhanya

It is one of the most important groups mentioned in Ayurvedic classical texts as it includes a major category of food ingredients. This group includes varieties of rice, wheat, millets, jowar, bajra, etc. Their names, properties, and actions are listed in **Table 264.1**.

Table 264.1 Properties and Actions of Various Shukadhanya

S. No.	Names/Varieties	Properties	Actions
1	Shali dhanya: Rakt shali, maha shali, kalam, shuknahat, turnak, gaurdhanya, panduk, langul, deerghashook, saugandhik, lohvaal, sariva, pramodak, patang, tapniya	Snigdha, madhura rasa, madhura vipaka, sheet virya	Shukral, mutral, brihmaniya, malabadhkrit, and slightly aggravates vata dosha. Among all these, Rakta shali is the best because it has tridoshahara and trishnaghna properties
2	Shastika dhanya	Aguru, snigdha, madhura rasa, sheet virya	Grahi, tridoshahara, and sthiratmaka. Gaur shastika dhanya is better in comparison to asita shastika
3	Varak, Udalaka, Cheen, Sharad, Ujjwal, Gandhna, Durdar, Kurvind	They are less potent than shastika dhanya	
4	Brihi dhanya	Guru, madhura rasa, amla vipaka, ushna virya	Pittavardhak, bahumutrapurisha. Among these, patal is tridoshahara
5	Mukund, Priyangu, Kordush, Shyamak	Laghu, madhura, kashaya rasa, sheet virya	Vata vardhak, kapha pittaghna, param sangrahi, and shoshaka
6	Yava	Laghu, ruksha, madhura, kashaya rasa, sheet virya	Vata purisha vardhak, stharyakrit, balya, kaphashamak
7	Venu Yava	Ruksha, madhura rasa, kashaya anurasa	Kapha pittahara, balya, medohara, krimighna, vishaghna
8	Godhuma	Guru, snigdha, madhura rasa, madhura vipaka, sheet virya	Jeevaniya, vrishya, brihmaniya, sthairyakrit, Sandhankrit, and vatahara. Its varieties: Nandimukhi and Madhuli are madhura, snigdha, sheet, and pathya in properties
9	Trinadhanya (Kangu, Kodrav, Neevar, Shyamak)	Laghu, sheeta virya	Vatakrit, kapha pittahara, and lekhan
10	Trinadhanya (Priyangu) (A.H. 6/11)	Guru	Brihmaniya and bhagnasandhankrit

Points to Ponder

- *Charaka samhita and Vagbhatta have described 15 and 26 varieties of rice, respectively.*
- *Sushruta has described Kodo, Shyamak, Varak, Priyangu, Madhuli, Nandimukhi, Venu yava, Gavedhuk, and Kurvinda in Kudhanya varga, whereas Shali, Shastik, and Brihi dhanya in Shali varga.*
- *Bhavamishra mentioned dhanya panchaka which includes Shali dhanya, Brihi dhanya, Shuka dhanya, Shimbi dhanya, and Kshudra dhanya.*

265. Taila Varga

Acharya Charak did not make a separate varga for taila. All the oils are described under Aharayogi varga.

General Properties of Oils

Shukshm, vyavayi, madhura rasa, kashaya anurasa, ushna virya, vataghna, aggravates pitta but doesn't aggravate kapha, balya, twachya, chakshushya, medhya, agnivardhaka, badhvinmutra, yonishodhaka, krimighna, and has the property to cure all the diseases by virtue of its samyog sanskara. It is used to reduce weight in obese person and to increase weight in lean thin individuals (C.S.S. 13/12). Its properties, actions, and uses are listed in **Table 265.1**.

Table 265.1 Properties, Actions, and Uses of Various Tailas

S. No.	Name of the Oil	Properties	Actions	Indications
1	Erand taila	Guru, tikshan, sara, shukshma, madhura rasa, katu, kashaya anurasa, madhur vipaka, ushna virya	Twachya, vrishya, deepan, shrotoshodhan, vyasthapana, yoni and shukravishodhaka, medha, kanti, smriti, bal vardhaka, adhobhagdoshhara **Rakta erand**—Ushna, tikshan, picchila, vishra	Considered as best oil for virechana karma. It is used in amavata, vatarakta, gulma, hridaya roga, jeerna jwar, vardhm, udar roga, and to reduce pain and inflammation of kati, prisht, guhya, and koshta region
2	Tila taila	Ushna, tikshan, guru, sara, shukshma, vishad, vyavayi, vikasi, madhura rasa, tikta, kashaya anurasa, madhur vipaka	Brihmaniya, preenan, vrishya, twakprasadana, garbhashya shodhak, chakshushya, lekhan, badhmutra, pachana, krimighna, medhya, balya, varnya, kaphavatahara, pittajanan, yoni, shira, karna shool prasasmana	Used in abhyanga, parishek and avagahana. Among the sthavara, sneha, it is considered best for balya karma
3	Sarshapa taila	Laghu, tikshna, katu rasa, katu vipaka, ushna virya	Rakta pitta pradoshak, kapha, meda, shukra anil hara, lekhan, deepan	Kandu, kotha, kushta, arsha, vrana, krimi
4	Priyala	Guru, madhur, Naatiushna	Kaphavardhak	Vata pittaj diseases
5	Atasi	Guru, snigdh, madhura, amla rasa, katu vipaka, ushna virya	Rakta pitta prakopaka, vata hara, bala nashak, achakshushya	Vatakapha roga, krimi, kushta, prameha, shiraroga
6	Kusumbh	Guru, vidahi, tikshna, katu vipaka, ushna virya	Rakta pitta kara, sarvadoshaprakopak, achakshushya, vidahi	Vatakapha roga, krimi, kushta, prameha, shiraroga

(Continued)

Table 265.1 *(Continued)* Properties, Actions, and Uses of Various Tailas

S. No.	Name of the Oil	Properties	Actions	Indications
7	Bibhitaki taila	Guru, madhura rasa, sheet virya	Keshya, vata pittahara	Vatapitta roga, premature graying of hair
8	Nimba taila	Natya ushna, tikta rasa	Kapha hara	Krimi, kushta
9	Ingudi taila	Laghu, tikta rasa	Krimighna, drishti, shukra, balanashaka	Kushta, krimi
10	Tuvraka and Bhallataka	Madhura, kashaya, tikta anurasa, ushna virya	Kusthaghna, krimighna, kandughna, deepan, medohara, vranashothahara	Kushta, medoroga, prameha, krimi
11	Saral, Devdaru, Gandeer, Aguru, and Shinshipa taila	Tikta, katu, kashaya rasa	Dushta vrana shodhaka, kapha vatahara	Kushta, krimi, vrana
12	Ingudi taila	Laghu, ishat tikta	Krimighna reduces the power of dristi, decreases bala and shukra	Cures krimi, kushta

Points to Ponder

- *All types of oil has vatashaman properties but til tail (sesame oil) is considered as best for vatashaman.*
- *Old pakwa or apakwa taila (processed oil or nonprocessed oil) has more medicinal properties than the fresh one.*

Frequently Asked Questions

Long Answer Questions (15 marks)

1. Write the external morphology and action of the following drugs.
   - Parpata
   - Ativisha
   - Eranda
2. Explain the Rasapanchaka and phytoconstituents of the following drugs.
   - Guduchi
   - Arjuna
   - Nimba
3. Explain the synonyms, family, morphology, Rasapanchaka, action, uses, indication, parts used, doses, and important formulations of Gokshura.
4. Write the Latin name, Rasapanchaka, action, parts used, methods of application, and doses of three important drugs that are specifically indicated for Amavata.
5. Provide detailed descriptions about the general identity, properties, actions, parts used, and doses of the following drugs.
   - Tagara
   - Musali
   - Amragandhi Haridra
6. Write the name, Rasapanchaka, actions, and methods of application of three important drugs which are specifically indicated for Shwasa Roga.
7. Provide detailed descriptions about synonyms, chemical constituents, Rasapanchaka, parts used, doses, and indications of the drug Sarpagandha.
8. Write the name, Rasapanchaka, actions, and methods of application of three important drugs which are used for Prameha (diabetes).
9. Describe the synonyms, gana, morphology, Rasapanchaka, parts used, doses, and indications of the drug Vidanga.
10. Describe the synonyms, morphology, habitat, types, Rasapanchaka, parts used, doses and indications, and important formulations of the drug Guggulu.
11. Describe the synonyms, gana, morphology, habitat, types, Rasapanchaka, parts used, doses and indications, and important formulations of the drug Haritaki.
12. Describe the synonyms, gana, morphology, habitat, Rasapanchaka, parts used, doses and uses, therapeutic indications, and important formulations of the drug Guduchi.
13. Describe the synonyms, gana, morphology, habitat, Rasapanchaka, parts used, doses and uses, purification methods, and important formulations of the drug Bhallatak.
14. Describe the synonyms, gana, morphology, habitats, Rasapanchaka, parts used, doses and uses, purification methods, and important formulations of the drug Kupilu.
15. Describe the synonyms, gana, morphology, habitats, parts used, doses and uses, and important formulations of the drug Ashwagandha.

Short Answer Questions (5 marks)

1. List down the types and uses of Jeeraka and Punarnava.
2. List down the botanical names, useful parts, and formulations of (a) Bilva and (b) Trivrut.
3. List down the botanical names, indications, and parts used of (a) Pushkaramula and (b) Tulasi.
4. List down the botanical names, actions, and uses of (a) Shirisha and (b) Vidanga.
5. List down the types and uses of Guggulu.
6. List down the botanical names and indications of (a) Lajjalu, (b) Danti, (c) Babbula, (d) Amra, and (e) Aswattha.
7. List down the botanical names and habitats of (a) Vruddadaru, (b) Puga, (c) Sarja, (d) Sarala, and (e) Kasamarda.
8. List down the botanical names and useful parts of (a) Snuhi, (b) Surana, (c) Tagara, (d) Vata and (e) Vrikshamla.
9. List down the botanical names and families of (a) Ishvari, (b) Dronapushpi, (c) Mahanimba, (d) Kusha, and (e) Japa
10. Justify the uses of paryaya in the identification of Guduchi.
11. Write about the external morphology, useful parts, and indications of Palasha.

12. Write about the shodhana of Chitraka and Vatsanabha.
13. List down the botanical sources and two important therapeutic uses of the following plants:
    (a) Bhringaraja
    (b) Katuki
    (c) Musta
    (d) Khadira.
14. Write about the guna karma of Pippali.
15. List down the useful parts, doses, formulations, and uses of Jatiphala.
16. Write about Madhu and its different uses.
17. List down the therapeutic uses, parts used, and doses of Bilwa.
18. List down the types and uses of Chitraka.
19. What is Kasturi? Write its types, guna karma, and uses.
20. List down the parts used, doses, and uses of Patola and Saptachakra.
21. List down the Latin names and families of (a) Kampillaka, (b) Kanchanara, (c) Shallaki, and (d) Yavani.
22. List down the specific karmas of (a) Ashoka, (b) Apamarga, (c) Jyotishmati, and (d) Ushira.
23. Write two specific dravyas for (a) Keshya, (b) Medhya, (c) Vrushya, (d) Varnya, and (e) Kantya.
24. Write any one shodhana procedure of (a) Dhatura, (b) Langali, (c) Jayapala, (d) Gunja, and (e) Karavira.
25. Write about the indications and contraindications of Haritaki.
26. Describe the officinal parts used in case of Yasthi, Vidanga, Maricha, and Palasha, and their therapeutic uses.
27. Write the synonyms of Gokshura, Kapikacchu, Vasa, and Guduchi.
28. Write the basonyms of Bhishakmata, Vaajigandha, Tishyaphala, Ramatha, and Ghrithakanya.
29. Write the guna karma of Mandukaparni and Varuna and their therapeutic uses.
30. Write the vishishta yogas of Guggulu, Punarnava, Jeeraka, and Haridra.

Very Short Answers Questions (3 marks)

1. Write the botanical names of (a) Indravaruni and (b) Atasi.
2. Write the family names of (a) Amragandhi Haridra and (b) Palandu.
3. Write the swarupas of (a) Bhumyamalaki and (b) Dhanyaka.
4. List down the parts used and uses of Agasthya.
5. List down the parts used and uses of Varuna.
6. List down the parts used and uses of Ajamoda.
7. List down the parts used and uses of Parijata.
8. List down the parts used and uses of Amlavetasa.
9. List down the parts used and uses of Lajjalu.
10. List down the parts used and uses of Jatiphala.
11. Write the uses and Latin names of Changeri and Tagara.
12. Write the Rasapanchaka of Haritaki and (b) Baladwaya.
13. Write the synonyms and ganas of Vidanga.
14. Write the prashasta of Chandan.
15. Write the types of (a) Jeeraka and (b) Punarnava.
16. Write the botanical names and useful parts of (a) Bilva and (b) Trivrut.
17. Write the botanical names and indications of (a) Pushkaramula and (b) Tulasi.
18. Write the botanical names and agrya karmas of (a) Shirisha and (b) Vidanga.
19. Write the botanical names, families, and habitats of (a) Matulunga and (b) Parnayavani.
20. Write the botanical names, families, and useful parts of (a) Mayaphala and (b) Bola.
21. Write the botanical name, families, and indications of (a) Shati and (b) Kulattha.
22. Write the botanical names and families of (a) Changeri and (b) Mulaka.
23. Write the purification methods of Vatsanabha.
24. Write the purification methods of Bhallataka.
25. Write the types of Haritaki.
26. Write the Rasapanchaka of Lasuna.
27. Write the chemical constituents of Vacha.
28. Write the parts used and indications of Kasni.
29. Write the parts used and indications of Gokshur.

Bibliography

A Handbook of Dravyaguna by Prof. J. K. Ojha. New Delhi: Chaukhamba Sanskrit Bhawan; 2004

Astanga Hridaya, Nirmala Hindi Commentary by Brahmanand Tripathy. Varanasi: Choukhambha Sanskrit Pratisthan; 2009

Astanga Sangraha, Indu Commentary Sashilekha vyakhya by Brahmanand Tripathy. Varanasi: Choukhambha Sanskrit Series office; 2008

Ayurvedokta Oushadha Niruktamala English, Hindi Translation by J.L.N. Sastry, Varanasi. India: Chaukhamba & Sanskrit Bhawan

Bhaisajya Ratnavali, Vidyotini Hindi Commentary by Kaviraj Shree Ambikadatta Shastri. Varanasi: Chaukhambha Prakashana; 2010

Bhava Prakash, Vidyotini namikaya Commentary by Brahma Shankara Mishra, Uttarardha. Edition. Varanasi: Choukhambha Sanskrit Bhavan; 2015

Bhavaprakasha Nighantu of Shri Bhava Mishra by Krushna Chandra Chunekar. Varanasi: Chaukhambha Bharati Academy; 2010

Bhela Samhita, Hindi Commentary by Abhaya Katyayan. Varanasi: Chaukhambha Surbharati Prakashan; 2009

Chakra Dutta, Vaidaya prabha vyakhya by Dr. Indra Deva Tripathy. Varanasi: Chaukhambha Sanskrit Bhawan; 2010

Charaka Samhita, Vidyotinee Hindi Commentary by Pt.Kashinath Shastri and Dr.Gorakshanath Charurvedi Vol-1 and 2. Varanasi: Choukhambha Bharati Academy; 2019

Classical Uses of Medicinal Plants by Priya Vrata Sharma. Varanasi: Chaukhambha Vishvabharati; 2004

Compendium of Indian Medicinal Plant by Ram P. Rastogi. B.N. Mehrotra, Vol-2, 3, 4, 5. Lucknow: Central Drug Research Institute and New Delhi: National Institute of Science Communication and Information Resources; 2006

Database on Indian medicinal plants used in Ayurveda & Siddha, Volume1-8; Department of AYUSH Ministry of Health & Family Welfare Government of India: CCRAS; 2008

Definitional Dictionary of Ayurveda (Sanskrit-English-Hindi), Commission for Scientific and Technical Terminology, Ministry of Human Resource Development (Department of Higher Education), Government of India; 2016

Dhanwantari Nighantu by Guru Prasad Sharma, Priya Vrata Sharma. Varanasi: Chaukhambha oriental.

Dravyaguna Hastamlaka by Banavari Lal Mishra. Jaipur: Sharan Book Deport; 2006

Dravyaguna Vijnana by K. Nishteswar. Koppula Hemadri. Delhi: Chaukhambha Sanskrit Pratisthan; 2010

Dravyaguna Vijnana by Priya Vrata Sharma. Vol-2. Varanasi: Chaukhambha Bharati Academy; 2009

Dravyaguna Vijnana, by Manasi Makarand Deshpandey, Aravind P. Deshpandey. Delhi: Chaukhambha Sanskrit Pratishthan; 2009. Dravyaguna-Vijnana- Study of Dravya-Materia Medica by D. Shanth Kumar Lucas. Varanasi: Chaukhambha Visvabharati; 2013

Fundamental Glossary of Ayurveda (Clinical). (Sanskrit-English-Hindi),Commission for Scientific and Technical Terminology, Ministry of Human Resource Development (Department of Higher Education), Government of India; 2016

Glossary of Vegetable drugs in Brihatrayee By Thakur Balwant Singh and Dr.K.C.Chunekar. Varanasi, India: Chakhamba Amarbharati Prakashan; Revised edition-2018.

Handbook of Medicinal plants by Prajapati &Purohit. Vranasi, India: Chaukhamba Publication; 2006

Harita Samhita text with Nirmala Hindi Commentary byVaidya Jaymini Pandey. Varanasi, India: Chaukhambha Visvabharati; reprint-2016.

Indian Medical Plants a compendium of 500 species by PS Varier's, Vol-1-5. Arya Vaidya Sala, Kottakkal: orient longman limited; 2013.

Indian Medicinal Plants by Kirtikar KR. Basu BD, Vol-1-4. Delhi: Periodical Experts Book Agency, Edition; 2012

Indian Medicinal Plants, An Illustrated Dictionary With Pictures of Crude Herbs by C.P.Khare, SpringerScience+BusinessMedia, LLC; 2007

Kaiyadeva Nighantuh by Guru Prasad Sharma, Priya Vrata Sharma. Varanasi: Chaukhambha oriental; 2013

Kashyap Samhita, English translation and Commentary by Prem Vati Tewari. Varanasi: Choukhamba Visvabharati; 2013

Madanapal Nighantu with Hari hindi commentary by Pandit Hariharprasad Tripathy. Varanasi, India: Chaukhamba Krishnadas Academy; 2018

Namarupajnanam by Acharya Priyavrat Sharma. Varanasi, India: Chaukhambha Vishvabharati; reprint-2011.

Nighantu Aadarsh Vol-1 and 2 by Bapalal G. Vaidya. Varanasi, India: Chaukhambha Bharati Academy; 1998

Priya Nighantu by Acharya Priyavrat Sharma. Varanasi, India: Chaukhamba Surabharati Prakashan; 2004

Quality Standard of Indian Medicinal Plants by A. K Gupta, Tandon Neeraj, Madhu Sharma, Vol-6. New Delhi: Medicinal Plants Unit, Indian Council of Medical Research; 2008

Raj Nighantu of Pandit Narahari by Indra Dev Tripathy. Varanasi: Chowkhamba Krishnadas Academy; 2006

Sarangadhara Samhita, Dipika Hindi Commentary by Brahmanand Tripathy, Purvakhanda. Varanasi: Chaukhambha Subharati Prakashan; 2011

Some Controversial Drugs in Indian Medicine by Bapalal G.Vaidya. Varanasi, India: Chaukhamba & Sanskrit Bhawan; 2008

Sushruta Samhita, Ayurveda Tatwa Sandeepika Hindi Commentary by Kaviraj Ambikadutta Shastri, Vol-1 and 2.Varanasi: Choukhambha Sankrit Sansthan; 2012

The Ayurvedic Pharmacopoeia of India; Part-I, Volume-I-VI, Government of India ministry of Health and Family welfare Department of Health; (1989- 2008).

The Treatise on Indian Medicinal Plants by Asima Chatterjee, Satyesh Chandra Pakrashi, Vol-1-6. New Delhi: National Institute of Science Communication and Information Resources, CSIR; 2006

The Wealth of India, (Raw materials) all Volume, Council of Scientific & Industrial Research; New Delhi(1946-76).

Vangasen Samhita, Chikitsasara Sangraha by Rajiv Kumar Roy. Varanasi: Prachya Prakashan; 2010

Yoga Ratnakara, Vyodotinee Hindi Commentary by Vaidya shree Laxmi Pati Shastri, Uttarardha. Varanasi: Choukhambha Prakashan; 2012.

Index